THE OXFORD HANDBOOK OF

ATTENTION

T0202142

Anna Christina (Kia) Nobre is the Chair in Translational Cognitive Neuroscience at the University of Oxford, where she heads the Department of Experimental Psychology and directs the Oxford Centre for Human Brain Activity. She received her PhD (1992) from Yale University and completed postdoctoral training at Yale and Harvard Medical School before moving to Oxford (1994). Dr Nobre uses a multi-methodological approach to investigate how perception and cognition are modulated according to task goals, expectations, and memories; and to understand how these dynamic regulatory mechanisms are affected by ageing, psychiatric conditions, and neurodegenerative disorders. She has published more than 200 articles in journals and books. She is a Fellow of the British Academy and a Member of the Academia Europaea.

Sabine Kastner is Professor of Neuroscience and Psychology at Princeton University, where she directs Princeton's neuroimaging facility and heads the Neuroscience of Attention and Perception Laboratory in the Princeton Neuroscience Institute and Department of Psychology. She earned an M.D. (1993) and PhD (1994) degree and received postdoctoral training at the Max-Planck-Institute for Biophysical Chemistry and NIMH before joining the faculty at Princeton University in 2000. Dr Kastner studies the neural basis of visual perception, attention, and awareness in healthy humans, patients with brain lesions and animal models and has published more than 100 articles in journals and books. Dr Kastner's contributions to the field of cognitive neuroscience were recognized with the Young Investigator Award from the Cognitive Neuroscience Society in 2005.

THE OXFORD HANDBOOK OF

ATTENTION

Edited by

ANNA C. NOBRE

Department of Experimental Psychology
Oxford Centre for Human Brain Activity
University of Oxford

and

SABINE KASTNER

Department of Psychology
Princeton Neuroscience Institute
Princeton University

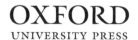

OXFORD
UNIVERSITY PRESS

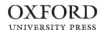

Great Clarendon Street, Oxford, OX2 6DP,
United Kingdom

Oxford University Press is a department of the University of Oxford.
It furthers the University's objective of excellence in research, scholarship,
and education by publishing worldwide. Oxford is a registered trade mark of
Oxford University Press in the UK and in certain other countries

First published 2014
First published in paperback 2018
Impression: 1

Published in the United States of America by Oxford University Press
198 Madison Avenue, New York, NY 10016, United States of America

British Library Cataloguing in Publication Data
Data available

Library of Congress Cataloging in Publication Data
Data available

ISBN 978–0–19–967511–1 (Hbk.)
ISBN 978–0–19–882467–1 (Pbk.)

Printed in Great Britain by
Ashford Colour Press Ltd, Gosport, Hampshire

Dedicated to the memory of our
friend and colleague Jon Driver (1962–2011)

ACKNOWLEDGEMENTS

The editors would like to thank all the authors of the Handbook for their erudite, comprehensive, and up-to-date contributions. We are also indebted to Charlotte Green and Jaimee Biggins at OUP for all their support and skill in stewarding the Handbook through its complex voyage from drafts to in-print and on-line. The inception of the project also benefited from sharp and constructive comments from anonymous reviewers of our initial proposal.

Kia, as ever, is pinching herself trying to understand if she's really that lucky. Thank you, Luciano, for giving meaning and bringing happiness to my life. And for tolerating that I go beyond breaking point on OTT projects like this.

Sabine, on the other hand, clearly lives in a dream. Thank you, Michael, for your incredible patience, and for the love and peace that you have brought to our journey. My contributions to the book are dedicated to Sarah and Benjamin, who show me the true meaning of life through the love and happiness that we experience together every day.

CONTENTS

PART C SPATIAL ATTENTION

PART D NON-SPATIAL ATTENTION

PART E INTERACTIONS BETWEEN ATTENTION & OTHER PSYCHOLOGICAL DOMAINS

NOTES ON CONTRIBUTORS

Dr Lorella Battelli Harvard Medical School, USA and Italian Institute of Technology, Italy

Professor Diane M. Beck Department of Psychology, Beckman Institute, University of Illinois, USA

Dr Nadia Bolognini Department of Psychology, University of Milano-Bicocca, and IRCCS Istituto Auxologico Italiano, Milan, Italy

Dr Valerie Bonnelle Department of Experimental Psychology, University of Oxford, UK

Dr Ali Borji University of Southern California, USA

Professor Claus Bundesen Department of Psychology, University of Copenhagen, Denmark

Dr Timothy J. Buschman Department of Psychology, Princeton Neuroscience Institute, Princeton University, USA

Professor Marisa Carrasco Department of Psychology and Department of Neural Science, New York University, USA

Professor Patrick Cavanagh Vision Sciences Laboratory, Harvard University and Laboratoire Psychologie de la Perception, Université Paris Descartes, Paris, France

Professor Marvin M. Chun Department of Psychology, Yale University, USA

Dr Kelsey L. Clark Department of Neurobiology, Stanford University School of Medicine, USA and Howard Hughes Medical Institute, Stanford, USA

Dr Marlene R. Cohen Department of Neuroscience, University of Pittsburgh and the Center for the Neural Basis of Cognition, USA

Dr Polly Dalton Department of Psychology, Royal Holloway, University of London, London, UK

Professor Heiner Deubel Department of Psychology, Ludwig-Maximilians-Universität, Munich, Germany

Professor John Duncan Medical Research Council Cognition and Brain Sciences Unit, Cambridge, UK

Dr Tobias Egner Center for Cognitive Neuroscience and Department of Psychology & Neuroscience, Duke University, USA

Professor Martin Eimer Department of Psychological Sciences, Birkbeck College, University of London, UK

Dr Edward F. Ester Department of Psychology University of California, San Diego, USA

Professor Adam Gazzaley Department of Neurology and Physiology, Keck Center for Integrative Neuroscience, University of California, San Francisco, USA

Professor Jacqueline Gottlieb Mahoney Center for Brain and Behavior, Center for Neurobiology and Behavior, Columbia University College of Physicians and Surgeons, and the New York State Psychiatric Institute, USA

Dr Thomas Habekost Department of Psychology, University of Copenhagen, Denmark

Dr Saskia Haegens Nathan Kline Institute for Psychiatric Research, Department of Psychiatry, Columbia University College of Physicians and Surgeons, USA

Dr Simon Hanslmayr School of Psychology, University of Birmingham, UK

Dr Jose L. Herrero Nathan Kline Institute for Psychiatric Research, Department of Psychiatry, Columbia University College of Physicians and Surgeons, USA

Dr Alex O. Holcombe School of Psychology, University of Sydney, Australia

Professor Glyn W. Humphreys Department of Experimental Psychology, University of Oxford, UK

Professor Masud Husain Department of Experimental Psychology and Nuffield Department of Clinical Neurosciences, University of Oxford, UK

Professor Laurent Itti Computer Science Department, University of Southern California, USA

Professor Sabine Kastner Department of Psychology, Princeton Neuroscience Institute, Princeton University, USA

Professor Richard J. Krauzlis Systems Neurobiology Laboratory, Salk Institute for Biological Studies, La Jolla, California, USA

Dr Brice A. Kuhl Department of Psychology, New York University, USA

Professor Nilli Lavie Department of Psychology and Institute for Cognitive Neuroscience, University College London, UK

Dr Sanjay Manohar Department of Experimental Psychology and Nuffield Department of Clinical Neurosciences, University of Oxford, UK

Professor John H. R. Maunsell Department of Neurobiology, Harvard Medical School, USA

Professor M. Marsel Mesulam Cognitive Neurology and Alzheimer's Disease Center, Northwestern University, Chicago, USA

Professor Earl K. Miller The Picower Institute for Learning and Memory and Department of Brain and Cognitive Sciences, Massachusetts Institute of Technology, USA

Professor Tirin Moore Department of Neurobiology, Stanford University School of Medicine and Howard Hughes Medical Institute, Stanford, USA

Professor Anna C. Nobre Department of Experimental Psychology, Oxford Centre for Human Brain Activity, University of Oxford, UK

Dr Behrad Noudoost Department of Neurobiology, Stanford University School of Medicine, and Howard Hughes Medical Institute, Stanford, USA

Dr Redmond G. O'Connell School of Psychology and Trinity College Institute of Neuroscience, Trinity College Dublin, Ireland

Professor Luiz Pessoa Department of Psychology, University of Maryland, USA

Professor Michael I. Posner Department of Psychology, University of Oregon, USA

Professor T. W. Robbins Department of Psychology and Behavioural and Clinical Neuroscience Institute, University of Cambridge, UK

Professor Ian H. Robertson School of Psychology and Trinity College Institute of Neuroscience, Trinity College Dublin, Ireland

Professor Lynn C. Robertson Helen Wills Neuroscience Institute, University of California, Berkeley, and Veterans Administration, Martinez, California, USA

Dr Gustavo Rohenkohl Department of Experimental Psychology and Oxford Centre for Human Brain Activity, University of Oxford, UK

Professor Mary K. Rothbart Department of Psychology, University of Oregon, USA

Dr M. Rosario Rueda Department of Experimental Psychology, University of Granada, Spain

Dr Yuri B. Saalmann Center for the Study of Brain, Mind and Behavior and Department of Psychology, Princeton Neuroscience Institute, Princeton University, USA

Dr Gaia Scerif Department of Experimental Psychology, University of Oxford, UK

Dr Robert J. Schafer Department of Neurobiology, Stanford University School of Medicine, and Howard Hughes Medical Institute, Stanford, USA

Dr Charles E. Schroeder Nathan Kline Institute for Psychiatric Research, Department of Psychiatry, Columbia University College of Physicians and Surgeons, USA

Dr Miranda Scolari Princeton Neuroscience Institute, Princeton University, San Diego, USA

Dr John T. Serences Department of Psychology, University of California, USA

Professor Kimron Shapiro School of Psychology, University of Birmingham, UK

Dr David Soto Department of Medicine, Imperial College, London, UK

Professor Charles Spence Department of Experimental Psychology and Oxford Centre for Human Brain Activity University of Oxford, UK

Dr Mark Stokes Department of Experimental Psychology, University of Oxford, UK

Dr Christopher Summerfield Department Experimental Psychology, University of Oxford, UK

Professor Jan Theeuwes Department of Cognitive Psychology, Vrije Universiteit, Amsterdam, the Netherlands

Professor Stefan Treue Department of Cognitive Neuroscience, University of Göttingen, Germany

Professor Giuseppe Vallar Department of Psychology, University of Milano-Bicocca and Neuropsychological Laboratory, S. Luca Hospital, Italian Auxological Institute, Milan, Italy

Professor Jeremy M. Wolfe Visual Attention Lab, Brigham and Women's Hospital, Harvard Medical School, USA

Dr Rachel Wu Department of Brain and Cognitive Sciences, University of Rochester, New York, USA

Professor Angela J. Yu Department of Cognitive Science, University of California, San Diego, USA

Dr Theodore P. Zanto Departments of Neurology and Physiology, University of California, San Francisco, USA

PART A

INTRODUCTION

CHAPTER 1

···

GUIDES TO THE STUDY
OF ATTENTION

···

MICHAEL I. POSNER

This volume presents a modern look at the field of attention. The identities of the editors of this volume suggest why it and they can serve as guides to current and future research. Kia Nobre is a leader in the use of neuroimaging to study attention largely in humans, while Sabine Kastner bridges neuroimaging approaches in both humans and monkeys to the cellular approach of neurophysiology. These two methods are increasingly integrated in empirical research and theory in the field. They have selected a very strong set of authors to provide guidance on theory and empirical research on attention. In this foreword I try to trace the background of these methods within the field of attention, look briefly at the current state of integration as represented by the chapters of this Handbook, and speculate on future developments.

HISTORICAL BACKGROUND

···

In the mid-twentieth century Moruzzi and Magoun (1949) began using animal models to explore aspects of attention. They studied the midbrain reticular system as the mechanism of arousal. In their work attention involved a state in which the animal was aroused from coma or sleep and then demonstrated both spontaneous integrated activity and processing of sensory stimuli.

Hubel and Wiesel (1968) used microelectrodes to probe the structure of the visual system. Before this method could be applied to attention, however, it was necessary to adapt the microelectrode technique to alert animals. This was accomplished in the early 1970s and applied by Mountcastle (1978) and Wurtz, Goldberg, and Robinson (1980) to examine mechanisms of orienting to visual objects in the superior colliculus and parietal lobe. Their findings suggested the importance of both of these areas to a shift of visual attention. It had been known for many years that patients with lesions of the right parietal lobe could suffer from a profound neglect of space opposite the lesion. The findings of 'attention-related cells' in the posterior parietal lobe of alert monkeys suggested that these cells might be responsible for the clinical syndrome of neglect.

An impressive result from the microelectrode work was that the time course of parietal cell activity seemed to follow a visual stimulus by 80–100 ms. Beginning in the 1970s, Hillyard (van Voorhis and Hillyard 1977) and other investigators explored the use of scalp electrodes to examine time differences in neural activity between attended and unattended visual locations. They found that early parts of the visual event-related potential (ERP) showed changes due to attention starting at about 100 ms after input. These findings showed likely convergence of the latency of psychological processes as measured by ERPs in human subjects and cellular processes measured in alert monkeys. These results were an important development for mental chronometry (i.e. the study of the time course of information processing in the human brain) because they suggested that scalp recordings could accurately reflect the underlying temporal structure of brain activity.

In the late 1980s, the Washington University School of Medicine was developing a centre for neuroimaging using positron emission tomography (PET). The centre was led by Marc Raichle. These studies helped establish neuroimaging as a means of exploring brain activity during cognitive functions in general and attention in particular (Corbetta and Shulman 2002; Posner and Raichle 1994, 1998). In general, these studies showed that most cognitive tasks, including those that are designed to explore mechanisms of attention, have activated a small number of widely scattered neural areas.

The findings from neuroimaging that cognitive tasks involve a number of different anatomical areas led to an emphasis on tracing the time dynamics of these areas during tasks involving attention. Because shifts of attention can be so rapid, it is difficult to follow them with hemodynamic imaging. To fill this role, algorithms were developed (Scherg and Berg 1993) to relate the scalp distribution recorded from high density electrical or magnetic sensors on or near the skull to brain areas active during hemodynamic imaging (see Dale et al. 2000, for a review). In some areas of attention there has been extensive validation of these algorithms (Heinze et al. 1994), and they allow precise data on the sequence of activations during the selection of visual stimuli (see Hillyard, Di Russo, and Martinez 2004, for a review). The combination of spatial localization with hemodynamic imaging and temporal precisions from electrical or magnetic recording has provided an approach to revealing the dynamic operations of the networks underlying attention in humans that fit very well with the use of cellular recording in monkeys. In current research these methods have become increasingly integrated as made clear by this Handbook.

CURRENT STATE OF RESEARCH

Theory

This volume presents nine chapters on theory related to attention. The chapters include world leaders in the field. The first six chapters (section B; Chs. 2–7) are mainly in verbal form while the remaining three (section F; Chs. 38–40) are computational. Taken together these chapters develop theoretical methods that summarize empirical findings and data concerning the localization, connectivity, and time course of a wide variety of attentional tasks. The chapters present a comprehensive view of the current state of theory in this field.

Empirical studies

This volume makes a distinction between orienting towards locations in empty space (section B; Chs. 8–19) and orienting to objects that occupy that space (section C; Chs. 21–25). Sections B and C summarize major results in this field. While it is unusual for people to operate in a space without objects, the empty fields discussed in section B allow one to concentrate on the mechanisms of top-down influence without having to consider at the same time the structure of the perceptual field. Section C provides the important constraints that a context of multiple distractors and multiple targets provide.

Section D deals with how attention relates to voluntary control of motor activity (Ch. 26), working memory (Ch. 30), executive functions (Chs. 28–29), emotion (Ch. 27), and consciousness (Ch. 31). These are all important functions of cognition in which attention is involved along with other brain systems. It is not always easy to disentangle these multiple processes within complex task, but these chapters provide a summary of current efforts to do so.

Development and disorders

Although our chapter on development of attention networks is in section B (Ch. 20) and section E has chapters on ageing (Ch. 36) and developmental disorders (Ch. 37), the three can be put together as a summary of lifespan typical and atypical development. While very early development depends heavily on spatial orienting, it is clear that what develop in childhood are more general control networks that allow for self-regulation. The developmental process continues throughout life so that it is probably not completely appropriate to consider ageing as a disorder, although declines in function are clearly involved.

Disorders ought to be viewed in relation to typical development. Three chapters in section D deal mainly with neurological disorders (Chs. 32–34). Disorders involving clear cases of brain injury from stroke, tumour, or closed head injury provide important clues to critical brain areas important for attention.

FUTURE OF RESEARCH

Although the job of predicting the future of the field is mainly left to Ch. 41 in section H, here I provide some speculations on developments towards the integration between cellular and systems approaches.

Networks

New methods have greatly reduced the gap between cellular and synaptic mechanisms and systems approaches to the field of attention. On the one hand, imaging reveals the brain areas and connections important at rest and during cognitive activity, while on the other hand multiple electrodes allow simultaneous recording from many neurons and brain areas. This has allowed modern theories to concentrate on a detailed account of how networks control the flow of information.

It is altogether likely that new methods will be developed. For example, within the last few years magnetic resonance imaging has been expanded to view white matter connections (Behrens and Sporns 2012) and to reveal networks active during the resting state (Raichle 2009).

The development of optogenetic methods provides the opportunity to view and manipulate cells at the millisecond level in appropriate organisms (Deisseroth 2011). This invasive technology is not appropriate for humans, but starting with algae it has progressed to primates. Further ingenious application of genomics to imaging may eventually allow the complete integration of cellular with systems level analysis even within the human brain.

A fascinating new method with interesting links to the study of attention involves the use of video games to open the critical period usually involved in vision (Li, Ngo, Nguen, and Levi 2011). For many years it was believed that there is an early period in which visual input is needed in order to avoid loss of function. The video games may have increased cholinergic activity associated with visual orienting thus allowing better plasticity beyond the critical period. This has led to speculations that cholinergic agonists might help improve plasticity of visual function (Rokem and Silver 2010).

Evolution

Currently the cellular versus systems approach overlaps somewhat with human versus animal studies. While there is convincing evidence that some forms of attention are present in fruit flies (Miller, Ngo, and van Swinderen 2012) and thus likely throughout the animal kingdom, many forms (e.g. control of language) are unique or are nearly unique to humans. In areas such as orienting to visual objects monkeys and even rodents have been important for understanding the anatomy and neurochemistry of attention.

Even when human control is less similar to animal models the studies may provide an important perspective on where human abilities come from. An important current case is the role of Von Economo cells present in the human insula and anterior cingulate in top-down control of emotion and cognition (Seeley et al. 2012). The evolution of these cells in social animals and non-human primates may provide an important perspective on the development of self-regulation in humans. With new knowledge of genetics the evolutional approach will doubtless advance in the future.

Individuality

Most work on attention and most of the chapters of this volume deal with the forms of attention common to all people. However, the network approach does provide a natural link between universal properties of attention and individual differences.

The efficiency of the neural network underlying attention may be the reason that individuals differ in attention. In part, these differences in efficiency are due to genetic polymorphisms (see chapter 20 for a current discussion). The interaction of these polymorphisms with training and other environmental influences may provide new insight into how various forms of training may change gene expression and thus the efficiency of attention networks. Already it is possible to change connectivity with some forms of training (Tang and Posner 2009) and thus the interaction of training with genetics is likely to provide important future perspectives on child rearing and education (van Ijzendoorn et al. 2011).

References

Behrens, T. E. and Sporns, O. (2012). Human connectomics. *Current opinion in neurobiology* 22(1): 144–153.

Corbetta, M. and Shulman, G. L. (2002). Control of goal-directed and stimulus-driven attention in the brain. *Nature Reviews Neuroscience* 3: 201–215.

Dale, A. M., Liu, A. K., Fischi, B. R., Buckner, R., Beliveau, J. W., Lewine, J. D., and Halgren, E. (2000). Dynamic statistical parameter mapping: Combining fMRI and MEG for high resolution cortical activity. *Neuron* 26: 55–67.

Deisseroth, K. (2011). Optogenetics. *Nature Methods* 8: 26–29. doi: 10.1038/nmeth.f.324.

Heinze, H. J., Mangun, G. R., Burchert, W., Hinrichs, H., Scholtz, M., Muntel, T. F., Gosel, A., Scherg, M., Johannes, S., Hundeshagen, H., Gazzaniga, M. S., and Hillyard, S. A. (1994). Combined spatial and temporal imaging of brain activity during visual selective attention in humans. *Nature* 372: 543–546.

Hillyard, S. A., Di Russo, F., and Martinez, A. (2004). The imaging of visual attention. In N. Kanwisher and J. Duncan (eds.), *Attention and Performance XX: Functional Neuroimaging of Visual Cognition* (pp. 381–390). New York: Oxford University Press.

Hubel, D. and Wiesel, T. N. (1968). Receptive field and functional architecture of the monkey striate cortex. *Journal of Physiology* 195: 215–243.

Li, R. W., Ngo, C., Nguyen, J., and Levi, D. M. (2011). Video-game play induces plasticity in the visual system of adults with amblyopia. *PLoS Biology* 9: e1001135. doi: 10.1371/journal. pbio.1001135.

Miller, S. M., Ngo, T. T., and van Swinderen, B. (2012). Attentional switching in humans and flies: Rivalry in large and miniature brains. *Frontiers in Human Neuroscience* 5: 188. doi: 10.3389/fnhum.2011.00188.

Moruzzi, G. and Magoun, H. W. (1949). Brain stem reticular formation and activation of the EEG. *Electroencephalography and Clinical Neurophysiology* 1: 455–473.

Mountcastle, V. M. (1978). The world around us: Neural command functions for selective attention. *Neuroscience Research Progress Bulletin* 14(Suppl.): 1–47.

Posner, M. I. and Raichle, M. E. (1994). *Images of Mind*. New York: Scientific American Library.

Posner, M. I. and Raichle, M. E. (1998). The neuroimaging of human brain function. *Proceedings of the National Academy of Sciences USA* 95: 763–764.

Raichle, M. E. (2009). A paradigm shift in functional imaging. *Journal of Neuroscience* 29: 12729–12734.

Rokem, A. and Silver, M. A. (2010). Cholinergic enhancement augments magnitude and specificity of visual perceptual learning in healthy humans. *Current Biology* 20: 1723–1728.

Scherg, M. and Berg, P. (1993). *Brain Electrical Source Analysis*. Version 2.0. NeuroScan, Herndon, Va. <http://www.besa.de/products/besa_mri/>.

Seeley, W. W., Merkle, F. T., Gaus, S. E., Craig, A. D., Allman, J. M., and Hof, P. R. (2012). Distinctive neurons of the anterior cingulate and fronto-insular cortex: A historical perspective. *Cerebral Cortex* 22: 245–250.

Tang, Y. and Posner, M. I. (2009). Attention training and attention state training. *Trends in Cognitive Sciences* 13: 222–227.

van Ijzendoorn, M. H., Bakermans-Kranenburg, M. J., Belsky, J., Beach, S., Brody, G., Dodge, K. A., Greenberg, M., Posner, M., and Scott, S. (2011). Gene-by-environment experiments: A new approach to finding the missing heritability. *Nature Reviews Genetics* 12: 881. doi: 10.1038/nrg2764-c1.

van Voorhis, S. T. and Hillyard, S. A. (1977). Visual evoked potentials and selective attention to points in space. *Perception & Psychophysics* 22: 54–62.

Wurtz, R. H., Goldberg, E., and Robinson, D. L. (1980). Behavioral modulation of visual responses in monkey: Stimulus selection for attention and movement. *Progress in Psychobiology and Physiological Psychology* 9: 43–83.

PART B

THEORETICAL MODELS OF ATTENTION

CHAPTER 2

APPROACHES TO VISUAL SEARCH: FEATURE INTEGRATION THEORY AND GUIDED SEARCH

JEREMY M. WOLFE

INTRODUCTION

THE visual world is full of objects and it is an interesting fact that we can see more of that world than we can understand at any given moment. Thus, looking at this picture of a park just off Market St in San Francisco (Fig.2.1), you immediately see a rectangle filled with visual stuff but you do not immediately know the answer to fairly basic questions that one might ask about the objects in the scene. What colour is the bus? (white). Are there any people present? (no). This chapter will be devoted to the investigation of these limits on our perception through the theoretical lenses of Feature Integration Theory (Treisman 1988; Treisman and Gelade 1980) and Guided Search Theory (Wolfe 1994, 2007; Wolfe, Cave, and Franzel 1989). The chapter will be organized around the four terms that make up the names of the theories. **Features:** What are the basic features that are seen immediately in that rectangle of an image? **Integration:** How are those features combined into object representations? In particular, we will focus on the need for attention-demanding feature 'binding' in object recognition. **Guidance:** How can unbound features be used to guide **Search** for those objects or properties of a scene that are not immediately available to us when we look at a scene?

VISUAL SEARCH

Most of the work discussed in this chapter will involve the visual search paradigm in which an observer looks for one or more targets in a display containing some distractor

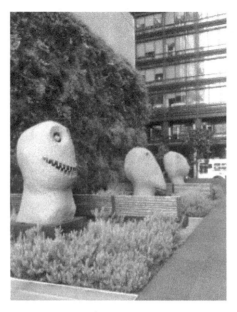

FIGURE 2.1 A park in San Francisco.

items. Search tasks are ubiquitous in daily life. Where is my coffee cup, the cellphone, the keyboard, the mouse, etc.? Such searches are typically concluded so quickly that we do not even register them as searches. We notice when the search is more prolonged. Where on stage is my child amidst the rest of the school choir? Moreover, our civilization has created socially important search tasks from airport baggage security (Gale, Mugglestone, Purdy, and McClumpha 2000; Rubenstein 2001) to medical image perception (Berbaum et al. 1998; Krupinski, Berger, Dallas, and Roehrig 2003; Kundel and Nodine 2004; Nodine, Krupinski, and Kundel 1993). These typically require trained expert searchers.

Beyond its face validity as a task that we perform all the time, visual search is a useful paradigm in the lab because it gives us a way to quantify the capacity limitations described in our initial example. With the San Francisco image, we can assert that you were not immediately aware of the presence of the bus or the absence of humans. With stimuli like those in Fig. 2.2, we can measure that.

Suppose that we showed observers a succession of displays like this and asked them to press one key if a red square was present and another if no red square was present. We could measure reaction time (or 'response time'—in either case, abbreviated 'RT') and/ or accuracy as a function of 'set size', the number of items in the display. We would find, to a first approximation, that the set size did not matter. Observers would be as fast and accurate with the 33-item display on the right as they are with the 9-item display on the left. The slope of the RT x set size function will be near zero. We can call such searches 'efficient' searches. In contrast, if observers were asked to find the item of medium size amidst the large and small items of Fig.2.2, we would obtain a very different pattern of results. RTs would increase roughly linearly with set size. The slope of the RT x set size function would probably be in the range of 20–40 msec/item for trials having

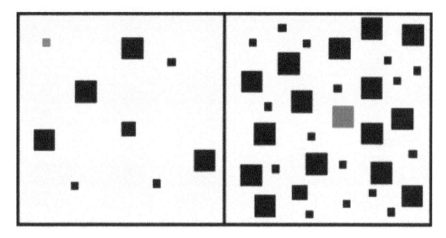

FIGURE 2.2 Search tasks: in each display, there are two targets; one, rather obviously, is red. The other is the square of medium size.

a medium-sized target. For target-absent trials, the slope would be roughly twice the target-present slope. (In fact, the ratio of absent to present slopes in an experiment with targets on 50% of trials appears to be reliably a bit more than 2:1—a fact that has theoretical importance, to be discussed below (Wolfe 1998).) If the display was presented only briefly or the observer was forced to respond by some very short deadline, we would find that the error rate for the 33-item display would be higher than the error rate for the 9-item display in the medium-target task but not in the red-target task. These speed–accuracy trade-off methods can be powerful tools in theoretical analysis of search tasks (Dukewich and Klein 2009; Guest and Lamberts 2011; McElree and Carrasco 1999). We can call tasks producing these sorts of results 'inefficient'.

FEATURE INTEGRATION THEORY

The distinction between what we are calling 'efficient' (Neisser 1963) and 'inefficient' (Atkinson, Holmgren, and Juola 1969) was central to the development of Treisman's Feature Integration Theory (Treisman and Gelade 1980). She argued that there was a limited set of basic features that could be processed 'preattentively', in parallel. In Fig. 2.2, colour is the example of such a feature. A target, defined by a unique basic feature would 'pop out' of a display. It would be available to awareness and for action without apparent capacity limitations. In contrast, many other search tasks, even if they involved quite simple perceptual discriminations (e.g. the distinction between big, medium, and small) showed a pattern of search results that Treisman argued was consistent with a serial self-terminating search; a search that proceeded one item after another until the target was discovered or the search was terminated—in the simplest case, after examining every item and determining that each was not the target. In a serial, self-terminating search,

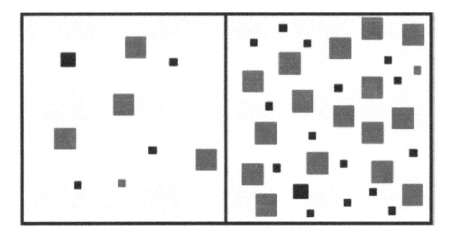

FIGURE 2.3 Conjunction search: look for the small red items.

observers would need to examine half of the items, on average, when the target was present and all of the items when it was absent. This predicted a 2:1 slope ratio between target-absent and target-present RT x set size functions; hence, the theoretical significance of the finding that those slope ratios may be reliably greater than 2:1.

The description of search tasks as 'parallel' and 'serial' has proven enduringly popular—to the distress of theoreticians who note that the patterns of results can be explained in many ways (Townsend 1971, 1990; Townsend and Wenger 2004; J. Palmer 1995; J. Palmer and McLean 1995). It is to avoid those theoretical commitments that we use the theory-neutral terms 'efficient' and 'inefficient'.

Conjunction searches like the one illustrated in Fig. 2.3 were critical to Treisman's originally dichotomous view of search. In Fig. 2.3, the target is defined by the conjunction of two features. It is the small red item. A sole small item in a field of large items or a sole red item in a field of black items would pop out. However, the small red item did not. The phenomenal experience of conjunction search was not a pop-out experience, and in a large body of Treisman's data, the RT x set size functions had slopes in the inefficient range. Treisman's conclusion was that while basic features were processed in parallel across the field, serial deployment of attention was required to integrate two or more features together. To change the language a little, serial attention was needed to 'bind' features to object representations. This was Treisman's solution to the 'binding problem'. There are multiple definitions of the problem (Treisman 1996). A useful way to think about it is in neural terms. If we stay with Fig. 2.3, there would be neurons that respond to an item's size and others that respond to its colour. How would one know which colours went with which size? Having higher-order cells for all possible combinations of all features at all locations seems implausible. Thus, there was a problem, and a limited-capacity, attention-directed binding process was the solution in Feature Integration Theory.

Here we are talking about the binding of two properties of one object, colour and size. However, as Treisman (2006) explains, binding is a more general issue. She identifies no fewer than seven types of binding. Some of these are conceptually quite similar to 'property binding' (her name in this paper for the binding of basic features like colour and size). For instance, knowing that two parts belong to one object is also a binding problem. Other forms could be similar at an abstract or computational level while being rather different phenomenologically. For instance, she notes that the fine discrimination of specific orientations (e.g. 22 deg. from 26 deg.) is thought to rely on ratios of two or more broadly tuned orientation channels (Olzak and Thomas 1986). So, in some sense, the outputs of those two coarse channels must be bound to produce the fine resolution. Unlike the binding of colour and size, the unbound components are not introspectively available in this case of what Treisman calls 'range binding'.

For those forms of binding, where the unbound properties are available, illusory conjunctions have been an important phenomenon, marshalled in support of Feature Integration Theory. The phenomenon is not easily demonstrated on the static page, but take a quick glance at Fig. 2.4 and then cover it up so that you cannot see it before returning to this text.

If you followed instructions, you are probably in a good position to list many of the colours and shapes that are present in the figure. You are probably quite sure that there was a diamond and, if asked, you are quite sure that there was no circle present. You are in a less confident position to report the conjunctions of colour and shape. What colour was the diamond? Odds are that you would not say 'blue' since nothing in the image was blue. However, Treisman found that there was quite a good chance that you would report seeing the diamond in the colour of one of the other shapes (Treisman and Schmidt 1982), perhaps yellow. It was as if the colours and shapes were floating free at some level in your visual system and, especially once the image was no longer present to provide a clear answer, those features could bind to form illusory conjunctions.

The original idea was that features were completely free-floating, but even in the first glimpse, the world doesn't look like a soup of loose features, and subsequent work reveals a role for location (Prinzmetal and Keysar 1989; Hazeltine, Prinzmetal, and Elliot 1997). The illusory conjunction phenomenon went well beyond simple shapes and colours to include, for example, letters and words (Prinzmetal 1991; Treisman and Souther 1986; Virzi and Egeth 1984) and clock times (Goolkasian 1988). Thus, basic features were not

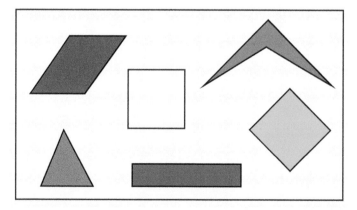

FIGURE 2.4 Stimuli for an illusory conjunction demonstration. Take a quick glance at the figure, cover it up, and return to the text.

the only units involved. It has been argued that illusory conjunctions are basically a phenomenon of memory (Briand and Klein 1989; Tsal 1989a, 1989b) and, indeed, memory for basic features can be quite terrible. In one experiment, Wolfe et al. showed observers an array of 20+ red and green dots. At one moment, signalled by a tone, one of the dots brightened and either did or did not change colour from red to green or green to red. Observers were close to chance performance when asked if the new colour was the same as the old one (Wolfe, Reinecke, and Brawn 2006). Observers knew that they had been looking at red and green dots, but the binding of colour to dot was clearly very fragile.

Still, binding errors need not be entirely in the remembered past tense. When items are relatively close to each other, especially in the periphery, observers experience 'crowding' phenomena (Levi 2008; Pelli and Tillman 2008) in which it may be possible to see features but not know how those features are bound together or even how they are bound to a location. That is, you might know there is a line at a location but you may be unable to determine its orientation. As Treisman would predict, attention allows illusory conjunctions to be resolved (Scolari, Kohnen, Barton, and Awh 2007) but the spatial grain of attention in the periphery is coarse (S. He, Cavanagh, and Intriligator 1996; Intriligator and Cavanagh 2001). So, away from fixation, illusory conjunctions may be a fact of life, even when the image remains continuously visible. Rosenholtz et al. talk about 'mongrels' that are created in the periphery by a system with weak spatial localization abilities and in which image statistics (e.g. average orientation) are calculated over multiple items. Portilla and Simoncelli (2000) developed a method for generating natural-looking textures from a set of image statistics. That is, if you took a picture of a forest, extracted the Portilla and Simoncelli statistics, and then synthesized a new image from those statistics, it would not be the original image but it would look forest-like. Rosenholtz et al. note that if this process is run over a standard search display like a search for a T among Ls, it creates new images in which some of the Ls have come to look like Ts. Arguing that this is the situation for vision away from the point of fixation, they have used the phenomenon to develop a theory of search performance (Rosenholtz, Chan, and Balas 2009). Even if crowding and mongrels are not quite the same things as illusory conjunctions, the problem of jumbled, possibly misbound features is similar. Attention-demanding binding is the Feature Integration solution to that problem (or, in more recent formulations, a leading solution among several—Treisman 2006).

INTEGRATION: IS ATTENTIVE BINDING REALLY NECESSARY?

Various challenges have been presented to the idea that binding requires attention and that binding is required for object identification. Quite early, Houck and Hoffman did an experiment with the McCollough Effect (Houck and Hoffman 1986). The McCollough effect is an orientation-contingent, colour after-effect based on adapting to, say, red vertical and green horizontal gratings. After adaptation, black and white vertical gratings would look greenish while black and white horizontal gratings would look pink (McCollough 1965). Houck and Hoffman found that the effect could be produced without attention to the adapting stimuli even though the effect clearly requires some sort of association of orientation and colour. If attention is required to bind colour to orientation, how could orientation-contingent colour adaptation occur without attention? One could attack the notion of 'without attention'. It is remarkably difficult to guarantee that a stimulus is unattended and it is virtually impossible to convince reviewers of this claim. As a consequence, more recent papers often refer to the 'near-absence' of attention (Reddy and Koch 2006; Reddy, Wilken, and Koch 2004).

Putting aside that methodological issue, there are situations where simple spatial co-occurrence of two features is all that is needed for the task at hand. Houck and Hoffman show one such case. A similar account could be invoked to explain other situations where conjunctive properties influence behaviour, apparently without attentive binding (Mordkoff, Yantis, and Egeth 1990). A particularly interesting case has to do with our remarkable ability to determine if humans or animals are present in scenes apparently without directing attention to the target object (VanRullen and Thorpe 2001; Kirchner and Thorpe 2006; Evans and Treisman 2005).

It may be that loose collections of unbound features are adequate to discriminate animal from non-animal (Treisman 2006), as is cartooned in Fig. 2.5.

Figure 2.5 is a cartoon because we cannot easily list or portray unbound 'animal' or 'oven' features but the point is that some discriminations in laboratory tasks will not require binding. Co-occurrence may be enough, though it must be confessed that other results such as the ability to identify a face in the 'near-absence' of attention are harder to explain with this unbound bundle of features idea (Reddy and Koch 2006).

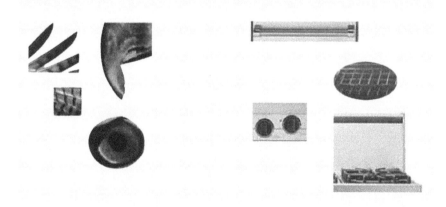

FIGURE 2.5 An unbound collection of features might be all that is required to determine if the 'animal' is on the left or right. This is only a cartoon as we do not know exactly what those 'unbound features' would look like.

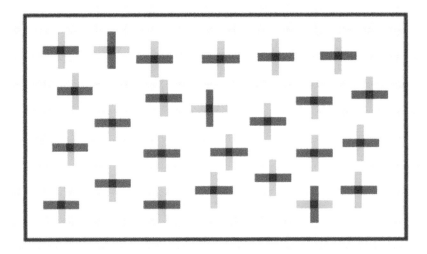

FIGURE 2.6 Search for the pluses with purple vertical and green horizontal components. Before attention arrives, all of these items are unbound collections of the same green, purple, vertical, and horizontal features.

Perhaps the best way to demonstrate the critical role of attentive binding is to create simple stimuli that eliminate the effectiveness of spatial co-occurrence of features. Figure 2.6 shows an example. You are a looking for 'pluses' with purple vertical and green horizontal components. You will find that this is an inefficient search. (There are three targets. Did you find them all?) Wolfe and Bennett (1997) argued that this was hard because before the arrival of attention, each one of these items was an unbound collection of purple, green, vertical, and horizontal features. As all the features of one item are in more or less the same location, associated with the same object, attention and binding are required before it can be determined if purple goes with vertical or horizontal.

One could object that, in fact, a purple-vertical-green-horizontal plus is just a green-vertical-purple-horizontal plus, rotated 90 degrees and, as a consequence, it is not surprising that one is hard to find amidst the other. Figure 2.7 shows stimuli intended to counter that argument. Here the targets and distractors are clearly very different objects. The targets look like puzzle pieces and the distractors look like some unusually rectangular, single-celled organism with a flagellum. These are designed to have very similar preattentive, unbound features. Each has a closed region and some straight and curved lines. The result, in the upper of the two search displays of Fig. 2.7, is a relatively inefficient search (Wolfe and Bennett 1997). Very similar stimuli produce an easier search in the second example because the targets are now the only items with the preattentively available attribute of 'closure' (Chen 1982; Elder and Zucker 1993, 1998).

Treisman's fundamental point about binding seems to be valid. If you eliminate the usefulness of spatial co-occurrence and if no basic feature distinguishes targets from distractors, an inefficient search is going to be required as the observer binds one item after another in the effort to identify a target.

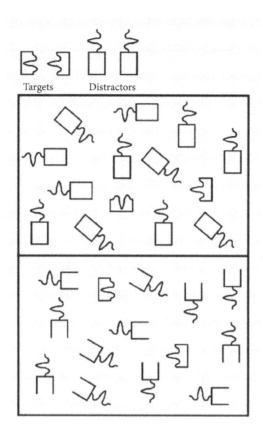

Targets   Distractors

FIGURE 2.7 A search for something like puzzle pieces among distractors with tails. This is easier in the lower panel because there the targets are the only items exhibiting 'closure'.

GUIDANCE: EFFICIENT CONJUNCTION SEARCH AND THE ROLE OF GUIDANCE

While it may be true that binding requires attention, it turns out not to be true that search tasks fall into two neat categories; efficient feature, 'pop-out' searches that do not require binding and can be done in parallel and all other searches that do require binding and are thus inefficient. While Treisman's original data were broadly consistent with this view, it rapidly became clear that conjunction searches, in particular, did not need to be inefficient. In the 1980s, exceptions started to appear (Alkhateeb, Morland, Ruddock, and Savage 1990; Dehaene 1989; McLeod, Driver, and Crisp, 1988; Nakayama and Silverman 1986; Sagi 1988; Zohary and Hochstein 1989). At first, it seemed like there might be a set of exceptions to the general rule, rather like irregular verb forms. Maybe stereopsis (Nakayama and Silverman 1986) or motion (McLeod et al. 1988) were special

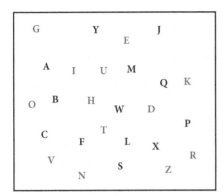

FIGURE 2.8 If you search for the red 'K', you will guide attention to red items and away from black. Reproduced from Egeth, H. E., Virzi, R. A. & Garbart, H. Searching for conjunctively defined targets. *Journal of Experimental Psychology: Human Perception and Performance*, 10, 32–39 © 1984, American Psychological Association.

features that operated under different rules of binding. However, by 1989, Wolfe et al. had data showing quite efficient search for colour x orientation searches and enough other examples had surfaced that it was time for a modification of the basic Feature Integration story (Wolfe, Cave, and Franzel 1989).

In retrospect, the key idea was made obvious by Egeth et al. (1984) and illustrated in Fig. 2.8. If you are asked to search for the letter 'V', you will perform some sort of relatively inefficient search. (It is complicated because letters are complicated bundles of features.) If you are asked to look for a red 'T', you will, again, perform some sort of relatively inefficient search, but this time only through the red items. A black item is simply never going to be a red T and you can use that knowledge about the basic features of the target to *guide* attention to items that have the features that make them more likely to be the target. If half of the items were red in this example, then the slope of the RT x set size function would be half that of an unguided letter search because half of the letters could be eliminated without ever being attended. The key observation of Guided Search (Wolfe et al. 1989) was that this could be a general property of search tasks. If observers were asked to search for a red vertical item among red horizontals and green verticals, preattentive, basic feature information could be used to guide attention toward red items and toward vertical items. The intersection of the sets of red and vertical items would be an excellent place to look for a red vertical target. Indeed, were guidance perfect, search for a basic conjunction of two features like colour and orientation should have been perfectly efficient. Such searches are more efficient than original Feature Integration Theory predicted but the slopes are greater than zero. We will return to the apparent imperfection of guidance later. For the present, where Feature Integration Theory saw two types of search—parallel and serial—Guided Search saw two ends of a continuum of guidance. Efficient 'parallel' search tasks were those where guidance was adequate to allow the deployment of attention to the target item first time, every time. Inefficient searches were those where no guidance was possible beyond guidance to the presence of an object in a location. Each of these items needed to be attended to, one after the other, until the target was found or the search was abandoned. In between were guided searches, where some basic feature information could be used to prioritize some items as more worthy of attention than others. The slope of the RT x set size function, in this view, becomes an estimate of the percentage of items that remain candidate targets even after guidance has done its work. If unguided, inefficient search has a standard slope of, say, 40 msec/item, then a search task producing a slope of 10 msec/item would imply that guidance could eliminate 3/4 of the items from consideration.

Working out the details of this straightforward idea is not entirely straightforward. The remainder of this chapter will discuss the nature of guiding features and the mechanics of Guided Search. While this chapter will focus on Guided Search, it is worth noting that there is a family of models that share aspects of Feature Integration and/or Guided Search architecture to greater or lesser extent (Cave 1999; Tsotsos 2011; E. Cohen and Ruppin 1999; Vidyasagar 1999; Hubner 2001; Lee, Buxton, and Feng 2005; Mozer and Baldwin 2008).

FEATURES

The nature of guiding features

In Treisman's original formulation, 'the visual scene is initially coded along a number of separable dimensions, such as color, orientation, spatial frequency, brightness, direction of movement' (Treisman and Gelade 1980). In her terminology, 'colour' would be a 'dimension' and 'red' a feature within that dimension. We often use the term 'attribute' for 'dimension' since dimension also gets used to talk about depth—which is a preattentive attribute. The cognitive architecture for early Feature Integration and early Guided Search was something like what is shown in Fig. 2.9. (It might or might not map directly onto neural structures.)

The stimulus was decomposed into a set of basic features. With the deployment of selective attention, the features of a particular object could be bound into a recognizable object with bound features in a particular location. In early Guided Search, the main addition to the standard Feature Integration story would be the idea that information about the decomposed features could be used to guide the deployment of attention. Thus, in Fig. 2.9, an intention to look for something horizontal would make use of the orientation map to deploy attention toward items showing some horizontal-ness in that map.

The architecture of the current version of Guided Search is somewhat different. The important change is that the representation that guides attention has been pulled out of the path from early vision to bound, recognized objects. This change was made when it became clear that the properties of the guiding representation were not the same as the building blocks of perception. Guidance is based on representations that do not 'see' the world as we experience it. This point is discussed more extensively elsewhere

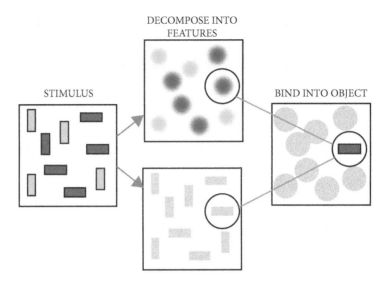

FIGURE 2.9 Cartoon of the cognitive architecture for early Feature Integration Theory and early Guided Search.

(Wolfe 2005, 2007, 2012; Wolfe and Horowitz 2004; Wolfe, Reijnen, Van Wert, and Kuzmova 2009). A single example will suffice here (Lindsey et al. 2010).

Suppose that your task is to search for desaturated targets. In the example in Fig. 2.10, the distractors would be fully saturated reds or blues and unsaturated whites. The targets would be pinkish on the left and pale blue on the right. This electronic or printed figure will not be colourmetrically precise, but the stimuli in the experiment were designed so that the targets lay perceptually exactly halfway between the distractors (details in Lindsey et al. 2010). This was done for a wide range of colours. Interestingly, searches for

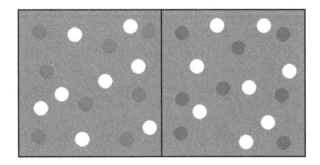

FIGURE 2.10 Search for the desaturated targets among saturated and achromatic distractors. Adapted from Lindsey, D. T., Brown, A. M., Reijnen, E., Rich, A. N., Kuzmova, Y., and Wolfe, J. M. , Color Channels, not Color Appearance or Color Categories, Guide Visual Search for Desaturated Color Targets, *Psychological Science*, 21 (9) pp. 225–31, copyright © 2010 by SAGE Publications. Reprinted by Permission of SAGE Publications.

the pinkish (maybe 'skin-coloured') targets were hundreds of msec faster than searches for other desaturated colours. In perceptual space, the distance from blue to pale blue might be the same as the distance from red to pale red. However, in the guiding representation, the red–pale red difference is, apparently, much more significant.

Consequently, the current version of Guided Search adopts an architecture like that cartooned in Fig. 2.11. Between early visual processes and bound representations of objects, there is a tight bottleneck. Access to that bottleneck is gated by a guiding representation that is itself an abstraction from early vision and, as noted, does not 'see' the world exactly as we see it. Once an object is selected, re-entrant processes (Di Lollo, Enns, and Rensink 2000; Hochstein and Ahissar 2002) reach back to make contact with the perceptual properties of the object. Treisman's current thinking also holds that re-entry is required for binding (Bouvier and Treisman 2010).

What are the features? (Wolfe and Horowitz 2004—revised)

A great deal of work has gone into defining the set of stimulus attributes that guide attention. Not all of this work is done by people who have adopted a Guided Search viewpoint, so in different papers, these attributes might be described as preattentive dimensions, pop-out features, etc. The goal is to determine the set of attributes that support efficient search and the guidance of attention.

Wolfe and Horowitz (2004) created a list of guiding attributes. Here that list is updated in a set of five annotated tables. Tables 1–3 1.1–1.3 rank candidates into categories of the 'undoubted', the 'probable and possible', and the 'doubtful' attributes. In addition, Table 2.4 is reserved for 'complicated' attributes and Table 2.5 introduces the idea of

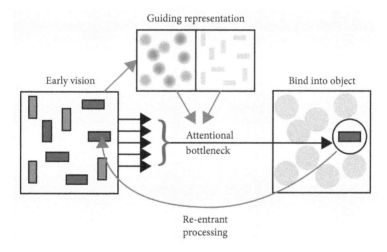

FIGURE 2.11 Guided Search architecture with the 'guiding representation' pulled out of the main path from early vision to perception.

Table 2.1 The Undoubted Feature Dimensions: 'Undoubted' means that the status of these properties is attested by a large body of work with converging methods

	The Undoubted Feature Dimensions	Notes
Colour	Bauer, Jolicoeur, & Cowan 1998; Bauer, Jolicoeur, & Cowan 1996; Brawn & Snowden 1999; Carter 1982; D'Zmura 1991; Daoutis, Pilling, & Davies 2006; Duncan 1988; Farmer & Taylor 1980; Green & Anderson 1956; Lindsey et al. 2010; Monnier & Nagy 2001; Nagy & Sanchez 1990; Nagy, Young, & Neriani 2004; Smith 1962; Treisman & Gormican 1988; Treisman & Souther 1985	1
Motion	Braddick & Holliday 1991; Burr, Baldassi, Morrone, & Verghese 2009; Dick, Ullman, & Sagi 1987; Horowitz, Wolfe, DiMase, and Klieger 2007; Kawahara 1993; McLeod et al. 1988; Muhlenen & Muller 1999; Nakayama & Silverman 1986; Nothdurft 1993b; Rosenholtz 2001a; Takeuchi 1997	2
Orientation	Bergen & Julesz 1983; Cavanagh, Arguin, & Treisman 1990; Foster & Ward 1991a, 1991b; Moraglia 1989a; Sagi 1990; Wolfe & Friedman-Hill 1992; Wolfe, Friedman-Hill, Stewart, & O'Connell 1992; Wolfe, Klempen, & Shulman 1999	
Size (incl. length & spatial freq.)	Cavanagh et al. 1990; Found & Muller 2001; Moraglia 1989b; D. Sagi 1988; Stuart 1993; Treisman & Gormican 1988; Verghese & Nakayama 1994; Verghese & Pelli 1994; L. G. Williams 1966	3

Notes:
1. Colour is certainly a feature. The currently interesting questions have to do with what aspects of colour signals guide attention as noted in the example in Fig. 2.10.
2. It is possible that motion could be decomposed into separate attributes of speed and direction (Driver, McLeod, & Dienes 1992).
3. We are calling this dimension 'size' but it covers a number of properties that, again, might be treated separately. It is possible that spatial frequency should be treated as its own dimension (Bilsky & Wolfe 1995), especially considering its possible role in guidance in scenes (Oliva, Torralba, Castelhano, & Henderson 2003). See also Alvarez & Cavanagh 2008.

Table 2.2 Probable and possible feature dimensions: The items can make a reasonable case for their status as guiding attributes. However, more data would be needed to address dissenting opinions or the possibility of alternative explanations

	Probable and Possible Feature Dimensions	Notes
Luminance onset (flicker)	Spalek, Kawahara, & Di Lollo 2009; Theeuwes 1995; Yantis & Jonides 1990	
Luminance polarity	Gilchrist, Humphreys, & Riddoch 1996; Theeuwes & Kooi 1994	4
Vernier offset	Fahle 1991a, 1991b	5
Stereoscopic depth & tilt	Z. J. He & Nakayama 1992; Holliday & Braddick 1991; McSorley & Findlay 2001; Moore, Elsinger, & Lleras 2001; Nakayama & Silverman 1986; O'Toole & Walker 1997; Sousa, Brenner, & Smeets 2009	6,7
Pictorial depth cues	Aks & Enns 1993; Enns & Rensink 1990, 1993; Enns, Rensink, & Douglas 1990; Epstein, Babler, & Bownds 1992; Sun & Perona 1996a; Von Grünau & Dubé 1994	6,7
Shape	Bergen & Julesz 1983; Cheal & Lyon 1992; Chen 1982, 1990; Kristjánsson & Tse 2001; Pilon & Friedman 1998; Pomerantz & Pristach 1989; Treisman & Gormican 1988; Tsal, Meiran, & Lamy 1995; Wolfe & Bennett 1997	8

Table 2.2 (continued)

	Probable and Possible Feature Dimensions	Notes
Line termination	Donnelly, Humphreys, & Riddoch 1991; Julesz & Bergen 1983; Taylor & Badcock 1988	8
Closure	Chen 1982; Elder & Zucker 1994, 1998; Enns 1986; Kanbe 2009; Kovacs & Julesz 1993; Treisman & Souther 1985; D. Williams & Julesz 1992	8
Topological status	Chen 1982, 1990, 2005; Rubin & Kanwisher 1985	8
Curvature	Fahle 1991b; Foster & Savage 2002; Gurnsey, Humphrey, & Kapitan 1992; Sakai, Morishita, & Matsumoto 2007; Treisman & Gormican 1988; Wolfe, Yee, & Friedman-Hill 1992	8
Lighting direction (shading)	Adams 2008; Aks & Enns 1992; Braun 1993; Kleffner & Ramachandran 1992; Ostrovsky, Cavanagh, & Sinha 2004; Ramachandran 1988; Sun & Perona 1996a, 1996b; Symons, Cuddy, & Humphrey 2000	9
Glossiness (lustre)	Wolfe & Franzel 1988	10
Expansion/looming	Braddick & Holliday 1991; Franconeri & Simons 2003; Skarratt, Cole, & Gellatly 2009; Takeuchi 1997	11
Number	Reijnen, Krummenacher, & Wolfe 2011; Taylor & Badcock 1988; Treisman & Gormican 1988	12
Aspect ratio	Treisman & Gormican 1988	

Notes:

4. Luminance polarity clearly supports efficient search but it might be nothing more than the black-white or luminance axis of a 3D colour space. Thus it could be grouped with colour.
5. The difficulty with Vernier as a guiding property in its own right is that it might be reducible to an orientation cue (Findlay 1973; Fahle & Harris 1998).
6. The taxonomy of depth cues as guiding attributes is not clear. Maybe it is a single, broad dimension of something like 3D layout (cf. Oliva & Torralba 2001) combining a variety of depth cues including stereopsis, the various pictorial depth cues, and shading into a representation of the 3D world. The relevant experiments would combine different guiding depth cues in a single display in order to see if they could act independently.
7. Depth guides attention in the sense that a 'near' item will pop out among far, for example. However, it also acts to modulate features like size. An item that is little in the image may be big in the world if it is far away. See 'modulators' in Table 5.
8. Rather like depth, it is not clear if 'shape' is one guiding dimension or many. Here we hedge our bets, listing shape and a collection of other properties that might be part of a family of shape attributes. To see the problem, consider line termination, closure, and curvature. Each supports efficient search, but are they actually independent attributes? Do an 'O' and a 'C' differ in closure or line termination or both? The issue has been complicated by the failure to settle on a generally accepted set of shape features (Kourtzi & Connor 2011; Logothetis, Pauls, & Poggio 1995; Yamane, Carlson, Bowman, Wang, & Connor 2008; Zhang et al. 2011).
9. The earlier evidence for guidance by shading (e.g. Ramachandran's 'eggs': Ramachandran 1988) has been undermined somewhat by later work (Cavanagh 1999; Ostrovsky et al. 2004). It is possible that shading information should be grouped with other cues like stereopsis, as part of one, omnibus 3D depth property.
10. The evidence for shininess or gloss comes from a single experiment on binocular lustre (Wolfe & Franzel 1988). Unpublished work in our lab casts doubt on the generality of the finding.
11. 'Expansion' and/or 'looming' cues are somewhat problematic because they might be decomposed into a depth cue, a size cue, a motion cue, or some combination of these, though an ability to deploy attention to something that might hit you in the head seems like a good idea.
12. Recent evidence shows that numerosity (does this cluster contain more dots than the other clusters?) is, at best, a rather weak feature, requiring large (>3:1) ratios between target and distractor numerosities (Reijnen et al. 2011).

Table 2.3 Doubtful cases and probable non-features: These are the proposed preattentive features where the preponderance of data seems to argue against their role as guiding features. It must be acknowledged that other authors would come to different conclusions about some of these attributes. Moreover, some attributes have their status on the basis of single experiments and would benefit from further study

	Doubtful cases & probable non-features	Notes
Novelty	Flowers & Lohr 1985; Frith 1974; Johnston, Hawley, & Farnham 1993; Q. Wang, Cavanagh, & Green 1994; Wolfe 2001; Zhaoping & Frith 2011	13
Learned features (e.g. letters)	Atkinson et al. 1969; Golcu & Gilbert 2009; Grice & Canham 1990; Kinchla 1974; Kinchla & Collyer 1974; Shiffrin & Gardner 1972	14
Alphanumeric category	Brand 1971; Duncan 1983; Jonides & Gleitman 1972; Krueger 1984	15
Intersection	Bergen & Adelson 1988; Bergen & Julesz 1983; Julesz 1981, 1984; Julesz & Bergen 1983; Julesz & Krose 1988; Nothdurft 1991; Wolfe & DiMase 2003	16
Optic flow	Braddick & Holliday 1991; Bravo 1998; Royden, Wolfe, & Klempen 2001, but see Rushton, Bradshaw, & Warren 2007	
Colour change	Theeuwes 1995	
3D volumes (e.g. geons)	J. M. Brown, Weisstein, & May 1992; Pilon & Friedman 1998	
Luminosity	Correani, Scot-Samuel, & Leonards 2006	17
Material type	Wolfe & Myers 2010	
Scene category	Greene & Wolfe 2011	
Duration	Morgan, Giora, & Solomon 2008	
Stare-in-crowd	Doi & Ueda 2007; Palanica & Itier 2011; M. A. Williams, Moss, & Bradshaw 2002; Von Grünau & Anston 1995	18
Eye of origin/ binocular rivalry	Paffen, Hooge, Benjamins, & Hogendoorn 2011; Shneor & Hochstein 2006; Wolfe & Franzel 1988; Zhaoping 2008	19
Your name	Bundesen, Kyllingsbaek, Houmann, & Jensen 1997	
Threat	Batty, Cave, & Pauli 2005; Lipp 2006; Notebaert, Crombez, Van Damme, De Houwer, & Theeuwes 2011; Öhman, Flykt, & Esteves 2001; Soares, Esteves, Lundqvist, & Ohman 2009; Tipples, Young, Quinlan, Broks, & Ellis 2002	20
Biological motion	Pratt, Radulescu, Guo, & Abrams 2010; L. Wang, Zhang, He, & Jiang 2010	21

Notes:

13. There are various claims for a guiding role for novelty and/or familiarity. The phenomena seem to be rather weak. For instance, as a general rule, a basic feature will continue to guide attention in the presence of some distractor heterogeneity in an irrelevant attribute. Thus, vertical will pop out among horizontal even if all the items are of different colour. However, while a novel mirror-reversed N might pop out among Ns (Wang et al. 1994), it is not clear that it would pop out among a heterogeneous set of normal letters.
14. Is it possible to learn a new preattentive feature? This is a long-standing question in visual search. Much of the work involves alphanumeric characters as over-learned sets of stimuli (Caerwinski, Lightfoot, & Shiffrin 1992; Malinowski & Hübner 2001; Sigman & Gilbert 2000; Sireteanu & Rettenbach 1995). The problem is that it is very hard to tell the difference between learning a new feature and learning to better exploit existing signals (e.g. line terminations, closure, etc.). This is a case where reasonable researchers could and do disagree (Shiffrin & Schneider 1977).

Table 2.3 (continued)

15. It was thought that a letter might pop out among numbers and vice versa but these results (e.g. the 'zero-oh' effect) have been hard to replicate.
16. Intersection once seemed to be a good candidate for feature status but more recent results have demoted it to 'unlikely' status (Wolfe & DiMase 2003).
17. People have a strong belief that they can detect when someone is staring at them. They even believe that they can detect someone staring at them from behind them (Simons & Chabris 2010). However, while we are very good at assessing someone else's gaze direction, especially if it is toward us (Watt, Craven, & Quinn 2007), we are probably not able to do so in a search setting and/or without attending to that person—but see Stein, Senju, Peelen, & Sterzer 2011.
18. Correani et al. (2006) found that luminosity did support efficient search. However, a series of control experiments showed this to be attributable to local luminance effects and not to luminosity itself.
19. Wolfe and Franzel (1988) had argued that eye-of-origin information and binocular rivalry signals were not available to guide search. However, more recent results suggest some sensitivity to those signals.
20. There is little question that threatening stimuli elicit threat-specific responses as seen, for example, in the responses of phobics to snakes or spiders (LoBue & DeLoache 2008; Rakison & Derringer 2008; Reinecke, Rinck, & Becker 2006). However, there does not appear to be a specific role for 'threat' in guiding search once other features are controlled (e.g. snakes have thin, curvy, and pointed attributes as well as possibly frightening ones).
21. Biological motion is a special stimulus (Blake 1993; Blake & Shiffrar 2007; Johansson 1973), but to date there is not a convincing demonstration that it is capable of supporting efficient visual search. It is possible that motion that implies animacy will have feature status (Gao, McCarthy, & Scholl 2010; Gao, Newman, & Scholl 2009; Gao & Scholl 2011).

Table 2.4 Complicated cases

Complicated		Notes
Faces (familiar, upright, angry, real, schematic, etc.)	D. V. Becker, Anderson, Mortensen, Neufield, & Neel 2011; S. I. Becker, Horstmann, & Remington 2011; Devue, Van der Stigchel, Brèdart, & Theeuwes 2009; Doi & Ueda 2007; Eastwood, Smilek, & Merikle 2001; Frischen, Eastwood, & Smilek 2008; Von Grünau & Anston 1995; Hansen & Hansen 1988; Hershler & Hochstein 2005, 2006; Horstmann, Bergmann, Burghaus, & Becker 2010; Langton, Law, Burton, & Schweinberger 2008; Nothdurft 1993c; D. G. Purcell, Stewart, & Skov 1996; Suzuki & Cavanagh 1995; Tong & Nakayama 1999; VanRullen 2006; M. A. Williams et al. 2002)	22
Other semantic categories (e.g. 'animal')	Levin, Takarae, Miner, & Keil 2001	

Notes:
22. No candidate features have generated more controversy than the family of face features. There are many demonstrations of apparently efficient search for real faces, schematic faces, angry faces, happy faces, and so forth. There are also many papers pointing to feature confounds in these stimuli. There are good reviews in some recent articles on the topic (S. I. Becker et al. 2011; Frischen et al. 2008). In previous versions of this list, faces were placed in the unlikely category (Wolfe and Horowitz 2004) but the literature is so large and so persistent that it seems best to describe the case as 'complicated' and leave its resolution to the future.

Table 2.5 Modulators

Modulators		23
Cast shadows	Rensink & Cavanagh 2004	
Amodal completion	Rensink & Enns 1998; Wolfe et al. 2011	
Apparent depth	Aks & Enns 1996; Champion & Warren 2008; Wheatley, Cook, & Vidyasagar 2004	

Notes:

23. The entries under this category do not appear to be preattentive features in their own right. However, they are properties that seem to be computed prior to the deployment of attention and that have an influence on other basic features. Thus, apparent depth can change the apparent size of an item and it is the apparent size, rather than the retinal or image size, that is critical in search (Aks & Enns 1996). The amodal completion of contours behind occluders can disrupt a feature. Rensink and Enns (1998) showed that the size of an element in the image could be lost when that element was tied to another element by amodal completion. On the other hand, it is possible to create oriented items that are only oriented if unoriented elements are tied together by amodal completion. Though these oriented bars are visually compelling, this orientation feature does not guide attention (Wolfe et al. 2011).

preattentive properties that modulate other guiding attributes without guiding attention in their own right. The referencing is extensive but not exhaustive.

To summarize, there appear to be one to two dozen guiding attributes. Some of these are more powerful directors of attention than others. It seems clear that attributes like colour and motion guide easily and effectively while an attribute like numerosity may guide but only rather weakly. It would be wonderful if we could rank order attributes in terms of their effectiveness. However, while some direct comparison between features has been done (Nothdurft 1993a), a comprehensive hierarchy does not exist. There are hierarchies within dimensions as well. Red really does seem to be a particularly powerful guiding colour, but again, there is a vast amount we do not know, including why a feature like red should be more effective than some other colour. There is plenty of interesting speculation (Changizi, Zhang, and Shimojo 2006).

Guidance by scene-based features: The next frontier

For all the detail and complexity of the feature list already presented, it has become increasingly clear that these features are not the whole story when it comes to describing sources of guidance. This can be illustrated if you look for people in Fig. 2.12. You will not search randomly and you will rapidly find the man on the sidewalk, halfway down the street. Eye movement data indicate that you will search first in locations where people are likely to be (Ehinger, Hidalgo-Sotelo, Torralba, and Oliva 2009; Torralba, Oliva, Castelhano, and Henderson 2006). People are on horizontal surfaces. They do not generally float. In addition, you know something about the size of people. Because you can very rapidly extract the spatial layout of a scene (Greene and Oliva 2009), you should

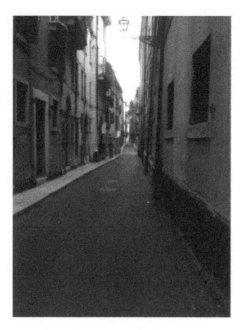

FIGURE 2.12 Find the two people in this scene. Which one did you find first, and why?

be able to determine if an object is a candidate human on the basis of the interaction of the size of an object in the image and its apparent depth (Sherman, Greene, and Wolfe 2011). Both of these factors may have kept you from noticing the other man, apparently very small and perched on the ledge of the first window on the right. The pixels and the rough local contrast are the same for each man (courtesy of Photoshop) but one target is far more plausible. If you found the plausible target first, it was probably scene guidance that directed your attention. While the classical features can be useful, the apparent efficiency of search in real-world scenes cannot be based on those features alone (Vickery, King, and Jiang 2005; Wolfe, Alvarez, Rosenholtz, Kuzmova, and Sherman 2011).

Our understanding of scene guidance is relatively young but it seems clear that observers make use of what can be called scene semantic guidance (forks are likely to be next to plates) and scene syntactic guidance (paintings hang on walls) (Castelhano and Heaven 2010; Henderson, Brockmole, Castelhano, and Mack 2007; Henderson and Ferreira 2004; Neider and Zelinsky 2006; Vo and Henderson 2009). Some of this guidance is probably relatively slow. After all, you cannot look for forks next to plates until you have identified the plates. However, the guidance that is based on scene structure and category can be based on information that is available very quickly from the global processing of the 'gist' of a scene (Fei-Fei, Iyer, Koch, and Perona 2007; Kirchner and Thorpe 2006; Oliva 2005; Sanocki and Epstein 1997). It is possible to know that you are viewing a man-made, navigable, urban scene before you have selectively attended to the various objects that make up that scene (Greene and Oliva 2009).

Two paths to awareness

The ability to extract some information from scenes without selective attention to objects reflects the working of a non-selective pathway from the stimulus to visual awareness (Wolfe, Vo, Evans, and Greene 2011). The capabilities of this pathway should not be overstated. You will not recognize specific objects without selective attention and binding. However, a non-selective pathway is a useful addition to the diagram in Fig. 2.11. This elaboration is shown in Fig. 2.13. Early visual processing of a scene feeds a non-selective pathway that can provide some information about spatial layout and the gist of the scene. It also feeds the Guiding Representation, here represented by colour, shape, and now gist—a scene guidance component. Finally, early vision provides the input to the selective pathway that supports object recognition. It has a selective attentional bottleneck whose selections are modulated by the Guiding Representation.

At any given moment, the contents of visual awareness include visual 'stuff' at all locations, provided by the non-selective pathway and one (or perhaps a few) bound objects, provided by the selective pathway. A more detailed account of this two-pathway architecture can be found in Wolfe et al. (2011).

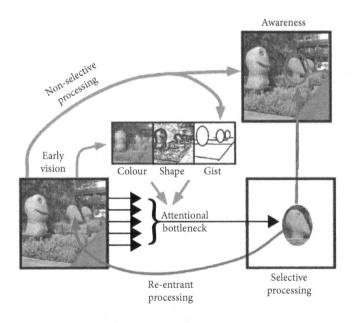

FIGURE 2.13 Guided Search architecture with the addition of a non-selective pathway. The non-selective pathway supports awareness of visual 'stuff' across the entire visual field in parallel. It is capable of limited semantic processing (e.g. of scene 'gist'). It is not subject to the attentional bottleneck and it is not capable of most acts of recognition.

GUIDANCE: THE RULES

The ability of a preattentive feature to guide attention is highly rule-governed. There are general rules that appear to operate over all dimensions and rules specific to a single dimension.

1. The greater the difference, along a preattentive dimension, between the target and the distractors, the more efficient the search (Duncan and Humphreys 1989). Thus, it will be easier to find vertical among 30 deg. tilted items than among 15 deg. tilted items.

2. The greater the differences between the distractors (distractor heterogeneity), the less efficient the search (Duncan and Humphreys 1989). Thus, it may be harder to find vertical among a mix of 15 and 30 deg. tilted distractors than among homogeneous 15 deg. distractors, even though the average difference between target and distractors is greater for the heterogeneous example (Rosenholtz 2001b).

3. The minimum target–distractor difference required to produce efficient search will be much greater than the just noticeable difference for those stimuli. Thus, with attentional scrutiny, it is possible to tell the difference between a vertical line and one tilted 1–2 deg. from vertical. It is not possible to search efficiently for vertical among 2 deg. distractors. Efficient search will require something more like 10 to 15 deg. differences (Foster and Ward 1991b; Foster and Westland 1998).

4. For purposes of guidance, differences are greater across categorical boundaries. It will be easier to find a steep item among shallow items than to find the steepest item among other steep items even if the angular differences are the same in the two conditions (Wolfe, Friedman-Hill, et al. 1992).

5. The detailed properties of guiding attributes need to be worked out separately for each attribute and are not necessarily predicted from conscious perception of the attribute. As noted earlier, for purposes of guidance, pink/peach/skin(?) colours seem to have special status (Lindsey et al. 2010). As another example, in orientation, one might wonder if guidance is represented in a 90 deg. or 180 deg. framework. Obviously, a simple line has the same orientation after a 180 deg. rotation but a polar object (e.g. a Christmas tree or sailboat) does not have the same appearance after a 180 deg. rotation. Visual search ignores object polarity. The biggest orientation difference is 90 deg., not 180 deg. (Wolfe et al. 1999).

6. Guidance will be stronger if the observer sees the actual guiding feature (e.g. the colour 'red') rather than merely the name of the feature (e.g. the word 'red') just prior to the appearance of the search display. This priming can be produced by a deliberate cue before the onset of the trial (Wolfe, Horowitz, Kenner, Hyle, and Vasan 2004). Similarly, finding the target on one trial effectively

primes that feature for the next (Kristjánsson and Driver 2008; Maljkovic and Nakayama 1994).

7. It is easier to find the presence of a feature than to find its absence. This is the root of many search asymmetries (Treisman and Gormican 1988; Treisman and Souther 1985) in which the search for A among B is notably more efficient than the search for B among A. Thus, it is easier to find the presence of a moving target among stationary distractors than to find a stationary target among moving distractors (Dick et al. 1987; Royden et al. 2001; Horowitz et al. 2007). There is a great deal more to be said about asymmetries (Wolfe 2001), much of it first said by Treisman, as noted above. Rosenholtz has noted that the designs of asymmetry experiments are sometimes themselves asymmetrical (Rosenholtz 2001a) and this is worth keeping in mind when evaluating search asymmetry results.

8. Not all search asymmetries are evidence for the preattentive processing of the stimulus property under study. Sometimes it is easier to find A among B than B among A, not because A pops out, but because it is easier to reject a succession of Bs as distractors. In these cases, both A vs B and B vs A tend to produce inefficient slopes. Thus, for example, if there is a real 'anger superiority effect' (Hansen and Hansen 1988), it may not be that 'angry' pops out, but rather that angry faces hold attention, making it harder to move through them when they are the distractors. As a result, search for an angry target among easily dismissed, happy distractors is more efficient than search for a happy target among hard-to-dismiss, angry distractors, but neither of these searches will be efficient.

9. It is possible to guide by more than one feature at a time. In Guided Search, this is how relatively efficient conjunction search is accomplished. If there are several target features, you can guide your attention to all of them. Indeed, higher-order conjunctions with three or even six defining features can be easier than the classic two-feature conjunction search (Wolfe et al. 1989; Wolfe 2010). There is a debate about how this is accomplished. We have argued that it is possible to simultaneously guide to multiple features (Friedman-Hill and Wolfe 1995). Huang and Pashler argue that guidance to multiple features must be done in a series of nested steps. For example, one might select all red items and then select the vertical items within the red set (Huang and Pashler 2007, 2012).

10. It is not possible to guide to two features from the same dimension/attribute at the same time. Conjunctions of two colours or two orientations are inefficient (Wolfe et al. 1990). Even though it is easy to identify an item that is red and yellow, it is not efficient to search for that item among red/blue and blue/yellow distractors.

11. It is relatively efficient to search for a conjunction of an item of one colour with a part of another colour. (Find the red thing with a yellow part among red things with blue parts and blue things with yellow parts.) This suggests that the

preattentive representations of objects have some part–whole structure to them (Wolfe, Friedman-Hill, and Bilsky 1994). Interestingly, search for orientation x orientation conjunctions of items with part–whole structure is not efficient. The vertical item with an oblique part is relatively hard to find amidst vertical items with horizontal parts and horizontal items with oblique parts (Bilsky and Wolfe 1995). The difference between colour and orientation could be due to different susceptibility to rotation. If you tilt your head, a red thing with a yellow part is still a red thing with a yellow part. A vertical thing with a horizontal part might not be rotationally invariant in the same way.

GUIDED SEARCH 2013: HOW DO WE SEARCH?

Figure 2.14 elaborates on Fig. 2.13 to provide a roadmap of the steps in visual search as imagined by the 2013 incarnation of the Guided Search model. Sections below refer to the letters on the figure:

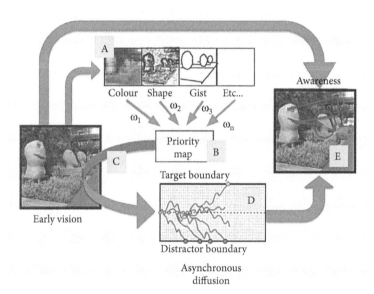

FIGURE 2.14 Guided Search 2013: A. A set of attributes, including scene-based attributes like gist, is derived from early visual processing. B. A priority map is created from a weighted average of those sources of guidance. C. The priority map controls selection of items, one after another, for binding and recognition. D. Binding and recognition are modelled as a diffusion process. Since the diffusion takes longer than the time between attentional selections, the result is an asynchronous diffusion with multiple items in process at the same time. See text for further details.

A. As described in the figure, a set of basic attributes is extracted from the early stages of visual processing. For each attribute, two forms of guidance are possible. *Bottom-up guidance* is stimulus-driven, based on local differences. Bottom-up guidance is essentially the same as 'salience' (Nothdurft 2000; Donk and van Zoest 2008; Lamy and Zoaris 2009). *Top-down guidance* is user-driven, based on what the observer's current understanding of the task demands. Thus, returning to Fig. 2.8, if you are looking for a red T, colour guidance will be directed to red. If you are looking for a black T, guidance will be directed to black. Nothing has changed in the stimulus or in the bottom-up salience of items. It is the top-down guidance that changes in this case. When neurophysiological studies refer to attention to multiple items in parallel (e.g. enhancing neural responses of all red items), they are generally describing what we refer to as top-down guidance (Bichot, Rossi, and Desimone 2005; Treue and Trujillo 1999; Carrasco, Eckstein, Verghese, Boynton, and Treue 2009).

The top-down/bottom-up terminology is not entirely unambiguous. Consider priming effects. Exposure to red will speed subsequent search for red. We have described this as a form of implicit top-down guidance (Wolfe et al. 2004) because something about the observer—in this case, their history—has changed the guidance of attention. Response to the same stimulus would be different if the observer's history was different. Others see priming as an automatic process that should be considered to be 'bottom-up' (Kristjánsson and Campana 2010).

B. Guidance by different attributes is combined into a 'priority map'. In the first versions of Guided Search this was called an 'activation map'. 'Priority map' (Serences and Yantis 2006) better captures the role of this representation, which is to prioritize items in the visual input for selective attention, binding, and recognition. In the absence of top-down guidance, a priority map built from pure bottom-up signals would be a 'salience map' (Koch and Ullman 1985; Itti and Koch 2000; Parkhurst, Law, and Niebur 2002). Each attribute makes a weighted contribution to the priority map. Thus, if you are looking for red vertical items, the weights on colour and orientation will be set high and other attributes will be de-emphasized. In order to guide to 'red', one can imagine either setting a high weight for a separate feature, 'red', or enhancing red within the colour module and setting a high weight for guidance by colour. See the work on 'dimension weighting' for more detail on this issue (Found and Muller 1996; Muller, Reimann, and Krummenacher 2003; Zehetleitner, Krummenacher, Geyer, Hegenloh, and Müller 2011).

Weights can be adjusted but not to the full extent that the user might wish. Notably, it does not seem possible to set the weight on bottom-up salience signals to zero. There has been a long-standing debate about what sorts of salient signals capture attention. Claims have been made for luminance onsets (Jonides and Yantis 1988; Yantis and Jonides 1990), new objects (Yantis 1993), and for many specific attributes (Franconeri and Simons 2003; Rauschenberger 2003; Turatto and Glafano 2000; Pratt, Radulescu, Guo, and Abrams 2010). There are generally counterclaims (Gibson and Kelsey 1998), but on balance, it seems that a highly salient signal from an irrelevant attribute will have some influence on the course of search, regardless of the desires of the searcher.

Some researchers are not fond of the idea of a priority map (Chan and Hayward 2009; Huang and Pashler 2012). However, while the details vary, some version of such a map is a part of many models of search and has been the subject of much neurophysiological investigation (Bisley and Goldberg 2010; Fecteau and Munoz 2006; Gottlieb, Balan, Oristaglio, and Schneider 2009; Li 2002; Thompson and Bichot 2004).

C. The priority map is so named because its role is to prioritize the selection of items. Since Koch and Ullman (1985), it has been proposed that something like a winner-take-all operation selects the next item for attention. This is straightforward for the first selection in an image but what about subsequent selections? The critical question is whether attention ever revisits the same location/item during the course of a search. The original assumption was that items were not revisited. This was the assumption of Feature Integration and the first versions of Guided Search. The phenomenon of 'Inhibition of Return' (IOR) seemed to provide a mechanism to prevent resampling from the display (Klein 1988; Posner 1980) since IOR showed that it was harder to get attention back to a previously attended item than to direct attention to a previously unattended item. However, subsequent results suggested that IOR probably only marked the most recently attended items (Abrams and Pratt 1996; Pratt and Abrams 1995; Tipper, Weaver, and Watson 1996) making it hard to see how this mechanism could prevent revisitations once the set size becomes large.

Horowitz and Wolfe did a series of experiments designed to directly test if items were being sampled with or without replacement during visual search and came to the conclusion that 'visual search has no memory' (Horowitz and Wolfe 1998, 2003)—at least, no memory for the deployments of covert attention. Their data were consistent with sampling with replacement, giving no role to IOR or other means of preventing revisitation. Other evidence suggested that this claim might be too strong (Peterson, Kramer, Wang, Irwin, and McCarley 2001; Shore and Klein 2000; Takeda 2004). Over the short timescale required for many standard laboratory search tasks, it seems most likely that neither extreme position is correct. Items are not sampled entirely without regard to the prior history of search but neither are they inhibited in a manner that can prevent some resampling. In Klein's words, inhibition of return appears to be a 'foraging facilitator' (Klein and MacInnes 1999), one of several mechanisms that bias attention toward new items during search (Klein 2009).

When search is more prolonged, as it is in many real-world tasks, strategic plans can play a role in preventing revisiting. Reading is a simple example. If you search this page of text for the word 'covert', you will most likely start at the top left and read the page in a manner that eliminates most resampling from the display without requiring specific inhibition of or memory for rejected items. Your prospective plan of search serves the role that memory would serve (McDaniel, Robinson-Riegler, and Einstein 1998). Similar factors are probably at work in many real-world searches (Hollingworth 2009; Hollingworth and Henderson 2002).

D. In the 2013 version of Guided Search, the recognition/classification of an object is modelled as a diffusion process (Ratcliff 1978). While we have used a Ratcliff-style diffuser, there is, at present, no reason to choose between any particular member of the class of models in which information accumulates toward a threshold over time (Brown and Heathcote 2008; Donkin, Brown, Heathcote, and Wagenmakers 2011; Purcell et al. 2010). The unique aspect of the Guided Search version is that it proposes an *asynchronous* diffusion process. That is, items are selected one at a time and begin diffusing toward a target or distractor boundary once they are selected. Since the rate of selection (say, 20–40 Hz) is faster than the time required to identify an item (say, 150–300 msec), multiple items are diffusing at the same time. Metaphorically, this can be seen as a 'pipeline' or a 'carwash' (Moore and Wolfe 2001; Wolfe 2003), albeit a carwash in which one car could enter second and leave first.

This architecture is a hybrid of serial and parallel processing (E. Cohen and Ruppin 1999; Herd and O'Reilly 2005; Thornton and Gilden 2007; Townsend and Wenger 2004; Verghese 2001). Selection is imagined to be strictly serial though nothing very dramatic would change if a small number of items could be selected at one time. Diffusion is parallel in the sense that multiple items are undergoing the process of binding and recognition at the same time.

Diffusion models produce the positively skewed reaction time distributions that are characteristic of visual search (E. M. Palmer, Horowitz, Torralba, and Wolfe 2011; Wolfe, Palmer, and Horowitz 2010). Errors are produced when a distractor reaches the target boundary or a target reaches the distractor boundary. An error could also be generated if the search was terminated with a guess (see next section). Changes in the parameters of the diffuser can be used to model various effects seen in the data. Thus, if the boundaries are brought closer together, the error rate will rise and the RTs will decline; a speed-accuracy trade-off. False alarms and miss errors can be traded off against each other by changing the starting point of the diffuser.

When do we stop?

The architecture of Fig. 2.14 makes the process of finding a target reasonably clear. With some preattentive guidance, items are selected into the diffuser and search ends when one of those items goes over the target boundary. But what happens if there is no target or if no item reaches the target boundary or if there are an unknown number of targets in the display? At some point, search must end. When is it time to quit? Feature Integration assumed that observers would quit when all items had been examined on target absent trials (or almost all, with miss errors produced when observers quit without checking the target). Early versions of Guided Search argued that observers searched through all items that received guiding activation above some threshold. Neither of these accounts works well if distractors are not perfectly tracked during search. Moreover, in real scenes, it is completely unclear what the 'set size' might be or what it would mean to attend to all items (Wolfe, Alvarez, et al. 2011).

A different approach adds another diffuser to the model. In this diffuser, a signal accumulates over time and the trial is terminated when that signal crosses a quitting threshold. The threshold is set dynamically, based on the observer's experience. After quitting correctly, the quitting threshold moves down, causing the observer to quit more quickly. After an error, it rises and the observer becomes more cautious about quitting. This adjustment can be observed in the pattern of RTs in search experiments (Chun and Wolfe 1996; Ishibashi, Kita, and Wolfe 2012).

Experiments that manipulate target prevalence are useful in constraining models of quitting behaviour in search (Colquhoun and Baddeley 1967; Fleck and Mitroff 2007; Wolfe, Horowitz, and Kenner 2005; Wolfe et al. 2007; Wolfe and VanWert 2010). When targets are rare, miss errors rise, false alarms fall, and RTs become shorter. If targets are common, miss errors fall, false alarms rise, and RTs become longer. To see this full pattern of behaviour, it is important to use stimuli that are ambiguous enough to produce false-alarm errors. Classic search experiments (find the T among Ls, etc.) tend not to produce false alarms. In contrast, real-world tasks like breast cancer screening (Wolfe, Birdwell, and Evans 2011) or airport baggage screening are characterized by ambiguous stimuli and very low prevalence. Wolfe and VanWert (2010) found that the effects of prevalence could be modelled as a change in criterion (which would be represented by a change in the starting point of the diffuser in Fig. 2.14) and a concurrent change in a quitting threshold. At low prevalence, the starting point moves toward the distractor bound, making miss errors more common, and the quitting threshold drops, making RTs shorter (and also increasing miss errors, if one assumes an 'absent' response when the quitting threshold is reached). Models that adjust only the starting point or only the quitting threshold, fail to capture the pattern of the data. It should be noted that search termination remains a complex and underinvestigated topic.

What We Didn't Discuss

Having discussed search termination, it is time to consider chapter termination. Before ending, it is worth noting that there are a number of important topics that have been largely omitted here. Some of these will be discussed elsewhere in this volume. Any complete account of search would include some treatment of:

Eye movements: What is the relationship between covert deployments of attention and overt deployments of the eyes (Hwang, Wang, and Pomplun 2011; Kowler 2011; Malcolm and Henderson 2010; Neider, Boot, and Kramer 2010).

The psychophysics of simple searches: There is an important body of work on the fine-grained details of simple searches. The tasks used in these studies permit a degree of control that is not common in standard search tasks and not possible in real-world search tasks (Najemnik and Geisler 2005; J. Palmer, Verghese, and Pavel, 2000; Cameron, Tai, Eckstein, and Carrasco 2004; Dosher, Han, and Lu 2010; Baldassi and Verghese 2002).

Memory in repeated search: What happens when the same scene is searched more than once? Contextual cueing shows learning (Brockmole and Henderson 2006; Chun and

Jiang 1998; Kunar, Flusberg, Horowitz, and Wolfe 2007). Repeated searches through simple, laboratory-style search displays do not produce an improvement in search efficiency (Wolfe, Klempen, and Dahlen 2000) but there is learning in repeated search through real scenes (Hollingworth 2009; Hollingworth and Henderson 2002; Vo and Wolfe 2012).

The neural basis of search: What might be the neural locus and operation of a priority map (Serences and Yantis 2006; Shipp 2004; Bisley and Goldberg 2010) or a diffuser (Ratcliff, Philiastides, and Sajda 2009) or a serial selection process (Buschman and Miller 2009; Chelazzi 1999) or set size effects (J. Y. Cohen, Heitz, Woodman, and Schall 2009)?

Of course, this is merely a sampling of the topics that have been studied from a neural perspective and a sampling of the topics, important to search, that have been omitted from this chapter.

BIBLIOGRAPHY

Abrams, R. A. and Pratt, J. (1996). Spatially diffuse inhibition affects multiple locations: A reply to Tipper, Weaver, and Watson (1996). *Journal of Experimental Psychology: Human Perception and Performance* 22(5): 1294–1298.

Adams, W. J. (2008). Frames of reference for the light-from-above prior in visual search and shape judgements. *Cognition* 107(1): 137–150.

Aks, D. J. and Enns, J. T. (1992). Visual search for direction of shading is influenced by apparent depth. *Perception & Psychophysics* 52(1): 63–74.

Aks, D. J. and Enns, J. T. (1993). Early vision's analysis of slant-from-texture. *Investigative Ophthalmology and Visual Science* 34(4): 1185.

Aks, D. J. and Enns, J. T. (1996). Visual search for size is influenced by a background texture gradient. *Journal of Experimental Psychology: Human Perception and Performance* 22(6): 1467–1481.

Alkhateeb, W. F., Morland, A. B., Ruddock, K. H., and Savage, C. J. (1990). Spatial, colour, and contrast response characteristics of mechanisms which mediate discrimination of pattern orientation and magnification. *Spatial Vision* 5(2): 143–157.

Alvarez, G. A. and Cavanagh, P. (2008). Visual short-term memory operates more efficiently on boundary features than on surface features. *Perception & Psychophysics* 70(2): 346–364.

Atkinson, R. C., Holmgren, J. E., and Juola, J. F. (1969). Processing time as influenced by the number of elements in a visual display. *Perception & Psychophysics* 6(6A): 321–326.

Baldassi, S. and Verghese, P. (2002). Comparing integration rules in visual search. *Journal of Vision* 2(8): 559–570.

Batty, M. J., Cave, K. R., and Pauli, P. (2005). Abstract stimuli associated with threat due to conditioning cannot be detected preattentively. *Emotion* 5(4): 418–430.

Bauer, B., Jolicoeur, P., and Cowan, W. B. (1996). Visual search for colour targets that are or are not linearly-separable from distractors. *Vision Research* 36(10): 1439–1466.

Bauer, B., Jolicoeur, P., and Cowan, W. B. (1998). The linear separability effect in color visual search: Ruling out the additive color hypothesis. *Perception & Psychophysics* 60(6): 1083–1093.

Becker, D. V., Anderson, U. S., Mortensen, C. R., Neufield, S. L., and Neel, R. (2011). The Face in the Crowd Effect unconfounded: Happy faces, not angry faces, are more efficiently detected in single- and multiple-target visual search tasks. *JEP: General* 140(4): 637–659.

Becker, S. I., Horstmann, G., and Remington, R. W. (2011). Perceptual grouping, not emotion, accounts for search asymmetries with schematic faces. *Journal of Experimental Psychology: Human Perception and Performance* 37(6): 1739–1757.

Berbaum, K. S., Franken, E. A., Jr., Dorfman, D. D., Miller, E. M., Caldwell, R. T., Kuehn, D. M., et al. (1998). Role of faulty visual search in the satisfaction of search effect in chest radiography. *Academic Radiology* 5(1): 9–19.

Bergen, J. R. and Julesz, B. (1983). Rapid discrimination of visual patterns. *IEEE Transactions on Systems, Man, and Cybernetics SMC-13*: 857–863.

Bergen, J. R. and Adelson, E. H. (1988). Early vision and texture perception. *Nature 333*: 363–364.

Bichot, N. P., Rossi, A. F., and Desimone, R. (2005). Parallel and serial neural mechanisms for visual search in macaque area V4. *Science 308*(5721): 529–534.

Bilsky, A. A. and Wolfe, J. M. (1995). Part–whole information is useful in size X size but not in orientation X orientation conjunction searches. *Perception & Psychophysics* 57(6): 749–760.

Bisley, J. W. and Goldberg, M. E. (2010). Attention, intention, and priority in the parietal lobe. *Annual Review of Neuroscience* 33(1): 1–21.

Blake, R. (1993). Cats perceive biological motion. *Psychological Science* 4(1): 54–57.

Blake, R. and Shiffrar, M. (2007). Perception of human motion. *Annual Review of Psychology* 58: 47–73.

Bouvier, S. and Treisman, A. (2010). Visual feature binding requires reentry. *Psychological Science* 21(2): 200–204.

Braddick, O. J. and Holliday, I. E. (1991). Serial search for targets defined by divergence or deformation of optic flow. *Perception* 20(3): 345–354.

Brand, J. (1971). Classification without identification in visual search. *Quarterly Journal of Experimental Psychology* 23: 178–186.

Braun, J. (1993). Shape-from-shading is independent of visual attention and may be a texton. *Spatial Vision* 7(4): 311–322.

Bravo, M. J. (1998). A global process in motion segregation. *Vision Research* 38(6): 853–864.

Brawn, P. and Snowden, R. J. (1999). Can one pay attention to a particular color? *Perception & Psychophysics* 61(5): 860–873.

Briand, K. A. and Klein, R. M. (1989). Has feature integration come unglued? A reply to Tsal. *Journal of Experimental Psychology: Human Perception and Performance* 15(2): 401–406.

Brockmole, J. R. and Henderson, J. M. (2006). Using real-world scenes as contextual cues for search. *Visual Cognition* 13(1): 99–108.

Brown, J. M., Weisstein, N., and May, J. G. (1992). Visual search for simple volumetric shapes. *Perception & Psychophysics* 51(1): 40–48.

Brown, S. D. and Heathcote, A. (2008). The simplest complete model of choice response time: Linear ballistic accumulation. *Cognitive Psychology* 57(3): 153–178.

Bundesen, C., Kyllingsbaek, S., Houmann, K. J., and Jensen, R. M. (1997). Is visual attention automatically attracted by one's own name? *Perception & Psychophysics* 59(5): 714–720.

Burr, D. C., Baldassi, S., Morrone, M. C., and Verghese, P. (2009). Pooling and segmenting motion signals. *Vision Research* 49(10): 1065–1072.

Buschman, T. J. and Miller, E. K. (2009). Serial, covert shifts of attention during visual search are reflected by the frontal eye fields and correlated with population oscillations. *Neuron* 63: 386–396.

Caerwinski, M., Lightfoot, N., and Shiffrin, R. (1992). Automatization and training in visual search. *American Journal of Psychology* 105(2): 271–315.

Cameron, E. L., Tai, J. C., Eckstein, M. P., and Carrasco, M. (2004). Signal detection theory applied to three visual search tasks—identification, yes/no detection and localization. *Spatial Vision* 17(4–5): 295–325.

Carrasco, M., Eckstein, M., Verghese, P., Boynton, G., and Treue, S. (2009). Visual attention: Neurophysiology, psychophysics and cognitive neuroscience. *Vision Research* 49(10): 1033–1036.

Carter, R. C. (1982). Visual search with color. *Journal of Experimental Psychology: Human Perception and Performance* 8: 127–136.

Castelhano, M. S. and Heaven, C. (2010). The relative contribution of scene context and target features to visual search in scenes. *Attention, Perception, & Psychophysics* 72(5): 1283–1297.

Cavanagh, P., Arguin, M., and Treisman, A. (1990). Effect of surface medium on visual search for orientation and size features. *Journal of Experimental Psychology: Human Perception and Performance* 16(3): 479–492.

Cavanagh, P. (1999). Pictorial art and vision. In R. A. Wilson and Frank C. Keil (eds.), *MIT Encyclopedia of Cognitive Science* (pp. 648–651). Cambridge, Mass.: MIT Press.

Cave, K. (1999). The FeatureGate model of visual selection. *Psychological Research* 62(2–3): 182–194.

Champion, R. A. and Warren, P. A. (2008). Rapid size scaling in visual search. *Vision Research* 48(17): 1820–1830 [doi: 10.1016/j.visres.2008.05.012].

Chan, L. K. H. and Hayward, W. G. (2009). Feature integration theory revisited: Dissociating feature detection and attentional guidance in visual search. *Journal of Experimental Psychology: Human Perception and Performance* 35(1): 119–132.

Changizi, M. A., Zhang, Q., and Shimojo, S. (2006). Bare skin, blood and the evolution of primate colour vision. *Biology Letters* 2(2): 217–221.

Cheal, M. and Lyon, D. (1992). Attention in visual search: Multiple search classes. *Perception & Psychophysics* 52(2): 113–138.

Chelazzi, L. (1999). Serial attention mechanisms in visual search: A critical look at the evidence. *Psychological Research* 62(2–3): 195–219.

Chen, L. (1982). Topological structure in visual perception. *Science* 218: 699–700.

Chen, L. (1990). Holes and wholes: A reply to Rubin and Kanwisher. *Perception & Psychophysics* 47: 47–53.

Chen, L. (2005). The topological approach to perceptual organization. *Visual Cognition* 12(4): 553–637.

Chun, M. M. and Wolfe, J. M. (1996). Just say no: How are visual searches terminated when there is no target present? *Cognitive Psychology* 30: 39–78.

Chun, M. M. and Jiang, Y. (1998). Contextual cueing: Implicit learning and memory of visual context guides spatial attention. *Cognitive Psychology* 36: 28–71.

Cohen, E. and Ruppin, E. (1999). From parallel to serial processing: A computational study of visual search. *Perception & Psychophysics* 61(7): 1449–1461.

Cohen, J. Y., Heitz, R. P., Woodman, G. F., and Schall, J. D. (2009). Neural basis of the set-size effect in frontal eye field: Timing of attention during visual search. *Journal of Neurophysiology* 101(4): 1699–1704.

Colquhoun, W. P. and Baddeley, A. D. (1967). Influence of signal probability during pretraining on vigilance decrement. *Journal of Experimental Psychology* 73(1): 153–155.

Correani, A., Scot-Samuel, N., and Leonards, U. (2006). Luminosity—a perceptual 'feature' of light-emitting objects? *Vision Research* 46(22): 3915–3925.

D'Zmura, M. (1991). Color in visual search. *Vision Research* 31(6): 951–966.

Daoutis, C. A., Pilling, M., and Davies, I. R. L. (2006). Categorical effects in visual search for colour. *Visual Cognition* 14(2): 217–240.

Dehaene, S. (1989). Discriminability and dimensionality effects in visual search for featural conjunctions: A functional pop-out. *Perception & Psychophysics* 46(1): 72–80.

Devue, C., Van der Stigchel, S., Brèdart, S., and Theeuwes, J. (2009). You do not find your own face faster; you just look at it longer. *Cognition* 111(1): 114–122.

Di Lollo, V., Enns, J. T., and Rensink, R. A. (2000). Competition for consciousness among visual events: The psychophysics of reentrant visual processes. *Journal of Experimental Psychology: General* 129: 481–507.

Dick, M., Ullman, S., and Sagi, D. (1987). Parallel and serial processes in motion detection. *Science* 237: 400–402.

Doi, H. and Ueda, K. (2007). Searching for a perceived stare in the crowd. *Perception* 36(5): 773–780.

Donk, M. and van Zoest, W. (2008). Effects of salience are short-lived. *Psychological Science* 19(7): 733–739.

Donkin, C., Brown, S., Heathcote, A., and Wagenmakers, E.-J. (2011). Diffusion versus linear ballistic accumulation: Different models but the same conclusions about psychological processes? *Psychonomic Bulletin & Review* 18(1): 61–69.

Donnelly, N., Humphreys, G. W., and Riddoch, M. J. (1991). Parallel computation of primitive shape descriptions. *Journal of Experimental Psychology: Human Perception and Performance* 17(2): 561–570.

Dosher, B. A., Han, S., and Lu, Z.-L. (2010). Information-limited parallel processing in difficult heterogeneous covert visual search. *Journal of Experimental Psychology: Human Perception and Performance* 36(5): 1128–1144.

Driver, J., McLeod, P., and Dienes, Z. (1992). Are direction and speed coded independently by the visual system? Evidence from visual search. *Spatial Vision* 6(2): 133–147.

Dukewich, K. R. and Klein, R. M. (2009). Finding the target in search tasks using detection, localization, and identification responses. *Canadian Journal of Experimental Psychology/ Revue canadienne de psychologie expérimentale* 63(1): 1–7.

Duncan, J. (1983). Category effects in visual search: A failure to replicate the 'oh-zero' phenomenon. *Perception & Psychophysics* 34(3): 221–232.

Duncan, J. (1988). Boundary conditions on parallel processing in human vision. *Perception* 17: 358.

Duncan, J. and Humphreys, G. W. (1989). Visual search and stimulus similarity. *Psychological Review* 96: 433–458.

Eastwood, J. D., Smilek, D., and Merikle, P. M. (2001). Differential attentional guidance by unattended faces expressing positive and negative emotion. *Perception & Psychophysics* 63(6): 1004–1013.

Egeth, H. E., Virzi, R. A., and Garbart, H. (1984). Searching for conjunctively defined targets. *Journal of Experimental Psychology: Human Perception and Performance* 10: 32–39.

Ehinger, K. A., Hidalgo-Sotelo, B., Torralba, A., and Oliva, A. (2009). Modelling search for people in 900 scenes: A combined source model of eye guidance. *Visual Cognition* 17(6): 945–978.

Elder, J. and Zucker, S. (1993). The effect of contour closure on the rapid discrimination of two-dimensional shapes. *Vision Research* 33(7): 981–991.

Elder, J. and Zucker, S. (1994). A measure of closure. *Vision Research* 34(24): 3361–3369.

Elder, J. and Zucker, S. (1998). Evidence for boundary-specific grouping. *Vision Research* 38(1): 142–152.

Enns, J. (1986). Seeing textons in context. *Perception & Psychophysics* 39(2): 143–147.

Enns, J. T. and Rensink, R. A. (1990). Sensitivity to three-dimensional orientation in visual search. *Psychological Science* 1(5): 323–326.

Enns, J. T., Rensink, R. A., and Douglas, R. (1990). The influence of line relations on visual search. *IOVS (Supplement)* 31(4): 105.

Enns, J. T. and Rensink, R. A. (1993). A model for the rapid discrimination of line drawing in early vision. In D. Brogan, A. Gale, and K. Carr (eds.), *Visual Search 2* (pp. 73–89). London: Taylor & Francis.

Epstein, W., Babler, T., and Bownds, S. (1992). Attentional demands of processing shape in three-dimensional space: Evidence from visual search and precuing paradigms. *Journal of Experimental Psychology: Human Perception and Performance* 18(2): 503–511.

Evans, K. K. and Treisman, A. (2005). Perception of objects in natural scenes: Is it really attention-free? *Journal of Experimental Psychology: Human Perception and Performance* 31(6): 1476–1492.

Fahle, M. (1991a). A new elementary feature of vision. *Investigative Ophthalmology and Visual Science* 32(7): 2151–2155.

Fahle, M. (1991b). Parallel perception of vernier offsets, curvature, and chevrons in humans. *Vision Research* 31(12): 2149–2184.

Fahle, M. and Harris, J. P. (1998). The use of different orientation cues in vernier acuity. *Perception & Psychophysics* 60(3): 405–426.

Farmer, E. W. and Taylor, R. M. (1980). Visual search through color displays: Effects of target-background similarity and background uniformity. *Perception & Psychophysics* 27: 267–272.

Fecteau, J. H. and Munoz, D. P. (2006). Salience, relevance, and firing: A priority map for target selection. *Trends in Cognitive Sciences* 10(8): 382–390.

Fei-Fei, L., Iyer, A., Koch, C., and Perona, P. (2007). What do we perceive in a glance of a real-world scene? *Journal of Vision* 7(1): 10.

Findlay, J. M. (1973). Feature detectors and vernier acuity. *Nature* 241(5385): 135–137.

Fleck, M. S. and Mitroff, S. R. (2007). Rare targets rarely missed in correctable search. *Psychological Science* 18(11): 943–947.

Flowers, J. H. and Lohr, D. J. (1985). How does familiarity affect visual search for letter strings? *Perception & Psychophysics* 37: 557–567.

Foster, D. H. and Ward, P. A. (1991a). Asymmetries in oriented-line detection indicate two orthogonal filters in early vision. *Proceedings of the Royal Society (London B)* 243: 75–81.

Foster, D. H. and Ward, P. A. (1991b). Horizontal-vertical filters in early vision predict anomalous line-orientation frequencies. *Proceedings of the Royal Society (London B)* 243: 83–86.

Foster, D. H. and Westland, S. (1998). Multiple groups of orientation-selective visual mechanisms underlying rapid oriented-line detection. *Proceedings of the Royal Society (London B)* 265: 1605–1613.

Foster, D. H. and Savage, C. J. (2002). Uniformities and asymmetries of rapid curved-line detection explained by parallel categorical coding of contour. *Vision Research* 42: 2163–2175.

Found, A. and Muller, H. J. (1996). Searching for unknown feature targets on more than one dimension: Investigating a 'dimension weighting' account. *Perception & Psychophysics* 58(1): 88–101.

Found, A. and Muller, H. J. (2001). Efficient search for size targets on a background texture gradient: Is detection guided by discontinuities in the retinal-size gradient of items? *Perception* 30(1): 21–48.

Franconeri, S. L. and Simons, D. J. (2003). Moving and looming stimuli capture attention. *Perception & Psychophysics* 65(7): 999–1010.

Friedman-Hill, S. R. and Wolfe, J. M. (1995). Second-order parallel processing: Visual search for the odd item in a subset. *Journal of Experimental Psychology: Human Perception and Performance* 21(3): 531–551.

Frischen, A., Eastwood, J. D., and Smilek, D. (2008). Visual search for faces with emotional expressions. *Psychological Bulletin* 134(5): 662–676.

Frith, U. (1974). A curious effect with reversed letters explained by a theory of schema. *Perception & Psychophysics* 16(1): 113–116.

Gale, A. G., Mugglestone, M. D., Purdy, K. J., and McClumpha, A. (2000). Is airport baggage inspection just another medical image? In E. A. Krupinski (ed.), *Medical Imaging 2000: Image Perception and Performance, Proceedings of SPIE*, vol. 3981 (pp. 184–192). Bellingham, Wash.: Society of Photo-Optical Instrumentation Engineers.

Gao, T., Newman, G. E., and Scholl, B. J. (2009). The psychophysics of chasing: A case study in the perception of animacy. *Cognitive Psychology* 59(2): 154–179.

Gao, T., McCarthy, G., and Scholl, B. J. (2010). The wolfpack effect: Perception of animacy irresistibly influences interactive behavior. *Psychological Science* 21(12): 1845–1853.

Gao, T. and Scholl, B. J. (2011). Chasing vs. stalking: Interrupting the perception of animacy. *Journal of Experimental Psychology: Human Perception and Performance* 37(3): 669–684.

Gibson, B. S. and Kelsey, E. M. (1998). Stimulus-driven attentional capture is contingent on attentional set for displaywide visual features. *Journal of Experimental Psychology: Human Perception and Performance* 24(3): 699–706.

Gilchrist, I. D., Humphreys, G. W., and Riddoch, M. J. (1996). Grouping and extinction: Evidence for low-level modulation of visual selection. *Cognitive Neuropsychology* 13(8): 1223–1249.

Golcu, D. and Gilbert, C. D. (2009). Perceptual learning of object shape. *Journal of Neuroscience* 29(43): 13621–13629.

Goolkasian, P. (1988). Illusory conjunctions in the processing of clock times. *Journal of General Psychology* 115(4): 341–353.

Gottlieb, J., Balan, P. F., Oristaglio, J., and Schneider, D. (2009). Task-specific computations in attentional maps. *Vision Research* 49(10): 1216–1226.

Green, B. F. and Anderson, L. K. (1956). Color coding in a visual search task. *Journal of Experimental Psychology* 51: 19–24.

Greene, M. R. and Oliva, A. (2009). The briefest of glances: The time course of natural scene understanding. *Psychological Science* 20(4): 464–472.

Greene, M. R. and Wolfe, J. M. (2011). Global image properties do not guide visual search. *Journal of Vision* 11(6): doi: 10.1167/11.6.18.

Grice, G. R. and Canham, L. (1990). Redundancy phenomena are affected by response requirements. *Perception & Psychophysics* 48(3): 209–213.

Guest, D. and Lamberts, K. (2011). The time course of similarity effects in visual search. *Journal of Experimental Psychology: Human Perception and Performance* 37(6): 1667–1688.

Gurnsey, R., Humphrey, G. K., and Kapitan, P. (1992). Parallel discrimination of subjective contours defined by offset gratings. *Perception & Psychophysics* 52(3): 263–276.

Hansen, C. H. and Hansen, R. D. (1988). Finding the face in the crowd: An anger superiority effect. *Journal of Personality and Social Psychology* 54(6): 917–924.

Hazeltine, R. E., Prinzmetal, W., and Elliot, K. (1997). If it's not there, where is it? Locating illusory conjunctions. *Journal of Experimental Psychology: Human Perception and Performance* 23(1): 263–277.

He, S., Cavanagh, P., and Intriligator, J. (1996). Attentional resolution and the locus of visual awareness. *Nature* 383(6598): 334–337.

He, Z. J. and Nakayama, K. (1992). Surfaces versus features in visual search. *Nature* 359: 231–233.

Henderson, J. M. and Ferreira, F. (2004). Scene perception for psycholinguists. In J. M. Henderson and F. Ferreira (eds.), *The Interface of Language, Vision, and Action: Eye Movements and the Visual World* (pp. 1–58). New York: Psychology Press.

Henderson, J. M., Brockmole, J. R., Castelhano, M. S., and Mack, M. (2007). Image salience versus cognitive control of eye movements in real-world scenes: Evidence from visual search. In R. van Gompel, M. Fischer, W. Murray, and R. Hill (eds.), *Eye Movement Research: Insights into Mind and Brain* (pp 537–562). Oxford: Elsevier.

Herd, S. and O'Reilly, R. (2005). Serial search from a parallel model. *Vision Research* 45(24): 2987–2992.

Hershler, O. and Hochstein, S. (2005). At first sight: A high-level pop-out effect for faces. *Vision Research* 45(13): 1707–1724.

Hershler, O. and Hochstein, S. (2006). With a careful look: Still no low-level confound to face pop-out. *Vision Research* 46(18): 3028–3035.

Hochstein, S. and Ahissar, M. (2002). View from the top: Hierarchies and reverse hierarchies in the visual system. *Neuron* 36: 791–804.

Holliday, I. E. and Braddick, O. J. (1991). Pre-attentive detection of a target defined by stereoscopic slant. *Perception* 20: 355–362.

Hollingworth, A. and Henderson, J. M. (2002). Accurate visual memory for previously attended objects in natural scenes. *Journal of Experimental Psychology: Human Perception and Performance* 28(1): 113–136.

Hollingworth, A. (2009). Two forms of scene memory guide visual search: Memory for scene context and memory for the binding of target object to scene location. *Visual Cognition* 17(1): 273–291.

Horowitz, T. S. and Wolfe, J. M. (1998). Visual search has no memory. *Nature* 394(6 August): 575–577.

Horowitz, T. S. and Wolfe, J. M. (2003). Memory for rejected distractors in visual search? *Visual Cognition* 10(3): 257–298.

Horowitz, T. S., Wolfe, J. M., DiMase, J., and Klieger, S. B. (2007). Visual search for type of motion is based on simple motion primitives. *Perception* 36: 1624–1634.

Horstmann, G., Bergmann, S., Burghaus, L., and Becker, S. (2010). A reversal of the search asymmetry favoring negative schematic faces. *Visual Cognition* 18(7): 981–1016.

Houck, M. R. and Hoffman, J. E. (1986). Conjunction of color and form without attention: Evidence from an orientation-contingent color after-effect. *Journal of Experimental Psychology: Human Perception and Performance* 12: 186–199.

Huang, L. and Pashler, H. (2007). A boolean map theory of visual attention. *Psychological Review* 114(3): 599–631.

Huang, L. and Pashler, H. (2012). Distinguishing different strategies of across-dimension attentional selection. *Journal of Experimental Psychology: Human Perception and Performance* 38(2): 453–464.

Hubner, R. (2001). A formal version of the Guided Search (GS2) model. *Perception & Psychophysics* 63(6): 945–951.

Hwang, A. D., Wang, H.-C., and Pomplun, M. (2011). Semantic guidance of eye movements in real-world scenes. *Vision Research* 51(10): 1192–1205.

Intriligator, J. and Cavanagh, P. (2001). The spatial resolution of visual attention. *Cognitive Psychology* 43(3): 171–216.

Ishibashi, K., Kita, S., and Wolfe, J. M. (2012). The effects of local prevalence and explicit expectations on search termination times. *Attention, Perception, & Psychophysics* 74: 115–123.

Itti, L. and Koch, C. (2000). A saliency-based search mechanism for overt and covert shifts of visual attention. *Vision Research* 40(10–12): 1489–1506.

Johansson, G. (1973). Visual perception of biological motion and a model for its analysis. *Perception & Psychophysics* 14: 201–211.

Johnston, W. A., Hawley, K. J., and Farnham, J. M. (1993). Novel popout: Empirical boundaries and tentative theory. *Journal of Experimental Psychology: Human Perception and Performance* 19(1): 140–153.

Jonides, J. and Gleitman, H. (1972). A conceptual category effect in visual search: O as letter or digit. *Perception & Psychophysics* 12: 457–460.

Jonides, J. and Yantis, S. (1988). Uniqueness of abrupt visual onset in capturing attention. *Perception & Psychophysics* 43: 346–354.

Julesz, B. (1981). A theory of preattentive texture discrimination based on first order statistics of textons. *Biological Cybernetics* 41: 131–138.

Julesz, B. and Bergen, J. R. (1983). Textons, the fundamental elements in preattentive vision and perceptions of textures. *Bell Systems Technical Journal* 62: 1619–1646.

Julesz, B. (1984). A brief outline of the texton theory of human vision. *Trends in Neurosciences*, 7(February): 41–45.

Julesz, B. and Krose, B. (1988). Features and spatial filters. *Nature* 333: 302–303.

Kanbe, F. (2009). Which is more critical in identification of random figures, endpoints or closures? *Japanese Psychological Research* 51(4): 235–245.

Kawahara, J. I. (1993). The effect of stimulus motion on visual search. *Japanese Journal of Psychology* 64(5): 396–400.

Kinchla, R. A. (1974). Detecting target elements in multielement arrays: A confusability model. *Perception & Psychophysics* 15(1): 149–158.

Kinchla, R. A. and Collyer, C. E. (1974). Detecting a target letter in briefly presented arrays: A confidence rating analysis in terms of a weighted additive effects model. *Perception & Psychophysics* 16(1): 117–122.

Kirchner, H. and Thorpe, S. J. (2006). Ultra-rapid object detection with saccadic eye movements: Visual processing speed revisited. *Vision Research* 46(11): 1762–1776.

Kleffner, D. A. and Ramachandran, V. S. (1992). On the perception of shape from shading. *Perception & Psychophysics* 52(1): 18–36.

Klein, R. (1988). Inhibitory tagging system facilitates visual search. *Nature* 334: 430–431.

Klein, R. M. and MacInnes, W. J. (1999). Inhibition of return is a foraging facilitator in visual search. *Psychological Science* 10(July): 346–352.

Klein, R. M. (2009). On the control of attention. *Canadian Journal of Experimental Psychology* 63(3): 240–252.

Koch, C. and Ullman, S. (1985). Shifts in selective visual attention: Towards the underlying neural circuitry. *Human Neurobiology* 4: 219–227.

Kourtzi, Z. and Connor, C. E. (2011). Neural representations for object perception: Structure, category, and adaptive coding. *Annual Review of Neuroscience* 34: 45–67.

Kovacs, I. and Julesz, B. (1993). A closed curve is much more than an incomplete one: Effect of closure in figure-ground segmentation. *Proceedings of the National Academy of Sciences USA* 90(16): 7495–7497.

Kowler, E. (2011). Eye movements: The past 25 years. *Vision Research* 51(13): 1457–1483.

Kristjánsson, A. and Tse, P. U. (2001). Curvature discontinuities are cues for rapid shape analysis. *Perception & Psychophysics* 63(3): 390–403.

Kristjánsson, A. and Driver, J. (2008). Priming in visual search: Separating the effects of target repetition, distractor repetition and role-reversal. *Vision Research* 48(10): 1217–1232.

Kristjánsson, A. and Campana, G. (2010). Where perception meets memory: A review of repetition priming in visual search tasks. *Attention, Perception, & Psychophysics* 72(1): 5–18.

Krueger, L. E. (1984). The category effect in visual search depends on physical rather than conceptual differences. *Perception & Psychophysics* 35(6): 558–564.

Krupinski, E. A., Berger, W. G., Dallas, W. J., and Roehrig, H. (2003). Searching for nodules: What features attract attention and influence detection? *Academic Radiology* 10(8): 861–868.

Kunar, M. A., Flusberg, S. J., Horowitz, T. S., and Wolfe, J. M. (2007). Does contextual cueing guide the deployment of attention? *Journal of Experimental Psychology: Human Perception and Performance* 33(4): 816–828.

Kundel, H. L. and Nodine, C. F. (2004). Modeling visual search during mammogram viewing. Paper presented at the conference Medical Imaging 2004: Image Perception, Observer Performance, and Technology Assessment.

Lamy, D. and Zoaris, L. (2009). Task-irrelevant stimulus salience affects visual search. *Vision Research* 49(11): 1472–1480.

Langton, S. R. H., Law, A. S., Burton, A. M., and Schweinberger, S. R. (2008). Attention capture by faces. *Cognition* 107(1): 330–342.

Lee, K. W., Buxton, H., and Feng, J. (2005). Cue-guided search: A computational model of selective attention. *IEEE Transactions on Neural Networks* 16(4): 910–924.

Levi, D. M. (2008). Crowding: An essential bottleneck for object recognition. A mini-review. *Vision Research* 48(5): 635–654.

Levin, D. T., Takarae, Y., Miner, A. G., and Keil, F. (2001). Efficient visual search by category: Specifying the features that mark the difference between artifacts and animals in preattentive vision. *Perception & Psychophysics* 63(4): 676–697.

Li, Z. (2002). A salience map in primary visual cortex. *Trends in Cognitive Sciences* 6(1): 9–16.

Lindsey, D. T., Brown, A. M., Reijnen, E., Rich, A. N., Kuzmova, Y. I., and Wolfe, J. M. (2010). Color channels, not color appearance or color categories, guide visual search for desaturated color targets. *Psychological Science* 21(9): 1208–1214.

Lipp, O. (2006). Of snakes and flowers: Does preferential detection of pictures of fear-relevant animals in visual search reflect on fear-relevance? *Emotion* 26(2): 296–308.

LoBue, V. and DeLoache, J. S. (2008). Detecting the snake in the grass: Attention to fear-relevant stimuli by adults and young children. *Psychological Science* 19(3): 284–289.

Logothetis, N. K., Pauls, J., and Poggio, T. (1995). Shape representation in the inferior temporal cortex of monkeys. *Current Biology* 5(5): 552–563.

Malcolm, G. L. and Henderson, J. M. (2010). Combining top-down processes to guide eye movements during real-world scene search. *Journal of Vision* 10(2): 1–11.

Malinowski, P. and Hübner, R. (2001). The effect of familiarity on visual-search performance: Evidence for learned basic features. *Perception & Psychophysics* 63(3): 458–463.

Maljkovic, V. and Nakayama, K. (1994). Priming of popout: I. Role of features. *Memory & Cognition* 22(6): 657–672.

McCollough, C. (1965). Color adaptation of edge-detectors in the human visual system. *Science* 149: 1115–1116.

McDaniel, M. A., Robinson-Riegler, B., and Einstein, G. O. (1998). Prospective remember-ing: Perceptually driven or conceptually drive processes? *Memory & Cognition* 26(1): 121–134.

McElree, B. and Carrasco, M. (1999). The temporal dynamics of visual search: Evidence for parallel processing in feature and conjunction searches. *Journal of Experimental Psychology: Human Perception and Performance* 25(6): 1517–1539.

McLeod, P., Driver, J., and Crisp, J. (1988). Visual search for conjunctions of movement and form is parallel. *Nature* 332: 154–155.

McSorley, E. and Findlay, J. M. (2001). Visual search in depth. *Vision Research* 41(25–26): 3487–3496.

Monnier, P. and Nagy, A. L. (2001). Uncertainty, attentional capacity and chromatic mecha-nisms in visual search. *Vision Research* 41(3): 313–328.

Moore, C. M., Elsinger, C. L., and Lleras, A. (2001). Visual attention and the apprehension of spatial relations: The case of depth. *Perception & Psychophysics* 63(4): 595–606.

Moore, C. M. and Wolfe, J. M. (2001). Getting beyond the serial/parallel debate in visual search: A hybrid approach. In K. Shapiro (ed.), *The Limits of Attention: Temporal Constraints on Human Information Processing* (pp. 178–198). Oxford: Oxford University Press.

Moraglia, G. (1989a). Display organization and the detection of horizontal lines segments. *Perception & Psychophysics* 45: 265–272.

Moraglia, G. (1989b). Visual search: Spatial frequency and orientation. *Perceptual & Motor Skills* 69(2): 675–689.

Mordkoff, J. T., Yantis, S., and Egeth, H. E. (1990). Detecting conjunctions of color and form in parallel. *Perception & Psychophysics* 48(2): 157–168.

Morgan, M. J., Giora, E., and Solomon, J. A. (2008). A single 'stopwatch' for duration estimation, a single 'ruler' for size. *Journal of Vision* 8(2): 14.1–14.8.

Mozer, M. C. and Baldwin, D. (2008). Experience-guided search: A theory of attentional con-trol. In D. K. J. Platt and Y. Singer (eds.), *Advances in Neural Information Processing Systems* (pp. 1033–1040). Cambridge, Mass.: MIT Press.

Muller, H. J., Reimann, B., and Krummenacher, J. (2003). Visual search for singleton feature tar-gets across dimensions: Stimulus- and expectancy-driven effects in dimensional weighting. *Journal of Experimental Psychology: Human Perception and Performance* 29(5): 1021–1035.

Nagy, A. L. and Sanchez, R. R. (1990). Critical color differences determined with a visual search task. *Journal of the Optical Society of America—A* 7(7): 1209–1217.

Nagy, A. L., Young, T., and Neriani, K. (2004). Combining information in different color-coding mechanisms to facilitate visual search. *Vision Research* 44(25): 2971–2980.

Najemnik, J. and Geisler, W. S. (2005). Optimal eye movement strategies in visual search. *Nature* 434(7031): 387–391.

Nakayama, K. and Silverman, G. H. (1986). Serial and parallel processing of visual feature con-junctions. *Nature* 320: 264–265.

Neider, M. B. and Zelinsky, G. J. (2006). Scene context guides eye movements during visual search. *Vision Research* 46(5): 614–621.

Neider, M. B., Boot, W. R., and Kramer, A. F. (2010). Visual search for real-world targets under conditions of high target–background similarity: Exploring training and transfer in younger and older adults. *Acta Psychologica* 34(1): 29–39.

Neisser, U. (1963). Decision time without reaction time: Experiments in visual scanning. *American Journal of Psychology* 76: 376–385.

Nodine, C. F., Krupinski, E. A., and Kundel, H. L. (1993). Visual processing and decision making in search and recognition of targets. In D. Brogan, A. Gale, and K. Carr (eds.), *Visual Search* 2 (pp. 239–249). London: Taylor & Francis.

Notebaert, L., Crombez, G., Van Damme, S., De Houwer, J., and Theeuwes, J. (2011). Signals of threat do not capture, but prioritize, attention: A conditioning approach. *Emotion* 11(1): 81–89.

Nothdurft, H.-C. (1991). Different effects from spatial frequency masking in texture segregation and text on detection tasks. *Vision Research* 31(2): 299–320.

Nothdurft, H.-C. (1993a). The role of features in preattentive vision: Comparison of orientation, motion and color cues. *Vision Research* 33(14): 1937–1958.

Nothdurft, H.-C. (1993b). The conspicuousness of orientation and visual motion. *Spatial Vision* 7(4): 341–366.

Nothdurft, H.-C. (1993c). Faces and facial expression do not pop-out. *Perception* 22: 1287–1298.

Nothdurft, H.-C. (2000). Salience from feature contrast: Additivity across dimensions. *Vision Research* 40: 1183–1201.

O'Toole, A. J. and Walker, C. L. (1997). On the preattentive accessibility of stereoscopic dispar-ity: Evidence from visual search. *Perception & Psychophysics* 59(2): 202–218.

Öhman, A., Flykt, A., and Esteves, F. (2001). Emotion drives attention: Detecting the snake in the grass. *Journal of Experimental Psychology: General* 130: 3.

Oliva, A. and Torralba, A. (2001). Modeling the shape of the scene: A holistic representation of the spatial envelope. *International Journal of Computer Vision* 42(3): 145–175.

Oliva, A., Torralba, A., Castelhano, M. S., and Henderson, J. M. (2003). Top-down control of visual attention in object detection. Paper presented at the Proceedings of the IEEE International Conference on Image Processing, 14–17 September, Barcelona, Spain.

Oliva, A. (2005). Gist of the scene. In L. Itti, G. Rees, and J. Tsotsos (eds.), *Neurobiology of Attention* (pp. 251–257). San Diego, Calif.: Academic Press/Elsevier.

Olzak, L. A. and Thomas, J. P. (1986). Seeing spatial patterns. In K. R. Boff, L. Kaufmann, and J. P. Thomas (eds.), *Handbook of Perception and Human Performance* (ch. 7). New York: Wiley & Sons.

Ostrovsky, Y., Cavanagh, P., and Sinha, P. (2004). Perceiving illumination inconsistencies in scenes. *Perception* 34: 1301–1314.

Paffen, C., Hooge, I., Benjamins, J., and Hogendoorn, H. (2011). A search asymmetry for interocular conflict. *Attention, Perception, & Psychophysics* 73(4): 1042–1053.

Palanica, A. and Itier, R. J. (2011). Searching for a perceived gaze direction using eye tracking. *Journal of Vision* 11(2): article 19. doi: 10.1167/11.2.19.

Palmer, E. M., Horowitz, T. S., Torralba, A., and Wolfe, J. M. (2011). What are the shapes of response time distributions in visual search? *Journal of Experimental Psychology: Human Perception and Performance* 37(1): 58–71.

Palmer, J. (1995). Attention in visual search: Distinguishing four causes of a set size effect. *Current Directions in Psychological Science* 4(4): 118–123.

Palmer, J. and McLean, J. (1995). Imperfect, unlimited-capacity, parallel search yields large set-size effects. Paper presented at the Society for Mathematical Psychology, Irvine, Calif.

Palmer, J., Verghese, P., and Pavel, M. (2000). The psychophysics of visual search. *Vision Research* 40(10–12): 1227–1268.

Parkhurst, D., Law, K., and Niebur, E. (2002). Modeling the role of salience in the allocation of overt visual attention. *Vision Research* 42(1): 107–123.

Pelli, D. G. and Tillman, K. A. (2008). The uncrowded window for object recognition. *Nature Neuroscience* 11(10): 1129–1135.

Peterson, M. S., Kramer, A. F., Wang, R. F., Irwin, D. E., and McCarley, J. S. (2001). Visual search has memory. *Psychological Science* 12(4): 287–292.

Pilon, D. and Friedman, A. (1998). Grouping and detecting vertices in 2-D, 3-D, and quasi-3-D objects. *Canadian Journal of Experimental Psychology* 52(3): 114–127.

Pomerantz, J. R. and Pristach, E. A. (1989). Emergent features, attention, and perceptual glue in visual form perception. *Journal of Experimental Psychology: Human Perception and Performance* 15(4): 635–649.

Portilla, J. and Simoncelli, E. P. (2000). A parametric texture model based on joint statistics of complex wavelet coefficients. *International Journal of Computer Vision* 40(1): 49–71.

Posner, M. I. (1980). Orienting of attention. *Quarterly Journal of Experimental Psychology* 32: 3–25.

Pratt, J. and Abrams, R. A. (1995). Inhibition of return to successively cued spatial locations. *Journal of Experimental Psychology: Human Perception and Performance* 21(6): 1343–1353.

Pratt, J., Radulescu, P. V., Guo, R. M., and Abrams, R. A. (2010). It's alive! Animate motion captures visual attention. *Psychological Science* 21(11): 1724–1730.

Prinzmetal, W. and Keysar, B. (1989). Functional theory of illusory conjunctions and neon colors. *Journal of Experimental Psychology: General* 118(2): 165–190.

Prinzmetal, W. (1991). Automatic processes in word perception: An analysis from illusory conjunctions. *Journal of Experimental Psychology: Human Perception and Performance* 17(4): 902–923.

Purcell, D. G., Stewart, A. L., and Skov, R. B. (1996). It takes a confounded face to pop out of a crowd. *Perception* 25(9): 1091–1108.

Purcell, B. A., Heitz, R. P., Cohen, J. Y., Schall, J. D., Logan, G. D., and Palmeri, T. J. (2010). Neurally constrained modeling of perceptual decision making. *Psychological Review* 117(4): 1113–1143.

Rakison, D. H. and Derringer, J. (2008). Do infants possess an evolved spider-detection mechanism? *Cognition* 107(1): 381–393.

Ramachandran, V. S. (1988). Perception of shape from shading. *Nature* 331: 163–165.

Ratcliff, R. (1978). A theory of memory retrieval. *Psychological Review* 85(2): 59–108.

Ratcliff, R., Philiastides, M. G., and Sajda, P. (2009). Quality of evidence for perceptual decision making is indexed by trial-to-trial variability of the EEG. *Proceedings of the National Academy of Sciences of the United States of America* 106(16): 6539–6544.

Rauschenberger, R. (2003). Attentional capture by auto- and allo-cues. *Psychonomic Bulletin & Review* 10(4): 814–842.

Reddy, L., Wilken, P., and Koch, C. (2004). Face-gender discrimination is possible in the near-absence of attention. *Journal of Vision* 4(2): 106–117.

Reddy, L. and Koch, C. (2006). Face identification in the near-absence of focal attention. *Vision Research* 46(15): 2336–2343.

Reijnen, E., Krummenacher, J., and Wolfe, J. M. (2011). Coarse guidance by numerosity in visual search. *Attention, Perception, & Psychophysics* 75(1): 16–28.

Reinecke, A., Rinck, M., and Becker, E. S. (2006). Spiders crawl easily through the bottleneck: Visual working memory for negative stimuli. *Emotion* 6(3): 438–449.

Rensink, R. A. and Enns, J. T. (1998). Early completion of occluded objects. *Vision Research* 38: 2489–2505.

Rensink, R. A. and Cavanagh, P. (2004). The influence of cast shadows on visual search. *Perception* 33(11): 1339–1358.

Rosenholtz, R. (2001a). Search asymmetries? What search asymmetries? *Perception & Psychophysics* 63(3): 476–489.

Rosenholtz, R. (2001b). Visual search for orientation among heterogeneous distractors: Experimental results and implications for signal-detection theory models of search. *Journal of Experimental Psychology: Human Perception and Performance* 27(4): 985–999.

Rosenholtz, R., Chan, S., and Balas, B. (2009). A crowded model of visual search. *Journal of Vision* 9(8): 1197–1197.

Royden, C. S., Wolfe, J., and Klempen, N. (2001). Visual search asymmetries in motion and optic flow fields. *Perception & Psychophysics* 63(3): 436–444.

Rubenstein, J. (2001). *Test and Evaluation Plan: X-ray Image Screener Selection Test* (No. DOT/ FAA/AR-01/47). Washington, D.C.: Office of Aviation Research.

Rubin, J. M. and Kanwisher, N. (1985). Topological perception: Holes in an experiment. *Perception & Psychophysics* 37: 179–180.

Rushton, S. K., Bradshaw, M. F., and Warren, P. A. (2007). The pop-out of scene-relative object movement against retinal motion due to self-movement. *Cognition* 105: 237–245.

Sagi, D. (1988). The combination of spatial frequency and orientation is effortlessly perceived. *Perception & Psychophysics* 43: 601–603.

Sagi, D. (1990). Detection of an orientation singularity in Gabor textures: Effect of signal density and spatial frequency. *Vision Research* 30(9): 1377–1388.

Sakai, K., Morishita, M., and Matsumoto, H. (2007). Set-size effects in simple visual search for contour curvature. *Perception* 36(3): 323–334.

Sanocki, T. and Epstein, W. (1997). Priming spatial layout of scenes. *Psychological Science* 8: 374–378.

Scolari, M., Kohnen, A., Barton, B., and Awh, E. (2007). Spatial attention, preview, and pop-out: Which factors influence critical spacing in crowded displays? *Journal of Vision* 7(2): 1–23.

Serences, J. T. and Yantis, S. (2006). Selective visual attention and perceptual coherence. *Trends in Cognitive Sciences* 10(1): 38–45.

Sherman, A. M., Greene, M. R., and Wolfe, J. M. (2011). Depth and size information reduce effective set size for visual search in real-world scenes. *Journal of Vision* 11(11): 1334.

Shiffrin, R. M. and Gardner, G. T. (1972). Visual processing capacity and attentional control. *Journal of Experimental Psychology* 93(1): 72–82.

Shiffrin, R. M. and Schneider, W. (1977). Controlled and automatic human information processing, II: Perceptual learning, automatic attending, and a general theory. *Psychological Review* 84: 127–190.

Shipp, S. (2004). The brain circuitry of attention. *Trends in Cognitive Sciences* 8(5): 223–230.

Shneor, E. and Hochstein, S. (2006). Eye dominance effects in feature search. *Vision Research* 46(25): 4258–4269.

Shore, D. I. and Klein, R. M. (2000). On the manifestations of memory in visual search. *Spatial Vision* 14(1): 59–75.

Sigman, M. and Gilbert, C. D. (2000). Learning to find a shape. *Nature Neuroscience* 3(3): 264–269.

Simons, D. J. and Chabris, C. F. (2010). *The Invisible Gorilla*. New York: Crown/Random House.

Sireteanu, R. and Rettenbach, R. (1995). Perceptual learning in visual search: Fast enduring but non-specific. *Vision Research* 35(14): 2037–2043.

Skarratt, P. A., Cole, G. G., and Gellatly, A. R. (2009). Prioritization of looming and receding objects: Equal slopes, different intercepts. *Attention, Perception, & Psychophysics* 71(4): 964–970.

Smith, S. L. (1962). Color coding and visual search. *Journal of Experimental Psychology* 64: 434–440.

Soares, S. C., Esteves, F., Lundqvist, D., and Ohman, A. (2009). Some animal specific fears are more specific than others: Evidence from attention and emotion measures. *Behaviour Research and Therapy* 47(12): 1032–1042.

Sousa, R., Brenner, E., and Smeets, J. B. J. (2009). Slant cue are combined early in visual processing: Evidence from visual search. *Vision Research* 49(2): 257–261.

Spalek, T. M., Kawahara, J., and Di Lollo, V. (2009). Flicker is a primitive visual attribute. *Canadian Journal of Experimental Psychology* 63(4): 319–322.

Stein, T., Senju, A., Peelen, M. V., and Sterzer, P. (2011). Eye contact facilitates awareness of faces during interocular suppression. *Cognition* 119(2): 307–311.

Stuart, G. W. (1993). Preattentive processing of object size: Implications for theories of size perception. *Perception* 22(10): 1175–1193.

Sun, J. and Perona, P. (1996a). Preattentive perception of elementary three-dimensional shapes. *Vision Research* 36(16): 2515–2529.

Sun, J. and Perona, P. (1996b). Where is the sun? *Investigative Ophthalmology and Visual Science* 37(3): S935.

Suzuki, S. and Cavanagh, P. (1995). Facial organization blocks access to low-level features: An object inferiority effect. *Journal of Experimental Psychology: Human Perception and Performance* 21(4): 901–913.

Symons, L. A., Cuddy, F., and Humphrey, K. (2000). Orientation tuning of shape from shading. *Perception & Psychophysics* 62(3): 557–568.

Takeda, Y. (2004). Search for multiple targets: Evidence for memory-based control of attention. *Psychonomic Bulletin & Review* 11(1): 71–76.

Takeuchi, T. (1997). Visual search of expansion and contraction. *Vision Research* 37(15): 2083–2090.

Taylor, S. and Badcock, D. (1988). Processing feature density in preattentive perception. *Perception & Psychophysics* 44: 551–562.

Theeuwes, J. and Kooi, J. L. (1994). Parallel search for a conjunction of shape and contrast polarity. *Vision Research* 34(22): 3013–3016.

Theeuwes, J. (1995). Abrupt luminance change pops out; abrupt color change does not. *Perception & Psychophysics* 57(5): 637–644.

Thompson, K. G. and Bichot, N. P. (2004). A visual salience map in the primate frontal eye field. *Progress in Brain Research* 147: 249–262.

Thornton, T. L. and Gilden, D. L. (2007). Parallel and serial process in visual search. *Psychological Review* 114(1): 71–103.

Tipper, S. P., Weaver, B., and Watson, F. L. (1996). Inhibition of return to successively cued spatial locations: Commentary on Pratt and Abrams (1995). *Journal of Experimental Psychology: Human Perception and Performance* 22(5): 1289–1293.

Tipples, J., Young, A., Quinlan, P., Broks, P., and Ellis, A. (2002). Searching for threat. *Quarterly Journal of Experimental Psychology* 55(3): 1007–1026.

Tong, F. and Nakayama, K. (1999). Robust representations for faces: Evidence from visual search. *Journal of Experimental Psychology: Human Perception and Performance* 25(4): 1016–1035.

Torralba, A., Oliva, A., Castelhano, M. S., and Henderson, J. M. (2006). Contextual guidance of eye movements and attention in real-world scenes: The role of global features on object search. *Psychological Review* 113(4): 766–786.

Townsend, J. T. (1971). A note on the identification of parallel and serial processes. *Perception & Psychophysics* 10: 161–163.

Townsend, J. T. (1990). Serial and parallel processing: Sometimes they look like Tweedledum and Tweedledee but they can (and should) be distinguished. *Psychological Science 1*: 46–54.

Townsend, J. T. and Wenger, M. J. (2004). The serial-parallel dilemma: A case study in a linkage of theory and method. *Psychonomic Bulletin & Review 11*(3): 391–418.

Treisman, A. M. and Gelade, G. (1980). A feature-integration theory of attention. *Cognitive Psychology 12*: 97–136.

Treisman, A. M. and Schmidt, H. (1982). Illusory conjunctions in the perception of objects. *Cognitive Psychology 14*: 107–141.

Treisman, A. M. and Souther, J. (1985). Search asymmetry: A diagnostic for preattentive processing of separable features. *Journal of Experimental Psychology: General 114*: 285–310.

Treisman, A. M. and Souther, J. (1986). Illusory words: The roles of attention and of top-down constraints in conjoining letters to form words. *Journal of Experimental Psychology: Human Perception and Performance 12*: 3–17.

Treisman, A. M. (1988). Features and objects: The 14th Bartlett memorial lecture. *Quarterly Journal of Experimental Psychology—A 40*: 201–237.

Treisman, A. M. and Gormican, S. (1988). Feature analysis in early vision: Evidence from search asymmetries. *Psychological Review 95*: 15–48.

Treisman, A. M. (1996). The binding problem. *Current Opinion in Neurobiology 6*: 171–178.

Treisman, A. M. (2006). How the deployment of attention determines what we see. *Visual Cognition 14*(4–8): 411–443.

Treue, S. and Trujillo, J. C. M. (1999). Feature-based attention influences motion processing gain in macaque visual cortex. *Nature 399*: 575–579.

Tsal, Y. (1989a). Do illusory conjunctions support feature integration theory? A critical review of theory and findings. *Journal of Experimental Psychology: Human Perception and Performance 15*(2): 394–400.

Tsal, Y. (1989b). Further comments on feature integration theory. A reply to Briand and Klein. *Journal of Experimental Psychology: Human Perception and Performance 15*(2): 407–410.

Tsal, Y., Meiran, N., and Lamy, D. (1995). Towards a resolution theory of visual attention. *Visual Cognition 2*(2/3): 313–330.

Tsotsos, J. (2011). *A Computational Perspective on Visual Attention*. Cambridge, Mass.: MIT Press.

Turatto, M. and Glafano, G. (2000). Color, form, and luminance capture attention in visual search. *Vision Research 40*(13): 1639–1643.

VanRullen, R. and Thorpe, S. J. (2001). Is it a bird? Is it a plane? Ultra-rapid visual categorisation of natural and artifactual objects. *Perception 30*(6): 655–668.

VanRullen, R. (2006). On second glance: Still no high-level pop-out effect for faces. *Vision Research 46*(18): 3017–3027.

Verghese, P. and Nakayama, K. (1994). Stimulus discriminability in visual search. *Vision Research 34*(18): 2453–2467.

Verghese, P. and Pelli, D. G. (1994). The scale bandwidth of visual search. *Vision Research 34*(7): 955–962.

Verghese, P. (2001). Visual search and attention: A signal detection approach. *Neuron 31*: 523–535.

Vickery, T. J., King, L.-W., and Jiang, Y. (2005). Setting up the target template in visual search. *Journal of Vision 5*(1): 81–92.

Vidyasagar, T. R. (1999). A neuronal model of attentional spotlight: Parietal guiding the temporal. *Brain Research Reviews 30*(1): 66–76.

Virzi, R. A. and Egeth, H. E. (1984). Is meaning implicated in illusory contours? *Journal of Experimental Psychology: Human Perception and Performance 10*: 573–580.

Vo, M. L.-H. and Henderson, J. M. (2009). Does gravity matter? Effects of semantic and syntactic inconsistencies on the allocation of attention during scene perception. *Journal of Vision* 9(3): 1–15.

Vo, M. L.-H. and Wolfe, J. M. (2012). When does repeated search in scenes involve memory? Looking at versus looking for objects in scenes. *Journal of Experimental Psychology: Human Perception and Performance* 38(1): 23–41.

Von Grünau, M. and Dubé, S. (1994). Visual search asymmetry for viewing direction. *Perception & Psychophysics* 56(2): 211–220.

Von Grünau, M. and Anston, C. (1995). The detection of gaze direction: A stare-in-the-crowd effect. *Perception* 24(11): 1297–1313.

von Muhlenen, A. and Muller, H. (1999). Visual search for motion-form conjunctions: Selective attention to movement direction. *Journal of General Psychology* 126: 289–317.

Wang, L., Zhang, K., He, S., and Jiang, Y. (2010). Searching for life motion signals: Visual search asymmetry in local but not global biological-motion processing. *Psychological Science* 21(8): 1083–1089.

Wang, Q., Cavanagh, P., and Green, M. (1994). Familiarity and pop-out in visual search. *Perception & Psychophysics* 56(5): 495–500.

Watt, R., Craven, B., and Quinn, S. (2007). A role for eyebrows in regulating the visibility of eye gaze direction. *Quarterly Journal of Experimental Psychology (Hove)* 60(9): 1169–1177.

Wheatley, C., Cook, M. L., and Vidyasagar, T. R. (2004). Surface segregation influences pre-attentive search in depth. *NeuroReport* 15(2): 303–305.

Williams, D. and Julesz, B. (1992). Perceptual asymmetry in texture perception. *Proceedings of the National Academy of Sciences USA* 89(14): 6531–6534.

Williams, L. G. (1966). The effect of target specification on objects fixed during visual search. *Perception & Psychophysics* 1: 315–318.

Williams, M. A., Moss, S. A., and Bradshaw, J. L. (2002). Searching for the eyes and mouth: Is the stare-in-the-crowd effect specific to the eyes? *Perception & Psychophysics*, MS 02–153.

Wolfe, J. M. and Franzel, S. L. (1988). Binocularity and visual search. *Perception & Psychophysics* 44: 81–93.

Wolfe, J. M., Cave, K. R., and Franzel, S. L. (1989). Guided Search: An alternative to the Feature Integration model for visual search. *Journal of Experimental Psychology: Human Perception and Performance* 15: 419–433.

Wolfe, J. M., Yu, K. P., Stewart, M. I., Shorter, A. D., Friedman-Hill, S. R., and Cave, K. R. (1990). Limitations on the parallel guidance of visual search: Color X color and orientation X orientation conjunctions. *Journal of Experimental Psychology: Human Perception and Performance* 16(4): 879–892.

Wolfe, J. M. and Friedman-Hill, S. R. (1992). Visual search for orientation: The role of angular relations between targets and distractors. *Spatial Vision* 6(3): 199–208.

Wolfe, J. M., Yee, A., and Friedman-Hill, S. R. (1992). Curvature is a basic feature for visual search. *Perception* 21: 465–480.

Wolfe, J. M., Friedman-Hill, S. R., Stewart, M. I., and O'Connell, K. M. (1992). The role of categorization in visual search for orientation. *Journal of Experimental Psychology: Human Perception and Performance* 18(1): 34–49.

Wolfe, J. M. (1994). Guided Search 2.0: A revised model of visual search. *Psychonomic Bulletin and Review* 1(2): 202–238.

Wolfe, J. M., Friedman-Hill, S. R., and Bilsky, A. B. (1994). Parallel processing of part/whole information in visual search tasks. *Perception & Psychophysics* 55(5): 537–550.

Wolfe, J. M. and Bennett, S. C. (1997). Preattentive object files: Shapeless bundles of basic features. *Vision Research* 37(1): 25–43.

Wolfe, J. M. (1998). What do 1,000,000 trials tell us about visual search? *Psychological Science* 9(1): 33–39.

Wolfe, J. M., Klempen, N. L., and Shulman, E. P. (1999). Which end is up? Two representations of orientation in visual search. *Vision Research* 39(12): 2075–2086.

Wolfe, J. M., Klempen, N., and Dahlen, K. (2000). Post-attentive vision. *Journal of Experimental Psychology: Human Perception and Performance* 26(2): 693–716.

Wolfe, J. M. (2001). Asymmetries in visual search: An Introduction. *Perception & Psychophysics* 63(3): 381–389.

Wolfe, J. M. (2003). Moving towards solutions to some enduring controversies in visual search. *Trends in Cognitive Sciences* 7(2): 70–76.

Wolfe, J. M. and DiMase, J. S. (2003). Do intersections serve as basic features in visual search? *Perception* 32(6): 645–656.

Wolfe, J. M., Horowitz, T., Kenner, N. M., Hyle, M., and Vasan, N. (2004). How fast can you change your mind? The speed of top-down guidance in visual search. *Vision Research* 44(12): 1411–1426.

Wolfe, J. M. and Horowitz, T. S. (2004). What attributes guide the deployment of visual attention and how do they do it? *Nature Reviews Neuroscience* 5(6): 495–501.

Wolfe, J. M. (2005). Guidance of visual search by preattentive information. In L. Itti, G. Rees, and J. Tsotsos (eds.), *Neurobiology of Attention* (pp. 101–104). San Diego, Calif.: Academic Press/Elsevier.

Wolfe, J. M., Horowitz, T. S., and Kenner, N. M. (2005). Rare items often missed in visual searches. *Nature* 435: 439–440.

Wolfe, J. M., Reinecke, A., and Brawn, P. (2006). Why don't we see changes? The role of attentional bottlenecks and limited visual memory. *Visual Cognition* 19(4–8): 749–780.

Wolfe, J. M. (2007). Guided Search 4.0: Current progress with a model of visual search. In W. Gray (ed.), *Integrated Models of Cognitive Systems* (pp. 99–119). New York: Oxford.

Wolfe, J. M., Horowitz, T. S., VanWert, M. J., Kenner, N. M., Place, S. S., and Kibbi, N. (2007). Low target prevalence is a stubborn source of errors in visual search tasks. *JEP: General* 136(4): 623–638.

Wolfe, J. M., Reijnen, E., VanWert, M. J., and Kuzmova, Y. (2009). In visual search, guidance by surface type is different than classic guidance. *Vision Research* 49(7): 765–773.

Wolfe, J. M. (2010). Bound to guide: A surprising, preattentive role for conjunctions in visual search. Paper presented at the Vision Science Society meeting: Naples, Fla, May 2010.

Wolfe, J. M. and Myers, L. (2010). Fur in the midst of the waters: visual search for material type is inefficient. *Journal of Vision* 10(9): 8.

Wolfe, J. M., Palmer, E. M., and Horowitz, T. S. (2010). Reaction time distributions constrain models of visual search. *Vision Research* 50: 1304–1311.

Wolfe, J. M. and VanWert, M. J. (2010). Varying target prevalence reveals two, dissociable decision criteria in visual search. *Current Biology* 20(2): 121–124.

Wolfe, J. M., Reijnen, E., Horowitz, T., Pedersini, R., Pinto, Y., and Hulleman, J. (2011). How does our search engine 'see' the world? The case of amodal completion. *Attention, Perception, & Psychophysics* 73(4): 1054–1064.

Wolfe, J. M., Alvarez, G. A., Rosenholtz, R., Kuzmova, Y. I., and Sherman, A. M. (2011). Visual search for arbitrary objects in real scenes. *Attention, Perception, & Psychophysics* 73(6): 1650–1671.

Wolfe, J. M., Birdwell, R. L., and Evans, K. K. (2011). If you don't find it often, you often don't find it: Disease prevalence is a source of miss errors in screening mammography. Paper presented at the Annual Radiological Society of North America meeting: Chicago, Ill., 30 November 2011.

Wolfe, J. M., Vo, M. L., Evans, K. K., and Greene, M. R. (2011). Visual search in scenes involves selective and nonselective pathways. *Trends in Cognitive Sciences* 15(2): 77–84.

Wolfe, J. M. (2012). The rules of guidance in visual search. *Lecture Notes in Computer Science*: 7143. Indo-Japan conference on Perception and Machine Intelligence, 1–10.

Yamane, Y., Carlson, E. T., Bowman, K. C., Wang, Z., and Connor, C. E. (2008). A neural code for three-dimensional object shape in macaque inferotemporal cortex. *Nature Neuroscience* 11(11): 1352–1360.

Yantis, S. and Jonides, J. (1990). Abrupt visual onsets and selective attention: Voluntary versus automatic allocation. *Journal of Experimental Psychology: Human Perception and Performance* 16(1): 121–134.

Yantis, S. (1993). Stimulus-driven attentional capture. *Current Directions in Psychological Science* 2(5): 156–161.

Zehetleitner, M., Krummenacher, J., Geyer, T., Hegenloh, M., and Müller, H. (2011). Dimension intertrial and cueing effects in localization: Support for pre-attentively weighted one-route models of saliency. *Attention, Perception, & Psychophysics* 73(2): 349–363.

Zhang, Y., Meyers, E. M., Bichot, N. P., Serre, T., Poggio, T. A., and Desimone, R. (2011). Object decoding with attention in inferior temporal cortex. *Proceedings of the National Academy of Sciences* 108(21): 8850–8855.

Zhaoping, L. (2008). Attention capture by eye of origin singletons even without awareness: A hallmark of a bottom-up saliency map in the primary visual cortex. *Journal of Vision* 8(5): 1–18.

Zhaoping, L. and Frith, U. (2011). A clash of bottom-up and top-down processes in visual search: The reversed letter effect revisited. *Journal of Experimental Psychology: Human Perception and Performance* 37(4): 997–1006.

Zohary, E. and Hochstein, S. (1989). How serial is serial processing in vision? *Perception* 18: 191–200.

CHAPTER 3

···

LOAD THEORY
OF ATTENTION AND
COGNITIVE CONTROL

···

NILLI LAVIE AND POLLY DALTON

Introduction
···

In order to achieve our goals successfully in today's busy world, we need to attend selectively to relevant information and avoid distraction by irrelevant information. To get a sense of the importance of this selective attention process, you only need to imagine trying to read this chapter in a busy city street, such as Oxford Street in central London. Without the ability to focus on the book, you would be faced with the challenge of understanding black letters on white paper amid a colourful clutter of sights and sounds (including jostling crowds, tempting shop windows, blaring sirens, and even a range of smells!) The ability to control your processing of the background information is essential if you are ever to get to the end of the chapter.

However, our everyday experience portrays a complex and somewhat puzzling picture of this ability. At times, we notice every little distraction, from the humming of the computer fan to the distant sound of people talking outside. At other times, we become so absorbed in a task that we may even miss someone talking directly to us. This everyday experience was reflected in the mixed pattern of empirical findings which emerged over decades of research starting in the 1950s: some experiments suggested that people could be highly selective, other experiments found high levels of distraction. Load theory set out to resolve this puzzle. What governs our ability to focus? Why are we sometimes highly distracted by information we wish to ignore when at other times we regrettably fail to notice important information? In this chapter we describe load theory and the evidence to support it, as well as reviewing the mechanisms that are proposed to underlie the observed load effects. We also highlight some of the theory's wider influences in areas as diverse as emotion processing, developmental psychology, and the understanding of psychological disorders. Although there is some interesting current work examining the effects of processing load as they might occur between and within sensory modalities other than vision, the current review focuses only on evidence from the visual domain.

BACKGROUND

Attention research began with Broadbent's (1958) seminal 'filter model' which proposed that the perceptual system has limited capacity and must therefore be protected from overload by an attentional filter that excludes unattended information at an early stage of processing, as soon as rudimentary analysis of the simple perceptual features of the input is complete. This was termed an 'early selection' model, because of the central claim that the filter acted relatively early in the processing stream. The model provided a good account for observations that people were often unable to report the contents of unattended information channels (for example, information presented to one ear while people attended to the other ear, e.g. Cherry 1953). However, it could not accommodate subsequent findings indicating that unattended information could in fact be perceived beyond the level of simple physical features. For example, messages to the participants that were inserted in the unattended channel (e.g. 'you may stop now') were sometimes perceived if they were preceded by the mention of the participant's own name (Moray 1959). This suggests that people were in fact able to process the semantic meaning of some of the ignored information (otherwise they would not have been able to recognize their name). These findings drove the development of a rival filter model, which proposed that attention acts at a much later stage of processing, filtering out irrelevant information from post-perceptual processes such as memory and overt responses, but allowing full perception of all information before unattended information is filtered out (Deutsch and Deutsch 1963). This was therefore termed a 'late-selection' model.

The stage was now set for a debate between the early and late selection positions which generated around forty years of research and discussion (see Driver 2001; Lavie 2006; Lavie and Tsal 1994, for more detailed overviews of this debate and its research). Load theory set out to provide a resolution between the two positions.

The central tenet of load theory (e.g. Lavie 1995, 2005, 2010) is that perceptual processing can only become selective when the limits of perceptual capacity are reached. If a task imposes sufficient demands to exceed capacity, task-irrelevant items are not processed and can therefore be successfully ignored (in other words, early selection can occur). By contrast, if a task imposes only low perceptual demands, the remaining capacity is automatically allocated to the processing of task-irrelevant items, which may then cause distraction (reflecting late selection). Load theory thus proposes a resolution for the early/late selection debate in suggesting that both types of selection can occur, depending on the perceptual demands of the task at hand. The theory also highlights the importance of higher-level cognitive mechanisms (such as working memory) that provide a form of 'executive' control in determining whether or not distraction can be avoided. These will be discussed later in the chapter.

PERCEPTUAL LOAD

Studies of perceptual load have used a range of load manipulations and a wide variety of measures of the extent to which irrelevant information is processed. Perceptual load can be manipulated through varying either the number of items in the display, or the perceptual similarity between the display items, or the processing requirements of the task. Irrelevant information processing can be measured either through behavioural indices of distractor interference (including response competition, negative priming, attentional capture, and so forth) or through reports about awareness of task-irrelevant items (or lack of it—a phenomenon known as inattentional blindness) or through neural measures of the brain response to the irrelevant stimuli. The studies reviewed below will provide examples of all these manipulations and measures.

The role of perceptual load in distractor interference

The first tests of the theory's predictions concerning perceptual load used the response competition paradigm: a well-established measure of distractor interference. In a typical task, participants make speeded responses according to which of two target letters (e.g. X or N) is present in a search array. An irrelevant distractor letter is also presented, typically in the periphery and well separated from the target. Distractor interference is assessed by measuring reaction times to the target as a function of the distractor's congruency with the target response. The distractor can either be congruent (e.g. X when the target is X), incongruent (e.g. X when the target is N), or neutral (e.g. the letter L which has no response associations in this example). Distractor interference is inferred from the slowing of reaction times in the presence of incongruent distractors as compared with congruent or neutral distractors. Distractor interference as measured in this way is typically reduced under high (vs low) perceptual load. For example, Lavie (1995) modified this response competition task to manipulate the level of perceptual load in the target processing. In some experiments, the target letter was presented in one of six central positions, either alone (low load) or among five other letters that were similar to the target (high load; see also Lavie and Cox 1997). In other experiments, load was manipulated by varying the processing requirements within the same target displays, requiring feature detection (e.g. blue or red) under low load or a complex feature conjunction discrimination (e.g. of colour, shape, and position) under high load. Regardless of the load manipulation used, distractor interference was reliably reduced under high (vs low) perceptual load, in support of the predictions of load theory.

One might ask, however, whether the reduced response competition effects seen under high load could in fact reflect an increase in active suppression of responses to the distractor under high load (i.e. a late-selection effect, whereby the distractor is perceived but the response towards it is inhibited), rather than the reduction in perceptual processing of the distractor (i.e. an early-selection effect) that load theory predicts. Lavie and Fox (2000) investigated this issue directly. They presented participants with pairs of letter search displays (a 'prime' display followed by a 'probe' display). On some trials, the letter that had served as the distractor in the prime display became the target in the subsequent probe display—a manipulation which would normally be expected to lead to negative priming (whereby people are slower to respond to a target if they have just ignored it on the previous trial). Since negative priming effects clearly indicate distractor perception, load theory predicts that they should only occur in conditions of low perceptual load. Indeed, these negative priming effects were observed as predicted under low perceptual load. However, across several experiments, negative priming was eliminated under high-load conditions. This rules out an account for perceptual load effects in terms of response inhibition, because an increase in inhibition of the distractor responses would lead to increased (rather than decreased) negative priming effects. Instead, the observed decrease in negative priming under high load provides additional support for perceptual load theory, in suggesting that perceptual processing of distractors is reduced under high perceptual load.

Interestingly, there is now evidence to suggest that the processing of potentially high-priority distractors can also be modulated by the perceptual load of the relevant task. For example, Beck and Lavie (2005) modified the response competition task described above in order to allow a comparison between processing of distractors presented in the periphery of the display and those presented at fixation (i.e. right where the participants were looking). Distractors at fixation caused twice the interference effects, reflecting their relative processing priority compared with distractors in the periphery. However, perceptual load modulated the interference from both types of distractor to similar extents, demonstrating that even high-priority distractors are subject to the influence of perceptual load. This claim is strengthened by a study of distraction by colourful and highly attention-capturing famous cartoon characters (e.g. Spiderman). Forster and Lavie (2008) presented the task-irrelevant characters alongside a letter search display and measured the extent to which they captured participants' attention (by comparing search reaction times when the characters were present vs absent). Despite being completely irrelevant to the task, the cartoon characters caused significant distraction, indicating that they were highly attention-capturing. However, even this interference by highly salient stimuli could be modulated by the perceptual load of the relevant task, indicating, in line with Beck and Lavie (2005), that even high-priority distractors can be rejected from processing under high perceptual load.

Whereas all the measures discussed above tested processing of externally generated stimuli, there is also evidence to suggest that perceptual load can modulate distraction by internally generated information, as measured in terms of task-unrelated thoughts (or 'mind wandering'). Forster and Lavie (2009) presented participants with a letter search task of either high or low perceptual load. Following each trial, participants were also asked to report whether their thoughts during performance had been related to the task (e.g. 'oops, I've pressed the wrong button') or unrelated to the task (e.g. 'I must stop by the supermarket on the way home'). Participants consistently reported lower levels of mind wandering under high (vs low) perceptual load, suggesting that even the processing of internally generated information may be dependent on the perceptual load of an ongoing task. Thus people's ability to avoid distraction from numerous sources depends on the level of demand imposed by the relevant task.

This conclusion has important applied implications. Perceptual load could improve performance in a range of everyday tasks, including, for example, learning and education, both in non-clinical populations and in people who may be more vulnerable to distraction (e.g. children with ADHD). Indeed, recent evidence suggests that people's performance is influenced by the effects of perceptual load regardless of their individual level of distractibility in everyday life. Forster and Lavie (2007) divided participants according to their responses on the Cognitive Failures Questionnaire (CFQ; Broadbent, Cooper, FitzGerald, and Parkes 1982), which is designed to measure individual differences in the extent to which people tend to become distracted during daily life. Under low perceptual load, the low-CFQ group experienced significantly more distractor interference in a standard response competition task than the high-CFQ group, but distractor processing was eliminated under high load for both CFQ groups. Thus even highly distractible people experience reduced distraction under high perceptual load. This finding highlights the important potential applications of this type of behavioural research to daily-life situations.

Overall, there is now broad agreement from a range of different behavioural studies that distractors interfere more under low perceptual load than under high load, supporting the central claim of load theory that successful selective attention can only be achieved if the demands of the relevant task are sufficient to exhaust perceptual capacity. It is particularly important to note that these behavioural findings have generalized across a number of different experimental designs when evaluating potential alternative claims. For example, the 'dilution account' (e.g. Tsal and Benoni 2010; Wilson, Muroi, and MacLeod 2011) suggests that distractor interference may be reduced in displays of larger (vs smaller) set size, not due to higher perceptual demands under the larger set size but due to 'dilution' of the distractor by the increased number of non-target items. Dayan and colleagues have made similar arguments in support of their Bayesian model of load effects within the response competition task, claiming that the additional noise from the non-targets under high load reduces the informative value of the large receptive fields containing the distractor and thus reduces their influence on inferences about the target identity (e.g. Dayan 2008). However, as described above, the effects of perceptual load have generalized across a range of different distractors, many of which do not share features with the targets and non-targets, meaning that their interference cannot be explained by either of these suggestions. For example, the large and colourful cartoon characters that were used as distractors by Forster and Lavie (2008) shared few features with the letters used in the relevant search task and were also far more salient than those letters. Thus the reduced influence of the distractors under high load in that study cannot be explained in terms of dilution of the large, colourful distractors by the extra letters present in the high-load display (see Lavie and Torralbo 2010, for a more detailed discussion). The lack of feature overlap also means that distractors such as these do not have any informative value with respect to the target and so cannot influence any inference regarding the target identity even in the low-load conditions in which target decisions are influenced by information processed within large receptive fields (as proposed by the Bayesian account). In addition, perceptual load has often been manipulated without any increase in the number of display items, giving rise to effects that cannot be explained by either of these alternative accounts. We describe such examples in more detail in the next section.

The role of perceptual load in visual perception

The distractor-interference measures described so far provide only an indirect test of the theory's claims concerning perceptual processing. This is because distractor-interference effects on reaction times may also be influenced by the additional processes occurring between perception and the eventual response (e.g. semantic processing and response-related decisions). A more straightforward test of the theory's predictions is provided by studies using direct measures of visual perception. This research has demonstrated that load plays a critical role in visual perception from the very early stages of visual processing (including those that are not yet conscious) to the higher-level processing that dictates our subjective visual awareness.

A clear example of the importance of load in determining whether stimuli are perceived comes from the phenomenon of inattentional blindness. The original findings were reported by Neisser and Becklen (1975) who superimposed two videos, one of a hand-shaking game and one of a ball game. Participants were asked to monitor one of the two videos (pressing a button in response to certain target events) while ignoring the other video. Most participants failed to notice unexpected events in the unattended episode (for example, only five of the twenty-four people attending to the hand game noticed that the original male players were replaced with female players!). These results provide indirect support for perceptual load theory, because the continuous video monitoring task is likely to have imposed high perceptual demands. This suggestion is supported more directly by a finding from the well-known recent demonstration of inattentional blindness, in which the attended event (a basketball game) and the unexpected event (the appearance of a person dressed as a gorilla) are presented within the same video (Simons and Chabris 1999). Participants in this study were more likely to notice the gorilla when performing an 'easy' task (counting the number of passes made) than when performing a more demanding task (maintaining two separate counts for the number of bounce passes and aerial passes). However, in both these studies, the task of monitoring the videos will have required eye movements pursuing the attended events, which is likely to have led to blurring of the unattended events on the retina. In other words, participants may have failed to report the ignored events not due to inattention but because they were in fact less visible due to a blurred image on the retina. This account could also be applied to the difficulty manipulation used in Simons and Chabris's (1999) study if one assumes that the hard task is likely to have required more eye movements than the easy task. In this case, the gorilla may have simply been less visible during performance of the hard task due to a greater rate of eye movements leading to increased retinal blurring under those conditions.

Cartwright-Finch and Lavie (2007) aimed to provide a clearer test of the prediction of load theory that awareness of task-irrelevant items should be reduced under high (vs low) load in a relevant task. They manipulated load within an inattentional blindness paradigm (originally developed by Mack and Rock 1998) in which display presentation is so brief that eye movements cannot occur during its duration. Participants carried out a visual discrimination task, determining either which line of a cross shape was blue (the horizontal or the vertical) or which of the cross lines was longer. Because the colour discrimination was very clear (one line was blue and the other was green) while the length difference was very subtle, the colour task involved low perceptual load and the length task involved high perceptual load for the very same stimulus. Participants were subsequently asked whether they noticed a small extra stimulus presented without warning in the periphery of the display on the last trial. Cartwright-Finch and Lavie found that participants in the high-load condition were much less likely to detect the unexpected peripheral stimulus than participants who were carrying out the low-load task. Since eye movements could not occur during the brief displays used, the inattentional blindness results are not open to alternative explanations in terms of blurring on the retina during eye movements. The findings thus provide strong support for the claim that perceptual load modulates people's susceptibility to inattentional blindness. Macdonald and Lavie (2011) have recently extended these findings to show that inattentional deafness (the failure to notice the appearance of an auditory stimulus while attending to an unrelated task) also depends on the level of visual perceptual load.

However, in all these studies awareness was measured retrospectively, by presenting participants with a surprise question about their noticing of an unexpected stimulus after the event. It is therefore possible that the failure to report this stimulus could reflect memory-related rather than perceptual processes (e.g. Wolfe 1999). This issue was addressed by Macdonald and Lavie (2008) in a modified inattentional blindness paradigm in which an expected task-irrelevant stimulus was presented on multiple trials. Participants were asked to make button-press responses whenever they noticed the stimulus, allowing Macdonald and Lavie to measure participants' sensitivity in detecting it. As predicted by load theory, detection sensitivity was reduced under high (vs low) perceptual load in a central letter search task, strengthening the claim that the effects of perceptual load on conscious awareness reflect perceptual rather than memory-related processes.

Studies that have established effects of perceptual load on early vision further support this interpretation. For example, Carmel et al. (2007) demonstrated that the fundamental ability to detect whether a point of light is flickering or continuous was significantly reduced under conditions of high (vs low) perceptual load in an unrelated visual task. Another study investigated the process whereby a peripheral visual stimulus presented against a background of dynamic visual noise tends to disappear from awareness after a few seconds' viewing. This process (referred to as 'filling in') was more likely to occur, and tended to occur more quickly, under low (vs high) perceptual load, indicating clear effects

(a)

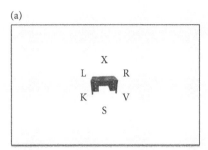

(b)

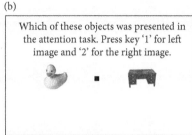

FIGURE 3.1 Examples of the stimuli used by Lavie et al. (2009, Experiment 5). Panel (a) shows a stimulus display from the high perceptual load condition. Participants were asked to report the identity (X or N) of the target letter (contained in the letter circle) while attempting to ignore the central distractor object. In the low perceptual load condition, the non-target letters were all Os. Panel (b) shows the surprise recognition test, presented after the selective attention task. Participants were asked to indicate which of the two objects had been presented as an irrelevant distractor during the attention task they had just performed. Recognition rates in the memory test were significantly higher under low perceptual load (M = 65%, SE = 3) than under high load (M = 50%, SE = 3.6), $t(11)$ = 3.170, p $\rangle$.01. Reproduced from Lavie, N., Lin, Z., Zokaei, N., Thoma, V., The role of perceptual load in object recognition, *Journal of Experimental Psychology: Human Perception and Performance*, 21, 42–57, experiment 5 © 2009, The American Psychological Association.

of attention on what might otherwise have appeared to be a low-level visual phenomenon (Weil et al. 2012). Using a similar logic, Lavie et al. (2009; see Fig. 3.1) demonstrated that recognition of distractor objects was reduced under high (vs low) perceptual load, casting doubt on earlier claims that view-dependent object representations are formed automatically and do not require attentional capacity (e.g. Hummel and Stankiewicz 1996).

Whereas all the studies described so far have measured processing of visible distractors, there is also evidence that perceptual load can even influence the processing of distractors that do not reach conscious awareness. For example, Bahrami et al. (2008) tested participants' adaptation to 'invisible' oriented gratings in the periphery (which were presented monocularly and masked by a simultaneous stimulus presented to the other eye at the same retinal location, so that the gratings did not reach conscious awareness). Successful adaptation was observed when a concurrent visual task at fixation was of low perceptual load, but adaptation was eliminated under high perceptual load, suggesting that even the unconscious processing of distractors that do not reach awareness can be modulated by the perceptual load of a relevant task.

Effects of perceptual load on neural processing

The load effects on perception described so far are underpinned by load modulations of sensory neural processing in visual cortex. These have been established in numerous fMRI studies where neural activity is measured in the precise sensory brain area that mediates perception of the particular distractor stimulus presented. Load theory predicts that high perceptual load will reduce the neural response to the distractor as measured in this way.

Rees, Frith, and Lavie (1997) tested this prediction using irrelevant motion distractors in order to take advantage of the fact that the neural markers of motion perception are very well delineated (for example, area V5/MT is known to respond selectively to moving (vs static) stimuli). Rees et al. asked participants to focus attention on written words presented one at a time at the centre of the screen. In the low-load condition they responded according to whether the words were presented in upper- or lower-case letters, whereas under high-load they discriminated bisyllabic words from mono- or trisyllabic words. The screen surround was filled in with dots which were either static or moving in a radially expanding pattern. As predicted, increased load in the word perception task reduced motion-related activity in V5/MT (as well as in the other motion-responsive areas, e.g. the superior colliculus).

Since then, a large number of studies of this type have identified clear modulation by perceptual load of neural responses to distractors throughout visual cortex and even in some subcortical areas. For example, it is well known that inferotemporal cortex mediates perception of meaningful visual objects. Pinsk, Doniger, and Kastner (2004) found that responses in this area to a wide variety of distractor images were drastically reduced under high (vs low) perceptual load in an attended task. Similarly, Yi et al. (2004) found that a brain area that is known to respond to places (known as the parahippocampal place area; Epstein and Kanwisher 1998) no longer responded to pictures of places under conditions of high (vs low) load in an attended task. Moreover, they found that the neural signature of adaptation to repeated stimuli (known as 'fMR adaptation', Grill-Spector and Malach 2001; or 'repetition suppression', Henson and Rugg 2003) was no longer seen under high load.

These demonstrations have now been extended to areas as early in the visual processing stream as V1 (e.g. Bahrami, Lavie, and Rees 2007; Schwartz et al. 2005; see Fig. 3.2) and even the subcortical lateral geniculate nucleus—the gateway to visual cortex (O'Connor et al. 2002). Sensory processing in these early visual areas is highly likely to reflect early perceptual processing that has not yet reached conscious awareness. Indeed, Bahrami, Lavie, and Rees (2007) directly addressed the effects of load on early unconscious processing. They used the continuous flash suppression method whereby a strong flashing mask presented to one eye suppresses awareness of stimuli presented to the other eye (rendering them literally invisible for periods as long as 20 seconds) and manipulated perceptual load for an attended stimulus that was presented centrally to both eyes. High perceptual load reduced V1 activity related to the invisible stimuli. This strongly suggests that perceptual load can affect neural processing even at these very early stages. Consistent with this conclusion, ERP studies have demonstrated modulations by perceptual load of relatively early components including the N1 (e.g. Fu et al. 2008) and, under some circumstances, the P1 (e.g. Handy and Mangun 2000).

Accounts of the neural mechanisms underpinning these load effects include the suggestion that perceptual load might modulate the neural excitability in visual cortex, such that increasing the demands on the neurons responding to the task stimuli reduces excitability in other populations of neurons that might compete for control of perception. For example, Muggleton et al. (2008) used transcranial magnetic stimulation (TMS) to measure

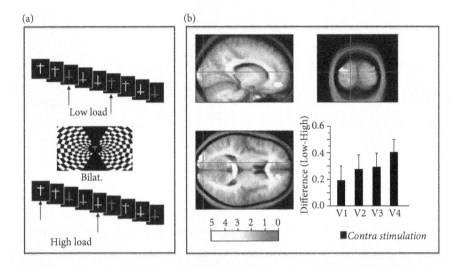

FIGURE 3.2   Stimuli and results from the perceptual load imaging experiment by Schwartz et al. (2005). Panel (a) shows the stimuli and procedure. A rapid stream of upright or inverted cross shapes of different colours was presented at fixation, accompanied by flickering checkerboards presented either on the left side, on the right side, on both sides (shown), or on neither side. Under low perceptual load, participants detected any red shape. Under high load, they detected specific conjunctions of colour and shape (e.g. yellow upright or green inverted). Panel (b) depicts the results. Visual cortex activity related to the checkerboards (pooled across unilateral and bilateral conditions) was greater under low (vs high) perceptual load, as shown in mid-saggital, coronal, and transverse sections. This difference increased across visual areas V1–V4, as shown in the bar graph. Reproduced from Schwartz, S., Vuilleumier, P., Hutton, C., Maravita, A., Dolan, R.J., and Driver, J., Attentional Load and Sensory Competition in Human Vision: Modulation of fMRI Responses by Load at Fixation during Task-irrelevant Stimulation in the Peripheral Visual Field, *Cerebral Cortex*, 15 (06), pp. 770–786 (c) 2005, Oxford University Press.

cortical excitability in area V5/MT as a function of the level of load in a static letter search task. When V5/MT is stimulated this can lead to the illusory percept of a moving flash of light (a moving phosphene). The intensity of stimulation required to elicit this percept can serve as an index of cortical excitability, such that a greater intensity is needed to elicit phosphene perception under reduced excitability. They found that high perceptual load in the letter search task increased the TMS intensity needed to elicit moving phosphenes, suggesting that the high-load task had indeed reduced excitability in V5/MT. This claim has received additional support from a recent demonstration of reduced sensory detection during the period of reduced cortical excitability under high load (Carmel et al. 2011).

Overall then, measures of neural processing have provided strong support for perceptual load theory in pinpointing the effects of load to the brain areas mediating sensory perception. Moreover, the extent of the modulations observed in these studies has important implications for real-world function. For example, the finding that the brain could not detect motion or novelty under high-load conditions has clear functional consequences due to the evolutionary importance of the detection of movement and change in the environment. Indeed, research in other species has demonstrated that birds can fail to detect even images that depict predators when pecking within a high-load seed array (Dukas and Kamil 2000).

Investigating automaticity

The manipulations that have been established through the study of perceptual load theory can also provide a method for examining the automaticity of particular cognitive processes. If processing of a certain type of stimulus remains unaffected by the level of perceptual load in an ongoing task, this might suggest that the stimulus can be processed 'automatically', regardless of the amount of capacity available. By contrast, if a particular process is shown to be eliminated under high (vs low) perceptual load, this can indicate that the process does in fact depend on limited-capacity resources.

The studies of the effects of perceptual load on early visual processing (described above) provide an example of this approach. Many aspects of early vision are considered to be automatic, in the sense that they are not under voluntary control and not subject to capacity limits. The findings described above suggest that while these processes are indeed not under voluntary control (and so proceed on all stimuli within capacity, including irrelevant stimuli that people wish to ignore), they do in fact have limited capacity and can therefore be reduced (or even eliminated) under high perceptual load.

The approach has also been applied to the study of emotion processing, which had often been argued to occur automatically (e.g. Dolan and Vuilleumier 2003)—an idea that is also intuitively appealing based on the high level of sociobiological significance that emotional stimuli are likely to possess. However, studies adopting perceptual load manipulations have challenged this viewpoint, demonstrating that the processing of emotional stimuli can be modulated by the perceptual load of the task at hand. For example, Yates, Ashwin, and Fox (2010) measured the interference caused by distractor pictures of angry faces that either had or had not been conditioned with an aversive noise under conditions of high and low load in a central letter search task. Under low load, they found more interference from fear-conditioned angry faces than from unconditioned angry faces or neutral faces. However, these effects were eliminated under high perceptual load, suggesting that attentional capture by fear-inducing stimuli is not fully automatic as may be assumed, but instead depends to some extent on attentional allocation (see also Mitchell et al. 2007).

Interestingly, famous faces are so far the only stimuli that have been shown to remain unaffected by the perceptual demands of an ongoing task, suggesting that some aspects of face processing may occur automatically. For example, Lavie, Ro, and Russell (2003) asked participants to search for names within displays of either high or low perceptual load, while ignoring peripheral distractor pictures of either famous faces or non-face objects. As predicted by load theory, congruency effects from non-face distractors were reduced under high (vs low) load. However, in a change from this normal pattern of findings, interference from distractor faces was unaffected by perceptual load. In contrast, perception of anonymous faces is significantly reduced under high perceptual load (He and Chen 2010; Jenkins, Lavie, and Driver 2005) suggesting that the automatic processing of famous faces relates to their high level of familiarity, rather than reflecting prioritized processing of faces in general.

Investigating people's perceptual capacity

The framework of load theory has also been used to study capacity differences between different groups of people. According to perceptual load theory, someone with a larger (vs smaller) perceptual processing capacity will require a more demanding perceptual task in order to exhaust their capacity and eliminate distractor processing. This approach has been useful both in developmental, ageing, and clinical contexts.

Many cognitive functions are known to develop through childhood and deteriorate in older age. What about perceptual capacity? Research using the load theory framework has shown that both children and older adults have reduced perceptual capacities compared with people in young to middle adulthood. For example, Maylor and Lavie (1998) asked groups of young and older adults to perform a version of the standard perceptual load flanker task. Under low load, the older participants demonstrated greater distractor interference than the younger participants. At the same time, the older group required a smaller increase in the search set size to prevent distractor processing compared to the younger group, suggesting that ageing reduces perceptual capacity. Similar effects have been found from studies of children's development, such that distractor–interference effects are eliminated at lower levels of perceptual load for children than for young adults, in line with the claim that perceptual capacity develops through childhood (Huang-Pollock, Carr, and Nigg 2002). Note that this research has in fact highlighted one positive consequence of reduced capacity: both the children and the older adults were less distracted by task-irrelevant stimuli compared to the young adults under intermediate levels of perceptual load. Studies using this approach have observed similar potentially beneficial effects of reduced capacity leading to reduced distraction under certain conditions (all involving lower levels of load than those needed to reduce distraction in healthy controls) in patients after parietal, frontal, and temporal brain lesions (Kumada and Humphreys 2002; Lavie and Robertson 2001) as well as in people with schizophrenia or high schizotypy (Ducato et al. 2008).

In contrast to this pattern of findings, research into autism spectrum disorder (ASD) suggests that adults with ASD might have larger perceptual capacity than typical adults. Remington et al. (2009) found that the level of perceptual load required to eliminate distractor processing in typical adults was not sufficient to prevent distractor processing in adults with ASD, and Remington, Swettenham, and Lavie (2012) showed that this pattern extends to visual detection abilities, such that adults with ASD exhibit superior detection to typical adults under higher levels of load. This confirms that ASD appears to involve enhanced perceptual capacity rather than increased vulnerability to irrelevant distraction. A recent study has made similar claims about people with high social anxiety, who also exhibited significant distractor processing under levels of perceptual load that were sufficient to extinguish distractor processing in people with low social anxiety (Moriya and Tanno 2010). Finally, similar findings from regular video game players have been used to underpin claims that they might have enhanced perceptual capacities compared with non-gamers (Green and Bavelier 2003).

EXECUTIVE CONTROL LOAD

Although load theory began with a focus on perceptual load, it was soon extended to address the role of load in another important determinant of selective attention, namely executive control (e.g. Lavie 2000; Lavie et al. 2004). Load theory stipulates that executive control functions such as working memory serve to maintain current stimulus processing and response priorities throughout task performance. The importance of these functions becomes particularly clear in task situations involving low perceptual load. While high perceptual load in a relevant task allows people to ignore irrelevant distractors simply by not perceiving them (early selection), low perceptual load allows the distractors to compete more effectively against the relevant stimuli (late selection). Nevertheless, people are still able to perform the task under low perceptual load, albeit less efficiently. This ability critically depends on the availability of executive control functions to actively maintain the current processing priorities. When executive control functions are loaded (for example, by asking participants to maintain additional information in working memory) they are no longer available to exert attentional control, resulting in greater processing of competing distractors. Thus the theory predicts that executive control load has the opposite effect to that of perceptual load, increasing distractor processing (rather than reducing it).

One happy side effect of these opposite predictions is that they provide a natural control for the effects of general task difficulty. Increased load, whether on perceptual or executive control processes, leads to increased task difficulty. Thus, if task difficulty were the critical determinant of distractor processing, the same effects should be seen under high executive control load as under high perceptual load. The fact that the two types of load are predicted to have opposite effects on distractor processing means that neither one can be explained in terms of task difficulty. Instead, the effects of load on distractor processing depend on the specific mental function that is loaded.

The role of executive control load in distractor interference

Behavioural studies of the impacts of executive control load have typically used a dual task design in which participants are asked to keep information in mind while also carrying out a selective attention task. For example, Lavie et al. (2004) used a standard flanker task (of low perceptual load) in which participants were asked to identify a target letter while ignoring a concurrently presented distractor letter (either congruent or incongruent with the target). Participants carried out this task under conditions of either high working memory load (where they were asked to remember six randomly chosen digits) or low working memory load (where they only had to remember one digit). Distractor congruency effects were greater under high (vs low) working memory load, supporting the claim that the availability of executive control functions is important for minimizing distractor interference.

This claim is supported by a study showing that people are more likely to experience attentional capture by salient (yet task-irrelevant) singleton distractors (e.g. a single red shape within a display of green shapes) under a high (vs low) concurrent working memory load (Lavie and de Fockert 2005; see Fig. 3.3). Notice that distractor interference in

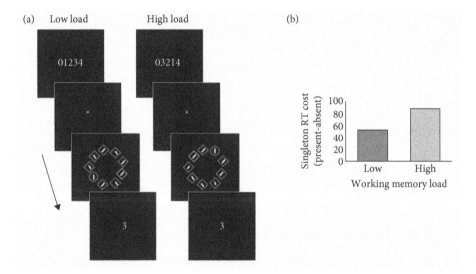

FIGURE 3.3   Examples of the stimuli and results from Lavie and de Fockert (2005, Experiment 2). Panel (a) shows the interleaving of the search task with the working memory task. Each trial began with presentation of a memory set. Under low working memory load, this consisted of the digits 0–4 in numerical order. Under high load, the sequence started with 0 but the remaining digits (1–4) were presented in random order. Participants were asked to hold the set in mind while they completed a search task. They searched for a red circle amid red diamonds, responding according to the orientation of the line contained within the circle. On some trials, one of the non-target diamonds was presented in green. Attentional capture by this unique and salient (yet task-irrelevant) 'singleton' item was measured in terms of the RT costs associated with its presence (vs absence). The trial ended with a memory probe task, in which participants named the digit from the original memory set that had followed the digit shown on screen, allowing confirmation that the set had been successfully maintained. As shown in panel (b), attentional capture by the task-irrelevant singleton in the search task was significantly larger under high (vs low) working memory load. Reproduced from *Psychonomic Bulletin and Review*, 12 (4), 2005 pp. 669–674, The role of working memory in attentional capture, Nilli Lavie and Jan De Fockert, experiment 2 © Springer Science and Business Media. With kind permission from Springer Science and Business Media.

this task was measured in terms of a general slowing in the presence (vs absence) of the singletons, which were not themselves associated with any response. Thus, the effects of working memory load are not confined to increased response competition but also appear to affect perceptual processing of distractors, as discussed further in the following section.

The role of executive control load in visual perception

Effects on reaction times cannot inform about the level of processing that was affected by load (as discussed earlier in this chapter). However, executive control load has also been shown to influence distractor processing in studies using more direct measures of visual perception and awareness. In line with this claim, people have been shown to be less susceptible to inattentional blindness (i.e. more likely to notice the task-irrelevant critical stimulus) under high (vs low) working memory load (e.g. de Fockert and Bremner 2011). A more direct test of visual perception including meaningful recognition (as opposed to detection of whether a stimulus was there or not, as measured in the typical inattentional blindness task) was offered by Carmel, Fairnie, and Lavie (2012). They asked participants to categorize written words while ignoring unfamiliar task-irrelevant faces presented in the periphery of the display. This task was carried out under high or low working memory load. After the final trial, participants were given a surprise recognition test measuring their identification of the irrelevant face that had been presented on that trial. Identification performance was better under high (vs low) working memory load, again suggesting that working memory plays an important role in determining distractor perception. There is also evidence that working memory load can influence people's susceptibility to the Ebbinghaus illusion (in which judgements about the size of a central circle are influenced by the sizes of the surrounding circles). De Fockert and Wu (2009) found that people experienced this illusion more strongly under high (vs low) concurrent working memory load, suggesting that a reduction in the availability of executive control functions for the illusion task led to increased processing of the task-irrelevant circles. Taken together, these studies confirm earlier findings from the distractor interference paradigm that people's ability to avoid distraction depends critically on the availability of executive control functions such as working memory. However, these studies go beyond those initial findings in demonstrating that executive control functions can affect distractor perception and awareness even in the absence of response competition.

Effects of executive control load on neural processing

The claim that executive control load can influence even sensory perceptual processing of distractors has also been supported by studies using neural measures. For example, de Fockert et al. (2001) varied working memory load while participants completed a selective attention task that required them to classify written names (as belonging to pop stars or politicians) while ignoring irrelevant distractor faces (which were also of pop stars or politicians). As predicted by load theory, cortical activity associated with the processing of distractor faces (e.g. in the fusiform face area; Kanwisher, McDermott, and Chun 1997) was significantly greater under conditions of high (vs low) working memory load, as was the behavioural interference caused by the face distractors. A more recent study has suggested that these high working memory load effects reflect a specific failure in the attenuation of distractor processing (rather than, for example, also including a reduction in the processing of relevant stimuli). Rissman, Gazzaley, and D'Esposito (2009) presented participants with sequences of four images (consisting of a mixture of scenes and faces) under both high and low working memory load. When the scenes were relevant to the task, the load manipulation had no effect on neural activity associated with scene processing. However, when the scenes were made irrelevant to the task, and people were asked to ignore them, activity in this area was greater under high (vs low) working memory load. This supports the findings of de Fockert et al. (2001) in demonstrating increased distractor processing under high working memory load. However, Rissman et al.'s work also extends those findings to suggest that working memory load does not appear to influence the processing of task-relevant items, thus linking the working memory effects specifically to distractor processing. A further study has demonstrated effects of working memory in areas as early in the visual processing stream as primary visual cortex (V1 and V2), suggesting that the availability of working memory during a selective attention task can affect even very early sensory processing of distractor stimuli (Kelley and Lavie 2010). Thus executive control functions appear to be important in minimizing the influence of competing distractors throughout the entire processing stream.

SUMMARY

A substantial body of evidence now agrees that the extent to which visual distractors are processed depends on the perceptual load of the task at hand. If a task imposes high perceptual demands, task-irrelevant distractors can often be ignored successfully. By contrast, if a task imposes only low perceptual demands, the distractors receive substantially more processing and are thus more likely to interfere with behaviour. These effects of perceptual load provide a resolution to the early- versus late-selection debate in demonstrating that selection can occur either earlier or later in processing, depending on the perceptual demands of the task at hand. Research has also converged to demonstrate that the effective prioritization of task-relevant stimuli in the face of competition from irrelevant distractors depends on the availability of executive control functions for active maintenance of the processing priorities. When these functions are highly loaded, the prioritization process is impaired and distractors compete more effectively for processing resources. The consistent convergence of the findings in support of these principles across a broad range of manipulations and measures rules out any specific task factors as alternative explanations for the load effects.

We began the chapter by considering the problem of how to read this book in the middle of Oxford Street. According to load theory, your ability to focus on the page while ignoring the many distractions of the bustling city scene will depend both on the perceptual demands of the reading task and on the level of executive control that you are able to summon. If the perceptual load of the reading task is high enough to exhaust your processing capacity, you are unlikely to process the surrounding scene very thoroughly and should therefore be able to avoid distraction. However, if the task imposes only a low perceptual load (for example, if you decide to check the formatting, rather than actually reading) your excess perceptual capacity will automatically be allocated to processing the background scene and you are more likely to become distracted. Under these circumstances, it is particularly important for you to be able to draw on executive control functions, to maintain your priority of focusing on the book. If you are able to dedicate your full executive capacity to this task (i.e. if your executive capacity is not highly loaded) then you should still be able to deprioritize the distractors and avoid too much interference. However, if you are unable to summon your full executive powers (for example, because you are also trying to remember a complicated to-do list for the day), you may lose your ability to control your attention, leaving you more susceptible to distraction.

REFERENCES

Bahrami, B., Lavie, N., and Rees, G. (2007). Attentional load modulates responses of human primary visual cortex to invisible stimuli. *Current Biology 17*: 509–513.

Bahrami, B., Carmel, D., Walsh, V., Rees, G., and Lavie, N. (2008). Unconscious orientation processing depends on perceptual load. *Journal of Vision 8*: 1–10.

Beck, D. and Lavie, N. (2005). Look here but ignore what you see: Effects of distractors at fixation. *Journal of Experimental Psychology: Human Perception and Performance 31*: 592–607.

Broadbent, D. E. (1958). *Perception and Communication*. Oxford: Oxford University Press.

Broadbent, D. E., Cooper, P. F., FitzGerald, P., and Parkes, K. R. (1982). The Cognitive Failures Questionnaire (CFQ) and its correlates. *British Journal of Clinical Psychology 21*: 1–16.

Carmel, D., Saker, P., Rees, G., and Lavie, N. (2007). Perceptual load modulates conscious flicker perception. *Journal of Vision 7*: 1–13.

Carmel, D., Thorne, J., Rees, G., and Lavie, N. (2011). Perceptual load alters visual excitability. *Journal of Experimental Psychology: Human Perception and Performance 37*: 1350–1360.

Carmel, D., Fairnie, J., and Lavie, N. (2012). Weight and see: Loading working memory improves incidental identification of irrelevant faces. *Frontiers in Psychology 3*: 286.

Cartwright-Finch, U. and Lavie, N. (2007). The role of perceptual load in inattentional blindness. *Cognition 102*: 321–340.

Cherry, E. C. (1953). Some experiments on the recognition of speech with one and with two ears. *Journal of the Acoustical Society of America 25*: 975–979.

Dayan, P. (2008). Load and attentional Bayes. Paper presented at the 22nd meeting of the Neural Information Processing Systems Foundation, Vancouver, Canada.

Deutsch, J. A. and Deutsch, D. (1963). Attention: Some theoretical considerations. *Psychological Review 87*: 272–300.

Dolan, R. J. and Vuilleumier, P. (2003). Amygdala automaticity in emotional processing. *Annals of the New York Academy of Sciences* 985: 348–355.

Driver, J. (2001). A selective review of selective attention research from the past century. *British Journal of Psychology* 92: 53–78.

Ducato, M.-G., Thomas, P., Monestes, J.-L., Despretz, P., and Boucart, M. (2008). Attentional capture in schizophrenia and schizotypy: Effect of attentional load. *Cognitive Neuropsychiatry* 13: 89–111.

Dukas, R. and Kamil, A. C. (2000). The cost of limited attention in blue jays. *Behavioral Ecology* 11: 502–506.

Epstein, R. and Kanwisher, N. (1998). A cortical representation of the local visual environment. *Nature* 392: 598–601.

Fockert, J. W. de, Rees, G., Frith, C., and Lavie, N. (2001). The role of working memory in visual selective attention. *Science* 291: 1803–1806.

Fockert, J. W. de and Wu, S. (2009). High working memory load leads to more Ebbinghaus illusion. *European Journal of Cognitive Psychology* 21: 961–970.

Fockert, J. W. de and Bremner, A. J. (2011). Release of inattentional blindness by high working memory load: Elucidating the relationship between working memory and selective attention. *Cognition* 121: 400–408.

Forster, S. and Lavie, N. (2007). High perceptual load makes everybody equal: Eliminating individual differences in distractibility with load. *Psychological Science* 18: 377–382.

Forster, S. and Lavie, N. (2008). Failures to ignore entirely irrelevant distractors: The role of load. *Journal of Experimental Psychology: Applied* 14: 73–83.

Forster, S. and Lavie, N. (2009). Harnessing the wandering mind: The role of perceptual load. *Cognition* 111: 345–355.

Fu, S., Zinni, M., Squire, P. N., Kumar, R., Caggiano, D. M., and Parasuraman, R. (2008). When and where perceptual load interacts with voluntary visuospatial attention: An event-related potential and dipole modeling study. *NeuroImage* 39: 1345–1355.

Green, C. S. and Bavelier, D. (2003). Action video games modify visual selective attention. *Nature* 423: 534–537.

Grill-Spector, K. and Malach, R. (2001). fMR-adaptation: A tool for studying the functional properties of human cortical neurons. *Acta Psychologica* 107: 293–232.

Handy, T. C. and Mangun, G. R. (2000). Attention and spatial selection: Electrophysiological evidence for modulation by perceptual load. *Perception & Psychophysics* 62: 175–186.

He, C. and Chen, A. (2010). Interference from familiar natural distractors is not eliminated by high perceptual load. *Psychological Research* 74: 268–276.

Henson, R. N. A. and Rugg, M. D. (2003). Neural response suppression, haemodynamic repetition effects and behavioural priming. *Neuropsychologia* 41: 263–270.

Huang-Pollock, C. L., Carr, T. H., and Nigg, J. T. (2002). Development of selective attention: Perceptual load influences early versus late attentional selection in children and adults. *Developmental Psychology* 38: 363–375.

Hummel, J. E. and Stankiewicz, B. J. (1996). An architecture for rapid, hierarchical structural description. In T. Inui and J. McClelland (eds.), *Attention and Performance, XVI: Information Integration in Perception and Communication* (pp. 93–121). Cambridge, Mass.: MIT Press.

Jenkins, R., Lavie, N., and Driver J. (2005). Recognition memory for distractor faces depends on attentional load at exposure. *Psychonomic Bulletin & Review* 12: 314–320.

Kanwisher, N., McDermott, J., and Chun, M. (1997). The fusiform face area: A module in human extrastriate cortex specialized for the perception of faces. *Journal of Neuroscience* 17: 4302–4311.

Kelley, T. A. and Lavie, N. (2010). Working memory load modulates distractor competition in primary visual cortex. *Cerebral Cortex* 21: 659–665.

Kumada, T. and Humphreys, G. W. (2002). Early selection induced by perceptual load in a patient with frontal lobe damage: External vs. internal modulation of processing control. *Cognitive Neuropsychology* 19: 49–65.

Lavie, N. and Tsal, Y. (1994). Perceptual load as a major determinant of the locus of selection in visual attention. *Perception & Psychophysics* 56: 183–197.

Lavie, N. (1995). Perceptual load as a necessary condition for selective attention. *Journal of Experimental Psychology: Human Perception and Performance* 21: 451–468.

Lavie, N. and Cox, S. (1997). On the efficiency of attentional selection: Efficient visual search results in inefficient rejection of distraction. *Psychological Science* 8: 395–398.

Lavie, N. (2000). Selective attention and cognitive control: Dissociating attentional functions through different types of load. In S. Monsell and J. Driver (eds.), *Attention and Performance XVIII* (pp. 175–194). Cambridge, Mass.: MIT Press.

Lavie, N. and Fox, E. (2000). The role of perceptual load in negative priming. *Journal of Experimental Psychology: Human Perception and Performance* 26: 1038–1052.

Lavie, N. and Robertson, I. (2001). The role of perceptual load in visual neglect: Rejection of ipsilesional distractors is facilitated with higher central load. *Journal of Cognitive Neuroscience* 13: 867–876.

Lavie, N., Ro, T., and Russell, C. (2003). The role of perceptual load in processing distractor faces. *Psychological Science* 14: 510–515.

Lavie, N., Hirst, A., Fockert, J. W. de, and Viding, E. (2004). Load theory of selective attention and cognitive control. *Journal of Experimental Psychology: General* 133: 339–354.

Lavie, N. (2005) Distracted and confused? Selective attention under load. *Trends in Cognitive Sciences* 9: 75–82.

Lavie, N. and Fockert, J. W. de (2005). The role of working memory in attentional capture. *Psychonomic Bulletin & Review* 12: 669–674.

Lavie, N. (2006). *Attention and Consciousness: The Blackwell Companion to Consciousness.* Oxford: Blackwell Publishing.

Lavie, N., Lin, Z., Zokaei, N., and Thoma, V. (2009). The role of perceptual load in object recognition. *Journal of Experimental Psychology: Human Perception and Performance* 21: 42–57.

Lavie, N. (2010). Attention, distraction and cognitive control under load. *Current Directions in Psychological Science* 19: 143–148.

Lavie, N. and Torralbo, A. (2010). Dilution: A theoretical burden or just load? A reply to Tsal and Benoni (2010). *Journal of Experimental Psychology: Human Perception and Performance* 36: 1657–1664.

Macdonald, J. and Lavie, N. (2008). Load-induced blindness. *Journal of Experimental Psychology: Human Perception and Performance* 34: 1078–1091.

Macdonald, J. and Lavie, N. (2011). Visual perceptual load induces inattentional deafness. *Attention, Perception, & Psychophysics* 73: 1780–1789.

Mack, A. and Rock, I. (1998). *Inattentional Blindness.* Cambridge, Mass.: MIT Press.

Maylor, E. and Lavie, N. (1998). The influence of perceptual load on age differences in selective attention. *Psychology and Aging* 13: 563–573.

Mitchell, D. G., Nakic, M., Fridberg, D., Kamel, N., Pine, D. S., and Blair, R. J. (2007). The impact of processing load on emotion. *NeuroImage* 34: 1299–1309.

Moray, N. (1959). Attention in dichotic listening: Affective cues and the influence of instructions. *Quarterly Journal of Experimental Psychology* 11: 56–60.

Moriya, J. and Tanno, Y. (2008). Attentional resources in social anxiety and the effects of perceptual load. *Cognition & Emotion 24*: 1329–1348.

Muggleton, N., Lamb, R., Walsh, V., and Lavie, N. (2008). Perceptual load modulates visual cortex excitability to magnetic stimulation. *Journal of Neurophysiology 100*: 516–519.

Neisser, U. and Becklen, R. (1975). Selective looking: Attending to visually specified events. *Cognitive Psychology 7*: 480–494.

O'Connor, D. H., Fukui, M. M., Pinsk, M. A., and Kastner, S. (2002). Attention modulates responses in the human lateral geniculate nucleus. *Nature Neuroscience 5*: 1203–1209.

Pinsk, M. A., Doniger, G. M., and Kastner, S. (2004). Push-pull mechanism of selective attention in human extrastriate cortex. *Journal of Neurophysiology 92*: 622–629.

Rees, G., Frith, C., and Lavie, N. (1997). Modulating irrelevant motion perception by varying attentional load in an unrelated task. *Science 278*: 1616–1619.

Remington, A. M., Swettenham, J. G., Campbell, R., and Coleman, M. (2009). Selective attention and perceptual load in autism spectrum disorder. *Psychological Science 20*: 1388–1393.

Remington, A. M., Swettenham, J. G., and Lavie, N. (2012). Lightening the load: Perceptual load impairs visual detection in typical adults but not in autism. *Journal of Abnormal Psychology 121*: 544–551.

Rissman, J., Gazzaley, A., and D'Esposito, M. (2009). The effect of non-visual working memory load on top-down modulation of visual processing. *Neuropsychologia 47*: 1637–1646.

Schwartz, S., Vuilleumier, P., Hutton, C., Maravita, A., Dolan, R. J., and Driver, J. (2005). Attentional load and sensory competition in human vision: Modulation of fMRI responses by load at fixation during task-irrelevant stimulation in the peripheral visual field. *Cerebral Cortex 15*: 770–786.

Simons, D. J. and Chabris, C. F. (1999). Gorillas in our midst: Sustained inattentional blindness for dynamic events. *Perception 28*: 1059–1074.

Tsal, Y. and Benoni, H. (2010). Diluting the burden of load: Perceptual load effects are simply dilution effects. *Journal of Experimental Psychology: Human Perception and Performance 36*: 1645–1656.

Weil, R. S., Wykes, V., Carmel, D., and Rees, G. (2012). Opposite effects of perceptual and working memory load on perceptual filling-in of an artificial scotoma. *Cognitive Neuroscience 3*: 36–44.

Wilson, D. E., Muroi, M., and MacLeod, C. M. (2011). Dilution, not load, affects distractor processing. *Journal of Experimental Psychology: Human Perception and Performance 37*: 319–335.

Wolfe, J. M. (1999). Inattentional amnesia. In V. Coltheart (ed.), *Fleeting Memories* (pp. 71–94). Cambridge, Mass.: MIT Press.

Yates, A., Ashwin, C., and Fox, E. (2010). Does emotion processing require attention? The effects of fear conditioning and perceptual load. *Emotion 10*: 822–830.

Yi, D.-J., Woodman, G. F., Widders, D., Marois, R., and Chun, M. M. (2004). Neural fate of ignored stimuli: Dissociable effects of perceptual and working memory load. *Nature Neuroscience 7*: 992–996.

CHAPTER 4

A MULTI-LEVEL ACCOUNT OF SELECTIVE ATTENTION

JOHN T. SERENCES AND SABINE KASTNER

INTRODUCTION

NEURAL information processing systems must overcome a series of bottlenecks that interrupt the sequence of events between sensory input and motor output. First, the sensory neurons that encode external stimuli are noisy. As a result, an identical stimulus will evoke a slightly different response pattern each time it is presented, and this instability can place limits on the amount of information that neurons can relay about stimulus features (Pouget, Dayan, and Zemel 2003; Seung and Sompolinsky 1993). Second, multiple items in the visual field compete for representation, and this competition must be resolved so that the most behaviourally relevant sensory stimuli are represented and allowed to guide goal-directed behaviour. Third, there are limits on the number of responses that can be selected simultaneously (Pashler 1994), and obvious limits on the number of simultaneous motor plans that can be executed. All of these factors restrict the speed and accuracy of sensory–response mappings, and at each stage, relevant stimuli must be prioritized over irrelevant distractors to ensure the successful completion of behavioural goals. The ability to prioritize relevant stimuli is generally referred to as *selective attention*, where the prefix *selective* is intentionally used to distinguish the term from changes in general arousal or states of consciousness.

There are three general mechanisms that support selection attention: signal enhancement, external and internal noise suppression, and selective read-out. The first two mechanisms influence selection by directly mediating the information content of neural representations as sensory signals are relayed and transformed across the processing hierarchy. Selective read-out is conceptually different, as it does not directly modify the quality of sensory representations. Instead, selective read-out influences the efficiency with which sensory information is used to inform decisions about the contents of the sensory array, either in the absence of or in combination with signal enhancement and noise suppression.

In this chapter, we focus on two general questions that have emerged over the last 50 years: *where* and *when* do these mechanisms of selective attention operate to enable efficient information processing? Such questions about the locus of selection are rooted in the classic debate between theories of early and late selection that have been actively pursued in the fields of cognitive psychology and cognitive neuroscience for decades. Early selection theories hold that attention filters sensory inputs based on simple low-level features (e.g. pitch of a sound, orientation of a line), whereas late selection theories hold that filtering occurs only after all basic features have been analysed and stimuli are semantically labelled. More recently, this early/late dichotomy has been subjected to increasingly sophisticated neuroscientific techniques that reveal signatures of selection in large-scale neural networks including the thalamus, sensory, and higher-order cortex. At different points in time and at different levels of the cortical hierarchy, selection can be implemented via signal enhancement, internal and external noise suppression, and the selective read-out of sensory signals. Moreover, these mechanisms operate in a complementary manner to facilitate information processing, with the relative contribution of each determined by behavioural demands and by the nature of the stimulus array.

We begin with a brief history of the early versus late selection debate, and then review current knowledge about *where* and *when* signal enhancement, noise suppression, and selective read-out exert their influence on information processing.

A Historical Perspective on Early Versus Late Selection Theories

One of the first clearly articulated theories concerning the locus of attentional selection was the filter model of Broadbent (Broadbent 1958). He posited that incoming stimuli were analysed to the level of basic features (e.g. pitch, location). Based on this information, one item at a time was then selected and brought into awareness. Critically, given the breakdown of information into basic components assumed in this model, selection must happen very early in the processing stream, before the level of semantic analysis. Thus, models of this type are termed *early selection* theories. Broadbent was primarily influenced by data from dichotic listening tasks, where subjects were presented with separate auditory input in each ear. In these classical studies, subjects were typically asked to shadow the input from one ear by repeating out loud. While this task is quite attentionally engaging, subjects have little problem selecting one of the two auditory streams to shadow based on low-level features such as the pitch of the speaker's voice or the ear of origin (location). Moreover, subjects typically report having little subjective awareness of the information presented in the unattended auditory channel, as reflected quantitatively in poor recognition memory performance (Cherry 1953; Moray 1959; Neisser and Becklen 1975). Nevertheless, subjects were still able to discriminate low-level stimulus attributes such as pitch in the unattended channel, supporting

Broadbent's notion that selection must be early, as these basic attributes appeared to be all that was retained from the unattended auditory stream.

Not long after Broadbent's seminal book, Moray (1959) demonstrated that selection was not always implemented by an early filtering mechanism, as he noted that about one-third of subjects detected their own name when it was inserted in the unattended stream, despite a general lack of awareness of the overall content of the message. In a related finding, Treisman (Treisman 1960) presented subjects with two coherent sentences, one in each ear, and subjects were instructed to shadow the input from one of the channels. When the flow of the prose from the shadowed channel changed to the other ear, subjects would often continue to shadow the same sentence, even though the words were now being presented in the to-be-ignored channel. This tendency to track a sentence from the attended to the unattended channel based on syntactic structure and semantic content suggests that the message in the unattended ear was processed to a far more advanced level of analysis than predicted by the original inception of Broadbent's early selection theory.

To account for the semantic processing of the unattended channel, Anthony and Diane Deutsch (Deutsch and Deutsch 1963) formalized a *late selection* theory of attentional selection. In stark contrast to Broadbent's early filter theory, the late selection account holds that all stimuli are analysed to the level of semantic description. Moreover, the mechanism that supports semantic analysis is not capacity limited and can thus process all perceptual inputs in parallel. After this analysis is complete, attention operates by selecting a subset of the items for further processing, such as encoding into working memory (Duncan 1980). Importantly, Deutsch and Deutsch did not imply that subjects necessarily had conscious access to these early semantic descriptions. Rather, awareness only occurred after the capacity-limited process of attentional selection, accounting for the commonly held notion that observers are only aware of a small subset of potential stimuli at any given moment in time.

After these two opposite views on the locus of selection had been established, a good deal of research over the next 30 years focused on attempting to critically discriminate between the competing models. While studies on dichotic listening remained prominent (e.g. Corteen and Wook 1972), many researchers turned to investigating early and late selection in the visual domain. The prototypical approach was to infer the locus of selection based on behavioural measures such as priming that reflect the extent to which unattended stimuli impacted performance. Instances in which unattended stimuli did not influence performance were taken as support for early selection. Conversely, the influence of unattended stimuli on performance was interpreted as evidence in favour of late selection. For instance, Eriksen and Eriksen (Eriksen and Eriksen 1974) had subjects report the identity of a target letter briefly presented in an attended location indicated by a pre-cue presented at the start of each trial. One of the two possible target letters was mapped to a button press with the index finger, and the other target letter was mapped to a button press with the middle finger. The target letter was flanked on either side by additional letters that were either mapped to the same response required by the target (termed *compatible flankers*) or to the opposite response (termed *incompatible flankers*). The main observation was that response times (RT) to the targets were slower when the target was accompanied by incompatible flankers as opposed to compatible flankers. The effect of flanker identity on RT supports the late selection tenet that items outside the locus of attention are processed at least to the level of semantic description despite the fact that subjects had perfect foreknowledge of the target's location and could presumably focus attention well in advance.

However, evidence of this sort is not undisputed. First, proponents of early selection can always assert that the behavioural tasks did not adequately engage the subject's attention, thus 'leakage' through an early perceptual filter might occur. Indeed, if attentional cues are made salient enough, then irrelevant flankers do not have a measurable effect on performance, as shown by Egeth and colleagues (Francolini and Egeth 1980; Yantis and Johnston 1990). Such observations undermine the strong form of the late selection account because late selection models clearly predict an effect of incompatible distractors, regardless of the attentional focus. However, it appears that these claims against late selection rest on the assumption that the dependent measure is sensitive to a subtle influence of distractors. Indeed, using a different behavioural measure, Tipper and Driver (Tipper and Driver 1988) found evidence that the distractors used by Egeth and colleagues were in fact processed to the level of semantic content, supporting a late selection account. Moreover, the view that a semantic description was formed and then suppressed prior to the response stage can always be asserted by supporters of late selection to countermand data consistent with early selection. The main conclusion of these behavioural studies, and many others like them, is that behavioural evidence in support of either early or late selection can be obtained using very similar experimental paradigms. Therefore, in this particular area of cognitive psychology, physiological metrics have had a great deal of influence, as they can provide more direct insight into the temporal dynamics of signal enhancement, noise suppression, and the level to which sensory information gets processed.

As with the behavioural studies reviewed above, the majority of neuroimaging and electrophysiology studies investigating the neural correlates underlying attentional selection have focused on the visual rather than the auditory domain. Thus, we will limit our discussion to studies on the visual system, first discussing issues pertaining to early and late selection in terms of 'where' within the visual processing hierarchy selection plays out and then asking 'when' these modulations occur.

The 'Where' of Selection via Signal Enhancement: Neural Evidence from Monkey Physiology and Human Neuroimaging

The first important question that emerges from the 'early' vs. 'late' selection debate that we will consider at the neural level is: where in the visual pathway does selective attention *first* affect neural processing? Early and late selection accounts appear to make straightforward predictions with respect to this question. An early selection theory would posit that selective attention should influence early stages of processing including primary visual cortex (striate cortex, or V1), where visual information is filtered based on basic features such as colour, motion, and orientation. In contrast, a late selection theory would predict no modulation at early processing stages, as information should be faithfully represented regardless of task demands (at least) up to stages where the visual information interfaces with other cognitive domains such as memory or action context.

The modulation of neural responses by spatially selective attention was originally demonstrated in the extrastriate cortex. In a seminal study, Moran and Desimone (Moran and Desimone 1985) recorded the activity of neurons in area V4 from monkeys trained to direct attention to a spatial location within a neuron's receptive field (RF). The target stimulus was either shown alone in the neuron's RF or in the presence of a nearby distractor. Attending to the target enhanced neural responses, but only when a competing stimulus was presented in the same RF as the target. These findings demonstrate that selective attention can gate the processing of behaviourally relevant information by effectively constricting the RF around the selected stimulus such that the distractor has little or no impact on the firing rate of the cell. Similar effects of attentional enhancement in area V4 have been demonstrated by several other groups (e.g. Connor, Preddie, Gallant, and Van Essen 1997; Haenny and Schiller 1988; McAdams and Maunsell 1999; Motter 1993), and have been found in several other extrastriate and parietal areas including V2 (Luck, Chelazzi, Hillyard, and Desimone 1997; Motter 1993), MT (e.g. Treue and Maunsell 1996) and LIP (e.g. Gottlieb, Kusunoki, and Goldberg 1998).

Despite the widespread and robust observation of attentional modulation in many areas of visual cortex, it was initially unclear if attention modulated activity in primary visual cortex. Several studies were unable to demonstrate such modulation (e.g. Luck et al. 1997), while others found relatively weak, but reliable effects (e.g. Motter 1993). While it was not clear what factors best accounted for these discrepant findings, there was an overall impression that attentional modulation at the earliest cortical processing stages may be highly dependent on task-related factors or the need to integrate information from beyond the classic RF (e.g. Ito and Gilbert 1999; Roelfsema, Lamme, and Spekreijse 1998). In either case, the few studies that recorded attention effects from different areas in the same animals (Cook and Maunsell 2002a, 2002b; Luck et al. 1997) showed that the magnitude of attentional modulation was stronger in more anterior extrastriate areas (e.g. V4) compared to more posterior areas such as V2. This graded effect was taken to suggest that attentional effects at earlier stages were caused by reactivation from higher-order extrastriate areas through cortico–cortical feedback connections, although a direct demonstration of this link has not been reported.

Thus, evidence from these initial physiology studies does not unequivocally support either early or late selection models. The finding of attentional modulation in relatively early cortical areas such as V2 and possibly even V1 is consistent with early selection accounts. However, the inconsistent observation of attention effects in V1, coupled with the possibility that these effects primarily reflect reactivation from higher-order areas, renders the evidence inconclusive. Thus, single unit recording data that emerged by the late 1990s did not clearly support either alternative, leaving the question far from being settled.

In the mid and late 1990s, the advent of functional magnetic resonance imaging (fMRI) enabled detailed studies of the human visual system and offered several advantages over previous approaches. In particular, human subjects can perform a wider range of tasks compared to non-human primates and activation changes tied to task manipulations can be examined across the entire brain (as opposed to monitoring single-unit activity in a single area). Soon, investigators had settled lingering questions about whether attention could modulate responses at the earliest anatomical levels of processing by showing response modulation in V1 with moving (Gandhi, Heeger, and Boynton 1999; Somers, Dale, Seiffert, and Tootell 1999) and stationary stimuli (Martinez et al. 1999). Even stronger evidence in support of early selection came from the subsequent demonstration of attention effects in the thalamus, i.e. the lateral geniculate nucleus (LGN) (O'Connor, Fukui, Pinsk, and Kastner 2002). The LGN is the thalamic component in the retinocortical projection and it is the first neural structure within the visual processing hierarchy that can be modulated by feedback input (via afferent input from the thalamic reticular nucleus, striate cortex, and the brainstem). Interestingly, attention effects in the LGN were found to be stronger than in area V1, more on the order of extrastriate areas such as V4 (O'Connor et al. 2002). Thus, these findings not only challenge the notion that cognitive processing primarily involves cortical networks, but also the notion that attentional modulation in early sensory areas can be explained solely by cortico–cortical re-entrant signals from later stages of the hierarchy, as such an account would have predicted smaller effects of attention in the LGN than in V1. Instead, fMRI signals may reflect the summed modulatory feedback that a given area receives from cortical, thalamic, and brainstem sources, as opposed to just local spiking activity. If this is indeed the case, then larger attentional modulation in LGN might be related to the larger number of afferent inputs that this region receives compared to primary visual cortex. Thus, fMRI evidence gathered over the last 15 years provides compelling support for anatomically early attention effects by demonstrating modulation in V1 and the LGN, the earliest stages of visual processing that receive feedback influences from other sources (see also chapters by Beck and Kastner, and Saalmann and Kastner).

The ability of fMRI measurements to index attentional modulation across the entire brain also provides key insights into how each area is driven by 'sensory-driven' or 'bottom-up' versus 'cognitively driven' or 'top-down' influences. For instance, sensory-driven population responses during passive viewing follow a characteristic pattern when measured with fMRI: the strongest responses are typically observed in early visual areas such as V1 and progressively weaker responses are observed at successively later stages of the hierarchy (see Fig. 4.1a). For example, 90% of the maximum response can be evoked in V1 by a simple visual stimulus, whereas the same input might evoke a modulation of only 10% in higher-order areas of parietal and frontal cortex (e.g. Treue 2003). On the other hand, the response modulation associated with deploying

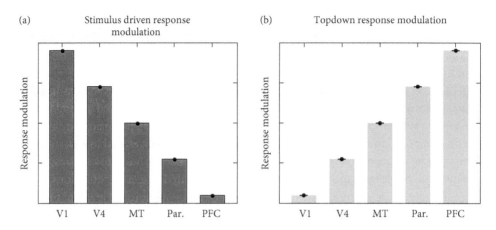

FIGURE 4.1 Schematic showing the relative magnitude of stimulus-driven and top-down modulation across the cortical hierarchy from occipital to parietal (Par.) to pre-frontal cortex (PFC). (a) The magnitude of sensory modulation gradually decreases. (b) In contrast, the magnitude of top-down modulations is largest in PFC and gradually decreases in earlier visual areas.

top-down attention to a fixed sensory stimulus exhibits the opposite pattern: a 90% increase in activation might be expected in areas of parietal and frontal cortex, whereas a modulation of 10% is expected in early visual cortex (see Fig. 4.1b).

Based on the neural evidence of attentional modulation at early processing stages, the preponderance of evidence seems to favour early selection as opposed to late selection accounts. However, several caveats should be noted. First, none of the studies reviewed thus far addressed the question of *what* was selected or what type of information was modulated at each processing stage. This is a critical issue, as the observation of an attentional modulation at a specific stage of the visual hierarchy does not speak to the issue of what kind of information is targeted by attention. For example, an increase in activation levels within a neural population that is thought to encode a certain feature—such as motion in area MT—does not necessarily mean that selective attention operates on the feature 'motion'. This is particularly true when neural effects are inferred based on fMRI measurements, as the blood oxygen level dependent (BOLD) signal reflects the aggregate activity across all neurons in a region and is generally insensitive to feature selective changes in population response profiles (see Serences and Saproo 2012). Thus, any attentional modulation that is measured within a given region may be targeted on any type of information processed in the area, or may simply reflect a general increase in the activity of all neurons within a region in a non-selective manner (i.e. analogous to a change in general arousal). Such effects may thus translate into a scaling of responses in a region without actually influencing the selectivity of the population response or the amount of stimulus-specific information that is encoded about relevant sensory stimuli. In addition, even though neuroimaging methods excel at pinpointing the anatomical locus of selection, fMRI does not have the temporal resolution to conclusively distinguish between modulations of afferent signals and modulations related to later re-entrant feedback. In contrast, electrophysiology studies that examine the temporal dynamics of the selection process have been able to shed more light on these issues by exploiting temporally precise markers that are thought to index the depth of information processing.

The 'When' of Selection via Signal Enhancement: the Temporal Dynamics of Selective Attention

As noted in the last section, the evidence is now compelling that attention can modulate neural activity very early in the visual processing stream (e.g. in LGN), consistent with early selection accounts. However, this is a necessary but not sufficient condition to support the early filtering of sensory information, as early selection also requires that the modulations occur early in *time*, before extensive processing has taken place at later stages. While still a matter of debate, studies that use human subjects and event-related potentials (ERPs) provide some of the most diagnostic information regarding the timing of attention effects.

The ERPs elicited by visual stimuli are generally decomposed into several components, the C1 (starting about 50–90 ms post-stimulus), the P1 (80–130 ms), and the N1 (140–200 ms). In a typical experimental paradigm, subjects are told to attend to a specific location in the visual field and a stimulus is either flashed at the attended location or at another, unattended, location. The classic finding is that the P1 and N1 components evoked by an attended stimulus are larger than the same components evoked by an unattended stimulus (see Mangun, Hillyard, and Luck 1993). Moreover, recent studies suggest that the earliest ERP component—the C1—can also be modulated by attentional factors, despite its onset as early as 50 ms after the presentation of a stimulus. Similarly early modulations have been shown in studies examining spatial attention (Kelly, Gomez-Ramirez, and Foxe 2008; Slotnick, Hopfinger, Klein, and Sutter 2002; Zhang, Zhaoping, Zhou, and Fang 2012—although see Martinez et al. 1999; Noesselt et al. 2002), auditory–visual coupling (Van der Burg, Talsma, Olivers, Hickey, and Theeuwes 2011), and in studies that examined the exogenous (or stimulus-driven) capture of attention to one of two superimposed visual surfaces (Khoe, Mitchell, Reynolds, and Hillyard 2005). Moreover, the C1 can be reasonably localized to V1 because the polarity of the response reverses when stimuli are presented in the upper and lower visual fields, consistent with the known anatomical layout and retinotopy of V1. Thus, the early onset of attention-related increases in response amplitude has led many researchers to conclude that attention modulates the afferent volley of sensory responses as they ascend the cortical hierarchy (Hillyard and Anllo-Vento 1998; Hillyard, Vogel, and Luck 1998). This evidence provides solid support for early selection, because strong forms of late selection cannot accommodate the differential processing of attended stimulus features during the initial feedforward sweep of sensory activity.

Taken together, the observation of enhanced early ERP responses suggests that attention mimics the effect of a physical increase in the salience of the sensory input (Hillyard and Anllo-Vento 1998; Hillyard et al. 1998). Importantly, early gain signals have also been associated with attention to basic features such as colour (Zhang and Luck 2009), which is consistent with Broadbent's original notion that early selection operates on basic stimulus features, not just on spatial locations. Importantly, these early amplitude modulations of ERP waveforms clearly violate assumptions made by pure late selection theories of attention that posit equivalent sensory analysis of all items present in the visual (or auditory) scene up to a relatively advanced levels of analysis. In addition, these early modulations are consistent with a recent line of work by Carrasco and co-workers, who have shown that attention actually increases the perceived salience of basic feature properties so that contrast becomes brighter, motion more salient, and so on (Carrasco 2009; Carrasco, Ling, and Read 2004; Carrasco and McElree 2001; Fuller, Park, and Carrasco 2009; Liu, Abrams, and Carrasco 2009; Liu, Fuller, and Carrasco 2006; see chapter by Carrasco; see also: Anton-Erxleben, Abrams, and Carrasco 2011; Carrasco, Fuller, and Ling 2008; Prinzmetal, Long, and Leonhardt 2008; Schneider 2006, 2011; Schneider and Komlos 2008). Collectively, these results support the intuitive notion that modulating the gain of responses in early visual areas should have a corresponding impact on the perceptual experience of attended features, contributing not only to increases in behavioural performance, but also to qualitative shifts in phenomenal experience.

Even though these results provide strong support for the feasibility of early selection accounts, there are several caveats. First, in order to directly compare responses evoked by attended and unattended stimuli, one must assume that the stimuli are processed in an identical manner except for the presence/absence of attentional gain. Presumably, if fundamentally different neural mechanisms were responsible for the observed differences in the response to attended and unattended stimuli, then the voltage distribution across the scalp would differ across these conditions. However, the voltage distribution across the scalp is nearly identical for attended and unattended stimuli (e.g. Mangun et al. 1993), suggesting that attention-related differences in ERP amplitude are indeed driven by changes in sensory gain and not by changes in the nature of the processing that is being carried out. Second, early sensory gain models predict that any amplitude and/or phase shifts due to attention should mirror those produced by actual changes in the physical attributes of the stimulus. In line with the predictions of early selection models, increasing stimulus brightness produces an increase in P1 and N1 amplitude that mirrors increases due to attention (particularly in the case of the P1; Johannes, Munte, Heinze, and Mangun 1995; Wijers, Lange, Mulder, and Mulder 1997).

Another key piece of evidence on the timing of attentional modulation comes from monkey single cell recording studies, which have demonstrated two patterns of neural activity that are consistent with early selection: an increase in spontaneous activity due to allocation of spatial attention and before the onset of a stimulus, and the rapid onset of a modulatory attention effect on visually evoked activity, presumably before recurrent feedback can influence the magnitude of spiking. Luck et al. (1997) were able to show both of these effects in single neurons recorded from the same animals (see also Kastner, Pinsk, De Weerd, Desimone, and Ungerleider 1999). In their paradigm, a monkey was trained to covertly attend to one of two spatial locations and to detect a pre-specified target at that location. In one condition, a single stimulus was presented within the RF of a V4 neuron and another stimulus was presented in the mirror symmetrical position across the vertical meridian (outside of the neuron's RF). When attention was directed inside the neuron's RF before the stimulus display was presented, there was an increase in the spiking rate of the neuron relative to when attention was directed to the other location outside of the RF. This divergence in activity, or *baseline shift*, was found during the 500 ms epochs before the onset of the stimulus display (see also Kastner et al. 1999; Ress, Backus, and Heeger 2000; Serences, Yantis, Culberson, and Awh 2004). Therefore, the observed modulation in spiking rate was not due to exogenous sensory stimulation. A second condition in the paradigm of Luck et al. (1997) evaluated the effects of attention on the post-stimulus activity of neurons in V4. To achieve maximum post-stimulus attention effects, both the target and the distractor were presented within the RF of a single V4 neuron (as in Moran and Desimone 1985). The monkey attended to one of the two possible stimulus locations, and spiking activity to the onset of a stimulus was recorded as a function of the locus of attention. Post-stimulus histograms revealed a clear separation of activity approximately 60 ms after stimulus onset such that attended stimuli evoked a larger response compared to unattended stimuli (see also Buffalo, Fries, Landman, Liang, and Desimone 2010). Similar results were also observed for single neurons in area V2, and are consistent with the similarly early modulation of the C1 ERP component measured from human subjects. Interestingly, however, no baseline shifts were observed in V1, perhaps because the RFs were too small to accommodate both attended and unattended stimuli.

Functional brain imaging studies in humans have extended these results by demonstrating increases in baseline activity not only at attended locations, but also in neural populations that respond preferentially to basic stimulus features such as motion (Chawla, Rees, and Friston 1999; Serences and Boynton 2007) and to more complex stimuli such as shapes (Stokes, Thompson, Nobre, and Duncan 2009) and objects (Peelen, Fei-Fei, and Kastner 2009). In these studies, baseline increases have been found at all stages of visual processing including the visual thalamus and striate cortex, which is somewhat inconsistent with reports from monkey physiology (which reported no baseline shifts in V1). One way to reconcile the apparent discrepancies between fMRI and physiology data is to consider the neural basis of the BOLD signal measured with fMRI. BOLD responses have been shown to more strongly correlate with local field potentials (LFPs) than with the action potentials that are typically recorded in physiology studies (Logothetis, Pauls, Augath, Trinath, and Oeltermann 2001; Logothetis and Wandell 2004). Critically, LFPs reflect multiple types of neuro-modulation including subthreshold changes in membrane potential, synaptic events, oscillatory activity, and after-potentials that follow action potentials. In addition, hemodynamic signals likely reflect the combined influence of small modulatory effects across large populations of neurons that may not be reliable at the level of single neuron recordings. Thus, BOLD fMRI might be more sensitive with respect to detecting the presence of an attentional modulation, at the expense of precise information about the origin of the modulatory signal.

The baseline shift and the early attentional modulation of stimulus-evoked responses represent complementary aspects of an early selection mechanism in monkey visual cortex. First, the baseline shift is consistent with a mechanism that increases the gain of the afferent volley of neural activity that is evoked by the presentation of a stimulus (Sylvester, Shulman, Jack, and Corbetta 2009). Thus, cells whose RFs correspond to an attended region of space already have a competitive advantage over cells whose RFs correspond to unattended regions of space, and they will tend to dominate the winner-take-all circuits posited by models such as biased competition (Desimone and Duncan 1995; Reynolds and Desimone 1999). Moreover, heightened spiking rates can be observed shortly after the presentation of an attended target, further amplifying the competitive advantage of relevant over irrelevant stimuli (e.g. Fig. 4.3a in Luck et al. 1997). Together, these findings are consistent with Broadbent's original conception that attention can use rudimentary qualities of the impinging sensory input such as location to influence attentional selection.

Taken at face value, the ERP, single cell, and fMRI studies reviewed in this section provide clear evidence for early signal gain in visual processing. Of course, these findings depend on linking propositions between observed neural activity and the ultimate behaviour of the organism that are often vague (Teller 1984). However, there is at least some evidence to support a correlation between enhanced sensory ERP components and decreased RTs in spatial cueing paradigms (e.g. Mangun et al. 1993; Zhang et al. 2012). While correlations cannot establish causal relationships, they substantially advance the argument that early modulation of neural activity directly contributes to behaviour. Moreover, caution must be exercised when interpreting the timing of the modulation effects. While it is widely accepted that the P1 and early modulations such as those documented by Luck et al. (1997) reflect feedforward processing, areas of parietal cortex (LIP) and frontal cortex can exert stimulus-driven responses with a latency on the order of 40–50 ms, raising the possibility that attentional feedback to early visual cortex could occur on an extremely short time scale (Bar et al. 2006; Bisley, Krishna, and Goldberg 2004). Nevertheless, it now seems clear that attentional modulation can occur well before the onset of neural markers that indicate more advanced neural processing, such as semantic analysis and the updating of information in working memory, processes that are typically thought to occur 300–400 ms post-stimulus (Kutas and Federmeier 2011; Kutas, Neville, and Holcomb 1987; Polich 2007).

Finally, it is important to point out that even though these studies are consistent with early selection accounts, they do not establish that early selection is the *only* mechanism of selective attention. Indeed, other ERP and single cell studies indicate that late selection can influence information processing as well. For example, early ERP components such as the P1 and N1 are similar for seen and unseen items in an attentional blink paradigm; however, large attenuations in later ERP components thought to index the updating of working memory are observed in the same context (Vogel, Luck, and Shapiro 1998). Thus, the emerging consensus from the cognitive neuroscience literature clarifies and solidifies earlier notions that both early and late selection can occur depending on task demands and are not mutually exclusive (Lavie and Tsal 1994; Vogel, Woodman, and Luck 2005; Yantis and Johnston 1990). However, the physiological evidence makes an especially compelling case indicating that pure inceptions of late selection theories can probably be entirely discarded.

WHERE AND WHEN OF NOISE SUPPRESSION VIA EXTERNAL DISTRACTOR EXCLUSION

Consider a classical visual search task, where subjects are presented with a display composed of green and red letters, e.g. T's and L's. The subject's task is to identify a target item composed of a conjunction of the two features present in the display, i.e. colour and shape (e.g. a red T) among the distractors (Treisman and Gelade 1980; see chapter by Wolfe). This type of task is designed to resemble real-world search situations, in which the visual system is constantly faced with an enormous amount of clutter from which behaviourally relevant information needs to be selected. Visual search entails at least two conceptually different processes: (i) the selection of the task-relevant stimulus and (ii) the filtering of multiple distractor stimuli that form the vast majority of information in the display. Thus far, we have focused almost exclusively on the anatomical and temporal properties of the target selection process. However, understanding the process of suppressing distractors is at least—if not more—important. Ultimately, these two processes are intimately linked, and there is now strong evidence that the neural mechanisms that support target selection and distractor exclusion interact to a high degree in visual cortex (e.g. Pinsk, Doniger, and Kastner 2004; Seidl, Peelen, and Kastner 2012). However, for reasons of clarity we will discuss the neural basis of distractor exclusion separately and without consideration of these interactions as they are not well understood at present.

The neural fate of unattended (distractor) information presents a second important question that arises from the early vs. late debate that we discussed above. Early selection accounts hold that unattended information should be mainly represented at early stages of processing, where the visual information is represented at a featural level, but not at later stages, where features are combined in complex ways to form objects and other semantically meaningful stimuli. In contrast, a late selection account would assume a neural representation at both early and advanced visual processing stages. Unfortunately, much less is known about the neural basis of distractor exclusion compared to the neural basis of target selection. This asymmetry is mainly due to the fact that most studies evaluate the effects of attention on a visual stimulus relative to a condition when the same stimulus is unattended. In this type of scenario, the effects of selective attention on unattended stimuli cannot be determined. Thus, some of the evidence discussed below will be indirect, but still important and telling about the mechanisms of distractor exclusion.

One example of such indirect evidence is the seminal work by Desimone and colleagues that led to the development of the biased competition model (Desimone and Duncan 1995; Kastner, De Weerd, Desimone, and Ungerleider 1998; Moran and Desimone 1985; Reynolds, Chelazzi, and Desimone 1999). As discussed above, the basic findings were two-fold. First, multiple stimuli appearing in a neuron's RF will interact in a mutually suppressive way suggesting that they are not processed independently. Instead, multiple stimuli engage in a competitive process that occurs automatically at the level of the RF. Second, when attention is allocated to one of two competing stimuli, the neural response to the attended stimulus is nearly as large as when the stimulus is presented in isolation (i.e. without the competing distractor). Thus, attention appears to restore the response of the attended stimulus and operates by counteracting the competing (suppressive) influence of the second stimulus. This finding suggests that attention not only boosts the response evoked by attended stimuli, but also acts to attenuate distractor interference by resolving competitive interactions between stimuli. Importantly, this mechanism of distractor exclusion has been shown to be tied to the RF and its immediate surround and scales with increasing RF size across the visual processing hierarchy (Kastner et al. 2001; Sundberg, Mitchell, and Reynolds 2009). However, as mentioned above, these studies did not directly measure the effects of attention on distractor stimuli, since only responses evoked by attended stimuli were considered. Thus, the conclusions drawn about the neural fate of distractor stimuli were based solely on changes in target-evoked responses as a function of different target–distractor configurations.

Recent studies using neuroimaging methods in human subjects have provided more direct evidence regarding the fate of unattended distractor stimuli. Some of the first evidence was obtained from studies in which the perceptual or cognitive load associated with a target stimulus was systematically and parametrically varied while responses evoked by the target and by distractors were separately assessed. In one study, the subject's attentional resources were parametrically modulated by manipulating the difficulty of a task at fixation while neural responses associated with an irrelevant and unattended peripheral motion stimulus were probed (Rees, Frith, and Lavie 1997) (see also chapter by Lavie). The response evoked by the unattended stimulus was significantly attenuated in motion-selective area MT when the task at fixation was difficult (high perceptual load) compared to when the task at fixation was easy (low perceptual load). O'Connor et al. (2002) extended these results by showing that responses evoked by an unattended visual stimulus also decreased in the thalamus, primary visual cortex, and extrastriate cortex depending on the load of a concurrent attentional task (see also Pinsk, et al. 2004; Schwartz et al. 2005). Interestingly, the load-dependent attenuation of distractor-related activity was strongest in the thalamus and extrastriate cortex and weaker in primary visual cortex, mirroring the pattern of effects observed for target-related attentional modulation (see section above, *The 'where' of selection via signal enhancement*). Thus, in addition to a gain control mechanism that modulates target-related neural signals throughout the visual processing hierarchy, active distractor suppression also appears to operate at multiple levels including the earliest stages of visual processing.

Corroborating evidence supporting an anatomically early locus of distractor suppression has also been found in studies of feature-based attention. One of the hallmarks of feature-based selection is that it operates by increasing neural responses to the selected feature (e.g. a particular direction of motion) regardless of spatial location, thus operating in a global manner across the visual field (Martinez-Trujillo and Treue 2004; Saenz, Buracas, and Boynton 2002; Serences and Boynton 2007; Treue and Martinez Trujillo 1999; see chapter by Scolari). In line with studies that examine the consequences of spatial selection on distractor processing, the response of neurons that are tuned to an attended feature (e.g. a direction of motion) are enhanced whereas the response of neurons tuned far from the attended feature are suppressed (Cohen and Maunsell 2011; Martinez-Trujillo and Treue 2004; Scolari, Byers, and Serences 2012; Serences, Saproo, Scolari, Ho, and Muftuler 2009). This joint enhancement and suppression occurs for all neurons that are sensitive to attended feature dimension, irrespective of whether the attended stimulus directly falls within their spatial receptive field. These results thus suggest that the exclusion of distractor information can happen at relatively early stages of sensory processing and that distractor suppression is not strictly tied to acts of selection based on spatial location.

In general, the spatial and feature-based suppression of distractor-related activity is more compatible with early selection accounts as it occurs at early stages of the visual hierarchy (although the timing of these effects is largely an open question). However, these studies all dealt with basic visual features as opposed to more complex objects and experimental settings that more closely resemble real-world search scenarios. Interestingly, and in line with studies that use basic visual features, most studies that examine the influence of attention on the processing of more complex objects reveal little representation of unattended distractor categories. In one classic study, a house and a face stimulus were presented simultaneously in separate hemifields and subjects were cued to attend either to the location of the face or to the location of the house (Serences, Schwarzbach, Courtney, Golay, and Yantis 2004; Wojciulik, Kanwisher, and Driver 1998). When subjects attended to the face stimuli, face-selective regions of ventral visual cortex were more responsive than house-selective regions of ventral visual cortex. The opposite was true when subjects attended to houses. More recent studies have extended these findings to more naturalistic and thus complex scenarios by showing that neural activity in object-selective cortex is entirely dominated by task-related demands when subjects extract categorical information from natural scenes. In one study, subjects attended to briefly presented street scenes and detected the presence of people or cars in the scenes. In object-selective ventral visual cortex, only task-relevant information was processed to the categorical level even when the relevant information was not spatially attended. In contrast, task-irrelevant information was not processed to the categorical level even when it was spatially attended (Peelen et al. 2009). Subsequent studies demonstrated that task-irrelevant objects can sometimes be processed up to the categorical level; however, their representation is weaker than that of task-relevant objects (Seidl

et al. 2012). In addition, distractors that were task-relevant in an immediately preceding trial that become task-irrelevant in the present trial are also actively suppressed
(Fig. 4.2). Together, these and other related findings strongly suggest that distractor
information is largely filtered out at the level of object-selective cortex, thereby further
supporting early selection accounts of attentional modulation.

    While the pattern of results regarding the fate of distractors is largely consistent across
single-unit and neuroimaging studies, results from patient literature are more mixed
with respect to early and late selection accounts. For example, the BOLD response
evoked by faces and by common objects in patients suffering from visuo-spatial hemineglect was similar when the stimuli were presented to the neglected hemifield and
when the stimuli were presented to the intact hemifield (Rees et al. 2000; Vuilleumier
et al. 2001). The similarity in magnitude of the response suggests that even unattended

FIGURE 4.2 Object category-based selection from natural scenes. In the scene
(a), people are the category that is relevant to ongoing behaviour (i.e. target
category), and cars are the object category that was previously relevant but
is presently not relevant (i.e. distractor
category), whereas all other object categories present in the scene are never
task-relevant (i.e. neutral category, such
as trees or houses). Visual search in natural scenes is accomplished through a
combination of enhancing task-relevant
information and suppressing a previous
attentional set relative to processing of
neutral categories. The resulting representation of object categories in object-
selective cortex is schematically shown
in the modified scene (b) relative to the
original scene (a). (A) Adapted from
Seidl, K. N., Peelen, M. V., and Kastner,
S., Neural evidence for distractor suppression during visual search in real-
world scenes, *Journal of Neuroscience*,
32, pp. 11812–11819 © 2012, The Society
for Neuroscience.

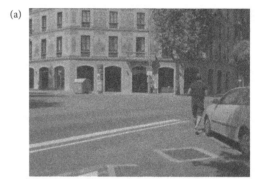

(a)

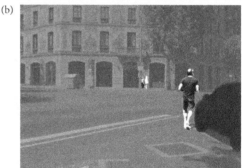

(b)

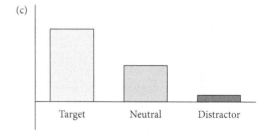

(c)

Target   Neutral   Distractor

stimuli undergo processing to a relatively advanced stage of processing, perhaps even to the level of category-specific object representations. However, in light of previous findings suggesting that object-based selection operates in a spatially global manner (similar to feature-based attention, e.g. Peelen et al. 2009), it is possible that objects presented in the intact hemifield heavily influenced the representation in the lesioned hemisphere. On this account, object identity was never represented in the lesioned hemisphere. Instead, activation observed in the lesioned hemisphere may have been related to the global processing of the attended target. Other lesion work suggests that neglected— and thus unattended—stimuli undergo significant processing, at least to the point at which they can influence behaviour (Marshall and Halligan 1988). For instance, neglect patients show behavioural interference effects tied to the presentation of incompatible distractors in their neglected hemifield, even though they report little awareness of the competing distractors (Shomstein, Kimchi, Hammer, and Behrmann 2010). Thus, it appears that at least some information about stimuli from the neglected hemifield can be processed; however, the depth of processing is not entirely clear, nor is the influence of parametric manipulations of task difficulty. Future studies will be required to determine the extent to which these late selection effects are still observed when sufficient attentional resources are allocated to the non-neglected side of space.

While relatively little is known about the fate of unattended distractor stimuli, even less is known about the temporal dynamics of distractor exclusion (or the 'when' of distractor exclusion). One possibility is that the processing of target-related information is simply sped up relative to the processing of distractor information. Such changes in the efficiency of processing may be reflected in the latency at which the target and distractor-evoked responses are registered in the visual system. To evaluate this possibility, several single-unit recording studies examined the response latency associated with identical stimuli when they were attended or unattended. With the exception of one study, the results suggest that attention does not significantly alter the response latency of single neurons (Bisley et al. 2004; Cook and Maunsell 2004; Lee, Williford, and Maunsell 2007; Reynolds, Pasternak, and Desimone 2000). In the one study that did find a positive effect, the latency shift was found both at the level of single neurons and at the level of local populations (Sundberg, Mitchell, Gawne, and Reynolds 2012), and was on the order of 1–2 msec. Despite this relatively modest shift, the decreased response latency may still have a significant impact on the computations performed by a network or neurons given that much of the information in a neural code likely depends on spike timing. Furthermore, small differences measured at the single cell or local population level can easily translate into more robust differences when averaged across larger neuronal populations, such as those observed using scalp EEG or electrocorticography (ECoG). Interestingly, a recent ERP study demonstrated that the enhancement of target-related activity measured over visual cortex started 220 msec after the onset of an attentional cue, whereas the suppression of distractor-evoked responses lagged by an additional 130 msec (Andersen and Muller 2010). Thus, while the temporal dynamics of distractor suppression are still not well understood, both of these studies highlight the importance of addressing the interaction between the facilitatory and suppressive effects of selective attention.

WHERE AND WHEN OF ATTENTION-RELATED INTERNAL NOISE REDUCTION

Signal enhancement can be used to efficiently encode relevant stimuli and to attenuate the influence of external distractors on information processing. In addition, recent research—primarily using single-unit physiology—also demonstrates that selective attention can reduce the intrinsic internal noise observed in spiking activity as quantified by a reduction in the ratio of the mean response to the variance of the response (termed the *Fano Factor*; Mitchell, Sundberg, and Reynolds 2007). Such internal noise reduction likely plays a complementary role to signal enhancement, as the signal-to-noise ratio (SNR) of neurons increases with gain and also with a reduction in noise (Fig. 4.3). This may be particularly important in light of neurobiologically observed

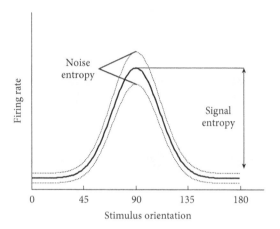

FIGURE 4.3 The amount of information that a sensory neuron encodes about sensory features depends on both response gain and response variance. Depicted here is a cartoon schematic of the tuning function of a simple cell in primary visual cortex that responds maximally to a 90° oriented bar of light. Mutual Information (or MI; Shannon 1949) is a useful metric for quantifying how much information about a sensory stimulus can be gained by measuring the response of this neuron to a visual stimulus. MI is, intuitively speaking, the difference between the signal entropy—or the amount of variance in the neural response that is systematically related to changes in the stimulus—and the noise entropy—or the amount of variance in the neural response that is unrelated to changes in the stimulus (i.e. 'noise'). Increasing the gain of sensory neurons will increase the signal entropy by increasing the range over which responses vary as a function of the stimulus. All else being equal, this will increase the MI between neural responses and the stimulus features being encoded. Alternatively, decreasing the variability of a neuron (i.e. decreasing the Fano Factor) will reduce the amount of variability in neural responses that is unrelated to changes in the stimulus. All else being equal, this will also increase the MI between neural responses and the stimulus features being encoded.

neuronal noise, which often far exceeds the typical assumption of a Poisson distribution (where the variance is equivalent to the mean; Anderson, Mitchell, and Reynolds 2011). In extreme cases where the Poisson expectation is far exceeded, increasing gain will have little effect on the information conveyed by a single unit about an attended stimulus feature because the noise will increase at a fast enough rate to offset any gain-related improvements in SNR. In these situations, reducing the variability of single unit responses may be a critical component to ensuring that relevant sensory stimuli get processed more efficiently than irrelevant distractors.

Even though attention can attenuate trial-by-trial variability in single-unit responses, a considerable amount of noise remains in the system. Thus, some pooling or averaging of responses is required to form stable representations of relevant sensory features. However, averaging cannot remove noise that is correlated between similarly tuned neurons, thus placing a limit on the precision of sensory representations that are based on population codes (Abbott and Dayan 1999; Averbeck, Latham, and Pouget 2006; Averbeck and Lee 2006; Bair, Zohary, and Newsome 2001; Johnson 1980; Kohn and Smith 2005; Mitchell et al. 2007; Shadlen, Britten, Newsome, and Movshon 1996; Shadlen and Newsome 1994). Given the potential limits imposed by correlated noise, several recent studies have focused on uncovering the role of attention in decreasing shared noise between similarly tuned neurons to improve the efficacy of pooling sensory signals. For example, Mitchell and co-workers (Mitchell, Sundberg, and Reynolds 2009) demonstrated that spatial attention can attenuate correlated noise, particularly low-frequency noise, in mid-level area V4. Assuming a simple population read-out rule that is based on averaging responses across all neurons tuned to the attended stimulus, the observed decorrelations can lead to an estimated 40% improvement in the SNR of the neuronal population, as compared to an estimated 10% improvement in SNR due solely to increases in gain (Mitchell et al. 2009). While the exact benefit in terms of SNR needs further exploration under different task conditions and assumptions about how population codes are used to information perceptual decisions, this asymmetry highlights the powerful role that changes in variability and covariance can play in influencing the quality of sensory representations. Further underscoring the importance of noise correlations, Cohen and Maunsell (Cohen and Maunsell 2009, 2010, 2011) demonstrated decorrelations related to both space- and feature-based attention in areas V4 and MT. Importantly, the degree of decorrelation predicted trial-by-trial fluctuations in behavioural performance.

While this field of inquiry is nascent, and attention-mediated changes in variability and covariance have only been documented in a few mid-level structures, even less is known about the time course of these modulations. In one relevant experiment, Mitchell et al. (2007, 2009) used a stimulus that moved into the receptive field of a V4 neuron for 1000 ms before leaving the receptive field. Thus, the authors could examine changes in the Fano Factor and in covariance across counting windows that varied in size from approximately 10 msec to 400 msec. They observed that both the attention-related reduction in the Fano Factor and the attention-related reduction in covariance onset quite rapidly. In fact, spatial attention seemed to anticipate the trajectory of the moving stimulus, and significant decreases in internal noise were already evident at the point that the stimulus entered a neuron's RF. This onset latency is early enough in time to influence decision-making in speeded perceptual tasks, consistent with the documented relationship between covariability and accuracy on a cueing task (Cohen and Maunsell 2009, 2011). In addition, the magnitude of attention-related reductions in variance and covariance increased as the size of the counting window increased, suggesting that attention had the largest modulatory impact on low-frequency noise.

Collectively, these studies thus suggest that attention improves the efficiency of information processing in large part via changes in the variance and covariance of neurons in mid-level visual areas. Moreover, the temporally early onset of these effects suggests that changes in the noise characteristics of sensory neurons might operate relatively early in information processing during the extraction of basic low-level features. However, given that only a handful of studies have been done in this area there is still much to learn about the anatomical extent of these noise modulations as well as their onset time and the temporal window over which they operate.

LATE SELECTION VIA THE EFFICIENT READ-OUT OF SENSORY SIGNALS

Although most of the discussion surrounding early versus late selection has centred on the anatomical locus, timing, and nature of sensory gain modulations, a parallel line of reasoning proposes that many of the effects attributed to selective attention can be explained without invoking either early or late modulations in early sensory regions. Instead, these *selective read-out* models posit that decision mechanisms can pool responses selectively from neurons that are optimally tuned to discriminate the attended stimulus, and that this selective pooling is sufficient to improve information processing even in the complete absence of sensory gain modulations (Dosher, Liu, Blair, and Lu 2004; Eckstein, Peterson, Pham, and Droll 2009; Eckstein, Thomas, Palmer, and Shimozaki 2000; Palmer, Verghese, and Pavel 2000; Shaw 1984). While it is clear that sensory gain modulations do occur as the result of attention, these models nevertheless make a critical, and often overlooked, point about the importance of maximizing the efficiency of how populations of sensory neurons are read out during decision-making (Fig. 4.4).

The power of selective read-out is perhaps most evident when considering how attention can greatly attenuate—or sometimes even eliminate—the influence of irrelevant distracting items that compete with relevant stimuli (Palmer and Moore 2009; Yigit-Elliott, Palmer, and Moore 2011). Since these models posit that decision mechanisms only read out responses from sensory neurons that are optimally tuned to make the relevant discrimination, the influence of irrelevant distracting items is automatically attenuated as responses associated with these stimuli have no impact whatsoever on the decision process. In this manner, selective read-out mechanisms can efficiently shunt

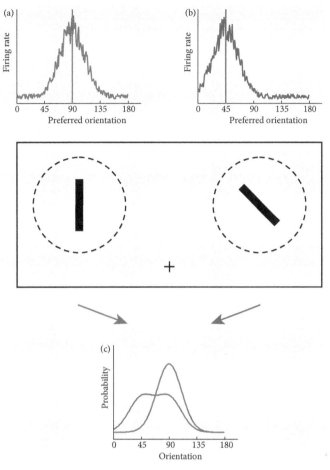

FIGURE 4.4 Selectively basing perceptual decisions on neural populations that are most sensitive to the relevant stimulus can improve the speed and accuracy of behavioural responses. (bottom panel) Schematic of a stimulus display presented briefly to a subject. The subject's task is to report, as quickly and accurately as possible, whether or not a vertical line is present in the display. (a) The response profile evoked by the vertical 90° stimulus across a population of sensory neurons that are maximally responsive (i.e. 'tuned to') different orientations and that have a spatial receptive field in the left hemifield. (b) The response profile evoked by a 45° stimulus across a different population of sensory neurons that have a spatial receptive field in the right hemifield. (c—Magenta line) If the subject has no advance knowledge about where the vertical line might appear, then they might reasonably pool responses across both neural populations before assessing the likelihood that a vertical line was present. This will lead to a relatively blurred and imprecise estimate of the stimulus features that gave rise to the sensory responses profiles show in panels a and b. (c—Red line) In contrast, if the subject knows in advance that the vertical line, if present, will appear in the left hemifield, then they need only base their likelihood estimate on the output of the neurons that have a spatial receptive field in the left hemifield (the neural response profile depicted in panel (a)). A comparison of the magenta and red lines suggests that inferences in this case will be more precise because irrelevant information provided by the neurons shown in panel b is not allowed to influence decision-making. Thus, selectively basing decisions on the most sensitive neurons can improve the efficiency of information processing, even in the absence of any direct modulation of sensory responses (e.g. gain or variance modulation).

interference from sensory neurons that encode irrelevant features, thereby increasing the discriminability of neural signals associated with attended stimuli.

While the selective read-out framework is appealing because complex modulations of sensory responses are not required, most of the work in this field is based on pure theory and mathematical models. Thus, even though selective read-out models can account for a variety of observed attentional modulations without recourse to sensory gain, this usually amounts to a proof of concept as opposed to a proof of existence. However, one recent neuroimaging study provides direct evidence that selective read-out plays an important role in implementing efficient information processing. Pestilli and co-workers (Pestilli, Carrasco, Heeger, and Gardner 2011) had observers search for a target embedded in a set of distractors, and demonstrated that sensory gain alone was not sufficient to account for the observed improvement in behaviour with attention. Instead, the data suggest that decision mechanisms over-weighted sensory responses associated with the attended stimulus and under-weighted responses associated with unattended distractors. This biased read-out process thereby ensured that signals associated with the attended stimulus dominated the decision process whereas signals associated with distractors had little or no impact. Again, the key element of this account is that selection occurs when sensory signals are integrated and evaluated by late-stage decision mechanisms, long after basic stimulus features are fully analyzed.

Related work has been done in the context of perceptual learning, where improvements in behaviour with practice are often thought to involve changes in the optimality of sensory read-out (Law and Gold 2008, 2009; Petrov, Dosher, and Lu 2005). For instance, Law and Gold (2008) found that firing rates in MT neurons did not significantly change after extensive training on a motion discrimination task. However, there were concurrent changes in the firing rates of the neurons in the lateral intraparietal area (LIP), an area implicated in accumulating sensory evidence during decision-making (Law and Gold 2008; see also Gold and Shadlen 2007). These data suggest that read-out from informative sensory neurons plays a more important role—at least in their task— than changes in sensory gain. In addition, even though the study ostensibly examined perceptual learning, Law and Gold (2008) used a motion stimulus that moved in a direction that was tailored to the tuning preference of the MT cells that they isolated each day. Thus, their task deviates from classic studies of learning that use a fixed stimulus feature, and may more closely resemble a more general perceptual task used in many attention studies (e.g. Treue and Maunsell 1996). The results are also consistent with some models of selective attention (Palmer and Moore 2009; Palmer et al. 2000), in which the most sensitive MT responses are pooled with linear weights and uninformative neurons are filtered out, leading to lower discrimination thresholds (Gold, Law, Connolly, and Bennur 2010; Law and Gold 2009).

While these empirical studies and the associated theories provide evidence for the importance of biased read-out as a mechanism of late selection, many important questions remain. For example, it seems likely that the importance of selective read-out depends critically on the number of competing items in the display. If only one item is present, then there is no need to selectively read out signals from only the attended item, so increasing the gain of sensory responses should be adequate to achieve what-ever signal-to-noise ratio is required to perform the required perceptual task. However, the benefits of sensory gain will likely decrease as the number of competing distractors increases, at least under the reasonable assumption that gain cannot be increased indefi-nitely. In this situation, shunting the influence of distractors by discounting their impact on a late decision mechanism is a computationally and metabolically efficient way to implement selection and to ensure that only the most relevant sensory stimuli influence working memory and subsequent behavioural responses. Selective read-out therefore provides an example of a robust late-selection mechanism that, especially when com-bined with early sensory gain, highlights the increasingly accepted idea that selection is achieved through a combination of mechanisms that simultaneously operate at nearly all stages of information processing.

Conclusions

Over the last several decades, data from neuroimaging and electrophysiology studies have shown that the neural mechanisms of selective attention operate at almost all stages of the visual system, as well as in many areas outside of classically defined visual cortex. When viewed together, these studies firmly establish that selection is neither early nor late. Instead, the locus of selection, both in terms of anatomy and time, flexibly depends on the demands placed on sensory processing machinery by the behavioural goals of an observer. Tasks that require highly focused attention on a specific location or feature will encourage early selection, whereas less demanding tasks that can be performed with a more diffuse attentional focus will accommodate late selection. Finally, a complete understanding of selective information processing is not all about understanding where and when the gain of sensory neurons is modulated: emerging evidence suggests equally important roles for modulating the variance and covariance of sensory neurons, and for selectively reading out information from only the most informative sensory neurons.

Moving ahead, the major challenge for future investigators is to meld the multiple mechanisms that support selective attention into a unified framework. For instance, it is well accepted that each stage of the visual processing hierarchy contributes differ-ently to visual perception. Therefore, it also seems likely that selective attention imple-ments different functions in different visual areas, and that each function is determined by the specific processing capabilities of a region. For example, at the thalamic level, attention may serve to control neural response gain. At early cortical processing stages, attention may influence feature and context selective responses, which may facilitate the basic mechanisms of scene segmentation and grouping (e.g. Ito and Gilbert 1999). At intermediate cortical processing stages where multiple stimuli often fall within a single RF, attention may mediate the filtering of unwanted information through internal and external noise reduction (i.e. distractor exclusion). These diverse modulatory processes appear to be controlled by a higher-order fronto-parietal network of brain areas that may coordinate large-scale attentional modulation via subcortical structures such as the superior colliculus (Zenon and Krauzlis 2012; see chapter by Krauzlis) and the pulvinar nucleus of the thalamus (Saalmann, Pinsk, Wang, Li, and Kastner 2012; see chapter by Saalmann). Ultimately, however, these brain systems cooperate to select relevant visual information for further processing in memory and other cognitive systems in order to guide actions. In this respect, attention can be described as a multi-level selection process that operates by integrating information across multiple anatomical and temporal scales to achieve behavioural goals in a flexible and adaptive manner.

ACKNOWLEDGEMENTS

Supported by NIH R01-MH092345 and a James S. McDonnell Foundation Scholar Award to J.T.S. and by NIH RO1-MH64043, RO1-EY017699, R21-EY0211078, and NSF BCS-1025149 to S.K.

REFERENCES

Abbott, L. F. and Dayan, P. (1999). The effect of correlated variability on the accuracy of a population code. *Neural Computation 11*: 91–101.

Andersen, S. K. and Muller, M. M. (2010). Behavioral performance follows the time course of neural facilitation and suppression during cued shifts of feature-selective attention. *Proceedings of the National Academy of Sciences USA 107*: 13878–13882.

Anderson, E. B., Mitchell, J. F., and Reynolds, J. H. (2011). Attentional modulation of firing rate varies with burstiness across putative pyramidal neurons in macaque visual area V4. *Journal of Neuroscience 31*: 10983–10992.

Anton-Erxleben, K., Abrams, J., and Carrasco, M. (2011). Equality judgments cannot distinguish between attention effects on appearance and criterion: A reply to Schneider (2011). *Journal of Vision 11*. doi: 10.1167/11.13.8.

Averbeck, B. B., Latham, P. E., and Pouget, A. (2006). Neural correlations, population coding and computation. *Nature Reviews Neuroscience 7*: 358–366.

Averbeck, B. B. and Lee, D. (2006). Effects of noise correlations on information encoding and decoding. *Journal of Neurophysiology 95*: 3633–3644.

Bair, W., Zohary, E., and Newsome, W. T. (2001). Correlated firing in macaque visual area MT: Time scales and relationship to behavior. *Journal of Neuroscience 21*: 1676–1697.

Bar, M., Kassam, K. S., Ghuman, A. S., Boshyan, J., Schmid, A. M., Dale, A. M., Hamalainen, M. S., Marinkovic, K., Schacter, D. L., Rosen, B. R., and Halgren, E. (2006). Top-down facilitation of visual recognition. *Proceedings of the National Academy of Sciences USA 103*: 449–454.

Bisley, J. W., Krishna, B. S., and Goldberg, M. E. (2004). A rapid and precise on-response in posterior parietal cortex. *Journal of Neuroscience 24*: 1833–1838.

Broadbent, D. (1958). *Perception and Communication*. London: Pergamon.

Buffalo, E. A., Fries, P., Landman, R., Liang, H., and Desimone, R. (2010). A backward progression of attentional effects in the ventral stream. *Proceedings of the National Academy of Sciences USA 107*: 361–365.

Carrasco, M. (2009). Cross-modal attention enhances perceived contrast. *Proceedings of the National Academy of Sciences USA 106*: 22039–22040.

Carrasco, M., Fuller, S., and Ling, S. (2008). Transient attention does increase perceived contrast of suprathreshold stimuli: A reply to Prinzmetal, Long, and Leonhardt (2008). *Perception & Psychophysics 70*: 1151–1164.

Carrasco, M., Ling, S., and Read, S. (2004). Attention alters appearance. *Nature Neuroscience 7*: 308–313.

Carrasco, M. and McElree, B. (2001). Covert attention accelerates the rate of visual information processing. *Proceedings of the National Academy of Sciences USA 98*: 5363–5367.

Chawla, D., Rees, G., and Friston, K. J. (1999). The physiological basis of attentional modulation in extrastriate visual areas. *Nature Neuroscience 2*: 671–676.

Cherry, E. C. (1953). Some experiments on the recognition of speech, with one and with two ears. *Journal of Acoustic Society of America 25*: 975–979.

Cohen, M. R. and Maunsell, J. H. (2009). Attention improves performance primarily by reducing interneuronal correlations. *Nature Neuroscience 12*: 1594–1600.

Cohen, M. R. and Maunsell, J. H. (2010). A neuronal population measure of attention predicts behavioral performance on individual trials. *The Journal of Neuroscience: The Official Journal of the Society for Neuroscience 30*: 15241–15253.

Cohen, M. R. and Maunsell, J. H. (2011). Using neuronal populations to study the mechanisms underlying spatial and feature attention. *Neuron 70*: 1192–1204.

Connor, C. E., Preddie, D. C., Gallant, J. L., and Van Essen, D. C. (1997). Spatial attention effects in macaque area V4. *Journal of Neuroscience 17*: 3201–3214.

Cook, E. P. and Maunsell, J. H. (2002a). Attentional modulation of behavioral performance and neuronal responses in middle temporal and ventral intraparietal areas of macaque monkey. *Journal of Neuroscience 22*: 1994–2004.

Cook, E. P. and Maunsell, J. H. (2002b). Dynamics of neuronal responses in macaque MT and VIP during motion detection. *Nature Neuroscience 5*: 985–994.

Cook, E. P. and Maunsell, J. H. (2004). Attentional modulation of motion integration of individual neurons in the middle temporal visual area. *Journal of Neuroscience 24*: 7964–7977.

Corteen, R. S. and Wook, B. (1972). Autonomic responses to shock-associated words in an unattended channel. *Journal of Experimental Psychology 94*: 308–313.

Desimone, R. and Duncan, J. (1995). Neural mechanisms of selective visual attention. *Annual Review of Neuroscience 18*: 193–222.

Deutsch, J. and Deutsch, D. (1963). Attention: Some theoretical considerations. *Psychological Review 70*: 80–90.

Dosher, B. A., Liu, S. H., Blair, N., and Lu, Z. L. (2004). The spatial window of the perceptual template and endogenous attention. *Vision Research 44*: 1257–1271.

Duncan, J. (1980). The locus of interference in the perception of simultaneous stimuli. *Psychological Review 87*: 272–300.

Eckstein, M. P., Peterson, M. F., Pham, B. T., and Droll, J. A. (2009). Statistical decision theory to relate neurons to behavior in the study of covert visual attention. *Vision Research 49*: 1097–1128.

Eckstein, M. P., Thomas, J. P., Palmer, J., and Shimozaki, S. S. (2000). A signal detection model predicts the effects of set size on visual search accuracy for feature, conjunction, triple conjunction, and disjunction displays. *Perception & Psychophysics 62*: 425–451.

Eriksen, B. A. and Eriksen, C. W. (1974). Effects of noise letters upon the identification of a target letter in a nonsearch task. *Perception & Psychophysics 16*: 143–149.

Francolini, C. M. and Egeth, H. E. (1980). On the nonautomaticity of 'automatic' activation: Evidence of selective seeing. *Perception & Psychophysics 27*: 331–342.

Fuller, S., Park, Y., and Carrasco, M. (2009). Cue contrast modulates the effects of exogenous attention on appearance. *Vision Research 49*: 1825–1837.

Gandhi, S. P., Heeger, D. J., and Boynton, G. M. (1999). Spatial attention affects brain activity in human primary visual cortex. *Proceedings of the National Academy of Sciences USA 96*: 3314–3319.

Gold, J. I., Law, C. T., Connolly, P., and Bennur, S. (2010). Relationships between the threshold and slope of psychometric and neurometric functions during perceptual learning: Implications for neuronal pooling. *Journal of Neurophysiology 103*: 140–154.

Gold, J. I. and Shadlen, M. N. (2007). The neural basis of decision making. *Annual Review of Neuroscience 30*: 535–574.

Gottlieb, J. P., Kusunoki, M., and Goldberg, M. E. (1998). The representation of visual salience in monkey parietal cortex. *Nature 391*: 481–484.

Haenny, P. E. and Schiller, P. H. (1988). State dependent activity in monkey visual cortex. I: Single cell activity in V1 and V4 on visual tasks. *Experimental Brain Research/Experimentelle Hirnforschung/Experimentation Cerebrale 69*: 225–244.

Hillyard, S. A. and Anllo-Vento, L. (1998). Event-related brain potentials in the study of visual selective attention. *Proceedings of the National Academy of Sciences USA 95*: 781–787.

Hillyard, S. A., Vogel, E. K., and Luck, S. J. (1998). Sensory gain control (amplification) as a mechanism of selective attention: Electrophysiological and neuroimaging evidence. *Philosophical Transactions of the Royal Society of London B: Biological Sciences 353*: 1257–1270.

Ito, M. and Gilbert, C. D. (1999). Attention modulates contextual influences in the primary visual cortex of alert monkeys. *Neuron 22*: 593–604.

Johannes, S., Munte, T. F., Heinze, H. J., and Mangun, G. R. (1995). Luminance and spatial attention effects on early visual processing. *Brain Research: Cognitive Brain Research 2*: 189–205.

Johnson, K. O. (1980). Sensory discrimination: Decision process. *Journal of Neurophysiology 43*: 1771–1792.

Kastner, S., De Weerd, P., Desimone, R., and Ungerleider, L. G. (1998). Mechanisms of directed attention in the human extrastriate cortex as revealed by functional MRI. *Science 282*: 108–111.

Kastner, S., De Weerd, P., Pinsk, M. A., Elizondo, M. I., Desimone, R., and Ungerleider, L. G. (2001). Modulation of sensory suppression: Implications for receptive field sizes in the human visual cortex. *Journal of Neurophysiology 86*: 1398–1411.

Kastner, S., Pinsk, M. A., De Weerd, P., Desimone, R., and Ungerleider, L. G. (1999). Increased activity in human visual cortex during directed attention in the absence of visual stimulation. *Neuron 22*: 751–761.

Kelly, S. P., Gomez-Ramirez, M., and Foxe, J. J. (2008). Spatial attention modulates initial afferent activity in human primary visual cortex. *Cerebral Cortex 18*: 2629–2636.

Khoe, W., Mitchell, J. F., Reynolds, J. H., and Hillyard, S. A. (2005). Exogenous attentional selection of transparent superimposed surfaces modulates early event-related potentials. *Vision Research 45*: 3004–3014.

Kohn, A. and Smith, M. A. (2005). Stimulus dependence of neuronal correlation in primary visual cortex of the macaque. *Journal of Neuroscience 25*: 3661–3673.

Kutas, M. and Federmeier, K. D. (2011). Thirty years and counting: Finding meaning in the N400 component of the event-related brain potential (ERP). *Annual Review of Psychology 62*: 621–647.

Kutas, M., Neville, H. J., and Holcomb, P. J. (1987). A preliminary comparison of the N400 response to semantic anomalies during reading, listening and signing. *Electroencephalography and Clinical Neurophysiology. Supplement 39*: 325–330.

Lavie, N. and Tsal, Y. (1994). Perceptual load as a major determinant of the locus of selection in visual attention. *Perception & Psychophysics* 56: 183–197.

Law, C. T. and Gold, J. I. (2008). Neural correlates of perceptual learning in a sensory-motor, but not a sensory, cortical area. *Nature Neuroscience* 11: 505–513.

Law, C. T. and Gold, J. I. (2009). Reinforcement learning can account for associative and perceptual learning on a visual-decision task. *Nature Neuroscience* 12: 655–663.

Lee, J., Williford, T., and Maunsell, J. H. (2007). Spatial attention and the latency of neuronal responses in macaque area V4. *Journal of Neuroscience* 27: 9632–9637.

Liu, T., Abrams, J., and Carrasco, M. (2009). Voluntary attention enhances contrast appearance. *Psychological Science: A Journal of the American Psychological Society/APS* 20: 354–362.

Liu, T., Fuller, S., and Carrasco, M. (2006). Attention alters the appearance of motion coherence. *Psychonomic Bulletin & Review* 13: 1091–1096.

Logothetis, N. K., Pauls, J., Augath, M., Trinath, T., and Oeltermann, A. (2001). Neurophysiological investigation of the basis of the fMRI signal. *Nature* 412: 150–157.

Logothetis, N. K. and Wandell, B. A. (2004). Interpreting the BOLD signal. *Annual Review of Physiology* 66: 735–769.

Luck, S. J., Chelazzi, L., Hillyard, S. A., and Desimone, R. (1997). Neural mechanisms of spatial selective attention in areas V1, V2, and V4 of macaque visual cortex. *Journal of Neurophysiology* 77: 24–42.

McAdams, C. J. and Maunsell, J. H. (1999). Effects of attention on orientation-tuning functions of single neurons in macaque cortical area V4. *Journal of Neuroscience* 19: 431–441.

Mangun, G. R., Hillyard, S. A., and Luck, S. J. (1993). Electrocortical substrates of visual selective attention. In D. Meyer and S. Kornblum (eds.), *Attention and Performance* (vol. 14, pp. 219–243). Cambridge, Mass.: MIT Press.

Marshall, J. C. and Halligan, P. W. (1988). Blindsight and insight in visuo-spatial neglect. *Nature* 336: 766–767.

Martinez, A., Anllo-Vento, L., Sereno, M. I., Frank, L. R., Buxton, R. B., Dubowitz, D. J., Wong, E. C., Hinrichs, H., Heinze, H. J., and Hillyard, S. A. (1999). Involvement of striate and extrastriate visual cortical areas in spatial attention. *Nature Neuroscience* 2: 364–369.

Martinez-Trujillo, J. C. and Treue, S. (2004). Feature-based attention increases the selectivity of population responses in primate visual cortex. *Current Biology: CB* 14: 744–751.

Mitchell, J. F., Sundberg, K. A., and Reynolds, J. H. (2007). Differential attention-dependent response modulation across cell classes in macaque visual area V4. *Neuron* 55: 131–141.

Mitchell, J. F., Sundberg, K. A., and Reynolds, J. H. (2009). Spatial attention decorrelates intrinsic activity fluctuations in macaque area V4. *Neuron* 63: 879–888.

Moran, J. and Desimone, R. (1985). Selective attention gates visual processing in the extrastriate cortex. *Science* 229: 782–784.

Moray, N. (1959). Attention in dichotic listening: Affective cues and the influence of instructions. *Quarterly Journal of Experimental Psychology* 11: 56–60.

Motter, B. C. (1993). Focal attention produces spatially selective processing in visual cortical areas V1, V2, and V4 in the presence of competing stimuli. *Journal of Neurophysiology* 70: 909–919.

Neisser, U. and Becklen, R. (1975). Selective looking: Attending to visually specified events. *Cognitive Psychology* 7: 480–494.

Noesselt, T., Hillyard, S. A., Woldorff, M. G., Schoenfeld, A., Hagner, T., Jancke, L., Tempelmann, C., Hinrichs, H., and Heinze, H. J. (2002). Delayed striate cortical activation during spatial attention. *Neuron* 35: 575–587.

O'Connor, D. H., Fukui, M. M., Pinsk, M. A., and Kastner, S. (2002). Attention modulates responses in the human lateral geniculate nucleus. *Nature Neuroscience* 5: 1203–1209.

Palmer, J. and Moore, C. M. (2009). Using a filtering task to measure the spatial extent of selective attention. *Vision Research* 49: 1045–1064.

Palmer, J., Verghese, P., and Pavel, M. (2000). The psychophysics of visual search. *Vision Research* 40: 1227–1268.

Pashler, H. (1994). Dual-task interference in simple tasks: Data and theory. *Psychological Bulletin* 116: 220–244.

Peelen, M. V., Fei-Fei, L., and Kastner, S. (2009). Neural mechanisms of rapid natural scene categorization in human visual cortex. *Nature* 460: 94–97.

Pestilli, F., Carrasco, M., Heeger, D. J., and Gardner, J. L. (2011). Attentional enhancement via selection and pooling of early sensory responses in human visual cortex. *Neuron* 72: 832–846.

Petrov, A. A., Dosher, B. A., and Lu, Z. L. (2005). The dynamics of perceptual learning: An incremental reweighting model. *Psychological Review* 112: 715–743.

Pinsk, M. A., Doniger, G. M., and Kastner, S. (2004). Push–pull mechanism of selective attention in human extrastriate cortex. *Journal of Neurophysiology* 92: 622–629.

Polich, J. (2007). Updating P300: An integrative theory of P3a and P3b. *Clinical Neurophysiology* 118: 2128–2148.

Pouget, A., Dayan, P., and Zemel, R. S. (2003). Inference and computation with population codes. *Annual Review of Neuroscience* 26: 381–410.

Prinzmetal, W., Long, V., and Leonhardt, J. (2008). Involuntary attention and brightness contrast. *Perception & Psychophysics* 70: 1139–1150.

Rees, G., Frith, C. D., and Lavie, N. (1997). Modulating irrelevant motion perception by varying attentional load in an unrelated task. *Science* 278: 1616–1619.

Rees, G., Wojciulik, E., Clarke, K., Husain, M., Frith, C., and Driver, J. (2000). Unconscious activation of visual cortex in the damaged right hemisphere of a parietal patient with extinction. *Brain* 123(Pt 8): 1624–1633.

Ress, D., Backus, B. T., and Heeger, D. J. (2000). Activity in primary visual cortex predicts performance in a visual detection task. *Nature Neuroscience* 3: 940–945.

Reynolds, J. H., Chelazzi, L., and Desimone, R. (1999). Competitive mechanisms subserve attention in macaque areas V2 and V4. *Journal of Neuroscience* 19: 1736–1753.

Reynolds, J. H. and Desimone, R. (1999). The role of neural mechanisms of attention in solving the binding problem. *Neuron* 24: 19–29, 111–125.

Reynolds, J. H., Pasternak, T., and Desimone, R. (2000). Attention increases sensitivity of V4 neurons. *Neuron* 26: 703–714.

Roelfsema, P. R., Lamme, V. A., and Spekreijse, H. (1998). Object-based attention in the primary visual cortex of the macaque monkey. *Nature* 395: 376–381.

Saalmann, Y. B., Pinsk, M. A., Wang, L., Li, X., and Kastner, S. (2012). The pulvinar regulates information transmission between cortical areas based on attention demands. *Science* 337: 753–756.

Saenz, M., Buracas, G. T., and Boynton, G. M. (2002). Global effects of feature-based attention in human visual cortex. *Nature Neuroscience* 5: 631–632.

Schneider, K. A. (2006). Does attention alter appearance? *Perception & Psychophysics* 68: 800–814.

Schneider, K. A. (2011). Attention alters decision criteria but not appearance: A reanalysis of Anton-Erxleben, Abrams, and Carrasco (2010). *Journal of Vision* 11: 7. doi: 10.1167/11.13.7.

Schneider, K. A. and Komlos, M. (2008). Attention biases decisions but does not alter appearance. *Journal of Vision* 8: 3.1–10.

Schwartz, S., Vuilleumier, P., Hutton, C., Maravita, A., Dolan, R. J., and Driver, J. (2005). Attentional load and sensory competition in human vision: Modulation of fMRI responses by load at fixation during task-irrelevant stimulation in the peripheral visual field. *Cerebral Cortex 15*: 770–786.

Scolari, M., Byers, A., and Serences, J. T. (2012). Optimal deployment of attentional gain during fine discriminations. *Journal of Neuroscience 32*: 7723–7733.

Seidl, K. N., Peelen, M. V., and Kastner, S. (2012). Neural evidence for distractor suppression during visual search in real-world scenes. *Journal of Neuroscience 32*: 11812–11819.

Serences, J. T. and Boynton, G. M. (2007). Feature-based attentional modulations in the absence of direct visual stimulation. *Neuron 55*: 301–312.

Serences, J. T. and Saproo, S. (2012). Computational advances towards linking BOLD and behavior. *Neuropsychologia 50*: 435–446.

Serences, J. T., Saproo, S., Scolari, M., Ho, T., and Muftuler, L. T. (2009). Estimating the influence of attention on population codes in human visual cortex using voxel-based tuning functions. *NeuroImage 44*: 223–231.

Serences, J. T., Schwarzbach, J., Courtney, S. M., Golay, X., and Yantis, S. (2004). Control of object-based attention in human cortex. *Cerebral Cortex 14*: 1346–1357.

Serences, J. T., Yantis, S., Culberson, A., and Awh, E. (2004). Preparatory activity in visual cortex indexes distractor suppression during covert spatial orienting. *Journal of Neurophysiology 92*: 3538–3545.

Seung, H. S. and Sompolinsky, H. (1993). Simple models for reading neuronal population codes. *Proceedings of the National Academy of Sciences USA 90*: 10749–10753.

Shadlen, M. N., Britten, K. H., Newsome, W. T., and Movshon, J. A. (1996). A computational analysis of the relationship between neuronal and behavioral responses to visual motion. *Journal of Neuroscience 16*: 1486–1510.

Shadlen, M. N. and Newsome, W. T. (1994). Noise, neural codes and cortical organization. *Current Opinion in Neurobiology 4*: 569–579.

Shannon, S. E. (1949). *A Mathematical Theory of Communication*. Urbana, Ill. University of Illinois Press.

Shaw, M. L. (1984). Division of attention among spatial locations: A fundamental difference between detection of letters and detection of luminance increments. In H. Bouma and D. G. Bouwhais (eds.), *Attention and Performance* (vol. 10, pp. 109–121). Hillsdale, N.J.: Lawrence Erlbaum Associates.

Shomstein, S., Kimchi, R., Hammer, M., and Behrmann, M. (2010). Perceptual grouping operates independently of attentional selection: Evidence from hemispatial neglect. *Attention, Perception, & Psychophysics 72*: 607–618.

Slotnick, S. D., Hopfinger, J. B., Klein, S. A., and Sutter, E. E. (2002). Darkness beyond the light: Attentional inhibition surrounding the classic spotlight. *NeuroReport 13*: 773–778.

Somers, D. C., Dale, A. M., Seiffert, A. E., and Tootell, R. B. (1999). Functional MRI reveals spatially specific attentional modulation in human primary visual cortex. *Proceedings of the National Academy of Sciences USA 96*: 1663–1668.

Stokes, M., Thompson, R., Nobre, A. C., and Duncan, J. (2009). Shape-specific preparatory activity mediates attention to targets in human visual cortex. *Proceedings of the National Academy of Sciences USA 106*: 19569–19574.

Sundberg, K. A., Mitchell, J. F., Gawne, T. J., and Reynolds, J. H. (2012). Attention influences single unit and local field potential response latencies in visual cortical area V4. *Journal of Neuroscience 32*: 16040–16050.

Sundberg, K. A., Mitchell, J. F., and Reynolds, J. H. (2009). Spatial attention modulates center-surround interactions in macaque visual area V4. *Neuron 61*: 952–963.

Sylvester, C. M., Shulman, G. L., Jack, A. I., and Corbetta, M. (2009). Anticipatory and stimulus-evoked blood oxygenation level-dependent modulations related to spatial attention reflect a common additive signal. *Journal of Neuroscience 29*: 10671–10682.

Teller, D. Y. (1984). Linking propositions. *Vision Research 24*: 1233–1246.

Tipper, S. P. and Driver, J. (1988). Negative priming between pictures and words in a selective attention task: Evidence for semantic processing of ignored stimuli. *Memory & Cognition 16*: 64–70.

Treisman, A. M. (1960). Contextual cues in selective listening. *Quarterly Journal of Experimental Psychology 12*: 242–248.

Treisman, A. M. and Gelade, G. (1980). A feature-integration theory of attention. *Cognitive Psychology 12*: 97–136.

Treue, S. (2003). Climbing the cortical ladder from sensation to perception. *Trends in Cognitive Sciences 7*: 469–471.

Treue, S. and Martinez-Trujillo, J. C. (1999). Feature-based attention influences motion processing gain in macaque visual cortex. *Nature 399*: 575–579.

Treue, S. and Maunsell, J. H. (1996). Attentional modulation of visual motion processing in cortical areas MT and MST. *Nature 382*: 539–541.

Van der Burg, E., Talsma, D., Olivers, C. N., Hickey, C., and Theeuwes, J. (2011). Early multisensory interactions affect the competition among multiple visual objects. *NeuroImage 55*: 1208–1218.

Vogel, E. K., Luck, S. J., and Shapiro, K. L. (1998). Electrophysiological evidence for a post-perceptual locus of suppression during the attentional blink. *Journal of Experimental Psychology: Human Perception and Performance 24*: 1656–1674.

Vogel, E. K., Woodman, G. F., and Luck, S. J. (2005). Pushing around the locus of selection: Evidence for the flexible-selection hypothesis. *Journal of Cognitive Neuroscience 17*: 1907–1922.

Vuilleumier, P., Sagiv, N., Hazeltine, E., Poldrack, R. A., Swick, D., Rafal, R. D., and Gabrieli, J. D. (2001). Neural fate of seen and unseen faces in visuospatial neglect: A combined event-related functional MRI and event-related potential study. *Proceedings of the National Academy of Sciences USA 98*: 3495–3500.

Wijers, A. A., Lange, J. J., Mulder, G., and Mulder, L. J. (1997). An ERP study of visual spatial attention and letter target detection for isoluminant and nonisoluminant stimuli. *Psychophysiology 34*: 553–565.

Wojciulik, E., Kanwisher, N., and Driver, J. (1998). Covert visual attention modulates face-specific activity in the human fusiform gyrus: fMRI study. *Journal of Neurophysiology 79*: 1574–1578.

Yantis, S. and Johnston, J. C. (1990). On the locus of visual selection: Evidence from focused attention tasks. *Journal of Experimental Psychology: Human Perception and Performance 16*: 135–149.

Yigit-Elliott, S., Palmer, J., and Moore, C. M. (2011). Distinguishing blocking from attenuation in visual selective attention. *Psychological Science: A Journal of the American Psychological Society/APS 22*: 771–780.

Zenon, A. and Krauzlis, R. J. (2012). Attention deficits without cortical neuronal deficits. *Nature 489*: 434–437.

Zhang, W. and Luck, S. J. (2009). Feature-based attention modulates feedforward visual processing. *Nature Neuroscience 12*: 24–25.

Zhang, X., Zhaoping, L., Zhou, T., and Fang, F. (2012). Neural activities in V1 create a bottom-up saliency map. *Neuron 73*: 183–192.

CHAPTER 5

LARGE-SCALE NETWORKS FOR ATTENTIONAL BIASES

ANNA C. NOBRE AND M. MARSEL MESULAM

THE core concept of 'attention' is a fundamental principle of cognition—the adaptive and proactive selectivity of our interface with the surrounding environment. Contrary to our intuition, we do not apprehend the complete and continuous stream of events unfolding around us. Instead, at any given moment we sample a handful of details that happen to be relevant or interesting within our current context and motivational state. Attention refers to the set of mechanisms that tune psychological and neural processing in order to identify and select the relevant events against all the competing distractions. This type of definition casts attention as function rather than as representation or as state. It is about orienting, focusing, and selecting.

SOME HISTORY

Some of the earliest known empirical studies of selective attention were by Herman von Helmholtz (1867). He built an apparatus akin to a tachistoscope, which could illuminate a display containing several letters for a fraction of a second (Fig. 5.1). Using it, he confronted the severe limitations in our perceptual abilities, noting that it was impossible to view all the letters simultaneously in a single glance. He then demonstrated our ability to orient attention to specific spatial locations at will, while still maintaining visual fixation on a single point. By orienting attention covertly to different locations of the array in turn, over multiple iterations, he could reconstitute the entire array. Summarizing early seminal experimental work and using introspective methods, William James (1890) provided insightful and lucid descriptions of varieties, effects, and mechanisms of attention, which remain rich and contemporary. According to James, attention is a pervasive faculty that shapes conscious experience: 'My experience is what I agree to attend to' (James 1890/1950: 403). At any given moment, the span of consciousness is limited to a single object or thought, attended to reflexively or voluntarily, due to immediate (intrinsic) or derived (associated) relevance. Focusing attention by anticipatory preparation

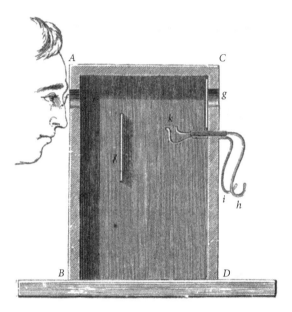

FIGURE 5.1 Apparatus built by Helmholtz to investigate the scope of perception while avoiding ocular movements. A drawing was fastened (at position g) to the back of a hollow box painted black inside. The observer maintained fixation on a small hole pierced in the drawing that was visible at all times. The image was illuminated by making contact between two electrical wires (I and h), triggering a spark illuminating the drawing. A white piece of cardboard (l) protected the observer's eye while also reflecting the light from the spark onto the drawing. 'The sparks were produced by a large Ruhmkorff induction coil connected with the terminals of a Leyden jar. The contact in the primary coil was made or broken by hand' Reproduced from von Helmholtz, *Treatise on Physiological Optics, Volume III*, figure 32 © 2005, Dover Publications.

using ideational centres concerned with the object to which the attention is paid results in adjustments in sense organs so that objects (or ideas of objects) are better perceived, conceived, distinguished, remembered, or more readily reacted to (James 1890/1950).

The early twentieth century witnessed a polarization of psychology between the psychoanalysts, who overemphasized the power of mental phenomena, and the behaviourists, who discredited it. The empirical study of attention regained a more balanced approach in the 1950s, when it became incorporated in the emerging 'information-processing' paradigm. Starting from the premise that our information-processing abilities are severely limited, the initial major experimental questions addressed the locus of the bottleneck. Experimental tasks were developed to test the consequences of focusing versus dividing attention in the presence of two or more competing streams (Cherry 1953). Opposing categorical views were put forward, which placed the information-processing limits at extremes of the information-processing stream: at very early, perceptual stages (Broadbent 1958) versus at late post-perceptual stages following semantic evaluation of stimuli (Deutsch and Deutsch 1963). The evidence was inconclusive in arbitrating between 'early selection' and 'late selection' theories, showing that it was possible to focus effectively on one stream of information based on physical characteristics of stimuli so that competing distractors generally did not reach awareness (compatible with early selection), but that high-level semantic or associative features of the unattended stream could nevertheless influence behaviour and occasionally break through into awareness (compatible with late selection; Treisman 1960) (for further discussion of this debate see Serences and Kastner (in chapter 4), this volume). A cogent theoretical model incorporating elements of both early and late selection was proposed by Anne Treisman (1960, 1969), in which modulatory mechanisms operating at perceptual levels attenuate processing of irrelevant material rather than blocking it completely, and in which stimulus representations have different thresholds of activation depending on their personal significance, conditional probability, or other contextual constraints (Treisman 1960). Nilli Lavie's 'perceptual-load theory' is another, contemporary hybrid model, which holds that a perceptual bottleneck only occurs when the perceptual demands of a task are high (Lavie 1995), see Lavie and Dalton (in chapter 3), this volume).

The present-day scene of attention research opens around the 1970s and 1980s as spectacular technological advances enabled increasingly sophisticated anatomical and functional brain studies in humans and non-human primates. The classical questions about the locus of capacity limitations quickly became obsolete, replaced by the clear realization that modulatory mechanisms operate at multiple levels of analysis in a distributed fashion in the brain (Nobre 2004; Nobre et al. 2011). Current research is directed toward characterizing the control and modulatory mechanisms of attention at the levels of individual neurons, neural systems, and large-scale networks. Orienting visual spatial attention according to task goals is the most widely investigated and, therefore, the most well understood paradigm.

Scope of the Chapter

The main focus of this chapter is to consider the mechanisms of attentional control, with particular emphasis on the process of top-down signals biasing information processing. Starting from the paradigmatic case of visual spatial attention, we will present a theoretical account suggesting that attention is controlled by a large-scale 'frontoparietal' network of brain areas that combines representational mapping of physically salient and relevant events, motor programs for intended actions, and motivational factors. We will summarize some principles emerging from a network approach to the control of attention. We will review evidence refining the characterization of the functional anatomy of the network, and supporting its critical role in modulating information processing.

Stepping outside the well-trodden terrain of visual spatial attention, we reflect on the scope of attentional control mechanisms more broadly. We examine the various possible '*sources*' of biases that can prepare perceptual mechanisms to improve interactions with the environment. In addition to the recognized effects of task goals, we entertain other possible potent modulators of ongoing information processing, such as long-term memories and motivational factors associated with anticipated events. We move on to consider the different '*types*' of biases that can operate upon information processing. Whereas studies in the literature have probed how biases can facilitate neural processing according to receptive-field properties of neurons, it is clear that it is possible to anticipate stimulus properties that may not be easily mapped onto receptive fields, such as the timing of events or the meaning of words. Finally, we show that attention can act upon multiple '*slates*' of information processing. We thus return to an old conception put forward by William James (1890) that attention is not restricted to operate upon objects from the sensory stream, but can also prioritize and select objects of thought. We describe a new body of work showing how attentional biases can act within representations maintained in visual short-term memory. To conclude, we discuss how this plurality of sources, types, and slates for attentional biases invites a reconsideration of the conceptualization of attention.

Modulatory Biases

One of the more influential theoretical models for modulatory mechanisms of attention is the 'biased competition model' (Desimone and Duncan 1995). According to this model, the limits of perception arise because of the inherently competitive organization of perceptual systems. Through the visual hierarchy, convergence of inputs from afferent areas leads to increasingly complex receptive-field properties with increasingly lower spatial and temporal resolution. At downstream areas, such as in inferior temporal (IT) cortex, multiple objects or attributes can fall within the receptive field of the same neuron. Averaging the response across all the stimuli impinging on the receptive field would conflate the coding of the various stimuli and abolish discriminability. To be informative, the neuron should respond according to one of the multiple competing stimulus sources. To be adaptive, the neuron should respond according to the most relevant stimulus source.

   One of the primary functions of attention is to set preparatory *biases* to influence the competitive interaction among multiple inputs in favour of the most behaviourally relevant stimulus. Biasing competitive interactions in this way facilitates selection of the attributes of relevant objects, and filtering out of irrelevant attributes, across populations of neurons. Interactions among neurons with spatially and temporally correlated activity further aid co-selection and integration of the features of the relevant objects (Desimone and Duncan 1995). Thus, as a corollary, such biasing signals are likely to play a major role in solving the difficult 'binding problem', by helping to reconstitute features of relevant events that may come to occupy awareness (Reynolds and Desimone 1999).

Our understanding of the cellular mechanisms for biasing neuronal activity, selecting target-related attributes, and integrating them into objects to guide awareness and action remains incomplete, but progress in this area is impressive, and several pieces of the puzzle are coming into view. Competitive interactions among neurons have been well described (Reynolds et al. 1999), as well as the influence of spatial (Moran and Desimone 1985), object-based (Chelazzi et al. 1993, 1998), and feature-based (Treue and Martinez Trujillo 1999) attention in resolving competitive interactions within multiple brain areas. For detailed accounts of the mechanisms being characterized, the reader is directed to the many excellent contemporary reviews of this literature (Reynolds and Chelazzi 2004). Although most experiments have concentrated on visual areas, there is clear evidence that analogous biasing mechanisms operate across sensory areas in other modalities (Mehta et al. 2000), as well as in motor (Cisek 2007; Pastor-Bernier and Cisek 2011) regions of the brain. The findings, therefore, argue against fixed points of limited capacity, and indicate instead that selective biasing mechanisms operate at multiple stages. Furthermore, the sites and temporal characteristics of modulatory mechanisms are likely to be highly task-dependent, and to be influenced by the specific types of features that need to be discriminated and the number of competing response tendencies that need to be handled for accurate task performance (Stokes et al. 2009) (for an early articulation of this flexible proposal see Kahneman and Treisman 1984).

CONTROL MECHANISMS

What are the sources of these modulatory biases that play such a fundamental role in guiding perception and action? One generally accepted distinction is that between 'exogenous' and 'endogenous' shifts of attention. These are also referred to as 'reflexive' or 'automatic' and 'voluntary' or 'effortful' respectively. The distinction dates back at least to James, who separated passive/reflexive/non-voluntary/effortless from active/voluntary attention (James 1890/1950).

In exogenous shifts, physically salient stimuli attract attention. Biases are set 'bottom-up' by sensory-driven mechanisms that prioritize neural processing of events rendered conspicuous by virtue of their higher stimulus energy or local contrast (e.g. bigger, brighter, or faster) (Yantis and Jonides 1984; see Theeuwes (in chapter 8), this volume). These stimuli have acquired an edge through the evolution of our perceptual systems, and carry their own intrinsic biases to the competitive perceptual mechanisms. Their dominance can be considered a natural consequence of competitive interactions among unequal stimuli. Interestingly, however, these perceptually salient stimuli also leave a modulatory trail. They 'prime' their location, facilitating detection and discrimination of other events occurring at the same location over very brief intervals (Posner 1978, 1980). Unless the location turns out to be relevant or informative, the transient facilitation is subsequently replaced by suppression, thus freeing the system to explore other locations (Posner and Cohen 1984; Klein 2000; Chica et al. 2006; Lupiañez 2010).

In endogenous shifts, focus is directed voluntarily to a location of choice. Biases operate 'top-down', driven by endogenous (mental) factors computed in high-level, associative areas, and influencing perceptual processing through feedback connections. Different scholars have emphasized different mechanisms of regulation for top-down biases. The biased-competition model proposes that top-down biasing signals are primarily mediated through working-memory representations of task-relevant items (Desimone and Duncan 1995). The alternative 'premotor theory' of attention emphasizes the role of motor intention, and proposes that computations in the oculomotor, as well as other sensorimotor systems, modulate perceptual analysis through feedback connections (Rizzolatti et al. 1987; Rizzolatti and Craighero 1998). Mesulam suggested a broader conceptualization, in which sensory, representational; motor, exploratory; and limbic, motivational biases combine to direct spatial attention through the action of a large-scale frontoparieto-cingulate attentional network (Mesulam 1981, 1990, 1999).

LARGE-SCALE NETWORK FOR ATTENTION

Original description

Everyone now agrees that the control of spatial attention depends on a large-scale network of brain areas. The first network model for attention was proposed by Mesulam in 1981, and subsequently refined and extended over the years (Mesulam 1990, 1999, 2005). The original proposed network architecture was based on clinical observations of patients with hemispatial neglect as well as on multiple sources of convergent data in non-human primates (Fig. 5.2). Four sets of brain areas, three cortical and one subcortical, constituted major nodes, each introducing a different functional specialization so that spatial attention emerged as a property of the network as a whole.

In the macaque, the three cortical nodes of this network were located in the dorsolateral portion of the inferior parietal lobule and lateral bank of the intraparietal sulcus (LIP) (area PG of von Bonin and Bailey, 7a of Brodmann), frontal eye fields (FEF) (area 8 of Brodmann), and the cingulate gyrus (areas 23–24 of Brodmann and the retrosplenial cortex). Anatomical tracer studies had shown these nodes to be monosynaptically interconnected (Mesulam et al. 1977). The parietal node was proposed to provide a multisensory perceptual map of the extrapersonal space weighted by physical salience and relevance of stimuli. The frontal node provided a hub for motor integration, which contained representations of motor programs for the distribution of exploratory actions. The cingulate node acted as a region for integration of limbic signals, assigning motivational relevance to events based on previous experience and current needs. Experimental lesions to any of these cortical nodes resulted in attention-related deficits akin to neglect (Bianchi 1895; Kennard 1939; Denny-Brown and Chambers 1958; Welch and Stuteville 1958; Heilman et al. 1970; Cowey and Latto 1971; Watson et al.

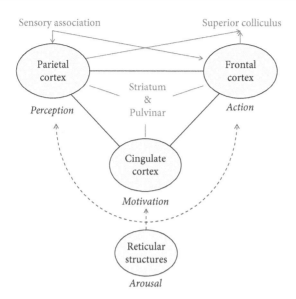

FIGURE 5.2 Large-scale network for orienting visual spatial attention proposed by Mesulam (1981, 1990, 1999, 2005). Parietal, frontal, and cingulate cortices are the three primary cortical nodes. These act as local hubs for organizing and integrating signals related to perception, exploratory action, and motivation, respectively. The three cortical nodes are directly inter-connected with one another, and are additionally interconnected through participating sub-cortical hubs in the striatum and the pulvinar nucleus of the thalamus. In addition to their intrinsic connections, the cortical and subcortical nodes also have connections to other areas with specialized sensory, limbic, and motor functions. The main nodes of the large-scale network each also receive modulatory reticular input from brainstem nuclei.

1973) and single-unit recordings showed modulation of neuronal activity by the rel-evance of the stimulus and nature of orienting responses it elicited (Hyvarinen and Poranen 1974; Mountcastle et al. 1975; Lynch et al. 1977; Bushnell et al. 1981). Each of these interconnected nodes had its own pattern of connections with functionally related areas, such as sensory association areas in the case of the parietal cortex, motor and pre-motor regions in the case of frontal eye fields, and other limbic nuclei in the case of the cingulate cortex. In addition, all three areas receive reticular input from a common set of thalamic, basal forebrain, and brainstem nuclei (see Mesulam 1990). These subcortical inputs comprised the fourth functional node of the network, and were proposed to play a central role in regulating the state of arousal, which underpins and interacts strongly with the selective control of spatial attention (Hecaen et al. 1956). Brainstem reticular lesions have long been known to cause severe deficits in arousal and awareness, and lesions of the intralaminar thalamic nucleus in monkeys have been observed to result in neglect (Watson et al. 1974, 1978).

The network approach is intermediary to centrist approaches, in which complex functions are supported by exclusively dedicated brain areas (Spurzheim 1825), and holistic approaches, in which complex functions are equipotentially distributed across areas (Lashley 1950). It has several noteworthy properties. According to the large-scale network approach, individual cognitive domains are enabled through the interaction of interconnected areas, each with a relative specialization for a component function of that domain. Having a network of areas supporting a complex function means that impairments can arise from different lesion sites. The network also provides some protective compensatory mechanisms, so that severe and lasting impairments may not arise unless multiple nodes are damaged. The presence of multiple nodes with distinct functional specializations can also help explain the variety of deficits that arise from lesions to the different nodes, their interconnections, or their connections to other regions (see Geschwind 1965a, 1965b).

The interactions among the areas in an integrated system can blur the categorical distinctions between the functional specializations contributed by the different nodes. For example, the distinction between sensory and motor contributions across parietal and frontal nodes in the attention network was considered to be relative, with sensory and motor functions observable in each of these areas. Such a proposal, of course, is perfectly acceptable nowadays with our growing exposure to the sensory properties of neurons in the motor system, as in mirror neurons (di Pellegrino et al. 1992), and to increasing proposals of action-based active sensing mechanisms in perceptual systems (Fortuyn 1979; Schroeder et al. 2010).

Another feature of the large-scale network model is that brain areas with a given functional specialization need not be exclusively dedicated to one network. Conceivably, the same physiological specialization could underlie multiple complex functions. For example, similar neuronal profiles in posterior parietal cortex have been implicated in spatial attention, oculomotor control (Colby and Duhamel 1996; Snyder et al. 2000; Bisley and Goldberg 2010), decision-making (Leon and Shadlen 1998; Gold and Shadlen 2007; Gould et al. 2012), working memory (LaBar et al. 1999; Todd and Marois 2004; Buschman et al. 2011), and long-term memory (Wagner et al. 2005; Cabeza et al. 2008). The nodes of large-scale networks also add flexibility by acting as portals of interactions with other brain areas so as to integrate attention control with other complex functions, such as language, working memory, and long-term memory.

Imaging the attentional network

Over subsequent years, the large-scale model of attention was amply vindicated. Refinements to the model came from continued characterization of neglect symptoms and their dissociations, and from increasing knowledge about physiological properties and connectivity of brain areas (Mesulam 1990, 1999; Mesulam et al. 2005). The development of positron-emission tomography (PET), and then functional magnetic-resonance imaging (fMRI) methods, introduced a wealth of new information on the attentional network. Non-invasive brain imaging enabled the testing and extending of the network model, by mapping its constituent critical nodes and revealing areas that participate without being critical to spatial orienting. The core cortical parietal, frontal, and cingulate nodes were recognized to comprise functional mosaics of multiple areas with distinct but interrelated contributions to representational, intentional, and motivational functions. Other, highly related cortical areas for attention were also proposed to participate in some spatial attention functions, such as in the medial parietal cortex, supplementary eye fields (SEF), premotor areas in the case of orienting attention to near space, dorsolateral prefrontal cortex (BA 46), and possibly parts of temporal cortex. Also stressed was the role of subcortical areas, in particular the superior colliculus, striatum, and pulvinar nucleus of the thalamus (see also Saalmann and Kastner (in chapter 14), this volume).

The first visualization of the network for controlling spatial attention in the human brain came from studies using PET using an adaptation of Posner's visuospatial orienting task over a group of participants (Corbetta et al. 1993, 1995) (Fig. 5.3). We extended

(a) Corbetta et al. 1993   (b) Nobre et al. 1997   (c) Kim et al. 1999   (d) Silver & Kastner 2009

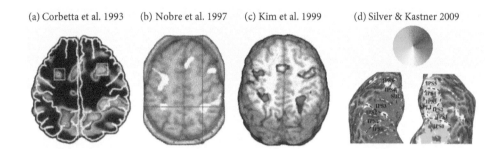

FIGURE 5.3 Imaging the cortical areas involved in the control of visual spatial attention with increasing resolution. All images are from an axial perspective with the posterior part of the brain on the bottom and the right hemisphere on the right. (a) The seminal study by Corbetta et al. (1993) used positron emission tomography (PET) and relied on patterns of activation across a small group of participants. Data from Corbetta, M., Miezin, F. M., Shulman, G. L. and Petersen, S. E., A PET study of visuospatial attention. *Journal of Neuroscience*, 13, pp. 1202–26 © 2003, Society for Neuroscience. (b) Nobre et al. (1997) used PET to image the network in individual participants as well as in groups. It became possible to localize cortical activations to the intraparietal sulcus, frontal eye fields, and anterior cingulate cortices. Data from Nobre, A. C., Sebestyen, G. N., Gitelman, D. R., Mesulam, M. M., Frackowiak, R. S. and Frith, C. D., Functional localization of the system for visuospatial attention using positron emission tomography, *Brain*, 120 (Pt 3), pp. 515–33 © 1997, Oxford University Press. (c) Functional magnetic-resonance imaging greatly increased the functional anatomical resolution for investigating the spatial attention networks in groups and individuals in tasks with much greater experimental control. The example illustrated is from the study by Kim et al. (1999), showing the overlap in brain areas activated by voluntary/endogenous spatial orienting based on informative central cues and by automatic/exogenous spatial orienting based on non-informative peripheral cues. Data from Kim, Y. H., Gitelman, D. R., Nobre, A. C., Parrish, T. B., LaBar, K. S. and Mesulam, M. M., The large-scale neural network for spatial attention displays multifunctional overlap but differential asymmetry. *Neuroimage*, 9 (3), 269–77 © 1999, Elsevier. (d) By adapting procedures for retinotopic mapping to produce spatiotopic maps, it has become possible to subdivide the nodes of the spatial attention networks into multiple constituent functional regions. The example shows the subdivision of posterior parietal cortex into multiple functional regions with spatial specificity. Reproduced from Silver, M. A. and Kastner, S., Topographic maps in human frontal and parietal cortex, *Trends in Cognitive Sciences*, 13 (11), 488–95, © 2009, Elsevier.

this work with the first functional anatomical characterization of the human 'frontopa-rietal network' using PET at the individual-subject level, which strongly supported Mesulam's model (Nobre et al. 1997). Three cortical areas were implicated in orient-ing spatial attention: posterior parietal cortex, straddling the intraparietal sulcus; dor-sal premotor/posterior prefrontal cortex (in both lateral and medial Brodmann area 6); and anterior cingulate cortex (Brodmann area 24). We replicated these sites of activa-tion with greater spatial resolution in an fMRI study using single-subject analyses and stringent behavioural controls (Gitelman et al. 1999). Studies investigating activity of spatial cues in isolation, separately from processing of subsequent targets, have verified that multiple brain areas participate in controlling spatial attention (Kastner et al. 1999; Corbetta et al. 2000; Hopfinger et al. 2000; Nobre et al. 2004; Woldorff et al. 2004).

By now, activation around the intraparietal sulcus and in dorsal premotor/prefron-tal areas has been replicated by dozens of spatial attention imaging studies across labs worldwide (Vandenberghe et al. 1996; Fink et al. 1997; Kim et al. 1999; Hopfinger et al. 2000; Kastner and Ungerleider 2000; Corbetta and Shulman 2002; Giesbrecht et al. 2003; Pollmann et al. 2003; Woldorff et al. 2004; Molenberghs et al. 2007). Involvement of cingulate cortex in top-down regulation of behaviour according to motivational fac-tors has also been convincingly demonstrated (Isomura and Takada 2004; Rushworth et al. 2007, 2011; Liu et al. 2011; Wallis and Kennerley 2011), and specifically noted in tasks involving spatial attention (Mesulam et al. 2001; Small et al. 2003, 2005; Dean et al. 2004; Mohanty et al. 2008; Kaping et al. 2011). Successive imaging stud-ies have achieved increasing spatial and functional characterization of the mosaic of parietal and frontal cortical areas, as well as of the subcortical areas involved (e.g. Vandenberghe et al. 2001; O'Connor et al. 2002; Astafiev et al. 2004; Kastner et al. 2007; Kelley et al. 2008; Konen and Kastner 2008; Molenberghs et al. 2008; Silver and Kastner 2009; Szczepanski et al. 2010; Saalmann and Kastner 2011; Serences 2011; Scolari et al. 2012).

Relationship between visuospatial attention and oculomotor control

In our original PET study (Nobre et al. 1997), the parietal and frontal areas were noted to resemble those highlighted by imaging studies of oculomotor control (Melamed and Larsen 1979; Fox et al. 1985; Petit et al. 1993; Anderson et al. 1994; Darby et al. 1996; Paus 1996), and were proposed to include the human homologues of macaque lateral intraparietal area (LIP), frontal eye fields (FEF), and supplementary eye fields (SEF). The strong functional interrelationship between visuospatial orienting and oculomotor control had been, and continues to be, suggested by a number of behavioural (Allport 1987; Sheliga et al. 1994) and neurophysiological (e.g. Colby and Duhamel 1996; Snyder et al. 1997, 1998; Gottlieb et al. 1998; Kusunoki et al. 2000) studies (see Deubel (in chapter 30), this volume). Human imag-ing studies comparing activations during spatial orienting of attention in the absence of eye movements (covert attention) and saccade generation confirmed a high degree of overlap in activated brain areas (Corbetta et al. 1998; Rosen et al. 1999; Nobre et al. 2000a; Perry and Zeki 2000; Van der Stigchel et al. 2006). Contemporary research continues to explore the nature and degree of functional and neural overlap between eye movements and attention, as well as the mechanisms which enable the two functions to be dissociated during covert attention (e.g. Juan et al. 2004; Cohen et al. 2009; Khan et al. 2009; Lawrence and Snyder 2009; Bisley and Goldberg 2010; see also Deubel (in chapter 30), this volume, Theeuwes (in chapter 8), this volume; Gottlieb and Balan 2010; Wardak et al. 2011; Belopolsky and Theeuwes 2012; Gregoriou et al. 2012). Although oculomotor circuits may play a primary role in the network for spatial attention, studies have suggested that other sensorimotor circuits, specialized for different forms of spatially guided action (e.g. reaching or point-ing movements), also display similar attentional modulations (e.g. Snyder et al. 1997, 1998; Astafiev et al. 2003; Van Der Werf et al. 2010; Deubel (in chapter 30), this volume).

Endogenous versus exogenous spatial orienting

The different characteristics of endogenous versus exogenous spatial shifts of attention (see Posner 1978, 1980; Posner et al. 1982, 1984; Müller and Rabbitt 1989; Friedrich et al. 1998; Losier and Klein 2001; Berger et al. 2005; Sieroff et al. 2007; Lakatos et al. 2008; Wright and Ward 2008; Chica et al. 2013) have led to numerous brain-imaging studies comparing the neural systems involved in these two types of orienting.

Initial studies used blocked designs to contrast experimental conditions with high versus low requirement for voluntary orienting under well controlled stimulus con-ditions (Nobre et al. 1997), or to contrast conditions using symbolic cues that predict subsequent target location versus non-predictive transient peripheral cues (Kim et al. 1999; Koski et al. 1999; Rosen et al. 1999; Peelen et al. 2004). Surprisingly, the patterns of activations in endogenous and exogenous conditions reported were very similar, and consistent with engagement of the dorsal frontoparietal network in both cases (see Fig. 5.3c). These studies therefore suggested that endogenous and exogenous shifts of attention rely on the same general network of brain areas (Posner 1978; Jonides and Irwin 1981; Yantis 1998), though they could be supported by different dynamics and mechanisms within a common network.

In contrast to these findings and interpretations, Corbetta and colleagues proposed that different circuits supported endogenous versus exogenous orienting of spatial attention (Corbetta et al. 2000; Corbetta and Shulman 2002). They proposed that the dorsal frontoparietal network mediated voluntary, endogenous shifts of spatial atten-tion; whereas a ventral network, comprising the temporal parietal junction (including supramarginal gyrus and superior temporal gyrus) and inferior frontal gyrus, mediated reflexive, exogenous shifts. Their proposal was based on the different patterns of activa-tions triggered by spatial cues versus subsequent targets in event-related fMRI tasks. In agreement with the previous literature (Kastner et al. 1999), spatial cues activated dorsal parietal and premotor/prefrontal cortices. Targets, on the other hand. engaged a more widespread network of areas, including the temporal parietal junction and infe-rior frontal gyrus, in addition to dorsal frontoparietal areas. Furthermore, the ventral parietal and frontal regions responded more strongly to targets that had been invalidly cued, appearing at unexpected locations. Corbetta and colleagues reasoned that unex-pected (e.g. invalidly cued) targets trigger predominantly exogenous shifts of attention to their location, and do more so when voluntary attention had been directed some-where else by the preceding cue. Their findings, but even more so their interpretations, led to their influential subdivision of attention into two functionally distinct 'dorsal' and 'ventral' attention networks (shortened to DAN and VAN respectively) (Corbetta and Shulman 2002).

The strict correspondence of the ventral network to exogenous orienting, however, could be challenged. The account does not explain the consistent similarity of cortical activation patterns between blocked endogenous versus exogenous attentional shifts (Kim et al. 1999; Koski et al. 1999; Rosen et al. 1999; Peelen et al. 2004). Furthermore, comparing the processing of unexpected targets to informative cues is not the same as comparing exogenous to endogenous orienting. The appearance of an invalidly cued target may trigger disengagement of attention from its previous site and a reflexive shift toward its location, but it may also engage a number of other processes: e.g. signalling a mismatch between current expectations about stimulus contingencies to direct action, updating learning of stimulus contingencies, switching stimulus–response associations between expected and novel patterns, as well as the motivational and emotional factors of violated expectations (see Nobre et al. 1999). The conceptualization of the 'ventral attention network' therefore conflates various putative factors that are not restricted to the control of attention (for further discussion on the 'VAN', see also Beck and Kastner (in chapter 9), this volume).

The conditions in which ventral parietal and frontal areas become activated have become better characterized through careful subsequent experiments. Findings argue clearly against the hypothesis that ventral frontoparietal regions play a special role in directing exogenous shifts of attention (Kincade et al. 2005). Using an ingenious and well controlled design, Corbetta's group compared activations triggered by predictive central cues versus non-predictive peripheral cues, as well as by validly versus invalidly cued targets in the endogenous and exogenous cueing contexts (Kincade et al. 2005). As expected, endogenous spatial cues activated the dorsal frontoparietal network. Contrary to their predictions, however, exogenous cues did not activate either dorsal or ventral frontoparietal areas. Valid and invalid targets in both endogenous and exogenous cue-ing conditions activated both dorsal and ventral frontoparietal regions. Furthermore, higher activation for invalid targets compared to valid targets only occurred in endog-enous cueing conditions, when spatial expectations were breached. These occurred in some of the dorsal (e.g. FEF) as well as ventral (e.g. supramarginal gyrus) regions. Targets at an invalid location after a non-informative cue did not recruit frontoparietal areas (for related results see Peelen et al. 2004; Natale et al. 2009). Additional experi-ments have also shown that irrelevant salient events fail to engage frontoparietal areas; only task-relevant target events, or distractors sharing target features, occurring at unattended or unpredicted locations engage ventral parietal and frontal regions (Serences et al. 2005; Indovina and Macaluso 2007; Serences and Yantis 2007).

Taken as a whole, the evidence shows that the 'ventral attention network' is a misnomer. Ventral parietal and frontal areas do not participate directly in shifting attention exogenously or in resetting attentional weights. These areas are not engaged by stimuli that trigger exogenous shifts of spatial attention, such as transient non-informative cues. Instead, they are activated by the appearance of imperative target stimuli (or distractor stimuli sharing target features), which require decisions or responses; and their activation is enhanced when target appearance is unexpected. Elucidating the precise functional roles these areas play will require continued experimentation. Though the functions are likely to interact closely with the control of attention in spatial orienting tasks, they should not be construed as spatial attention functions in their own right. Many possibilities remain, such as functions related to motivational or emotional responses to breaches in expectation, sensory prediction-error signals, and/or updating representations of stimulus contingencies relevant to behaviour. Dropping the misleading nomenclature is an important first step in achieving clarity and making progress in understanding the nature of and interrelationship among the various types of control functions.

Temporal dynamics within the attention network

The high degree of interaction among nodes of the frontoparietal network has been fully supported by studies of functional connectivity in humans and macaques. The similarity in functional profiles of areas like FEF and LIP has long been noted (e.g. Chafee and Goldman-Rakic 1998), and indeed it is difficult to distinguish them other than in a relative way (e.g. Lawrence and Snyder 2009; Muggleton et al. 2011; Wardak et al. 2011). During tasks requiring spatial attention, correlations have been noted to increase among network areas (e.g. Buchel and Friston 1997; Gitelman et al. 2002; Buschman and Miller 2007; Vincent et al. 2008; Ozaki 2011; Vossel et al. 2012).

A key question in this field concerns the identity of the prime mover in shifting the focus of spatial attention. Given the high degree of proposed interaction and coordination across the nodes of the large-scale network for attention, it is unlikely that a clear and consistent temporal hierarchy of contributions can be identified. Hemodynamic imaging methods lack the resolution to measure timing differences at the scale necessary to resolve a sequence of events across the network of attention. Studies using event-related potentials show that lateralization of cortical activity triggered by predictive spatial cues starts posteriorly, suggestive of a parietal origin, and then progresses anteriorly, suggestive of frontal engagement (Harter et al. 1989; Hopf and Mangun 2000; Nobre et al. 2000b; but see van Velzen and Eimer 2003; Praamstra et al. 2005; Murray et al. 2011). A similar posterior-to-anterior progression is observed in non-lateralized brain activity triggered by cues that instruct a shift of spatial attention versus maintenance of attention at the same locations (Talsma et al. 2005, 2011;

Brignani et al. 2009), though spatial shifts compared to a cued rest period elicit a different pattern (Grent-'t-Jong and Woldorff 2007). Stepping back, it is important to realize that the sequence of effects within the attention network may largely depend on what triggers a spatial shift—an instructional cue, a working-memory representation of an anticipated target, or a salient perceptual event. Buschman and Miller (2007) neatly demonstrated this context dependency of the temporal hierarchy among spatial attention control areas. Recording simultaneously from different brain areas in the macaque, they showed that LIP was the first to signal a target within a search array when it popped out based on sensory features; but that FEF and lateral prefrontal areas took the lead when target detection required effortful matching of the target to a template held in working memory.

Interactions between the attention network and visual areas

The large-scale network for spatial attention—bringing together perceptual representations, intentions, and motivations—is proposed to act as the main source of spatial biases to prioritize the selection and integration of relevant events during the competitive processing in visual, and other sensory areas (Hopfinger et al. 2000; Kastner and Ungerleider 2000; Mendenorp et al. 2011). Single-unit and local field-potential recordings taken from multiple brain regions simultaneously in macaques show task-related correlations between visual areas and FEF and LIP (Buschman and Miller 2007; Saalmann et al. 2007; Gregoriou et al. 2009). In humans, analyses of functional interactions among brain areas using fMRI (Buchel and Friston 1997; Gillebert et al. 2012) or MEG (Siegel et al. 2008) also show enhanced coupling between frontoparietal nodes and visual areas with attention. Strong confirmation that frontal and parietal areas play a causal role in modulating excitability of visual neurons has come from studies using interference methods to change activity in FEF or posterior parietal areas while simultaneously measuring visual activity. Pioneering studies by Moore and colleagues showed that microstimulation of FEF neurons led to changes in the firing rate of V4 neurons with compatible receptive fields, and improved visual discriminability of targets therein (Moore and Armstrong 2003; Moore and Fallah 2004; Armstrong et al. 2006; Armstrong and Moore 2007). In humans, studies using transcranial magnetic stimulation (TMS) to FEF or posterior parietal areas while simultaneously measuring visual activity using fMRI or EEG have confirmed that frontal and parietal areas play a causal role in modulating visual excitability (e.g. Paus et al. 1997; Ruff et al. 2006, 2008; Taylor et al. 2007; Capotosto et al. 2009; Blankenburg et al. 2010; Driver et al. 2010).

These studies provide convincing evidence that the frontoparietal network acts as a source of top-down signals to influence perceptual analysis at sensory sites. Future work combining interference and correlational methods should help describe differences in the types and timings of top-down influences originating from different areas within the large-scale attention network. It will be equally important to test for alterations in visual excitability in patients who have sustained focal cortical lesions to different functional regions within posterior parietal, frontal, and cingulate areas (see Knight et al. 1980; Woods and Knight 1986; Woods et al. 1993; Vandenberghe et al. 2012).

The network for visuospatial attention and hemispatial neglect

Neglect, a neurological syndrome of disrupted spatial attention, is often associated with parietal lesions (Brain 1941; Vallar and Bolognini (in chapter 33), this volume), but can also occur after frontal, temporal, thalamic, or striatal damage (Karnath et al. 2002; Husain and Rorden 2003). This multiplicity of neglect-causing lesion sites is incorporated into the large-scale network model of spatial attention (Mesulam 1981, 1999). However, the fit between the location of neglect-causing lesions in neurological patients and of areas activated by attentional tasks in healthy subjects is far from perfect. Human brain-imaging studies of visuospatial attention have implicated parietal areas around the middle segment of the intraparietal sulcus (Nobre et al. 1997, 2003, 2004; Kastner and Ungerleider 2000; Nobre 2000; Corbetta and Shulman 2002; Giesbrecht et al. 2003; Woldorff et al. 2004), in the posterior segment of the intraparietal sulcus (Vandenberghe et al. 1997, 2005; Silver and Kastner 2009), and in the superior parietal lobule (Vandenberghe et al. 2001; Yantis et al. 2002; Molenberghs et al. 2007; Serences and Yantis 2007). In contrast, 'parietal' lesions, which are the most common cause for neglect, occur at more inferior locations such as the angular gyrus (Vallar and Perani 1986; Hillis et al. 2005; Verdon et al. 2010; Vossel et al. 2011), supramarginal gyrus (Committeri et al. 2007; Golay et al. 2008), the temporal–parietal junction (Driver and Vuilleumier 2001), or the posterior superior temporal gyrus (Karnath et al. 2001; Hillis et al. 2005; Verdon et al. 2010).

This potential mismatch can be partially resolved by considering that neglect is caused by lesions disconnecting the communication between network nodes or between the network and input and output areas (see Geschwind 1965a, 1965b; Gaffan and Hornak 1997; Thiebaut de Schotten et al. 2005; Bartolomeo et al. 2007). Studies using diffusion-tensor imaging methods to measure damage of white matter tracts in patients with and without neglect symptoms have confirmed that structural damage to the superior longitudinal fasciculus (SLF), linking parietal and frontal nodes of the attention network, contributes significantly in determining the occurrence of persistent neglect symptoms (Doricchi and Tomaiuolo 2003; Doricchi et al. 2008; Urbanski et al. 2008, 2011; Ciaraffa et al. 2013). In a similar vein, it has also been proposed that effective lesions exert their influence remotely (Corbetta et al. 2005; He et al. 2007; Corbetta and Shulman 2011).

Whereas it is easy to imagine how differences in the prevalence of certain brain lesions, consequences of disconnection, and remote effects could have led to the current picture of clinic-pathological associations, it remains important to verify whether lesions to the areas implicated in spatial attention functions by imaging and neurophysiology studies impair spatial attention. An early study testing patients with parietal lesions in a simple spatial orienting task suggested a role for dorsal parietal cortex in orienting attention to a spatially unpredicted stimulus (Posner et al. 1984, 1987), but methods were not available at the time to perform accurate lesion localization. A subsequent study using the same experimental task but improved lesion localization separated a group of fifteen patients according to whether they had lesions to the temporal–parietal junction including the superior temporal gyrus, or lesions involving the parietal but not the superior temporal region (Friedrich et al. 1998). Extinction-like spatial orienting deficits were specific to patients in the temporal–parietal junction group. These data have been very influential in framing the thinking about the critical parietal areas for mediating shifts of attention. However, as recently pointed out by Vandenberghe and colleagues (2012), the patient groupings in the study by Friedrich and colleagues (1998) were potentially misleading in titrating the contributions of superior parietal versus inferior parietotemporal areas.

In a series of elegant and methodologically rigorous studies, Vandenberghe's group has investigated the effects of focal parietal lesions that spare white matter on visuospatial orienting functions. They used an adaptation of the Posner spatial orienting task in which unilateral targets appear at correctly spatially cued positions most of the time. On remaining trials, unilateral targets appear at the non-cued side, requiring reorienting of spatial attention; or bilateral targets appear, requiring filtering of the irrelevant item. In initial group studies, they showed that lesion overlap included inferior parietal, temporal–parietal, and intraparietal regions (Molenberghs et al. 2008; Gillebert et al. 2011). When locations of effective lesions were compared to brain activations in a group of control participants performing the same task, there was clear overlap between lesion and activation sites in the intraparietal sulcus (Molenberghs et al. 2008). In order to test whether intraparietal lesions alone can disrupt spatial orienting, studies were carried out on individual patients with rare, small, circumscribed lesions (Gillebert et al. 2011). A lesion to the left posterior intraparietal cortex resulted in large deficits to detect contralesional targets when these were invalidly cued or accompanied by an ipsilesional distractor. A lesion confined to the right middle intraparietal area showed a similar pattern of effects, though with a more distributed reorienting deficit to both contralesional and ipsilesional targets. Functional MRI measures of these patients showed no abnormalities in the activity of more inferior parietal regions, ruling out explanations based on remote effects of the dorsal lesions. A patient with a small bilateral lesion of the medial wall of the SPL was described separately (Vandenberghe et al. 2012). In this case large bilateral deficits in reorienting attention, but no deficits in filtering were observed. Corroborating results came from a study correlating different types of spatial attention deficits with location of lesion using a region-of-interest approach in twenty neglect patients (Ptak and Schnider 2011). Though the maximum lesion overlap was in the temporal–parietal junction, spatial orienting effects were more strongly associated with damage to the intraparietal sulcus. Studies such as these raise caution about overrating centres of lesion overlap, which may primarily reflect vascular variables rather than any measure of the brain–behaviour relationships of interest.

This rigorous experimental approach involving combined behavioural and imaging measurements in patients with focal and informative lesions, and comparison of results to those obtained on healthy volunteers, is redressing the apparent inconsistency between the neuropsychological and imaging literatures. Future work of this kind should continue to add clarity and important insights to the study of spatial attention.

Lateralization in lesion and imaging studies

Clinico-pathological observations of patients with neglect suggest that the network for spatial attention displays a strong right-hemisphere dominance (Heilman and Van Den Abell 1980; Mesulam 1981; Weintraub and Mesulam 1987). Neglect is much more frequent and severe following right-hemisphere lesions in humans (Mesulam 1981; Weintraub and Mesulam 1987), an asymmetry which is not observed in non-human primates. Mesulam (1981) proposed a model by which each hemisphere controlled attention toward the contralateral hemispace, but in which the right hemisphere dedicated more synaptic space to attentional functions and additionally controlled attention to the ipsilateral hemispace.

Some spatial attention imaging studies have reported larger or stronger activations in the right hemisphere (e.g. Corbetta et al. 1993; Nobre et al. 1997; Gitelman et al. 1999; Hopfinger et al. 2010), but this pattern has not been consistently observed (e.g. Sommer et al. 2008; Shulman et al. 2010). Instead, studies mapping the spatiotopic organization of parietal and frontal areas suggest symmetrical involvement of the hemispheres in directing attention to the contralateral space (Kastner et al. 2007; Konen and Kastner 2008; Silver and Kastner 2009; Szczepanski et al. 2010; Szczepanski and Kastner 2013), in line with the simpler inter-hemispheric competition account of spatial attention and neglect (Kinsbourne 1977). In particular, studies by Szczepanski and colleagues combined sustained spatial attention manipulations with spatiotopic mapping to investigate the degree of inter-hemispheric bias in the different functional regions in the posterior parietal cortex (Szczepanski et al. 2010; Szczepanski and Kastner 2013). Different regions showed different patterns of bias, though across the network of areas the biases were well balanced across participants (Szczepanski et al. 2010). The degree of overall inter-hemispheric spatial biases varied among individual participants and correlated with performance measures on an independent test of spatial bias. Furthermore, applying to topographically identified areas consistently shifted the spatial bias toward the ipsilesional visual field (Szczepanski and Kastner 2013) (for further discussion of hemispheric dominance in spatial attention, see also Beck and Kastner (in chapter 9), this volume).

There may be multiple ways to reconcile these apparently discrepant findings. It is possible that specific functional regions with systematic hemispheric biases contribute disproportionately to spatial deficits in neglect. Alternatively, the balance of spatial biases within the frontoparietal network may be disrupted by remote lesions. Corbetta and his colleagues have proposed that neglect occurs as a result of damage to the right temporal parietal junction creating a hemispheric imbalance in activity within the dorsal frontoparietal network (Corbetta et al. 2005; He et al. 2007; Corbetta and Shulman 2011). Finally, it may be prudent to conceptualize neglect as a syndrome to which multiple deficits may contribute, in addition to those involved in orienting spatial attention. Patients with verified visuospatial orienting deficits do not always fulfil the criteria for neglect (e.g. Posner et al. 1984; Gillebert et al. 2011). Other deficits may interact with spatial deficits and play an important role in determining the range, severity, and duration of neglect, such as problems with alerting, sustaining attention, or maintaining information in working memory (Robertson 2001; Husain and Rorden 2003).

It is also important to bear in mind the limits of imaging methods to reveal the mechanisms of hemispheric dominance. Hemodynamic imaging methods may lack the temporal resolution to reveal short-lived neural mechanisms that may contribute to hemispheric dominance. Even if activity occurs bilaterally, activity in one hemisphere may lead in time or last longer. For example, asymmetries have been noted in event-related potentials linked to attention control and modulation (e.g. Nobre et al. 2000a; Miniussi et al. 2002). Structural imaging methods may also provide clues. Structural diffusion-imaging tractography has recently revealed hemispheric differences in the branches of the superior longitudinal fasciculus, with variability in the lateralization of one of the branches correlating with performance in line bisection performance and speed of target detection across the visual fields (Thiebaut de Schotten et al. 2011). The substrate of hemispheric asymmetry in spatial attention may therefore involve fibre pathways as well as cortical activation patterns.

Correlational methods alone, however, will ultimately be insufficient to reveal asymmetries in the causal influence of spatial attention areas on sensory processing. By combining TMS with fMRI, Ruff and colleagues (2009) were able to demonstrate different patterns of visual modulation when stimulating left versus right frontal or intraparietal sulcus. For example, in parietal areas, only right stimulation led to changes in hemodynamic activity in visual areas. The powerful combination of interference (TMS or lesions) and correlational (fMRI or MEG/EEG) methods may be the most effective way to make headway on this intriguing question of hemispheric asymmetry in spatial attention in humans (see also Blankenburg et al. 2010; Driver et al. 2010; Heinen et al. 2011).

EXPANDING THE SCOPE OF ATTENTION

Whereas the bulk of attention research has considered spatial or object-based attention operating within vision or other perceptual domains, the scope of attention is much wider. The essence of selective attention is the biasing of neural activity to favour selection and integration of items that are relevant and adaptive within the current context. This definition leaves open several aspects, regarding what constitutes the sources of bias, what type of information they may carry, the representational slates upon which they can operate, and what behavioural purpose they ultimately support.

SOURCES OF BIAS

In most attention studies, it is the current *task goal* that guides attention. Perceptual cues are typically used to define the target events or to predict their location (e.g. Hillyard et al. 1973; Posner 1980).[1] Depending on the theoretical account, these perceptual cues in turn establish task-relevant working-memory representations (Desimone and Duncan 1985), action intentions (Rizzolatti et al. 1987; Rizzolatti and Craighero 1998), or predictive priors (Rao and Ballard 1999; Feldman and Friston 2010), which serve as sources of top-down signals to influence neural activity within sensory areas or further along the processing stream.

Guidance by long-term memory

Experimental paradigms using perceptual cues have served as powerful platforms for dissecting the mechanisms of attention control and modulation, but they also leave out arguably the most common source of attentional biases: those coming from prior experience and stored as long-term memory (LTM). The critical role memory plays in guiding perception has been long recognized (al-Haytham 1021/1989; Helmholtz 1867). According to Helmholtz, perception is a process of unconscious inference, arising from testing predictions acquired through experience against incoming stimulation. A contemporary and computational articulation of these notions is found in Friston's Free Energy Principle (Friston 2009; Feldman and Friston 2010).

Contemporary attention research is repossessing the notion of memory-guided attention and beginning to reveal the neural mechanisms involved (see also Kuhl and Chun (in chapter 28), this volume). The most established paradigm is that of 'contextual cueing' within visual search (Chun and Jiang 1998, 2003). Response times to identify targets within search arrays decrease as the same spatial configurations of distractors repeat through the experiment, even when participants are unaware of these contingencies (Chun and Jiang 1998, 2003). Associative links between objects in a search array can also affect performance during visual search (Moores et al. 2003). Contextual cueing effects are particularly strong when rich and naturalistic scenes provide the contextual background to guide target identification (Brockmole et al. 2006; see also Becker and Rasmussen 2008), and when the contextual information is presented ahead of the search array, providing time for memory-based guidance to develop (Kunar et al. 2008). Critically, LTM has extremely high storage capacity, greatly outperforming working memory in the number of specific contextual, object, and spatial associations that can be used to guide perception (Brady et al. 2008; Stokes et al. 2012).

Nobre's laboratory has recently adapted contextual cueing tasks to investigate the neural mechanisms of memory-guided orienting of attention (Fig. 5.4). The experimental paradigm is designed to separate mechanisms related to learning context-target

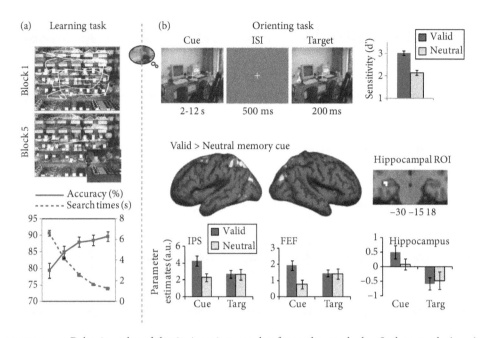

FIGURE 5.4 Behavioural and brain-imaging results from the study by Stokes et al. (2011) showing orienting of spatial attention based on long-term contextual spatial memories. (a) Leftmost panel illustrates the pattern of eye movements (yellow lines on the scene pictures) as participants search for the location of a small pre-designated target stimulus (a key) within 192 complex scenes. Half of the scenes contained a target and the other half did not (counterbalanced). Over five blocks of searching, participants become proficient at finding keys. Whereas they search extensively in the first block, eye movements and the duration of search are greatly reduced by the final block. The bottom graph plots the systematic increase in the number of targets found (solid line) and the decreasing response times to find the target over the successive experimental blocks. Data from Stokes, M. G., Atherton, K., Patai, E. Z. and Nobre, A. C., Long-term memory prepares neural activity for perception, *Proceedings of the National Academy of Sciences of the USA*, 109, E360–7 © 2012, the National Academy of Sciences. (b) The orienting task was performed on the following day during fMRI scanning. Studied scenes (without any target) were presented as cues. Cue duration was lengthy and jittered in order to enable analysis of cue-related fMRI responses. After a brief interval, the scene was repeated briefly with or without an embedded target. Participants were required to make a speeded, forced-choice discrimination response. Scenes in which participants had successfully located the target during the learning session acted as 'valid memory cues', providing 100% predictive information about the spatial location of the upcoming target when present. Scenes in which no targets had been present in the previous learning task acted as 'neutral memory cues', providing no specific information about the likely upcoming target location. The perceptual sensitivity (d') graph shows that participants were reliably better at discriminating the presence of a target after valid memory cues. Equivalent results are obtained when the pacing of the task is quicker and cue durations are reduced to 200 ms (not shown). Brain-imaging results are taken from the simple contrast of cue-related activations when these were 'valid memory cues' compared to when they were 'neutral memory cues'. Memory cues carrying valid predictive information were reliably associated with higher levels of activation in a network of

associations, orienting attention based on learned contexts, and identifying and selecting target items within contexts (Summerfield et al. 2006). In an initial session, participants learn to locate target items across a large set of complex scenes until they reach a stable and high level of performance. On a subsequent day, they perform a memory-guided spatial orienting task, in which the familiar scenes are used as attention cues. Scenes are presented briefly before the appearance of the target item, requiring a detection or discrimination response. Performance is compared for targets appearing at the remembered location from the learning task (valid), a location different to that learned (invalid), or in a scene in which no target location had been learned (neutral). Behavioural measures show reliable benefits of memory-guided orienting on response speed (Summerfield et al. 2006, 2011) and perceptual discrimination (Patai et al. 2012; Stokes et al. 2012; Doallo et al. 2013). The effects develop surprisingly rapidly, being reliably observable at 100 ms cue–target intervals (Summerfield et al. 2006). Electrophysiological recordings during the orienting task show that memory cues induce lateralized alpha-band modulations in anticipation of the target, in a similar pattern to that observed during perceptual visual spatial orienting tasks (Summerfield et al. 2011; Stokes et al 2012). Recordings during target processing reveal modulation of early visual potentials, but also raise the possibility that some of the modulatory mechanisms may differ from those arising from perceptual cues (Summerfield et al. 2011; Patai et al. 2012; Doallo et al. 2012). For instance, contrary to what is observed during visual spatial cueing (Leblanc et al. 2008; Seiss et al. 2009; Brignani et al. 2010; Schankin and Schubo 2010), the N2PC potential related to detecting a target within a visual search array is reliably attenuated by memory cues (Doallo et al. 2012; Patai et al. 2012). fMRI studies show that memory cues trigger activity in the hippocampus as well as in dorsal frontoparietal areas involved in visual spatial attention (Summerfield et al. 2006; Stokes et al. 2012). Ongoing studies continue to characterize the network and dynamics involved in top-down biasing of perception by LTM. One intuitive possibility is that neural mechanisms associated with externally cued attentional orienting are also co-opted for biasing perception according to past experience stored in LTM, with the hippocampus and possibly other areas participating in spatial contextual memories serving as a critical link. Alternatively, activity in brain areas related to spatial contextual memories could influence early visual or other sensory areas directly through feedback, re-entrant connections, independently of the frontoparietal network. Both types of mechanisms could also coexist. The use of interference methods, such as TMS or lesions, will be of crucial importance to determine the extent of overlap and interaction between memory and dorsal frontoparietal attention systems in the dynamic modulation of perception.

---

frontoparietal regions linked to visual spatial attention (see Fig. 5.3). Plots show that the enhanced activations in frontoparietal regions and in the hippocampus are specific to the cue period. Data from Summerfield, J. J., Lepsien, J., Gitelman, D. R., Mesulam, M. M. & Nobre, A. C., Orienting attention based on long-term memory experience, *Neuron*, 49 (6), pp. 905–16 © 2006, Elsevier.

Guidance by motivation

Another widely recognized source of adaptive behavioural control relates to the attainment of rewards and fulfilment of motivational drives (Thorndike 1901). A network of cortical and subcortical areas is thought to guide decision-making and behavioural responses through reinforcement learning, including the ventral tegmental area of the midbrain, the nucleus accumbens in the ventral striatum, and prefrontal and cingulate cortices (O'Doherty 2004). During reinforcement learning, several factors may contribute to behaviour, such as the value and quantity of predicted and obtained reward, action representations, and utility functions.

Research is being increasingly aimed at revealing whether and how motivation and reward-related functions are capable of biasing perceptual functions (see Pessoa (in chapter 25), this volume). So far, results have demonstrated improved perceptual discrimination of stimuli that are motivationally significant, through physiological or monetary reward associations or incentives (e.g. Della Libera and Chelazzi 2006, 2009; Engelmann and Pessoa 2007; Engelmann et al. 2009; Raymond and O'Brien 2009; Kristjansson et al. 2010; Piech et al. 2010; Rutherford et al. 2010; Della Libera et al. 2011). Reward incentives or prior history have also been shown to enhance excitability in visual areas (Serences 2008; Engelmann et al. 2009; Hickey et al. 2010a; Baines et al. 2011; Tosoni et al. 2012).

Understanding whether reward-related influences necessarily occur through the spatial attention network is of major interest. Direct connections between the reward network and sensory areas, such as those between the amygdala and extrastriate cortex, could mediate reward-based perceptual biases originating from areas such as the orbitofrontal cortex (OFC) (Kringelbach and Rolls 2004). Alternatively, reward and motivation could act through the attention-control system (e.g. Padmala and Pessoa 2011), through linking points such as the posterior cingulate (Mesulam et al. 2005) or intraparietal sulcus (Gottlieb and Balan 2010; see Gottlieb (in chapter 12), this volume). A combination of both routes may also occur, and their interaction may depend on the interplay between voluntary and instinctive factors. Separating the functional contributions of reward associations and task goals within a given task can be challenging. These are conflated in many common task designs (see Maunsell 2004), and it may be difficult to prevent voluntary shifts of attention to stimuli with motivational relevance even in designs that formally orthogonalize these factors (see Hickey et al. 2010a, 2010b).

Behavioural and neural measures in humans (Kiss et al. 2009; Hickey et al. 2010a, 2010b, 2011; Anderson et al. 2011a, 2011b; Krebs et al. 2011; Anderson and Yantis 2012; Hickey and van Zoest 2012) and non-human primates (Peck et al. 2009; Gottlieb and Balan 2010) show that stimuli with reward value capture attention automatically, even when task-irrelevant or distracting. Brain-imaging studies combining manipulations of spatial attention and reward incentives have shown that reward incentives can enhance activity in areas involved in control of spatial attention as well as recruit activation in additional limbic regions (Small et al. 2005; Mohanty

et al. 2008, 2009; Engelmann et al. 2009; Tosoni et al. 2012). Studies also implicate posterior cingulate cortex and its connection to parietal cortex as candidates
for mediating the interaction between attention and motivation, though there are
different interpretations regarding the extent to which this region carries primarily reward-related signals (Tosoni et al. 2012) or also contributes to the integration
of reward and spatial orienting functions (Mesulam et al. 2005; Small et al. 2005;
Mohanty et al. 2008).

Both additive and interactive effects have been noted between attention and motivation (see Pessoa and Engelmann 2010; Pessoa (in chapter 25), this volume). By
comparing effects during manipulations of reward incentives versus the requirement
to shift attention in control areas, Tosoni and colleagues (2012) have concluded that
the two sources of control may operate largely independently. Single-unit studies in
area LIP of macaques have also revealed largely independent effects of reward and
spatial orienting (Bendiksby and Platt 2006). Direct comparisons of visual responses
according to manipulations of attention versus reward incentives also show that
modulatory mechanisms are not coextensive, and that reward-related changes in
visual excitability may occur independently of spatial or object-based attention
(Serences and Saproo 2010; Baines et al. 2011).

Multiple sources of bias

In real life motivational signals are often bound to memories. The reward outcomes
of experiences play an important role in shaping what we will approach or avoid in
the future (Shohamy and Adcock 2010). In order to start unravelling how memories of past reward outcomes influence ongoing perceptual processing, Doallo and
colleagues (2013) manipulated reward outcomes during the learning phase of the
memory-based orienting task (Summerfield et al. 2006; Patai et al. 2012). They found
that even one single exposure to a monetary reward outcome after learning a spatial contextual association for a target was sufficient to enhance subsequent behavioural and neural markers of memory-based orienting. The experimental paradigm
provides a way to start investigating the interplay between motivation, memory, and
task goals in shaping perception.

Future work should continue to explore the multiplicity of sources of top-down biasing mechanisms. Are top-down biases from various types of sources such as task goals,
memories, and motivation consistently funnelled through a common large-scale frontoparietal attentional network? Or, are there various lines of bias that can interact with
one another or act independently to influence perception? The latter possibility may call
into question the existence of 'attention' as an autonomous psychological domain, and
instead reveal the selective biasing of information processing as a general property of
cognitive systems.

TYPES OF BIAS

In most, if not all, contemporary theories, attentional biases operate upon receptive-field properties. Anticipatory signals increase spontaneous firing levels of neurons coding the relevant or predicted location or features. Prioritized selection of these attributes in turn leads to suppression of activity in neurons coding other, competing locations or features (Desimone and Duncan 1995; Driver and Frith 2000; Reynolds and Heeger 2009). Understanding how assemblies of neurons with spatially congruent receptive fields can come to be selected to integrate representations of spatially attended objects is intuitive (e.g. Treisman and Gelade 1980; Koch and Ullman 1985) even if figuring out the implementation details is far from trivial. Understanding how feature-based attention can organize cell assemblies (see Chelazzi, et al. 1998; Stokes, et al. 2009) is more difficult, given the lack of clear anatomical segregation according to features within visual areas and the lack of feature-based organization of connections between areas. Nevertheless, it is possible to imagine how flexible, adaptive coding mechanisms (Duncan 2001; Freedman et al. 2001) can set up coalitions of neurons with relevant receptive-field properties and tune excitability through some kind of reverberating (Hebb 1949) or oscillatory activity (Grossberg 1982; Fries 2005).

Ultimately, however, attention models based on prioritization of receptive field properties are insufficient to explain the varieties of attention. Clearly we are able to anticipate and prioritize events based on information that does not map directly onto receptive field properties. Let us illustrate what we ____. Presumably the reader was able to anticipate an end to the previous statement.

Semantic expectations

Seminal early work by Anne Treisman demonstrated that semantic context effects can override selection based on simple features to drive disambiguation and interpretation of stimuli within dichotic listening paradigms (Treisman 1960). Using an orienting paradigm, Neely, and Posner and Snyder, showed that it was possible to direct attention voluntarily to semantic categories of words (Posner and Snyder 1975a 1975b; Neely 1976). Building on this work, Nobre and colleagues compared neural mechanisms of orienting attention to semantic categories versus location of words (see also Moores et al. 2003). An ERP study showed that similar patterns of behavioural facilitation arise from very different modulatory mechanisms (Cristescu and Nobre 2008). fMRI showed selective activation of brain areas involved in semantic analysis (see Gough et al. 2005) when orienting attention to semantic categories, in addition to recruitment of the dorsal frontoparietal network associated with control of spatial attention (Cristescu et al. 2006). Following a similar approach, Miniussi and colleagues (2005) showed behavioural benefits of anticipating different—spatial or verbal—task sets brought about through different modulatory mechanisms. These studies indicate that theoretical and computational models of attention modulation will need to move beyond simple receptive-field biases to take into account the ability to focus selectively on high-level, associative types of representations that are likely to be coded in large populations of neurons across multiple brain regions.

Temporal expectations

Another critical dimension framing our behaviour missing from current models is the 'timing' of events. Building on early work showing facilitation of behaviour by alertness (Posner and Boies 1971) and by predictable intervals between events (foreperiods) (Woodrow 1914; Alegria and Delhaye-Rembaux 1975; Niemi and Näätänen 1981), Nobre and colleagues have demonstrated our ability to orient attention voluntarily and flexibly to predicted or relevant times of target events (Coull and Nobre 1998; Nobre et al. 2011; see Nobre and Rohenkohl (in chapter 24), this volume) (Fig. 5.5). Temporal orienting of attention has proven to be a robust phenomenon, observed in different sensory modalities and across many types of experimental paradigms (see Nobre et al. 2007; Nobre and Rohenkohl (in chapter 24), this volume). Regular rhythmic patterns of stimulation also lead to strong benefits in behavioural performance and perceptual discrimination of target events (Jones 1976; Rohenkohl et al. 2012). The investigation of temporal orienting mechanisms has intensified, and is beginning to tackle the puzzling question of how temporal predictions can be coded and influence perceptual analysis in the absence of temporal receptive fields. Studies comparing temporal versus spatial orienting of attention under controlled experimental conditions show that similar magnitudes of behavioural facilitation come about through distinct modulatory mechanisms (Griffin et al. 2002; Doherty et al. 2005). In addition, when both temporal and spatial expectations are present, these two types of biases can interact synergistically to enhance modulatory mechanisms based on spatial receptive fields (Doherty et al. 2005; Rohenkohl and Nobre 2011). Current research indicates that oscillatory brain activity may play an important role as a conduit for temporal expectations to regulate neural excitability (Lakatos et al. 2008; Schroeder and Lakatos 2009).

SLATES FOR BIASES

There is no single locus at which attention operates. Most attention researchers investigate its effects within vision. Even within the narrow confines of visual perception, modulations can occur at multiple levels of processing (see Serences and Kastner (in chapter 4), this volume) depending on the features that discriminate targets from distractors, the types of attentional biases available, and the requirements of the task. Beyond visual perception, we know attention operates across the different sensory modalities (Spence

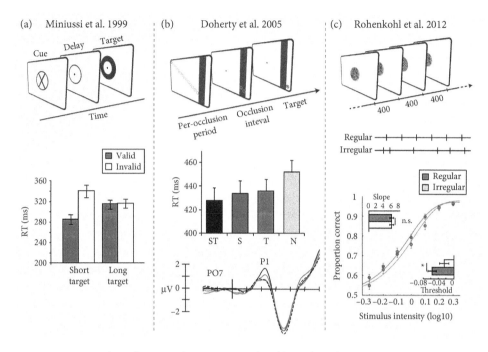

FIGURE 5.5 Examples of temporal orienting tasks. (a) Task and reaction-time results in the study by Miniussi et al. (1999). Foveally presented symbolic cues predicted (80% validity) whether the target would appear after a short (600 ms) or long (1400 ms) interval after cue onset. Targets were easy to discriminate and required a simple speeded detection response (there were 10% of catch trials containing no target). Data from Miniussi, C., Wilding, E. L., Coull, J. T., and Nobre A C. D., Orienting attention in time. Modulation of brain potentials, *Brain*, 122 (Pt 8), pp. 1507–18 © 1999, Oxford University Press http://brain.oxfordjournals.org/. (b) Task and results from Doherty et al. (2005). Spatial and temporal expectations were manipulated orthogonally, according to the spatial and temporal regularity with which a disc traversed the monitor in discrete jumps before it disappeared under an occluding band. Participants had to discriminate whether a small dot appeared with the disc on its reappearance after occlusion, and make a go/no-go response accordingly. Plot of reaction times shows that participants were significantly faster to detect targets appearing at predictable spatial locations (S) or temporal intervals (T) compared to the non-predictive condition (N). Effects of spatial and temporal expectations on reaction times were additive, leading to even faster response times when participants had combined spatio-temporal expectations (ST). Visual event-related potentials over contralateral visual electrodes (plotted for PO7) revealed a marked interaction between spatial and temporal expectations during early visual processing. The early visual P1 potential elicited by targets in the temporal-expectation condition (plotted in red) was no different than the P1 elicited for targets in the non-predictive condition (plotted in dashed line). Targets occurring at predicted spatial locations elicited an enhanced P1 potential (plotted in blue). When combined with spatial expectations, temporal expectations (ST, plotted in black) significantly boosted the gain modulation of the visual P1. Data from Doherty, J. R., Rao, A., Mesulam, M. M. & Nobre, A. C., Synergistic effect of combined temporal and spatial expectations on visual attention, *Journal of Neuroscience*, 25, pp. 8259–66 © 2005, Society for Neuroscience. (c) Task and results by Rohenkohl et al. (2012) showing modulation of perceptual processing by temporal expectations under the right

and Driver 2004) and upon motor representations (Rushworth et al. 1997, 2001) to facilitate our interface with the boundless incoming sensory stream. But, attention does not only face the incoming sensory stream. In fractionating the 'varieties of attention', James suggested a subdivision between 'sensorial attention', directed toward objects of sense, and 'intellectual attention', directed at ideal or represented objects.

Certainly, intuition suggests an ability to orient attention to selective aspects of internalized memory representations that can be independent of continual sensory stimulation. For some time, however, it appeared this intuition was wrong. Early empirical work suggested that the ability to orient spatial attention to memory was confined to fractions of a second, when representations were said to be in an 'iconic' state (Sperling 1960; Averbach and Coriell 1961). Spatial cues prompting selective retrieval (post-cues) after this brief iconic period were found to be ineffective at improving performance (Phillips and Baddeley 1971; Phillips 1974). The more enduring form of visual short-term memory (VSTM) is highly limited in capacity, and is usually considered the result of attention operating on the sensory stream to direct selective encoding and to support maintenance (Cowan 1995; Awh and Jonides 2001; Postle 2006). Its contents were considered not to be susceptible to further selective modulation (Sperling 1960; Sternberg 1966).

Two groups of researchers independently re-examined the question of attentional control over the contents of VSTM (Griffin and Nobre 2003; Landman et al. 2003). They presented cues in the period during which a memory array was being maintained in VSTM indicating the location of the item from the memory array that was likely to be required for a subsequent memory-based judgement (Fig. 5.6). These retrodictive cues (retro-cues), enabling orienting of spatial attention to selective locations of VSTM representations, conferred clear behavioural advantages. Retro-cueing effects are robust and by now are firmly established through numerous replications (see Nobre and Stokes 2011; Gazzaley and Nobre 2012; Stokes and Nobre 2012; Kuhl and Chun (in chapter 28), this volume).

◄───

experimental conditions. Gaussian noise-patch stimuli occurred in a temporally predictive, rhythmic stream (50 ms duration, 400 ms onset asynchrony) (shown) or in a non-predictive, arrhythmic stream (50 ms duration, 200–600 onset asynchrony). Target Gabor patches were superimposed on a minority (10%) of the noise patches. These were indicated by a pink surrounding placeholder, which prompted participants to make a forced-choice discrimination about the clockwise or counter-clockwise orientation of the target. Targets appeared at one of seven luminance contrast levels, anchored to individuals' 75% accuracy performance in a previous session. The intervals surrounding the targets were kept exactly the same for the regular and irregular condition. Performance was significantly improved for the predictive, regular condition (plotted in red) than in the non-predictive, irregular condition (grey). The psychometric function shows enhanced contrast sensitivity levels, with improved threshold levels, for the regular condition. The slope of the psychometric function remained unchanged. Response times were also significantly and consistently improved for the regular condition (not shown). Modelling (not shown) suggested that rhythmic temporal expectation in this task enhanced the signal-to-noise gain of the sensory evidence upon which decisions were made Data from Rohenkohl, G., Cravo, A. M., Wyart, V., and Nobre, A. C., Temporal expectation improves the quality of sensory information, *Journal of Neuroscience*, 32, pp. 8424–8 © 2012, Society for Neuroscience.

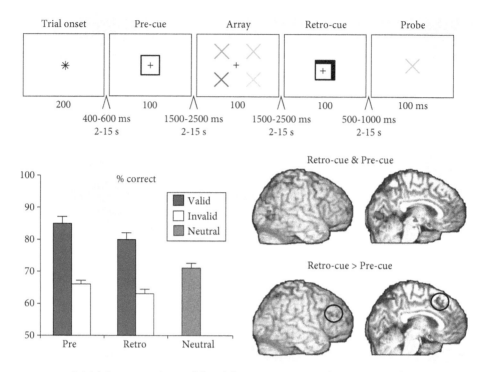

FIGURE 5.6 Initial demonstrations of the ability to orient spatial attention within arrays maintained in visual short-term memory. The top panel illustrates the behavioural task used in Griffin and Nobre (2003, Experiment 1) and adapted for fMRI in the study by Nobre et al. (2004). Intervals for blank displays in between the trial events were shorter in the task used for the behavioural study (top row) than for the fMRI study (bottom row). In the behavioural study, participants viewed an array of four different colours. At the end of the trial they viewed a probe array and made a forced-choice response to indicate whether the probe had been present or absent in the previous array (50% likelihood). Spatially predictive cues (80% valid) were presented either before (pre-cue) or after (retro-cue) the array. In the example shown, a valid retro-cue points to the location in which the target was present. The accuracy plot shows that participants are more accurate when predictive spatial cues are provided compared to trials in which only neutral cues are presented. Their accuracy is significantly worse when spatial cues are misleading (invalid). Interestingly, the magnitude of the cueing effects was similar for retro-cues and pre-cues. In the imaging study, pre-cues and retro-cues cues were imperative, and participants judged whether the probe matched the cued item. The imaging results show activations specific for spatial pre-cues and retro-cues (compared to non-spatial cues at the same trial frame). Both types of spatial cues activated a similar frontoparietal network of regions, including the intraparietal sulcus and the frontal eye fields, as shown in the conjunction analysis (retro-cue and pre-cue). Retro-cues showed enhanced activations in some of the parietal areas and engaged additional lateral and medial prefrontal regions (circled). Data from Nobre, A. C., Coull, J. T., Maquet, P., Frith, C. D., Vandenberghe, R., and Mesulam, M. M., Orienting attention to locations in perceptual versus mental representations, *Journal of Cognitive Neuroscience*, 16, pp. 363–73 © 2004, Massachusetts Institute of Technology.

Retro-cues are different from post-cues. They do not prompt immediate retrieval, but instead trigger top-down biasing mechanisms that operate on representations being maintained in VSTM to guide subsequent performance. The mechanisms by which attentional orienting can facilitate maintenance and/or retrieval of representations in VSTM are still being detailed. Brain-imaging studies so far suggest involvement of similar control mechanisms as during orienting to perceptual representations with possible recruitment of additional, selective regulatory mechanisms mediated by prefrontal areas (Nobre et al. 2004; Lepsien and Nobre 2007; Bledowski et al. 2009; Nee and Jonides 2009; Lepsien et al. 2011; Tamber-Rosenau et al. 2011). Modulation of visual processing similar to that which occurs during perceptual orienting has also been observed (Lepsien and Nobre 2007; Sligte et al. 2009; Higo et al. 2011), although it is sometimes challenging to separate modulation of maintenance-related activity in posterior visual areas participating in VSTM from modulation related to anticipating the subsequent probe stimulus (Lepsien and Nobre 2007; Lepsien et al. 2011). Similar behavioural and neural patterns of effects have also been observed after cues prompting participants to refresh their current focus in VSTM by thinking back to a specific previously viewed item (Johnson et al. 2007; Yi et al. 2008; Johnson and Johnson 2009).

The existence of a form of James' 'intellectual' attention has thus been confirmed. Prioritization and selection of information is not confined to operate upon the incoming sensory stream and immediate perception–action cycle. Instead, selective attention can also operate on internalized, 'off-line' representations that are no longer supported by sensory stimulation to facilitate behaviour.

A natural extension of 'off-line' attention is to consider its putative role in the voluntary retrieval of selective long-term memories (see Nobre and Stokes 2012; Kuhl and Chun (in chapter 28), this volume; Kuhl et al. 2012). A recent model, for example, proposes that mechanisms of endogenous versus exogenous orienting of attention mediate voluntary and spontaneous long-term memory retrieval respectively (Cabeza et al. 2008). Others suggest that separate functional anatomical mechanisms mediate perceptual attention control and memory retrieval (Hutchinson et al. 2009; Sestieri et al. 2010), which may be in competition with one another (Guerin et al. 2012). This is clearly a fascinating area of fundamental interest, which deserves further investigation (see Kuhl and Chun (in chapter 28), this volume).

Summary

Bringing together goals, expectations, intentions, memories, and motivations to guide our perception, choices, actions, and memories through biases about the locations, features, timings, and associations of anticipated events, the functions of attention pervade every aspect of our cognitive life. This plurality of sources, slates, and types of attentional biases invites a reconsideration of the very conceptualization of attention. It may be time to do away with narrow views of 'attention' that delimit it as an independent domain within cognition operating through a set of consistent modulatory mechanisms, and instead embrace the notion that selective biasing is a hallmark embedded property of information processing throughout cognitive functions. Through mechanisms of voluntary control 'each of us literally chooses, by his ways of attending to things, what sort of a universe he shall appear to himself to inhabit' (James 1890/1950: 425–426).

NOTE

1. Task relevance and likelihood of events are, of course, conceptually separable and can be manipulated independently (Summerfield and Egner 2009). However, in practice, these two types of manipulations are often combined or used interchangeably to prompt shifts in spatial or object-based attention. It could be argued that these constructs go hand-in-hand, and show a large degree of interaction. In the limit, it may seem absurd to set goals about highly unlikely or impossible events, and wasteful to generate expectations about any and all possible irrelevant events. Nevertheless, the mechanisms that underpin these different types of biasing signals may rely on fundamentally different neural mechanisms. It will be interesting and important to characterize each of these in turn, as well as how they interact, in order to understand the repertoire of attention mechanisms and their implications in psychological, neuropsychiatric, and neurological disorders. Initial investigations along these lines are beginning to yield alluring findings (Wyart et al. 2012). *Proceedings of the National Academy of Sciences USA.*

REFERENCES

al-Haytham, A. I. (1021/1989). *The Optics of Ibn al-Haytham: Books I–III: On Direct Vision.* London: Warburg Institute.

Alegria, J. and Delhaye-Rembaux, M. (1975). Sequential effects of foreperiod duration and conditional probability of the signal in a choice reaction time task. *Acta Psychologica 39*: 321–328.

Allport, A. (1987). Selection for action: Some behavioral and neurophysiological considerations of attention and action. In H. Heuer and A. F. Sanders (eds.), *Perspectives on Perception and Action* (pp. 395–419). Hillsdale, N.J.: Lawrence Erlbaum Associates.

Anderson, B. A., Laurent, P. A., and Yantis, S. (2011a). Learned value magnifies salience-based attentional capture. *PLoS One 6*: e27926.

Anderson, B. A., Laurent, P. A., and Yantis, S. (2011b). Value-driven attentional capture. *Proceedings of the National Academy of Sciences USA 108*: 10367–10371.

Anderson, B. A. and Yantis, S. (2012). Value-driven attentional and oculomotor capture during goal-directed, unconstrained viewing. *Attention, Perception, & Psychophysics 74*: 1644–1653.

Anderson, T. J., Jenkins, I. H., Brooks, D. J., Hawken, M. B., Frackowiak, R. S., and Kennard, C. (1994). Cortical control of saccades and fixation in man: A PET study. *Brain 117*(Pt 5): 1073–1084.

Armstrong, K. M., Fitzgerald, J. K., and Moore, T. (2006). Changes in visual receptive fields with microstimulation of frontal cortex. *Neuron 50*: 791–798.

Armstrong, K. M. and Moore, T. (2007). Rapid enhancement of visual cortical response discriminability by microstimulation of the frontal eye field. *Proceedings of the National Academy of Sciences USA 104*: 9499–9504.

Astafiev, S. V., Shulman, G. L., Stanley, C. M., Snyder, A. Z., Van Essen, D. C., and Corbetta, M. (2003). Functional organization of human intraparietal and frontal cortex for attending, looking, and pointing. *Journal of Neuroscience* 23: 4689–4699.

Astafiev, S. V., Stanley, C. M., Shulman, G. L., and Corbetta, M. (2004). Extrastriate body area in human occipital cortex responds to the performance of motor actions. *Nature Neuroscience* 7: 542–548.

Averbach, E. and Coriell, A. S. (1961). Short term memory in vision. *Bell Systems Technical Journal* 40: 309–328.

Awh, E. and Jonides, J. (2001). Overlapping mechanisms of attention and spatial working memory. *Trends in Cognitive Sciences* 5: 119–126.

Baines, S., Ruz, M., Rao, A., Denison, R., and Nobre, A. C. (2011). Modulation of neural activity by motivational and spatial biases. *Neuropsychologia* 49: 2489–2897.

Bartolomeo, P., Thiebaut de Schotten, M., and Doricchi, F. (2007). Left unilateral neglect as a disconnection syndrome. *Cerebral Cortex* 17: 2479–2490.

Becker, M. W. and Rasmussen, I. P. (2008). Guidance of attention to objects and locations by long-term memory of natural scenes. *Journal of Experimental Psychology: Learning, Memory, and Cognition* 34: 1325–1338.

Belopolsky, A. V. and Theeuwes, J. (2012). Updating the premotor theory: The allocation of attention is not always accompanied by saccade preparation. *Journal of Experimental Psychology: Human Perception and Performance* 38: 902–914.

Bendiksby, M. S. and Platt, M. L. (2006). Neural correlates of reward and attention in macaque area LIP. *Neuropsychologia* 44: 2411–2420.

Berger, A., Henik, A., and Rafal, R. (2005). Competition between endogenous and exogenous orienting of visual attention. *Journal of Experimental Psychology: General* 134: 207–221.

Bianchi, L. (1895). The functions of the frontal lobes. *Brain* 18: 497–522.

Bisley, J. W. and Goldberg, M. E. (2010). Attention, intention, and priority in the parietal lobe. *Annual Review of Neuroscience* 33: 1–21.

Blankenburg, F., Ruff, C. C., Bestmann, S., Bjoertomt, O., Josephs, O., Deichmann, R., and Driver, J. (2010). Studying the role of human parietal cortex in visuospatial attention with concurrent TMS–fMRI. *Cerebral Cortex* 20: 2702–2711.

Bledowski, C., Rahm, B., and Rowe, J. B. (2009). What 'works' in working memory? Separate systems for selection and updating of critical information. *Journal of Neuroscience* 29: 13735–13741.

Brady, T. F., Konkle, T., Alvarez, G. A., and Oliva, A. (2008). Visual long-term memory has a massive storage capacity for object details. *Proceedings of the National Academy of Sciences USA* 105: 14325–14329.

Brain, W. R. (1941). A form of visual disorientation resulting from lesions of the right cerebral hemisphere: Section of neurology. *Proceedings of the Royal Society of Medicine* 34: 71–76.

Brignani, D., Guzzon, D., Marzi, C. A., and Miniussi, C. (2009). Attentional orienting induced by arrows and eye-gaze compared with an endogenous cue. *Neuropsychologia* 47: 370–381.

Brignani, D., Lepsien, J., and Nobre, A. C. (2010). Purely endogenous capture of attention by task-defining features proceeds independently from spatial attention. *NeuroImage* 51: 859–866.

Broadbent, D. E. (1958). *Perception and Communication*. New York: Pergamon Press.

Brockmole, J. R., Castelhano, M. S., and Henderson, J. M. (2006). Contextual cueing in naturalistic scenes: Global and local contexts. *Journal of Experimental Psychology: Learning, Memory, and Cognition* 32: 699–706.

Buchel, C. and Friston, K. J. (1997). Modulation of connectivity in visual pathways by attention: Cortical interactions evaluated with structural equation modelling and fMRI. *Cerebral Cortex* 7: 768–778.

Buschman, T. J. and Miller, E. K. (2007). Top-down versus bottom-up control of attention in the prefrontal and posterior parietal cortices. *Science* 315: 1860–1862.

Buschman, T. J., Siegel, M., Roy, J. E., and Miller, E. K. (2011). Neural substrates of cognitive capacity limitations. *Proceedings of the National Academy of Sciences USA* 108: 11252–11255.

Bushnell, M. C., Goldberg, M. E., and Robinson, D. L. (1981). Behavioral enhancement of visual responses in monkey cerebral cortex. I: Modulation in posterior parietal cortex related to selective visual attention. *Journal of Neurophysiology* 46: 755–772.

Cabeza, R., Ciaramelli, E., Olson, I. R., and Moscovitch, M. (2008). The parietal cortex and episodic memory: An attentional account. *Nature Reviews Neuroscience* 9: 613–625.

Capotosto, P., Babiloni, C., Romani, G. L., and Corbetta, M. (2009). Frontoparietal cortex controls spatial attention through modulation of anticipatory alpha rhythms. *Journal of Neuroscience* 29: 5863–5872.

Chafee, M. V. and Goldman-Rakic, P. S. (1998). Matching patterns of activity in primate prefrontal area 8a and parietal area 7ip neurons during a spatial working memory task. *Journal of Neurophysiology* 79: 2919–2940.

Chelazzi, L., Duncan, J., Miller, E. K., and Desimone, R. (1998). Responses of neurons in inferior temporal cortex during memory-guided visual search. *Journal of Neurophysiology* 80: 2918–2940.

Chelazzi, L., Miller, E. K., Duncan, J., and Desimone, R. (1993). A neural basis for visual search in inferior temporal cortex. *Nature* 363: 345–347.

Cherry, E. C. (1953). Some experiments on the recognition of speech with one and with two ears. *Journal of the Acoustical Society of America* 25: 975–979.

Chica, A. B., Bartolomeo, P., and Lupiañez, J. (2013). Two cognitive and neural systems for endogenous and exogenous spatial attention. *Behavioural Brain Research* 237: 107–123.

Chica, A. B., Lupiañez, J., and Bartolomeo, P. (2006). Dissociating inhibition of return from endogenous orienting of spatial attention: Evidence from detection and discrimination tasks. *Cognitive Neuropsychology* 23: 1015–1034.

Chun, M. M. and Jiang, Y. (1998). Contextual cueing: Implicit learning and memory of visual context guides spatial attention. *Cognitive Psychology* 36: 28–71.

Chun, M. M. and Jiang, Y. (2003). Implicit, long-term spatial contextual memory. *Journal of Experimental Psychology: Learning, Memory, and Cognition* 29: 224–234.

Ciaraffa, F., Castelli, G., Parati, E. A., Bartolomeo, P., and Bizzi, A. (2013). Visual neglect as a disconnection syndrome? A confirmatory case report. *Neurocase* 19: 351–359.

Cohen, J. Y., Pouget, P., Heitz, R. P., Woodman, G. F., and Schall, J. D. (2009). Biophysical support for functionally distinct cell types in the frontal eye field. *Journal of Neurophysiology* 101: 912–916.

Colby, C. L. and Duhamel, J. R. (1996). Spatial representations for action in parietal cortex. *Brain Research: Cognitive Brain Research* 5: 105–115.

Committeri, G., Pitzalis, S., Galati, G., Patria, F., Pelle, G., Sabatini, U., Castriota-Scanderbeg, A., Piccardi, L., Guariglia, C., and Pizzamiglio, L. (2007). Neural bases of personal and extrapersonal neglect in humans. *Brain* 130: 431–441.

Corbetta, M., Akbudak, E., Conturo, T. E., Snyder, A. Z., Ollinger, J. M., Drury, H. A., Linenweber, M. R., Petersen, S. E., Raichle, M. E., Van Essen, D. C., and Shulman, G. L. (1998). A common network of functional areas for attention and eye movements. *Neuron* 21: 761–773.

Corbetta, M., Kincade, M. J., Lewis, C., Snyder, A. Z., and Sapir, A. (2005). Neural basis and recovery of spatial attention deficits in spatial neglect. *Nature Neuroscience* 8: 1603–1610.

Corbetta, M., Kincade, J. M., Ollinger, J. M., McAvoy, M. P., and Shulman, G. L. (2000). Voluntary orienting is dissociated from target detection in human posterior parietal cortex. *Nature Neuroscience* 3: 292–297.

Corbetta, M., Miezin, F. M., Shulman, G. L., and Petersen, S. E. (1993). A PET study of visuospatial attention. *Journal of Neuroscience* 13: 1202–1226.

Corbetta, M. and Shulman, G. L. (2002). Control of goal-directed and stimulus-driven attention in the brain. *Nature Reviews Neuroscience* 3: 201–215.

Corbetta, M. and Shulman, G. L. (2011). Spatial neglect and attention networks. *Annual Review of Neuroscience* 34: 569–599.

Corbetta, M., Shulman, G. L., Miezin, F. M., and Petersen, S. E. (1995). Superior parietal cortex activation during spatial attention shifts and visual feature conjunction. *Science* 270: 802–805.

Coull, J. T. and Nobre, A. C. (1998). Where and when to pay attention: The neural systems for directing attention to spatial locations and to time intervals as revealed by both PET and fMRI. *Journal of Neuroscience* 18: 7426–7435.

Cowan, N. (1995). Sensory memory and its role in information processing. *Electroencephalography and Clinical Neurophysiology Supplement* 44: 21–31.

Cowey, A. and Latto, R. M. (1971). Effects of frontal eye-field ablation on visual fields and on fixation in rhesus monkeys. *Brain Research* 31: 375–376.

Cristescu, T. C., Devlin, J. T., and Nobre, A. C. (2006). Orienting attention to semantic categories. *NeuroImage* 33: 1178–1187.

Cristescu, T. C. and Nobre, A. C. (2008). Differential modulation of word recognition by semantic and spatial orienting of attention. *Journal of Cognitive Neuroscience* 20: 787–801.

Darby, D. G., Nobre, A. C., Thangaraj, V., Edelman, R., Mesulam, M. M., and Warach, S. (1996). Cortical activation in the human brain during lateral saccades using EPISTAR functional magnetic resonance imaging. *NeuroImage* 3: 53–62.

Dean, H. L., Crowley, J. C., and Platt, M. L. (2004). Visual and saccade-related activity in macaque posterior cingulate cortex. *Journal of Neurophysiology* 92: 3056–3068.

Della Libera, C. and Chelazzi, L. (2006). Visual selective attention and the effects of monetary rewards. *Psychological Science* 17: 222–227.

Della Libera, C. and Chelazzi, L. (2009). Learning to attend and to ignore is a matter of gains and losses. *Psychological Science* 20: 778–784.

Della Libera, C., Perlato, A., and Chelazzi, L. (2011). Dissociable effects of reward on attentional learning: from passive associations to active monitoring. *PLoS One* 6: e19460.

Denny-Brown, D. and Chambers, R. A. (1958). The parietal lobe and behavior. *Research Publications: Association for Research in Nervous and Mental Disease* 36: 35–117.

Desimone, R. and Duncan, J. (1995). Neural mechanisms of selective visual attention. *Annual Review of Neuroscience* 18: 193–222.

Deutsch, J. A. and Deutsch, D. (1963). Attention: Some theoretical considerations. *Psychological Review* 87: 272–300.

di Pellegrino, G., Fadiga, L., Fogassi, L., Gallese, V., and Rizzolatti, G. (1992). Understanding motor events: A neurophysiological study. *Experimental Brain Research* 91: 176–180.

Doallo, S., Patai, E. Z., and Nobre, A. C. (2013). Reward associations magnify memory-based biases on perception. *Journal of Cognitive Neuroscience* 25: 245–257.

Doherty, J. R., Rao, A., Mesulam, M. M., and Nobre, A. C. (2005). Synergistic effect of combined temporal and spatial expectations on visual attention. *Journal of Neuroscience* 25: 8259–8266.

Doricchi, F., Thiebaut de Schotten, M., Tomaiuolo, F., and Bartolomeo, P. (2008). White matter (dis)connections and gray matter (dys)functions in visual neglect: Gaining insights into the brain networks of spatial awareness. *Cortex 44*: 983–995.

Doricchi, F. and Tomaiuolo, F. (2003). The anatomy of neglect without hemianopia: A key role for parietal-frontal disconnection? *NeuroReport 14*: 2239–2243.

Driver, J., Blankenburg, F., Bestmann, S., and Ruff, C. C. (2010). New approaches to the study of human brain networks underlying spatial attention and related processes. *Experimental Brain Research 206*: 153–162.

Driver, J. and Frith, C. (2000). Shifting baselines in attention research. *Nature Reviews Neuroscience 1*: 147–148.

Driver, J. and Vuilleumier, P. (2001). Perceptual awareness and its loss in unilateral neglect and extinction. *Cognition 79*: 39–88.

Duncan, J. (2001). An adaptive coding model of neural function in prefrontal cortex. *Nature Reviews Neuroscience 2*: 820–829.

Engelmann, J. B., Damaraju, E., Padmala, S., and Pessoa, L. (2009). Combined effects of attention and motivation on visual task performance: Transient and sustained motivational effects. *Frontiers in Human Neuroscience 3*: 4.

Engelmann, J. B. and Pessoa, L. (2007). Motivation sharpens exogenous spatial attention. *Emotion 7*: 668–674.

Feldman, H. and Friston, K. J. (2010). Attention, uncertainty, and free-energy. *Frontiers in Human Neuroscience 4*: 215.

Fink, G. R., Dolan, R. J., Halligan, P. W., Marshall, J. C., and Frith, C. D. (1997). Space-based and object-based visual attention: Shared and specific neural domains. *Brain 120*(Pt 11): 2013–2028.

Fortuyn, J. D. (1979). On the neurology of perception. *Clinical Neurology and Neurosurgery 81*: 97–107.

Fox, P. T., Raichle, M. E., and Thach, W. T. (1985). Functional mapping of the human cerebellum with positron emission tomography. *Proceedings of the National Academy of Sciences USA 82*: 7462–7466.

Freedman, D. J., Riesenhuber, M., Poggio, T., and Miller, E. K. (2001). Categorical representation of visual stimuli in the primate prefrontal cortex. *Science 291*: 312–316.

Friedrich, F. J., Egly, R., Rafal, R. D., and Beck, D. (1998). Spatial attention deficits in humans: A comparison of superior parietal and temporal-parietal junction lesions. *Neuropsychology 12*: 193–207.

Fries, P. (2005). A mechanism for cognitive dynamics: Neuronal communication through neuronal coherence. *Trends in Cognitive Sciences 9*: 474–480.

Friston, K. (2009). The free-energy principle: A rough guide to the brain? *Trends in Cognitive Sciences 13*: 293–301.

Gaffan, D. and Hornak, J. (1997). Visual neglect in the monkey: Representation and disconnection. *Brain 120*(Pt 9): 1647–1657.

Gazzaley, A. and Nobre, A. C. (2012). Top-down modulation: Bridging selective attention and working memory. *Trends in Cognitive Sciences 16*: 129–135.

Geschwind, N. (1965a). Disconnexion syndromes in animals and man. I. *Brain 88*: 237–294.

Geschwind, N. (1965b). Disconnexion syndromes in animals and man. II. *Brain 88*: 585–644.

Giesbrecht, B., Woldorff, M. G., Song, A. W., and Mangun, G. R. (2003). Neural mechanisms of top-down control during spatial and feature attention. *NeuroImage 19*: 496–512.

Gillebert, C. R., Dyrholm, M., Vangkilde, S., Kyllingsbaek, S., Peeters, R., and Vandenberghe, R. (2012). Attentional priorities and access to short-term memory: Parietal interactions. *NeuroImage 62*: 1551–1562.

Gillebert, C. R., Mantini, D., Thijs, V., Sunaert, S., Dupont, P., and Vandenberghe, R. (2011). Lesion evidence for the critical role of the intraparietal sulcus in spatial attention. *Brain* 134: 1694–1709.

Gitelman, D. R., Nobre, A. C., Parrish, T. B., LaBar, K. S., Kim, Y. H., Meyer, J. R., and Mesulam, M. (1999). A large-scale distributed network for covert spatial attention: Further anatomical delineation based on stringent behavioural and cognitive controls. *Brain* 122(Pt 6): 1093–1106.

Gitelman, D. R., Parrish, T. B., Friston, K. J., and Mesulam, M. M. (2002). Functional anatomy of visual search: Regional segregations within the frontal eye fields and effective connectivity of the superior colliculus. *NeuroImage* 15: 970–982.

Golay, L., Schnider, A., and Ptak, R. (2008). Cortical and subcortical anatomy of chronic spatial neglect following vascular damage. *Behavioral and Brain Functions* 4: 43.

Gold, J. I. and Shadlen, M. N. (2007). The neural basis of decision making. *Annual Review of Neuroscience* 30: 535–574.

Gottlieb, J. and Balan, P. (2010). Attention as a decision in information space. *Trends in Cognitive Sciences* 14: 240–248.

Gottlieb, J. P., Kusunoki, M., and Goldberg, M. E. (1998). The representation of visual salience in monkey parietal cortex. *Nature* 391: 481–484.

Gould, I. C., Nobre, A. C., Wyart, V., and Rushworth, M. F. (2012). Effects of decision variables and intraparietal stimulation on sensorimotor oscillatory activity in the human brain. *Journal of Neuroscience* 32: 13805–13818.

Gregoriou, G. G., Gotts, S. J., and Desimone, R. (2012). Cell-type-specific synchronization of neural activity in FEF with V4 during attention. *Neuron* 73: 581–594.

Gregoriou, G. G., Gotts, S. J., Zhou, H., and Desimone, R. (2009). High-frequency, long-range coupling between prefrontal and visual cortex during attention. *Science* 324: 1207–1210.

Grent-'t-Jong, T. and Woldorff, M. G. (2007). Timing and sequence of brain activity in top-down control of visual-spatial attention. *PLoS Biology* 5: e12.

Griffin, I. C., Miniussi, C., and Nobre, A. C. (2002). Multiple mechanisms of selective attention: Differential modulation of stimulus processing by attention to space or time. *Neuropsychologia* 40: 2325–2340.

Griffin, I. C. and Nobre, A. C. (2003). Orienting attention to locations in internal representations. *Journal of Cognitive Neuroscience* 15: 1176–1194.

Grossberg, S. (1982). *Studies of Mind and Brain: Neural Principles of Learning, Perception, Development, Cognition, and Motor Control*. Dordrecht: Springer.

Guerin, S. A., Robbins, C. A., Gilmore, A. W., and Schacter, D. L. (2012). Interactions between visual attention and episodic retrieval: Dissociable contributions of parietal regions during gist-based false recognition. *Neuron* 75: 1122–1134.

Harter, M. R., Anllo-Vento, L., and Wood, F. B. (1989). Event-related potentials, spatial orienting, and reading disabilities. *Psychophysiology* 26: 404–421.

He, B. J., Snyder, A. Z., Vincent, J. L., Epstein, A., Shulman, G. L., and Corbetta, M. (2007). Breakdown of functional connectivity in frontoparietal networks underlies behavioral deficits in spatial neglect. *Neuron* 53: 905–918.

Hebb, D. O. (1949). *The Organization of Behavior: A Neuropsychological Theory*. New York: John Wiley.

Hecaen, H., Penfield, W., Bertrand, C., and Malmo, R. (1956). The syndrome of apractognosia due to lesions of the minor cerebral hemisphere. *AMA Archives of Neurology and Psychiatry* 75: 400–434.

Heilman, K. M., Pandya, D. N., and Geschwind, N. (1970). Trimodal inattention following parietal lobe ablations. *Transactions of the American Neurological Association* 95: 259–261.

Heilman, K. M. and Van Den Abell, T. (1980). Right hemisphere dominance for attention: The mechanism underlying hemispheric asymmetries of inattention (neglect). *Neurology* 30: 327–330.

Heinen, K., Ruff, C. C., Bjoertomt, O., Schenkluhn, B., Bestmann, S., Blankenburg, F., Driver, J., and Chambers, C. D. (2011). Concurrent TMS–fMRI reveals dynamic interhemispheric influences of the right parietal cortex during exogenously cued visuospatial attention. *European Journal of Neuroscience* 33: 991–1000.

Helmholtz, H. von (1867). *Handbuch der physiologischen Optik*. Leipzig: L. Voss.

Hickey, C., Chelazzi, L., and Theeuwes, J. (2010a). Reward changes salience in human vision via the anterior cingulate. *Journal of Neuroscience* 30: 11096–11103.

Hickey, C., Chelazzi, L., and Theeuwes, J. (2010b). Reward guides vision when it's your thing: Trait reward-seeking in reward-mediated visual priming. *PLoS One* 5: e14087.

Hickey, C., Olivers, C., Meeter, M., and Theeuwes, J. (2011). Feature priming and the capture of visual attention: Linking two ambiguity resolution hypotheses. *Brain Research* 1370: 175–184.

Hickey, C. and van Zoest, W. (2012). Reward creates oculomotor salience. *Current Biology* 22: R219–R220.

Higo, T., Mars, R. B., Boorman, E. D., Buch, E. R., and Rushworth, M. F. (2011). Distributed and causal influence of frontal operculum in task control. *Proceedings of the National Academy of Sciences USA* 108: 4230–4235.

Hillis, A. E., Newhart, M., Heidler, J., Barker, P. B., Herskovits, E. H., and Degaonkar, M. (2005). Anatomy of spatial attention: Insights from perfusion imaging and hemispatial neglect in acute stroke. *Journal of Neuroscience* 25: 3161–3167.

Hillyard, S. A., Hink, R. F., Schwent, V. L., and Picton, T. W. (1973). Electrical signs of selective attention in the human brain. *Science* 182: 177–180.

Hopf, J. M. and Mangun, G. R. (2000). Shifting visual attention in space: An electrophysiological analysis using high spatial resolution mapping. *Clinical Neurophysiology* 111: 1241–1257.

Hopfinger, J. B., Buonocore, M. H., and Mangun, G. R. (2000). The neural mechanisms of top-down attentional control. *Nature Neuroscience* 3: 284–291.

Husain, M. and Rorden, C. (2003). Non-spatially lateralized mechanisms in hemispatial neglect. *Nature Reviews Neuroscience* 4: 26–36.

Hutchinson, J. B., Uncapher, M. R., and Wagner, A. D. (2009). Posterior parietal cortex and episodic retrieval: Convergent and divergent effects of attention and memory. *Learning & Memory* 16: 343–356.

Hyvarinen, J. and Poranen, A. (1974). Function of the parietal associative area 7 as revealed from cellular discharges in alert monkeys. *Brain* 97: 673–692.

Indovina, I. and Macaluso, E. (2007). Dissociation of stimulus relevance and saliency factors during shifts of visuospatial attention. *Cerebral Cortex* 17: 1701–1711.

Isomura, Y. and Takada, M. (2004). Neural mechanisms of versatile functions in primate anterior cingulate cortex. *Review of Neuroscience* 15: 279–291.

James, W. A. (1890/1950). *The Principles of Psychology*. New York: Dover.

Johnson, M. R. and Johnson, M. K. (2009). Top-down enhancement and suppression of activity in category-selective extrastriate cortex from an act of reflective attention. *Journal of Cognitive Neuroscience* 21: 2320–2327.

Johnson, M. R., Mitchell, K. J., Raye, C. L., D'Esposito, M., and Johnson, M. K. (2007). A brief thought can modulate activity in extrastriate visual areas: Top-down effects of refreshing just-seen visual stimuli. *NeuroImage* 37: 290–299.

Jones, M. R. (1976). Time, our lost dimension: Toward a new theory of perception, attention, and memory. *Psychological Review* 83: 323–355.

Jonides, J. and Irwin, D. E. (1981). Capturing attention. *Cognition 10*: 145–150.

Juan, C. H., Shorter-Jacobi, S. M., and Schall, J. D. (2004). Dissociation of spatial attention and saccade preparation. *Proceedings of the National Academy of Sciences USA 101*: 15541–15544.

Kahneman, D. and Treisman, A. (1984). Changing views of attention and automaticity. In R. Parasuraman and R. Davies (eds.), *Varieties of Attention* (pp. 29–61). New York: Academic Press.

Kaping, D., Vinck, M., Hutchison, R. M., Everling, S., and Womelsdorf, T. (2011). Specific contributions of ventromedial, anterior cingulate, and lateral prefrontal cortex for attentional selection and stimulus valuation. *PLoS Biology 9*: e1001224.

Karnath, H. O., Ferber, S., and Himmelbach, M. (2001). Spatial awareness is a function of the temporal not the posterior parietal lobe. *Nature 411*: 950–953.

Karnath, H. O., Himmelbach, M., and Rorden, C. (2002). The subcortical anatomy of human spatial neglect: Putamen, caudate nucleus and pulvinar. *Brain 125*: 350–360.

Kastner, S., DeSimone, K., Konen, C. S., Szczepanski, S. M., Weiner, K. S., and Schneider, K. A. (2007). Topographic maps in human frontal cortex revealed in memory-guided saccade and spatial working-memory tasks. *Journal of Neurophysiology 97*: 3494–3507.

Kastner, S., Pinsk, M. A., De Weerd, P., Desimone, R., and Ungerleider, L. G. (1999). Increased activity in human visual cortex during directed attention in the absence of visual stimulation. *Neuron 22*: 751–761.

Kastner, S. and Ungerleider, L. G. (2000). Mechanisms of visual attention in the human cortex. *Annual Review of Neuroscience 23*: 315–341.

Kelley, T. A., Serences, J. T., Giesbrecht, B., and Yantis, S. (2008). Cortical mechanisms for shifting and holding visuospatial attention. *Cerebral Cortex 18*: 114–125.

Kennard, M. A. (1939). Alterations in response to visual stimuli following lesions of frontal lobe in monkey. *Archives of Neurology & Psychiatry 41*: 1153–1165.

Khan, A. Z., Blohm, G., McPeek, R. M., and Lefevre, P. (2009). Differential influence of attention on gaze and head movements. *Journal of Neurophysiology 101*: 198–206.

Kim, Y. H., Gitelman, D. R., Nobre, A. C., Parrish, T. B., LaBar, K. S., and Mesulam, M. M. (1999). The large-scale neural network for spatial attention displays multifunctional overlap but differential asymmetry. *NeuroImage 9*: 269–277.

Kincade, J. M., Abrams, R. A., Astafiev, S. V., Shulman, G. L., and Corbetta, M. (2005). An event-related functional magnetic resonance imaging study of voluntary and stimulus-driven orienting of attention. *Journal of Neuroscience 25*: 4593–4604.

Kinsbourne, M. (1977). Hemi-neglect and hemisphere rivalry. *Advances in Neurology 18*: 41–49.

Kiss, M., Driver, J., and Eimer, M. (2009). Reward priority of visual target singletons modulates event-related potential signatures of attentional selection. *Psychological Science 20*: 245–251.

Klein, R. M. (2000). Inhibition of return. *Trends in Cognitive Sciences 4*: 138–147.

Knight, R. T., Hillyard, S. A., Woods, D. L., and Neville, H. J. (1980). The effects of frontal and temporal-parietal lesions on the auditory evoked potential in man. *Electroencephalography and Clinical Neurophysiology 50*: 112–124.

Koch, C. and Ullman, S. (1985). Shifts in selective visual attention: Towards the underlying neural circuitry. *Human Neurobiology 4*: 219–227.

Konen, C. S. and Kastner, S. (2008). Representation of eye movements and stimulus motion in topographically organized areas of human posterior parietal cortex. *Journal of Neuroscience 28*: 8361–8375.

Koski, L., Paus, T., Hofle, N., and Petrides, M. (1999). Increased blood flow in the basal ganglia when using cues to direct attention. *Experimental Brain Research 129*: 241–246.

Krebs, R. M., Boehler, C. N., Egner, T., and Woldorff, M. G. (2011). The neural underpinnings of how reward associations can both guide and misguide attention. *Journal of Neuroscience* 31: 9752–9759.

Kringelbach, M. L. and Rolls, E. T. (2004). The functional neuroanatomy of the human orbitofrontal cortex: Evidence from neuroimaging and neuropsychology. *Progress in Neurobiology* 72: 341–372.

Kristjansson, A., Sigurjonsdottir, O., and Driver, J. (2010). Fortune and reversals of fortune in visual search: Reward contingencies for pop-out targets affect search efficiency and target repetition effects. *Attention, Perception, & Psychophysics* 72: 1229–1236.

Kuhl, B. A., Bainbridge, W. A., and Chun, M. M. (2012). Neural reactivation reveals mechanisms for updating memory. *Journal of Neuroscience* 32: 3453–3461.

Kunar, M. A., Flusberg, S. J., and Wolfe, J. M. (2008). Time to guide: Evidence for delayed attentional guidance in contextual cueing. *Visual Cognition* 16: 804–825.

Kusunoki, M., Gottlieb, J., and Goldberg, M. E. (2000). The lateral intraparietal area as a salience map: The representation of abrupt onset, stimulus motion, and task relevance. *Vision Research* 40: 1459–1468.

LaBar, K. S., Gitelman, D. R., Parrish, T. B., and Mesulam, M. (1999). Neuroanatomic overlap of working memory and spatial attention networks: A functional MRI comparison within subjects. *NeuroImage* 10: 695–704.

Lakatos, P., Karmos, G., Mehta, A. D., Ulbert, I., and Schroeder, C. E. (2008). Entrainment of neuronal oscillations as a mechanism of attentional selection. *Science* 320: 110–113.

Landman, R., Spekreijse, H., and Lamme, V. A. (2003). Large capacity storage of integrated objects before change blindness. *Vision Research* 43: 149–164.

Lashley, K. S. (1950). In search of the engram. In J. F. Danielli and R. Brown (eds.), *Physiological Mechanisms in Animal Behaviour* (pp. 454–482). New York: Academic Press.

Lavie, N. (1995). Perceptual load as a necessary condition for selective attention. *Journal of Experimental Psychology: Human Perception and Performance* 21: 451–468.

Lawrence, B. M. and Snyder, L. H. (2009). The responses of visual neurons in the frontal eye field are biased for saccades. *Journal of Neuroscience* 29: 13815–13822.

Leblanc, E., Prime, D. J., and Jolicoeur, P. (2008). Tracking the location of visuospatial attention in a contingent capture paradigm. *Journal of Cognitive Neuroscience* 20: 657–671.

Leon, M. I. and Shadlen, M. N. (1998). Exploring the neurophysiology of decisions. *Neuron* 21: 669–672.

Lepsien, J. and Nobre, A. C. (2007). Attentional modulation of object representations in working memory. *Cerebral Cortex* 17: 2072–2083.

Lepsien, J., Thornton, I., and Nobre, A. C. (2011). Modulation of working-memory maintenance by directed attention. *Neuropsychologia* 49: 1569–1577.

Liu, X., Hairston, J., Schrier, M., and Fan, J. (2011). Common and distinct networks underlying reward valence and processing stages: A meta-analysis of functional neuroimaging studies. *Neuroscience & Biobehavioral Reviews* 35: 1219–1236.

Losier, B. J. and Klein, R. M. (2001). A review of the evidence for a disengage deficit following parietal lobe damage. *Neuroscience & Biobehavioral Reviews* 25: 1–13.

Lupiañez, J. (2010). Inhibition of return. In A. C. Nobre and J. T. Coull (eds.), *Attention and Time* (pp. 17–34). Oxford: Oxford University Press.

Lynch, J. C., Mountcastle, V. B., Talbot, W. H., and Yin, T. C. (1977). Parietal lobe mechanisms for directed visual attention. *Journal of Neurophysiology* 40: 362–389.

Maunsell, J. H. (2004). Neuronal representations of cognitive state: Reward or attention? *Trends in Cognitive Sciences 8*: 261–265.

Mehta, A. D., Ulbert, I., and Schroeder, C. E. (2000). Intermodal selective attention in monkeys. I: Distribution and timing of effects across visual areas. *Cerebral Cortex 10*: 343–358.

Melamed, E. and Larsen, B. (1979). Cortical activation pattern during saccadic eye movements in humans: Localization by focal cerebral blood flow increases. *Annals of Neurology 5*: 79–88.

Mesulam, M. M. (1981). A cortical network for directed attention and unilateral neglect. *Annals of Neurology 10*: 309–325.

Mesulam, M. M. (1990). Large-scale neurocognitive networks and distributed processing for attention, language, and memory. *Annals of Neurology 28*: 597–613.

Mesulam, M. M. (1999). Spatial attention and neglect: Parietal, frontal and cingulate contributions to the mental representation and attentional targeting of salient extrapersonal events. *Philosophical Transactions of the Royal Society of London B: Biological Sciences 354*: 1325–1346.

Mesulam, M. M. (2005). Imaging connectivity in the human cerebral cortex: The next frontier? *Annals of Neurology 57*: 5–7.

Mesulam, M. M., Nobre, A. C., Kim, Y. H., Parrish, T. B., and Gitelman, D. R. (2001). Heterogeneity of cingulate contributions to spatial attention. *NeuroImage 13*: 1065–1072.

Mesulam, M. M., Van Hoesen, G. W., Pandya, D. N., and Geschwind, N. (1977). Limbic and sensory connections of the inferior parietal lobule (area PG) in the rhesus monkey: A study with a new method for horseradish peroxidase histochemistry. *Brain Research 136*: 393–414.

Mesulam, M., Weintraub, S., Parrish, T., and Gitelman, D. (2005). Primary progressive aphasia: Reversed asymmetry of atrophy and right hemisphere language dominance. *Neurology 64*: 556–557.

Miniussi, C., Marzi, C. A., and Nobre, A. C. (2005). Modulation of brain activity by selective task sets observed using event-related potentials. *Neuropsychologia 43*: 1514–1528.

Miniussi, C., Rao, A., and Nobre, A. C. (2002). Watching where you look: Modulation of visual processing of foveal stimuli by spatial attention. *Neuropsychologia 40*: 2448–2460.

Mohanty, A., Egner, T., Monti, J. M., and Mesulam, M. M. (2009). Search for a threatening target triggers limbic guidance of spatial attention. *Journal of Neuroscience 29*: 10563–10572.

Mohanty, A., Gitelman, D. R., Small, D. M., and Mesulam, M. M. (2008). The spatial attention network interacts with limbic and monoaminergic systems to modulate motivation-induced attention shifts. *Cerebral Cortex 18*: 2604–2613.

Molenberghs, P., Gillebert, C. R., Peeters, R., and Vandenberghe, R. (2008). Convergence between lesion–symptom mapping and functional magnetic resonance imaging of spatially selective attention in the intact brain. *Journal of Neuroscience 28*: 3359–3373.

Molenberghs, P., Mesulam, M. M., Peeters, R., and Vandenberghe, R. R. (2007). Remapping attentional priorities: Differential contribution of superior parietal lobule and intraparietal sulcus. *Cerebral Cortex 17*: 2703–2712.

Moore, T. and Armstrong, K. M. (2003). Selective gating of visual signals by microstimulation of frontal cortex. *Nature 421*: 370–373.

Moore, T. and Fallah, M. (2004). Microstimulation of the frontal eye field and its effects on covert spatial attention. *Journal of Neurophysiology 91*: 152–162.

Moores, E., Laiti, L., and Chelazzi, L. (2003). Associative knowledge controls deployment of visual selective attention. *Nature Neuroscience 6*: 182–189.

144   ANNA C. NOBRE AND M. MARSEL MESULAM

Moran, J. and Desimone, R. (1985). Selective attention gates visual processing in the extrastriate cortex. *Science* 229: 782–784.

Mountcastle, V. B., Lynch, J. C., Georgopoulos, A., Sakata, H., and Acuna, C. (1975). Posterior parietal association cortex of the monkey: Command functions for operations within extrapersonal space. *Journal of Neurophysiology* 38: 871–908.

Muggleton, N. G., Kalla, R., Juan, C. H., and Walsh, V. (2011). Dissociating the contributions of human frontal eye fields and posterior parietal cortex to visual search. *Journal of Neurophysiology* 105: 2891–2896.

Müller, H. J. and Rabbitt, P. M. (1989). Spatial cueing and the relation between the accuracy of 'where' and 'what' decisions in visual search. *Quarterly Journal of Experimental Psychology A: Human Experimental Psychology* 41: 747–773.

Murray, A. M., Nobre, A. C., and Stokes, M. G. (2011). Markers of preparatory attention predict visual short-term memory performance. *Neuropsychologia* 49: 1458–1465.

Natale, E., Marzi, C. A., and Macaluso, E. (2009). fMRI correlates of visuo-spatial reorienting investigated with an attention shifting double-cue paradigm. *Human Brain Mapping* 30: 2367–2381.

Nee, D. E. and Jonides, J. (2009). Common and distinct neural correlates of perceptual and memorial selection. *NeuroImage* 45: 963–975.

Neely, J. H. (1976). Semantic priming and retrieval from lexical memory: Evidence for facilitatory and inhibitory processes. *Memory & Cognition* 4: 648–654.

Niemi, P. and Näätänen, R. (1981). Foreperiod and simple reaction time. *Psychological Bulletin* 89: 133–162.

Nobre, A. C. (2000). Review of The Autonomous Brain: Peter D. Milner. *Neuropsychologia* 38: 906.

Nobre, A. C. (2004). Probing the flexibility of attentional orienting in the human brain. In M. I. Posner (ed.), *Cognitive Neuroscience of Attention*, 1st edn. (pp. 157–179). New York: Guilford Press.

Nobre, A. C., Correa, A., and Coull, J. (2007). The hazards of time. *Current Opinion in Neurobiology* 17: 465–470.

Nobre, A. C., Coull, J. T., Frith, C. D., and Mesulam, M. M. (1999). Orbitofrontal cortex is activated during breaches of expectation in tasks of visual attention. *Nature Neuroscience* 2: 11–12

Nobre, A. C., Coull, J. T., Maquet, P., Frith, C. D., Vandenberghe, R., and Mesulam, M. M. (2004). Orienting attention to locations in perceptual versus mental representations. *Journal of Cognitive Neuroscience* 16: 363–373.

Nobre, A. C., Coull, J. T., Walsh, V., and Frith, C. D. (2003). Brain activations during visual search: Contributions of search efficiency versus feature binding. *NeuroImage* 18: 91–103.

Nobre, A. C., Gitelman, D. R., Dias, E. C., and Mesulam, M. M. (2000a). Covert visual spatial orienting and saccades: Overlapping neural systems. *NeuroImage* 11: 210–216.

Nobre, A. C., Rohenkohl, G., and Stokes, M. G. (2011). Nervous anticipation: Top-down biasing across space and time. In M. I. Posner (ed.), *Cognitive Neuroscience of Attention*, 2nd edn. (pp. 159–186). New York: Guilford Press.

Nobre, A. C., Sebestyen, G. N., Gitelman, D. R., Mesulam, M. M., Frackowiak, R. S., and Frith, C. D. (1997). Functional localization of the system for visuospatial attention using positron emission tomography. *Brain* 120(Pt 3): 515–533.

Nobre, A. C., Sebestyen, G. N., and Miniussi, C. (2000b). The dynamics of shifting visuospatial attention revealed by event-related potentials. *Neuropsychologia* 38: 964–974.

Nobre, A. C. and Stokes, M. G. (2011). Attention and short-term memory: Crossroads. *Neuropsychologia 49*: 1391–1392.

O'Connor, D. H., Fukui, M. M., Pinsk, M. A., and Kastner, S. (2002). Attention modulates responses in the human lateral geniculate nucleus. *Nature Neuroscience 5*: 1203–1209.

O'Doherty, J. P. (2004). Reward representations and reward-related learning in the human brain: Insights from neuroimaging. *Current Opinion in Neurobiology 14*: 769–776.

Ozaki, T. J. (2011). Frontal-to-parietal top-down causal streams along the dorsal attention network exclusively mediate voluntary orienting of attention. *PLoS One 6*: e20079.

Padmala, S. and Pessoa, L. (2011). Reward reduces conflict by enhancing attentional control and biasing visual cortical processing. *Journal of Cognitive Neuroscience 23*: 3419–3432.

Patai, E. Z., Doallo, S., and Nobre, A. C. (2012). Long-term memories bias sensitivity and target selection in complex scenes. *Journal of Cognitive Neuroscience 24*: 2281–2291.

Paus, T. (1996). Location and function of the human frontal eye-field: A selective review. *Neuropsychologia 34*: 475–483.

Paus, T., Jech, R., Thompson, C. J., Comeau, R., Peters, T., and Evans, A. C. (1997). Transcranial magnetic stimulation during positron emission tomography: A new method for studying connectivity of the human cerebral cortex. *Journal of Neuroscience 17*: 3178–3184.

Peck, C. J., Jangraw, D. C., Suzuki, M., Efem, R., and Gottlieb, J. (2009). Reward modulates attention independently of action value in posterior parietal cortex. *Journal of Neuroscience 29*: 11182–11191.

Peelen, M. V., Heslenfeld, D. J., and Theeuwes, J. (2004). Endogenous and exogenous attention shifts are mediated by the same large-scale neural network. *NeuroImage 22*: 822–830.

Perry, R. J. and Zeki, S. (2000). The neurology of saccades and covert shifts in spatial attention: An event-related fMRI study. *Brain 123*(Pt 11): 2273–2288.

Pessoa, L. and Engelmann, J. B. (2010). Embedding reward signals into perception and cognition. *Frontiers in Neuroscience 4*: 17.

Petit, L., Orssaud, C., Tzourio, N., Salamon, G., Mazoyer, B., and Berthoz, A. (1993). PET study of voluntary saccadic eye movements in humans: Basal ganglia-thalamocortical system and cingulate cortex involvement. *Journal of Neurophysiology 69*: 1009–1017.

Phillips, W. A. (1974). Distinction between sensory storage and short-term visual memory. *Perception & Psychophysics 16*: 283–290.

Phillips, W. A. and Baddeley, A. D. (1971). Reaction time and short-term visual memory. *Psychonomic Science 22*: 73–74.

Piech, R. M., Lewis, J., Parkinson, C. H., Owen, A. M., Roberts, A. C., Downing, P. E., and Parkinson, J. A. (2010). Neural correlates of affective influence on choice. *Brain and Cognition 72*: 282–288.

Pollmann, S., Weidner, R., Humphreys, G. W., Olivers, C. N., Müller, K., Lohmann, G., Wiggins, C. J., and Watson, D. G. (2003). Separating distractor rejection and target detection in posterior parietal cortex: An event-related fMRI study of visual marking. *NeuroImage 18*: 310–323.

Posner, M. I. (1978). *Chronometric Explorations of Mind: The Third Paul M. Fitts Lectures*, delivered at the University of Michigan, September 1976. Hillsdale, N.J.: Lawrence Erlbaum Associates.

Posner, M. I. (1980). Orienting of attention. *Quarterly Journal of Experimental Psychology 32*: 3–25.

Posner, M. I. and Boies, S. J. (1971). Components of attention. *Psychological Review 78*: 391–408.

Posner, M. I. and Cohen, Y. (1984). Components of visual orienting. In H. Bouma and D. Bonwhuis (eds.), *Attention and Performance X: Control of Language Processes* (pp. 531–556). Hillsdale, N.J.: Lawrence Erlbaum Associates.

Posner, M. I., Cohen, Y., and Rafal, R. D. (1982). Neural systems control of spatial orienting. *Philosophical Transactions of the Royal Society of London B: Biological Sciences* 298: 187–198.

Posner, M. I. and Snyder, C. R. (1975a). Attention and cognitive control. In R. L. Solso (ed.), *Information Processing and Cognition* (pp. 55–85). Hillsdale, N.J.: Lawrence Erlbaum Associates.

Posner, M. I. and Snyder, C. R. (1975b). Facilitation and inhibition in the processing of signals. In P. M. A. Rabbitt (ed.), *Attention and Performance V* (pp. 669–682). London: Academic Press.

Posner, M. I., Walker, J. A., Friedrich, F. J., and Rafal, R. D. (1984). Effects of parietal injury on covert orienting of attention. *Journal of Neuroscience* 4: 1863–1874.

Posner, M. I., Walker, J. A., Friedrich, F. A., and Rafal, R. D. (1987). How do the parietal lobes direct covert attention? *Neuropsychologia* 25: 135–145.

Postle, B. R. (2006). Working memory as an emergent property of the mind and brain. *Neuroscience* 139: 23–38.

Praamstra, P., Boutsen, L., and Humphreys, G. W. (2005). Frontoparietal control of spatial attention and motor intention in human EEG. *Journal of Neurophysiology* 94: 764–774.

Ptak, R. and Schnider, A. (2011). The attention network of the human brain: Relating structural damage associated with spatial neglect to functional imaging correlates of spatial attention. *Neuropsychologia* 49: 3063–3070.

Rao, R. P. and Ballard, D. H. (1999). Predictive coding in the visual cortex: A functional interpretation of some extra-classical receptive-field effects. *Nature Neuroscience* 2: 79–87.

Raymond, J. E. and O'Brien, J. L. (2009). Selective visual attention and motivation: The consequences of value learning in an attentional blink task. *Psychological Science* 20: 981–988.

Reynolds, J. H. and Chelazzi, L. (2004). Attentional modulation of visual processing. *Annual Review of Neuroscience* 27: 611–647.

Reynolds, J. H., Chelazzi, L., and Desimone, R. (1999). Competitive mechanisms subserve attention in macaque areas V2 and V4. *Journal of Neuroscience* 19: 1736–1753.

Reynolds, J. H. and Desimone, R. (1999). The role of neural mechanisms of attention in solving the binding problem. *Neuron* 24: 19–29, 111–125.

Reynolds, J. H. and Heeger, D. J. (2009). The normalization model of attention. *Neuron* 61: 168–185.

Rizzolatti, G. and Craighero, L. (1998). Spatial attention: Mechanisms and theories. In M. Sabourin and F. Craik (eds.), *Advances in Psychological Science, Vol. 2: Biological and Cognitive Aspects* (pp. 171–198). Hove, UK: Psychology Press.

Rizzolatti, G., Riggio, L., Dascola, I., and Umiltá, C. (1987). Reorienting attention across the horizontal and vertical meridians: Evidence in favor of a premotor theory of attention. *Neuropsychologia* 25: 31–40.

Robertson, I. H. (2001). Do we need the 'lateral' in unilateral neglect? Spatially nonselective attention deficits in unilateral neglect and their implications for rehabilitation. *NeuroImage* 14: S85–S90.

Rohenkohl, G., Cravo, A. M., Wyart, V., and Nobre, A. C. (2012). Temporal expectation improves the quality of sensory information. *Journal of Neuroscience* 32: 8424–8428.

Rohenkohl, G. and Nobre, A. C. (2011). Alpha oscillations related to anticipatory attention follow temporal expectations. *Journal of Neuroscience* 31: 14076–14084.

Rosen, A. C., Rao, S. M., Caffarra, P., Scaglioni, A., Bobholz, J. A., Woodley, S. J., Hammeke, T. A., Cunningham, J. M., Prieto, T. E., and Binder, J. R. (1999). Neural basis of endogenous and exogenous spatial orienting: A functional MRI study. *Journal of Cognitive Neuroscience* 11: 135–152.

Ruff, C. C., Bestmann, S., Blankenburg, F., Bjoertomt, O., Josephs, O., Weiskopf, N., Deichmann, R., and Driver, J. (2008). Distinct causal influences of parietal versus frontal areas on human visual cortex: Evidence from concurrent TMS–fMRI. *Cerebral Cortex 18*: 817–827.

Ruff, C. C., Blankenburg, F., Bjoertomt, O., Bestmann, S., Freeman, E., Haynes, J. D., Rees, G., Josephs, O., Deichmann, R., and Driver, J. (2006). Concurrent TMS–fMRI and psychophysics reveal frontal influences on human retinotopic visual cortex. *Current Biology 16*: 1479–1488.

Ruff, C. C., Driver, J., and Bestmann, S. (2009). Combining TMS and fMRI: From 'virtual lesions' to functional-network accounts of cognition. *Cortex 45*: 1043–1049.

Rushworth, M. F., Behrens, T. E., Rudebeck, P. H., and Walton, M. E. (2007). Contrasting roles for cingulate and orbitofrontal cortex in decisions and social behaviour. *Trends in Cognitive Sciences 11*: 168–176.

Rushworth, M. F., Nixon, P. D., Renowden, S., Wade, D. T., and Passingham, R. E. (1997). The left parietal cortex and motor attention. *Neuropsychologia 35*: 1261–1273.

Rushworth, M. F., Noonan, M. P., Boorman, E. D., Walton, M. E., and Behrens, T. E. (2011). Frontal cortex and reward-guided learning and decision-making. *Neuron 70*: 1054–1069.

Rushworth, M. F., Paus, T., and Sipila, P. K. (2001). Attention systems and the organization of the human parietal cortex. *Journal of Neuroscience 21*: 5262–5271.

Rutherford, H. J., O'Brien, J. L., and Raymond, J. E. (2010). Value associations of irrelevant stimuli modify rapid visual orienting. *Psychonomic Bulletin & Review 17*: 536–542.

Saalmann, Y. B. and Kastner, S. (2011). Cognitive and perceptual functions of the visual thalamus. *Neuron 71*: 209–223.

Saalmann, Y. B., Pigarev, I. N., and Vidyasagar, T. R. (2007). Neural mechanisms of visual attention: How top-down feedback highlights relevant locations. *Science 316*: 1612–1615.

Schankin, A. and Schubo, A. (2010). Contextual cueing effects despite spatially cued target locations. *Psychophysiology 47*: 717–727.

Schroeder, C. E. and Lakatos, P. (2009). Low-frequency neuronal oscillations as instruments of sensory selection. *Trends in Neurosciences 32*: 9–18.

Schroeder, C. E., Wilson, D. A., Radman, T., Scharfman, H., and Lakatos, P. (2010). Dynamics of active sensing and perceptual selection. *Current Opinion in Neurobiology 20*: 172–176.

Scolari, M., Byers, A., and Serences, J. T. (2012). Optimal deployment of attentional gain during fine discriminations. *Journal of Neuroscience 32*: 7723–7733.

Seiss, E., Kiss, M., and Eimer, M. (2009). Does focused endogenous attention prevent attentional capture in pop-out visual search? *Psychophysiology 46*: 703–717.

Serences, J. T. (2008). Value-based modulations in human visual cortex. *Neuron 60*: 1169–1181.

Serences, J. T. (2011). Mechanisms of selective attention: Response enhancement, noise reduction, and efficient pooling of sensory responses. *Neuron 72*: 685–687.

Serences, J. T., Liu, T., and Yantis, S. (2005). Parietal mechanisms of switching and maintaining attention to locations, objects, and features. In L. Itti, G. Rees, and J. Tsotsos (eds.), *Neurobiology of Attention* (pp. 35–41). New York: Academic Press.

Serences, J. T. and Saproo, S. (2010). Population response profiles in early visual cortex are biased in favor of more valuable stimuli. *Journal of Neurophysiology 104*: 76–87.

Serences, J. T. and Yantis, S. (2007). Spatially selective representations of voluntary and stimulus-driven attentional priority in human occipital, parietal, and frontal cortex. *Cerebral Cortex 17*: 284–293.

Sestieri, C., Shulman, G. L., and Corbetta, M. (2010). Attention to memory and the environment: Functional specialization and dynamic competition in human posterior parietal cortex. *Journal of Neuroscience 30*: 8445–8456.

Sheliga, B. M., Riggio, L., and Rizzolatti, G. (1994). Orienting of attention and eye movements. *Experimental Brain Research* 98: 507–522.

Shohamy, D. and Adcock, R. A. (2010). Dopamine and adaptive memory. *Trends in Cognitive Sciences* 14: 464–472.

Shulman, G. L., Pope, D. L., Astafiev, S. V., McAvoy, M. P., Snyder, A. Z., and Corbetta, M. (2010). Right hemisphere dominance during spatial selective attention and target detection occurs outside the dorsal frontoparietal network. *Journal of Neuroscience* 30: 3640–3651.

Siegel, M., Donner, T. H., Oostenveld, R., Fries, P., and Engel, A. K. (2008). Neuronal synchronization along the dorsal visual pathway reflects the focus of spatial attention. *Neuron* 60: 709–719.

Sieroff, E., Decaix, C., Chokron, S., and Bartolomeo, P. (2007). Impaired orienting of attention in left unilateral neglect: A componential analysis. *Neuropsychology* 21: 94–113.

Silver, M. A. and Kastner, S. (2009). Topographic maps in human frontal and parietal cortex. *Trends in Cognitive Sciences* 13: 488–495.

Sligte, I. G., Scholte, H. S., and Lamme, V. A. (2009). V4 activity predicts the strength of visual short-term memory representations. *Journal of Neuroscience* 29: 7432–7438.

Small, D. M., Gitelman, D. R., Gregory, M. D., Nobre, A. C., Parrish, T. B., and Mesulam, M. M. (2003). The posterior cingulate and medial prefrontal cortex mediate the anticipatory allocation of spatial attention. *NeuroImage* 18: 633–641.

Small, D. M., Gitelman, D., Simmons, K., Bloise, S. M., Parrish, T., and Mesulam, M. M. (2005). Monetary incentives enhance processing in brain regions mediating top-down control of attention. *Cerebral Cortex* 15: 1855–1865.

Snyder, L. H., Batista, A. P., and Andersen, R. A. (1997). Coding of intention in the posterior parietal cortex. *Nature* 386: 167–170.

Snyder, L. H., Batista, A. P., and Andersen, R. A. (1998). Change in motor plan, without a change in the spatial locus of attention, modulates activity in posterior parietal cortex. *Journal of Neurophysiology* 79: 2814–2819.

Snyder, L. H., Batista, A. P., and Andersen, R. A. (2000). Intention-related activity in the posterior parietal cortex: a review. *Vision Research* 40: 1433–1441.

Sommer, W. H., Kraft, A., Schmidt, S., Olma, M. C., and Brandt, S. A. (2008). Dynamic spatial coding within the dorsal frontoparietal network during a visual search task. *PLoS One* 3: e3167.

Spence, C. and Driver, J. (2004). *Crossmodal Space and Crossmodal Attention*. Oxford: Oxford University Press.

Sperling, G. (1960). The information available in brief visual presentations. *Psychological Monographs* 74: 1–29.

Spurzheim, J. G. (1825). *Phrenology, or, The Doctrine of the Mind*. London: Treuttel, Wurtz & Richter.

Sternberg, S. (1966). High-speed scanning in human memory. *Science* 153: 652–654.

Stokes, M. G., Atherton, K., Patai, E. Z., and Nobre, A. C. (2012). Long-term memory prepares neural activity for perception. *Proceedings of the National Academy of Sciences USA* 109: E360–E367.

Stokes, M. G. and Nobre, A. C. (2012). Top-down biases in visual short-term memory. In G. R. Mangun (ed.), *Neuroscience of Attention: Attentional Control and Selection* (pp. 209–229). New York: Oxford University Press.

Stokes, M., Thompson, R., Nobre, A. C., and Duncan, J. (2009). Shape-specific preparatory activity mediates attention to targets in human visual cortex. *Proceedings of the National Academy of Sciences USA* 106: 19569–19574.

Summerfield, C. and Egner, T. (2009). Expectation (and attention) in visual cognition. *Trends in Cognitive Sciences 13*: 403–409.

Summerfield, J. J., Lepsien, J., Gitelman, D. R., Mesulam, M. M., and Nobre, A. C. (2006). Orienting attention based on long-term memory experience. *Neuron 49*: 905–916.

Summerfield, J. J., Rao, A., Garside, N., and Nobre, A. C. (2011). Biasing perception by spatial long-term memory. *Journal of Neuroscience 31*: 14952–14960.

Szczepanski, S. M. and Kastner, S. (2013). Shifting attentional priorities: Control of spatial attention through hemispheric competition. *Journal of Neuroscience 33*: 5411–5421.

Szczepanski, S. M., Konen, C. S., and Kastner, S. (2010). Mechanisms of spatial attention control in frontal and parietal cortex. *Journal of Neuroscience 30*: 148–160.

Talsma, D., Sikkens, J. J., and Theeuwes, J. (2011). Stay tuned: What is special about not shifting attention? *PLoS One 6*: e16829.

Talsma, D., Slagter, H. A., Nieuwenhuis, S., Hage, J., and Kok, A. (2005). The orienting of visuospatial attention: An event-related brain potential study. *Brain Research: Cognitive Brain Research 25*: 117–129.

Tamber-Rosenau, B. J., Esterman, M., Chiu, Y. C., and Yantis, S. (2011). Cortical mechanisms of cognitive control for shifting attention in vision and working memory. *Journal of Cognitive Neuroscience 23*: 2905–2919.

Taylor, P. C., Nobre, A. C., and Rushworth, M. F. (2007). FEF TMS affects visual cortical activity. *Cerebral Cortex 17*: 391–399.

Thiebaut de Schotten, M., Dell'Acqua, F., Forkel, S. J., Simmons, A., Vergani, F., Murphy, D. G., and Catani, M. (2011). A lateralized brain network for visuospatial attention. *Nature Neuroscience 14*: 1245–1246.

Thiebaut de Schotten, M., Urbanski, M., Duffau, H., Volle, E., Levy, R., Dubois, B., and Bartolomeo, P. (2005). Direct evidence for a parietal-frontal pathway subserving spatial awareness in humans. *Science 309*: 2226–2228.

Thorndike, E. L. (1901). Adaptation in vision. *Science 14*: 221.

Todd, J. J. and Marois, R. (2004). Capacity limit of visual short-term memory in human posterior parietal cortex. *Nature 428*: 751–754.

Tosoni, A., Shulman, G. L., Pope, A. L., McAvoy, M. P., and Corbetta, M. (2012). Distinct representations for shifts of spatial attention and changes of reward contingencies in the human brain. *Cortex 49*: 1733–1749.

Treisman, A. (1960). Contextual cues in selective listening. *Quarterly Journal of Experimental Psychology 12*: 242–248.

Treisman, A. M. (1969). Strategies and models of selective attention. *Psychological Review 76*: 282–299.

Treisman, A. M. and Gelade, G. (1980). A feature-integration theory of attention. *Cognitive Psychology 12*: 97–136.

Treue, S. and Martinez Trujillo, J. C. (1999). Feature-based attention influences motion processing gain in macaque visual cortex. *Nature 399*: 575–579.

Urbanski, M., Thiebaut de Schotten, M., Rodrigo, S., Catani, M., Oppenheim, C., Touze, E., Chokron, S., Meder, J. F., Levy, R., Dubois, B., and Bartolomeo, P. (2008). Brain networks of spatial awareness: Evidence from diffusion tensor imaging tractography. *Journal of Neurology, Neurosurgery & Psychiatry 79*: 598–601.

Urbanski, M., Thiebaut de Schotten, M., Rodrigo, S., Oppenheim, C., Touze, E., Meder, J. F., Moreau, K., Loeper-Jeny, C., Dubois, B., and Bartolomeo, P. (2011). DTI-MR tractography of white matter damage in stroke patients with neglect. *Experimental Brain Research 208*: 491–505.

Vallar, G. and Perani, D. (1986). The anatomy of unilateral neglect after right-hemisphere stroke lesions: A clinical/CT-scan correlation study in man. *Neuropsychologia* 24: 609–622.

Van der Stigchel, S., Meeter, M., and Theeuwes, J. (2006). Eye movement trajectories and what they tell us. *Neuroscience & Biobehavioral Reviews* 30: 666–679.

Van Der Werf, J., Jensen, O., Fries, P., and Medendorp, W. P. (2010). Neuronal synchronization in human posterior parietal cortex during reach planning. *Journal of Neuroscience* 30: 1402–1412.

van Velzen, J. and Eimer, M. (2003). Early posterior ERP components do not reflect the control of attentional shifts toward expected peripheral events. *Psychophysiology* 40: 827–831.

Vandenberghe, R., Duncan, J., Dupont, P., Ward, R., Poline, J. B., Bormans, G., Michiels, J., Mortelmans, L., and Orban, G. A. (1997). Attention to one or two features in left or right visual field: A positron emission tomography study. *Journal of Neuroscience* 17: 3739–3750.

Vandenberghe, R., Dupont, P., De Bruyn, B., Bormans, G., Michiels, J., Mortelmans, L., and Orban, G. A. (1996). The influence of stimulus location on the brain activation pattern in detection and orientation discrimination: A PET study of visual attention. *Brain* 119(Pt 4): 1263–1276.

Vandenberghe, R., Geeraerts, S., Molenberghs, P., Lafosse, C., Vandenbulcke, M., Peeters, K., Peeters, R., Van Hecke, P., and Orban, G. A. (2005). Attentional responses to unattended stimuli in human parietal cortex. *Brain* 128(Pt 12): 2843–2857.

Vandenberghe, R., Gitelman, D. R., Parrish, T. B., and Mesulam, M. M. (2001). Functional specificity of superior parietal mediation of spatial shifting. *NeuroImage* 14: 661–673.

Vandenberghe, R., Molenberghs, P., and Gillebert, C. R. (2012). Spatial attention deficits in humans: The critical role of superior compared to inferior parietal lesions. *Neuropsychologia* 50: 1092–1103.

Verdon, V., Schwartz, S., Lovblad, K. O., Hauert, C. A., and Vuilleumier, P. (2010). Neuroanatomy of hemispatial neglect and its functional components: A study using voxel-based lesion-symptom mapping. *Brain* 133(Pt 3): 880–894.

Vincent, J. L., Kahn, I., Snyder, A. Z., Raichle, M. E., and Buckner, R. L. (2008). Evidence for a frontoparietal control system revealed by intrinsic functional connectivity. *Journal of Neurophysiology* 100: 3328–3342.

Vossel, S., Eschenbeck, P., Weiss, P. H., Weidner, R., Saliger, J., Karbe, H., and Fink, G. R. (2011). Visual extinction in relation to visuospatial neglect after right-hemispheric stroke: Quantitative assessment and statistical lesion-symptom mapping. *Journal of Neurology, Neurosurgery & Psychiatry* 82: 862–868.

Vossel, S., Weidner, R., Driver, J., Friston, K. J., and Fink, G. R. (2012). Deconstructing the architecture of dorsal and ventral attention systems with dynamic causal modeling. *Journal of Neuroscience* 32: 10637–10648.

Wagner, A. D., Shannon, B. J., Kahn, I., and Buckner, R. L. (2005). Parietal lobe contributions to episodic memory retrieval. *Trends in Cognitive Sciences* 9: 445–453.

Wallis, J. D. and Kennerley, S. W. (2011). Contrasting reward signals in the orbitofrontal cortex and anterior cingulate cortex. *Annals of the New York Academy of Sciences* 1239: 33–42.

Wardak, C., Olivier, E., and Duhamel, J. R. (2011). The relationship between spatial attention and saccades in the frontoparietal network of the monkey. *European Journal of Neuroscience* 33: 1973–1981.

Watson, R. T., Heilman, K. M., Cauthen, J. C., and King, F. A. (1973). Neglect after cingulectomy. *Neurology* 23: 1003–1007.

Watson, R. T., Heilman, K. M., Miller, B. D., and King, F. A. (1974). Neglect after mesencephalic reticular formation lesions. *Neurology 24*: 294–298.

Watson, R. T., Miller, B. D., and Heilman, K. M. (1978). Nonsensory neglect. *Annals of Neurology* 3: 505–508.

Weintraub, S. and Mesulam, M. M. (1987). Right cerebral dominance in spatial attention. Further evidence based on ipsilateral neglect. *Archives of Neurology 44*: 621–625.

Welch, K. and Stuteville, P. (1958). Experimental production of unilateral neglect in monkeys. *Brain 81*: 341–347.

Woldorff, M. G., Hazlett, C. J., Fichtenholtz, H. M., Weissman, D. H., Dale, A. M., and Song, A. W. (2004). Functional parcellation of attentional control regions of the brain. *Journal of Cognitive Neuroscience 16*: 149–165.

Woodrow, H. (1914). The measurement of attention. *Psychological Monographs 17*(5, whole no. 76): 1–158.

Woods, D. L. and Knight, R. T. (1986). Electrophysiologic evidence of increased distractibility after dorsolateral prefrontal lesions. *Neurology 36*: 212–216.

Woods, D. L., Knight, R. T., and Scabini, D. (1993). Anatomical substrates of auditory selective attention: Behavioral and electrophysiological effects of posterior association cortex lesions. *Brain Research: Cognitive Brain Research 1*: 227–240.

Wright, R. D. and Ward, L. M. (2008). *Orienting of Attention*. Oxford and New York: Oxford University Press.

Wyart, V., Nobre, A. C., and Summerfield, C. (2012). Dissociable prior influences of signal probability and relevance on visual contrast sensitivity. *Proceedings of the National Academy of Sciences USA 109*: 3593–3598.

Yantis, S. (1998). Control of visual attention. In H. Pashler (ed.), *Attention* (pp. 223–256). Hove, UK: Psychology Press.

Yantis, S. and Jonides, J. (1984). Abrupt visual onsets and selective attention: Evidence from visual search. *Journal of Experimental Psychology: Human Perception and Performance 10*: 601–621.

Yantis, S., Schwarzbach, J., Serences, J. T., Carlson, R. L., Steinmetz, M. A., Pekar, J. J., and Courtney, S. M. (2002). Transient neural activity in human parietal cortex during spatial attention shifts. *Nature Neuroscience 5*: 995–1002.

Yi, D. J., Turk-Browne, N. B., Chun, M. M., and Johnson, M. K. (2008). When a thought equals a look: Refreshing enhances perceptual memory. *Journal of Cognitive Neuroscience 20*: 1371–1380.

···

CHAPTER 6

DYNAMIC BRAIN STATES FOR PREPARATORY ATTENTION AND WORKING MEMORY

···

MARK STOKES AND JOHN DUNCAN

IN this chapter we consider how dynamic brain states continuously fine-tune processing to accommodate changes in behavioural context and task goals. First, we review the extant literature suggesting that content-specific patterns of preparatory activity bias competitive processing in visual cortex to favour behaviourally relevant input. Next, we consider how higher-level brain areas might provide a top-down attentional signal for modulating baseline visual activity. Extensive evidence suggests that working memory representations in prefrontal cortex are especially important for generating and maintaining biases in preparatory visual activity via modulatory feedback. Although it is often proposed that such working memory representations are maintained via persistent prefrontal activity, we review more recent evidence that rapid short-term synaptic plasticity provides a common substrate for maintaining the content of past experience and the rules for guiding future goal-directed processing.

NEURAL COMPETITION

Neural processing is inherently competitive: simultaneous input competes for driving the neural response, and ultimately for guiding behaviour. For example, in early visual cortex, individual neurons are tuned to specific types of stimuli presented at specific locations. Combined, these response properties define the cell's preference and receptive field. By definition, the cell responds maximally when the preferred stimulus is presented in its receptive field, but minimally to a non-preferred stimulus. Importantly, if both preferred and non-preferred stimuli are presented simultaneously within the cell's receptive field, the output response reflects a combination of the two. In effect, both the preferred and non-preferred stimuli compete for determining how the cell responds to the content of its receptive field (Reynolds, Chelazzi, and Desimone 1999). Importantly, attention directed to one or other item within the receptive field modulates these competitive interactions (see Fig. 6.1a). If attention is directed to the preferred stimulus, the cell responds as if only the preferred stimulus was presented. Conversely, if attention is directed to the non-preferred stimulus, the cell responds as if only the non-preferred stimulus were driving the response (Moran and Desimone 1985). Effectively, attention biases competition in favour of the attended item (Desimone and Duncan 1995).

Neural competition is likely to take many forms throughout the central nervous system (Duncan 1998). Lateral inhibition is a particularly well-studied form of competition within a spatial frame of reference; however, similar principles are likely to generalize to non-spatial features, such as orientation, colour, shape, etc. Such competitive mechanisms display important self-organizing qualities. For example, popular neural network models often exploit an architecture based on self-excitation with surround inhibition to implement winner(s)-take-all behaviour (see Itti and Borji (in chapter 38), this volume and Koch 2001). Although the inherent architecture of sensory cortex is presumably important for shaping self-organizing selectivity, stimulus-driven competitive dynamics are not sufficiently flexible to accommodate moment-to-moment changes in task goals that must also underlie attentional competition. This chapter focuses on preparatory mechanisms that underlie such attentional modulations, particularly focusing on selective changes in baseline visual activity and preparatory states in prefrontal cortex.

PREPARATORY ACTIVITY IN VISUAL CORTEX

Luck and colleagues (Luck, Chelazzi, Hillyard, and Desimone 1997) were the first to demonstrate that covert allocation of spatial attention is associated with an increase in the baseline firing rates of neurons that are important for processing the anticipated target. They recorded from single cells in visual cortex (V1, V2, and V4) while monkeys attended to a specific spatial location for a target stimulus (Luck et al. 1997). They found that when attention was directed to a location within the cell's receptive field, the baseline firing rate increased relative to when attention was directed outside the receptive field (Fig. 6.1b, left panel). Because this attention-related effect was observed *prior* to target presentation, the relative shift in baseline firing rate could be attributed to an extrinsic top-down modulation that selectively enhances activity for spatially specific neurons in preparation for target processing at the attended location.

Since these highly influential findings, spatially specific preparatory modulation has also been observed in human visual cortex using fMRI (Kastner et al. 1999; Ress, Backus, and Heeger 2000; Silver, Ress, and Heeger 2007). For example, Kastner and colleagues recorded increased preparatory visual activity within areas of visual cortex representing the attended location (Fig. 6.1b, right panel). As in Luck et al. (1997), these

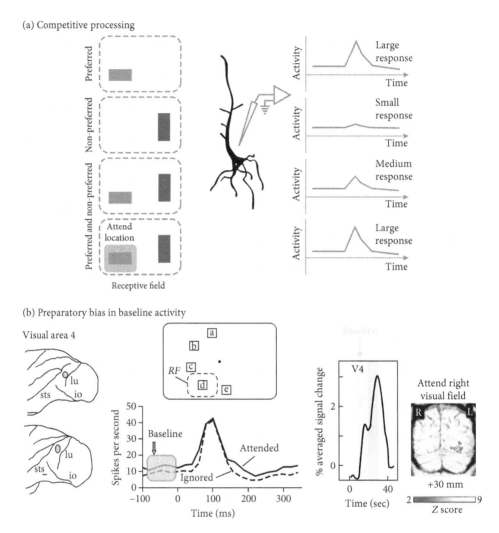

FIGURE 6.1 Preparatory activity biases competitive processing in visual cortex. (a) Illustration of stimulus competition within the receptive field of an example neuron. The preferred stimulus (blue horizontal bar) elicits a strong response, whereas a non-preferred stimulus (red vertical bar) elicits a weak response. If both preferred and non-preferred stimuli are presented simultaneously within the receptive field, the response lies between these two extremes, as if both the preferred and non-preferred are competing for influence over the cell's output response. If attention is directed to the preferred stimulus, the output resembles the response driven by the preferred stimulus alone, as if the influence of the unattended non-preferred stimulus has been suppressed. For relevant empirical results, see Moran and Desimone (1985); Reynolds, Chelazzi, and Desimone (1999). (b) Preparatory spatial attention modulates baseline activity before the presentations of the target, shown here in monkey visual area V4 and human V4. Monkey: Adapted from *Journal of Neurophysiology*, 77 (1), Steven J. Luck, Leonardo Chelazzi, Steven A. Hillyard, and Robert Desimone, pp. 24–42 © 1997, The American Physiological Society. Human: Reprinted from *Neuron*, 22 (4), Sabine Kastner, Mark A. Pinsk, Peter De Weerd, Robert Desimone, and Leslie G. Ungerleider, Increased Activity in Human Visual Cortex during Directed Attention in the Absence of Visual Stimulation, pp. 751–61, Copyright (1999), with permission from Elsevier.

studies demonstrate that task goals can modulate activity in visual cortex independently of stimulus-driven input, presumably via top-down feedback mechanisms.

THE 'BIAS' IN A BIASED COMPETITION MODEL OF ATTENTION

Spatially specific shifts in the baseline firing rate could reflect a fundamental neurophysiological state for preparatory attention. According to the biased competition model of attention (Desimone and Duncan 1995), selective pre-activation of neurons that code specific attended features (e.g. location, shape, colour) could help resolve competition at subsequent processing stages, thereby biasing processing in favour of task-relevant sensory input.

Consistent with this proposal, the relative magnitude of preparatory activity in retinotopically specific subregions of early visual cortex turns out to predict perceptual sensitivity for stimuli presented within the attended visual field (Ress, Backus, and Heeger 2000; Serences, Yantis, Culberson, and Awh 2004). Trial-by-trial coupling between brain activity and behaviour provides important evidence that increased baseline activity is indeed functionally relevant. More recent evidence further suggests that the trial-wise variations in preparatory activity directly relate to fluctuations in the target-related evoked response (Sylvester, Shulman, Jack, and Corbetta 2009). This coupling between preparatory activity and the stimulus-driven response is consistent with the proposal that changes in the baseline directly influence the response sensitivity for attended representations. That is, the response to visual stimulation co-depends on the input and the preparatory state of the visual system, here defined according to baseline levels of activity.

NON-SPATIAL PREPARATORY ACTIVATION IN VISUAL CORTEX

Spatial attention provides a convenient model for exploring preparatory attention in the visual system. For neurophysiological studies (e.g. Luck et al. 1997), it is relatively easy to define the receptive field for individual neurons, and for fMRI studies (e.g. Kastner et al. 1999), the macro-scale topographical organization of visual cortex allows researchers to differentiate spatially specific brain areas. Experimenters can then selectively measure activity in neurons, and/or neural populations, that correspond to the focus of attention.

However, task-relevance is often defined by non-spatial features. During visual search, for example, the task-relevant feature may be a specific shape, colour, and/or line orientation (Wolfe 2003). In many real world situations, we typically know more about what we are looking for than where to find it. Examples might include searching a crowd for a friend's face, or a cluttered office for your favourite coffee mug.

In contrast to the relatively ordered spatiotopic organization of visual cortex, coding for non-spatial features is distributed amongst other neural populations that code for other features within the same dimension. For example, in early visual cortex, cells tuned to a specific orientation are distributed throughout the retinotopic map (see schematic in Fig. 6.2a, adapted from Serences and Saproo 2012). Similarly, neurons coding for a specific colour are densely intermingled with neurons coding other colours (e.g. in V4; Tanigawa, Lu, and Roe 2010), and higher in the visual system, neural populations that code for a specific shape are mixed up with neurons coding other shapes (e.g. Haxby et al. 2001).

Chelazzi and colleagues provided initial evidence suggesting that non-spatial preparatory attention is mediated via a similar mechanism to spatial attention (Fig. 6.2b; Chelazzi, Duncan, Miller, and Desimone 1998; Chelazzi, Miller, Duncan, and Desimone 1993). Each trial of their memory-guided search task began with the presentation of the search target item, then after a brief delay one or two stimuli were presented at unpredictable locations. The task was to execute an eye-movement (i.e. saccade) to the target item if it was present within the search array. Recording from single units in primate inferior temporal (IT) cortex, they found that neurons that were initially selective for the cue stimulus remained active throughout the delay period, even though the driving stimulus was no longer present in the display. The authors reasoned that this sustained stimulus-specific response reflects the maintenance of the search target in working memory, which results in a selective increase in baseline activity across the population of cells that code the task-relevant information. As a consequence of this baseline shift, the response to subsequent sensory input interacts with this elevated activity state, resulting in a selective increase in firing for sensory input that matches the search template.

However, in this experiment, the elevated baseline during the pre-stimulus period could have been dependent on the initial presentation of the cue stimulus. Because the target-selective neurons were already activated by the cue stimulus, the visual system need only maintain the pattern of activity already triggered at the start of the trial. Therefore, top-down modulation may not have been strictly necessary to generate the precise pattern of baseline activity in this variant of a memory guided search task. A more general signal could have been sufficient to preserve the pattern of activity triggered by the cue stimulus.

Long-term memory experiments have shown that target-related neurons can, in principle, be activated by association rather than direct sensory stimulation (Miyashita 2004). For example, Naya, Sakai, and Miyashita (1996) taught monkeys arbitrary pairings between shape stimuli. After training, monkeys performed either a standard delayed match to sample task, or a paired associate task in which the animal's task was to detect the stimulus associated to the initial sample. Importantly, they found that neurons in anterior IT anticipate the presentation of the associated stimulus, even though it was not initially presented to the visual system (Naya et al. 1996). However, these associations are learned over a long training regime; therefore, this kind of preparatory activity might depend on local associative connections (e.g. Hebb 1949) rather than flexible top-down input (but see Tomita et al. 1999).

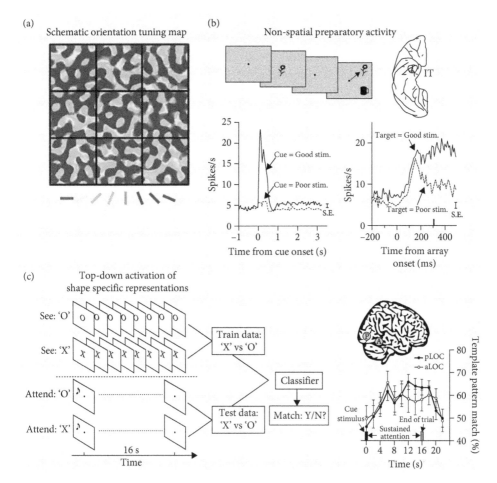

FIGURE 6.2 Non-spatial preparatory attention modulates baseline activity in visual cortex. (a) Schematic of distributed coding for orientation, Adapted from *Neuropsychologia*, 50 (4), John T. Serences and Sameer Saproo, Computational advances towards linking BOLD and behavior, pp. 435–46, Copyright (2012), with permission from Elsevier. (b) Evidence for maintenance of shape-specific neural activity in the delay period of a memory-guided search task in monkey inferior temporal (IT) cortex (upper panels). Neurons selective for the cue stimulus maintain an elevated firing rate during the delay period, in anticipation of the target stimulus (lower panels; Adapted from *Journal of Neurophysiology*, 80 (6), Leonardo Chelazzi, John Duncan, Earl K. Miller, and Robert Desimone, pp. 2918–2940 © 1998, The American Physiological Society.) (c) Multivariate pattern analysis of functional magnetic resonance imaging data reveals how top-down mechanisms pre-activate shape-specific representations in human visual cortex (in posterior/anterior lateral occipital complex: pLOC/aLOC) during preparatory attention. Adapted from Stokes, M., Thompson, R., Nobre, A. C., & Duncan, J., Shape-specific preparatory activity mediates attention to targets in human visual cortex, *Proceedings of the National Academy of Sciences of the United States of America*, 104(46), pp. 19569–19574 © 2009, The National Academy of Sciences.

Experiments in humans are more readily suited for exploring flexible attentional control, yet attempts to identify top-down modulation of non-spatial preparatory activity in human visual cortex have yielded mixed results. Non-invasive brain imaging methods lack the spatial resolution to measure specific neurons with well-defined stimulus selectivity (as studied in Chelazzi et al. 1998). Consequently, many human studies of non-spatial preparatory attention have explored activity biases between brain areas that are selective for different feature dimensions, such as colour and motion processing areas (e.g. Chawla, Rees, and Friston 1999). The underlying logic is straightforward: directing attention to colour should increase the baseline firing rate of neurons that process colour, whereas directing attention to motion should increase the baseline firing rate of neurons specialized for processing motion. Because these neural populations can be measured more or less independently with standard human brain imaging methods (e.g. fMRI; Tootell et al. 1995), it should be relatively straightforward to detect preparatory activation for non-spatial attentional bias.

While some studies reported positive evidence for selective shifts in baseline activity between feature dimensions (Chawla et al. 1999; Giesbrecht, Weissman, Woldorff, and Mangun 2006), others have found only modest (Fannon, Saron, and Mangun 2007; Shulman, d'Avossa, Tansy, and Corbetta 2002) and/or transient changes (Shibata et al. 2008), or none at all (McMains, Fehd, Emmanouil, and Kastner 2007). Indeed, the inconsistencies in the literature have led some authors to propose that preparatory attention is fundamentally limited to spatial attention (McMains et al. 2007).

These inconsistencies are perhaps not surprising if we consider that cueing attention between distinct feature dimensions may not be particularly important for resolving competition in the visual system (cf. Desimone and Duncan 1995). The paradigmatic example of competition in the visual system is between preferred and non-preferred feature values within a particular coding dimension of the neural population (Navalpakkam and Itti 2007), such as selecting a stimulus with a specific orientation relative to other orientations (Moran and Desimone 1985) or a specific target shape among distractor shapes (Chelazzi et al. 1993, 1998). Indeed, feature values from different feature dimensions are more likely to cooperate than compete (Duncan 1998), especially when they belong to the same object (e.g. O'Craven, Downing, and Kanwisher 1999).

Consequently, the use of dimensions that are easily separable for neuroimaging purposes might have inadvertently undermined the actual attentional manipulation of interest. Although it may be possible to globally up-regulate activity in visual brain areas that are selective for processing information within a specific dimension (e.g. Chawla et al. 1999), if there is little advantage to this kind of bias then empirical results are likely to be highly variable (e.g. Shulman et al. 2002) and not well linked to behaviour (as in Fannon et al. 2007).

It is therefore important that preparatory attention is manipulated between feature values, rather than between feature dimensions. However, this raises a non-trivial practical challenge for human brain imaging studies. As noted above, non-spatial features are not well defined by cortical topography. Whereas some feature dimensions are topographically separable, feature values are typically represented across spatially overlapping neural populations that are more or less evenly distributed throughout the relevant processing area. The average activity profile within the visual area of interest cannot, therefore, distinguish between activation of one or other overlapping neural population coding specific feature values.

In recent years, multivariate pattern analysis (MVPA) has emerged as a powerful method for differentiating activation of two or more functionally distinct neural populations, even if they are spatially overlapping (Haynes and Rees 2006; Norman, Polyn, Detre, and Haxby 2006). Borrowing from methods developed for machine learning, Kamitani and Tong (2005) first demonstrated the feasibility of differentiating the pattern of responses elicited by specific orientations in visual cortex (see also Haynes and Rees 2005). Specifically, they used a pattern classification method known as the support vector machine (Vapnik 1998) to read out orientation-specific information from activity patterns distributed across the overall population response. This was the first non-invasive study to be able to selectively measure activity associated with spatially overlapping, but functionally distinct, neural populations.[1]

This methodological development has dramatically changed the brain-imaging field. Rather than being just a new application for esoteric machine learning tools, the popularization of multivariate analyses approaches to fMRI was an important conceptual development. Essentially, MVPA provides a more general approach for mapping information in brain imaging data by pooling across multiple measures, irrespective of the specific direction of the preference (Kriegeskorte, Goebel, and Bandettini 2006). For example, if half the voxels within a given area respond maximally to condition A, and the other half to condition B, the averaged response would not differ between the two conditions. If the information can be pooled in such a way that preserves the magnitude of activity differences between conditions, irrespective of the sign, the overall condition-specificity of the potentially heterogeneous set of measures can be expressed as a single estimate of multivariate difference. In practice, this can be achieved using sophisticated machine-learning classification approaches (Kamitani and Tong 2005), but also with difference measures that are directly analogous to standard univariate tests (Kriegeskorte et al. 2006). The precise method used is relatively unimportant; what matters most is that the *pattern* of activity is preserved in the ensemble metric.

Recently we exploited this development in the human brain imaging literature to measure top-down pre-activation of specific feature values (Stokes, Thompson, Nobre, and Duncan 2009b). The overall procedure is illustrated in Fig. 6.2c. The perceptual task was to detect low contrast shapes (X or O) embedded in dynamic noise. At the start of each trial, an auditory cue indicated which stimulus was the current target. Target and/or non-target stimuli could be presented at any time during the 16s trial to encourage participants to maintain an active attentional template for the duration of the trial. On some trials, no letter stimulus was presented, only the background noise. The aim of the experiment was to test whether preparatory activity reflects an increase in baseline activity for the cued target stimulus.

To define target-related patterns, we first trained linear classifiers to discriminate between stimulus-driven activation patterns associated with the two shape stimuli. Using independent data, we first verified that these classifiers could accurately differentiate the stimulus-driven response to the shape stimuli in regions of higher visual cortex.

Having established the sensitivity and specificity of the pattern analytic approach, we were then able to show that these stimulus-specific patterns re-emerged following the corresponding cue in the attention task. Specifically, we found that the patterns of activity elicited by the attention cue in lateral occipital complex matched the corresponding stimulus-driven patterns. This response was sustained throughout the duration of the attention trial, thereby tracking the duration of the preparatory attentional state. Moreover, the degree of pattern match between preparatory activity and corresponding stimulus-driven activity correlated with individual differences in the perceptual task. Participants who were able to maintain an accurate representation of the target in visual cortex were also better at detecting the target stimulus when it was presented.

Because there was no difference in the visual stimulation between the cueing conditions of the attention task, we could conclude that extrinsic top-down feedback selectively modulated overlapping populations representing the target shapes. Moreover, top-down control in this task was necessarily flexible: the association between the auditory cue and visual target was randomly assigned at the start of the experiment, and also reversed halfway through the experiment. Therefore, the association between the two stimuli was presumably mediated via feedback connections from higher regions such as prefrontal cortex (see below). Similar results have also been observed for object categories in ventral visual cortex (Peelen and Kastner 2011), confirming the important role for preparatory activation of search templates in the visual system.

Top-Down Feedback

As reviewed above, the extant evidence indicates that preparatory attention shapes baseline activity in visual cortex to optimize processing of task-relevant input. Foreknowledge of the most likely location of a target stimulus results in a selective up-regulation of neurons that represent the attended location, relative to unattended locations (Kastner et al. 1999; Luck et al. 1997). Similarly, attending for a specific shape generates a selective bias in visual cortex that matches the neural representation of the search target (Chelazzi et al. 1998; Stokes et al. 2009b). Crucially, these preparatory biases do not depend on visual input, but can be established using arbitrarily assigned symbolic non-visual cues that convey task-relevant information (Stokes et al. 2009b; Sylvester et al. 2009). This implies an extrinsic process for controlling preparatory biases in visual cortex. A likely candidate is top-down feedback from prefrontal cortex (PFC).

Prefrontal cortex is an ideal piece of hardware for computing task relevance. Diverse input connections deliver information about the external environment derived from the senses along with internal variables such as reward values, abstract rules, and long-term goals (Fuster 1997). Moreover, extensive output connections also place PFC in an ideal neuroanatomical position to modulate processing in other brain areas according to the product of external and internal variables.

In a series of microstimulation studies in non-human primates, Moore, Armstrong, and colleagues have revealed the important role of the frontal eye fields (FEF) in generating spatially specific biases in visual cortex (Armstrong, Fitzgerald, and Moore 2006; Armstrong and Moore 2007; Moore and Armstrong 2003). Neurons tuned to specific spatial locations for eye-movement planning in FEF modulate corresponding spatially specific neurons in V4 (for a review, see Moore 2006). Analogous studies using non-invasive methods for simultaneous FEF stimulation and recording visual responses have confirmed that similar mechanisms operate in the human brain (Ruff et al. 2006; Taylor, Nobre, and Rushworth 2007). Further research implicates similar links between intraparietal sulcus (IPS) and visual cortex (Heinen et al. 2011), although this pathway has received much less attention to date (but see Cutrell and Marrocco 2002).

In lateral PFC, cells are not tuned to fixed stimulus features, but appear to adapt their tuning profile to represent currently relevant information (Freedman and Asaad 2006; Freedman, Riesenhuber, Poggio, and Miller 2001; see below for more discussion). This variability in neural tuning clearly demands an extremely flexible mapping between PFC and visual cortex. Recently, it has been proposed that high-frequency oscillations (e.g. in the gamma band, ~40–80 Hz) could be important for functionally modulating pre-existing connection pathways (Fries 2009). Interregional coherence, therefore, could help establish functional pathways by rapidly facilitating, or 'switching on', specific neuroanatomical tracts (Gregoriou, Gotts, and Desimone 2012). Future research on this intriguing possibility will help determine whether high-frequency coupling helps establish temporary connections between visual cortex and higher brain areas for preparatory attention.

A WORKING MEMORY BASIS FOR PREPARATORY ATTENTION

Preparatory attention typically implies memory: a preparatory attentional state is only useful for as long as it can be held in mind. Correspondingly, it is widely accepted that working memory is important for maintaining the behaviourally relevant information that determines the focus of attention. However, the link between working memory and attention could run even deeper. Indeed, it has even been proposed that working memory representations could constitute the basic substrate of top-down bias (Desimone and Duncan 1995).

Extensive behavioural evidence suggests a strong coupling between attention and working memory (Awh and Jonides 2001). For example, Awh and colleagues showed that memory for a specific location facilitates simple detection of a choice stimulus presented at the memory location during the retention interval (Awh, Jonides, and Reuter-Lorenz 1998). In a similar vein, Soto, Humphreys and colleagues have demonstrated that non-spatial features in working memory also capture attention (Soto,

Heinke, Humphreys, and Blanco 2005; Soto and Humphreys 2007, 2009). In their dual task scenario, participants are presented with a number of items to remember, and then during the maintenance interval, there is an additional search task. On valid trials, the target item in the search array shares a feature (e.g. colour) with the item in working memory, but on invalid trials the mnemonic feature is shared with a non-target item. For a baseline comparison, neutral trials contain no match between the features in memory and features in the search array. Search times are faster on valid trials and slower on invalid trials, relative to neutral trials. This effect persists even when participants should, if possible, decouple working memory from attentional control. That is, attention is still drawn to the memory feature even when participants can expect the memory feature to match a non-target item (Soto and Humphreys 2009). These results suggest that, at least under these experimental conditions, working memory representations are sufficient for biasing visual processing (but see Peters, Goebel, and Roelfsema 2009).

WORKING MEMORY REPRESENTATIONS IN PFC

Since the 1970s, it has been widely accepted that cells in PFC maintain information in working memory through sustained firing. In one of the earliest experiments, Fuster and Alexander (1971) found that activity in some prefrontal cells co-varied with the mnemonic demands imposed by a delayed reaching task. Activity increased for the duration that response-related information needed to be held in mind, and returned to baseline after the response was executed, that is, when memory for the response was no longer required (Fuster and Alexander 1971). Sustained activity in dedicated memory cells could reflect the active maintenance of the appropriate motor command throughout the experimentally imposed delay period (see also Kubota and Niki 1971).

More recent studies suggest that a similar scheme underlies the active maintenance of perceptual information. For example, Miller and colleagues (Miller, Erickson, and Desimone 1996) identified neurons within the PFC that responded selectively to visual memoranda with an elevated firing rate. Similar to the behaviour of memory cells in the delayed reaching task (Fuster and Alexander 1971), prefrontal activity also co-varied with the duration of maintenance in working memory. Moreover, some cells even maintained memory specificity after the presentation of distracting items, indicating a potential correlate of distractor-resistant working memory (Miller et al. 1996). Similarly, in the human PFC, delay activity corresponds closely to working memory demands (for reviews, see Curtis and D'Esposito 2003; Passingham and Sakai 2004). Such findings have been extremely influential, and have motivated numerous conceptual and computational models of working memory based on actively maintained persistent firing of

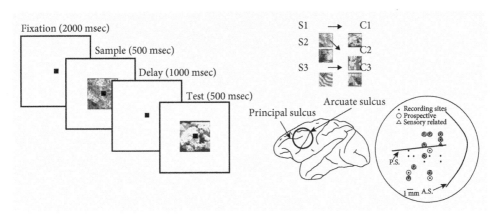

FIGURE 6.3 A prospective coding model of working memory. In this experiment, monkeys were trained on a paired association task in which an initial sample stimulus is paired with a specific target. By varying the perceptual similarity between the sample stimuli, and between target stimuli, Rainer and colleagues (1999) showed that delay activity is more selective for the expected target than the previous sample. These results highlight how the principal goal of working memory is to use recent past experiences to guide future behaviour. Adapted from Rainer, G., Rao, S. C., and Miller, E. K., Prospective coding for objects in primate prefrontal cortex, *Journal of Neuroscience*, 19(13), pp. 5493–5505 © 1999, The Society for Neuroscience.

stimulus-specific neurons in PFC (Curtis and D'Esposito 2003; Goldman-Rakic 1995; Wang 2001). Although other candidate mechanisms are emerging (discussed in more detail below), persistent delay activity continues to dominate in most models for sustaining information in PFC.

A prospective coding model of working memory further proposes that active representations in PFC primarily code for the expected target (Rainer, Rao, and Miller 1999), rather than previous input. Rainer et al. (1999) used a paired-associate working memory task to test whether selectively the PFC differentiates previous or anticipated stimuli (see Fig. 6.3). By independently varying the perceptual similarity between sample stimuli, and perceptual similarity between the associated test stimuli, they found that firing during the delay period reflected the similarity between the anticipated test stimuli, rather than the preceding sample.

Rainer and colleagues (1999) argue that the primary goal of working memory is to maintain information from recent past experience to guide future behaviour. Accordingly, activity in PFC constitutes a forward model based on expected task demands (Friston 2010), rather than a buffer for maintaining previous input. Importantly, this prospective coding model conceptually integrates working memory and preparatory attention, as pre-activation of target-related neurons could provide a basic neurophysiological mechanism for the biased competition model of attention (Desimone and Duncan 1995). Raising the baseline firing rate of target-related neurons in PFC could bias target-related processing, as described above for the visual system.

DYNAMIC POPULATION CODING:
A PROBLEM FOR STABLE ACTIVITY STATES?

Working memory is very often viewed as a persistent activity state that is maintained via self-excitatory re-entrant connections (Goldman-Rakic 1995; Wang 2001). However, recent studies highlight the dynamic behaviour of neural representation in various brain areas (Buonomano and Maass 2009), including parietal (Crowe, Averbeck, and Chafee 2010) and prefrontal cortex (Meyers et al. 2008). In this section we consider new evidence for dynamic population coding in prefrontal cortex, and the implications for working memory and preparatory attention.

Some of the most detailed studies of dynamic population coding have been performed in the olfactory system of the locust (Laurent 2002). For example, Mazor and Laurent (2005) demonstrated that specific odours trigger a series of activity patterns within antennal lobe projection neurons (Mazor and Laurent 2005). Although the population eventually returns to a stable low energy state (i.e. low mean firing rate), the most discriminative information for odour classification is actually observed along the dynamic trajectory through the activity state-space. Neurons that receive output signals from these projection neurons respond most vigorously during the most dynamic phase of the response. In contrast, activity is relatively mute in these putative readout neurons after the projection cells have returned to a relatively stable state.

Importantly, these dynamics are not specific to locust olfaction, but are likely to constitute a general property of neural processing (Buonomano and Maass 2009). Of particular interest here, dynamic population coding has also been observed in primate parietal (Crowe et al. 2010) and prefrontal cortex (Meyers et al. 2008). It is therefore important to reconcile dynamic population coding with theoretical accounts that highlight stationary activity states, such as sustained activity for working memory and preparatory attention.

We recently explored population coding dynamics in primate prefrontal cortex during a cued target detection task (Stokes et al. 2013). As shown in Fig. 6.4a, a cue stimulus at the start of each experimental trial determined which stimulus was the current target. After a series of 0–3 non-targets, the cued target was presented and followed by a behavioural response (saccade at target offset). Non-targets were either a stimulus serving as a target on other trials ('distractor'), or as never a target ('neutral' stimulus). For accurate behavioural performance in this task, cue context must be maintained across the various delays and distractions.

Using similar pattern analytic methods to previous fMRI studies (schematized in Fig. 6.4b; see also Stokes, Saraiva, Rohenkohl, and Nobre 2011; Stokes, Thompson, Cusack, and Duncan 2009a; Stokes et al. 2009b), we were able to classify cue identity from the population response 100ms after cue onset (Fig. 6.4c). Toward the end of the cue-stimulation period, classification performance decreased, but remained above chance throughout the following memory delay. It is important to note that this

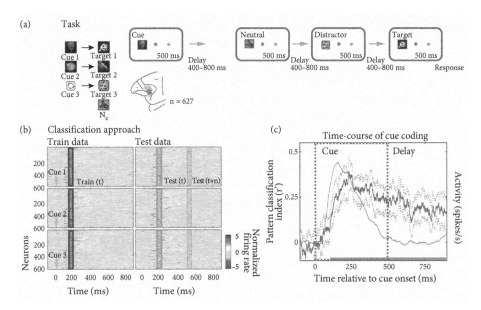

FIGURE 6.4 Population-level analyses of task-relevant coding during a cued target detection task. (a) In this task, the cue stimulus determines which choice stimulus is currently relevant. The monkey is only rewarded for responding to the cued target, the trial is aborted for all other responses. Consequently, the cue context must be maintained throughout the duration of the trial. Data were analysed from 627 randomly sampled neurons in prefrontal cortex. (b) Pattern classification was performed over the full population of recorded neurons. The classifiers were trained to discriminate cue type at time t in a training data set: Train(t). Classification performance could then be assessed on independent data taken from either the same time point in the test data set [Test(t), within-time classification] or at different times [Test(t+n): cross-temporal classification]. (c) The time-course of cue coding was estimated by performing within-time classification during the presentation of the cue and subsequent memory delay period (blue trace). For reference, the mean firing rate of the population is presented in grey. Reprinted from *Neuron*, 78 (2), Mark G. Stokes, Makoto Kusunoki, Natasha Sigala, Hamed Nili, David Gaffan, and John Duncan, Dynamic Coding for Cognitive Control in Prefrontal Cortex, pp. 364–75, Copyright (2013), with permission from Elsevier.

time-resolved pattern analytic approach tests only for consistency, or decodability, of the neural patterns within a specific time point. Consequently, we can infer that a specific pattern of activity differentiates cue type at time point A, and similarly for time point B, but we cannot tell if it is the same neural code (or similar codes) underlying discrimination across time points (also see Rainer et al. 1999).

To answer this question, we extended the pattern analytic approach to test for cross-generalization between different time points within the trial (see schematic, Fig. 6.4b). By decoupling train/test temporal windows, we could assess whether a classifier trained on data from one time window can accurately classify patterns observed at other times (see also Crowe et al. 2010; Meyers et al. 2008). If accurate generalization is observed across time (train at time t, test at time t + *n*), we can infer that the population code that differentiates cue type at time t is significantly similar to the coding scheme at time t + n. In other words, if the coding schemes are stable across time, pattern classification should not be sensitive to which time points are used for test or train. Conversely, if classifiers trained at time t are unable to decode patterns observed at time t + n, then we can conclude that population coding is time-specific.

The results of this cross-temporal analysis are summarized in Fig. 6.5. In the upper panel, different colour traces represent classification performance for classifiers trained on data from corresponding shaded time windows, and tested throughout the remainder of the trial. For reference, the within-time pattern analysis is shown in grey in each plot to illustrate the envelope of cue-related differences in the population response, i.e. the maximal cue-related information at each time point.

Evidence for time-specific coding is most apparent for the earliest training epoch (see Fig. 6.5a). Classifiers trained on data from 100–150ms post-cue onset (in red) can only successfully discriminate between cue-type for test data sampled from the equivalent and closely neighbouring time windows (e.g. 100ms to 200ms). For data sampled at further times, classification is no better than chance. This failure cannot be attributed to a more general lack of discriminative information at these subsequent time points following cue onset. On the contrary, within-time classification actually peaks at around 250ms (see grey trace, and also Fig. 6.4c). Temporal specificity is also evident at the next training window (200–250ms), albeit with a broader window of above-chance classification (from 150 to 300ms). This increase in tolerance implies a greater degree of time stability, although cross-generalization still returns to chance levels by the delay period.

These results do not easily fit within a persistent activation hypothesis model of working memory (e.g. Goldman-Rakic 1995; Wang 2001). The pattern of activity that drives the most robust classification during cue processing does not persist into the delay period. Rather, the pattern seems to evolve along a specific but complex trajectory and, like the locust olfactory system, the informational content peaks during the most dynamic phase of the trajectory. This relationship between the information content and the system dynamics is most evident in reference to the state-space velocity plot shown in Fig. 6.5b.

From a prospective coding framework, dynamic changes in population coding could reflect remapping from the cue representation to a representation of the anticipated target stimulus. Accordingly, the network would be expected to settle into a pattern that reflects pre-activation of the anticipated target stimulus. To test this prediction directly, we extended the cross-temporal analysis to the presentation of the target (right panels in Fig. 6.5a). Although the population response contains rich information about the identity of the target stimulus (grey trace), there was no evident relationship between neural patterns coding the target and the population response observed during cue and/ or delay periods.

These observed dynamics suggest that stimulus processing is associated with a complex spatiotemporal trajectory through multidimensional state space (see schematic in Fig. 6.6a, adapted from Stokes 2011a). Although the path through state space is reliable

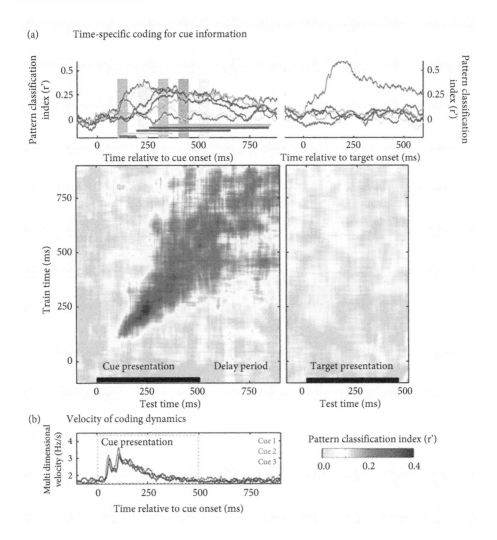

FIGURE 6.5 Dynamic population coding of task-relevant information in prefrontal cortex. (a) Each colour trace in the upper panel plots the discrimination accuracy of classifiers trained on data from the corresponding colour-coded time window, and tested at all other time points indicated along the x-axis during the cue, delay (left) and target period (right). Horizontal significance bars indicate periods of significant cross-temporal classification. For reference, the within-time classification performance is shown in grey to indicate the upper bound classification performance. The full cross-temporal matrix is shown in the lower panel, with the reliability of classification colour-coded from green (low) to red (high). (b) The velocity of dynamic coding was assessed by calculating the rate of change of the population response in the multidimensional activity state space. Reprinted from *Neuron*, 78 (2), Mark G. Stokes, Makoto Kusunoki,Natasha Sigala, Hamed Nili, David Gaffan, and John Duncan, Dynamic Coding for Cognitive Control in Prefrontal Cortex, Pages 364–75, Copyright (2013), with permission from Elsevier.

across trials, there is little evidence for a robust time-stable code. Activity seems to travel through a continuous series of states rather than maintaining a fixed 'memory' or 'anticipation' state.

Buonomano and Maass (2009) argue that these complex population dynamics could result from the evolution of state-dependent processing that is determined by a cascading interaction between past and current input. According to their framework, the response sensitivity, or hidden state, of a neural network necessarily reflects the previous stimulation history at various timescales. Consequently, the response profile of the network is in constant flux. Stimulus driven activity alters the response to subsequent stimulation (e.g. through short-term synaptic facilitation/depression), so that subsequent input will trigger a unique response pattern reflecting the new hidden state. Moreover, this new pattern will further modulate the hidden state of the system, thus determining the response to the next input, and so on (see schematic in Fig. 6.6b, adapted from Buonomano and Maass 2009). The reciprocal interaction between the activation state and the hidden state of the network would result in a complex spatiotemporal trajectory through state space (Crowe et al. 2010; Meyers et al. 2008). The full trajectory is reproducible across trials to the extent that the hidden state returns to the baseline connective state, established through longer-term plasticity (i.e. long-term potentiation/depression).

It has recently been proposed that such hidden states could be used to maintain information in working memory (Mongillo, Barak, and Tsodyks 2008). Because the hidden state is shaped by past experience (i.e. previous activation history), it constitutes a memory by definition. The duration of this mnemonic trace depends on the time-constants of the biophysical factors that shape the hidden state. Recently, Mongillo and colleagues highlight calcium kinetics as an ideal candidate for shaping the hidden state of the network at a timescale suitable for working memory. According to their synaptic model of working memory, spike history determines the residual Ca+ concentrations at synaptic terminals, which in turn modulate synaptic efficacy. Numerous other biophysical mechanisms result in activity-dependent modulation of synaptic efficacy over a range of timescales, from tens of milliseconds to minutes (Zucker and Regehr 2002). Moreover, such short-term synaptic modulations may be as robust as long-term potentiation (Marder and Buonomano 2003), the canonical memory trace that underpins long-term memory.

Computational models demonstrate that information can be efficiently read out of a hidden state comprised of temporarily tuned network weights (Deco, Rolls, and Romo 2010; Sugase-Miyamoto et al. 2008). Because memory readout is computed by the weighted sum of input from the retrieval cue (i.e. match-filter, in Sugase-Miyamoto et al. 2008), there is no need to explicitly compare the similarity between two activity patterns representing the previous and current input to decide if a stimulus matches expectation. In these respects, working memory could share fundamental characteristics with long-term memory (Nairne 2002). The repertoire of possible memories is coded in an effectively dormant state of network weights. These representations are only active when necessary, for example during retrieval (e.g. Nairne 2002), and/or preparation for retrieval (Lepsien, Thornton, and Nobre 2011; Lewis-Peacock, Drysdale, Oberauer, and Postle 2012), and/or active rehearsal (Awh et al. 1998). Otherwise the memory trace remains silent, hidden

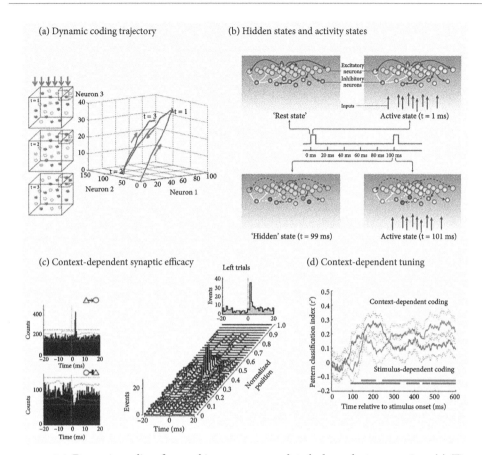

FIGURE 6.6 Dynamic coding for working memory and task-dependent processing. (a) Time-specific population coding implies that activity moves through a continuous series of states, rather than maintaining a fixed 'memory' or 'anticipation' state. Adapted from Stokes, M., The spatiotemporal structure of population coding in monkey parietal cortex. *The Journal of Neuroscience*, 31(4), pp. 1167–1169 © 2011, The Society for Neuroscience. (b) Complex spatiotemporal dynamics can be accounted for by the interaction between the activation state of the system, and the underlying hidden state. Input activity triggers a patterned response in the network that is governed by the configuration of synaptic connections (i.e. hidden state). Because this patterned response temporarily alters the hidden state according to various biophysical mechanisms for activity-dependent short-term synaptic plasticity (see text), subsequent input will trigger a different patterned response in the network, which in turn will result in a different pattern of changes to the hidden state, and so on. Consequently, even identical input will result in a dynamic trajectory of time-specific coding, as the hidden state that determines the response of the network is constantly modulated by on-going activity. Reprinted by permission from Macmillan Publishers Ltd: *Nature Reviews Neuroscience*, 10 (2), State-dependent computations: spatiotemporal processing in cortical networks, Dean V. Buonomano and Wolfgang Maass, pp. 113–25, copyright © 2009, Nature Publishing Group. (c) The hidden state of the network can be inferred from a proxy measure of pair-wise synaptic connections. An increase in the relative probability that neuron A fires directly after neuron B (~3ms) suggests that neuron B is excitatory and monosynaptically connected to neuron A (upper example pair). Conversely, a relative decrease in probability that neuron A fires directly after neuron B suggests that neuron B is inhibitory and monosynaptically connected to neuron A (lower example pair). Fujisawa and colleagues (2008) found that indices for such

from activity-dependent measures such as readout performed by downstream detectors ('reader-actuator' mechanisms in Buzsaki 2010), or the curious neuroscientist.

A temporary assembly of synaptic weights, or 'synapsemble' (Buzsaki 2010), could be a more effective neurophysiological implementation of working memory than sustained activity patterns (Mongillo et al. 2008). Assuming that working memory is in constant use (i.e. constructing and maintaining an up-to-date world model of the contents of the environment and the rules that govern them), a silent memory code could provide a more general and metabolically efficient solution than persistent spiking activity. Moreover, because memories are stored in a format that is qualitatively different from perceptual representations, their informational content could be more resistant to interference from, and/or confusion with, other activity-based representations (Olivers, Peters, Houtkamp, and Roelfsema 2011). Finally, temporary synaptic weight changes could be more stable than reverberatory mechanisms (Wang 2001), as positive feedback systems are inherently prone to noise amplification (Buonomano and Maass 2009).

As described above, dynamic coding trajectories are a predicted consequence of constantly evolving hidden states (Buonomano and Maass 2009). However, more direct evidence that working memory is mediated via temporary synaptic weight changes would depend on accurate *in vivo* measures of synaptic efficacy during maintenance in working memory. Though this is not yet feasible, Fujisawa and colleagues (Fujisawa, Amarasingham, Harrison, and Buzsaki 2008) provide indirect but compelling evidence for context-dependent modulation of synaptic connections using a proxy measure of synaptic efficacy in rat prefrontal cortex. Specifically, they computed the cross-correlation in firing between simultaneously recorded pairs of neurons in search of distinct peaks at a timing lag that is consistent with monosynaptic transmission (~3ms). This work-around solution provides an indirect measure of the direction, sign (facilitation/inhibition), and strength of the synaptic connections between candidate pairs of connected neurons (see Fig. 6.6c, left panel). Consistent with a synaptic model of working memory (e.g. Mongillo et al. 2008), they found that the pattern of effective synaptic connections was dynamically modulated during a working memory dependent maze task (see Fig. 6.6c, right panel).

---

connections in rat prefrontal cortex vary with the working memory state. Reprinted by permission from Macmillan Publishers Ltd: *Nature Neuroscience*, 11 (7), Behavior-dependent short-term assembly dynamics in the medial prefrontal cortex, Shigeyoshi Fujisawa, Asohan Amarasingham, Matthew T Harrisonand, and György Buzsákipp. 823–833, copyright © 2008, Nature Publishing Group. (d) According to an adaptive coding model of prefrontal cortex, temporary synaptic weight changes established during cue encoding and maintained during the memory delay constitute the task-dependent rules that determine how the network will respond to subsequent input. Here we show that choice stimuli from the experiment described in Figs. 6.4 and 6.5 are initially coded according to stimulus-driven differences (image 1 vs image 2 vs image 3, in blue), but context dependent coding rapidly dominates in prefrontal cortex (target vs non-target, in red; Reprinted from *Neuron*, 78 (2), Mark G. Stokes, Makoto Kusunoki, Natasha Sigala, Hamed Nili, David Gaffan, and John Duncan, Dynamic Coding for Cognitive Control in Prefrontal Cortex, pp. 364–75, Copyright (2013), with permission from Elsevier.)

Formal computational models predict that the hidden state of a network can be read out via undifferentiated input activity (Deco et al. 2010; Mongillo et al. 2008). The guiding concept here is that any input will trigger a unique pattern that depends on the initial state of the system (Buonomano and Maass 2009). Thus, even an identical stimulus input can result in robust differences in the elicited activity patterns depending on the current hidden state of the system. Borrowing from signal-processing terminology, we can consider this the impulse response function of the system. In Stokes et al. (2013), the impulse response function of the cue-configured network can be approximated by measuring the population response to the fixed neutral stimulus (Fig. 6.4a). Although the stimulus was identical across conditions, the pattern of activity elicited in PFC differentiated the cue state, exactly as expected of a cue-specific hidden state (Buonomano and Maass 2009; Mongillo et al. 2008). Because the patterned response reliably discriminates between the memory states, a similar impulse response could be used by the system for reading out the contents of working memory during retrieval (Mongillo et al. 2008; Nairne 2002).

Empirical evidence suggests that even random input can generate a reliable patterned response that reflects the hidden network state. For example, in cat visual cortex, the response to a randomly selected stimulus drives a patterned response that reflects both the previous and current stimuli (Nikolic, Hausler, Singer, and Maass, 2009). Thus, diverse input is also able to drive a patterned response that betrays the hidden state of the network. It is possible that a similar phenomenon is responsible for memory-specific activity patterns in the delay period. On average, spontaneous neural activity could drive a consistent pattern that reflects the connective state. In this respect, the hidden state is not necessarily silent, as random spontaneous activity still drives a differential response. This kind of reflected pattern could explain previous reports of sustained activity in PFC that differentiates the memory state (Miller et al. 1996; Rainer et al. 1999), but according to different coding preferences than an activity state that matches either the previous or anticipated stimulus.

Super-Rapid Adaptive Coding in PFC

Although state-dependent processing could be a general property for many brain areas, short-term synaptic dynamics in PFC could be especially important for guiding flexible behaviour. At the apex of the processing hierarchy (e.g. Fuster 1997), input to PFC is already highly filtered for behavioural relevance (e.g. via mechanisms in visual cortex described above), so that information driving changes to the network is already likely to be task-relevant. In contrast, similar changes in lower brain areas, such as perceptual cortex (Nikolic et al. 2009), could reflect less selective forms of memory (e.g. iconic memory, Jaaskelainen et al. 2011). Moreover, because perceptual areas are constantly updated by new input, temporary state changes may be particularly vulnerable to overwriting, thus limiting the durability and life span of non-prefrontal memory traces (Sligte, Scholte, and Lamme 2008).

According to an adaptive coding model of PFC, flexible goal-oriented behaviour is mediated via dynamic changes to prefrontal tuning properties (Duncan 2001). Within this perspective, PFC constitutes a flexible pool of neural resources that can be recruited on the fly to represent whatever information is currently most relevant for achieving behavioural goals. One of the most striking findings in prefrontal neurophysiology is the number of cells that seem to respond selectively in any given task (Duncan 2001). Any random sample of PFC neurons typically yields a high proportion of cells that seem especially tuned for representing the various parameters of current behaviour. Similarly, in the fMRI literature, PFC is conspicuously active across a broad range of possible tasks (Duncan 2010; Duncan and Owen 2000).

It is implausible that PFC is hardwired to perform all these functions, but more likely, tuning in PFC adapts rapidly to current task demands. Ultimately, the tuning profile of any neuron is determined by the input it receives via synaptic connections: thus, flexible tuning implies short-term synaptic plasticity. Extending directly on synaptic models of working memory (Mongillo et al. 2008), we suggest that activity-dependent changes in prefrontal connectivity rapidly tune prefrontal cells to respond selectively to information that is currently relevant to goal-directed behaviour.

If we consider again the cued target-detection task, adaptive coding would strongly predict that the response to choice stimuli should be determined by the cue state. Again, using population-level decoding methods, we find that the initial population response codes the physical properties of the input, but trajectories then rapidly diverge according to task-relevance (Fig. 6.6d). Depending on the cue state, in other words, quite different sensory inputs lead to similar final 'target' or 'non-target' representations. This is consistent with the hypothesis that the cue stimulus establishes a context-specific tuning profile in prefrontal cortex that is able to classify the cue-associated choice stimulus as a target, and all other choice stimuli as currently task-irrelevant.

Essentially, this framework builds on the prospective coding model described above, although preparation in prefrontal cortex does not depend on the activity state per se, but rather the hidden state that determines the tuning profile. Essentially, this account preserves the integration of memory and preparatory attention (i.e. working memory as a forward model for guiding future action), but implemented according to a different neurophysiological mechanism. Perhaps a more important conceptual advance is that a dynamic coding perspective also naturally integrates maintenance of content as well as rules. In fact, the content in working memory is actually coded in the rules that map subsequent input to the patterned output. As described above, this could mediate a matched filter process (Sugase-Miyamoto et al. 2008), and/or a more general retrieval based re-instantiation of a memory-specific pattern (e.g. Nairne 2002). Fundamentally, however, dynamic tuning also constitutes a context-dependent rule for defining the current input/output behaviour of the network. This kind of flexible mapping is fundamental to adaptive goal-directed behaviour (Duncan 2001; Miller 2000; Miller and Cohen 2001).

Relationship between Dynamic Coding and Preparatory Activity in Visual Cortex

At the beginning of this chapter, we considered how preparatory attention could be mediated via feedback connections to perceptual cortex, ultimately to bias baseline levels of activity in favour of task-relevant input. We have also considered the relationship between maintaining preparatory attentional states and working memory processes in PFC. Some researchers have suggested that maintenance in working memory is necessary and sufficient for biasing attention (e.g. Soto, Hodsoll, Rotshtein, and Humphreys 2008). A slightly modified account further differentiates states within working memory (Olivers et al. 2011): only one item at any given time occupies the privileged status to bias attention (Cowan 2001; Oberauer 2003). Other items in working memory do not bias attention, even though they can be successfully maintained.

A similar division between maintenance and bias was recently proposed by Lewis-Peacock and colleagues. In a human fMRI study, they used MVPA to show that delay activity in perceptual cortex was specific to the item in working memory that was in the focus of attention (Lewis-Peacock et al. 2012). They found no evidence for memory selective delay activity for unattended items, even though the unattended information was still successfully recalled at the end of the trial. They conclude that selective increases in baseline activity reflect preparation for the expected probe stimulus (see also Lepsien et al. 2011; Stokes 2011b). In contrast, working memory does not require sustained delay activity, but can be re-instantiated when necessary. This conclusion is consistent with the silent working memory hypothesis discussed above, and also evidence that increases in baseline activity in visual cortex during working memory delay periods reflect attentional preparation for the memory probe (Offen, Schluppeck, and Heeger 2009).

If task-relevant information is stored in silent memory codes, as proposed in this chapter, it would be maximally efficient to reactivate and use this information, for example to generate activity biases in visual cortex, only when necessary. This might happen, for example, when critical visual stimuli are expected to be accompanied by distractors, or to be embedded in visual noise (e.g. Chelazzi et al. 1998; Stokes et al. 2009b).Active use of working memory codes might also be restricted to the expected time of target presentation; in this respect, preparatory attention essentially implies temporal expectation. Exactly how temporal expectation is coordinated remains a significant problem to solve, though several candidate mechanisms have been identified and explored (see Nobre and Coull 2010). For example, state-dependent processing dynamics could be important for some forms of time keeping (Buonomano and Maass 2009). Similarly, circular dynamics, such as low-frequency neural oscillations, could also be useful for time-structuring neural activity.

Temporal organization of preparatory activity accords with Nobre's synergistic model of attention (Doherty, Rao, Mesulam, and Nobre 2005; Nobre, Correa, and Coull 2007), in which the specificity of attentional biases varies along three principal dimensions: what, when, and where. For example, consider a real world vigilance task in which an airport security officer monitors an X-ray screen for many hours looking for ill-defined targets (i.e. anything suspicious). This is presumably extremely taxing, and probably alarmingly ineffective. However, the cognitive demand could be dramatically reduced, and/or success rate increased, if attention were cued to a specific moment in time (i.e. the next few bags are very likely to contain something suspicious), and/or to a specific item (i.e. only look for handguns), and/or a specific location within the bag. Or even better: 'the next bag is likely to have a gun in the upper left hand corner'. The attention gain is best conceived by the synergistic dependencies (Nobre, Rohenkohl, and Stokes 2012; Nobre and Rohenkohl (chapter 24), this volume). It may make little sense to consider the isolated effect of temporal, spatial, or feature attention on neural activity that is driven by the combined presence of a particular feature at a particular position in time and space.

Summary

In this chapter, we review evidence that preparatory attention increases baseline activity in neurons responsive to the attended stimulus, including both spatial (Kastner et al. 1999; Luck et al. 1997) and non-spatial features (Chelazzi et al. 1998; Stokes et al. 2009b). According to a biased competition model of attention, these changes in baseline activity could favour processing of input that matches the attentional template (Desimone and Duncan 1995). Such preparatory states can be instantiated via symbolic and/or non-visual cues (e.g. Stokes et al. 2009b), directly implicating top-down modulation from control areas higher along the processing hierarchy, especially prefrontal cortex.

Prefrontal cortex has long been associated with working memory (Fuster and Alexander 1971), and working memory is at least necessary (Desimone and Duncan 1995), and perhaps even sufficient (Soto et al. 2008), for maintaining a preparatory attentional state. Although it is often assumed that working memory and/or preparatory attention are instantiated through persistent activation of task-relevant representations in PFC (Miller et al. 1996; Rainer et al. 1999), in this chapter we further develop an alternative proposal that is more consistent with a dynamic view of neural coding (Buonomano and Maass 2009) and adaptive coding for task-relevant information in PFC (Duncan 2001). We present recent evidence that is broadly consistent with rapid, yet temporary, synaptic changes in PFC that mediate goal-directed behaviour. We predict that further methodological developments in the near future will allow researchers to directly measure temporary synaptic changes during complex, goal-directed behaviour.

Acknowledgements

This work was supported by Queen's College, Oxford (Extraordinary Junior Research Fellowship, to MS) and MRC intramural programme MC-A060-5PQ10.

Note

1. Similar inferences were previously made using adaptation fMRI (Tootell et al. 1998), but methodological constraints limit the application of this approach across different experimental contexts (Krekelberg, Boynton, and van Wezel 2006). Most importantly, release from adaption is inferred by changes in the presentation sequence (i.e. repetition vs change), which is likely to influence attentional factors as well (Summerfield and Egner 2009).

References

Armstrong, K. M., Fitzgerald, J. K., and Moore, T. (2006). Changes in visual receptive fields with microstimulation of frontal cortex. *Neuron 50*(5): 791–798.

Armstrong, K. M. and Moore, T. (2007). Rapid enhancement of visual cortical response discriminability by microstimulation of the frontal eye field. *Proceedings of the National Academy of Sciences USA 104*(22): 9499–9504.

Awh, E. and Jonides, J. (2001). Overlapping mechanisms of attention and spatial working memory. *Trends in Cognitive Sciences 5*(3): 119–126.

Awh, E., Jonides, J., and Reuter-Lorenz, P. A. (1998). Rehearsal in spatial working memory. *Journal of Experimental Psychology: Human Perception and Performance 24*(3): 780–790.

Buonomano, D. V. and Maass, W. (2009). State-dependent computations: spatiotemporal processing in cortical networks. *Nature Reviews Neuroscience 10*(2): 113–125.

Buzsaki, G. (2010). Neural syntax: Cell assemblies, synapsembles, and readers. *Neuron 68*(3): 362–385.

Chawla, D., Rees, G., and Friston, K. J. (1999). The physiological basis of attentional modulation in extrastriate visual areas. *Nature Neuroscience 2*(7): 671–676.

Chelazzi, L., Duncan, J., Miller, E. K., and Desimone, R. (1998). Responses of neurons in inferior temporal cortex during memory-guided visual search. *Journal of Neurophysiology 80*(6): 2918–2940.

Chelazzi, L., Miller, E. K., Duncan, J., and Desimone, R. (1993). A neural basis for visual search in inferior temporal cortex. [Research Support, Non-U.S. Gov't Research Support, U.S. Gov't, Non-P.H.S.] *Nature 363*(6427): 345–347.

Cowan, N. (2001). The magical number 4 in short-term memory: A reconsideration of mental storage capacity. *Behavioral and Brain Sciences 24*(1): 87–114.

Crowe, D. A., Averbeck, B. B., and Chafee, M. V. (2010). Rapid sequences of population activity patterns dynamically encode task-critical spatial information in parietal cortex. *Journal of Neuroscience 30*(35): 11640–11653.

Curtis, C. E. and D'Esposito, M. (2003). Persistent activity in the prefrontal cortex during working memory. *Trends in Cognitive Sciences 7*(9): 415–423.

Cutrell, E. B. and Marrocco, R. T. (2002). Electrical microstimulation of primate posterior parietal cortex initiates orienting and alerting components of covert attention. [Research Support, Non-U.S. Gov't Research Support, U.S. Gov't, P.H.S.] *Experimental Brain Research* 144(1): 103–113.

Deco, G., Rolls, E. T., and Romo, R. (2010). Synaptic dynamics and decision making. *Proceedings of the National Academy of Sciences USA* 107(16): 7545–7549.

Desimone, R. and Duncan, J. (1995). Neural mechanisms of selective visual attention. *Annual Review of Neuroscience* 18: 193–222.

Doherty, J. R., Rao, A., Mesulam, M. M., and Nobre, A. C. (2005). Synergistic effect of combined temporal and spatial expectations on visual attention. [Research Support, Non-U.S. Gov't.] *Journal of Neuroscience* 25(36): 8259–8266.

Duncan, J. (1998). Converging levels of analysis in the cognitive neuroscience of visual attention. *Philosophical Transactions of the Royal Society of London B: Biological Sciences* 353(1373): 1307–1317.

Duncan, J. (2001). An adaptive coding model of neural function in prefrontal cortex. *Nature Reviews Neuroscience* 2(11): 820–829.

Duncan, J. (2010). The multiple-demand (MD) system of the primate brain: Mental programs for intelligent behaviour. [Research Support, Non-U.S. Gov't Review.] *Trends in Cognitive Sciences* 14(4): 172–179.

Duncan, J. and Owen, A. M. (2000). Common regions of the human frontal lobe recruited by diverse cognitive demands. *Trends in Neurosciences* 23(10): 475–483.

Fannon, S. P., Saron, C. D., and Mangun, G. R. (2007). Baseline shifts do not predict attentional modulation of target processing during feature-based visual attention. *Frontiers in Human Neuroscience* 1: 7. doi: 10.3389/neuro.09.007.2007.

Freedman, D. J. and Asaad, W. F. (2006). Experience-dependent representation of visual categories in parietal cortex. *Nature* 443(7): 85–88.

Freedman, D. J., Riesenhuber, M., Poggio, T., and Miller, E. K. (2001). Categorical representation of visual stimuli in the primate prefrontal cortex. *Science* 291(5502): 312–316.

Fries, P. (2009). Neuronal gamma-band synchronization as a fundamental process in cortical computation. *Annual Review of Neuroscience* 32: 209–224.

Friston, K. (2010). The free-energy principle: A unified brain theory? *Nature Reviews Neuroscience* 11(2): 127–138.

Fujisawa, S., Amarasingham, A., Harrison, M. T., and Buzsaki, G. (2008). Behavior-dependent short-term assembly dynamics in the medial prefrontal cortex. *Nature Neuroscience* 11(7): 823–833.

Fuster, J. M. (1997). *The Prefrontal Cortex: Anatomy, Physiology, and Neuropsychology of the Frontal Lobe*. New York: Raven Press.

Fuster, J. M. and Alexander, G. E. (1971). Neuron activity related to short-term memory. *Science* 173(3997): 652–654.

Giesbrecht, B., Weissman, D. H., Woldorff, M. G., and Mangun, G. R. (2006). Pre-target activity in visual cortex predicts behavioral performance on spatial and feature attention tasks. *Brain Research* 1080(1): 63–72.

Goldman-Rakic, P. S. (1995). Cellular basis of working memory. *Neuron* 14(3): 477–485.

Gregoriou, G. G., Gotts, S. J., and Desimone, R. (2012). Cell-type-specific synchronization of neural activity in FEF with V4 during attention. [Research Support, N.I.H., Extramural Research Support, N.I.H., Intramural.] *Neuron* 73(3): 581–594.

Haxby, J. V., Gobbini, M. I., Furey, M. L., Ishai, A., Schouten, J. L., and Pietrini, P. (2001). Distributed and overlapping representations of faces and objects in ventral temporal cortex. *Science* 293(5539): 2425–2430.

Haynes, J.-D. and Rees, G. (2005). Predicting the orientation of invisible stimuli from activity in human primary visual cortex. *Nature Neuroscience* 8(5): 686–691.

Haynes, J.-D. and Rees, G. (2006). Decoding mental states from brain activity in humans. *Nature Reviews Neuroscience* 7(7): 523–534.

Hebb, D. O. (1949). *The Organization of Behavior: A Neuropsychological Theory.* New York: Wiley.

Heinen, K., Ruff, C. C., Bjoertomt, O., Schenkluhn, B., Bestmann, S., Blankenburg, F., et al. (2011). Concurrent TMS–fMRI reveals dynamic interhemispheric influences of the right parietal cortex during exogenously cued visuospatial attention. [Research Support, Non-U.S. Gov't.] *European Journal of Neuroscience* 33(5): 991–1000.

Itti, L. and Koch, C. (2001). Computational modelling of visual attention. *Nature Reviews Neuroscience* 2(3): 194–203.

Jaaskelainen, I. P., Ahveninen, J., Andermann, M. L., Belliveau, J. W., Raij, T., and Sams, M. (2011). Short-term plasticity as a neural mechanism supporting memory and attentional functions. [Research Support, N.I.H., Extramural Research Support, Non-U.S. Gov't Review.] *Brain Research* 1422: 66–81.

Kamitani, Y. and Tong, F. (2005). Decoding the visual and subjective contents of the human brain. *Nature Neuroscience* 8(5): 679–685.

Kastner, S., Pinsk, M. A., De Weerd, P., Desimone, R., and Ungerleider, L. G. (1999). Increased activity in human visual cortex during directed attention in the absence of visual stimulation. *Neuron* 22(4): 751–761.

Krekelberg, B., Boynton, G. M., and van Wezel, R. J. (2006). Adaptation: From single cells to BOLD signals. [Research Support, N.I.H., Extramural Research Support, Non-U.S. Gov't Review.] *Trends in Neurosciences* 29(5): 250–256.

Kriegeskorte, N., Goebel, R., and Bandettini, P. (2006). Information-based functional brain mapping. *Proceedings of the National Academy of Sciences USA* 103(10): 3863–3868.

Kubota, K. and Niki, H. (1971). Prefrontal cortical unit activity and delayed alternation performance in monkeys. *Journal of Neurophysiology* 34(3): 337–347.

Laurent, G. (2002). Olfactory network dynamics and the coding of multidimensional signals. [Research Support, Non-U.S. Gov't Research Support, U.S. Gov't, Non-P.H.S. Research Support, U.S. Gov't, P.H.S. Review.] *Nature Reviews Neuroscience* 3(11): 884–895.

Lepsien, J., Thornton, I., and Nobre, A. C. (2011). Modulation of working-memory maintenance by directed attention. *Neuropsychologia* 49(6): 1569–1577.

Lewis-Peacock, J. A., Drysdale, A. T., Oberauer, K., and Postle, B. R. (2012). Neural evidence for a distinction between short-term memory and the focus of attention. [Research Support, N.I.H., Extramural.] *Journal of Cognitive Neuroscience* 24(1): 61–79.

Luck, S. J., Chelazzi, L., Hillyard, S. A., and Desimone, R. (1997). Neural mechanisms of spatial selective attention in areas V1, V2, and V4 of macaque visual cortex. *Journal of Neurophysiology* 77(1): 24–42.

McMains, S. A., Fehd, H. M., Emmanouil, T.-A., and Kastner, S. (2007). Mechanisms of feature- and space-based attention: Response modulation and baseline increases. *Journal of Neurophysiology* 98(4): 2110–2121.

Marder, C. P. and Buonomano, D. V. (2003). Differential effects of short- and long-term potentiation on cell firing in the CA1 region of the hippocampus. [Research Support, Non-U.S. Gov't Research Support, U.S. Gov't, Non-P.H.S. Research Support, U.S. Gov't, P.H.S.] *Journal of Neuroscience* 23(1): 112–121.

Mazor, O. and Laurent, G. (2005). Transient dynamics versus fixed points in odor representations by locust antennal lobe projection neurons. [Research Support, N.I.H., Extramural.] *Neuron* 48(4): 661–673.

Meyers, E. M., Freedman, D. J., Kreiman, G., Miller, E. K., and Poggio, T. (2008). Dynamic population coding of category information in inferior temporal and prefrontal cortex. *Journal of Neurophysiology* 100(3): 1407–1419.

Miller, E. K. (2000). The prefrontal cortex and cognitive control. *Nature Reviews Neuroscience* 1(1): 59–65.

Miller, E. K. and Cohen, J. D. (2001). An integrative theory of prefrontal cortex function. *Annual Review of Neuroscience* 24: 167–202.

Miller, E. K., Erickson, C. A., and Desimone, R. (1996). Neural mechanisms of visual working memory in prefrontal cortex of the macaque. *Journal of Neuroscience* 16(16): 5154–5167.

Miyashita, Y. (2004). Cognitive memory: Cellular and network machineries and their top-down control. [Research Support, Non-U.S. Gov't Review.] *Science* 306(5695): 435–440.

Mongillo, G., Barak, O., and Tsodyks, M. (2008). Synaptic theory of working memory. *Science* 319(5869): 1543–1546.

Moore, T. (2006). The neurobiology of visual attention: Finding sources. *Current Opinion in Neurobiology* 16(2): 159–165.

Moore, T. and Armstrong, K. M. (2003). Selective gating of visual signals by microstimulation of frontal cortex. *Nature* 421(6921): 370–373.

Moran, J. and Desimone, R. (1985). Selective attention gates visual processing in the extrastriate cortex. *Science* 229(4715): 782–784.

Nairne, J. S. (2002). Remembering over the short-term: The case against the standard model. *Annual Review of Psychology* 53: 53–81.

Navalpakkam, V. and Itti, L. (2007). Search goal tunes visual features optimally. *Neuron* 53(4): 605–617.

Naya, Y., Sakai, K., and Miyashita, Y. (1996). Activity of primate inferotemporal neurons related to a sought target in pair-association task. [Research Support, Non-U.S. Gov't.] *Proceedings of the National Academy of Sciences USA* 93(7): 2664–2669.

Nikolic, D., Hausler, S., Singer, W., and Maass, W. (2009). Distributed fading memory for stimulus properties in the primary visual cortex. *PLoS Biology* 7(12): e1000260. doi: 10.1371/journal.pbio.1000260.

Nobre, A. C., Correa, A., and Coull, J. (2007). The hazards of time [Review]. *Current Opinion in Neurobiology* 17(4): 465–470.

Nobre, A. C. and Coull, J. T. (2010). *Attention and Time*. Oxford and New York: Oxford University Press.

Nobre, A. C., Rohenkohl, G., and Stokes, M. (eds.) (2012). *Nervous Anticipation: Top-down Biasing across Space and Time*. New York: Guilford Press.

Norman, K. A., Polyn, S. M., Detre, G. J., and Haxby, J. V. (2006). Beyond mind-reading: Multi-voxel pattern analysis of fMRI data. *Trends in Cognitive Sciences* 10(9): 424–430.

Oberauer, K. (2003). Selective attention to elements in working memory. *Experimental Psychology* 50(4): 257–269.

O'Craven, K. M., Downing, P. E., and Kanwisher, N. (1999). fMRI evidence for objects as the units of attentional selection. *Nature* 401(6753): 584–587.

Offen, S., Schluppeck, D., and Heeger, D. J. (2009). The role of early visual cortex in visual short-term memory and visual attention. *Vision Research* 49(10): 1352–1362.

Olivers, C. N., Peters, J., Houtkamp, R., and Roelfsema, P. R. (2011). Different states in visual working memory: When it guides attention and when it does not. [Research Support, Non-U.S. Gov't Review.] *Trends in Cognitive Sciences* 15(7): 327–334.

Passingham, D. and Sakai, K. (2004). The prefrontal cortex and working memory: Physiology and brain imaging. *Current Opinion in Neurobiology* 14(2): 163–168.

Peelen, M. V. and Kastner, S. (2011). A neural basis for real-world visual search in human occipitotemporal cortex. [Research Support, N.I.H., Extramural Research Support, U.S. Gov't, Non-P.H.S.] *Proceedings of the National Academy of Sciences USA 108*(29): 12125–12130.

Peters, J. C., Goebel, R., and Roelfsema, P. R. (2009). Remembered but unused: The accessory items in working memory that do not guide attention. [Research Support, Non-U.S. Gov't.] *Journal of Cognitive Neuroscience 21*(6): 1081–1091.

Rainer, G., Rao, S. C., and Miller, E. K. (1999). Prospective coding for objects in primate prefrontal cortex. *Journal of Neuroscience 19*(13): 5493–5505.

Ress, D., Backus, B. T., and Heeger, D. J. (2000). Activity in primary visual cortex predicts performance in a visual detection task. *Nature Neuroscience 3*(9): 940–945.

Reynolds, J. H., Chelazzi, L., and Desimone, R. (1999). Competitive mechanisms subserve attention in macaque areas V2 and V4. *Journal of Neuroscience 19*(5): 1736–1753.

Ruff, C. C., Blankenburg, F., Bjoertomt, O., Bestmann, S., Freeman, E., Haynes, J.-D., et al. (2006). Concurrent TMS–fMRI and psychophysics reveal frontal influences on human retinotopic visual cortex. *Current Biology 16*(15): 1479–1488.

Serences, J. T. and Saproo, S. (2012). Computational advances towards linking BOLD and behavior. [Research Support, N.I.H., Extramural Review.] *Neuropsychologia 50*(4): 435–446.

Serences, J. T., Yantis, S., Culberson, A., and Awh, E. (2004). Preparatory activity in visual cortex indexes distractor suppression during covert spatial orienting. [Research Support, U.S. Gov't, Non-P.H.S. Research Support, U.S. Gov't, P.H.S.] *Journal of Neurophysiology 92*(6): 3538–3545.

Shibata, K., Yamagishi, N., Goda, N., Yoshioka, T., Yamashita, O., Sato, M. A., and Kawato, M. (2008). The effects of feature attention on prestimulus cortical activity in the human visual system. [Research Support, Non-U.S. Gov't.] *Cerebral Cortex 18*(7): 1664–1675.

Shulman, G. L., d'Avossa, G., Tansy, A. P., and Corbetta, M. (2002). Two attentional processes in the parietal lobe. [Research Support, U.S. Gov't, P.H.S.] *Cerebral Cortex 12*(11): 1124–1131.

Silver, M. A., Ress, D., and Heeger, D. J. (2007). Neural correlates of sustained spatial attention in human early visual cortex. *Journal of Neurophysiology 97*(1): 229–237.

Sligte, I. G., Scholte, H. S., and Lamme, V. A. (2008). Are there multiple visual short-term memory stores? *PLoS One 3*(2): e1699. doi: 10.1371/journal.pone.0001699.

Soto, D., Heinke, D., Humphreys, G. W., and Blanco, M. J. (2005). Early, involuntary top-down guidance of attention from working memory. *Journal of Experimental Psychology: Human Perception and Performance 31*(2): 248–261.

Soto, D., Hodsoll, J., Rotshtein, P., and Humphreys, G. W. (2008). Automatic guidance of attention from working memory. *Trends in Cognitive Sciences 12*(9): 342–348.

Soto, D. and Humphreys, G. W. (2007). Automatic guidance of visual attention from verbal working memory. *Journal of Experimental Psychology: Human Perception and Performance 33*(3): 730–737.

Soto, D. and Humphreys, G. W. (2009). Automatic selection of irrelevant object features through working memory: Evidence for top-down attentional capture. *Experimental Psychology 56*(3): 165–172.

Stokes, M. (2011a). The spatiotemporal structure of population coding in monkey parietal cortex. *Journal of Neuroscience 31*(4): 1167–1169.

Stokes, M. (2011b). Top-down visual activity underlying VSTM and preparatory attention. *Neuropsychologia 49*(6): 1425–1427.

Stokes, M., Kusunoki, M., Sigala, N., Nili, H., Gaffan, D., and Duncan, J. (2013). Dynamic coding for working memory and attention in prefrontal cortex. *Neuron 78*(2): 364–375.

Stokes, M., Saraiva, A., Rohenkohl, G., and Nobre, A. C. (2011). Imagery for shapes activates position-invariant representations in human visual cortex. *NeuroImage* 56(3): 1540–1545.

Stokes, M., Thompson, R., Cusack, R., and Duncan, J. (2009a). Top-down activation of shape-specific population codes in visual cortex during mental imagery. *Journal of Neuroscience* 29(5): 1565–1572.

Stokes, M., Thompson, R., Nobre, A. C., and Duncan, J. (2009b). Shape-specific preparatory activity mediates attention to targets in human visual cortex. *Proceedings of the National Academy of Sciences USA* 106(46): 19569–19574.

Sugase-Miyamoto, Y., Liu, Z., Wiener, M. C., Optican, L. M., and Richmond, B. J. (2008). Short-term memory trace in rapidly adapting synapses of inferior temporal cortex. [Research Support, N.I.H., Intramural.] *PLoS Computational Biology* 4(5): e1000073. doi: 10.1371/journal.pcbi.1000073.

Summerfield, C. and Egner, T. (2009). Expectation (and attention) in visual cognition. *Trends in Cognitive Sciences* 13(9): 403–409.

Sylvester, C. M., Shulman, G. L., Jack, A. I., and Corbetta, M. (2009). Anticipatory and stimulus-evoked blood oxygenation level-dependent modulations related to spatial attention reflect a common additive signal. *Journal of Neuroscience* 29(34): 10671–10682.

Tanigawa, H., Lu, H. D., and Roe, A. W. (2010). Functional organization for color and orientation in macaque V4. [Comparative Study Research Support, N.I.H., Extramural Research Support, Non-U.S. Gov't.] *Nature Neuroscience* 13(12): 1542–1548.

Taylor, P. C., Nobre, A. C., and Rushworth, M. F. (2007). FEF TMS affects visual cortical activity. *Cerebral Cortex* 17(2): 391–399.

Tomita, H., Ohbayashi, M., Nakahara, K., Hasegawa, I., and Miyashita, Y. (1999). Top-down signal from prefrontal cortex in executive control of memory retrieval. *Nature* 401(6754): 699–703.

Tootell, R. B., Hadjikhani, N. K., Vanduffel, W., Liu, A. K., Mendola, J. D., Sereno, M. I., and Dale, A. M. (1998). Functional analysis of primary visual cortex (V1) in humans. [Research Support, Non-U.S. Gov't Research Support, U.S. Gov't, P.H.S. Review.] *Proceedings of the National Academy of Sciences USA* 95(3): 811–817.

Tootell, R. B., Reppas, J. B., Kwong, K. K., Malach, R., Born, R. T., Brady, T. J., et al. (1995). Functional analysis of human MT and related visual cortical areas using magnetic resonance imaging. [Research Support, Non-U.S. Gov't Research Support, U.S. Gov't, P.H.S.] *Journal of Neuroscience* 15(4): 3215–3230.

Vapnik, V. N. (1998). *Statistical Learning Theory*. New York: Wiley.

Wang, X. J. (2001). Synaptic reverberation underlying mnemonic persistent activity. *Trends in Neurosciences* 24(8): 455–463.

Wolfe, J. M. (2003). Moving towards solutions to some enduring controversies in visual search. *Trends in Cognitive Sciences* 7(2): 70–76.

Zucker, R. S. and Regehr, W. G. (2002). Short-term synaptic plasticity. *Annual Review of Physiology* 64: 355–405.

PART C

SPATIAL
ATTENTION

CHAPTER 7

···

SPATIAL COVERT ATTENTION: PERCEPTUAL MODULATION

···

MARISA CARRASCO

ATTENTION IS A SELECTIVE PROCESS
···

EACH time we open our eyes we are confronted with an overwhelming amount of information. Despite this, we experience a seemingly effortless understanding of our visual world. Attention allows us to selectively process the vast amount of information with which we are confronted, prioritizing some aspects of information while ignoring others by focusing on a certain location or aspect of the visual scene.

Attention is a selective process. Selection is necessary because there are severe limits on our capacity to process visual information. These limits are likely imposed by the fixed amount of overall energy available to the brain and by the high energy cost of the neuronal activity involved in cortical computation. Given that the amount of overall energy consumption available to the brain is essentially constant, the high bioenergetic cost of spikes requires the use of efficient representational codes relying on a sparse collection of active neurons, as well as the flexible allocation of metabolic resources according to task demands. These energy limitations, which allow only a small fraction of the machinery to be engaged concurrently, provide a neurophysiological basis for the idea that selective attention arises from the brain's limited capacity to process information (Lennie 2003).

The notion that stimuli compete for limited resources (Broadbent 1958; Kinchla 1980, 1992; Neisser 1967; Treisman 1960) is supported by electrophysiological, neuroimaging, and behavioural studies (for reviews see Beck and Kastner 2009; Desimone and Duncan 1995; Reynolds and Chelazzi 2004; Carrasco 2011). According to the biased-competition hypothesis, stimuli in the visual field activate populations of neurons that engage in competitive interactions, most likely at the intracortical level. When observers attend to visual stimulation at a given location, such competition is biased in favour of the neurons encoding information at the attended area. Thus, neurons with receptive fields at that location become more active while others are suppressed.

Changing an observer's attentional state while keeping the retinal image constant can affect perceptual performance and the activity of 'sensory' neurons throughout visual cortex. In the 1980s and 1990s, there was much interest in categorizing mechanisms of vision as preattentive or attentive. The interest in that distinction has waned as many studies have shown that attention actually affects many tasks that were once considered preattentive, such as contrast discrimination, acuity, and texture segmentation.

SPATIAL COVERT ATTENTION

Knowledge and assumptions about the world, the behavioural state of the organism, and the (sudden) appearance of possibly relevant information in the environment, facilitate the processing of sensory input. Attention can be allocated by moving one's eyes toward a location (overt attention) or by attending to an area in the periphery without actually directing one's gaze toward it (covert attention). The deployment of covert attention aids us in monitoring the environment and can inform subsequent eye movements. Humans deploy covert attention routinely in many everyday situations, such as searching for objects, driving, crossing the street, playing sports, and dancing. Moreover, covert attention plays an important role in social situations, when moving the eyes provides a cue to intentions that the individual wishes to conceal. Covert attention allows us to monitor the environment and guides our eye movements (overt attention) to locations of the visual field where salient and/or relevant information is likely to be.

The focus of spatial attention has been likened to a spotlight (Posner 1980), a zoom lens (Eriksen, Webb, and Fournier 1990), or a Gaussian gradient (Downing and Pinker 1985), which enhances processing of visual stimuli within a confined region of space. The size of this attended region may be adjusted voluntarily. When attention is distributed over a larger region of the visual field, rather than being focused on one location, there is a loss in spatial resolution and processing efficiency for any given subregion of the attended region (Eriksen, Webb, and Fournier 1990; Castiello and Umiltà 1990, 1992; Eriksen and Murphy 1987; Eriksen and Schultz 1979; Eriksen and St James 1986; Eriksen and Yeh 1985; Shulman and Wilson 1987).

Often we think of the need to selectively process information in cluttered displays with different colours and shapes (i.e. in 'Where's Wally'-like displays). Even with very simple displays, however, attention is involved in distributing resources across the visual field. There are processing trade-offs for simple, non-cluttered displays, in which only two stimuli are competing for processing; the benefit at the attended location for contrast sensitivity and acuity has a concomitant cost at the unattended location (Herrmann, Montaser-Kouhsari, Carrasco, and Heeger 2010; Montagna, Pestilli, and Carrasco 2009; Pestilli and Carrasco 2005; Pestilli, Viera, and Carrasco 2007; Barbot, Landy, and Carrasco 2011). These findings are inconsistent with the idea that perceptual processes have unlimited capacity (Eckstein, Thomas, Palmer, and Shimozaki 2000; Palmer, Verghese, and Pavel 2000; Solomon 2004), or that attentional selection is required only once the perceptual load exceeds the capacity limit of the system (Lavie 1995). Rather, they suggest that trade-offs are a characteristic of attentional allocation, which has a general effect across different tasks.

Here I review studies that deal with the effects of covert attention—endogenous or exogenous—on perceptual performance of many detection, discrimination, and localization tasks mediated by early visual processing, e.g. contrast sensitivity and spatial resolution. Attention can affect perception by altering performance—how accurately and quickly we perform on a given task—and/or by altering the subjective appearance of a stimulus or object. Most of the studies described in this review deal with discrimination tasks, because they depend on attention more than detection judgements do (Bashinski and Bacharach 1980; Bonnel and Miller 1994; Bonnel, Stein, and Bertucci 1992; Downing 1988; Muller and Findlay 1987; Shaw 1984). The perceptual distinction between larger or smaller sensory signals (detection) poses a much simpler problem for the visual system than the distinction between sensory signals that are equally large but differ in qualitative ways (discrimination).

Types of covert spatial attention: Endogenous and exogenous

William James (1890) described two different kinds of attention; one is passive, reflexive, and involuntary, whereas the other is active and voluntary. We now refer to these as exogenous/transient attention and endogenous/sustained attention. A growing body of behavioural evidence has demonstrated that these two covert attention systems facilitate processing and select information. The endogenous system corresponds to our ability to voluntarily monitor information at a given location; the exogenous system corresponds to an involuntary, automatic orienting response to a location where sudden stimulation has occurred. Due to their temporal nature, endogenous attention is also known as 'sustained' attention and exogenous attention is also known as 'transient' attention. It takes ~300 ms for observers to deploy endogenous attention, and they can sustain it voluntarily for as long as is needed to perform a task; the involuntary deployment of attention is transient: it rises and decays quickly, peaking at about 100–120 ms (Cheal, Lyon, and Hubbard 1991; Hein, Rolke, and Ulrich 2006; Ling and Carrasco 2006a, 2006b; Liu, Stevens, and Carrasco 2007; Muller and Rabbitt 1989a; Nakayama and Mackeben 1989; Remington, Johnston, and Yantis 1992). In line with these studies, a single-unit recording study has demonstrated that in macaque area MT exogenous attention has a faster time course than endogenous attention (Busse, Katzner, and Treue 2008).[1]

A seminal task in the study of attention is the Posner cueing task, in which observers have to respond as quickly as possible to a peripheral target, which is preceded by a central or peripheral cue (Posner 1980). This paradigm allows the comparison of performance in conditions where attention is deliberately directed to either a given location (attended condition), away from that location (unattended condition), or distributed across the display (neutral or control condition). I explain this cueing procedure in detail below (see the third part of this section). Whereas the shifts of attention prompted by central/sustained cues appear to be under conscious control and observers can allocate resources according to cue validity (Kinchla 1980; Giordano, McElree, and Carrasco 2009; Mangun and Hillyard 1990; Sperling and Melchner 1978), it is extremely difficult for observers to ignore peripheral/transient cues (Cheal, Lyon, and Hubbard 1991; Nakayama and Mackeben 1989; Giordano, McElree, and Carrasco 2009; Jonides 1981; Yantis and Jonides 1996). Involuntary transient shifts of attention occur even when the cues are known to be uninformative and irrelevant (Montagna, Pestilli, and Carrasco 2009; Pestilli and Carrasco 2005; Pestilli, Viera, and Carrasco 2007; Barbot, Landy, and Carrasco 2011; Muller and Rabbitt 1989b; Prinzmetal, McCool, and Park 2005; Yeshurun and Rashal 2010), and when they impair performance (Eriksen, Webb, and Fournier 1990; Hein, Rolke, and Ulrich 2006; Carrasco, Loula, and Ho 2006; Talgar and Carrasco 2002; Yeshurun 2004; Yeshurun and Carrasco 1998, 2000; Yeshurun and Levy 2003; Yeshurun, Montagna, and Carrasco 2008).

Endogenous attention and exogenous attention show some common (Montagna, Pestilli, and Carrasco 2009; Hikosaka, Miyauchi, and Shimojo 1993; Suzuki and Cavanagh 1997) and some unique perceptual effects. For instance, with peripheral cues, but not with central cues, the effects of attention are larger for a conjunction search than for a feature search in a letter search task (Hikosaka, Miyauchi, and Shimojo 1993; Suzuki and Cavanagh 1997; Briand 1998; Briand and Klein 1987). Furthermore, transient attention improves performance in a texture segmentation task at peripheral locations but impairs it at central locations (Carrasco, Loula, and Ho 2006; Talgar and Carrasco 2002; Yeshurun and Carrasco 1998; Yeshurun and Carrasco 2000; Yeshurun and Carrasco 2008), whereas sustained attention improves performance at all eccentricities (Yeshurun, Montagna, and Carrasco 2008).

Endogenous and exogenous attention also show differential effects regarding contrast sensitivity to texture patterns (Barbot, Landy, and Carrasco 2012), temporal order judgement (Hein, Rolke, and Ulrich 2006), vigilance (Maclean et al. 2009), and inhibition of return (Chica and Lupiañez 2009). Furthermore, a study employing a speed–accuracy trade-off procedure, which enables conjoint measures of discriminability and temporal dynamics, showed that the attentional benefits of endogenous attention increased with cue validity while costs remained relatively constant. However, the benefits and the costs of exogenous attention in discriminability and temporal dynamics were similar across a wide range of cue validities (Giordano, McElree, and Carrasco 2009).

The different temporal characteristics and degrees of automaticity of these attentional systems suggest that they may have evolved at different times and for different purposes—the exogenous system may be phylogenetically older, allowing us to respond automatically and quickly to stimuli that may provide behaviourally relevant information.

Mechanisms of covert attention

Although it is well established that covert attention improves performance in various visual tasks, the nature of the attentional mechanisms and the levels of processing at which they modulate visual activity are not yet well understood. Explanations of how attention improves perception range from proposals maintaining that the deployment of attention enhances the signal, to those stating that attention improves sensitivity by reducing external noise, to those proposing that the effects are due to observers' decision criteria and/or reduction in spatial uncertainty. Sensory enhancement, noise reduction, and efficient selection are not mutually exclusive; rather, all three are likely to contribute to the computational processes by which attention improves performance (Pestilli and Carrasco 2005; Eckstein, Thomas, Palmer, and Shimozaki 2000; Palmer, Verghese, and Pavel 2000; Lu and Dosher 1998, 2000; Pestilli, Carrasco, Heeger, and Gardner 2011).

The signal enhancement hypothesis proposes that attention improves the quality of the stimulus representation by increasing the gain on the signal within the locus of attentional selection (Bashinski and Bacharach 1980; Downing 1988; Ling and Carrasco 2006a; Lu and Dosher 1998, 2000; Cameron, Tai, and Carrasco 2002; Carrasco, Penpeci-Talgar, and Eckstein 2000; Carrasco, Williams, and Yeshurun 2002; Dosher and Lu 2000a, 2000b; Luck, Hillyard, Mouloua, and Hawkins 1996; Morrone, Denti, and Spinelli 2002; Muller et al. 1998). The external noise reduction hypothesis has two distinct, not mutually exclusive, formulations—noise exclusion and distractor suppression—that suggest different underlying computations. With noise exclusion, attention changes the properties of perceptual filters, enhancing the signal portion of the stimulus and mitigating the noise (e.g. Lu and Dosher 1998; Dosher and Lu 2000a, 2000b; Lu, Lesmes, and Dosher 2002). Attention acts like a filter at a specific location, only letting specific information pass; different filters process information outside the attention filter (i.e. distractors at other locations). With distractor suppression, attention enables the observer to utilize a specific filter and to disregard information outside the focus of attention. Noise-limited models of distractor suppression incorporate internal noise arising from sources such as spatial and temporal uncertainty of targets and distractors, as well as external noise resulting from distractors and masks. Several studies have attributed attentional facilitation to reduction of external noise, either because a near-threshold target presented alone could be confused with empty locations (spatial uncertainty) or because a suprathreshold target could be confused with suprathreshold distractors. According to these models, performance decreases as spatial uncertainty and the number of distractors increase, because the noise they introduce can be confused with the target signal (Kinchla 1992; Baldassi and Burr 2000; Cameron, Tai, Eckstein, and Carrasco 2004; Morgan, Ward, and Castet 1998; Shiu and Pashler 1994; Solomon, Lavie, and Morgan 1997). Presumably, precues allow observers to monitor only the relevant location(s) instead of all possible ones, reducing statistical noise with respect to the target location. This is known as reduction of spatial uncertainty (Kinchla 1992; Eckstein, Thomas, Palmer, and Shimozaki 2000; Shiu and Pashler 1994; Davis,

Kramer, and Graham 1983; Nachmias 2002; Palmer 1994; Sperling and Dosher 1986; Verghese 2001). A comprehensive study describes physiological measures and behavioural predictions distinguishing reduction of spatial uncertainty from increased sensitivity models (Eckstein, Peterson, Pham, and Droll 2009).

Methodological considerations in behavioural studies of covert attention

As mentioned, the Posner cueing task (Posner 1980) is a seminal task in the study of attention. This paradigm allows us to compare performance when attention is directed to the target location (attended condition), away from that location (unattended condition) or distributed across the display (neutral or control condition). For endogenous attention, a central cue indicates the most likely location of the subsequent target with a given cue probability (e.g. 70%). Central cues are typically small lines presented at fixation that point to particular locations of the visual field (e.g. upper left quadrant; Fig. 7.1); symbolic cues include different numbers or coloured shapes that indicate

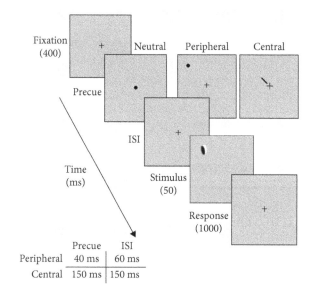

FIGURE 7.1 Sequence of events in a trial. Observers perform a two-alternative forced-choice (2AFC) orientation discrimination task on a tilted target Gabor patch, which appears at one of four isoeccentric locations. The target is preceded by a central cue (instructing observers to deploy their endogenous attention to the upcoming target location), a peripheral cue (reflexively capturing attention to the upcoming target location), or a neutral cue (baseline). The cue in this example is valid. The timing (precue and interstimulus interval) for endogenous and exogenous conditions differs (along with their respective neutral conditions), in order to maximize the effectiveness of the cues.

different locations where the observer is to attend (e.g. a green triangle or number 1 indicates upper left quadrant, a red triangle or number 4 indicates lower right quadrant). For exogenous attention, a brief peripheral cue, typically a dot or a small bar, is presented adjacent to one of the target locations, and is often not predictive of the subsequent target location. Peripheral cues attract spatial attention in an automatic, stimulus-driven manner within ~100 ms.

In the neutral trials, a small disk or bar appears in the centre of the display (central neutral cue) or several small bars appear at the centre pointing to or at all possible target locations (distributed neutral cue for endogenous and exogenous, respectively), or two long lines encompass the whole display (distributed neutral cue), indicating display onset and that the target is equally likely to occur at any possible location. Performance is comparable with these different types of neutral cues in acuity (Carrasco, Williams, and Yeshurun 2002), texture segmentation (Yeshurun and Carrasco 2008), letter identification (Talgar, Pelli, and Carrasco 2004), and temporal resolution (Yeshurun 2004). Many studies discussed in the third and fourth sections below use the Posner paradigm or a variant of it.

The following are some critical methodological issues to be considered when using spatial cues to test for sensory effects of attention.

To investigate covert attention, it is necessary to ensure that observers' eyes remain fixated at one location and to keep both the task and stimuli constant across conditions while manipulating attention. Given that ~200–250 ms are needed for goal-directed saccades to occur (Mayfrank, Kimmig, and Fischer 1987), the stimulus onset asynchrony (SOA) for the endogenous cue may allow observers to make an eye movement towards the cued location. Thus, to verify that the outcome of this manipulation is due to covert attention, it is necessary to monitor with an eye-tracker whether central fixation is maintained.

Spatial cues should convey only information that is orthogonal to the task, e.g. in a discrimination task they could indicate probable target location but not the correct response (e.g. the orientation of a stimulus; Fig. 7.2). Many experiments manipulate endogenous attention in detection tasks with cues indicating that a certain location has a given probability of containing the target. Although a high probability encourages observers to direct their attention to a particular location, it is unclear whether the enhanced detection is due to facilitation of information coding at that location, to probability matching, or to a decision mechanism, i.e. the higher probability encourages observers to assign more weight to information extracted from that probability location (Kinchla 1992). By using a two-alternative forced choice (2AFC) in which the observers discriminate stimuli preceded by a cue (e.g. stimulus orientation: left vs right), even when the cue is 100% valid in terms of location, it conveys no information as to the correct response. Thus, we can assess whether a cueing effect reflects changes in sensory discriminability (e.g. with the help of the d' index), rather than decisional (criterion), processes.

Another critical factor is that of spatial uncertainty. According to noise-limited models, performance decreases as spatial uncertainty increases because the empty locations introduce noise that can be confused with the target signal. For instance, a spatial uncertainty effect is present for low-contrast pedestals but not for high-contrast pedestals (Foley 1998). Uncertainty about the target location produces a more noticeable degradation at low than at high performance levels (Eckstein and Whiting 1996; Pelli 1985), and uncertainty is larger for less discriminable stimuli (Pelli 1985; Cohn 1981; Nachmias and Kocher 1970). Thus, uncertainty models predict that the cueing effect would be greater for low-contrast stimuli and when localization performance is poor (Carrasco, Penpeci-Talgar, and Eckstein 2000; Carrasco, Williams, and Yeshurun 2002; Pelli 1985; Cohn 1981; Nachmias and Kocher 1970). Some studies have evaluated whether attention effects go beyond uncertainty reduction, considered to be a benchmark (e.g. Carrasco, Penpeci-Talgar, and Eckstein 2000; Carrasco, Williams, and Yeshurun 2002; Morgan, Ward, and Castet 1998; Eckstein, Shimozaki, and Abbey 2002). Physiological measures and behavioural predictions can distinguish uncertainty vs increased sensitivity models (Eckstein, Peterson, Pham, and Droll 2009).

COVERT ATTENTION AND CONTRAST SENSITIVITY

Many studies described in this section involve an orientation discrimination task because this dimension has been well characterized both psychophysically and neurophysiologically, and a link between findings obtained with these two approaches has been well established (De Valois and De Valois 1988; Graham 1989; Regan and Beverley 1985; Ringach, Hawken, and Shapley 1997). In addition, orientation discrimination is used to assess the effect of attention on stimulus contrast because performance on this task improves with increasing contrast (Nachmias 1967; Skottun et al. 1987), and because fMRI response increases monotonically with stimulus contrast (Boynton, Demb, Glover, and Heeger 1999). Moreover, the shared non-linearity between the contrast response function and the magnitude of the attentional modulation across different areas of the dorsal and ventral visual pathways indicates a close link between attentional mechanisms and the mechanisms responsible for contrast encoding (Martinez Trujillo and Treue 2005; Reynolds 2005).

The effect of attention on contrast sensitivity has been well documented with studies employing an array of attention manipulations (e.g. Barbot, Landy, and Carrasco 2011; Solomon 2004; Barbot, Landy, and Carrasco 2012; Lu and Dosher 1998, 2000; Cameron, Tai, and Carrasco 2002; Carrasco, Penpeci-Talgar, and Eckstein 2000; Dosher and Lu 2000a, 2000b; Solomon, Lavie, and Morgan 1997; Foley 1998; Huang and Dobkins 2005; Lee, Itti, Koch, and Braun 1999; Lee, Koch, and Braun 1997; Morrone, Denti, and Spinelli 2004; Smith, Wolfgang, and Sinclair 2004). Psychophysical studies have shown that contrast sensitivity for the attended stimulus is enhanced in the presence of competing stimuli (e.g. Lu and Dosher 1998; Dosher and Lu 2000a, 2000b; Solomon, Lavie, and Morgan 1997; Foley 1998; Huang and Dobkins 2005; Lee, Itti, Koch, and Braun 1999; Lee, Koch, and Braun 1997; Morrone, Denti, and Spinelli 2004; Carrasco and McElree 2001). In some studies, the target is displayed simultaneously with distractors and observers indicate whether the target has an increment or decrement in contrast. Performance deteriorates as number of stimuli increases. However, a cue improves performance and this effect increases with number of distractors (Cameron, Tai, Eckstein, and Carrasco 2004; Morgan, Ward, and Castet 1998; Foley 1998; Carrasco and McElree 2001; Carrasco, Giordano, and McElree 2006). These findings are attributed to result from spatial uncertainty reduction (Kinchla 1992; Shaw 1984; Solomon, Lavie, and Morgan 1997; Palmer 1994; Eckstein, Peterson, Pham, and Droll 2009; Foley 1998).

Other studies have shown that attentional benefits go beyond what is predicted by uncertainty reduction (Ling and Carrasco 2006a; Lu and Dosher 1998; Carrasco, Penpeci-Talgar, and Eckstein 2000; Carrasco, Williams, and Yeshurun 2002; Dosher and Lu 2000a, 2000b; Morgan, Ward, and Castet 1998; Lee, Koch, and Braun 1997). For instance, Lee et al. (1997) measured contrast and orientation thresholds, which are well characterized under normal viewing conditions (Rovamo and Virsu 1979; Virsu and Rovamo 1979), in the 'near absence of attention'. They asked observers to carry out two concurrent visual tasks, one of them highly demanding of attention ('primary task'), in which optimal performance is reached only when attention is fully focused, and thus almost completely withdrawn from the other task ('secondary task'). This paradigm ensures that less attention is devoted to the latter, thus the term 'near absence of attention' (Braun and Julesz 1998; Braun 1994). Performing a concurrent task increased both orientation and contrast thresholds, and the effect was more pronounced for the former than the latter (Lee, Koch, and Braun 1997).

Signal enhancement and external noise reduction

There are a number of mechanisms proposed to explain how attention may affect perception, many of which can be indexed within the perceptual template model (PTM). The PTM provides a theoretical and empirical framework to assess the mechanisms of attention by systematically manipulating the amount and/or characteristics of external noise added to stimuli and measuring modulation of perceptual discriminability.

According to the PTM, a signal is analysed by a perceptual template. There are three characteristic mechanisms by which attention can interact with the perceptual template to improve performance: (1) Stimulus enhancement, by which attention turns up the gain on the perceptual template, improving performance through amplification of the signal stimulus. It is mathematically equivalent to internal additive noise reduction (Fig. 7.2a). Increased gain helps to overcome internal noise in low-noise displays, but has little effect in high external noise because the external noise and signal stimulus are amplified equally (Fig. 7.2b). (2) External noise exclusion reduces the effects of external noise through filtering (Fig. 7.2c), by focusing the perceptual template on the appropriate spatial region or content characteristics of the stimulus.

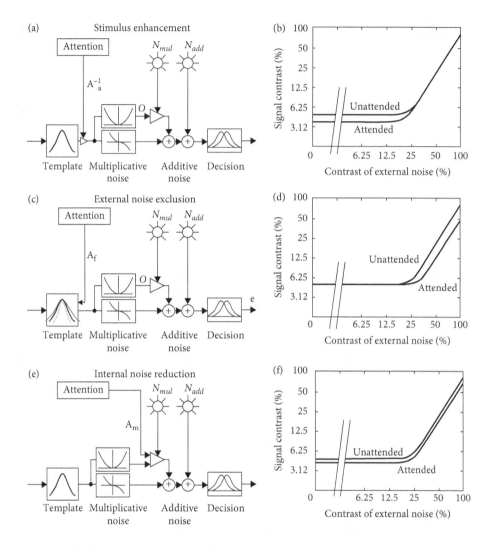

FIGURE 7.2 (a) Stimulus enhancement affects both the signal and the external noise in the input stimulus in the same way; thus, there is no retuning of the perceptual template entering the decision. (b) Stimulus enhancement has an effect at low but not high levels of external noise. (c) External noise exclusion reduces the effects of external noise through filtering, or retuning of the perceptual template that enters in the decision. (d) External noise exclusion improves performance in the region of high external noise, where there is external noise to exclude. (e) Internal noise reduction. Multiplicative noise increases with increasing contrast in the stimulus display. (f) Performance improves across all levels of external noise. Reprinted from *Vision Research*, 49 (10), Zhong-Lin Lu, Hennis Chi-Hang Tse, Barbara Anne Dosher, Luis A Lesmes, Christian Posner, and Wilson Chu, Intra- and cross-modal cuing of spatial attention: Time courses and mechanisms, pp. 1081–96, Copyright (2009), with permission from Elsevier.

Excluding external noise improves performance only when there is significant external noise in the stimulus to filter out (Fig. 7.2d). (3) Multiplicative internal noise reduction (Fig. 7.2e) impacts performance across all levels of external noise with slightly larger effects in high external noise. This pattern is rarely observed. The magnitude of the attention effect is the same (on the log contrast axis) at different performance levels (e.g. 75% and 85% performance threshold) for signal enhancement (Fig. 7.2a) or external noise exclusion (Fig. 7.2b), but not for multiplicative noise reduction. Thus, were there an effect across all levels of external noise, testing at two performance levels would disambiguate a combination of both stimulus enhancement and external noise reduction from multiplicative noise reduction. In the first case, the effect would scale, whereas in the second case it would not.

The PTM is an extension of models of the human observer (Burgess, Wagner, Jennings, and Barlow 1981; Pelli and Farell 1999) that incorporates known qualities of the visual system (for a review see Lu and Dosher 2008). Accuracy is constrained by internal limitations (receptor sampling errors, noise in neural responses, information loss during neural transmission) and external noise in the stimulus. Performance in d' (or % correct) for psychometric functions or contrast threshold from threshold versus contrast (TvC) functions is measured as a function of task, attention, external noise, and contrast. The parameters of the PTM model are estimated from psychometric functions (Dosher and Lu 2000a, 2000b; Lu and Dosher 2008) or from TvC functions from two or three measured threshold levels (Dosher and Lu 1998; Lu and Dosher 1999).

Using an external noise paradigm, cueing attention to a spatial location has revealed external noise exclusion and signal enhancement as the primary and secondary mechanisms underlying spatial attention. In the absence of uncertainty, one of the primary roles of spatial attention is to exclude external noise in the target region (Lu and Dosher 2000; Dosher and Lu 2000a, 2000b; Lu, Lesmes, and Dosher 2002). Transient attention increases contrast sensitivity in conditions of low noise, indicative of signal enhancement, and also improves performance in high-noise conditions, indicative of external noise reduction (Lu and Dosher 1998, 2000). However, these authors have attributed sustained attention effects exclusively to external noise reduction (Lu and Dosher 2000; Dosher and Lu 2000a, 2000b; Lu, Lesmes, and Dosher 2002); but see Ling and Carrasco (2006a). Figure 7.3 illustrates a trial sequence to manipulate sustained attention via a central precue. In this example the precue is invalid, because it cues a location away from the stimulus. The bottom panel shows that for this sample observer, the precue lowered the contrast threshold for high but not low levels of external noise, i.e. the signature of external noise reduction.

External noise paradigms have been widely used to probe different levels of visual processing and examine properties of detection and discrimination mechanisms. These paradigms assume that signal processing is noise-invariant: i.e. external noise adds to the variance of a single perceptual template, but that that filter remains unperturbed with different levels of external noise. Some recent findings, however, question this key assumption (Abbey and Eckstein 2009; Allard and Cavanagh 2011).

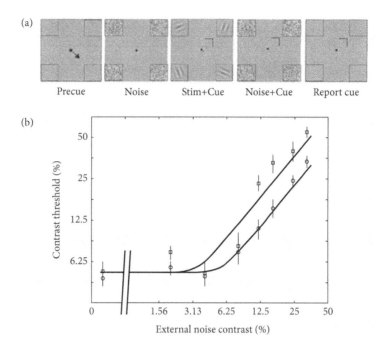

FIGURE 7.3 (a) Trial sequence illustrating an invalid cue: a central cue indicates a location; the stimulus and the response cue appear simultaneously indicating to the observer the target location. (b) Contrast threshold versus external noise contrast data from a sample observer. Endogenous attention reduces contrast thresholds at high noise levels but not at low noise levels, suggesting tuning of the perceptual template to exclude external noise. Reprinted from *Vision Research*, 40 (10–12), Barbara Anne Dosher and Zhong-Lin Lu, Mechanisms of perceptual attention in precuing of location, pp. 1269–92, Copyright (2000), with permission from Elsevier.

Exogenous attention and contrast sensitivity

To assess the conditions for which the effect of attention can be attributed to signal enhancement, it is necessary to ensure that a performance benefit occurs under conditions that exclude all variables that the external noise reduction models hold to be responsible for the attentional effect (Lu and Dosher 2000; Dosher and Lu 2000a, 2000b; Baldassi and Burr 2000; Morgan, Ward, and Castet 1998; Solomon, Lavie, and Morgan 1997; Davis, Kramer, and Graham 1983; Nachmias 2002). That is, the target should be suprathreshold (to reduce spatial uncertainty) and presented alone, without distractors or masks (Ling and Carrasco 2006a; Cameron, Tai, and Carrasco 2002; Carrasco, Penpeci-Talgar, and Eckstein 2000; Carrasco, Williams, and Yeshurun 2002; Golla, Ignashchenkova, Haarmeier, and Thier 2004).

A study with these experimental conditions evaluated whether the effect of attention on contrast sensitivity could be mediated by signal enhancement. For a wide range of spatial frequencies, contrast threshold was lower when the target location was preceded by a peripheral cue than by a neutral cue. A signal detection theory (SDT) model of external noise reduction could account for the cueing benefit in an easy discrimination task (vertical vs horizontal Gabor patches), but not when location uncertainty was reduced (by increasing stimulus contrast to enable fine discriminations of slightly tilted suprathreshold stimuli, or presenting a local post-mask). An SDT model that incorporates intrinsic uncertainty (the observers' inability to perfectly use information about the elements' spatial or temporal positions, sizes, or spatial frequencies) revealed that the cueing effect exceeded the one predicted by uncertainty reduction. Given that the attentional benefits occurred under conditions that exclude all variables predicted by the external noise reduction model, the results support the signal enhancement model of attention (Carrasco, Penpeci-Talgar, and Eckstein 2000). This finding is consistent with those of the low-noise conditions in the external noise plus attention paradigm (Lu and Dosher 1998, 2000).

Another study showed that transient attention decreased the threshold for contrast sensitivity in an orientation discrimination task across the contrast psychometric function (Cameron, Tai, and Carrasco 2002). Two control experiments assessed the role of spatial uncertainty. First, attention increased performance to the same extent in conditions with different uncertainty levels, even though observers required higher stimulus contrasts to perform the discrimination task with a small than with a large tilt. Second, for a large tilt discrimination and localization performance were tightly coupled, but performance on the localization task was much better than on the discrimination task with a small tilt, and yet the attentional effect was comparable for both orientation conditions. Thus, given that there was no added external noise and spatial uncertainty cannot explain the cue effect on contrast threshold, the observed attentional benefit is consistent with a signal enhancement mechanism (Cameron, Tai, and Carrasco 2002).

Attention improves performance at the attended location, but how sensitive to contrast are observers at the unattended locations? To assess contrast sensitivity at both cued and uncued locations, observers were asked to discriminate the orientation of one of two Gabor patches simultaneously presented left and right of fixation. A response cue was presented after the Gabor stimuli, indicating which Gabor to respond to; in valid trials, the cue location and response cue match and in invalid trials, they do not match (Fig. 7.4a). The response cue equates location uncertainty across conditions (Montagna, Pestilli, and Carrasco 2009; Pestilli and Carrasco 2005; Pestilli, Viera, and Carrasco 2007; Barbot, Landy, and Carrasco 2011; Ling and Carrasco 2006b; Barbot, Landy, and Carrasco 2012; Lu and Dosher 2000; Eckstein, Shimozaki, and Abbey 2002). Contrast sensitivity was measured at the valid cue and invalid cue locations, and compared with the contrast sensitivity obtained at the same locations when the target was preceded by a neutral cue. Observers were told that the peripheral cue was uninformative: that it preceded the target or the distractor with the same probability.

Despite the simplicity of the display, there is a performance trade-off: the cue increases sensitivity at the cued location (benefit) and impairs it at the uncued location (cost), as compared to the neutral condition (Fig. 7.4b; Pestilli and Carrasco 2005); see also (Pestilli, Viera, and Carrasco 2007). Given that for an ideal observer the uninformative cue would not reduce uncertainty, this finding supports sensitivity-based explanations,

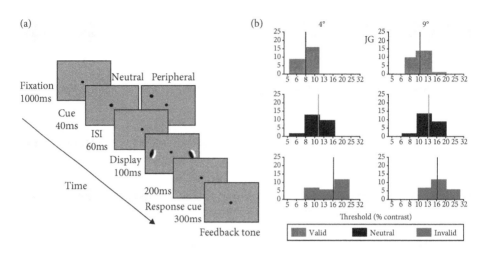

FIGURE 7.4 (a) A trial sequence. Following a fixation point, a cue appears either above one of the two Gabor locations (peripheral cue) or at fixation (neutral cue). After an ISI, two Gabor stimuli are simultaneously presented (randomly oriented to the left or to the right) on the horizontal meridian. Then a response cue appears at fixation to indicate the target Gabor for which the observer had to report the orientation. On one third of the trials the response cue points to a precued Gabor (valid cue). On another third of the trials it points to the Gabor that was not precued (invalid cue). In the remaining trials the precue is presented in the centre of the screen and the response cue is equally likely to indicate the Gabor to the right or to the left of fixation (neutral cue). (b) The histograms represent the distribution of the measured thresholds obtained for an individual observer in each cue condition at 4° and 9° of eccentricity. Top row—valid cue; middle row—neutral cue; bottom row—invalid cue. Dashed vertical lines indicate the median values. Reprinted from *Vision Research*, 45 (14), Franco Pestilli and Marisa Carrasco, Attention enhances contrast sensitivity at cued and impairs it at uncued locations, pp. 1867–75, Copyright (2005), with permission from Elsevier.

i.e. signal enhancement at the cued location and external noise reduction at the uncued location. This study provides evidence that exogenous attention affects visual processing in an automatic fashion (Cheal, Lyon, and Hubbard 1991; Muller and Rabbitt 1989a; Nakayama and Mackeben 1989; Yantis and Jonides 1996).

A performance trade-off has also been obtained for an intermediate stage of processing—second-order contrast (Barbot, Landy, and Carrasco 2011). Much of the early system, from the retina to the primary visual cortex, is dedicated to detecting changes in luminance (first-order information). However, humans are also sensitive to patterns defined only by spatial variations of textural attributes (second-order information). Texture patterns can be homogeneous in terms of average luminance, but have different regions segregated by means of their global grouping characteristics—regional similarity, spatial frequency, or orientation (Fig. 7.5b). Naturally occurring edges are usually defined by spatially coincident changes in both luminance and texture information (Johnson and Baker 2004). However, luminance-defined information generally originates from non-uniform surface illumination that does not correspond to object

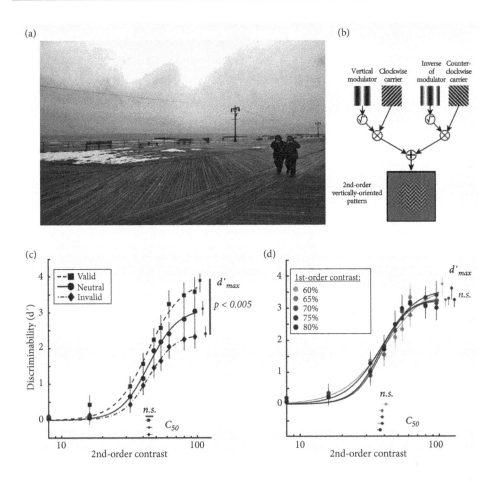

FIGURE 7.5 (a) Natural scene containing 1st- and 2nd-order boundaries. The boundary between the pedestrians and the walkway in the lower right is defined by a change in luminance (1st-order information); the boundaries between the different regions of the walkway are defined by changes in textural attributes (i.e. local orientation) without any changes in luminance (2nd-order information). (b) Texture patterns constructed by spatially modulating two orthogonal gratings (1st-order carriers ±45°) using a second horizontal or vertical grating with lower spatial frequency (2nd-order modulator). (c) Effects of exogenous attention, and (d) Effects of change in 1st-order peak luminance contrast, on performance (d') across observers as a function of 2nd-order modulator contrast. Psychometric functions and parameter estimates (c_{50}: 2nd-order contrast yielding half-maximum performance; d'_{max}: asymptotic performance) for each cueing condition (C, peak luminance carrier contrast was 70%, and D, for different 1st-order carrier contrast values). Adapted from *Vision Research*, 51 (9) Antoine Barbot, Michael S. Landy, and Marisa Carrasco, Exogenous attention enhances 2nd-order contrast sensitivity, pp. 1086–98, Copyright (2011), with permission from Elsevier.

boundaries (Schofield, Hesse, Rock, and Georgeson 2006; Sun and Schofield 2011). Consequently, by increasing the sensitivity to second-order information, attention may considerably improve object detection.

Like first-order luminance filters, second-order channels are tuned for orientation (Arsenault, Wilkinson, and Kingdom 1999; Dakin, Williams, and Hess 1999; Graham and Wolfson 2001) and spatial frequency (Landy and Oruc 2002; Scott-Samuel and Georgeson 1999), but have wider bandwidths (Landy and Oruc 2002). Exogenous attention also affects contrast sensitivity for second-order, texture-defined, information (Barbot, Landy, and Carrasco 2011). Specifically, attention increases second-order contrast sensitivity at the attended location, while decreasing it at unattended locations, relative to a neutral condition (Fig. 7.5c). A recent study shows that endogenous attention also alters second-order contrast sensitivity (Barbot, Landy, and Carrasco 2012). These effects of attention on second-order contrast sensitivity could not be explained by changes in first-order luminance contrast because discriminability is the same at a wide range of contrasts (Fig. 7.5d). Together with the effects of covert attention on first-order contrast sensitivity reviewed above, this study suggests that attention aids in the segmentation of the retinal image by increasing both first- and second-order sensitivity at the attended location.

In a study using a different attention manipulation, thresholds were compared when observers performed various tasks with full attention and transient attention focusing elsewhere on a concurrent, secondary task (Lee, Itti, Koch, and Braun 1999). The measurements included a dipper curve (contrast detection and contrast increment detection), contrast-masking thresholds (for masks of different orientations and spatial frequencies), orientation discrimination thresholds, and spatial-frequency discrimination thresholds. Based on the psychophysical results and modelling ('linear-filter-population-interacting-through-divisive-normalization'), the authors concluded that transient attention has a generic effect, that it boosts both excitatory and suppressive inputs prior to the divisive normalization, and that the final effect on the population response depends on the relative strength of target and distractor stimuli.

Endogenous attention and contrast sensitivity

Using an external noise procedure, Lu and Dosher reported that exogenous attention is mediated by signal enhancement (at low levels of external noise) and external noise reduction (at high levels of external noise), whereas endogenous attention is only mediated by external noise reduction (Dosher and Lu 2000a, 2000b; Lu, Lesmes, and Dosher 2002; Lu, Liu, and Dosher 2000). This result is surprising given that electrophysiological studies have reported facilitation effects of attention in conditions of low noise. Ling and Carrasco (2006a) compared these two types of covert attention using the same task, stimuli, and observers. They evaluated whether a signal enhancement mechanism underlies both types of attention and investigated the neural model underlying signal enhancement by measuring the psychometric functions for both types of attention to assess whether they have similar or different effects on the contrast response function. Observers performed a 2AFC orientation discrimination task on a slightly tilted Gabor patch.

Results indicated that both endogenous and exogenous attention have a similar effect on performance; both types of attention increase contrast sensitivity under zero-noise conditions (the display contained nothing to be suppressed because there was no added external noise). Hence, both attentional systems can be mediated by a signal enhancement mechanism. However, they have different effects on the contrast response function: endogenous attention seemed to operate via contrast gain, i.e. a shift in threshold, whereas exogenous attention seemed to operate via response gain, i.e. a shift in asymptote (Pestilli, Viera, and Carrasco 2007; Pestilli, Ling, and Carrasco 2009), but see Herrmann, Montaser-Kouhsari, Carrasco, and Heeger (2010).

These results cannot be explained by an uncertainty reduction model, which would predict that the attention effect should be most prominent with low-contrast stimuli (Pelli 1985) for both types of attention. Ling and Carrasco (2006a) proposed that the short 150 ms SOA may have precluded an emergence of the signal enhancement mechanism in the Dosher and Lu studies (Dosher and Lu 2000a, 2000b). As mentioned, it takes ~300 ms for endogenous attention to be deployed (e.g. Liu, Stevens, and Carrasco 2007; Muller and Rabbitt 1989a; Nakayama and Mackeben 1989).

A population coding model based on few biological-plausible assumptions and only two free parameters—threshold and asymptote of the contrast response function—estimated attentional effects on population contrast response given psychophysical data (including those of Ling and Carrasco 2006a). According to this model, whereas endogenous attention changes population contrast response via contrast gain, exogenous attention changes population contrast response via response gain (Pestilli, Ling, and Carrasco 2009; Fig. 7.6).

With a dual-task paradigm, a sustained attention task was used to investigate the independence of the attentional resources on the processing of luminance- and chromatic-modulated stimuli. Observers' threshold vs contrast (TvC) functions were measured under conditions of full or poor attention. The effect of attention was constant at pedestal contrasts above 0%, consistent with a response gain model (Morrone, Denti, and Spinelli 2004). Similar results have been obtained with visually evoked potentials (Di Russo, Spinelli, and Morrone 2001). Based on the findings that there was interference only when both stimuli involved luminance or colour contrast, the authors concluded that the two attributes are processed separately and that they engage different attentive resources. However, this conclusion is controversial; the attentional demand of the central task may have been higher for the same contrast than the different contrast conditions (Huang and Dobkins 2005; Pastukhov, Fischer, and Braun 2009).

Using a similar dual-task paradigm, a subsequent study found evidence for both contrast gain and response gain, and proposed a hybrid model in which attention first undergoes contrast gain, followed by a later-stage response gain modulation (Huang and Dobkins 2005). The authors attributed the differing findings to experimental parameters; they state that the contrasts they tested captured the entire response functions better, and that the dual task used by Morrone et al. may have not been demanding enough.

Whereas the dual-task paradigm has the advantage of eliminating location uncertainty reduction as an alternative explanation, it also has drawbacks. Dual-task paradigms do not control the deployment of attention well, and make it hard to isolate the source of possible processing differences (Sperling and Dosher 1986; Pashler and Johnston 1998).

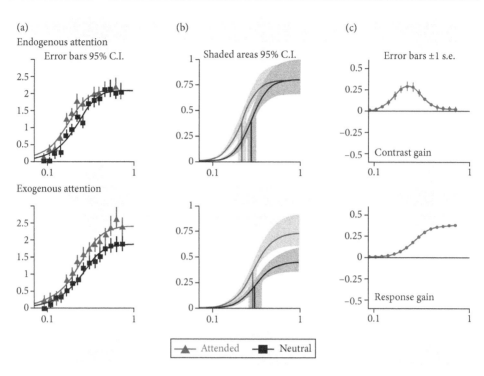

FIGURE 7.6 (a) Model fits and averaged psychometric data for attended (red) and neutral attention (black) conditions with endogenous (top panel) and exogenous (bottom panel) attention. (b) Normalized population contrast-response functions (pCRF) for contrast and response gain. The best model for endogenous attention is contrast gain; attention shifts the pCRF horizontally towards lower contrast. The best model for exogenous attention is response gain; attention increases pCRF incrementally from low to high contrast (bottom panel). (c) Average difference in responses (from b): neutral-minus-attended (blue) across all observers. Error bars in (a) are 95% confidence intervals (C.I.), obtained by non-parametric bootstrap. Shaded areas in (B) show model parameters' (C_{50} and Rmax) variability obtained by fitting the model to each one of the bootstrapped samples within the 95% C.I. in (a). Reprinted from *Vision Research*, 49 (10), Franco Pestilli, Sam Ling, and Marisa Carrasco, A population-coding model of attention's influence on contrast response: Estimating neural effects from psychophysical data, pp. 1144–53, Copyright (2009), with permission from Elsevier.

Ling and Carrasco (2006a) speculate that the difference in results with those obtained by Huang and Dobkins (2005) and Morrone et al. (2002, 2004) may be due to the way in which attention was manipulated. In dual-task paradigms, attention is not directed to a specific location, but the amount of resources being spread to all locations is manipulated. (For an alternative explanation for these differences, see the next section.)

A selective adaptation procedure, which assesses the spatiotemporal properties of the visual system, has also been used to further investigate the effects of endogenous attention on contrast sensitivity. Prolonged exposure to a stimulus reduces sensitivity to it and to similar stimuli, thus allowing for the selective adaptation of a particular feature, such as spatial frequency or orientation (Graham 1989; Blakemore and Campbell 1969;

Movshon and Lennie 1979). Capitalizing on this procedure, and on the finding that the magnitude of adaptation increases with the intensity of the adaptor stimulus (Langley 2002), the time course of attention's effects on contrast sensitivity was assessed. Given that attention boosts signal strength, it initially enhances contrast sensitivity, but over time sustaining endogenous attention to an adapting pattern actually impairs sensitivity because the adapting signal is stronger at the attended location. Conversely, contrast sensitivity at an unattended location is impaired at short adapting times, but this effect reverses with time, because the adapting signal is weaker at unattended locations (Ling and Carrasco 2006b).

A recent experiment has investigated the effect of attention (relevance) and expectation (probability) on contrast sensitivity by using a signal detection task in conjunction with reverse correlation (Wyart, Nobre, and Summerfield 2012). The authors manipulated independently relevance and probability using two cues and showed that they produce dissociable effects on contrast sensitivity. Both attention and expectation influence energy sensitivity, but they do so in a different way (Fig. 7.7): attention increases energy sensitivity mainly for signal-present stimuli (hits) whereas expectation increases the frequency and energy sensitivity mainly for signal-absent stimuli (false alarms). Based on a computational model, the authors propose that attention suppresses internal noise during signal processing via a multiplicative mechanism, consistent with electrophysiological findings showing that attention reduces interneuronal correlations (Cohen and Maunsell 2009; Mitchell, Sundberg, and Reynolds 2009; see Maunsell's chapter in Kastner and Nobre, forthcoming). Further, by comparing two models in which signal probability facilitates signal detection either at the input stage or at the response stage, the authors concluded that probability biases signal detection by increasing the baseline activity of signal-selective units, in agreement with 'predictive-coding' models of perception (Rao and Ballard 1999).

Model of enhanced contrast: The Normalization Model of Attention

A recent model, the Normalization Model of Attention, was proposed to reconcile previous, seemingly contradictory findings on the effects of visual attention, to unify alternative models on attention, and to offer a computational framework to simulate new research questions (Reynolds and Heeger 2009). Based on the model (Fig. 7.8), spatial attention can be characterized with an attention field selective for a given spatial location, but not selective (constant) across features of a dimension (e.g. orientation). The stimulus drive is multiplied with the attention field and then normalized, such that the extent of the stimulus and the relative extent of the attention field can shift the balance between excitation and suppression. Thus, the model can exhibit different effects of attentional modulation, described in the literature, such as response gain changes that increase firing rates by a multiplicative scale factor without changing the shape or width of neuronal tuning (McAdams and Maunsell 1999; Treue and Maunsell 1999); contrast

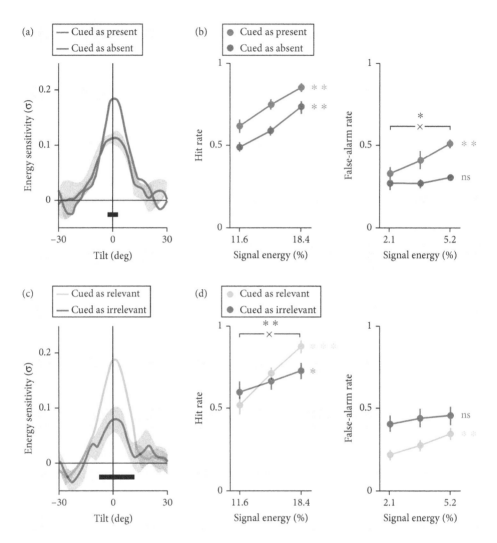

FIGURE 7.7 (a) Signal probability and (c) signal relevance increase the energy-sensitive profile at the target orientation. However, they do so in a dissociable manner: Signal probability increases primarily sensitivity of false alarms (b), but signal relevance increases predominantly the sensitivity of hits (d), to parametric changes in signal energy. Reprinted from *Proceedings of the National Academy of Sciences of the United States of America*, 109 (9), Wyart, V., A. C. Nobre, and C. Summerfield, Dissociable prior influences of signal probability and relevance on visual contrast sensitivity, pp. 1594–600, figure 3, Copyright (2012), with permission from The National Academy of Sciences.

gain changes that increase responses, multiplying the stimulus contrast by a scale factor (Martinez-Trujillo and Treue 2002; Reynolds, Pasternak, and Desimone 2000); a combination of both response gain and contrast gain changes (Williford and Maunsell 2006); or sharpening of neuronal tuning (Martinez-Trujillo and Treue 2004; Spitzer, Desimone, and Moran 1988).

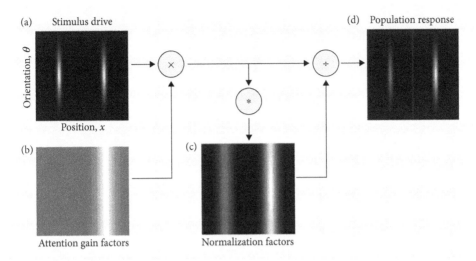

FIGURE 7.8 The Normalization Model of Attention. Stimuli, presented as input to the model, were two spatially noncontiguous locations identical in contrast, one of which was attended. (a) depicts the stimulus drive for a population of neurons with various receptive field centres (horizontal) and orientation preferences (vertical). Brightness at each location in the image corresponds to the stimulus drive to a single neuron. (b) shows the attention field when attending to the right location. Grey indicates a value of 1 and white indicates an attentional gain factor >1. The attention field is multiplied point-by-point with the stimulus drive. (c) The normalization factors are computed by the product of the stimulus drive and the attention field, and then pooled over space and orientation through convolution with the suppressive field. (d) Neural image depicting the output firing rates of the population of simulated neurons, computed by dividing the stimulus drive by the normalization factors. The stimulus drive, attention field, and normalization factor all had Gaussian profiles in space and orientation. Reprinted by permission from Macmillan Publishers Ltd: *Nature Reviews Neuroscience*, 13 (1), Matteo Carandini and David J. Heeger, Normalization as a canonical neural computation, pp. 51–62, © 2012, Nature Publishing Group.

A key prediction of this model is that the effect of attention can systematically shift from a change in response gain to contrast gain with smaller stimuli and a broader attention field. This prediction was recently confirmed by using spatial uncertainty to manipulate attention field size (Herrmann, Montaser-Kouhsari, Carrasco, and Heeger 2010). When the stimuli are large and the size of the window is small, both exogenous (Fig. 7.9a) and endogenous (Fig. 7.9b) attention yield response gain. However, when the stimuli are small and the size of the window is large, both exogenous (Fig. 7.9c) and endogenous (Fig. 7.9d) attention yield contrast gain.

An fMRI experiment showed that the attention field was larger with spatial uncertainty than without it. As predicted by the Normalization Model of Attention, attention modulates activity in visual cortex in a manner that can resemble either a change in response gain or contrast gain, depending on stimulus size and attention field size.

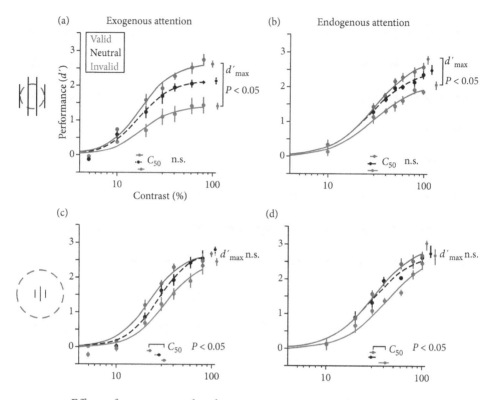

FIGURE 7.9 Effects of exogenous and endogenous attention on performance (d') as a function of contrast. (a, b) Large stimulus with small attention field. (c, d) Small stimulus with large attention field. Exogenous attention is shown in (a, c). Endogenous attention is shown in (b, d). Shown are plots of psychometric functions for each attentional condition (valid, neutral, and invalid precues) and parameter estimates (c50, contrast yielding half-maximum performance; d' max, asymptotic performance at high contrast). Each data point represents the mean across four observers. Error bars on data points are ±, i.e. error bars on parameter estimates are confidence intervals obtained by bootstrapping. Reprinted by permission from Macmillan Publishers Ltd: *Nature Neuroscience*, 13 (12), Herrmann, K., L. Montaser-Kouhsari, M. Carrasco, and D. J. Heeger, When size matters: attention affects performance by contrast or response gain, pp. 1554–9, © 2010, Nature Publishing Group.

Thus, differences in the experimental protocols may also explain previous discrepancies among psychophysical studies (Pestilli and Carrasco 2005; Pestilli, Viera, and Carrasco 2007; Ling and Carrasco 2006a; Morrone, Denti, and Spinelli 2002, 2004; Di Russo, Spinelli, and Morrone 2001). With constant stimulus size, some studies have found that exogenous attention alters performance via a response gain change, whereas endogenous attention does so via a contrast gain change (Pestilli and Carrasco 2005; Pestilli, Viera, and Carrasco 2007; Ling and Carrasco 2006a; Huang and Dobkins 2005; Di Russo, Spinelli, and Morrone 2001). A response gain change could have been elicited by brief peripheral cues nearby the stimulus, whereas a contrast gain change could have resulted from endogenous cues at fixation, rather than cues adjacent to the stimulus, which may have encouraged a narrower or larger attention field, respectively. Moreover, the different results seem to be related to differences in stimulus size; for endogenous attention, response gain changes were reported with the largest stimuli (Morrone, Denti, and Spinelli 2002, 2004), a combination of contrast and response gain changes was observed with intermediate stimulus sizes (Huang and Dobkins 2005) and contrast gain changes were reported with smaller stimuli (Ling and Carrasco 2006a).

Attention, contrast, and appearance

From psychophysical and neurophysiological evidence indicating that covert attention increases contrast sensitivity, one might infer that attention changes contrast appearance. But does attention alter appearance? Whether attention can actually affect the perceived intensity of a stimulus has been a matter of debate dating back to the founding fathers of experimental psychology and psychophysics—Helmholtz (1866/1911), James, and Fechner. Surprisingly, until the last decade, very little direct empirical evidence has addressed the issue (Prinzmetal, Amiri, Allen, and Edwards 1998; Prinzmetal et al. 1997; Tsal, Shalev, Zakay, and Lubow 1994) and some methodological issues questioned the results of these studies (Carrasco, Ling, and Read 2004; Treue 2004). To investigate this issue further, Carrasco, Ling, and Read (2004) implemented a novel paradigm that assesses the effects of spatial cueing on appearance and tests subjective contrast, while circumventing methodological limitations of previous studies.

To test subjective perception, a paradigm has been developed in which observers perform a task contingent upon a comparative judgement between two stimuli, while an uninformative cue directs spatial attention to one of the stimuli (Carrasco, Ling, and Read 2004). For example, observers are asked to report the orientation of the higher-contrast stimulus. With one response, observers convey information regarding both properties, and implicitly report their subjective experience of contrast. Changes in apparent contrast are measured in terms of shifts of the point of subjective equality (PSE), at which the two stimuli appear equal. An additional advantage of this 2X2 alternative forced choice (AFC) paradigm is that it provides concurrent assessment of appearance and performance: in addition to altering appearance, attention improves performance at the cued location, indicating that attention has been successfully manipulated. This AFC paradigm enables an objective and rigorous study of attention and subjective experience (Treue 2004; Luck 2004).

Exogenous attention significantly increased perceived contrast. When a Gabor stimulus was peripherally cued, the point of subjective equality (PSE) was shifted—the apparent contrast of the attended stimulus was higher than for the other Gabor. Thus, when observers attend to a stimulus, they perceive it to be of significantly higher contrast than when they perceive it without attention (Carrasco, Ling, and Read 2004). An attentional effect consistent with these findings has been obtained using low-contrast sine-wave gratings (Hsieh, Caplovitz, and Tse 2005).

Multiple control experiments have ruled out alternative accounts of these findings based on cue bias or response bias with regard to perceived contrast (Carrasco, Ling, and Read 2004; Carrasco, Fuller, and Ling 2008; Fuller, Rodriguez, and Carrasco 2008; Ling and Carrasco 2007), as well as with regard to the effects of exogenous attention on the subjective perception of other dimensions, such as spatial frequency (Gobell and Carrasco 2005), saturation (Fuller and Carrasco 2006), motion coherence (Liu, Fuller, and Carrasco 2006), stimulus size of a moving object (Anton-Erxleben, Henrich, and Treue 2007), flicker rate (Montagna and Carrasco 2006), and speed (Fuller, Park, and Carrasco 2009; Turatto, Vescovi, and Valsecchi 2007). A bias should be of similar magnitude independent of:

(1) The temporal order of cue and stimulus; however, the effect disappears when the order of cue and stimulus is reversed (postcue) (Carrasco, Fuller, and Ling 2008; Gobell and Carrasco 2005; Anton-Erxleben, Henrich, and Treue 2007; Fuller, Park, and Carrasco 2009; Liu, Pestilli, and Carrasco 2005).
(2) The interval between cue and stimulus; however, when it is lengthened to 500 ms, the cue effect disappears, consistent with the transient timing of exogenous attention (Carrasco, Ling, and Read 2004; Ling and Carrasco 2007; Liu, Fuller, and Carrasco 2006; Turatto, Vescovi, and Valsecchi 2007).
(3) Stimulus properties; however, attention increases perceived saturation but not apparent hue, even though it improves performance in both cases (Fuller and Carrasco 2006).
(4) Visual field location; however, the attention effect on apparent contrast is greater at the lower than at the upper vertical meridian (Fuller, Rodriguez, and Carrasco 2008).
(5) The direction of the question; however, when observers are asked to report the orientation of the stimulus of lower, rather than higher, contrast, they choose the cued test stimulus less frequently (Carrasco, Ling, and Read 2004; Ling and Carrasco 2007; Gobell and Carrasco 2005; Fuller and Carrasco 2006; Montagna and Carrasco 2006; Fuller, Park, and Carrasco 2009; Turatto, Vescovi, and Valsecchi 2007; Liu, Abrams, and Carrasco 2009).

Notwithstanding all these controls, alternative explanations have been proposed for the effects of exogenous attention on perceived contrast (Schneider 2006) and reply by Ling and Carrasco (2007), Prinzmetal, Long, and Leonhardt (2008) and reply by Carrasco, Fuller, and Ling (2008), Schneider and Komlos (2008) and reply by Anton-Erxleben, Abrams, and Carrasco (2010).

It has been proposed that the observed increase in apparent contrast is largely due to sensory interactions occurring between the precue and stimulus, rather than to attention (Schneider 2006). This study reports that cueing effects only occur at contrasts near detection threshold, and that there are confounding sensory interactions between the cue and stimulus at suprathreshold detection contrasts. In a reply to this study, Ling and Carrasco first outlined the key methodological differences between Carrasco et al.'s (2004) original study and Schneider's study that are likely to account for the different results, and explained how the sensory interaction explanation of the cue had been ruled out. Furthermore, they directly tested the prediction put forth by Schneider: if the effects were due to sensory interactions, reversing the luminance polarity of the precue should lead to differential cueing effects. Ling and Carrasco's results (Carrasco, Ling, and Read 2004) replicated their original findings—an increase in apparent contrast of a high-contrast stimulus when it was precued. Moreover, they found that the black cue and the white cue had the same effect, thus ruling out the alternative explanation proposed by Schneider.

Prinzmetal et al. (2008) suggested that for stimuli of low visibility, observers may bias their response toward the cued location, and proposed a cue-bias explanation for previous studies. In a reply to that study, Carrasco, Fuller, and Ling (2008) concluded that a cue-bias hypothesis is a plausible explanation for Prinzmetal et al.'s results given the characteristics of their stimuli, but that such an explanation had no bearing on the studies by Carrasco and colleagues in which the stimuli were suprathreshold. Furthermore, an increase in apparent contrast for high-contrast stimuli when a stimulus was precued, but not when it was postcued (Carrasco, Fuller, and Ling 2008), further supported the claim that attention alters the contrast appearance of suprathreshold stimuli.

Lastly, Schneider and Komlos (2008) have argued that in a comparative paradigm, PSE and criterion are confounded, whereas in an equality judgement the PSE is independent of criterion shifts. Using the equality task, in which observers report whether two stimuli are the same or different in contrast, they did not find a significant effect of attention on contrast appearance and thus concluded that the effects of attention in previous studies were due to a bias. Their null results with the equality paradigm and their positive result with the comparative paradigm led them to argue that attention increases stimulus saliency, biasing decisions rather than altering perception. These conclusions are unwarranted for three reasons: (1) the inconsistent theoretical relation among salience, perception, and attention; (2) issues with criteria in the equality paradigm; and (3) the difficulty in interpreting their null results (Abrams, Barbot, and Carrasco 2010).

In an experimental reply to Schneider and Komlos (2008), the sensitivity of equality and comparative judgements of perceived contrast were compared with regard to physical contrast differences and attentional modulation (Anton-Erxleben, Abrams, and Carrasco 2010). Questioning the assumption of equal sensitivity of both types of judgements and an absence of bias from the equality judgement (Schneider and Komlos 2008), the reply study demonstrates several methodological limitations of the equality paradigm, which may contribute to decrease the reliability of PSE estimation and render the equality judgement less sensitive to shifts in perceived contrast. Notwithstanding these methodological limitations, in this study both paradigms revealed that attention enhances apparent contrast (Anton-Erxleben, Abrams, and Carrasco 2010).

A study investigating the effect of exogenous attention on contrast appearance with concurrent electrophysiological and behavioural measures (Stormer, McDonald, and Hillyard 2009) has lent further support to the view that attention enhances apparent contrast. Cross-modal spatial cueing of attention increased perceived contrast of the stimulus at the attended location concurrent with an amplified neural response in the contralateral visual cortex. Specifically, cueing attention to one of two identical stimuli boosted early processing (100–140 ms) of the attended stimulus in the ventral occipitotemporal visual cortex. Moreover, the amplitude of the enhanced neural response correlated positively with the perceived contrast of the cued stimulus, which provides converging evidence that contrast appearance arises from early cortical processing of visual stimuli. Crucially, the cueing of attention enhanced neural processing in the same ventral regions of the visual cortex that are responsive to physical differences in contrast. These results contradict the hypothesis that the effect of attention is due to a decisional bias (Schneider and Komlos 2008). By providing converging evidence from human electrophysiology and behaviour, this study demonstrates that the enhanced perceived contrast at the cued location is attributable to an effect of attention on early visual processing (Stormer, McDonald, and Hillyard 2009).

The appearance paradigm has been adapted to investigate the effect of endogenous attention, which also increases perceived contrast (Liu, Abrams, and Carrasco 2009). Thus, many studies provide evidence consistent with the 'linking hypothesis', which states that the attentional enhancement of neural firing is interpreted as if the stimulus had a higher contrast (Reynolds and Chelazzi 2004; Treue 2004). This proposal is supported by converging evidence from neurophysiological, psychophysical, and neuroimaging studies (for a review, see Carrasco 2011).

Another study has shown that endogenous attention can also modulate perceived brightness (Tse 2005). The author proposes that understanding this phenomenon may require new models that include higher-level mechanisms than gain control, such as surface, boundary formation, and inhibition among higher-level surfaces or objects.

The studies showing that attention alters appearance exemplify how the visual system operates on the retinal image to maximize its usefulness to the perceiver, often producing non-veridical percepts. The visual system does not provide an internal one-to-one copy of the external visual world; rather, it optimizes processing resources. Attention is a pervasive example of this perceptual optimization: attention augments perception by optimizing our representation of sensory input and by emphasizing relevant details at the expense of a faithful representation (Treue 2004; Carrasco, Fuller, and Ling 2008; Fuller, Rodriguez, and Carrasco 2008; Carrasco 2009). The biophysical machinery of the brain engenders our phenomenological experience of the world: attention, both intra-modal and cross-modal, affects not only how we perform in a visual task but also what we see and experience (Carrasco 2011, 2009).

COVERT ATTENTION INCREASES SPATIAL RESOLUTION

Spatial resolution, our ability to discriminate fine patterns, decreases with eccentricity. Signals from the central parts of the visual field are processed with greater accuracy and faster reaction times (Cannon 1985; Carrasco, Evert, Chang, and Katz 1995; Rijsdijk, Kroon, and van der Wildt 1980). In many tasks, these performance differences are eliminated when stimulus size is enlarged according to the cortical magnification factor which equates the size of the cortical representation for stimuli presented at different eccentricities (Rovamo and Virsu 1979; Virsu and Rovamo 1979). However, there are also qualitative differences in neural processing between central and peripheral vision. Thus, compensating for cortical magnification does not eliminate all differences (for a review see Kitterle 1986). Moreover, spatial resolution is not uniform across iso-eccentric locations. It is better along the horizontal meridian than the vertical one and better in the lower region than in the upper region of the vertical meridian (Talgar and Carrasco 2002; Fuller, Rodriguez, and Carrasco 2008; Abrams, Nizam, and Carrasco 2011; Montaser-Kouhsari and Carrasco 2009).

Several factors contribute to differences in spatial resolution across eccentricities. A greater proportion of cortex is devoted to processing input from the centre of the visual field than the periphery (cortical magnification). In area V1, approximately 25% of cortex is devoted to processing the central 2.5 deg. of visual angle (De Valois and De Valois 1988). Neuronal RF sizes increase with eccentricity, as the RF density decreases. Thus, as eccentricity increases, information is pooled over a larger area, diminishing sensitivity to fine patterns. Moreover, the visual system's peak sensitivity to spatial frequencies decreases with eccentricity (De Valois and De Valois 1988; Kitterle 1986).

A series of psychophysical studies provides evidence for the 'resolution hypothesis', which states that attention can enhance spatial resolution, and that the magnitude of such an effect increases with eccentricity (Carrasco, Williams, and Yeshurun 2002; Carrasco and Yeshurun 1998). When spatial attention is directed to a given location, performance improves in visual search, acuity, texture segmentation (unless resolution is already too high for the task at hand; see below), and crowding tasks, which are mediated by spatial resolution.

Attention and visual search

In a visual search task, observers are typically required to detect the presence of a predefined target appearing among other irrelevant items; for instance, a red vertical line appearing among red tilted lines in a feature search, or a red vertical line appearing among red tilted and blue vertical lines in a conjunction search (e.g. Treisman 1985). Performance typically decreases with the number of distractors (the set size effect) for conjunction search, whereas for feature search it does not. However, there are exceptions to both: there are feature searches yielding a set size effect (Carrasco and Frieder 1997; Carrasco, McLean, Katz, and Frieder 1998; Dosher, Han, and Lu 2004) and conjunction searches that do not (Duncan and Humphreys 1989; Carrasco, Ponte, Rechea, and Sampedro 1998; McLeod, Driver, and Crisp 1988; Nakayama and Silverman 1986).

Performance in visual search tasks deteriorates as the target is presented at farther peripheral locations (Carrasco, Evert, Chang, and Katz 1995; Carrasco and Frieder 1997; Carrasco, McLean, Katz, and Frieder 1998; Carrasco and Chang 1995). This reduction in performance has been attributed to the poorer spatial resolution at the periphery because performance is constant across eccentricity when stimulus size is enlarged according to the cortical magnification factor (Carrasco and Frieder 1997; Carrasco, McLean, Katz, and Frieder 1998), but see Wolfe, O'Neill, and Bennett (1998). Similarly, a study in which attention was manipulated via a peripheral cue showed that attention eliminates the eccentricity effect for both features and conjunctions (Carrasco and Yeshurun 1998). These results support the resolution hypothesis; by improving performance more at peripheral than at central locations, attention can minimize resolution differences between the fovea and the periphery.

The idea that attention enhances spatial resolution was also supported by a study in which orientation thresholds were assessed in a visual search task (Morgan, Ward, and Castet 1998). The authors reported that when distractors were present, indicating the target location with a peripheral cue reduces orientation thresholds to the level found when the target was presented alone. The authors interpreted these effects to suggest that attention reduces the scale over which an image is analysed. Similarly, orientation discrimination thresholds increased with set size but cueing the target location eliminated this effect (Baldassi and Burr 2000). These results are also consistent with a reduction of spatial scale of processing and distractor exclusion.

Attention and acuity tasks

Acuity tasks are designed to measure the observer's ability to resolve fine details. Performance in some of these tasks, e.g. detection of a small gap in a Landolt square, is limited by the retinal mosaic, whereas in other tasks, e.g. identification of offset direction with Vernier targets, performance is hyperacute and limited by cortical processes (Levi, Klein, and Aitsebaomo 1985; Thomas and Olzak 1986). Directing transient attention to the target location improves performance in both acuity and hyperacuity tasks. A peripheral cue improved observers' performance and the magnitude of this improvement increased with eccentricity. Similarly, directing attention to the location of a Vernier target allowed observers to identify smaller horizontal offsets (Yeshurun and Carrasco 1999). The same pattern of results emerged when all sources of added external noise were eliminated from the display; i.e. local masks, global masks, and distractors (Carrasco, Williams, and Yeshurun 2002). Consistent findings emerged from a comparative study that evaluated the effects of covert attention on Landolt acuity in humans and non-human primates (Golla, Ignashchenkova, Haarmeier, and Thier 2004). Acuity was enhanced when the target location was precued and the attentional effect increased with eccentricity in both human and non-human primates (Fig. 7.10). Moreover, cueing the location of a line enabled observers to better detect when the gap was present and to localize its location (Shalev and Tsal 2002). All these findings further support the idea that attention enhances spatial resolution.

Increased spatial acuity at the attended location is coupled with decreased acuity at unattended locations (Montagna, Pestilli, and Carrasco 2009). For exogenous attention,

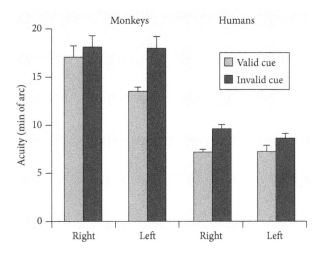

FIGURE 7.10 Means and standard errors of acuity thresholds at 9° horizontal retinal eccentricity for monkeys and humans under the valid (75% of trials) and invalid (25%) cueing conditions. Reprinted from *Vision Research*, 44 (13), Heidrun Golla, Alla Ignashchenkova, Thomas Haarmeier, and Peter Thier, Improvement of visual acuity by spatial cueing: a comparative study in human and non-human primates, pp. 1589–1600, Copyright (2004), with permission from Elsevier.

observers were explicitly told that the peripheral cue was uninformative, i.e. not predictive of target location or gap side. For endogenous attention, observers were informed that the cue would indicate the target location, but not the gap side, on 70% of the central-cue trials. For both exogenous and endogenous attention, gap-size thresholds were lower in the cued and higher in the uncued condition compared to the neutral baseline condition (Fig. 7.11). The fact that acuity trade-offs emerge for very simple, non-cluttered displays, supports the idea that covert spatial attention helps regulate the expenditure of cortical computation.

The improved performance in acuity tasks could only be accounted for by the resolution hypothesis—attention enhances spatial resolution at attended locations. Note that these attention effects could not be accounted for by any of the alternative hypotheses regarding attentional mechanisms—shifts in the decisional criterion, location uncertainty reduction, or reduction of external noise (see section 'Mechanisms of covert attention')—for the following reasons: (a) the peripheral cue only conveyed information regarding the target location, or conveyed no information regarding either the correct response or the target location; (b) the peripheral cue did not associate a higher probability with one of the responses and observers could not rely on its presence to reach a discrimination decision; (c) a suprathreshold target could not be confused with the blank at the other locations and was presented alone, without other items to introduce external noise; (d) similar results were obtained when two suprathreshold targets were presented at fixed locations, which could not be confused with the blank at other locations; and (e) similar results were found with and without a local post-mask.

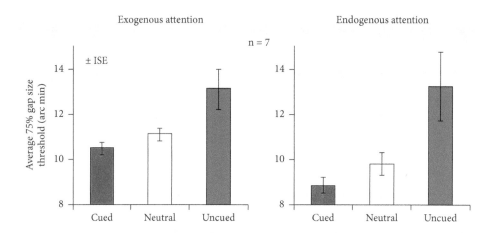

FIGURE 7.11 Average gap-size thresholds (75% localization accuracy) for both exogenous (top-left panel) and endogenous (top-right panel) attention for the cued, neutral, and uncued conditions. Error bars show +/− 1 SE. Reprinted from *Vision Research*, 49 (7), Barbara Montagna, Franco Pestilli, and Marisa Carrasco, Attention trades off spatial acuity, pp. 735–45, Copyright (2009), with permission from Elsevier.

Attention and temporal resolution

Transient attention can alter temporal processing as it alters spatial processing. Given the trade-off between spatial and temporal resolution, enhancing the former necessarily results in degrading the latter (Yeshurun 2004; Yeshurun and Levy 2003; Yeshurun and Hein 2011; Yeshurun and Marom 2008). Several studies have found an impaired temporal resolution at the attended location suggesting that transient attention degrades temporal segregation. For instance, a peripheral cue diminishes observers' ability to indicate whether a target is continuous or flickering at the attended location (Yeshurun 2004; Yeshurun and Levy 2003; Rolke, Dinkelbach, Hein, and Ulrich 2008), but see Chica and Christie (2009). When observers are cued to a specific location, they improve at spatial-gap detection, but worsen at temporal-gap detection (Fig. 7.12). Similarly, automatic orienting of attention impairs discrimination of the temporal order of two dots (Hein, Rolke, and Ulrich 2006). Furthermore, in apparent motion tasks, an attentional cue decreases observers' accuracy, when indicating the motion direction of an apparently moving rectangle (Yeshurun and Hein 2011). Finally, transient attention leads to longer temporal integration (Megna, Rocchi, and Baldassi 2012) and prolongs perceived duration (Yeshurun and Marom 2008).

Yeshurun and colleagues have proposed that these results can be explained by an attentional mechanism that facilitates spatial segregation and temporal integration but impairs their counterparts—spatial integration and temporal segregation—due to perceptual trade-offs. They further suggested that a possible physiological implementation of such mechanism is attentional favouring of parvocellular over magnocellular activity.

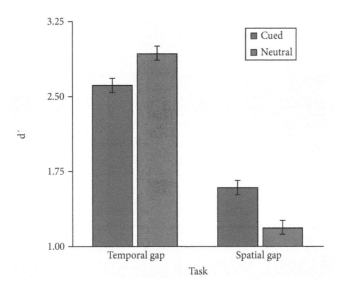

FIGURE 7.12 Performance (data averaged across observers) for detection tasks of a temporal gap (left panel) and a spatial gap (right panel). A peripheral cue improves performance in a spatial-gap task but impairs it in a temporal-gap task. Adapted from Yaffa Yeshurun and Liat Levy, Transient Spatial Attention Degrades Temporal Resolution, *Psychological Science*, 14 (3) pp. 225–31, copyright © 2003 by SAGE Publications. Reprinted by Permission of SAGE Publications.

Parvocellular neurons have higher spatial resolution and longer temporal integration than magnocellular neurons, but their temporal resolution is low. An attentional facilitation of parvocellular activity on the expense of magnocellular activity could, therefore, account for these various effects of attention (Yeshurun 2004; Yeshurun and Levy 2003; Yeshurun and Hein 2011; Yeshurun and Marom 2008; Yeshurun and Sabo 2012). Also consistent with this hypothesis is the finding that attention benefits discrimination of high- but not of low-spatial frequencies (Srinivasan and Brown 2006).

Attention and texture segmentation

Heightened resolution benefits many everyday tasks, such as reading or discriminating objects. However, in certain situations resolution enhancement is not beneficial; for example, when a global assessment of a scene is required (e.g. when seeing a whole tree rather than its individual leaves) or when navigating under poor atmospheric conditions (e.g. fog or haze). The fact that increasing spatial resolution can be detrimental in tasks in which performance is diminished by heightened resolution enabled a crucial test of the resolution hypothesis. If attention enhanced resolution, performance at the attended location should be impaired rather than improved in such a task (Yeshurun and Carrasco 1998). A basic texture segmentation task was used in which a to-be-detected texture target was embedded in a background of an orthogonal orientation. Observers' performance is highest at mid-peripheral locations, and drops as the target appears at more central or farther peripheral locations. This 'central performance drop' (CPD) is attributed to a mismatch between the average size of spatial filters at the fovea and the scale of the texture (Gurnsey, Pearson, and Day 1996; Kehrer 1997). The size of these filters at the fovea is too small for the scale of the texture and spatial resolution would be too high for the task. The filters' average size increases gradually with eccentricity and is optimal around the performance peak. At farther locations, performance decreases because the filters are too big and the resolution is too low for the task. Thus, enlarging the scale of the texture shifts the performance peak to farther locations, whereas decreasing this scale shifts the peak towards the centre (Gurnsey, Pearson, and Day 1996; Kehrer 1997; Joffe and Scialfa 1995).

If attention enhances spatial resolution, attending to the target location should improve performance at the periphery where the resolution is too low, but should impair performance at the fovea where the resolution is already too high for the task (Yeshurun and Carrasco 1998). Accuracy was higher for the peripherally cued than the neutral trials at peripheral locations, but was lower at central locations (Fig. 7.13a). The size of the scale of the texture was manipulated by viewing distance. Attention impaired performance in a larger range of eccentricities with a larger scale of the texture. Conversely, with a smaller texture scale, performance was impaired at a smaller range of eccentricities. Thus, transient attention improves performance when it is limited by resolution that is too low, but hinders performance when it is limited by resolution that is too high for the task. The scale of the texture and the average size of the filters at a given eccentricity determine whether attention helps or hinders performance. The finding that attention affects performance even at the fovea is in accord with a study that demonstrated that targets that occur unexpectedly at fixation capture attention in a stimulus-driven manner similar to attentional capture in the periphery (Coull, Frith, Buchel, and Nobre 2000). The impairment at central locations is predicted by the resolution hypothesis; no other model can predict these impairments (Yeshurun and Carrasco 1998). Shifts in the decisional criterion, location uncertainty reduction, or reduction of external noise would predict a benefit on performance throughout all eccentricities.

To test the hypothesis that covert attention enhances spatial resolution by increasing sensitivity to high spatial frequencies, a peripheral cueing procedure was employed in conjunction with selective adaptation to spatial frequency (Carrasco, Loula, and Ho 2006). The selective adaptation procedure is used to assess the spatiotemporal properties of the visual system (Graham 1989; Blakemore and Campbell 1969; Movshon and Lennie 1979). While keeping the stimulus content identical, the availability of spatial frequency information was manipulated by reducing observers' sensitivity to a range of frequencies. Hence, by adapting to high spatial frequencies, the non-optimal filters would be removed from the normalization process and the magnitude of the CPD would be diminished. Furthermore, were the central attentional impairment due to an increased sensitivity to high frequencies and a reduced sensitivity to lower frequencies, adapting to high spatial frequencies should eliminate the attentional impairment at central locations and diminish the benefit in the peripheral locations. The results confirmed these predictions, indicating that the CPD is primarily due to the predominance of high

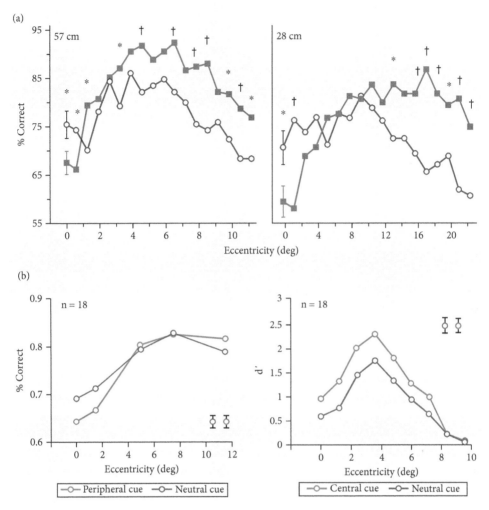

FIGURE 7.13 Observers' performance as a function of target eccentricity and cueing condition for (a) transient attention, the two viewing distances (indicated on each panel). Because viewing distance varied, the eccentricity values (abscissa) differ in the two top panels. Adapted with permission from Macmillan Publishers Ltd: *Nature*. 396 (6706), Yaffa Yeshurun and Marisa Carrasco, Attention improves or impairs visual performance by enhancing spatial resolution, pp. 72–5 © 1998, Nature Publishing Group. (b) transient (left panel) and sustained (right panel) attention. Adapted from *Vision Research*, 48 (1), Yaffa Yeshurun, Barbara Montagna, and Marisa Carrasco, On the flexibility of sustained attention and its effects on a texture segmentation task, pp. 80–95, Copyright (2008), with permission from Elsevier.

spatial frequency responses, and that covert attention enhances spatial resolution by increasing sensitivity to higher spatial frequencies (Carrasco, Loula, and Ho 2006).

When this texture is presented along the vertical meridian, performance peaks at farther eccentricities in the lower than in the upper vertical meridian, consistent with the resolution being higher in the lower meridian (Montaser-Kouhsari and Carrasco 2009), but the attention benefit and cost are the same in both regions of the vertical meridian (Talgar and Carrasco 2002). These findings indicate that the vertical meridian asymmetry is limited by visual rather than attentional factors, and support the hypothesis that attention enhances spatial resolution at the attended location.

At the level of the visual cortex, texture segmentation theoretically involves passage of visual input through two layers of spatial linear filters, separated by a pointwise non-linearity. The first-order linear filters perform a more local analysis of spatial frequency and orientation, and are thought to reflect the activity of simple cortical cells in area V1. The second-order linear filters which are of a larger scale perform a more global analysis on the output of the first-order filters plus the intermediate non-linearity (Bergen and Landy 1991; Graham, Beck, and Sutter 1992; Sutter, Beck, and Graham 1989). To assess the level of processing at which transient attention affects spatial resolution, textures composed of narrow-band stimuli were used to ensure that first- or second-order filters of various specific scales would be differentially stimulated. For both first-order low- and high-frequency conditions, accuracy was higher for cued than neutral trials at more peripheral eccentricities, but it was lower at central locations. In contrast, the attentional effect differed as a function of the second-order spatial frequency content: attention impaired performance in a greater range of eccentricities for the low- than the high-frequency condition, and an attentional benefit emerged only for the high-frequency condition. These findings suggest that attention operates at the second stage of filtering, possibly by reducing the size of the second-order filters (Yeshurun and Carrasco 2000).

The texture segmentation studies described thus far show that transient attention increases spatial resolution even when this is detrimental. Would the pattern of results be the same with sustained attention, which is considered to be more flexible and capable of adapting to task demands? A central cue was used to test whether the attentional effect would be similar to that found with peripheral cues (Yeshurun, Montagna, and Carrasco 2008). Unlike transient attention, sustained attention improves performance in texture segmentation tasks at all eccentricities (Fig. 7.13b). The finding that performance improves at fovea is in agreement with behavioural and neurophysiological enhancements at the fovea for focused versus distributed attention (Miniussi, Rao, and Nobre 2002). By comparing the effect of precues and postcues, the authors showed that the benefit of the central precue went well beyond the mere effect of location uncertainty at the decisional stage (Yeshurun, Montagna, and Carrasco 2008).

The improvement at all eccentricities is consistent with the idea that sustained attention is more flexible than transient attention, and suggests that sustained attention may increase the resolution at peripheral locations but decrease the resolution at central locations where an increase would be detrimental. Alternatively, the findings may be explained by an attentional mechanism that improves the signal to noise ratio at all eccentricities through reduction of external noise at early levels of processing (Dosher and Lu 2000a; Lu and Dosher 2004), possibly via distractor suppression (Shiu and Pashler 1994). A recent study has shown that sustained attention improves performance at central locations by decreasing the sensitivity of high-spatial frequency filters, thus decreasing resolution (Barbot, Montagna, and Carrasco 2012).

Attention, spatial resolution, and appearance

The studies discussed above show that spatial resolution is enhanced by exogenous/ transient attention, regardless of whether this helps or hinders performance, and by endogenous/sustained attention when such an enhancement improves performance, but not when it would be detrimental. Does attention also affect appearance of the types of stimuli used to assess spatial resolution?

Using the paradigm developed to assess the effects of attention on contrast appearance (Carrasco, Ling, and Read 2004), it has been shown that exogenous attention increases both perceived spatial frequency and Landolt-square gap size (Gobell and Carrasco 2005). In line with this study, it has been found that exogenous attention also increases the perceived size of moving visual patterns (Fig. 7.14a) (Anton-Erxleben, Henrich, and Treue 2007). These authors attribute their findings to the fact that spatial attention shifts receptive fields in monkey extrastriate visual cortex toward the focus of attention (Womelsdorf, Anton-Erxleben, Pieper, and Treue 2006), so that they respond to a new location closer to the attentional focus, but without updating the position label

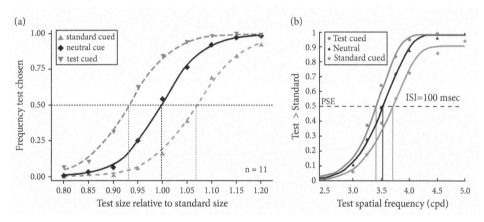

FIGURE 7.14 (a) Average data across observers for test-cued, neutral, and standard-cued trials. Percentage of trials in which observers responded that the test stimulus was bigger than the standard stimulus, as a function of test size. Data are averaged across observers and then fitted with a psychometric function using iterative likelihood maximization. Reprinted from *Journal of Vision*, 7 (11), Anton-Erxleben, K., C. Henrich, and S. Treue, Attention changes perceived size of moving visual patterns, p. 1–9, figure 2a © 2007, with permission from the Association for Research in Vision and Opthalmology. (b) Psychometric functions showing the proportion of trials on which the observers chose the test stimulus to be of higher spatial frequency than the standard stimulus, as a function of the physical spatial frequency of the test stimulus. Reprinted from *Proceedings of the National Academy of Sciences of the United States of America*, 106(52), Stormer, V. S., J. J. McDonald, and S. A. Hillyard, Cross-modal cueing of attention alters appearance and early cortical processing of visual stimuli, pp. 22456–61, Copyright (2009), with permission from the National Academy of Sciences.

(according to a labelled-line code). Thus, this distortion in the retinotopic distribution of receptive fields may increase the perceived size of attended stimuli.

Similarly, a rapid serial visual presentation (RSVP) paradigm developed to assess endogenous attention and perceived contrast (Liu, Abrams, and Carrasco 2009) was adapted to investigate the effects of endogenous attention on spatial resolution, particularly on perceived spatial frequency. A demanding rapid serial visual presentation task was used to direct voluntary attention to a given location and perceived spatial frequency was measured at the attended and unattended locations (Abrams, Barbot, and Carrasco 2010). Attention increased the perceived spatial frequency of suprathreshold stimuli and also improved performance on a concurrent orientation discrimination task (Fig. 7.14b). These studies included a number of control experiments that rule out possible alternative interpretations of the findings of increased perceived spatial resolution, such as cue bias or response bias (see section above, 'Attention, contrast, and appearance').

A previous study had reported that sustained attention did not shift the mean apparent spatial frequency, but merely reduced the variance of the estimates (Prinzmetal, Amiri, Allen, and Edwards 1998). The discrepancy between this study and the studies reporting that attention increases perceived spatial frequency may result from methodological differences. In the study reporting no shift in appearance (Prinzmetal, Amiri, Allen, and Edwards 1998), the location of spatial attention was not manipulated; instead, a dual-task procedure was used, and the difficulty of the primary letter identification task (simultaneous vs sequential presentation) was varied to manipulate attentional deployment in the secondary appearance task. Furthermore, the results of this study are inconclusive because there was no independent measurement ensuring that attention had been deployed to the correct location.

Another line of studies supporting the view that attention affects appearance has shown that cueing the target location with a peripheral cue reduces perceived line length (Tsal and Shalev 1996). These authors proposed that the visual field consists of a grid of attentional receptive fields (ARFs), a hypothetical construct that operates as a functional receptive field, whose operation follows an all-or-none principle. Thus, when a stimulus appears within its boundaries, this unit signals its entire length to the central processor (Tsal, Meiran, and Lamy 1995). Moreover, because the ARFs are smaller at the attended than the unattended field, the attended line is systematically perceived as shorter than the unattended one (Tsal and Shalev 1996). The authors have proposed that smaller receptive fields increase spatial resolution, and have ruled out that spatial interactions between the cue and the target could affect line-length judgements (Tsal, Shalev, and Zakay 2005). Differences in the manipulation of attention and cueing parameters may explain the discrepancy with the results reported by others (Anton-Erxleben, Henrich, and Treue 2007).

Both endogenous attention and exogenous attention also affect perceived position by repelling briefly presented Vernier stimuli away from its focus. This repulsion effect illustrates that attention can distort the encoding of nearby positions and suggests an over-representation of space around the attended area (Suzuki and Cavanagh 1997); see also Wardak, Deneve, and Ben Hamed (2010). Spatial attention is also critical for observers' ability to accurately report the relative position of two stimuli. When attention is prevented from shifting to a target location by a concurrent task, performance on reporting relative position of two features falls to chance (Lee, Itti, Koch, and Braun 1999; Pastukhov, Fischer, and Braun 2009; Li, VanRullen, Koch, and Perona 2002). The performance drops are large and fit well with the hypothesis that attention enhances spatial resolution (for a review, see Carrasco and Yeshurun 2009), as well as the enhanced resolution models (Lee, Itti, Koch, and Braun 1999; Deco and Heinke 2007; Deco and Schurmann 2000; Salinas and Abbott 1997; Womelsdorf, Anton-Erxleben, and Treue 2008) and single-unit studies on attention and resolution (Womelsdorf, Anton-Erxleben, Pieper, and Treue 2006; Anton-Erxleben, Stephan, and Treue 2009; Moran and Desimone 1985).

Adapting the attention and appearance paradigm developed by Carrasco and colleagues (Carrasco, Ling, and Read 2004), a study has shown that attention also distorts perceived shape. Depending on cue placement inside or outside the contour of an oval, the aligned dimension (height or width) was perceived longer or shorter, respectively. Visual cues alter perceived shape so that the oval contours were repelled (Fortenbaugh, Prinzmetal, and Robertson 2011). These results are consistent with those of Anton-Erxleben et al. (2007) and with the explanation based on RF shifts they proposed to account for effects of attention on the size of an object.

CONCLUSION

This review includes psychophysical studies of visual attention that allow us to probe the human visual system. I have described the effects of spatial attention on perceptual effects mediated by early vision—contrast sensitivity and spatial resolution—for which the best mechanistic understanding has been achieved by the confluence of psychophysical, electrophysiological, neuroimaging, and computational studies. I have shown that trade-offs in processing result in increased performance at the attended location and decreased performance at unattended locations, consistent with a selective representation of the world. There is a fixed amount of overall energy available to the brain, and the cost of cortical computation is high. Attention is crucial in optimizing the system's limited resources. As a selective process, attention provides an organism with an optimized representation of the sensory input that emphasizes relevant details, at times even at the expense of a faithful representation of the sensory input.

NOTE

1. The terms endogenous attention and sustained attention have been used interchangeably or as synonyms. The term exogenous should be used only when the cue is uninformative regarding the target location, whereas the term transient does not necessarily imply that the cue is uninformative. Here I use the terms endogenous and exogenous, except in cases where the authors used a transient cue instead of an exogenous cue.

References

Abbey, C. K. and Eckstein, M. P. (2009). Frequency tuning of perceptual templates changes with noise magnitude. *Journal of the Optical Society of America A 26*(11): 72–83.

Abrams, J., Barbot, A., and Carrasco, M. (2010). Voluntary attention increases perceived spatial frequency. *Attention, Perception, & Psychophysics 72*(6): 1510–1521.

Abrams, J., Nizam, A., and Carrasco, M. (2011). Isoeccentric locations are not equivalent: The extent of the vertical meridian asymmetry. *Vision Research 52*(1): 70–78.

Allard, R. and Cavanagh, P. (2011). Crowding in a detection task: External noise triggers change in processing strategy. *Vision Research 51*(4): 408–416.

Anton-Erxleben, K., Henrich, C., and Treue, S. (2007). Attention changes perceived size of moving visual patterns. *Journal of Vision 7*(11): 1–9.

Anton-Erxleben, K., Stephan, V. M., and Treue, S. (2009). Attention reshapes center-surround receptive field structure in macaque cortical area MT. *Cerebral Cortex 19*(10): 2466–2478.

Anton-Erxleben, K., Abrams, J., and Carrasco, M. (2010). Evaluating comparative and equality judgments in contrast perception: Attention alters appearance. *Journal of Vision 10*(11): 1–22.

Arsenault, A. S., Wilkinson, F., and Kingdom, F. A. (1999). Modulation frequency and orientation tuning of second-order texture mechanisms. *Journal of the Optical Society of America A 16*(3): 427–435.

Baldassi, S. and Burr, D. C. (2000). Feature-based integration of orientation signals in visual search. *Vision Research 40*(10–12): 1293–1300.

Barbot, A., Landy, M. S., and Carrasco, M. (2011). Exogenous attention enhances 2nd-order contrast sensitivity. *Vision Research 51*(9): 1086–1098.

Barbot, A., Landy, M. S., and Carrasco, M. (2012). Differential effects of exogenous and endogenous attention on second-order texture contrast sensitivity. *Journal of Vision 12*(8): 1–15.

Barbot, A., Montagna, B., and Carrasco, M. (2012). Endogenous attention optimizes performance by adjusting spatial resolution: Evidence from selective adaptation. *Journal of Vision 12*(9): art. 387 [abstract].

Bashinski, H. S. and Bacharach, V. R. (1980). Enhancement of perceptual sensitivity as the result of selectively attending to spatial locations. *Perception & Psychophysics 28*(3): 241–248.

Beck, D. M. and Kastner, S. (2009). Top-down and bottom-up mechanisms in biasing competition in the human brain. *Vision Research 49*(10): 1154–1165.

Bergen, J. R. and Landy, M. S. (1991). *Computational Modeling of Visual Texture Segregation, in Computational Models of Visual Processing* (pp. 253–271). Cambridge, Mass.: MIT Press.

Blakemore, C. and Campbell, F. W. (1969). On the existence of neurones in the human visual system selectively sensitive to the orientation and size of retinal images. *Journal of Physiology 203*(1): 237–260.

Bonnel, A. M., Stein, J. F. and Bertucci, P. (1992). Does attention modulate the perception of luminance changes? *Quarterly Journal of Experimental Psychology A 44*(4): 601–626.

Bonnel, A. M. and Miller, J. (1994). Attentional effects on concurrent psychophysical discriminations: Investigations of a sample-size model. *Perception & Psychophysics 55*(2): 162–179.

Boynton, G. M., Demb, J. B., Glover, G. H., and Heeger, D. J. (1999). Neuronal basis of contrast discrimination. *Vision Research 39*(2): 257–269.

Braun, J. (1994). Visual search among items of different salience: removal of visual attention mimics a lesion in extrastriate area V4. *Journal of Neuroscience 14*(2): 554–567.

Braun, J. and Julesz, B. (1998). Withdrawing attention at little or no cost: Detection and discrimination tasks. *Perception & Psychophysics 60*(1): 1–23.

Briand, K. A. and Klein, R. M. (1987). Is Posner's 'beam' the same as Treisman's 'glue'? On the relation between visual orienting and feature integration theory. *Journal of Experimental Psychology: Human Perception and Performance* 13(2): 228–241.

Briand, K. A. (1998). Feature integration and spatial attention: More evidence of a dissociation between endogenous and exogenous orienting. *Journal of Experimental Psychology: Human Perception and Performance* 24(4): 1243–1256.

Broadbent, D. E. (1958). *Perception and Communication* (p. 340). Elmsford, N.Y.: Pergamon Press.

Burgess, A. E., Wagner, R. F., Jennings, R. J., and Barlow, H. B. (1981). Efficiency of human visual signal discrimination. *Science* 214(4516): 93–94.

Busse, L., Katzner, S., and Treue, S. (2008). Temporal dynamics of neuronal modulation during exogenous and endogenous shifts of visual attention in macaque area MT. *Proceedings of the National Academy of Sciences USA* 105(42): 16380–16385.

Cameron, E. L., Tai, J. C., and Carrasco, M. (2002). Covert attention affects the psychometric function of contrast sensitivity. *Vision Research* 42(8): 949–967.

Cameron, E. L., Tai, J. C., Eckstein, M. P., and Carrasco, M. (2004). Signal detection theory applied to three visual search tasks—identification, yes/no detection and localization. *Spatial Vision* 17(4–5): 295–325.

Cannon, M. W. (1985). Perceived contrast in the fovea and periphery. *Journal of the Optical Society of America A* 2(10): 1760–1768.

Carandini, M. and Heeger, D. J. (2011). Normalization as a canonical neural computation. *Nature Reviews Neuroscience* 13(1): 51–62.

Carrasco, M. and Chang, I. (1995). The interaction of objective and subjective organizations in a localization search task. *Perception & Psychophysics* 57(8): 1134–1150.

Carrasco, M., Evert, D. L., Chang, I., and Katz, S. M. (1995). The eccentricity effect: Target eccentricity affects performance on conjunction searches. *Perception & Psychophysics* 57(8): 1241–1261.

Carrasco, M. and Frieder, K. S. (1997). Cortical magnification neutralizes the eccentricity effect in visual search. *Vision Research* 37(1): 63–82.

Carrasco, M., McLean, T. L., Katz, S. M. and Frieder, K. S. (1998). Feature asymmetries in visual search: Effects of display duration, target eccentricity, orientation and spatial frequency. *Vision Research* 38(3): 347–374.

Carrasco, M., Ponte, D., Rechea, C., and Sampedro, M. J. (1998). 'Transient structures': The effects of practice and distractor grouping on within-dimension conjunction searches. *Perception & Psychophysics* 60(7): 1243–1258.

Carrasco, M. and Yeshurun, Y. (1998). The contribution of covert attention to the set-size and eccentricity effects in visual search. *Journal of Experimental Psychology: Human Perception and Performance* 24(2): 673–692.

Carrasco, M., Penpeci-Talgar, C., and Eckstein, M. (2000). Spatial covert attention increases contrast sensitivity across the CSF: Support for signal enhancement. *Vision Research* 40(10–12): 1203–1215.

Carrasco, M. and McElree, B. (2001). Covert attention accelerates the rate of visual information processing. *Proceedings of the National Academy of Sciences USA* 98(9): 5363–5367.

Carrasco, M., Williams, P. E., and Yeshurun, Y. (2002). Covert attention increases spatial resolution with or without masks: Support for signal enhancement. *Journal of Vision* 2(6): 467–479.

Carrasco, M., Ling, S., and Read, S. (2004). Attention alters appearance. *Nature Neuroscience* 7(3): 308–313.

Carrasco, M., Giordano, A. M., and McElree, B. (2006). Attention speeds processing across eccentricity: Feature and conjunction searches. *Vision Research* 46(13): 2028–2040.

Carrasco, M., Loula, F., and Ho, Y. X. (2006). How attention enhances spatial resolution: Evidence from selective adaptation to spatial frequency. *Perception & Psychophysics* 68(6): 1004–1012.

Carrasco, M., Fuller, S., and Ling, S. (2008). Transient attention does increase perceived contrast of suprathreshold stimuli: A reply to Prinzmetal, Long and Leonhardt. *Perception & Psychophysics* 70(7): 1151–1164.

Carrasco, M. (2009). Cross-modal attention enhances perceived contrast. *Proceedings of the National Academy of Sciences USA* 106(52): 22039–22040.

Carrasco, M. and Yeshurun, Y. (2009). Covert attention effects on spatial resolution. *Progress in Brain Research* 176: 65–86.

Carrasco, M. (2011). Visual attention: The past 25 years. *Vision Research* 51(13): 1484–1525.

Castiello, U. and Umiltà, C. (1990). Size of the attentional focus and efficiency of processing. *Acta Psychologica* 73(3): 195–209.

Castiello, U. and Umiltà, C. (1992). Splitting focal attention. *Journal of Experimental Psychology: Human Perception and Performance* 18(3): 837–848.

Cheal, M., Lyon, D. R., and Hubbard, D. C. (1991). Does attention have different effects on line orientation and line arrangement discrimination? *Quarterly Journal of Experimental Psychology A* 43(4): 825–857.

Chica, A. B. and Christie, J. (2009). Spatial attention does improve temporal discrimination. *Attention, Perception, & Psychophysics* 71(2): 273–280.

Chica, A. B. and Lupiañez, J. (2009). Effects of endogenous and exogenous attention on visual processing: An Inhibition of Return study. *Brain Research* 1278: 75–85.

Cohen, M. R. and Maunsell, J. H. (2009). Attention improves performance primarily by reducing interneuronal correlations. *Nature Neuroscience* 12(12): 1594–1600.

Cohen, M. R. and Maunsell, J. H. (forthcoming). Neuronal mechanisms of spatial attention in visual cerebral cortex. In S. Kastner and K. Nobre (eds.), *Handbook of Attention*. Oxford: Oxford University Press.

Cohn, T. E. (1981). Absolute threshold: Analysis in terms of uncertainty. *Journal of the Optical Society of America* 71(6): 783–785.

Coull, J. T., Frith, C. D., Buchel, C., and Nobre, A. C. (2000). Orienting attention in time: Behavioural and neuroanatomical distinction between exogenous and endogenous shifts. *Neuropsychologia* 38(6): 808–819.

Dakin, S. C., Williams, C. B., and Hess, R. F. (1999). The interaction of first- and second-order cues to orientation. *Vision Research* 39(17): 2867–2884.

Davis, E. T., Kramer, P., and Graham, N. (1983). Uncertainty about spatial frequency, spatial position, or contrast of visual patterns. *Perception & Psychophysics* 33(1): 20–28.

De Valois, R. L. and De Valois, K. K. (1988). *Spatial Vision*. New York: Oxford University Press.

Deco, G. and Schurmann, B. (2000). A hierarchical neural system with attentional top-down enhancement of the spatial resolution for object recognition. *Vision Research* 40(20): 2845–2859.

Deco, G. and Heinke, D. (2007). Attention and spatial resolution: A theoretical and experimental study of visual search in hierarchical patterns. *Perception* 36(3): 335–354.

Desimone, R. and Duncan, J. (1995). Neural mechanisms of selective visual attention. *Annual Review of Neuroscience* 18: 193–222.

Di Russo, F., Spinelli, D., and Morrone, M. C. (2001). Automatic gain control contrast mechanisms are modulated by attention in humans: Evidence from visual evoked potentials. *Vision Research* 41(19): 2435–2447.

Dosher, B. A. and Lu, Z. L. (1998). Perceptual learning reflects external noise filtering and internal noise reduction through channel reweighting. *Proceedings of the National Academy of Sciences USA* 95(23): 13988–13993.

Dosher, B. A. and Lu, Z. L. (2000a). Noise exclusion in spatial attention. *Psychological Science* 11(2): 139–146.

Dosher, B. A. and Lu, Z. L. (2000b). Mechanisms of perceptual attention in precuing of location. *Vision Research*, 40(10–12), 1269–1292.

Dosher, B. A., Han, S., and Lu, Z. L. (2004). Information-limited parallel processing in difficult heterogeneous covert visual search. *Journal of Experimental Psychology: Human Perception and Performance* 36(5): 1128–1144.

Downing, C. J. and Pinker, S. (1985). The spatial structure of visual attention. In M. I. Posner and O. S. M. Marin (eds.), *Attention and Performance XI* (pp. 171–188). Hillsdale, N.J.: Lawrence Erlbaum Associates.

Downing, C. J. (1988). Expectancy and visual-spatial attention: Effects on perceptual quality. *Journal of Experimental Psychology: Human Perception and Performance* 14(2): 188–202.

Duncan, J. and Humphreys, G. W. (1989). Visual search and stimulus similarity. *Psychological Review* 96(3): 433–458.

Eckstein, M. P. and Whiting, J. S. (1996). Visual signal detection in structured backgrounds. I. Effect of number of possible spatial locations and signal contrast. *Journal of the Optical Society of America A* 13(9): 1777–1787.

Eckstein, M. P., Thomas, J. P., Palmer, J., and Shimozaki, S. S. (2000). A signal detection model predicts the effects of set size on visual search accuracy for feature, conjunction, triple conjunction, and disjunction displays. *Perception & Psychophysics* 62(3): 425–451.

Eckstein, M. P., Shimozaki, S. S., and Abbey, C. K. (2002). The footprints of visual attention in the Posner cueing paradigm revealed by classification images. *Journal of Vision* 2(1): 25–45.

Eckstein, M. P., Peterson, M. F., Pham, B. T., and Droll, J. A. (2009). Statistical decision theory to relate neurons to behavior in the study of covert visual attention. *Vision Research* 49(10): 1097–1128.

Eriksen, C. W. and Schultz, D. W. (1979). Information processing in visual search: A continuous flow conception and experimental results. *Perception & Psychophysics* 25(4): 249–263.

Eriksen, C. W. and Yeh, Y. Y. (1985). Allocation of attention in the visual field. *Journal of Experimental Psychology: Human Perception and Performance* 11(5): 583–597.

Eriksen, C. W. and St James, J. D. (1986). Visual attention within and around the field of focal attention: A zoom lens model. *Perception & Psychophysics* 40(4): 225–240.

Eriksen, C. W. and Murphy, T. D. (1987). Movement of attentional focus across the visual field: A critical look at the evidence. *Perception & Psychophysics* 42(3): 299–305.

Eriksen, C. W., Webb, J. M., and Fournier, L. R. (1990). How much processing do nonattended stimuli receive? Apparently very little, but… *Perception & Psychophysics* 47(5): 477–488.

Foley, J. M. S. (1998). Spatial attention: Effect of position uncertainty and number of distractor patterns on the threshold-versus-contrast function for contrast discrimination. *Journal of the Optical Society of America A* 15(5): 1036–1047.

Fortenbaugh, F. C., Prinzmetal, W., and Robertson, L. C. (2011). Rapid changes in visual-spatial attention distort object shape. *Psychonomic Bulletin & Review* 18(2): 287–294.

Fuller, S. and Carrasco, M. (2006). Exogenous attention and color perception: Performance and appearance of saturation and hue. *Vision Research* 46(23): 4032–4047.

Fuller, S., Rodriguez, R. Z., and Carrasco, M. (2008). Apparent contrast differs across the vertical meridian: Visual and attentional factors. *Journal of Vision* 8(1): 1–16.

Fuller, S., Park, Y., and Carrasco, M. (2009). Cue contrast modulates the effects of exogenous attention on appearance. *Vision Research* 49(14): 1825–1837.

Giordano, A. M., McElree, B., and Carrasco, M. (2009). On the automaticity and flexibility of covert attention: A speed-accuracy trade-off analysis. *Journal of Vision* 9(3): 1–10.

Gobell, J. and Carrasco, M. (2005). Attention alters the appearance of spatial frequency and gap size. *Psychological Science* 16(8): 644–651.

Golla, H., Ignashchenkova, A., Haarmeier, T., and Thier, P. (2004). Improvement of visual acuity by spatial cueing: A comparative study in human and non-human primates. *Vision Research* 44(13): 1589–1600.

Graham, N. (1989). *Visual Pattern Analyzers*. New York: Oxford University Press.

Graham, N., Beck, J., and Sutter, A. (1992). Nonlinear processes in spatial-frequency channel models of perceived texture segregation: Effects of sign and amount of contrast. *Vision Research* 32(4): 719–743.

Graham, N. and Wolfson, S. S. (2001). A note about preferred orientations at the first and second stages of complex (second-order) texture channels. *Journal of the Optical Society of America A* 18(9): 2273–2281.

Gurnsey, R., Pearson, P., and Day, D. (1996). Texture segmentation along the horizontal meridian: Nonmonotonic changes in performance with eccentricity. *Journal of Experimental Psychology: Human Perception and Performance* 22(3): 738–757.

Hein, E., Rolke, B., and Ulrich, R. (2006). Visual attention and temporal discrimination: Differential effects of automatic and voluntary cueing. *Visual Cognition* 13(1): 29–50.

Helmholtz, H. von (1866/1911). *Treatise on Physiological Optics*. Rochester: Continuum.

Herrmann, K., Montaser-Kouhsari, L., Carrasco, M., and Heeger, D. J. (2010). When size matters: Attention affects performance by contrast or response gain. *Nature Neuroscience* 13(12): 1554–1559.

Hikosaka, O., Miyauchi, S., and Shimojo, S. (1993). Focal visual attention produces illusory temporal order and motion sensation. *Vision Research* 33(9): 1219–1240.

Hsieh, P. J., Caplovitz, G. P., and Tse, P. U. (2005). Illusory rebound motion and the motion continuity heuristic. *Vision Research* 45(23): 2972–2985.

Huang, L. and Dobkins, K. R. (2005). Attentional effects on contrast discrimination in humans: Evidence for both contrast gain and response gain. *Vision Research* 45(9): 1201–1212.

James, W. (1890). *The Principles of Psychology*. New York: Henry Holt.

Joffe, K. M. and Scialfa, C. T. (1995). Texture segmentation as a function of eccentricity, spatial frequency and target size. *Spatial Vision* 9(3): 325–342.

Johnson, A. P. and Baker, C. L., Jr (2004). First- and second-order information in natural images: A filter-based approach to image statistics. *Journal of the Optical Society of America A* 21(6): 913–925.

Jonides, J. (1981). Voluntary vs automatic control of the mind's eye's movement. In J. B. Long and A. Baddeley (eds.), *Attention and Performance IX* (pp. 187–204). Hillsdale, N.J.: Lawrence Erlbaum Associates.

Kehrer, L. (1997). The central performance drop in texture segmentation: A simulation based on a spatial filter model. *Biological Cybernetics* 77(4): 297–305.

Kinchla, R. A. (1980). The measurement of attention. In R. Nickerson (ed.), *Attention and Performance VIII* (pp. 213–238). Princeton, N.J.: Psychology Press.

Kinchla, R. A. (1992). Attention. *Annual Review of Psychology* 43: 711–742.

Kitterle, F. L. (1986). Psychophysics of lateral tachistoscopic presentation. *Brain and Cognition* 5(2): 131–162.

Landy, M. S. and Oruc, I. (2002). Properties of second-order spatial frequency channels. *Vision Research* 42(19): 2311–2329.

Langley, K. (2002). A parametric account of contrast adaptation on contrast perception. *Spatial Vision* 16(1): 77–93.

Lavie, N. (1995). Perceptual load as a necessary condition for selective attention. *Journal of Experimental Psychology: Human Perception and Performance* 21(3): 451–468.

Lee, D. K., Koch, C., and Braun, J. (1997). Spatial vision thresholds in the near absence of attention. *Vision Research* 37(17): 2409–2418.

Lee, D. K., Itti, L., Koch, C., and Braun, J. (1999). Attention activates winner-take-all competition among visual filters. *Nature Neuroscience* 2(4): 375–381.

Lennie, P. (2003). The cost of cortical computation. *Current Biology* 13(6): 493–497.

Levi, D. M., Klein, S. A., and Aitsebaomo A. P. (1985). Vernier acuity, crowding and cortical magnification. *Vision Research* 25(7): 963–977.

Li, F. F., VanRullen, R., Koch, C. and Perona, P. (2002). Rapid natural scene categorization in the near absence of attention. *Proceedings of the National Academy of Sciences USA* 99(14): 9596–9601.

Ling, S. and Carrasco, M. (2006a). Sustained and transient covert attention enhance the signal via different contrast response functions. *Vision Research* 46(8–9): 1210–1220.

Ling, S. and Carrasco, M. (2006b). When sustained attention impairs perception. *Nature Neuroscience* 9(10): 1243–1245.

Ling, S. and Carrasco, M. (2007). Transient covert attention does alter appearance: A reply to Schneider (2006). *Perception & Psychophysics* 69(6): 1051–1058.

Liu, T., Pestilli, F., and Carrasco, M. (2005). Transient attention enhances perceptual performance and FMRI response in human visual cortex. *Neuron* 45(3): 469–477.

Liu, T., Fuller, S., and Carrasco, M. (2006). Attention alters the appearance of motion coherence. *Psychonomic Bulletin & Review* 13(6): 1091–1096.

Liu, T., Stevens, S. T., and Carrasco, M. (2007). Comparing the time course and efficacy of spatial and feature-based attention. *Vision Research* 47(1): 108–113.

Liu, T., Abrams, J., and Carrasco, M. (2009). Voluntary attention enhances contrast appearance. *Psychological Science* 20(3): 354–362.

Lu, Z. L. and Dosher, B. A. (1998). External noise distinguishes attention mechanisms. *Vision Research* 38(9): 1183–1198.

Lu, Z. L. and Dosher, B. A. (1999). Characterizing human perceptual inefficiencies with equivalent internal noise. *Journal of the Optical Society of America A* 16(3): 764–778.

Lu, Z. L. and Dosher, B. A. (2000). Spatial attention: Different mechanisms for central and peripheral temporal precues? *Journal of Experimental Psychology: Human Perception and Performance* 26(5): 1534–1548.

Lu, Z. L., Liu, T., and Dosher, B. A. (2000). Attention mechanisms for multi-location first- and second-order motion perception. *Vision Research* 40(2): 173–186.

Lu, Z. L., Lesmes, L. A., and Dosher, B. A. (2002). Spatial attention excludes external noise at the target location. *Journal of Vision* 2(4): 312–323.

Lu, Z. L. and Dosher, B. A. (2004). Spatial attention excludes external noise without changing the spatial frequency tuning of the perceptual template. *Journal of Vision* 4(10): 955–966.

Lu, Z. L. and Dosher, B. A. (2008). Characterizing observers using external noise and observer models: assessing internal representations with external noise. *Psychological Review* 115(1): 44–82.

Lu, Z. L., Tse, H. C., Dosher, B. A., Lesmes, L. A., Posner, C., and Chu, W. (2009). Intra- and cross-modal cuing of spatial attention: Time courses and mechanisms. *Vision Research* 49(10): 1081–1096.

Luck, S. J., Hillyard, S. A., Mouloua, M., and Hawkins, H. L. (1996). Mechanisms of visual-spatial attention: Resource allocation or uncertainty reduction? *Journal of Experimental Psychology: Human Perception and Performance* 22(3): 725–737.

Luck, S. J. (2004). Understanding awareness: One step closer. *Nature Neuroscience* 7(3): 208–209.

Maclean, K. A., Aichele, S. R., Bridwell, D. A., Mangun, G. R., Wojciulik, E., and Saron, C. D. (2009). Interactions between endogenous and exogenous attention during vigilance. *Attention, Perception, & Psychophysics* 71(5): 1042–1058.

Mangun, G. R. and Hillyard, S. A. (1990). Allocation of visual attention to spatial locations: Tradeoff functions for event-related brain potentials and detection performance. *Perception & Psychophysics* 47(6): 532–550.

Martinez-Trujillo, J. C. and Treue, S. (2002). Attentional modulation strength in cortical area MT depends on stimulus contrast. *Neuron* 35(2): 365–370.

Martinez-Trujillo, J. C. and Treue, S. (2004). Feature-based attention increases the selectivity of population responses in primate visual cortex. *Current Biology* 14(9): 744–751.

Martinez Trujillo, J. C. and Treue, S. (2005). Attentional modulation of apparent stimulus contrast. In L. Itti, G. Rees, and J. Tsotsos (eds.), *Neurobiology of Attention* (p. 428). San Diego: Elsevier.

Mayfrank, L., Kimmig, H., and Fischer, B. (1987). The role of attention in the preparation of visually guided saccadic eye movements in man. In J. K. O'Regan and A. Levy-Schoen (eds.), *Eye Movements: From Pyschology to Cognition* (pp. 37–45). New York: North Holland.

McAdams, C. J. and Maunsell, J. H. (1999). Effects of attention on the reliability of individual neurons in monkey visual cortex. *Neuron* 23(4): 765–773.

McLeod, P., Driver, J., and Crisp, J. (1988). Visual search for a conjunction of movement and form is parallel. *Nature* 332(6160): 154–155.

Megna, N., Rocchi, F., and Baldassi, S. (2012). Spatio-temporal templates of transient attention revealed by classification images. *Vision Research* 54: 39–48.

Miniussi, C., Rao, A., and Nobre, A. C. (2002). Watching where you look: Modulation of visual processing of foveal stimuli by spatial attention. *Neuropsychologia* 40(13): 2448–2460.

Mitchell, J. F., Sundberg, K. A., and Reynolds, J. H. (2009). Spatial attention decorrelates intrinsic activity fluctuations in macaque area V4. *Neuron* 63(6): 879–888.

Montagna, B. and Carrasco, M. (2006). Transient covert attention and the perceived rate of flicker. *Journal of Vision* 6(9): 955–965.

Montagna, B., Pestilli, F., and Carrasco, M. (2009). Attention trades off spatial acuity. *Vision Research* 49(7): 735–745.

Montaser-Kouhsari, L. and Carrasco, M. (2009). Perceptual asymmetries are preserved in short-term memory tasks. *Attention, Perception, & Psychophysics* 71(8): 1782–1792.

Moran, J. and Desimone, R. (1985). Selective attention gates visual processing in the extrastriate cortex. *Science* 229(4715): 782–784.

Morgan, M. J., Ward, R. M., and Castet, E. (1998). Visual search for a tilted target: Tests of spatial uncertainty models. *Quarterly Journal of Experimental Psychology A* 51(2): 347–370.

Morrone, M. C., Denti, V., and Spinelli, D. (2002). Color and luminance contrasts attract independent attention. *Current Biology* 12(13): 1134–1137.

Morrone, M. C., Denti, V., and Spinelli, D. (2004). Different attentional resources modulate the gain mechanisms for color and luminance contrast. *Vision Research* 44(12): 1389–1401.

Movshon, J. A. and Lennie, P. (1979). Pattern-selective adaptation in visual cortical neurones. *Nature* 278(5707): 850–852.

Muller, H. J. and Findlay, J. M. (1987). Sensitivity and criterion effects in the spatial cuing of visual attention. *Perception & Psychophysics* 42(4): 383–399.

Muller, H. J. and Rabbitt, P. M. (1989a). Reflexive and voluntary orienting of visual attention: Time course of activation and resistance to interruption. *Journal of Experimental Psychology: Human Perception and Performance* 15(2): 315–330.

Muller, H. J. and Rabbitt, P. M. (1989b). Spatial cueing and the relation between the accuracy of 'where' and 'what' decisions in visual search. *Quarterly Journal of Experimental Psychology A* 41(4): 747–773.

Muller, M. M., Picton, T. W., Valdes-Sosa, P., Riera, J., Teder-Salejarvi, W. A., and Hillyard, S. A. (1998). Effects of spatial selective attention on the steady-state visual evoked potential in the 20–28 Hz range. *Cognitive Brain Research* 6(4): 249–261.

Nachmias, J. (1967). Effect of exposure duration on visual contrast sensitivity with square-wave gratings. *Journal of the Optical Society of America A* 57(3): 421–427.

Nachmias, J. and Kocher, E. (1970). Visual detection and discrimination of luminance increments. *Vision Research* 60: 382–389.

Nachmias, J. (2002). Contrast discrimination with and without spatial uncertainty. *Vision Research* 42(1): 41–48.

Nakayama, K. and Silverman, G. H. (1986). Serial and parallel processing of visual feature conjunctions. *Nature* 320(6059): 264–265.

Nakayama, K. and Mackeben, M. (1989). Sustained and transient components of focal visual attention. *Vision Research* 29(11): 1631–1647.

Neisser, U. (1967). *Cognitive Psychology*. East Norwalk, Conn.: Appleton Century Crofts.

Palmer, J. (1994). Set-size effects in visual search: the effect of attention is independent of the stimulus for simple tasks. *Vision Research* 34(13): 1703–1721.

Palmer, J., Verghese, P., and Pavel, M. (2000). The psychophysics of visual search. *Vision Research* 40(10–12): 1227–1268.

Pashler, H. and Johnston, J. C. (1998). Attentional limitations in dual-task performance. In H. Pashler (ed.), *Attention* (pp. 155–189). Hove: Psychology Press/Erlbaum (UK) Taylor & Francis.

Pastukhov, A., Fischer, L., and Braun, J. (2009). Visual attention is a single, integrated resource. *Vision Research* 49(10): 1166–1173.

Pelli, D. G. (1985). Uncertainty explains many aspects of visual contrast detection and discrimination. *Journal of the Optical Society of America A* 2(9): 1508–1532.

Pelli, D. G. and Farell, B. (1999). Why use noise? *Journal of the Optical Society of America A* 16(3): 647–653.

Pestilli, F. and Carrasco, M. (2005). Attention enhances contrast sensitivity at cued and impairs it at uncued locations. *Vision Research* 45(14): 1867–1875.

Pestilli, F., Viera, G., and Carrasco, M. (2007). How do attention and adaptation affect contrast sensitivity? *Journal of Vision* 7(7): 1–12.

Pestilli, F., Ling, S., and Carrasco, M. (2009). A population-coding model of attention's influence on contrast response: Estimating neural effects from psychophysical data. *Vision Research* 49(10): 1144–1153.

Pestilli, F., Carrasco, M., Heeger, D. J., and Gardner, J. L. (2011). Attentional enhancement via selection and pooling of early sensory responses in human visual cortex. *Neuron* 72(5): 832–846.

Posner, M. I. (1980). Orienting of attention. *Quarterly Journal of Experimental Psychology* 32(1): 3–25.

Prinzmetal, W., Nwachuku, I., Bodanski, L., Blumenfeld, L., and Shimizu, N. (1997). The phenomenology of attention, 2: Brightness and contrast. *Conscious Cognition* 6(2–3): 372–412.

Prinzmetal, W., Amiri, H., Allen, K., and Edwards, T. (1998). Phenomenology of attention, 1: Color, location, orientation and spatial frequency. *Journal of Experimental Psychology: Human Perception and Performance* 21(1): 261–282.

Prinzmetal, W., McCool, C., and Park, S. (2005). Attention: Reaction time and accuracy reveal different mechanisms. *Journal of Experimental Psychology: General* 134(1): 73–92.

Prinzmetal, W., Long, V., and Leonhardt, J. (2008). Involuntary attention and brightness contrast. *Perception & Psychophysics* 70(7): 1139–1150.

Rao, R. P. and Ballard, D. H. (1999). Predictive coding in the visual cortex: A functional interpretation of some extra-classical receptive-field effects. *Nature Neuroscience* 2(1): 79–87.

Regan, D. and Beverley, K. I. (1985). Postadaptation orientation discrimination. *Journal of the Optical Society of America A* 2(2): 147–155.

Remington, R. W., Johnston, J. C., and Yantis, S. (1992). Involuntary attentional capture by abrupt onsets. *Perception & Psychophysics* 51(3): 279–290.

Reynolds, J. H., Pasternak, T., and Desimone, R. (2000). Attention increases sensitivity of V4 neurons. *Neuron* 26(3): 703–714.

Reynolds, J. H. and Chelazzi, L. (2004). Attentional modulation of visual processing. *Annual Review of Neuroscience* 27: 611–647.

Reynolds, J. H. and Heeger, D. J. (2009). The normalization model of attention. *Neuron* 61(2): 168–185.

Reynolds, J. H. (2005). Visual cortical circuits and spatial attention. In L. Itti, G. Rees, and J. Tsotsos (eds.), *Neurobiology of Attention* (pp. 42–49). San Diego: Elsevier.

Rijsdijk, J. P., Kroon, J. N., and van der Wildt, G. J. (1980). Contrast sensitivity as a function of position on the retina. *Vision Research* 20(3): 235–241.

Ringach, D. L., Hawken, M. J., and Shapley, R. (1997). Dynamics of orientation tuning in macaque primary visual cortex. *Nature* 387(6630): 281–284.

Rolke, B., Dinkelbach, A., Hein, E., and Ulrich, R. (2008). Does attention impair temporal discrimination? Examining non-attentional accounts. *Psychological Research* 72(1): 49–60.

Rovamo, J. and Virsu, V. (1979). An estimation and application of the human cortical magnification factor. *Experimental Brain Research* 37(3): 495–510.

Salinas, E. and Abbott, L. F. (1997). Invariant visual responses from attentional gain fields. *Journal of Neurophysiology* 77(6): 3267–3272.

Schneider, K. A. (2006). Does attention alter appearance? *Perception & Psychophysics* 68(5): 800–814.

Schneider, K. A. and Komlos, M. (2008). Attention biases decisions but does not alter appearance. *Journal of Vision* 8(15): 1–10.

Schofield, A. J., Hesse, G., Rock, P. B., and Georgeson, M. A. (2006). Local luminance amplitude modulates the interpretation of shape-from-shading in textured surfaces. *Vision Research* 46(20): 3462–3482.

Scott-Samuel, N. E. and Georgeson, M. A. (1999). Does early non-linearity account for second-order motion? *Vision Research* 39(17): 2853–2865.

Shalev, L. and Tsal, Y. (2002). Detecting gaps with and without attention: Further evidence for attentional receptive fields. *European Journal of Cognitive Psychology* 14(1): 3–26.

Shaw, M. L. (1984). Division of attention among spatial locations: A fundamental difference between detection of letters and detection of luminance increments. In H. Bouma and D. G. Bouwhuis (eds.), *Attention and Performance X* (pp. 109–121). Hillsdale, N.J.: Lawrence Erlbaum Associates.

Shiu, L. and Pashler, H. (1994). Negligible effect of spatial precuing on identification of single digits. *Journal of Experimental Psychology: Human Perception and Performance* 20(5): 1037–1054.

Shulman, G. L. and Wilson, J. (1987). Spatial frequency and selective attention to spatial location. *Perception* 16(1): 103–111.

Skottun, B. C., Bradley, A., Sclar, G., Ohzawa, I., and Freeman, R. D. (1987). The effects of contrast on visual orientation and spatial frequency discrimination: A comparison of single cells and behavior. *Journal of Neurophysiology* 57(3): 773–786.

Smith, P. L., Wolfgang, B. J., and Sinclair, A. J. (2004). Mask-dependent attentional cuing effects in visual signal detection: The psychometric function for contrast. *Perception & Psychophysics* 66(6): 1056–1075.

Solomon, J. A., Lavie, N., and Morgan, M. J. (1997). Contrast discrimination function: Spatial cuing effects. *Journal of the Optical Society of America A* 14(9): 2443–2448.

Solomon, J. A. (2004). The effect of spatial cues on visual sensitivity. *Vision Research Special Issue: Visual Attention* 44(12): 1209–1216.

Sperling, G. and Dosher, B. A. (1986). Strategy and optimization in human information processing. In K. R. Boff, L. Kaufman, and J. P. Thomas (eds.), *Handbook of Perception and Human Performance* (pp. 1–65). New York: Wiley.

Sperling, G. and Melchner, M. J. (1978). The attention operating characteristic: Examples from visual search. *Science* 202(4365): 315–318.

Spitzer, H., Desimone, R., and Moran, J. (1988). Increased attention enhances both behavioral and neuronal performance. *Science* 240(4850): 338–340.

Srinivasan, N. and Brown, J. M. (2006). Effects of endogenous spatial attention on the detection and discrimination of spatial frequencies. *Perception* 35(2): 193–200.

Stormer, V. S., McDonald, J. J., and Hillyard, S. A. (2009). Cross-modal cueing of attention alters appearance and early cortical processing of visual stimuli. *Proceedings of the National Academy of Sciences USA* 106(52): 22456–22461.

Sun, P. and Schofield, A. J. (2011). The efficacy of local luminance amplitude in disambiguating the origin of luminance signals depends on carrier frequency: Further evidence for the active role of second-order vision in layer decomposition. *Vision Research* 51(5): 496–507.

Sutter, A., Beck, J., and Graham, N. (1989). Contrast and spatial variables in texture segregation: Testing a simple spatial-frequency channels model. *Perception & Psychophysics* 46(4): 312–332.

Suzuki, S. and Cavanagh, P. (1997). Focused attention distorts visual space: An attentional repulsion effect. *Journal of Experimental Psychology: Human Perception and Performance* 23(2): 443–463.

Talgar, C. P. and Carrasco, M. (2002). Vertical meridian asymmetry in spatial resolution: Visual and attentional factors. *Psychonomic Bulletin & Review* 9(4): 714–722.

Talgar, C. P., Pelli, D. G., and Carrasco, M. (2004). Covert attention enhances letter identification without affecting channel tuning. *Journal of Vision* 4(1): 22–31.

Thomas, J. P. and Olzak, L. A. (1986). Seeing spatial patterns. In K. R. Boff, L. Kaufman, and J. P. Thomas (eds.), *Handbook of Perception and Human Performance*, (vol. 1, pp. 1–65). New York: Wiley.

Treisman, A. M. (1960). Contextual cues in selective listening. *Quarterly Journal of Experimental Psychology* 12: 242–248.

Treisman, A. M. (1985). Preattentive processing in vision. *Computer Vision, Graphics, and Image Processing* 31: 156–177.

Treue, S. and Maunsell, J. H. (1999). Effects of attention on the processing of motion in macaque middle temporal and medial superior temporal visual cortical areas. *Journal of Neuroscience* 19(17): 7591–7602.

Treue, S. (2004). Perceptual enhancement of contrast by attention. *Trends in Cognitive Sciences* 8(10): 435–437.

Tsal, Y., Shalev, L., Zakay, D., and Lubow, R. E. (1994). Attention reduces perceived brightness contrast. *Quarterly Journal of Experimental Psychology A* 47(4): 865–893.

Tsal, Y., Meiran, N., and Lamy, D. (1995). Towards a resolution theory of visual attention. In C. Bundesen and H. Shibuya (eds.), *Visual Selective Attention* (special issue of *Visual Cognition*) 2(2–3): 313–330.

Tsal, Y. and Shalev, L. (1996). Inattention magnifies perceived length: The attentional receptive field hypothesis. *Journal of Experimental Psychology: Human Perception and Performance* 22(1): 233–243.

Tsal, Y., Shalev, L., and Zakay, D. (2005). The lengthening effect revisited: A reply to Prinzmetal and Wilson (1997) and Masin (1999). *Psychonomic Bulletin & Review* 12(1): 185–190.

Tse, P. U. (2005). Voluntary attention modulates the brightness of overlapping transparent surfaces. *Vision Research* 45(9): 1095–1098.

Turatto, M., Vescovi, M., and Valsecchi, M. (2007). Attention makes moving objects be perceived to move faster. *Vision Research* 47(2): 166–178.

Verghese, P. (2001). Visual search and attention: A signal detection theory approach. *Neuron* 31(4): 523–535.

Virsu, V. and Rovamo, J. (1979). Visual resolution, contrast sensitivity, and the cortical magnification factor. *Experimental Brain Research* 37(3): 475–494.

Wardak, C., Deneve, S., and Ben Hamed, S. (2010). Focused visual attention distorts distance perception away from the attentional locus. *Neuropsychologia* 49(3): 535–545.

Williford, T. and Maunsell, J. H. (2006). Effects of spatial attention on contrast response functions in macaque area V4. *Journal of Neurophysiology* 96(1): 40–54.

Wolfe, J. M., O'Neill, P., and Bennett, S. C. (1998). Why are there eccentricity effects in visual search? Visual and attentional hypotheses. *Perception & Psychophysics* 60(1): 140–156.

Womelsdorf, T., Anton-Erxleben, K., Pieper, F., and Treue, S. (2006). Dynamic shifts of visual receptive fields in cortical area MT by spatial attention. *Nature Neuroscience* 9(9): 1156–1160.

Womelsdorf, T., Anton-Erxleben, K., and Treue, S. (2008). Receptive field shift and shrinkage in macaque middle temporal area through attentional gain modulation. *Journal of Neuroscience* 28(36): 8934–8944.

Wyart, V., Nobre, A. C., and Summerfield, C. (2012). Dissociable prior influences of signal probability and relevance on visual contrast sensitivity. *Proceedings of the National Academy of Sciences USA* 109(9): 3593–3598.

Yantis, S. and Jonides, J. (1996). Attentional capture by abrupt onsets: New perceptual objects or visual masking? *Journal of Experimental Psychology: Human Perception and Performance* 22(6): 1505–1513.

Yeshurun, Y. and Carrasco, M. (1998). Attention improves or impairs visual performance by enhancing spatial resolution. *Nature* 396(6706): 72–75.

Yeshurun, Y. and Carrasco, M. (1999). Spatial attention improves performance in spatial resolution tasks. *Vision Research* 39(2): 293–306.

Yeshurun, Y. and Carrasco, M. (2000). The locus of attentional effects in texture segmentation. *Nature Neuroscience* 3(6): 622–627.

Yeshurun, Y. and Levy, L. (2003). Transient spatial attention degrades temporal resolution. *Psychological Science* 14(3): 225–231.

Yeshurun, Y. (2004). Isoluminant stimuli and red background attenuate the effects of transient spatial attention on temporal resolution. *Vision Research* 44(12): 1375–1387.

Yeshurun, Y. and Carrasco, M. (2008). The effects of transient attention on spatial resolution and the size of the attentional cue. *Perception & Psychophysics* 70(1): 104–113.

Yeshurun, Y. and Marom, G. (2008). Transient spatial attention and the perceived duration of brief visual events. *Visual Cognition* 16(6): 826–848.

Yeshurun, Y., Montagna, B., and Carrasco, M. (2008). On the flexibility of sustained attention and its effects on a texture segmentation task. *Vision Research* 48(1): 80–95.

Yeshurun, Y. and Rashal, E. (2010). Precueing attention to the target location diminishes crowding and reduces the critical distance. *Journal of Vision* 10(10): 16.

Yeshurun, Y. and Hein, E. (2011). Transient attention degrades perceived apparent motion. *Perception* 40(8): 905–918.

Yeshurun, Y. and Sabo, G. (2012). Differential effects of transient attention on inferred parvocellular and magnocellular processing. *Vision Research* 74: 21–29.

CHAPTER 8

....

SPATIAL ORIENTING AND ATTENTIONAL CAPTURE

....

JAN THEEUWES

As a metaphor, visual attention has been compared to a spotlight that selects parts of the visual world around us (e.g. Posner 1980). Visual attention allows people to select information that is relevant for their ongoing behaviour and ignore information that is irrelevant. The spotlight 'shines' on everything within the region covered by its beam. In its classic notion, information that is present within this region is processed and information outside the beam is ignored (Posner, Snyder, and Davidson 1980). Selection on the basis of location information is assumed to be superior relative to selection on the basis of other features (such as colour or shape) because the visual system is organized spatially (retino- and spatiotopically).

For several decades, there has been agreement that there are two functionally independent stages of visual processing (e.g. Broadbent 1958; Neisser 1967; Treisman and Gelade 1980). An early visual stage, sometimes referred to as preattentive, operates in parallel across the visual field; and a later stage, often referred to as attentive, can deal with only one or a few items at the same time. Even though the dichotomy between these two stages appears not to be as strict as originally assumed, this basic architecture is more or less still present in almost all past and present theories of visual attention (e.g. Itti and Koch 2001; Li 2002; Treue 2003; Wolfe 1994). Processing occurring during the initial wave of stimulation through the brain determines which element is selected and passed on to the second stage of processing. In line with the two-stage approach, passing on an item to the second stage of processing implies that this item has been selected for further processing (e.g. Broadbent 1958; Treisman and Gelade 1980).

Since the late 1970s and early 1980s, there has been agreement that visual selective attention can be directed to a non-fixated location in space (e.g. Eriksen and Hoffman 1973; Hoffman 1975; Posner, Snyder, and Davidson 1980). Providing information about the location of an upcoming target may enhance the efficiency of processing (e.g. Posner, Snyder, and Davidson 1980), reduce stimulus uncertainty (e.g. Eckstein, Shimozaki, and Abbey 2002; Palmer 1994), reduce interference from unattended locations (e.g. Theeuwes 1991a), or suppress masking at attended locations (Enns and Di Lollo 1997).

The effective utilization of spatial information is related to the attention mechanism that operates analogous to a beam of light. As a metaphor, Posner described visual selective attention as a 'spotlight that enhances the efficiency of the detection of events within its beam' (Posner 1980: 172).

When shifting attention from one location in space to another, the spotlight of attention 'highlights' the new location in the environment. Processing information at that location is then better than at the previous location or at any other of the non-attended locations. Shifts of attention are usually (but not necessarily) accompanied by eye movements. In some circumstances, you may want to attend to a person (i.e. shifting your attention towards that person) without directly looking at the person. In many cases, shifts of spatial attention are under the control of the observer, directing attention *at will* from one location to the next. In other circumstances, events in the environment (such as the sudden appearance of an object) may pull your attention towards the event, as if attention were automatically and reflexively controlled by the environment.

Shifts of spatial attention play a role in tasks in which observers are instructed to direct their attention to a particular location, for example, indicated by a cue (e.g. direct your attention to an object to the right of fixation). Shifting spatial attention also plays a role in visual search tasks, in which observers are instructed to look for a particular target object among multiple non-targets. On the basis of the classic work of Treisman and Gelade (1980), it was postulated that serial shifts of visuospatial attention are required when searching for a target defined by a conjunction of elementary features (such as colour, orientation, motion, etc.). Typically, the time to find a target increases with the number of elements in the display.

Once attention has shifted to a location, and the target is not present at that location, attention needs to be disengaged from that location and shifted to the next location. Disengagement of attention plays a role both in attentional cueing tasks as well as in tasks that involve visual search among multiple objects. Even though not extensively researched, it is likely that it is harder to disengage attention from an object that looks like the target than from an object that is dissimilar from the target (see for example, Theeuwes, Atchley, and Kramer 2000; Born, Kerzel, and Theeuwes 2011).

Spatial Orienting

Endogenous spatial orienting

It is possible to direct attention to a location in space 'at will'. For example, without moving the eyes, people are able to direct their attention to a non-fixated location in space. In the classic study by Posner, Nissen, and Ogden (1978), before display onset, observers received a central symbolic cue (e.g. an arrow) that indicated the location of the upcoming target with 80% validity. In other words, on 80% of trials the centrally presented

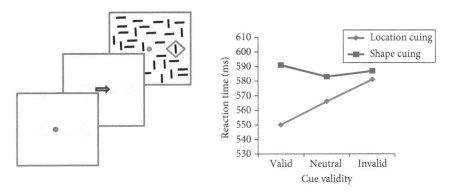

FIGURE 8.1 Stimuli and data from Theeuwes (1989). Left side: The central arrow indicated with a validity of 80% the location of the upcoming target. Observers responded to the orientation (horizontal or vertical) of the line segment presented within a target diamond or circle shape. Right side: Reaction time (RT) for cue-valid, neutral, and invalid conditions. Cueing the location resulted in clear performance costs and benefits. Cueing the shape of the target (whether it was a circle or a square) had no effect.

arrow pointed to the location where the target appeared. On 20% of the trials the target appeared at the 'invalid' location (i.e. at the location opposite to that indicated by the arrow). The results showed that observers were faster and more accurate when the target appeared at the cued location than when it occurred at an uncued location. Typically, relative to a neutral condition in which no information about the upcoming target is given, there are both performance benefits and costs. Posner, Nissen, and Ogden (1978) argued that in response to the cue, observers endogenously direct their attention to the cued location, suggesting that the focus of visual attention is shifted voluntarily. Crucially, in these types of experiments, the location to which observers are required to direct their attention varies from trial to trial, indicating that the focus of attention can be truly shifted 'at will' from one trial to the next, ruling out some type of location priming.

Theeuwes (1989) also investigated endogenous orienting by means of a central cue and compared it to cueing on the basis of shape information. If location information is no different from any other information that helps to separate the target from non-targets, then one would expect that cueing on the basis of shape should generate the same effects as those with location cueing. In Theeuwes (1989), observers made a speeded discrimination response to the orientation of a line segment positioned in either a circle or a diamond shape presented either to the left or right of fixation (see Fig. 8.1). The results showed clear costs and benefits for location cueing (see Fig. 8.1), but not shape cueing. The findings are consistent with a spotlight of attention model.

In a more recent study, Theeuwes and Van der Burg (2007) again investigated the efficiency of location cueing using dependent measures derived from signal detection theory. Unlike previous studies that typically use an arrow to direct attention to the location in space (Posner 1980), Theeuwes and Van der Burg employed a truly endogenous location cue in which the likely target position was indicated by a number corresponding to the hour indication of an analogue clock (e.g. 12 is the top location, 2 is the top-right location, etc.). Also, unlike earlier studies that used relatively short stimulus-onset asynchronies (SOAs) (typically from 300 to 600 ms) an SOA of more than 1.5 was used to allow observers to optimally, endogenously prepare for the upcoming target singleton. Again the results indicated that endogenous location cuing was very effective (A' = 0.90 for valid versus A' = 0.75 for invalidly cued location). This study shows that a location cue that is relatively abstract and cognitively complex also results in strong location cueing effects.

In sum, there have been numerous studies demonstrating that it is possible to direct attention 'at will' to a location in space without moving our eyes. Visual attention can be guided directly to the relevant spatial location. Attentional guidance by non-spatial features such as colour and shape is more controversial. Some claim that attention to non-spatial features may bias attention directly (e.g. Bundesen 1990) while others claim that, if anything, non-spatial guidance indirectly affects selection to the extent that it guides attention to the relevant locations (e.g. Awh, Belopolsky, and Theeuwes 2012; Theeuwes and Van der Burg 2007, 2011). According to this latter view, space is the ultimate attribute by which selective attention operates (Theeuwes, Van der Burg, and Belopolsky 2008).

Exogenous spatial orienting

Visual orienting may also occur in an automatic, bottom-up fashion controlled by events occurring in the external environment. In their classic paper, Posner and Cohen (1984) investigated the time course of attentional orienting of uninformative peripheral cues. The basic paradigm consisted of three horizontally aligned boxes. Observers had to fixate the central box. During a trial, the outline of one of the peripheral boxes was briefly brightened for 150 ms. At a variable SOA of 0, 50, 100, 200, 300, or 500 ms the target (a 0.1 degree filled square) was displayed inside one of the boxes and observers had to detect it as quickly as possible by pressing a single key. The results showed that responses were faster when the cue and target appeared at the same location than when the cue and target appeared at different locations but only when the cue–target SOA was less than 200 ms. With longer SOAs Posner and Cohen found the reverse: observers were now faster at the uncued than at the cued location. It was argued that with exogenous cues early facilitation was followed by inhibition. The inhibitory effect due to exogenous spatial orienting was named Inhibition of Return (IOR). IOR is typically only found when attention is exogenously captured by the onset. No IOR is found following endogenous spatial orienting.

Jonides (1981) also used peripheral cues with abrupt onsets to indicate the likely target position. The results indicated that such cues elicit an exogenous shift of attention to the indicated location. Jonides (1981) found that giving a concurrent memory load task only affected endogenous orienting in response to a central cue, whereas exogenous orienting in response to a peripheral cue was not affected. Because the attention-capturing power of the peripheral cue was unaffected by the increased task demands, Jonides argued that exogenous orienting is truly automatic.

Various studies have demonstrated that abrupt onsets have the ability to summon attention in a fast and reflexive way. For example, Yantis and Jonides (1984) showed that an item with abrupt onset was always processed first, resulting in a fast identification of onset stimuli compared to no-onset stimuli. These results were interpreted as evidence that an abrupt onset exerts control over the allocation of attention such that it draws attention to its location. Because in Jonides and Yantis the number of simultaneous no-onset items did not affect reaction time, it was claimed that an abrupt onset has an automatic orienting effect. Jonides and Yantis (1988; Yantis and Jonides 1984) have demonstrated that stimulus onset transients are capable of attracting attention. Theeuwes (1990, 1991a) showed that attention is not controlled by abrupt onset per se, but that all abrupt changes in the visual field (including offsets, and movement) are capable of attracting attention.

Typically, in exogenous spatial cueing tasks, observers are instructed to look for a particular target (e.g. a letter) and a completely irrelevant peripheral onset stimulus is presented somewhere in the visual field. If the target (in this example a letter) happens to be near the abrupt onset, the question is whether observers are quicker in finding the target than when the target is presented at an uncued location. If this is the case, it is argued that the irrelevant onset stimulus automatically and reflexively captured attention. The key aspect of the exogenous spatial cueing is that the location of the irrelevant onset cue is not predictive of where the target is going to be presented (which is unlike endogenous cueing where the cue is predictive) and that observers typically have no other goal than to search for a particular target.

Interactions between exogenous and endogenous spatial orienting

It is generally agreed that there are two distinct modes of spatial orienting. One voluntary, endogenous orienting mode in which the 'spotlight' is shifted in response to a central cue to a location in space at will, and one reflexive, exogenous orienting mode in which attention is captured by a peripheral onset cue. Several studies have looked at the interaction between exogenous and endogenous orienting.

Initially, it was assumed observers never could prevent the automatic orienting towards an abrupt onset. For example, even though Jonides (1981) instructed observers to ignore the peripheral onset cue, the results indicated that observers could not do so. Müller and Rabbitt (1989) instructed observers to attend a location cued by a central arrowhead. At various moments after the appearance of the arrowhead, a peripheral box surrounding one of the four possible target locations flashed for 50 ms. Even though voluntary allocation modulated the extent to which a peripheral flash captured attention, Müller and Rabbitt concluded that allocating

attention to a location could not prevent a shift of attention to the abruptly changing flash. Clearly, these results provide evidence for the claim that abrupt onsets are
genuinely automatic and reflexive.

Other studies provided evidence that focusing spatial attention in a top-down way to
a location in space prevents the capture of attention by abrupt onsets. For example, in
Theeuwes (1991a) a central arrowhead instructed observers to direct their attention to
one out of four placeholders presented equi-spaced in the periphery around the fixation
point. If observers directed their attention to one of the locations, an irrelevant abrupt
onset presented at one of the other locations had no measurable effect on performance.
Therefore, it was concluded that salient irrelevant abrupt onsets do not capture attention
if observers are focused in advance on a restricted area in space.

The difference between previous studies that showed that endogenous spatial orienting could not prevent attentional capture versus studies that shows that capture was prevented by endogenous orienting is related to the validity of the endogenous cue. Only
when the cue is 100% valid and observers exert a high attentional focus at the cued location can capture by an irrelevant onset be prevented. Overall, there is consensus that
when observers are in an unfocused state, abrupt onsets capture attention. When spatial attention is highly focused before display onset to a location in space, abrupt onsets
elsewhere in the visual field no longer capture attention. The extent to which observers are in a focused or diffused spatial attention state is under top-down control. More
specifically, Theeuwes (1994b) introduced the notion of the attentional window suggesting that observers can vary the extent to which they focus or spread attention in a
top-down way. The idea of the attentional window can explain why salient onsets may
fail to capture attention in some situations while they do capture attention in others (see
the 'Attentional window' section below).

Controversies and speculations regarding spatial orienting

Spatial attention and eye movements

Over the last twenty years or so, many studies have demonstrated a relationship between
spatial orienting and saccadic eye movements (e.g. Belopolsky and Theeuwes 2009;
Deubel and Schneider 1996; Hoffman and Subramaniam 1995; Godijn and Theeuwes
2002). As spatial orienting is metaphorically compared to a mental spotlight that illu-
minates a selected area, it is generally agreed that the eyes typically follow the mental
spotlight. In this view spatial orienting and saccades are functionally related as both
facilitate the processing of information located at the position of attention and the eyes
are shifted. Even though spatial overt orienting (eye movements) usually follows a shift
of spatial covert orienting, it is possible to dissociate them. One can direct spatial attention to a location in space without making an eye movement. However, the reverse is
not possible: one cannot make a saccade without first shifting attention to the saccade
target location (see also Deubel (chapter 30), this volume). According to the well-known

premotor theory (Rizzolatti, Riggio, Dascola, and Umiltà 1987; Rizzolatti, Riggio, and Sheliga 1994), a shift of spatial attention is 'nothing other' than the preparation of a saccadic eye movement. In this view spatial orienting attention is a by-product of the intention of making a saccade.

Even though the relationship between spatial orienting and saccadic eye movements has been relatively undisputed, a recent study showed that the relationship is more complicated than initially assumed. Belopolsky and Theeuwes (2009) used a task that allowed simultaneous measurement of attentional spatial orienting and saccade preparation, avoiding the typical problems of prioritizing one task over the other as often seen in dual-task studies. Belopolsky and Theeuwes (2009) showed that the premotor theory is partly correct: shifting spatial attention to a location in space will facilitate the execution of a saccade to that location. This is true for both exogenous and endogenous shifting of attention. However, maintaining (i.e. not shifting) endogenous attention at a location can either facilitate or suppress the initiation of a saccade to that location. The direction of this relationship depends on the probability of making a saccade to the attended location: when this probability is high, the oculomotor system is activated, but when this probability is low, the oculomotor system is suppressed.

It is clear that the results of Belopolsky and Theeuwes (2009) are not consistent with a classic version of the premotor theory. If allocation of attention is the same as programming a saccade, then allocation of attention would have to be associated with facilitation, not suppression, of overt orienting. When attention is shifted either exogenously or endogenously, the premotor theory holds; if attention is maintained endogenously at a location in space, spatial orienting and saccade preparation may be dissociated.

Subliminal location cueing

One intriguing question that was recently addressed is whether it is possible to obtain exogenous orienting to a location in space without awareness. Mulckhuyse, Talsma, and Theeuwes (2007) presented three placeholders (three discs) on the screen, one in the centre (at fixation) and one at the left and one at the right side of fixation, a set-up similar to the classic study of Posner and Cohen (1984). One of the three discs (either to the left or right of fixation) was presented just an instant earlier in time (16 ms) than the other two. The notion was that this disc would attract attention by its sudden onset and thereby serve as a cue. Because the other two discs followed immediately, it gave the impression that all three discs were presented simultaneously. Following the presentation of the three placeholder discs, a small black target circle was presented on top of the placeholder at one of peripheral locations either immediately following the cue (80 ms) or with an SOA of 1000 ms. Observers had to detect the presence of the small black target circle. The results showed that for the short SOA observers were faster when the target was presented at the cued location (i.e. the location having a placeholder that was presented slightly earlier in time than the other discs) than at the uncued location. Moreover, at the long SOA, the effect reversed, i.e. observers were slower at the cued than at the uncued location signifying the classic IOR effect.

Crucially, in a separate control experiment, observers were asked to indicate which of the placeholders was presented first. The results showed that none of the observers was able to indicate above chance which disc was presented first, indicating that they were not aware which placeholder was presented first. This implies that observers were not aware of the location of the cue.

Although the effects reported by Mulckhuyse et al. (2007) were not as pronounced as when visible cues were used, the classic biphasic effect of facilitation followed by inhibition was clearly observed. Previous studies using subliminal cues reported ambiguous results with respect to the occurrence of facilitation and inhibition (e.g. Ivanoff and Klein 2003; Ansorge and Neumann 2005), questioning the existence of subliminal cueing. The Mulckhuyse et al. (2007) study was the first to show the classic effect of facilitation followed by inhibition using subliminal cues. Since it is generally agreed that IOR is the product of reflexive, involuntary orienting, these findings provide evidence that subliminal cues can cause exogenous attentional orienting. Obviously, it is impossible to have subliminal cueing with endogenous cues because the very nature of this type of cueing (i.e. observers have to voluntarily direct attention) requires that observers are aware.

Is location information needed for detecting simple features?

It is clear that cueing the location of an upcoming target results in performance benefits and costs, even for a single target presented in an empty field (e.g. Van der Heijden, Schreuder, and Wolters 1985). However, there is controversy whether spatial attention is *needed* to detect simple features. According to the classic feature integration theory (Treisman and Gelade 1980), simple features are coded independently and in parallel across the visual field. Only when features of a particular object need to be combined, or when an object needs to be localized, must spatial attention be focused on that particular object (Treisman 1988).

Along these lines, it has been suggested that detecting a simple feature does not require spatial attention since its presence can be detected on the basis of a pooled response from the relevant feature map (e.g. Treisman 1988). Therefore detecting any activity in one of the feature maps should be enough to generate a response without any need for spatial attention. This is consistent with a neurophysiological perspective according to which spatial attention is only required when ambiguities in neural coding have to be resolved (see, e.g., Luck and Ford 1998). When multiple objects fall inside the large receptive fields of the ventral object recognition pathway, feature-specific neurons may respond, but because multiple objects are present inside the receptive field, it is unclear to which object the neurons have responded. Directing spatial attention to one object may resolve this ambiguity, because the neurons become responsive only to the features of the one object that is receiving.

According to other theories, before a response (even the simplest pop-out detection response) can be made, spatial attention needs to be directed to the location of the feature singleton (Joseph, Chun, and Nakayama 1997; Nothdurft 1999; Theeuwes 1992; Theeuwes, Reimann, and Mortier 2006). This viewpoint claims that post-selective processing is necessary for a detection response and occurs even in tasks in which identifying the target is not necessary.

Recently, Theeuwes, Van der Burg, and Belopolsky (2008) addressed this question again in a task in which observers had to detect the presence or absence of a single popping-out red element. They pressed one button when the red singleton was present and another when it was absent. The question was whether spatial attention was needed to perform this task. The popping-out red element was a letter, the identity of which could be repeated or not on the subsequent trial. The identity of the singleton letter was completely task-irrelevant, and only became available if spatial attention was directed to the letter location. Theeuwes et al. showed that repeating the letter of the singleton resulted in repetition priming on the next trial. Such repetition priming was not found when a non-singleton letter was repeated as the singleton. Crucially, they showed that the effect was equally strong in conditions of low and high perceptual load, suggesting that directing attention to the location of the singleton did not just occur because the load was too small, but instead that attention is always necessary for detection of even the simplest feature. This provides strong evidence for the notion that spatial attention plays a crucial role in the selection of objects.

Spatial cuing of the distractor location

As our review indicates, most studies have examined the costs and benefits of cueing the location of an upcoming target. Recently a few studies have examined the effects of cueing the location of a distractor (Ruff and Driver 2006; Munneke, Van der Stigchel, and Theeuwes 2008). The idea is that advance knowledge of the spatial location of an upcoming distractor may possibly help reduce the interference of this stimulus on target processing. It is thought that cueing a distractor location may help to inhibit this location such that this location no longer competes for the limited resources involved in target selection.

For example, Munneke et al. (2008) used a flanker-like task in which observers had to respond to one letter and ignore a flanking letter. The results showed that cueing the upcoming to-be-ignored flanker letter resulted in a reduced compatibility effect between the target and distractor. In other words, observers were able to reduce the effect of the flanker letter if its location was cued in advanced, providing evidence for the idea that it possible to inhibit locations that need to be ignored. The notion that it is possible to inhibit spatial locations is consistent with ERP data, which have shown that P1 and N1 modulations can occur independently of each other. This may suggest that spatial cueing invokes two separate attentional processes, one that suppresses information at unattended locations as reflected by a decrease in P1 amplitude and the other that enhances information processing at the attended location as reflected by a decrease in N1 amplitude (e.g. Mangun and Hillyard 1991).

Even though there are numerous studies that show that cueing the location of the target affects performance, there is now some evidence that observers can actively use a cue to inhibit locations that should not be selected.

ATTENTIONAL CAPTURE

Unlike spatial cueing in which observers receive spatial information about the upcoming target, attentional capture studies usually employ visual search as their principal paradigm. Typically, observers receive the instruction of look for a specific target (for example, the letter H, the red item, a face). In some trials, an additional object is presented that is irrelevant for the task, and one examines the performance in the presence and absence of this irrelevant element. If such an irrelevant element receives attentional priority independently of the observer's goals and beliefs, one refers to this as attentional capture (e.g. Theeuwes 1992, 1994a).

Even though the paradigms are different, it should be realized that attentional capture is in fact a specific form of exogenous spatial orienting. The idea is that the irrelevant object summons spatial attention (just like an exogenous onset cue). Even though the observer has the instruction to look for one particular target object, attention is exogenously drawn to the location of the irrelevant object such that performance in finding the target is hampered.

Stimulus-driven capture

In the early 1990s Theeuwes (1991a, 1992, 1994a) developed the so-called *additional singleton* task, which consisted of a visual search task in which observers had to search for one specific clearly defined salient target singleton. Simultaneously with this target singleton, another irrelevant singleton was also present. Figure 8.2 gives examples of the displays used in these types of studies. In one of the versions of this task, observers had to search consistently throughout the whole experiment for a green diamond singleton. In the distractor condition, one of the green circles was made red, constituting the colour distractor singleton. The crucial finding (see Fig. 8.2) was that reaction time (RT) was higher in the condition in which a uniquely coloured irrelevant distractor singleton was present (in this case the red circle) than when such a distractor was absent. It is important to note that the irrelevant singleton only caused an RT increase when it was more salient than the target. When the colour distractor was made less salient (see Fig. 8.2, right panels), its presence did not affect search for the diamond target anymore.

On the basis of these and related findings, Theeuwes (1991a, 1992, 1994a, 1994b, 2010a) formulated his notion of stimulus-driven capture, arguing that the bottom-up salience signal of the stimuli in the visual field determines the selection order. The increase in the time to find the target when the irrelevant singleton was present was explained in terms of attentional capture. Because the irrelevant colour singleton was selected even though observers were instructed to look for the diamond, it was argued that the irrelevant singleton summoned attention exogenously to its location. This erroneous capture of attention caused an increase in the time to find the target. Because the

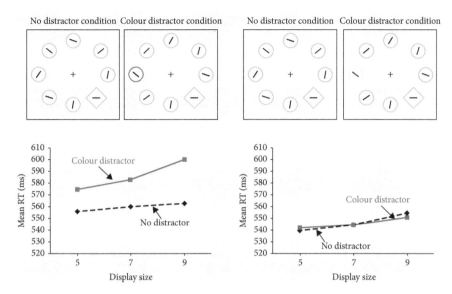

FIGURE 8.2 Stimuli and data from Theeuwes (1992). Observers searched for a green diamond presented among a variable number of circles and responded to the orientation (horizontal or vertical) of the line segment presented within the target diamond shape. Left side: The colour distractor singleton captured attention causing an increase in reaction time (RT) because the colour distractor was more salient than the target singleton (the green diamond). Right side: Finding the shape singleton is not affected by the presence of the colour singleton because the colour singleton was less salient than the target singleton (the green diamond).

order of selectivity was completely dependent on the relative salience of the target and distractor singleton, it was argued that initial selection was fully driven by bottom-up factors. The claim is that during the first sweep of information through the brain, the competition between the two salient objects was resolved by bottom-up salience signals (Mathôt, Hickey, and Theeuwes 2010).

It is important to note that in the additional singleton task, the irrelevant colour distractor was never the target, so there was no reason for observers to attend to it. If in this task the irrelevant singleton is selected first, it is a clear example of pure stimulus-driven capture. Moreover, observers also had a well-defined search goal: throughout the whole experiment observers consistently looked for the same target (a green diamond), allowing them to adopt a clear top-down search set. Note that observers searched for a particular target shape (a green diamond) but responded to the orientation of the line segment inside the target shape. This makes it possible to disentangle factors affecting the selection of the target from those affecting the response selection. As is clear from Fig. 8.2, search functions are flat, suggesting that this task involves a parallel pop-out detection task.

Since its introduction in 1991, the basic findings of the additional singleton paradigm (and variations of it) have been replicated by many labs using reaction time (Bacon and Egeth 1994; Kim and Cave 1999; Kumada 1999), d-prime (Theeuwes, Kramer, and

Kingstone 2004; Theeuwes and Chen 2005) and saccadic eye movements (Theeuwes et al. 1998). Even though the basic finding is undisputed, over the last twenty years or so, there has been a large controversy about the interpretation of performance decrement caused by the irrelevant distractor—that is, whether it reflects attentional capture at all. In a recent paper, Theeuwes (2010a) discussed these controversies in great detail and provided answers to the most pressing concerns (Theeuwes 2010b).

Contingent attentional capture

A notion that is completely diametrical to the stimulus-driven attentional capture account is the notion that all orienting is contingent on top-down control settings. According to this view, known as the contingent capture hypothesis (e.g. Folk et al. 1992, 1994), selection depends on the explicit or implicit goals held by the observer. In the original series of experiments, Folk et al. (1992) showed that visual selection depends critically on the top-down attentional set. Folk et al. used a spatial cueing paradigm in which a cue display was followed in rapid succession by a target display.

Figure 8.3 presents the basic paradigm. During a block of trials, observers either consistently looked for an onset target (top right) or, in another block, consistently looked for a colour target (bottom right). Observers had to identify the unique element

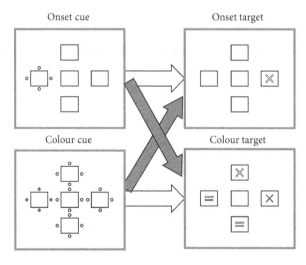

FIGURE 8.3 The spatial cuing paradigm of Folk, Remington, and Johnston (1992). Observers had to respond to a target letter (either an 'X' or an ' = ') which was defined as a singleton which either had a unique colour ('colour target' condition, bottom right) or was the only element presented as an onset ('onset target' condition, top right). Each type of target display was preceded by a cue display. The cue display consisted of either an onset cue (top left) or a colour cue (bottom left). All conditions were factorially combined. The important finding was that each cue type (onset versus colour cue) only captured attention when observers were set to look for it.

('X' or '='). There were two types of target displays. In the colour display the target was red while the other three elements were white. In the onset display, only one element was presented, and so the target was characterized as being the only element with an abrupt onset. Immediately preceding the target display at 150 ms SOA, a cue display was presented. Similar to the target displays, cue displays consisted of two types: the cue was either defined by colour (in which one location was surrounded by red dots and the other three locations were surrounded by white dots) or by onset (in which one location was surrounded by an abrupt onset of white dots and the remaining locations remained empty).

In the critical experiment, the cue that preceded the search display could either be valid (i.e. it appeared at the same location as the target), or invalid (i.e. it appeared at a different location as the target). Among the four possible target locations, the cue was valid on 25% of the trials and invalid on the remaining trials. Folk et al. reasoned that there was no incentive for observers to use the cue because it only indicated the location of the target at chance level (same reasoning as is used for 'classic' exogenous location cueing). The crucial finding was that observers who had to look for a target defined as an abrupt onset were fast on valid trials and slow on invalid trials, but only when the cue was defined by an onset. The same was found when observers searched for a target defined by colour: they were fast on valid and slow on invalid trials, but only when the cue was defined by colour. When the cue was defined by the feature that was not relevant during that block of trials (i.e. colour when looking for onset or the other way around), there was no measurable effect of the cue. Stated differently: only when the search display was preceded by a to-be-ignored featural singleton (the 'cue') that matched the singleton for which observers were searching did the cue capture attention.

To illustrate the working of contingent capture in more detail: in the example display shown in Fig. 8.3 this would mean that when searching for a red target singleton, attention automatically shifts to the location of the irrelevant red cue that preceded the search display while the irrelevant onset was completely ignored. The reasoning underlying contingent capture is that the top-down attentional set determines the selection priority: when set for a particular feature singleton, one will select each element that matches this top-down set; feature singletons that do not match top-down attentional sets will simply be ignored. Contingent capture claims that the attentional readiness adopted by the observer determines selection.

The findings of Folk have been replicated many times using various modifications of the classic paradigm (Folk, Remington, and Wright 1994; Folk and Remington 2006; Gibson and Amelio 2000; Remington, Folk, and McLean 2001; Pratt, Sekuler, and McAuliffe 2001; but see Yeh and Liao 2008).

Controversies regarding attentional capture

Over the last twenty years or so, there have been many controversies regarding the extent to which capture is fully bottom-up as advocated by Theeuwes (1992, 2010a) or completely top-down as advocated by Folk et al. (1992). In this section we briefly review some of the discussions. For a detailed discussion see Theeuwes (2010a, 2010b).

Non-spatial filtering costs

The basic finding of the additional singleton task is that reaction time increases when an irrelevant salient singleton is present (see Fig. 8.2). Theeuwes explained this effect in terms of attentional capture: spatial attention was exogenously attracted by the location of the salient singleton before it could move to the location of the (less salient) single-ton target. Folk and Remington (1998; Folk, Remington, and Wu 2009) suggested an alternative explanation for the increase in RT when the distractor was present. They argued that the interference was due to non-spatial filtering costs, a notion introduced by Kahneman, Treisman, and Burkell (1983) according to which irrelevant new objects that appear simultaneously with the target compete for attention and need to be filtered out. Filtering is assumed to be an effortful and time-consuming operation, which then will slow down the deployment of attention to the target. In this view, spatial attention is only deployed to the target in a truly top-down way but this deployment is slowed by the irrelevant singleton because filtering is needed. Clearly, this view does not assume a shift of spatial attention to the location of the irrelevant singleton (i.e. no attentional capture).

The exact mechanism underlying non-spatial filtering is unknown (for a discussion, see Schreij, Theeuwes, and Olivers 2010a, 2010b). For such an operation to work, one has to assume that it is possible to suppress information that is present at a particular location in space (in this case the location of the distractor) without a shift of spatial attention to that location. In fact, non-spatial filtering assumes that there is no spatial component whatsoever. Even though it is hard to conceptualize something like suppres-sion without spatial attention, over the years we have provided several different lines of evidence against the notion of non-spatial filtering.

The first approach we employed was to show that spatial attention did shift to the location of the irrelevant singleton. We used a technique labelled as 'identity intru-sion' (Theeuwes 1995; Theeuwes and Burger 1998; see also Gibson and Bryant 2008) in which we examined the congruency between the element presented inside the distrac-tor and the element presented inside the target, a technique reminiscent of the classic Eriksen and Eriksen (1974) flanker effect. For example, in Theeuwes (1995) observ-ers performed a typical additional singleton search as displayed in Fig. 8.2. Instead of a neutral element being presented inside the irrelevant singleton (a line segment), the congruency of the element inside the irrelevant singleton and the target singleton was manipulated. In half of the trials the character at the distractor location was associated with the same response as required by the target (for example, in both the target and distractor the letter 'R'), while in the other half of the trials it was the opposite (inside the distractor the letter 'R' and inside the target the letter 'L'). Theeuwes (1995) argued that the identity of the character at the location of the irrelevant singleton could only have an effect on responding if spatial attention were deployed to the location of the dis-tractor at some point. If, however, attention never went to the location of the irrelevant singleton, as assumed by the non-spatial filtering account, then no congruency effect was to be expected. Theeuwes (1995) did find a clear congruency effect, which provided strong evidence that spatial attention was directed to the location of the irrelevant singleton at some point before a response was given. This finding was completely in line with the notion that spatial attention was captured by the irrelevant singleton (but see Folk, Remington, and Wu 2009 for a different interpretation).

A second approach examining whether spatial attention is involved in stimulus-driven capture comes from studies using inhibition of return (IOR) as a marker for spatial attention. There is consensus that IOR is an attentional effect (Posner and Cohen 1984) resulting from an inhibition of returning attention to a location that was attended previously (see Klein 2000). An important hallmark of IOR is that it only follows for a location to which attention has shifted reflexively. IOR does not follow endogenous shifts of attention (Posner and Cohen 1984; Pratt, Sekuler, and McAuliffe 2001). Thus if IOR occurs, it can only be the result of a shift of spatial exogenous attention. In three different studies we have found IOR at the location of the irrelevant singleton. Theeuwes and Chen (2005) used d-prime as a dependent measure and showed that at the location of the irrelevant colour singleton, there was first an increased sensitivity (signifying attentional capture), which was followed by a reduced sensitivity (signifying IOR). Theeuwes and Godijn (2002) showed that observers were slower to detect a target presented at the location of the irrelevant singleton, relative to other locations (see Folk and Remington 2006 for a replication). Finally, when using the contingent capture task, Schreij, Theeuwes, and Olivers (2010a) showed that when observers are set for a colour singleton an irrelevant abrupt onset captures attention followed by IOR. Crucially, no IOR was found at the location of the colour cue, suggesting that what has been labelled as 'contingent capture' may in fact not be exogenous but instead may be the result of engaging attention in a top-down way to elements that fit the attentional set. According to this reasoning, contingent capture may not be about attentional capture, but instead about the endogenous orienting of attention, which may explain why no IOR is found in the spatial cueing paradigm by Folk et al. (see Schreij et al. 2010a,b).

Search modes

The stimulus-driven attentional capture account has also been challenged by claims that the observers choose to be distracted by the irrelevant singleton. In this sense, observers choose to search for a unique element (the so-called singleton detection mode) instead of searching for a particular singleton (the so-called feature search mode). The underlying idea is that if observers in the additional singleton task chose the so-called feature search mode, they would not be distracted by the irrelevant singleton. By definition, the act of choosing a specific search mode implies the involvement of top-down control over stimulus-driven capture.

This claim was made on the basis of a series of experiments by Bacon and Egeth (1994). They first replicated the additional singleton results (see Fig. 8.2) in which a colour singleton interfered with search for a shape singleton. In subsequent experiments, Bacon and Egeth added extra shapes to the display (i.e. squares and triangles) so that the shape singleton was no longer unique. In this condition the colour singleton did not interfere anymore. Bacon and Egeth reasoned that these conditions prevented observers from using 'uniqueness' to find the target. Instead, observers needed to switch to the 'feature search mode' in which they exclusively searched for one particular feature. In this condition, the irrelevant singletons no longer interfered. Bacon and Egeth (1994) concluded that 'goal-directed selection of a specific known featural singleton identity may override stimulus-driven capture by salient singletons' (p. 493). The idea of different search modes is compelling and intuitively plausible. However, Theeuwes (2004) challenged these ideas and argued that the Bacon and Egeth results may have been the outcome of the heterogeneity of the search displays (i.e. the stimulus) rather than the attentional state of the observers (i.e. top-down settings). The introduction of the additional shapes may have made the display more complex, which in turn may have forced observers to search in a more focused fashion. This focused mode precludes attentional capture (see the following section). When Theeuwes (2004) used the same displays as Bacon and Egeth (1994) with three different shape singletons (thus forcing observers to engage in a feature search mode), but at the same time increased the salience of target and distractor singletons (by adding more non-target elements), search became more efficient (flat search functions), and the interference caused by the colour singleton re-emerged.

The viability of the assumed search modes is still a matter of debate (see Theeuwes 2010b). One of the problems is that there is no independent evidence for the existence of these different modes of search. Also, it remains unclear why observers do not always simply choose a feature search mode as this will prevent erroneous capture by irrelevant singletons. For example, in one study, observers performed 1,800 trials and even after such a long training sequence a 'feature search mode' could not be instantiated as the irrelevant singleton kept interfering with search (Theeuwes 1992, experiment 2).

Attentional window

If search becomes slow and serial, irrelevant singletons no longer capture attention. For example, in a study by Proulx and Egeth (2006) the distraction caused by an irrelevant feature (a bright singleton) was modulated by target–non-target similarity. With increasing target–non-target similarity, search became more difficult, and with increasing search difficulty, the effect of the presence of the irrelevant bright singleton was reduced. This same reasoning holds for the more heterogeneous displays of Bacon and Egeth (1994).

Given the notion that inefficient search eliminates attentional capture, Theeuwes (1994b: 436) argued that 'top-down control over visual selection can be accomplished by endogenously varying the spatial attentional window'. According to this reasoning the attentional window adopted by observers could be one of the factors explaining why salient colour singletons fail to capture attention in some studies (as in Jonides and Yantis 1988; Bacon and Egeth 1994) while in other studies they do capture attention (as in Theeuwes 1992). Direct evidence for this notion was provided by Belopolsky et al. (2007) who adopted the original Jonides and Yantis (1988) paradigm, in which observers search serially for a particular target letter. Within each display one element had a unique colour. Importantly, the target letter had a unique colour at chance level, suggesting that observers had no incentive to selectively search for the unique colour. Typically, in this Jonides and Yantis task, observers ignored the salient singleton. Search was serial and started at any of the letters, not necessarily the salient one. Using this very same paradigm as Jonides and Yantis, Belopolsky et al. varied the size of the attentional window by asking observers to detect either a global (diffuse attention) or a local shape (focused attention) before starting the search for a non-singleton target. The results showed that when attention was initially focused in the centre (focused attention condition) the salient colour singleton was examined just as frequently as the other elements in the display, confirming the 'classic' finding of Jonides and Yantis (1988). However, when observers had to detect the global shape and attention was more diffusely distributed across the display, attention was frequently captured by the salient singleton. Belopolsky reasoned that when the attentional window is set wide, salient stimuli capture attention, but when it is small salient stimuli falling outside of the window can be ignored (see also Hernández, Costa, and Humphreys 2010 for a similar result).

In a more recent study, Belopolsky and Theeuwes (2010) tested the notion of the attentional window using the additional singleton task. They showed the classic attentional capture effect (see Fig. 8.2) when observers engaged in a diffuse attentional state. However, the very same capture effect was abolished when observers engaged in a focused attentional state before the presentation of the search display. If attention was not spread over the display, but instead focused at the centre, the presence of an irrelevant singleton no longer captured attention. This study provides strong evidence for the notion of the attentional window. Within the attentional window, salient singletons capture attention; when a salient event falls outside the narrow attentional window, it fails to compete for selection and no longer interferes (see also Joseph et al. 1997; Theeuwes 1991a). In a recent fMRI study, Mulckhuyse, Belopolsky, Heslenfeld, Talsma, and Theeuwes (2011) confirmed these findings, and showed that exogenous capture was associated with increased activity in visual area V3 but not in V2 and V1.

Contingent capture is nothing else than top-down orienting

Recent studies have challenged the notion of contingent capture. If only objects that fit the attentional set capture spatial attention then one would expect that observers could enable this top-down set from trial to trial. Belopolsky, Schreij, and Theeuwes (2010) tested this idea using the exact same spatial cueing paradigm as Folk, Remington, and Johnston (1992). (See Fig. 8.3.) Rather than keeping the target observers had to look for fixed over a whole block of trials (as was originally done in contingent capture experiments), observers had to adopt a top-down set before the start of each trial. More specifically, observers were cued on each trial to either look for a unique colour or a unique onset. If, as claimed by the contingent capture hypothesis, top-down attentional set determines which property captures attention, then one would expect that only properties that match the top-down set would capture attention. Belopolsky et al. showed that even though observers knew what the target would be on the upcoming trial, both relevant and irrelevant cue properties captured attention. In other words, there was no sign of contingent capture; instead both the relevant cue that matched the target as well as the irrelevant cue captured attention.

In several follow-up experiments, Belopolsky et al. (2010) had observers either choose themselves which feature they wanted to search for in that trial or had observers repeat out loud the chosen target feature until the search display appeared. These manipulations installed the strongest top-down set possible. With these measures it was ensured that in each trial observers established and maintained their top-down control for a specific feature. In these experiments, there was now a clear suppression of the cue that did not match the search feature. For example, when searching for an onset, observers were extremely slow when the target was presented at the location of the colour cue. Unlike in Folk et al.'s experiments, observers did not simply ignore the irrelevant cue; they actively suppressed it. Belopolsky et al. claimed that this top-down active suppression of the non-matching cue was the result of initial capture of attention to that location followed by active suppression.

In an additional analysis, Belopolsky et al. showed that results that have been traditionally attributed to contingent capture can, to a large extent, be explained by inter-trial priming. As outlined, in all contingent capture studies using the classic Folk et al. paradigm, observers searched throughout a whole block of trials for one particular target (a colour singleton or an onset). Such a set-up makes it very likely that inter-trial priming (and not so much top-down set) drives the contingent capture effect. As Belopolsky et al. showed that the attentional set cannot be changed on a trial-by-trial basis in the traditional Folk et al. paradigm, it is likely that bottom-up inter-trial priming is the underlying mechanism for what is known in the literature as top-down contingent capture (see also Theeuwes and Van der Burg 2011).

Overall Conclusions

The present paper argues that directing attention to a location in space is under top-down control. Observers are able to vary the extent to which they spread attention across the visual field. Within the attentional window, salient irrelevant events may capture attention. Outside the attentional window, salient information is simply ignored. We have argued that selection on the basis of location information is 'special' because it mediates selection directly. We have speculated that directing attention to a location in space is necessary even for the detection of simple features.

References

Ansorge, U. and Neumann, O. (2005). Intentions determine the effect of invisible metacontrast masked primes: Evidence for top-down contingencies in a peripheral cueing task. *Journal of Experimental Psychology: Human Perception and Performance* 31: 762–777.

Awh, E., Belopolsky, A. V., and Theeuwes, J. (2012). Top-down versus bottom-up attentional control: A failed theoretical dichotomy. *Trends in Cognitive Sciences* 16(8): 437–443.

Bacon, W. F. and Egeth, H. E. (1994). Overriding stimulus-driven attentional capture. *Perception & Psychophysics* 55: 485–496.

Belopolsky, A. V., Zwaan, L., Theeuwes, J., and Kramer, A. F. (2007). The size of an attentional window modulates attentional capture by color singletons. *Psychonomic Bulletin & Review* 14(5): 934–938.

Belopolsky, A. V. and Theeuwes, J. (2009). When are attention and saccade preparation dissociated? *Psychological Science* 20: 1340–1347.

Belopolsky, A., Schreij, D., and Theeuwes, J. (2010). What is top-down about contingent capture? *Attention, Perception, & Psychophysics* 72(2): 326–341.

Belopolsky, A. V. and Theeuwes, J. (2010). No capture outside the attentional window. *Vision Research* 50: 2543–2550.

Born, S., Kerzel, D., and Theeuwes, J. (2011). Evidence for a dissociation between the control of oculomotor capture and disengagement. *Experimental Brain Research* 208: 621–631.

Broadbent, D. E. (1958). *Perception and Communication*. Oxford: Pergamon Press.

Bundesen, C. (1990). A theory of visual attention. *Psychological Review* 97: 523–547.

Deubel, H. and Schneider, W. X. (1996). Saccade target selection and object recognition: Evidence for a common attentional mechanism. *Vision Research* 36: 1827–1837.

Eckstein, M. P., Shimozaki, S. S., and Abbey, C. K. (2002). The footprints of visual attention in the Posner cueing paradigm revealed by classification images. *Journal of Vision* 2: 25–45.

Enns, J. T. and Di Lollo, V. (1997). Object substitution: A new form of masking in unattended visual locations. *Psychological Science* 8: 135–139.

Eriksen, B. A. and Eriksen, C. W. (1974). Effects of noise letters upon the identification of a target letter in a nonsearch task. *Perception & Psychophysics* 16: 143–149.

Eriksen, C. W., and Hoffman, J. (1973). The extent of processing of noise elements during selective encoding from visual displays. *Perception & Psychophysics* 40: 225–240.

Folk, C. L., Remington, R. W., and Johnston, J. C. (1992). Involuntary covert orienting is contingent on attentional control settings. *Journal of Experimental Psychology: Human Perception and Performance* 18(4): 1030–1044.

Folk, C. L., Remington, R. W., and Wright, J. H. (1994). The structure of attentional control: Contingent attentional capture by apparent motion, abrupt onset, and color. *Journal of Experimental Psychology: Human Perception and Performance* 20: 317–329.

Folk, C. L. and Remington, R. W. (1998). Selectivity in distraction by irrelevant featural singletons: Evidence for two forms of attentional capture. *Journal of Experimental Psychology: Human Perception and Performance* 24(3): 847–858.

Folk, C. L. and Remington, R. (2006). Top-down modulation of preattentive processing: Testing the recovery account of contingent capture. *Visual Cognition* 14(4–8): 445–465.

Folk, C. L., Remington, R. W., and Wu, S. C. (2009). Additivity of abrupt onset effects supports nonspatial distraction, not the capture of spatial attention. *Attention, Perception, and Psychophysics* 71(2): 308–313.

Gibson, B. S. and Amelio, J. (2000). Inhibition of return and attentional control settings. *Perception & Psychophysics* 62(3): 496–504.

Gibson, B. S. and Bryant, T. A. (2008). The identity intrusion effect: Attentional capture or perceptual load? *Visual Cognition* 16(2–3): 182–199.

Godijn, R. and Theeuwes, J. (2002). Programming of endogenous and exogenous saccades: Evidence for a competitive integration model. *Journal of Experimental Psychology: Human Perception and Performance* 28(5): 1039–1054.

Hernández, M., Costa, A., and Humphreys, G. W. (2010). The size of an attentional window affects working memory guidance. *Attention, Perception, & Psychophysics* 72: 963–972.

Hoffman, J. E. (1975). Hierarchical stages in the processing of visual information. *Perception & Psychophysics* 18: 348–354.

Hoffman, J. E. and Subramaniam, B. (1995). The role of visual attention in saccadic eye movements. *Perception & Psychophysics* 57: 787–795.

Itti, L. and Koch, C. (2001). Computational modelling of visual attention. *Nature Reviews Neuroscience* 2(3): 194–203.

Ivanoff, J. and Klein, R. M. (2003). Orienting of attention without awareness is affected by measurement-induced attentional control settings. *Journal of Vision* 3: 32–40.

Jonides, J. (1981). Voluntary versus automatic control over the mind's eye's movement. In J. B. Long and A. D. Baddeley (eds), *Attention and Performance IX* (pp. 187–203). Hillsdale, N.J.: Erlbaum.

Jonides, J. and Yantis, S. (1988). Uniqueness of abrupt visual onset in capturing attention. *Perception & Psychophysics* 43: 346–354.

Joseph, J. S., Chun, M. M., and Nakayama, K. (1997). Attentional requirements in a 'preattentive' feature search task. *Nature* 387: 805–807.

Kahneman, D., Treisman, A., and Burkell, J. (1983). The cost of visual filtering. *Journal of Experimental Psychology: Human Perception and Performance* 9(4): 510–522.

Kim, M. S. and Cave, K. R. (1999). Top-down and bottom-up attentional control: On the nature of interference from a salient distractor. *Perception & Psychophysics* 61: 1009–1023.

Klein, R. (2000). Inhibition of return. *Trends in Cognitive Sciences* 4(4): 138–147.

Kumada, T. (1999). Limitations in attending to a feature value for overriding stimulus-driven interference. *Perception & Psychophysics* 61: 61–79.

Li, Z. (2002). A saliency map in primary visual cortex. *Trends in Cognitive Sciences* 6(1): 9–16.

Luck, S. J. and Ford, M. A. (1998). On the role of selective attention in visual perception. *Proceedings of the National Academy of Sciences* 95: 825–830.

Mangun G. R. and Hillyard S. A. (1991). Modulation of sensory-evoked brain potentials provide evidence for changes in perceptual processing during visual-spatial priming. *Journal of Experimental Psychology: Human Perception and Performance* 17: 1057–1074.

Mathôt, S., Hickey, C., and Theeuwes, J. (2010). From reorienting of attention to biased competition: Evidence from Hemifield effects. *Attention, Perception, & Psychophysics* 72(3): 651–657.

Mulckhuyse, M., Talsma, D., and Theeuwes, J. (2007). Grabbing attention without knowing: Automatic capture of attention by subliminal spatial cues. *Visual Cognition* 15: 779–788.

Mulckhuyse, M., Belopolsky, A. V., Heslenfeld, D. J., Talsma, D., and Theeuwes, J. (2011). Distribution of attention modulates salience signals in early visual areas. *PLoS One* 6(5): e20379.

Müller, H. J. and Rabbitt, P. M. A., 1989. Reflexive and voluntary orienting of visual attention: Time course of activation and resistance to interruption. *Journal of Experimental Psychology: Human Perception and Performance* 15: 315–330.

Munneke, J., Van der Stigchel, S., and Theeuwes, J. (2008). Cueing the location of a distractor: An inhibitory mechanism of spatial attention? *Acta Psychologica* 129: 101–107.

Neisser, U. (1967). *Cognitive Psychology*. New York: Appleton Century Crofts.

Nothdurft, H.-C. (1999). Focal attention in visual search. *Vision Research* 39: 2305–2310.

Palmer, J. (1994). Set-size effects in visual search: The effect of attention is independent of the stimulus for simple tasks. *Vision Research* 34: 1703–1721.

Posner, M. I., Nissen, M. J., and Ogden, W.C. (1978). Attended and unattended process-ing modes: The role of set for spatial location. In H. Pick and I. Saltzman (eds.), *Modes of Perceiving and Processing Information* (pp. 137–158). Hillsdale, N.J.: Erlbaum.

Posner, M. I. (1980). Orienting of attention: The Seventh Sir Frederic Bartlett Lecture. *Quarterly Journal of Experimental Psychology 32*: 3–25.

Posner, M. I., Snyder, C. R. R., and Davidson, B. J. (1980). Attention and the detection of signals. *Journal of Experimental Psychology: General 109*: 160–174.

Posner, M. I. and Cohen, Y. (1984). Components of visual orienting. In H. Bouma and D. G. Bouwhuis (eds.), *Attention and Performance X: Control of Language Processes* (pp. 531–556). Hillsdale, N.J.: Lawrence Erlbaum.

Pratt, J., Sekuler, A. B., and McAuliffe, J. (2001). The role of attentional set on attentional cueing and inhibition of return. *Visual Cognition 8*: 33–46.

Proulx, M. J. and Egeth, H. E. (2006). Target–nontarget similarity modulates stimulus-driven control in visual search. *Psychonomic Bulletin & Review 13*(3): 524–529.

Remington, R. W., Folk, C. L., and McLean, J. P. (2001). Contingent attentional capture or delayed allocation of attention? *Perception & Psychophysics 63*(2): 298–307.

Rizzolatti, G., Riggio, L., Dascola, I., and Umiltà, C. (1987). Reorienting attention across the horizontal and vertical meridians: Evidence in favor of a premotor theory of attention. *Neuropsychologia 25*: 31–40.

Rizzolatti, G., Riggio, L., and Sheliga, B. M. (1994). Space and selective attention. In C. Umiltà and M. Moscovitch (eds.), *Attention and Performance XV: Conscious and Nonconscious Information Processing* (pp. 231–265). Cambridge, Mass.: MIT Press.

Ruff, C. C. and Driver, J. (2006). Attentional preparation for a lateralized visual distrac-tor: Behavioral and fMRI evidence. *Journal of Cognitive Neuroscience 18*: 522–538.

Schreij, D., Theeuwes, J., and Olivers, C. N. L. (2010a). Irrelevant onsets cause inhibition of return regardless of attentional set. *Attention, Perception, & Psychophysics 72*: 1725–1729.

Schreij, D., Theeuwes, J., and Olivers, C. N. L. (2010b). Abrupt onsets capture attention inde-pendent of top-down control settings II: Additivity is no evidence for filtering. *Attention, Perception, & Psychophysics 72*: 672–682.

Theeuwes, J. (1989). Effects of location and form cueing on the allocation of attention in the visual field. *Acta Psychologica 72*(2): 177–192.

Theeuwes, J. (1990). Perceptual selectivity is task-dependent—Evidence from selective search. *Acta Psychologica 74*(1): 81–99.

Theeuwes, J. (1991a). Exogenous and endogenous control of attention—The effect of visual onsets and offsets. *Perception & Psychophysics 49*(1): 83–90.

Theeuwes, J. (1991b). Cross-dimensional perceptual selectivity. *Perception & Psychophysics 50*(2): 184–193.

Theeuwes, J. (1992). Perceptual selectivity for color and form. *Perception & Psychophysics 51*(6): 599–606.

Theeuwes, J. (1994a). Stimulus-driven capture and attentional set—Selective search for color and visual abrupt onsets. *Journal of Experimental Psychology: Human Perception and Performance 20*(4): 799–806.

Theeuwes, J. (1994b). Endogenous and exogenous control of visual selection. *Perception 23*(4): 429–440.

Theeuwes, J. (1995). Perceptual selectivity for color and form: On the nature of the interference effect. In A. F. Kramer, M. G. H. Coles, and G. D. Logan (eds.), *Converging Operations in the Study of Visual Attention* (pp. 297–314). Washington, DC: American Psychological Association.

Theeuwes, J. (2013). Feature-based attention: It is all bottom-up priming. *Philosophical Transactions of the Royal Society B: Biological Sciences 368*(1628): 20130055.

Theeuwes, J. and Burger, R. (1998). Attentional control during visual search: The effect of irrelevant singletons. *Journal of Experimental Psychology: Human Perception and Performance 24*(5): 1342–1353.

Theeuwes, J., Kramer, A. F., Hahn, S., and Irwin, D. E. (1998). Our eyes do not always go where we want them to go: Capture of the eyes by new objects. *Psychological Science 9*(5): 379–385.

Theeuwes, J., Atchley, P., and Kramer, A. F. (2000). On the time course of top-down and bottom-up control of visual attention. In S. M. J. Driver (ed.), *Attention and Performance*, XVIII (pp. 105–125). Cambridge, Mass.: MIT Press.

Theeuwes, J. and Godijn, R. (2002). Irrelevant singletons capture attention: Evidence from inhibition of return. *Perception & Psychophysics 64*(5): 764–770.

Theeuwes, J. (2004). Top-down search strategies cannot override attentional capture. *Psychonomic Bulletin & Review 11*(1): 65–70.

Theeuwes, J., Kramer, A. F., and Kingstone, A. (2004). Attentional capture modulates perceptual sensitivity. *Psychonomic Bulletin & Review 11*(3): 551–554.

Theeuwes, J. and Chen, C. Y. D. (2005). Attentional capture and inhibition (of return): The effect on perceptual sensitivity. *Perception & Psychophysics 67*(8): 1305–1312.

Theeuwes, J., Reimann, B., and Mortier, K. (2006). Visual search for featural singletons: No top-down modulation, only bottom-up priming. *Visual Cognition, 14*(4–8), 466–489.

Theeuwes, J. and Van der Burg, E. (2007). The role of spatial and nonspatial information in visual selection. *Journal of Experimental Psychology: Human Perception and Performance 33*(6): 1335–1351.

Theeuwes, J., Van Der Burg, E., and Belopolsky, A. (2008). Detecting the presence of a singleton involves focal attention. *Psychonomic Bulletin & Review 15*(3): 555–560.

Theeuwes, J. (2010a). Top-down and bottom-up control of visual selection. *Acta Psychologica 123*: 77–99.

Theeuwes, J. (2010b). Top-down and bottom-up control of visual selection: Reply to commentaries. *Acta Psychologica 123*: 133–139.

Theeuwes, J. and Van der Burg, E. (2011). On the limits of top-down control. *Attention, Perception & Psychophysics 73*: 2092–2103.

Treisman, A. M. and Gelade, G. (1980). A feature-integration theory of attention. *Cognitive Psychology 12*: 97–136.

Treisman, A. M. (1988). Features and objects: The Fourteenth Bartlett Memorial Lecture. *Quarterly Journal of Experimental Psychology 40A*: 201–237.

Treue, S. (2003). Visual attention: The where, what, how and why of saliency. *Current Opinion in Neurobiology 13*(4): 428–432.

Van der Heijden, A. H. C., Schreuder, R., and Wolters, G. (1985). Enhancing single-item recognition accuracy by cuing spatial locations in vision. *Quarterly Journal of Experimental Psychology 37A*: 427–434.

Wolfe, J. M. (1994). Guided Search 2.0. A revised model of visual search. *Psychonomic Bulletin & Review 1*: 202–238.

Yantis, S. and Jonides, J. (1984). Abrupt visual onsets and selective attention: Evidence from visual search. *Journal of Experimental Psychology: Human Perception and Performance 10*: 601–621.

Yeh, S. L. and Liao, H. I. (2008). On the generality of the contingent orienting hypothesis. *Acta Psychologica 129*(1): 157–165.

CHAPTER 9

NEURAL SYSTEMS FOR SPATIAL ATTENTION IN THE HUMAN BRAIN: EVIDENCE FROM NEUROIMAGING IN THE FRAMEWORK OF BIASED COMPETITION

DIANE M. BECK AND SABINE KASTNER

ALTHOUGH our retinas register information in parallel across the visual field, our visual experience is surprisingly more limited. We encounter this limited processing capacity whenever we view a complex scene containing multiple objects. We may be able to quickly infer the gist of the scene in a single glance (Potter 1976; Fei-Fei, Iyer et al. 2007), but extracting the details of any particular object or set of objects is a slower, more selective process; that is, we must selectively process some aspects of the scene at the expense of others (e.g. Broadbent 1958). There are a number of ways in which the visual system can selectively route information from a visual scene: it is possible to direct attention to a particular location (space-based attention), to a particular feature (e.g. anything red in the visual field, feature-based attention; see chapters by Treue, Serences) or to a set of features that comprise an object (object-based attention; see chapter by Serences). In this chapter, we will review the literature on space-based attention, the form of selective attention that is arguably the most well studied. Attentional mechanisms include both source and site signals; that is, control regions ('sources' of attention) in fronto-parietal cortex interact with and act on 'site' regions in the visual cortex and thalamus. We will summarize what is known from neuroimaging research in humans about both the sites and sources of space-based attention.

We will discuss a substantial amount of evidence in the framework of the biased competition theory of visual attention (Desimone and Duncan 1995). This theory attempts to conceptualize some very basic observations in attention research with a number of general principles that present testable hypotheses for neural function (Duncan 1996). Suppose that you are looking for a face in a crowd. Two basic phenomena occur while processing that scene. First, not all faces can be processed at the same time, that is, there is limited processing capacity. Second, while processing a particular face, one is able to filter out the unwanted information in the scene, that is, there is selectivity. These observations can be conceptualized by three general principles. First, of the many brain systems that represent visual information (sensory and motor, cortical and subcortical), most are *competitive*. Within each system, a gain of representation for a particular visual object will be at the expense of other objects' representations. Such competitive interactions among multiple objects (such as the faces in a crowd) occur automatically and operate in parallel across the visual field. Second, competition is *controlled* within and across brain systems. If one looks for a particular object (e.g. a friend's face), units matching the internal 'template' of that object will be pre-activated and therefore gain an advantage by receiving an increased processing weight. Thus, such top-down mechanisms introduce bias signals that help resolve the ongoing competition. The competition among multiple objects can also be biased by bottom-up mechanisms that separate figures from their background, or constitute objects by principles of perceptual organization. And third, the competition between systems is *integrated*. As a visual object gains dominance in representation within one system (e.g. visual cortex), it will tend to gain similar dominance in other systems (e.g. higher-order frontal and parietal areas). An example is given by representations of visual space. All units that represent a certain location in multiple spatial maps will be activated together, when the object at that location gains dominance in the system. In the following, we will provide the neural evidence in support of these principles outlined in biased competition theory, as it has emerged from human neuroimaging studies.

VISUAL CORTEX AND THALAMUS: THE 'SITE' OF ATTENTION

Directing attention to a spatial location increases the speed and accuracy with which a subject can detect a target at that location (Posner, Snyder et al. 1980), increases discrimination sensitivity (Lu and Dosher 1998), improves acuity (Yeshurun and Carrasco 1998; Carrasco, Loula et al. 2006), increases contrast sensitivity (Cameron, Tai et al. 2002; Carrasco, Ling et al. 2004), and reduces the interference caused by distractors (Shiu and Pashler 1995) (see chapter by Carrasco). In keeping with this improved sensitivity and performance for stimuli at an attended location, neural activity is enhanced throughout the visual cortex. Specifically, stimuli that are otherwise identical evoke greater activity when subjects direct attention towards it (attended condition) than when attention is directed away from the stimulus (unattended condition) (Fig. 9.1a, d). For example, O'Connor and colleagues (O'Connor, Fukui et al. 2002) used functional magnetic resonance imaging (fMRI) to measure activity evoked by flickering checkerboard stimuli presented to either the right or left visual field. Such stimuli evoke robust activity throughout the visual system, but this activity was greater still when subjects directed attention towards the checkerboard stimulus rather than when they ignored the stimulus and attended to a stream of letters presented at fixation. Specifically, mean BOLD signals evoked by the checkerboard stimulus increased significantly when attended in cortical areas V1, V2, V3, V4, TEO, V3a, and MT+. Interestingly, this effect of attentional response enhancement was also found in the visual thalamus, as we will discuss in a separate section below. Similar attention-related modulation of neural activity has been reported when subjects were asked to attend to one of two peripheral stimuli presented to the right or left visual field (Heinze, Luck et al. 1994; Heinze, Mangun et al. 1994; Tootell, Hadjikhani et al. 1998; Brefczynski and DeYoe 1999; O'Connor, Fukui et al. 2002). Attention-related enhancement has been observed throughout both ventral and dorsal visual areas, including retinotopic regions as well as more category-selective regions such as the fusiform face area (FFA), parahippocampal place area (PPA), and lateral occipital complex (LOC).

Interestingly, the effects of attention increase across the visual processing hierarchy (Kastner, De Weerd et al. 1998; Martinez, Anllo-Vento et al. 1999; O'Connor, Fukui et al. 2002; Beck and Kastner 2005; Bles, Schwarzbach et al. 2006; Beck and Kastner 2007; McMains and Kastner 2010; McMains and Kastner 2011), with small or non-existent effects in V1 and larger effects in intermediate and higher-order visual areas. Similar effects have been observed at a single-cell level in macaque visual cortex (e.g. Moran and Desimone 1985; Luck, Chelazzi et al. 1997; Mehta, Ulbert et al. 2000a; Mehta, Ulbert et al. 2000b). Such results suggest that fronto-parietal attention mechanisms, possibly in accord with the pulvinar of the thalamus (Saalmann, Pinsk et al. 2012), may act first on later cortical areas, with the effects of attention filtering back to earlier regions via feedback within the visual cortex (Martinez, Anllo-Vento et al. 1999). However, there is evidence that peak attention effects may be more flexibly determined by the properties of the attended stimulus (e.g. size) and its relationship (e.g. spacing) with other stimuli in the display (Buffalo, Bertini et al. 2005; Hopf, Boehler et al. 2006), raising the possibility that attention may in some circumstances act on intermediate or early visual areas first if the task requires resolving increasing small stimuli. We will return to this issue when we discuss the neural evidence in support of the biased competition theory of attention (Desimone and Duncan 1995). This theory posits that one of attention's primary roles is to resolve competitive interactions among stimuli at the level of the receptive field (RF) and thus not only predicts that attention effects should increase with increasing RF sizes in later areas but also that the locus of attention will vary with the size of the stimuli being attended. We will also discuss a number of alternative interpretations as to the flow of attention-related effects among cortical and thalamic visual areas in subsequent sections.

Neural gain control by spatial attention. The enhancement of the neural response to attended stimuli has typically been interpreted as reflecting neural gain control (e.g. Hillyard, Vogel et al. 1998). The nature of this gain, however, has been the subject of considerable debate. There is evidence in support of a multiplicative gain control mechanism, sometimes referred to as *response gain* due to the fact that the strength of such a gain is dependent on the initial response of the neuron (McAdams and Maunsell

Lateral geniculate nucleus

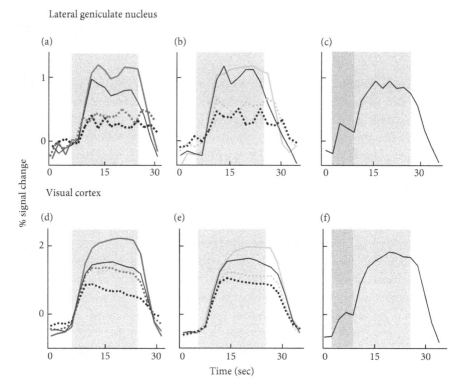

Visual cortex

FIGURE 9.1 *Time series of fMRI signals in the LGN and in visual cortex.* Group analysis (*n* = 4). Data from the LGN and visual cortex were combined across left and right hemispheres. Activity in visual cortex was pooled across areas V1, V2, V3/VP, V4, TEO, V3A, and MT/MST. (a, d) Attentional enhancement. During directed attention to the stimuli (red curves), responses to both the high-contrast stimulus (100%, solid curves) and low-contrast stimulus (5%, dashed curves) were enhanced relative to an unattended condition (black curves). (b, e) Attentional suppression. During an attentionally demanding 'hard' fixation task (black curves), responses evoked by both the high-contrast stimulus (100%, solid curves) and low-contrast stimulus (10%, dashed curves) were attenuated relative to an easy attention task at fixation (green curves). (c, f) Baseline increases. Baseline activity was elevated during directed attention to the periphery of the visual hemifield in expectation of the stimulus onset; the expectation period is indicated by the blue-grey rectangle. Grey rectangles indicate the checkerboard presentation periods. Reproduced with permission from Macmillan Publishers Ltd: *Nat Neurosci* 5(11), O'Connor, D. H., M. M. Fukui, et al., Attention modulates responses in the human lateral geniculate nucleus, pp. 1203–9 © 2002, Nature Publishing Group.

1999; Treue and Martinez Trujillo 1999). For example, McAdams and Maunsell (McAdams and Maunsell 1999) cued macaques to attend to a specific location and feature (e.g. orientation) in a delayed match-to-sample task. When, for instance, an oriented Gabor was attended, the response of a neuron increased for all orientations in a response-dependent way; that is, it was as though the neuron's response was multiplied by a constant resulting in the largest increases for orientations to which the neuron was most sensitive and the smallest increases for the orientations to which the neuron was least responsive (see chapter by Maunsell). Reynolds and colleagues (Reynolds, Chelazzi et al. 1999; Reynolds, Pasternak et al. 2000; Reynolds and Desimone 2003; Reynolds and Chelazzi 2004) also observed response-dependent modulations of attention but in contrast to a response gain these amplifications were better described as *contrast gain*; the effect of attention, like physical increases in contrast, saturated when stimulus contrast was already high. Thus, with the contrast gain control mechanism, the largest effects of attention occurred for low-contrast stimuli that the neurons were least responsive to while small, if any, effects were observed for high contrast stimuli that the neurons were strongly responsive to. Still other single-cell studies have suggested that both response gain and contrast gain mechanisms can occur in the same or different neurons (Williford and Maunsell 2006). Recent theoretical work by Reynolds and Heeger (Reynolds and Heeger 2009) has attempted to reconcile these models under a single normalization model of attention, in which varying task and stimulus parameters can result in different patterns of relative enhancement and suppression.

Neuroimaging studies, which indirectly measure neural activity from large populations of neurons, have also observed both multiplicative and contrast gain patterns under different task conditions and in different visual areas (Di Russo, Spinelli et al. 2001; Im, Gururajan et al. 2007; Li, Lu et al. 2008; Lauritzen, Ales et al. 2011). Interestingly, however, neuroimaging has produced yet a third gain model, a purely additive mechanism, which was initially observed in higher visual areas (Avidan, Harel et al. 2002; Murray and He 2006) but was later extended to V1, V2, and V3 (Buracas and Boynton 2007; Murray 2008). A similar additive effect of attention has since been observed in V1 using single-cell and multi-unit methods (Thiele, Pooresmaeili et al. 2009). Taken together, converging evidence from physiology and neuroimaging suggests that attentional response enhancement reflects a variety of gain control mechanisms that depend on the context and properties of the visual input.

Spatial specificity of attention. One of the most consistent effects of spatial attention on the visual system is its spatial specificity. Simple spatial cueing paradigms have not only demonstrated superior performance at cued locations, but reaction times typically increase with the distance between the cue and target (Eriksen and Hoffman 1973; Hoffman 1975; Posner, Nissen et al. 1978; LaBerge 1983; LaBerge and Brown 1986). Such data indicate that attention can be directed to a specific spatial location, albeit in a graded rather than discrete fashion, prompting researchers to use a 'spotlight' metaphor for the effects of spatial attention. Not surprisingly then, directing attention to a specific location in space results in a spatially specific signal in the visual cortex. An early ERP (event-related potential) and PET (positron emission tomography) study demonstrated spatially specific attention signals in the human brain (Heinze, Mangun et al. 1994). In particular, it was shown that activity increased 80–130 ms after stimulus onset in extrastriate regions contralateral to the attended visual field. Similar specific spatial attention effects were subsequently reported in each area of the visual system that contains an orderly representation of visual space, or a retinotopic map, using fMRI. With the advent of retinotopic mapping procedures (e.g. Sereno, Dale et al. 1995) it became possible not only to assess the effects of attention in different visual areas (e.g. V1–V4) but also to go beyond the visual field effects and more precisely map the effects of attention throughout the visual cortex. Striate and extrastriate cortices exhibit a clear retinotopic organization. Experiments comparing fMRI activity evoked by visual versus blank presentations and attended versus unattended visual presentation showed remarkable overlap (Tootell, Hadjikhani et al. 1998; Brefczynski and DeYoe 1999), that is, the effects of attention in the human visual cortex were shown to exhibit the same retinotopic specificity.

Neural competition and the need for selective attention. The need for selecting information represented by certain neural populations and not others becomes strikingly apparent when one considers a ubiquitous property of visual cortex; that is, single-cell physiology studies have shown that simultaneously presented stimuli are not processed independently but interact with each other. The response of a V1 cell, for instance, can be either facilitated or inhibited by the context of nearby stimuli located outside of the classic receptive field (RF) of the neuron (see Gilbert, Ito et al. 2000) for review). Although the majority of such contextual effects are due to interactions between neurons (Blakemore and Tobin 1972; Maffei and Fiorentini 1976; Knierim and van Essen 1992; Li and Li 1994; Kapadia, Ito et al. 1995; Lamme 1995; Sillito, Grieve et al. 1995; Kastner, Nothdurft et al. 1997; Polat, Mizobe et al. 1998; Kapadia, Westheimer et al. 1999; Bair, Cavanaugh et al. 2003), under the appropriate conditions a second stimulus can diminish the response of a neuron due to inhibitory interactions within a V1 RF (DeAngelis, Robson et al. 1992). In extrastriate cortex, multiple single-cell studies have shown that two stimuli presented simultaneously in an RF of a neuron evoke less activity than would be predicted by the response of the neuron to either stimulus presented alone (Snowden, Treue et al. 1991; Miller, Gochin et al. 1993; Recanzone, Wurtz et al. 1997; Reynolds, Chelazzi et al. 1999). In particular, responses to a pair of stimuli appeared to be a weighted average of the responses evoked by each of the individual stimuli (Luck, Chelazzi et al. 1997; Reynolds, Chelazzi et al. 1999). Such suppressive interactions among multiple stimuli have been found throughout the visual cortex of the macaque, including V2, V4, MT, MST, and IT (Snowden, Treue et al. 1991; Miller, Gochin et al. 1993; Recanzone, Wurtz et al. 1997; Reynolds, Chelazzi et al. 1999) and have been interpreted as competitive interactions among multiple stimuli for neural representation, thereby providing an example for the first general principle of biased competition theory (see above; Desimone and Duncan 1995). The idea that multiple objects are represented as a weighted average of individual responses in extrastriate cortex has also been corroborated by recent studies targeted at human object-selective cortex (Macevoy and Epstein 2009; Reddy, Kanwisher et al. 2009).

Similar competitive processes have been demonstrated across the visual cortex in a paradigm, in which four colourful visual stimuli, chosen to optimally activate ventral visual cortex, were presented to four nearby locations in the periphery of the visual field under two presentation conditions: sequential and simultaneous (Fig. 9.2a) (Kastner, De Weerd et al. 1998; Kastner, De Weerd et al. 2001; Beck and Kastner 2005; Beck and Kastner 2007; McMains and Kastner 2010; McMains and Kastner 2011). In the sequential presentation condition, each stimulus was presented alone, one after the other, in one of the four locations. In the simultaneous presentation condition, the same four stimuli appeared simultaneously in each of the four locations. Integrated over time, the

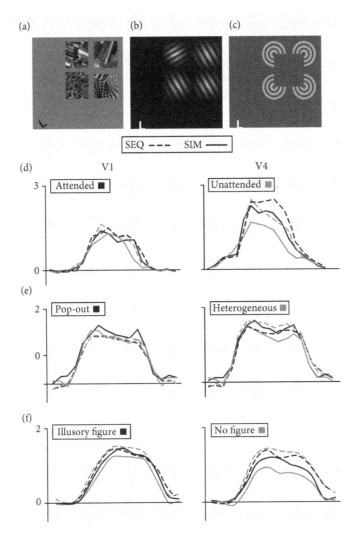

FIGURE 9.2 *Top-down and bottom-up biases in resolving neural competition in visual cortex.* In three experiments, competitive interactions among stimuli were assessed in the presence of top-down and bottom-up biases. Competition was measured by comparing fMRI responses to four stimuli presented either simultaneously (potentially competing; SIM) or sequentially (non-competing; SEQ). (a) In the study investigating top-down attention biases (Kastner, De Weerd et al. 1998), the four stimuli were complex coloured images. In the attended conditions, subjects monitored the lower left location for the appearance of a target stimulus, whereas in the unattended condition they ignored the colourful stimuli and instead detected targets at fixation. (b) In the bottom-up pop-out study (Beck and Kastner 2005), the stimuli were four Gabors that either all differed in colour and orientation (heterogeneous condition; not shown) or in which one Gabor differed in colour and orientation from the rest (pop-out condition; shown here without colour). (c) In the illusory contour study (McMains and Kastner 2009), four 'pacman' were aligned to form an illusory square (shown) or rotated such that no square was perceived. (d–e) Dashed curves indicate activity evoked by sequential presentations and solid curves indicated activity evoked by simultaneous presentations

physical stimulation parameters at each of the four locations were identical in the two presentation conditions. Critically, however, suppressive (competitive) interactions among stimuli could only take place in the simultaneous and not in the sequential presentation condition.

Consistent with the predictions from monkey physiology studies, simultaneous presentations evoked weaker responses than sequential presentations in V1 (Fig. 9.2d), V2/VP, V4 (Fig. 9.2d), TEO, V3A, and MT. Moreover, the response differences between simultaneous and sequential presentations were largest in regions with larger receptive fields (V4, TEO, MT, V3a) and decreased in magnitude in early visual cortex, with the smallest differences in V1. Importantly, the four peripheral stimuli were irrelevant to the subjects' task. Instead, subjects were asked to perform a demanding letter counting task in a stream of letters and symbols presented at fixation, which not only ensured subjects' fixation but also engaged subjects' attention at fixation away from the peripheral stimuli. Thus, the suppressive interactions observed occurred automatically and in the absence of attention, consistent with the idea that neural competition is a constant and ongoing process.

Top-down influences on competition. The competitive interactions among stimuli suggest that none of the stimuli is represented strongly at the neural level, and thus a constant state of competition would not be an optimal one for the visual system to be in. How might the visual system resolve this competition? Single-cell recording studies have shown that spatially directed attention represents one top-down mechanism that can bias the competition among multiple stimuli in favour of the attended stimulus and thus helps resolve the competition. When a monkey directed attention to one of two competing stimuli within an RF, the responses in areas V2, V4, and MT to the pair of stimuli were biased towards the response evoked by that same stimulus when presented alone (Reynolds, Chelazzi et al. 1999; Recanzone and Wurtz 2000); that is, it was as if the RF had shrunk around the attended stimulus and thus the attended stimulus dominated the response of the neuron.

A similar mechanism appears to operate in the human visual cortex. Kastner et al. (Kastner, De Weerd et al. 1998) studied the effects of spatially directed attention on competing visual stimuli in a variation of the paradigm described above. In addition to the two different presentation conditions, sequential and simultaneous, two different attentional conditions were tested, attended and unattended. During the unattended condition, attention was directed away from the peripheral visual display by having subjects count letters at fixation. In the attended condition, subjects were instructed to attend covertly to the peripheral stimulus location closest to fixation and to count the

for attention (d), pop-out (e), and illusory contour (f) studies. Black lines represent the conditions, in which a top-down or bottom-up bias was probed, while grey lines represent conditions during which stimuli were competing without any bias. For all three studies, competition was partially overcome in V4 when a bias was present (black curves), resulting in smaller differences in responses evoked by sequential and simultaneous presentations (dashed and solid curves). These effects were smaller (f) or non-existent in V1 (d, e).

occurrences of a target stimulus there. Although directing attention to this location led to greater activity for simultaneously and sequentially presented stimuli in areas V4 and TEO, the effect of attention was much larger for simultaneously presented than sequentially presented stimuli (Fig. 9.2d). In other words, directing attention to a single item in the display reduced the difference in evoked activity between simultaneous and sequential presentation conditions. Like the competition effects, the magnitude of these attention effects scaled with RF size, with no effect in V1 and the strongest reduction of suppression occurring in ventral extrastriate areas V4 and TEO (Fig. 9.2d; see also Bles, Schwarzbach et al. 2006). Taken together, directed attention appears to operate optimally on local networks that engage in competitive interactions, and is geared to route the information represented by the attended stimuli across cortex while filtering out the unwanted distractor information. This mechanism operates through resolving competitive interactions among neural populations representing preferred and non-preferred visual information and is scaled to RF sizes of neurons across the visual system that appear to be a neural substrate for the much acclaimed 'focus of attention' metaphor. These top-down effects on neural competition illustrate the second principle of biased competition theory, referring to the controlled nature of the process. Such control can also be exerted by the visual stimuli themselves through saliency or perceptual grouping.

Bottom-up influences on competition. Top-down attention is not the only mechanism that can resolve competition in visual cortex. Properties of the stimulus, that is, bottom-up stimulus-driven mechanisms have also been shown to modulate competition (Reynolds and Desimone 2003; Beck and Kastner 2005; Beck and Kastner 2007; McMains and Kastner 2010; McMains and Kastner 2011). For instance, in physiology studies, Reynolds and Desimone (Reynolds and Desimone 2003) found that the responses of V4 neurons to a pair of stimuli presented together in a neuron's RF were dominated by the higher contrast stimulus, suggesting that competition may have been biased in favour of the salient stimulus. In particular, they showed that as the contrast of a probe grating was decreased relative to the contrast of reference grating presented simultaneously in the RF, suppressive interactions among the stimuli were reduced. In other words, the response of the cell to the pair of stimuli increasingly resembled the response to the reference grating alone as the relative salience of the reference grating increased.

A similar effect was found in human visual cortex using colour-orientation pop-out displays (Fig. 9.2b; Beck and Kastner 2005) in a variation of the sequential/simultaneous fMRI paradigm, described above. Instead of the complex images used in the previous designs, four Gabor patches (each approximately $2 \times 2°$ in size) of different colours and orientations were presented in the upper right quadrant of the visual field. In addition to the sequential and simultaneous presentation conditions, the four stimuli appeared in two display contexts: pop-out displays, in which a single item differed from the others in colour and orientation, and heterogeneous displays, in which all items differed from each other in both dimensions. In accordance with previous findings, robust suppressive interactions among multiple stimuli were found in areas V2/VP and V4 when the stimuli were presented in the context of heterogeneous displays (Fig. 9.2e). However, this suppression was eliminated when the same stimuli were presented in the context of pop-out displays, consistent with the prediction that visual salience can bias competitive interactions among multiple stimuli in intermediate processing areas (Fig. 9.2e).

In addition to biasing competition in favour of a single item, other attributes of the physical stimuli can modulate competition. As originally noted by the Gestalt psychologists (e.g. Rubin 1915; Wertheimer 1923), multiple visual stimuli may be perceptually grouped according to their similarity, proximity, common fate, and other stimulus properties (Palmer 1992; Palmer and Rock 1994). The aggregation of nearby stimulus features by grouping mechanisms would seem at odds with the notion of competitive interactions. Interestingly, however, it has been shown that competitive interactions are actually modulated by perceptual grouping (Beck and Kastner 2007; McMains and Kastner 2010; McMains and Kastner 2011). In one study, suppressive interactions (using a sequential versus simultaneous fMRI paradigm) evoked by four identical items (homogeneous display) were compared to those induced by four heterogeneous stimuli that differed in both colour and orientation (heterogeneous display). In accordance with previous data, simultaneous presentation of four heterogeneous visual stimuli evoked significantly less activity in areas V2, VP, and V4 than the same stimuli presented sequentially, consistent with the idea that the stimuli were in competition for neural representation. However, when the four stimuli were identical, the suppression was considerably reduced relative to the heterogeneous conditions. This reduction was most evident in V4, but a similar pattern was found in V2 and VP. These results can be explained in terms of perceptual grouping and the competitive interaction expected to occur between items in that group: stimuli that form a better perceptual group might be expected to compete with each other less (Bundesen and Pedersen 1983; Desimone and Duncan 1995). Grouping may influence competitive interactions in two ways. Mechanisms from elsewhere in the cortex could boost the activity related to the set of stimuli as it enters V4, effectively counteracting any competition that may have occurred between stimuli. Such a perspective is consistent with effects of grouping and figure-ground segmentation found in early visual cortex (Kapadia, Ito et al. 1995; Lamme 1995; Kastner, Pinsk et al. 1999; Nothdurft, Gallant et al. 1999; Zhou, Friedman et al. 2000). Alternatively, this similarity grouping may be a consequence of the competitive interactions themselves. As mentioned, the response of V4 neurons to a pair of stimuli is best described as a weighted average of the responses to the two stimuli when presented alone (Luck, Chelazzi et al. 1997; Reynolds, Chelazzi et al. 1999). If the two stimuli that comprise the pair are identical, then the weighted-average model would predict that the response to the pair should be indistinguishable from the response to each of the individual stimuli (Reynolds, Chelazzi et al. 1999). Thus, it may not be necessary to appeal to additional grouping mechanisms to interpret these results. However, such an interpretation is only possible because the grouped stimuli are identical and grouping can and does occur for non-identical stimuli.

For example, McMains and Kastner (McMains and Kastner 2010) investigated competition among items that form the vertices of an illusory object in a variant of the

Kanizsa illusion (Kanizsa 1976). Four circular 'pacman' items, also called inducers, were aligned to form an illusory square (Fig. 9.2c) that is perceived as a single foreground object with the inducers lying behind it. The illusion occurs when the four inducers are rotated inward and aligned to form a common object, but not when they are rotated outward. Based on the hypothesis that the degree of perceptual organization in a visual display should determine the degree of competition, it was predicted that when the four pacmen were rotated inward such that they were perceived as part of a single object they should compete less with one another than when the four pacmen were oriented randomly, thereby disrupting the illusion. As predicted, the competitive interactions were significantly reduced across visual cortex, when the four inducers formed a single object, but not when they were oriented randomly as four separate items (Fig. 9.2f). Together these results suggest that although competition may occur between perceptual groups, it is reduced among elements within a perceptual group (Beck and Kastner 2007; McMains and Kastner 2010; McMains and Kastner 2011).

The interaction of top-down and bottom-up influences on competition. Given that competition is influenced by both top-down and bottom-up processes, it is important to ask how these two factors may interact. Are they independent, thus producing additive effects, or might they work in concert such that the strength of attention is constrained by the amount of competition left unresolved by bottom-up factors? McMains and Kastner (McMains and Kastner 2011) used the Kanizsa-like grouping stimuli just described except that they parametrically varied the degree to which the stimuli grouped by adding a third weakly grouped illusory figure condition (Weak Group) to the previous grouped (now called Strong Group) and ungrouped stimuli (No Group). Stimuli were again presented sequentially and simultaneously and attention was manipulated by asking subjects either to perform a demanding letter-detection task at fixation or attend the lower left inducer nearest to fixation and detect a brief dimming of the inducer. In accordance with the previous study, activity evoked by the simultaneously but not the sequentially presented stimuli decreased monotonically with increased perceptual grouping in V2, V3, and V4; the more the displays formed a coherent group the less competition occurred among its elements. Importantly, however, there was a significant interaction of perceptual group and attention in these same areas, such that the effects of attention were strongest when grouping was weakest and weakest when grouping was strongest. Furthermore, this interaction was only present for simultaneously and not sequentially presented stimuli, suggesting that attention resolves competitive interactions among multiple stimuli depending on the degree to which competitive interactions have been left unresolved by bottom-up grouping processes. Thus, the amount of attentional modulation appears to depend on the degree to which the stimuli compete in the first place (Kastner, De Weerd et al. 1998; Bles, Schwarzbach et al. 2006). This relationship between competition and attention suggests that similar or even the same neural circuits underlie both processes. Indeed, the circuits that mediate competition may provide an interface for attention to operate on. Von der Heydt and colleagues (Qiu, Sugihara et al. 2007) proposed a similar interface hypothesis in relation to attention and figure-ground processing.

We note that the increasing effects of attention as we ascend the visual pathway can also be accommodated by the interface hypothesis. If one of attention's primary functions is to resolve competitive interactions in favour of an attended item, and competitive interactions are themselves influenced by RF sizes, then attention will have its largest effects in regions where the competitive interactions are the strongest (Kastner, De Weerd et al. 1998; Martinez, Anllo-Vento et al. 1999; Kastner, De Weerd et al. 2001; O'Connor, Fukui et al. 2002; Beck and Kastner 2005; Bles, Schwarzbach et al. 2006; Beck and Kastner 2007; McMains and Kastner 2010; McMains and Kastner 2011). Furthermore, the effects of attention should be flexibly determined by the spatial scale of the displays. Large or spatially distant targets, for example, will compete in areas with larger RFs and thus the locus of attention should shift to more anterior extrastriate areas for large as opposed to smaller displays (Kastner, De Weerd et al. 2001; Buffalo, Bertini et al. 2005; Hopf, Boehler et al. 2006)

Attention-related baseline increases. Thus far, we have discussed the effects of attention on visually evoked activity; that is, attention can modulate the degree to which a visual stimulus evokes activity in visually responsive areas. However, it is also the case that effects of attention have been measured in these areas in absence of visual stimulation. Specifically, spontaneous firing rates, or so-called baseline responses, in V2 and V4 increased when an animal was cued to attend to the location within the cell's RF but before a visual stimulus actually appeared (Luck, Chelazzi et al. 1997; Lee, Williford et al. 2007). Similar baseline increases were observed in human visual cortex using fMRI (Kastner, Pinsk et al. 1999; O'Connor, Fukui et al. 2002; Muller, Bartelt et al. 2003; McMains, Fehd et al. 2007; Sylvester, Josephs et al. 2007). For example, to study baseline increases in the human, Kastner and colleagues (Kastner, Pinsk et al. 1999) added an 'expectation period' to their visual stimulation design. In particular, a delay of 11 seconds was added between the cue to attend to the target location and the presentation of the first visual stimulus, during which time subjects were required to covertly direct their attention to the target location and expect the visual presentations. Thus, the effects of attention could be assessed in the presence (ATT in Fig. 9.3c, see also grey-shaded area in Fig. 9.1c, f) and absence (EXP in Fig. 9.3c, see also blue-shaded area in Fig. 9.1c, f) of visual stimulation. As predicted on the basis of the single-cell data, fMRI signals increased during the expectation period in visual cortex, despite the fact that there was no visual presentation at that time. This baseline increase was then followed by a further increase in activity during stimulus presentations. In fact, every visual area that typically shows an effect of attention on visually evoked activity also showed a baseline increase (O'Connor, Fukui et al. 2002) (Fig. 9.1). These data, then, are consistent with the idea that baseline increases may be one mechanism by which activity in the visual system is biased in favour of an attended location. However, it is interesting to note that the magnitude of the baseline increases does not predict the size of the attention effect during visual presentations (McMains, Fehd et al. 2007; Luck, Chelazzi et al. 1997), indicating that the effects of attention on visually evoked activity are not simply the addition of a baseline increase but rather result from some non-linear interaction of the bias and the visually evoked activity. Indeed, because baseline increases occur in the absence of stimulation, they are by nature purely additive

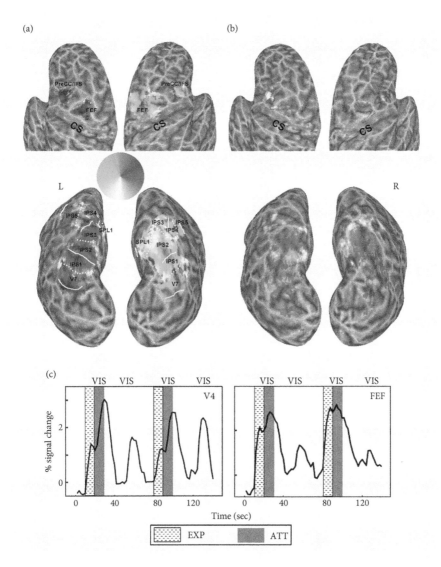

FIGURE 9.3 The fronto-parietal attention network. (a) Topographic organization of areas in frontal and parietal cortex. Using a memory-guided saccade task several areas with a systematic representation of the contralateral visual field were identified along the intraparietal sulcus (IPS1–5), adjacent superior parietal cortex (SPL1), and in superior (FEF) and inferior aspects of precentral cortex. (b) Attention-related activations within parietal and frontal cortex in a spatial attention task. There was significant overlap between attention-related activations and topographic representations in higher-order cortex. (c) Time series of fMRI signals in V4. Directing attention to a peripheral target location in the absence of visual stimulation led to an increase of baseline activity (textured blocks), which was followed by a further increase after the onset of the stimuli (grey shaded blocks). Baseline increases were found in both striate and extrastriate visual cortex. (d) Time series of fMRI signals in FEF. Directing attention to the peripheral target location in the absence of visual stimulation led to a stronger increase in baseline activity than in visual cortex; the further increase of activity after the onset of the stimuli was not significant.

gains. They cannot then account for multiplicative and contrast gain responses which, by definition, vary as a function of the visually evoked activity, although the baseline increases may still contribute to those gains.

Neural processing of unattended stimuli. One of the essential properties of selective attention is that, while a subset of the information present is selected for preferential processing, other unwanted information is filtered out. What, then, is the neural fate of the unattended information? Indeed, questions about the fate of unattended information not only sparked some of the earliest experiments in cognitive psychology (Cherry 1953; Broadbent 1958) but also generated a long-standing debate. In particular, some theorists argued that unattended information was excluded *early* in processing and thus had no effect on behaviour (Broadbent 1958; Treisman 1969), whereas others argued that unattended information was excluded much later in processing such that it could still influence behaviour (Deutsch and Deutsch 1963; Norman 1968; Duncan 1980; see chapter by Kastner and Serences). This debate was finally resolved, as many such debates are, by positing that both early and late selection could occur, but under different circumstances (see chapter by Lavie). According to perceptual load theory (Lavie and Tsal 1994; Lavie 1995), early selection occurs when the perceptual difficulty (or load) of the task is high, leaving no residual capacity for task-irrelevant information; whereas when the perceptual load of the task is low, spare capacity can then spill over to task-irrelevant, or distracting information. This theory makes a very specific neural prediction: as the perceptual difficulty of the attended task increases, the activity evoked by the attended information should increase while activity evoked by the unattended information should decrease. Such predictions were probed using fMRI (Rees, Frith et al. 1997; O'Connor, Fukui et al. 2002; Pinsk, Doniger et al. 2004; Schwartz, Vuilleumier et al. 2005), event-related potentials (Handy and Mangun 2000), and steady-state evoked potentials (Parks, Hilimire et al. 2010; Parks, Beck et al. (submitted)). Increasing the perceptual difficulty of the task not only resulted in greater target-related activity but also reduced distractor-related activity, and this was true even though the distracting stimuli were such visually salient stimuli as moving dots (Rees, Frith et al. 1997), colourful images (Pinsk, Doniger et al. 2004), and large flickering checkerboards (Fig. 9.1b, e; (O'Connor, Fukui et al. 2002; Schwartz, Vuilleumier et al. 2005; Parks, Hilimire et al. 2010; Parks, Beck et al. (submitted)). Moreover, this push–pull relationship between targets and distractors was found throughout visual system cortex (O'Connor, Fukui et al. 2002; Schwartz, Vuilleumier et al. 2005). Although perceptual load may be an important determinant of the suppression of unattended stimuli, the precise neural mechanisms underlying this process are not specified (although see Torralbo and Beck 2008). We will discuss more specific neural mechanisms of suppression in the context of biased competition theory below.

Dividing attention. The question of whether attention can be divided has been pondered by even the earliest of psychological thinkers (James 1890). Although feature-based attention (see chapters by Serences, Treue) can be applied in parallel across the visual field (Treue and Martinez Trujillo 1999; Saenz, Buracas et al. 2002; Bichot, Rossi et al. 2005; Serences and Boynton 2007; White and Carrasco 2011), when the task requires participants to bind multiple features together in a single object, attention appears much more limited (e.g. Treisman and Gelade 1980; Kleiss and Lane 1986; Duncan 1987). For instance, identification of complex stimuli presented simultaneously often suffers a cost relative to the same stimuli presented sequentially (Fisher 1984; Kleiss and Lane 1986; Duncan 1987). As described previously, an experimental design using sequential and simultaneous presentations was developed to assess competition, finding greater competition among simultaneously presented than sequentially presented stimuli. Indeed, such a similarity raises the possibility that competition among stimuli in visual cortex may be one of the limiting factors in attending to multiple items simultaneously.

Attending to multiple locations simultaneously not only results in poorer behavioural performance but it also evokes less activity than either alone (Muller, Bartelt et al. 2003; McMains and Somers 2005). Such a result is consistent with limited resource theories of attention in which the 'spotlight' or 'zoom lens' of attention has a fixed capacity that can then be directed towards either a single item or shared among many. However, reduced processing when attention is distributed among multiple items would also be predicted on the basis of neural competition. Although attending to a single item among many resolves competition in favour of the attended item, attending to multiple items simultaneously places the attended items back in competition with each other: attention can no longer boost the activity of one item at the expense of the others. Scalf and Beck (Scalf and Beck 2010) used the experimental paradigm of sequential and simultaneous presentations to assess whether the cost associated with divided attention among multiple objects was due to competition among attended stimuli in visual cortex. The paradigm was similar to those described above except that subjects were asked to attend to either one or three of five locations. To equate the physical stimulation and area of activation across the two conditions, activity for the attend-one location was compared under both the attend-one and attend-three conditions. In keeping with previous results, attending to three items evoked less activity during attend-three conditions than attend-one. Importantly, however, this was only true when the stimuli were presented simultaneously and thus could compete with each other. In a second experiment, the stimuli were presented simultaneously but the degree of competition was manipulated by placing them in the same or different hemispheres. Because competition is thought to occur locally among stimuli represented by a common cell population, competition between stimuli presented in different visual fields should compete less in areas in which the visual fields are represented separately (i.e. in V1 through V4). Again, in keeping with the prediction that it is competition that impedes attention to multiple items, the reduction in activity evoked by attend-three compared to attend-one conditions was only observed under conditions in which the stimuli could compete with each other: when all three attended stimuli fell within the same visual field. Together these results suggest that one of the reasons that make it difficult to attend to multiple items simultaneously is that competition prevents attention from acting as efficiently when it is directed towards multiple items as when it is directed towards a single item.

Interestingly, however, although attending to multiple stimuli cannot resolve competition among them, it is not the case that attention has no effect when it is directed towards multiple stimuli (Scalf, Basak et al. 2011). Multiple attended stimuli evoked more activity than when none of the peripheral sequential or simultaneously presented stimuli were attended (i.e. attention was directed towards a stream of rapidly presented visual items such as letters and numbers at fixation). However, the difference between sequential and simultaneous presentations was identical whether attention was directed to all five stimuli or towards fixation. In other words, although the attended stimuli did receive an overall boost (relative to being unattended), in keeping with previous results (Scalf and Beck 2010), this boost did not resolve competition. Such a result suggests that although they are related, the ability of attention to enhance activity is not limited to its ability to resolve competition among stimuli.

Subcortical structures: Lateral geniculate nucleus (LGN). Initially, attentional response modulation was demonstrated in extrastriate cortex (e.g. Moran and Desimone 1985) and subsequently also in striate cortex, where the modulation appears to depend more on task-related factors, such as the attentional demands of the task at hand or the need to integrate contextual information from areas beyond the classical receptive field (Motter 1993; Watanabe, Harner et al. 1998; Gandhi, Heeger et al. 1999; Ito and Gilbert 1999; Martinez, Anllo-Vento et al. 1999; Somers, Dale et al. 1999). These findings in combination with negative results failing to demonstrate attentional modulation at the thalamic stage of the retinocortical projection, the LGN, led to a notion that selective attention affects neural processing only at the cortical level (Mehta, Ulbert et al. 2000a; Mehta, Ulbert et al. 2000b; Bender and Youakim 2001). This notion has been thoroughly revised based on reports of attentional modulation in the human and macaque LGN (O'Connor, Fukui et al. 2002; McAlonan, Cavanaugh et al. 2008; Schneider and Kastner 2009). The first compelling evidence originated from a series of neuroimaging experiments showing that selective attention affects visual processing in at least three different ways, similar to the modulatory effects observed in visual cortex. First, LGN responses to attended visual stimuli increased relative to the same stimuli when unattended (Fig. 9.1b). This response enhancement was specific to the attended visual field location and occurred in both parvo- and magnocellular regions of the LGN. The attentional enhancement tended to be stronger in magnocellular regions (Schneider and Kastner 2009), consistent with a deoxyglucose study in macaques suggesting that attention had a larger influence on magnocellular LGN layers (Vanduffel, Tootell et al. 2000). Second, neural responses to unattended stimuli were attenuated depending on the load of attentional resources engaged elsewhere (Fig. 9.1c). Third, baseline activity increased when participants directed attention to a location in the absence of visual stimulation and in anticipation of the upcoming stimulus (Fig. 9.1d). All three attention effects tended to be larger in the LGN than in V1, with effects on the order of the attentional modulation typically observed in extrastriate areas such as V4. Thus, it is likely that feedback from V1 may only partly contribute to the attentional modulation of LGN responses, suggesting that additional sources such as the thalamic reticular nucleus (TRN) and brainstem cholinergic inputs may contribute as well (see chapter by Saalmann and Kastner for further details).

Subcortical structures: Superior colliculus and pulvinar. As for subcortical structures, effects of attention have not only been demonstrated in the LGN, but also in the thalamic reticular nucleus (McAlonan, Cavanaugh et al. 2006; McAlonan, Cavanaugh et al. 2008), superior colliculus (Robinson and Kertzman 1995; Gattass and Desimone 1996; Kustov and Robinson 1996; Fecteau, Bell et al. 2004; Ignashchenkova, Dicke et al. 2004; Lee and Keller 2006; Schneider and Kastner 2009), and the pulvinar nucleus of the thalamus (Petersen, Robinson et al. 1985; LaBerge and Buchsbaum 1990; Bender and Youakim 2001; Kastner, O'Connor et al. 2004; Smith, Cotton et al. 2009; Schneider 2011), raising the possibility that the initial effects of attention may precede V1. Indeed, single-cell data in the LGN and TRN suggest that attention has its first effects within 100 ms of the onset of a target stimulus (see chapter by Saalmann and Kastner for additional details). The effects of attention are similarly fast in the superior colliculus (SC), although the vast majority of attention studies in the SC use exogenous, reflexive, attention paradigms, in which the cue occurs at the target location (Robinson and Kertzman 1995; Gattass and Desimone 1996; Kustov and Robinson 1996; Bell, Fecteau et al. 2004; Fecteau, Bell et al. 2004; Ignashchenkova, Dicke et al. 2004). In fact, an early study suggested that activity in the SC was modulated by exogenous attention but not by top-down endogenous attention (Gattass and Desimone 1996), consistent with the idea that attention effects in the SC result from sensory interactions of the cue and target-related activity (Robinson and Kertzman 1995; Bell, Fecteau et al. 2004). However, a number of studies now suggest that the SC also plays a role in more cognitively mediated, top-down spatial attention. First, using an evoked-saccade paradigm, Kustov and Robinson (Kustov and Robinson 1996) showed that the SC is affected by both peripheral exogenous cues and central endogenous cues, although endogenous attention had both a later and less pronounced effect on saccades. Lee and Keller (Lee and Keller 2006) showed that the effect of exogenous cues (i.e. peripheral cues at the target location) in the SC could be modulated by endogenous attention (i.e. whether the peripheral cue was a cued colour or not). Finally, using fMRI, Schneider and Kastner (Schneider and Kastner 2009) showed that the human SC is modulated by endogenous and sustained spatial attention and this attentional enhancement effect is several times stronger in the SC than the LGN (measured in the same experiment). Taken together, these studies suggest an important role of the SC in stimulus-driven (exogenous) as well as internally generated (endogenous) allocation of spatial attention (see chapter by Krauzlis for further discussion).

There is corroborating evidence from physiology and neuroimaging studies showing that neural responses in the visual pulvinar reflect the behavioural relevance of stimuli (see chapter by Saalmann and Kastner for detailed discussion). In human neuroimaging studies, attention-related modulation of responses has been shown in several different parts of the human pulvinar, including dorso-medial and inferior regions, using selective attention tasks that emphasized directing attention to a spatial location (Kastner, O'Connor et al. 2004), filtering of unwanted information (LaBerge and Buchsbaum 1990), and shifts of attention across the visual field (Yantis, Schwarzbach et al. 2002). Because the pulvinar is heavily and topographically connected to the cerebral cortex, including striate and extrastriate areas as well as posterior parietal cortex, it has been proposed that it coordinates cortical activity, perhaps through corticothalamic synchronization (Shipp 2003; Saalmann and Kastner 2009, 2011), and thus may play a role in coordinating attention across various cortical maps (Saalmann, Pinsk et al., 2012). In that respect, the visual pulvinar, or at least parts of it, may play the role of a subcortical control structure, or that of a 'source' region generating modulatory signals, rather than that of a 'site' region that receives such signals. Since there is little known about the role of the pulvinar in spatial attention and other cognitive processing in the human brain, we will focus our discussion of attentional 'source' regions, or control structures, to higher-order fronto-parietal cortex (see chapter by Saalmann and Kastner for a discussion of the emerging control functions of the primate thalamus).

THE 'SOURCE' OF ATTENTION: EFFECTS OF ATTENTION ON FRONTAL AND PARIETAL CORTEX

Evidence for involvement of higher-order cortex in attentional selection. There is a long history indicating that unilateral brain lesions, especially of higher-order cortex, may cause impairment in spatially directing attention to the contralateral hemifield, a syndrome known as visuospatial hemineglect. In severe cases, patients suffering from neglect will completely disregard the visual hemifield contralateral to the side of the lesion (e.g. Bisiach and Vallar 1988; Heilman, Watson et al. 1993). Typical examples of their deficits are that these patients will read from only one side of a book, apply make-up to only one half of their face, or eat from only one side of a plate. In less severe cases, the deficit is more subtle, and becomes apparent only if the patient is confronted with competing stimuli, as in the case of visual extinction. In visual extinction, patients are able to orient attention to a single visual object presented to their impaired visual hemifield; however, if two stimuli are presented simultaneously, one in the impaired and the other in the intact hemifield, the patients will only detect the one presented to the intact side. These findings suggest that visual extinction reflects an attentional bias towards the intact hemifield in the presence of competing objects (Kinsbourne 1993; Duncan 1998).

Visuospatial neglect may follow unilateral lesions at different sites, including the parietal lobe and superior temporal cortex (e.g. Vallar and Perani 1987; Karnath, Ferber et al. 2001), regions of the frontal lobe (e.g. Damasio, Damasio et al. 1980), the anterior cingulate cortex (e.g. Janer and Pardo 1991), the basal ganglia (e.g. Damasio, Damasio et al. 1980), and the thalamus, in particular the pulvinar (e.g. Karnath, Himmelbach et al. 2002). The lesion sites that have been observed most frequently in visuospatial hemineglect are the parietal cortex, especially its inferior part as well as the temporo-parietal junction (Mort, Malhotra et al. 2003), and the superior temporal cortex (Karnath, Ferber et al. 2001). The issue of which of the two most prominent sites is critical for causing the syndrome is still heavily contested. Neglect occurs more often with right-sided lesions than with left-sided lesions, which has been taken as evidence for a specialized role for the right hemisphere in space-based attentional selection (Vallar 1993) (see chapter by Vallar for further discussion).

Models of space-based attention control. To account for the hemispheric asymmetry observed with the neglect syndrome, a 'hemispatial' theory has been proposed by Heilman and colleagues (Heilman and Van Den Abell 1980; see also Mesulam, 1981). In this account, the right hemisphere (RH) directs attention to both visual hemifields, whereas the left hemisphere (LH) directs attention to the right visual field only (see Rafal and Robertson 1995 for a related theory involving local and global attention biases). Thus, while LH damage can be compensated for by the right hemisphere, such compensation will not be possible with RH damage, thereby resulting in neglect of the left visual field. An alternative account, Kinsbourne's 'interhemispheric competition' theory, has proposed an opponent processor control system, in which each hemisphere directs attention towards the contralateral visual field with the left hemispheric processor being more powerful than the right hemispheric processor. In an intact system, the two hemispheric processors are balanced through mutual reciprocal inhibition, presumably through direct callosal connections. Alternatively, such inhibitory control could be achieved through cortico–subcortical interactions between parietal cortex and the superior colliculus (SC) (Sprague 1966). According to the interhemispheric competition account, neglect occurs as a consequence of an imbalanced system following damage to one of the processors, thereby resulting in a bias towards the ipsilesional visual field that is controlled by the remaining intact, unopposed processor (Kinsbourne 1977). Despite their differences, these accounts make at least two predictions that we will further discuss in the following sections: (i) higher-order cortex appears to be involved in controlling attentional operations throughout the visual field, and (ii) higher-order cortex may contain discrete representations of visual space.

Attention-related activations in higher-order cortex. In meeting the first prediction, functional brain imaging studies have identified areas in parietal and frontal cortex that are involved in the allocation of spatial attention. When subjects attend to a location in space in anticipation of the appearance of a stimulus, neural signals increase in a fronto-parietal network consisting of the superior parietal lobule (SPL), the frontal eye field (FEF), and the supplementary eye field (SEF) extending into the anterior cingulate cortex (Fig. 3b; for a meta-analysis, see Kastner and Ungerleider 2000). This so-called dorsal fronto-parietal attention network has been implicated in many visuospatial tasks, regardless of the specific task requirements, that is, when target stimuli were detected, discriminated, or tracked in visual space, to give just a few examples (e.g. Nobre, Sebestyen et al. 1997; Corbetta, Akbudak et al. 1998). Further, the fronto-parietal attention network is not limited to controlling spatial attention. It is also activated when subjects select non-spatial information (see chapter by Serences et al.).

In addition to activations within a dorsal fronto-parietal attention network, selective attention has also been shown to engage a ventral attention network consisting of regions in temporo-parietal cortex and inferior frontal cortex (Corbetta and Shulman 2002). This network is largely lateralized to the right hemisphere and does not appear to contribute to the maintenance of goal-directed behaviour in selecting relevant stimuli, but rather appears to be specialized for detecting behaviourally relevant information from the environment that is salient or occurs unexpectedly, thereby requiring a reorienting of spatial attention and a resetting of the attentional task to a new location in visual space. We will discuss the functions of the ventral attention network in more detail in a later section.

In the human brain, evidence that the fronto-parietal attention network is the source of the modulatory signals found in the visual system has been provided by imaging studies in which subjects were cued to direct attention to a location in the visual field, where a target stimulus would appear with a delay (Kastner, Pinsk et al. 1999; Hopfinger, Buonocore et al. 2000). In one study, it was shown that during directed attention to the target location in the delay period, thus in the absence of visual stimuli, there was a stronger increase in baseline activity in frontal and parietal areas of the attention network than in visual cortex. Importantly, there was no further increase in activity evoked by the attended stimulus presentations in these higher-order areas (Fig. 9.3c; Kastner, Pinsk et al. 1999). Rather, there was sustained activity throughout the expectation period and the attended presentations, indicating that the activity reflected the attentional operations of the task and not visual processing. This evidence has been elegantly corroborated by recent studies that combined transcranial magnetic stimulation (TMS) concurrently with fMRI, or EEG measurements (Ruff, Blankenburg et al. 2006; Taylor, Nobre et al. 2007). With TMS, a brief magnetic pulse is applied through the skull to an underlying brain region, which may cause a variety of phenomena depending on the specific brain region that is targeted, but importantly often includes interference with ongoing neural processing for a short period of time. Thus, this method provides a causal measure of brain–behaviour relationships. Stimulating the human FEF evoked a characteristic and topographic pattern of activity in early and intermediate visual cortex that was accompanied by alterations in visual perception (Ruff, Blankenburg et al. 2006), in keeping with single-cell work (Moore and Armstrong 2003; Armstrong, Fitzgerald et al. 2006; Armstrong and Moore 2007). These effects on neural activity occurred in the absence and in the presence of visual stimuli. TMS applied over parietal cortex also influenced neural activity in downstream visual areas (Ruff, Bestmann et al. 2008), and the pattern of activity changes was different from frontal stimulation, suggesting different roles for parietal and frontal cortex in cognitive control. Together, these findings have provided strong evidence in support of the notion that these parietal and frontal areas are the sources of feedback that generate the top-down biasing signals seen in visual cortex.

Topographic organization in parietal and frontal cortex. As mentioned earlier, the existence of topographic representations in sensory systems has greatly facilitated the study of functional specialization of cortical areas. The methods of measuring cortical fMRI responses under passive conditions in order to reveal retinotopic organization have recently been extended to a variety of more complex tasks and stimuli. Such 'cognitive mapping' approaches have revealed topographic organization in parietal and frontal cortex, thereby meeting the second prediction made by models of space-based attention control.

The first evidence of topographic organization within human parietal cortex was provided by Sereno and colleagues (Sereno, Pitzalis et al. 2001), employing a memory-guided saccade task in which the location of a target stimulus was remembered during a delay period, followed by a saccadic eye movement to the remembered location. The location of the target stimulus and saccade endpoint systematically traversed the visual field, and analysis of fMRI responses revealed a topographic map in posterior parietal cortex (PPC). Subsequent investigations used a variety of experimental paradigms including a visual spatial attention task (Silver, Ress et al. 2005), presentation of a colourful and dynamic periodic mapping stimulus (Swisher, Halko et al. 2007), and a variation of the memory-guided saccade task originally used by Sereno and colleagues (Schluppeck, Glimcher et al. 2005; Konen and Kastner 2008) to characterize topographic organization of responses in human PPC. Thus far, seven topographically organized parietal areas have been described: six of these areas form a contiguous band along the intraparietal sulcus (IPS0–IPS5), and one area branches off into the superior parietal lobule (SPL1) (Fig. 9.3a). Each of these topographic areas contains a continuous representation of the contralateral visual field and is separated from neighbouring areas by reversals in the orientation of the visual field representation. Boundaries between these areas correspond to alternating representations of the upper (denoted in blue in Fig. 9.3a) and lower (denoted in yellow) vertical meridian.

Topographic maps have also been discovered in frontal cortex in a variety of periodic tasks (Hagler and Sereno 2006; Kastner, DeSimone et al. 2007). One such map is located in the superior branch of precentral cortex (PreCC), in the approximate location of the human frontal eye field (FEF), and a second one in the inferior branch of PreCC (Fig. 9.3a). Both of these areas are also activated by visually guided saccadic eye movements (Kastner, DeSimone et al. 2007), and their topographic representations have several characteristic features. First, there is a bias towards a contralateral representation of both saccade directions and memorized locations in each area. Second, similar saccade directions and memorized locations are represented in common neighbouring locations of each topographic map. Finally, for each area, particular saccade directions or memorized locations are represented redundantly in several parts of the topographic map. Thus, the representation of visual space in these frontal maps appears to be different from the organization of occipital and parietal maps, which typically exhibit a one-to-one mapping between locations in visual space and locations on the cortical sheet. Remarkably, topographic representations in frontal cortex showed significant variability across subjects but were highly reproducible within subjects.

Importantly, there is a great amount of overlap between the attention-related activations discussed in the last section with topographically organized frontal and parietal areas (see Fig. 9.3a, b), which permits the systematic study of attention control systems as represented in topographically defined higher-order cortical areas in individual subjects. Such an approach promises to yield a more mechanistic understanding of the neural underpinnings of cognitive control processes related to selective attention as well as others than is currently known.

Defining control properties of the fronto-parietal attention network. Following such a research strategy, attention signals in topographic frontal and parietal areas were investigated in individual subjects in a study in which subjects were instructed to covertly

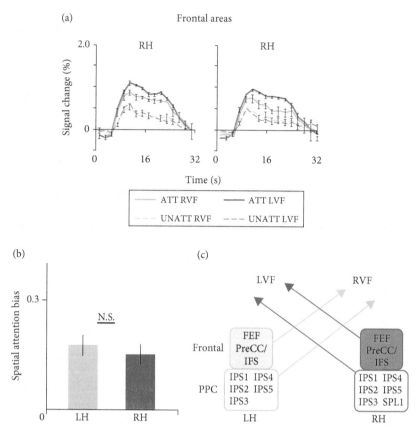

FIGURE 9.4 An inter-hemispheric competition model of spatial attention control. (a) Spatial attention signals averaged across subjects in topographic regions of frontal cortex ($n = 9$) are shown separately for each hemisphere. Solid curves indicate activity evoked by the attended conditions (ATT) and dashed curves indicate activity evoked by the unattended (UNATT) conditions. Red curves correspond to directed attention to the LVF, while blue curves correspond to directed attention to the RVF. Error bars indicate SEM across subjects. (b) Attention bias signals toward the right or left visual field were computed as index measures for each topographic area and averaged across topographic frontal and parietal areas within a hemisphere. The contralateral biases exerted by each hemisphere were similar, suggesting that the control of spatial attention across the visual field is exerted by a balanced competition of spatial biasing signals between the two hemispheres. (c) A model of spatial attention control is proposed, in which a number of topographically organized areas in fronto-parietal cortex bias attention to the contralateral visual field. Arrows towards the RVF or LVF denote the direction of attentional bias for each lobe (frontal cortex or PPC), while the thickness of each arrow refers to the strength of the attentional bias, or 'attentional weight'. LH = left hemisphere; RH = right hemisphere.

direct attention to a peripheral location in either the left or right visual hemifield and to detect targets embedded in a stream of visual stimuli (Szczepanski, Konen et al. 2010). Activity in most of the topographic PPC areas was found to be spatially specific, with stronger responses associated with directing attention to the contralateral as compared to the ipsilateral visual field, thereby generating a contralateral spatial biasing signal (Fig. 9.4a). With the exception of left SPL1, each topographic area in frontal and parietal cortex generated an individual contralateral spatial bias that was on average balanced between the two hemispheres (Fig. 9.4b). Importantly, two hemispheric asymmetries were noted (Szczepanski, Konen et al. 2010). First, right, but not left SPL1 carried spatial attention signals, as measured with fMRI. Second, left FEF and left IPS1/2 generated stronger contralateral biasing signals than their counterparts in the right hemisphere.

These results, based on data from the normal adult brain, potentially provide a neural basis for interhemispheric competition accounts of space-based attention control (Kinsbourne 1977; Smania, Martini et al. 1998). Specifically, with this account (Fig. 9.4c), each of the left hemisphere's and right hemisphere's areas contributes to the control of spatial attention across the visual field by generating a spatial bias, or 'attentional weight' (Duncan, Bundesen et al. 1999) towards the contralateral hemifield. The sum of the weights contributed by each area within a hemisphere constitutes the overall spatial bias that can be exerted over contralateral space. The net output of attentional weights generated by the two hemispheres is similar, indicating that the control system is normally balanced. This balance of attentional weights across the hemispheres may be achieved through reciprocal interhemispheric inhibition of corresponding areas (see He 2008). However, the higher-order control system appears to be complicated by right SPL1's unique role in spatial attention. The attentional weight generated by this area was not counteracted by left SPL1. Instead, left FEF and left IPS1/2 generated stronger attentional weights than their right-hemispheric counterparts, possibly to maintain a balanced distribution of attentional resources across the visual field. Thus, the left hemispheric control system requires the cooperation of several distributed subcomponents in order to balance the spatial biasing signals generated by the two hemispheres (Fig. 9.4c).

This empirical model of space-based attention control makes a number of predictions that can account for key findings from behavioural studies in neglect patients. First, the model predicts that dysfunction of right PPC (including right SPL1) will result in a spatial bias towards the right visual field and a neglect of the left visual field due to the shift of the residual attentional weights towards contralateral space. This is in agreement with data from visuospatial neglect patients with damage to right parietal cortex (Mesulam 1999). Second, the model predicts that if a portion of either PPC or FEF and surrounding frontal regions is dysfunctional in the left hemisphere, a strong neglect of the right visual field is less likely to result, since the intact portion of left frontal or parietal cortex may be able to compensate. Therefore, isolated dysfunction of left PPC or left FEF is *less* likely to cause a strong shift in the weights towards the left visual field. This is in agreement with observations that right visual field neglect occurs much less frequently with isolated frontal or parietal lesions. Therefore, together, the first two predictions are consistent with the notion of right hemispheric dominance of attention function (Heilman and Van Den Abell 1980; Mesulam 1981).

Third, the model predicts that both left frontal cortex and left PPC need to be dysfunctional before right neglect is strongly manifested. In general, too few studies have examined patients in great enough detail to determine the exact neural correlates of right neglect. However, interestingly and in accordance with the model predictions, right neglect has been reported to occur more frequently in patients with extensive left hemisphere damage covering frontal, parietal, and temporal cortex. Several studies have reported extensive lesions (Bartolomeo, Chokron et al. 2001) or tissue dysfunction (Kleinman, Newhart et al. 2007) of frontal, parietal, and temporal cortex in patients exhibiting right neglect. Beis et al. (Beis, Keller et al. 2004) compared a large number of patients with left and right neglect and found that those patients with large antero-posterior strokes, covering frontal and parietal cortex in the right or the left hemisphere, respectively, performed relatively similarly on a comprehensive battery of tests for unilateral neglect. Thus, these studies appear to provide at least some preliminary evidence in support of the model predictions regarding the occurrence of right neglect.

Importantly, studies in patients suffering from hemineglect following a stroke to the right hemisphere show reduced activity in the right relative to the left posterior parietal cortex, even though these brain regions are structurally intact (Corbetta, Kincade et al. 2005). Thus, the attentional deficits observed in these patients may be explained by a distal impact of the lesion, which typically includes inferior parts of the right parietal lobe and adjacent superior temporal cortex, on structurally intact brain issue in the right dorsal attention network, thereby resulting in an imbalance of attentional weights generated by each hemisphere to control contralateral space. This imbalance is also accompanied by a breakdown of functional connectivity within the dorsal network between the two hemispheres (He 2008).

Modelling the information flow through the attention network. While there is good evidence that areas in frontal and parietal cortex are the sources that generate modulatory signals for feedback to sensory processing areas, neuroimaging data have limitations in testing hypotheses about the directionality of the flow of information within the network and in deriving information in the time domain about the ongoing computations due to the sluggishness and poor temporal resolution of hemodynamic signals. Functional connectivity models have recently begun to tackle some of these issues and provide first evidence for a possible connectivity model of selective attention that will include the entire large-scale network that has been discussed in this chapter. Thus far, measures of Granger causality have confirmed greater influences in the 'top-down' direction, that is from FEF and regions within the IPS to intermediate and lower level tiers of visual cortex, than in the reverse direction (Bressler, Tang et al. 2008). Moreover, these studies suggest greater causal influences from FEF to IPS than from IPS to FEF, suggesting together with corroborating evidence from monkey physiology (Buschman and Miller 2007; Gregoriou, Gotts et al. 2009) that areas in frontal cortex are key nodes for attentional control within the rest of the network. Attention signals in parietal cortex appear to precede those in visual cortex by about 200 ms (Lauritzen,

D'Esposito et al. 2009). Future network modelling studies will be invaluable in understanding the involvement of certain nodes within a given task epoch and across different tasks as well as the directionality of the information flow within a network. Linking such models to individual behaviour will be particularly powerful in informing about brain–behaviour relationships at the network level.

The ventral attention network and its many functions. As mentioned earlier, selective attention appears to involve two large-scale networks that are spatially and functionally segregated, a dorsal fronto-parietal network that we have discussed thus far and a so-called 'ventral' fronto-parietal network, respectively. While the dorsal network engages both hemispheres with the few asymmetries that were noted above, the ventral network is largely lateralized to the right hemisphere and consists of areas in the region of the temporo-parietal junction (TPJ) and inferior frontal cortex (Corbetta and Shulman 2002). Since these areas are mainly located along the lateral and not on the ventral surface of the brain, as the term 'ventral' network suggests, it is worth noting that this terminology is somewhat misleading; the network has been termed 'ventral' relative to the more medial and dorsal regions of the parietal and superior frontal cortex. We will continue to use the established, albeit misleading nomenclature in this section. Studies investigating activity patterns during a resting state confirmed that the ventral and dorsal networks constitute separate entities that were identifiable by characteristic coherence of signal fluctuations during the resting state that can be used as neural signatures of functional connectivity within large-scale networks (He, Snyder et al. 2007).

Initial studies suggested that the ventral network reflected a reorienting of spatial attention to a new location in the visual field, where a stimulus had unexpectedly occurred (Corbetta, Kincade et al. 2000). Particularly, it was shown that the dorsal, but not the ventral network became activated when spatial attention was directed to and maintained at a cued location, thus when a specific attentional set was instantiated and maintained. In contrast, the ventral network was activated when spatial attention needed to be redirected to a location that was not previously cued, where a target had appeared unexpectedly. Subsequently it was shown that such activation did not require a spatial redirection of attention, but occurred also in so-called oddball tasks performed at a fixed spatial location, in which infrequently presented target stimuli had to be detected within a series of visual stimuli. Importantly, the ventral network is engaged during the detection of infrequently occurring target stimuli independent of their sensory modality, or the specific response demands of the task (Downar, Crawley et al. 2000). Together, these studies indicated that the ventral attention network constituted a general domain mechanism for the detection of salient and infrequently occurring events in the environment. It should be noted that the ventral attention network is considered a 'non-spatial' network, that is, a network that does not represent spatial information systematically. Indeed, topographic organization has not yet been identified in the brain regions that constitute the ventral attention network.

Importantly, it has been demonstrated that activation of the ventral attention network is enhanced with salient or infrequent sensory stimuli, particularly when they are relevant to the current task set (Downar, Crawley et al. 2001). Further, the TPJ has been shown to be deactivated depending on task relevance and subjects' focus (Shulman, Astafiev et al. 2007), which has been interpreted as a filter mechanism that prevents reorienting to unimportant sensory stimuli. Such deactivation of the ventral network may be controlled by the dorsal attention network to maintain and optimize its attentional task set.

The ventral attention network, and in particular the TPJ, has also been shown to be activated in a number of tasks that involve self-referencing and are important in social cognition. For example, the TPJ is involved in 'theory of mind' cognition; these are tasks during which subjects reason about other people's mental states (Fletcher, Happé et al. 1995; Gallagher and Frith 2003) or feel empathy for others (Decety and Lamm 2007). While it is not clear whether the same populations of neurons in the region of the TPJ are involved with tasks that involve redirecting attention versus those that involve referencing oneself to another person's state of mind, it is conceivable that the reorienting function of the TPJ is not restricted to sensory events in the environment, but can also be applied to changing a self-referential context (Graziano and Kastner 2011). Thus, the ventral network may be a general purpose network for re-referencing social context that could involve events driven by the environment as well as by cognitive states.

CONCLUSION

Evidence from functional brain imaging reveals that attention operates at various processing levels within the human visual system and beyond. These attention mechanisms appear to be controlled by a distributed network of higher-order areas in frontal and parietal cortex, which generate top-down signals that are transmitted via feedback connections to the visual system. Together, these widely distributed brain systems cooperate to mediate the selection of behaviourally relevant information that can be further utilized in other cognitive networks to ultimately guide goal-directed action.

ACKNOWLEDGEMENT

We gratefully acknowledge the support of the National Institutes of Health and the National Science Foundation in funding our research.

REFERENCES

Armstrong, K. M., Fitzgerald, J. K., and Moore, T. (2006). Changes in visual receptive fields with microstimulation of frontal cortex. *Neuron* 50(5): 791–798.

Armstrong, K. M. and Moore, T. (2007). Rapid enhancement of visual cortical response discriminability by microstimulation of the frontal eye field. *Proceedings of the National Academy of Sciences USA* 104(22): 9499–9504.

Avidan, G., Harel, M., Hendler, T., Ben-Bashat, D., Zohary, E., and Malach, R. (2002). Contrast sensitivity in human visual areas and its relationship to object recognition. *Journal of Neurophysiology* 87(6): 3102–3116.

Bair, W., Cavanaugh, J. R., and Movshon, J. A. (2003). Time course and time-distance relationships for surround suppression in macaque V1 neurons. *Journal of Neuroscience* 23(20): 7690–7701.

Bartolomeo, P., Chokron, S., and Gainotti, G. (2001). Laterally directed arm movements and right unilateral neglect after left hemisphere damage. *Neuropsychologia* 39(10): 1013–1021.

Beck, D. M. and Kastner, S. (2005). Stimulus context modulates competition in human extrastriate cortex. *Nature Neuroscience* 8(8): 1110–1116.

Beck, D. M. and Kastner, S. (2007). Stimulus similarity modulates competitive interactions in human visual cortex. *Journal of Vision* 7(2): 19.1–12.

Beis, J. M., Keller, C., Morin, N., et al. (2004). Right spatial neglect after left hemisphere stroke: Qualitative and quantitative study. *Neurology* 63(9): 1600–1605.

Bell, A. H., Fecteau, J. H., and Munoz, D. P. (2004). Using auditory and visual stimuli to investigate the behavioral and neuronal consequences of reflexive covert orienting. *Journal of Neurophysiology* 91(5): 2172–2184.

Bender, D. B. and Youakim, M. (2001). Effect of attentive fixation in macaque thalamus and cortex. *Journal of Neurophysiology* 85(1): 219–234.

Bichot, N. P., Rossi, A. F., and Desimone, R. (2005). Parallel and serial neural mechanisms for visual search in macaque area V4. *Science* 308(5721): 529–534.

Bisiach, E. and Vallar, G. (1988). Hemineglect in humans. In J. G. F. Boller (ed.), *Handbook of Neuropsychology* (vol. 1, pp. 195–222). Amsterdam: Elsevier.

Blakemore, C. and Tobin, E. A. (1972). Lateral inhibition between orientation detectors in the cat's visual cortex. *Experimental Brain Research* 15(4): 439–440.

Bles, M., Schwarzbach, J., De Weerd, P., Goebel, R., and Jansma, B. M. (2006). Receptive field size-dependent attention effects in simultaneously presented stimulus displays. *NeuroImage* 30(2): 506–511.

Brefczynski, J. A. and DeYoe, E. A. (1999). A physiological correlate of the 'spotlight' of visual attention. *Nature Neuroscience* 2(4): 370–374.

Bressler, S. L., Tang, W., Sylvester, C. M., Shulman, G. L., and Corbetta, M. (2008). Top-down control of human visual cortex by frontal and parietal cortex in anticipatory visual spatial attention. *Journal of Neuroscience* 28(40): 10056–10061.

Broadbent, D. E. (1958). *Perception and Communication*. Oxford: Oxford University Press.

Buffalo, E. A., Bertini, G., Ungerleider, L. G., and Desimone, R. (2005). Impaired filtering of distractor stimuli by TE neurons following V4 and TEO lesions in macaques. *Cerebral Cortex* 15(2): 141–151.

Bundesen, C. and Pedersen, L. F. (1983). Color segregation and visual search. *Perception & Psychophysics* 33(5): 487–493.

Buracas, G. T. and Boynton, G. M. (2007). The effect of spatial attention on contrast response functions in human visual cortex. *Journal of Neuroscience* 27(1): 93–97.

Buschman, T. J. and Miller, E. K. (2007). Top-down versus bottom-up control of attention in the prefrontal and posterior parietal cortices. *Science* 315(5820): 1860–1862.

Cameron, E. L., Tai, J. C., and Carrasco, M. (2002). Covert attention affects the psychometric function of contrast sensitivity. *Vision Research* 42(8): 949–967.

Carrasco, M., Ling, S., and Read, S. (2004). Attention alters appearance. *Nature Neuroscience* 7(3): 308–313.

Carrasco, M., Loula, F., and Ho, Y. X. (2006). How attention enhances spatial resolution: Evidence from selective adaptation to spatial frequency. *Perception & Psychophysics* 68(6): 1004–1012.

Cherry, E. C. (1953). Experiments on the recognition of speech with one and two ears. *Journal of the Acoustical Society of America* 25: 975–979.

Corbetta, M., Akbudak, E., Conturo, T. E., et al. (1998). A common network of functional areas for attention and eye movements. *Neuron* 21(4): 761–773.

Corbetta, M., Kincade, M. J., Lewis, C., Snyder, A. Z., and Sapir, A. (2005). Neural basis and recovery of spatial attention deficits in spatial neglect. *Nature Neuroscience* 8(11): 1603–1610.

Corbetta, M., Kincade, J. M., Ollinger, J. M., McAvoy, M. P., and Shulman, G. L. (2000). Voluntary orienting is dissociated from target detection in human posterior parietal cortex. *Nature Neuroscience* 3(3): 292–297.

Corbetta, M. and Shulman, G. L. (2002). Control of goal-directed and stimulus-driven attention in the brain. *Nature Reviews Neuroscience* 3(3): 201–215.

Damasio, A. R., Damasio, H., and Chui, H. C. (1980). Neglect following damage to frontal lobe or basal ganglia. *Neuropsychologia* 18(2): 123–132.

DeAngelis, G. C., Robson, J. G., Ohzawa, I., and Freeman, R. D. (1992). Organization of suppression in receptive fields of neurons in cat visual cortex. *Journal of Neurophysiology* 68(1): 144–163.

Decety, J. and Lamm, C. (2007). The role of the right temporoparietal junction in social interaction: How low-level computational processes contribute to meta-cognition. *Neuroscientist* 13(6): 580–593.

Desimone, R. and Duncan, J. (1995). Neural mechanisms of selective visual attention. *Annual Review of Neuroscience* 18: 193–222.

Deutsch, J. A. and Deutsch, D. (1963). Some theoretical considerations. *Psychological Review* 70: 80–90.

Di Russo, F., Spinelli, D., and Morrone, M. C. (2001). Automatic gain control contrast mechanisms are modulated by attention in humans: evidence from visual evoked potentials. *Vision Research* 41(19): 2435–2447.

Downar, J., Crawley, A. P., Mikulis, D. J., and Davis, K. D. (2000). A multimodal cortical network for the detection of changes in the sensory environment. *Nature Neuroscience* 3(3): 277–283.

Downar, J., Crawley, A. P., Mikulis, D. J., and Davis, K. D. (2001). The effect of task relevance on the cortical response to changes in visual and auditory stimuli: An event-related fMRI study. *NeuroImage* 14(6): 1256–1267.

Duncan, J. (1980). The locus of interference in the perception of simultaneous stimuli. *Psychological Review* 87(3): 272–300.

Duncan, J. (1987). Attention and reading: Wholes and parts in shape recognition—a tutorial review. In M. Coltheart (ed.), *Attention and Performance XII: The Psychology of Reading* (pp. 36–61). Hove, UK: Erlbaum.

Duncan, J. (1996). Cooperating brain systems in selective perception and action. In T. Inui and J. L. McClelland (eds.), *Attention and Performance XVI* (pp. 549–578). Cambridge, Mass.: MIT Press.

Duncan, J. (1998). Converging levels of analysis in the cognitive neuroscience of visual attention. *Philosophical Transactions of the Royal Society B: Biological Sciences* 353(1373): 1307–1317.

Duncan, J., Bundesen, C., Olson, A., Humphreys, G., Chavda, S., and Shibuya, H. (1999). Systematic analysis of deficits in visual attention. *Journal of Experimental Psychology: General* 128(4): 450–478.

Eriksen, C. W. and Hoffman, J. E. (1973). The extent of processing of noise elements during selective visual encoding from visual displays. *Perception & Psychophysics* 14: 155–160.

Fecteau, J. H., Bell, A. H., and Munoz, D. P. (2004). Neural correlates of the automatic and goal-driven biases in orienting spatial attention. *Journal of Neurophysiology* 92(3): 1728–1737.

Fei-Fei, L., Iyer, A., Koch, C., and Perona, P. (2007). What do we perceive in a glance of a real-world scene? *Journal of Vision* 7(1): 10.

Fisher, D. L. (1984). Central capacity limits in consistent mapping, visual search tasks: Four channels or more? *Cognitive Psychology* 16(4): 449–484.

Fletcher, P. C., Happé, F., Frith, U., Baker, S. C., Dolan, R. J., Frackowiak, R. S., and Frith, C. D. (1995). Other minds in the brain: A functional imaging study of 'theory of mind' in story comprehension. *Cognition* 57(2): 109–128.

Gallagher, H. L. and Frith, C. D. (2003). Functional imaging of 'theory of mind'. *Trends in Cognitive Sciences* 7(2): 77–83.

Gandhi, S. P., Heeger, D. J., and Boynton, G. M. (1999). Spatial attention affects brain activity in human primary visual cortex. *Proceedings of the National Academy of Sciences USA* 96(6): 3314–3319.

Gattass, R. and Desimone, R. (1996). Responses of cells in the superior colliculus during performance of a spatial attention task in the macaque. *Revista Brasileira de Biologia* 56 Supplement 1 Part 2: 257–279.

Gilbert, C., Ito, M., Kapadia, M., and Westheimer, G. (2000). Interactions between attention, context and learning in primary visual cortex. *Vision Research* 40(10–12): 1217–1226.

Graziano, M. S. and Kastner, S. (2011). Human consciousness and its relationship to social neuroscience: A novel hypothesis. *Cognitive Neuroscience* 2(2): 98–113.

Gregoriou, G. G., Gotts, S. J., Zhou, H., and Desimone, R. (2009). High-frequency, long-range coupling between prefrontal and visual cortex during attention. *Science* 324(5931): 1207–1210.

Hagler, D. J., Jr. and Sereno, M. I. (2006). Spatial maps in frontal and prefrontal cortex. *NeuroImage* 29(2): 567–577.

Handy, T. C. and Mangun, G. R. (2000). Attention and spatial selection: Electrophysiological evidence for modulation by perceptual load. *Perception & Psychophysics* 62(1): 175–186.

He, B. (2008). Functional neuroimaging of dynamic brain activation. *Conference Proceedings of the IEEE Engineering in Medicine and Biology Society 2008*: 3355.

He, B. J., Snyder, A. Z., Vincent, J. L., Epstein, A., Shulman, G. L., and Corbetta, M. (2007). Breakdown of functional connectivity in frontoparietal networks underlies behavioral deficits in spatial neglect. *Neuron* 53(6): 905–918.

Heilman, K. M. and Van Den Abell, T. (1980). Right hemisphere dominance for attention: The mechanism underlying hemispheric asymmetries of inattention (neglect). *Neurology* 30(3): 327–330.

Heilman, K. M., Watson, R. T., and Valenstein, E. (1993). Neglect and related disorders. In K. M. Heilman and E. Valenstein (eds.), *Clinical Neuropsychology* (pp. 279–336). Oxford: Oxford University Press.

Heinze, H. J., Luck, S. J., Münte, T. F., Gös, A., Mangun, G. R., and Hillyard, S. A. (1994). Attention to adjacent and separate positions in space: An electrophysiological analysis. *Perception & Psychophysics* 56(1): 42–52.

Heinze, H. J., Mangun, G. R., Burchert, W., et al. (1994). Combined spatial and temporal imaging of brain activity during visual selective attention in humans. *Nature* 372(6506): 543–546.

Hillyard, S. A., Vogel, E. K., and Luck, S. J. (1998). Sensory gain control (amplification) as a mechanism of selective attention: Electrophysiological and neuroimaging evidence. *Philosophical Transactions of the Royal Society B: Biological Sciences* 353(1373): 1257–1270.

Hoffman, J. E. (1975). Hierarchical stages in the processing of visual information. *Perception & Psychophysics* 18: 348–354.

Hopf, J. M., Boehler, C. N., Luck, S. J., Tsotsos, J. K., Heinze, H. J., and Schoenfeld, M. A. (2006). Direct neurophysiological evidence for spatial suppression surrounding the focus of attention in vision. *Proceedings of the National Academy of Sciences USA 103*(4): 1053–1058.

Hopfinger, J. B., Buonocore, M. H., and Mangun, G. R. (2000). The neural mechanisms of top-down attentional control. *Nature Neuroscience 3*(3): 284–291.

Ignashchenkova, A., Dicke, P. W., Haarmeier, T., and Their, P. (2004). Neuron-specific contribution of the superior colliculus to overt and covert shifts of attention. *Nature Neuroscience 7*(1): 56–64.

Im, C. H., Gururajan, A., Zhang, N., Chen, W., and He, B. (2007). Spatial resolution of EEG cortical source imaging revealed by localization of retinotopic organization in human primary visual cortex. *Journal of Neuroscience Methods 161*(1): 142–154.

Ito, M. and Gilbert, C. D. (1999). Attention modulates contextual influences in the primary visual cortex of alert monkeys. *Neuron 22*(3): 593–604.

James, W. (1890). *The Principles of Psychology*. New York: H. Holt and Company.

Janer, K. W. and Pardo, J. V. (1991). Deficits in selective attention following bilateral anterior cingulotomy. *Journal of Cognitive Neuroscience 3*: 231–241.

Kanizsa, G. (1976). Subjective contours. *Scientific American 234*(4): 48–52.

Kapadia, M. K., Ito, M., Gilbert, C. D., and Westheimer, G. (1995). Improvement in visual sensitivity by changes in local context: Parallel studies in human observers and in V1 of alert monkeys. *Neuron 15*(4): 843–856.

Kapadia, M. K., Westheimer, G., and Gilbert, C. D. (1999). Dynamics of spatial summation in primary visual cortex of alert monkeys. *Proceedings of the National Academy of Sciences USA 96*(21): 12073–12078.

Karnath, H. O., Ferber, S., and Himmelbach, M. (2001). Spatial awareness is a function of the temporal not the posterior parietal lobe. *Nature 411*(6840): 950–953.

Karnath, H. O., Himmelbach, M., and Rorden, C. (2002). The subcortical anatomy of human spatial neglect: Putamen, caudate nucleus and pulvinar. *Brain 125*(2): 350–360.

Kastner, S., DeSimone, K., Konen, C. S., Szczepanski, S. M., Weiner, K. S., and Schneider, K. A. (2007). Topographic maps in human frontal cortex revealed in memory-guided saccade and spatial working-memory tasks. *Journal of Neurophysiology 97*(5): 3494–3507.

Kastner, S., De Weerd, P., Desimone, R., and Ungerleider, L. G. (1998). Mechanisms of directed attention in the human extrastriate cortex as revealed by functional MRI. *Science 282*(5386): 108–111.

Kastner, S., De Weerd, P., Pinsk, M. A., Elizondo, M. I., Desimone, R., and Ungerleider, L. G. (2001). Modulation of sensory suppression: Implications for receptive field sizes in the human visual cortex. *Journal of Neurophysiology 86*(3): 1398–1411.

Kastner, S., Nothdurft, H. C., and Pigarev, I. N. (1997). Neuronal correlates of pop-out in cat striate cortex. *Vision Research 37*(4): 371–376.

Kastner, S., O'Connor, D. H., Fukui, M. M., Fehd, H. M., Herwig, U., and Pinsk, M. A. (2004). Functional imaging of the human lateral geniculate nucleus and pulvinar. *Journal of Neurophysiology 91*(1): 438–448.

Kastner, S., Pinsk, M. A., De Weerd, P., Desimone, R., and Ungerleider, L. G. (1999). Increased activity in human visual cortex during directed attention in the absence of visual stimulation. *Neuron 22*(4): 751–761.

Kastner, S. and Ungerleider, L. G. (2000). Mechanisms of visual attention in the human cortex. *Annual Review of Neuroscience 23*: 315–341.

Kinsbourne, M. (1977). Hemi-neglect and hemisphere rivalry. *Advances in Neurology 18*: 41–49.

Kinsbourne, M. (1993). Orientation bias model of unilateral neglect: Evidence from attentional gradients within hemispace. In I. H. Robertson and J. C. Marshall (eds.), *Unilateral Neglect: Clinical and Experimental Studies* (pp. 63–86). Hillsdale, N.J.: Erlbaum.

Kleinman, J. T., Newhart, M., Davis, C., Heidler-Gary, J., Gottesman, R. F., and Hillis, A. E. (2007). Right hemispatial neglect: Frequency and characterization following acute left hemisphere stroke. *Brain and Cognition* 64(1): 50–59.

Kleiss, J. A. and Lane, D. M. (1986). Locus and persistence of capacity limitations in visual information processing. *Journal of Experimental Psychology: Human Perception and Performance* 12(2): 200–210.

Knierim, J. J. and van Essen, D. C. (1992). Neuronal responses to static texture patterns in area V1 of the alert macaque monkey. *Journal of Neurophysiology* 67(4): 961–980.

Konen, C. S. and Kastner, S. (2008). Representation of eye movements and stimulus motion in topographically organized areas of human posterior parietal cortex. *Journal of Neuroscience* 28(33): 8361–8375.

Kustov, A. A. and Robinson, D. L. (1996). Shared neural control of attentional shifts and eye movements. *Nature* 384(6604): 74–77.

LaBerge, D. (1983). Spatial extent of attention to letters and words. *Journal of Experimental Psychology: Human Perception and Performance* 9(3): 371–379.

LaBerge, D. and Brown, V. (1986). Variations in size of the visual field in which targets are presented: An attentional range effect. *Perception & Psychophysics* 40(3): 188–200.

LaBerge, D. and Buchsbaum, M. S. (1990). Positron emission tomographic measurements of pulvinar activity during an attention task. *Journal of Neuroscience* 10(2): 613–619.

Lamme, V. A. (1995). The neurophysiology of figure-ground segregation in primary visual cortex. *Journal of Neuroscience* 15(2): 1605–1615.

Lauritzen, T. Z., Ales, J. M., and Wade, A. R. (2011). The effects of visuospatial attention measured across visual cortex using source-imaged, steady-state EEG. *Journal of Vision* 10(14): 39.1–17.

Lauritzen, T. Z., D'Esposito, M., Heeger, D. J., and Silver, M. A. (2009). Top-down flow of visual spatial attention signals from parietal to occipital cortex. *Journal of Vision* 9(13): 18.1–14.

Lavie, N. (1995). Perceptual load as a necessary condition for selective attention. *Journal of Experimental Psychology: Human Perception and Performance* 21(3): 451–468.

Lavie, N. and Tsal, Y. (1994). Perceptual load as a major determinant of the locus of selection in visual attention. *Perception & Psychophysics* 56(2): 183–197.

Lee, J., Williford, T., and Maunsell, J. H. R. (2007). Spatial attention and the latency of neuronal responses in macaque area V4. *Journal of Neuroscience* 27(36): 9632–9637.

Lee, K. M. and Keller, E. L. (2006). Symbolic cue-driven activity in superior colliculus neurons in a peripheral visual choice task. *Journal of Neurophysiology* 95(6): 3585–3595.

Li, C. Y. and Li, W. (1994). Extensive integration field beyond the classical receptive field of cat's striate cortical neurons—classification and tuning properties. *Vision Research* 34(18): 2337–2355.

Li, X., Lu, Z. L., Tjan, B. S., Dosher, B. A., and Chu, W. (2008). Blood oxygenation level-dependent contrast response functions identify mechanisms of covert attention in early visual areas. *Proceedings of the National Academy of Sciences USA* 105(16): 6202–6207.

Lu, Z. L. and Dosher, B. A. (1998). External noise distinguishes attention mechanisms. *Vision Research* 38(9): 1183–1198.

Luck, S. J., Chelazzi, L., Hillyard, S. A., and Desimone, R. (1997). Neural mechanisms of spatial selective attention in areas V1, V2, and V4 of macaque visual cortex. *Journal of Neurophysiology* 77(1): 24–42.

McAdams, C. J. and Maunsell, J. H. (1999). Effects of attention on orientation-tuning functions of single neurons in macaque cortical area V4. *Journal of Neuroscience* 19(1): 431–441.

McAlonan, K., Cavanaugh, J., and Wurtz, R. W. (2006). Attentional modulation of thalamic reticular neurons. *Journal of Neuroscience* 26(16): 4444–4450.

McAlonan, K., Cavanaugh, J., and Wurtz, R. W. (2008). Guarding the gateway to cortex with attention in visual thalamus. *Nature* 456(7220): 391–394.

Macevoy, S. P. and Epstein, R. A. (2009). Decoding the representation of multiple simultaneous objects in human occipitotemporal cortex. *Current Biology* 19(11): 943–947.

McMains, S. A., Fehd, H. M., Emmanouil, T.-A., and Kastner, S. (2007). Mechanisms of feature- and space-based attention: Response modulation and baseline increases. *Journal of Neurophysiology* 98(4): 2110–2121.

McMains, S. A. and Kastner, S. (2009). Neural basis of attention. In T. Bayne, A. Cleeremans, and P. Wilken (eds.), *The Oxford Companion to Consciousness* (pp. 79–84). Oxford: Oxford University Press.

McMains, S. A. and Kastner, S. (2010). Defining the units of competition: Influences of perceptual organization on competitive interactions in human visual cortex. *Journal of Cognitive Neuroscience* 22(11): 2417–2426.

McMains, S. and Kastner, S. (2011). Interactions of top-down and bottom-up mechanisms in human visual cortex. *Journal of Neuroscience* 31(2): 587–597.

McMains, S. A. and Somers, D. C. (2005). Processing efficiency of divided spatial attention mechanisms in human visual cortex. *Journal of Neuroscience* 25(41): 9444–94448.

Maffei, L. and Fiorentini, A. (1976). The unresponsive regions of visual cortical receptive fields. *Vision Research* 16(10): 1131–1139.

Martinez, A., Anllo-Vento, L., Sereno, M. I., et al. (1999). Involvement of striate and extrastriate visual cortical areas in spatial attention. *Nature Neuroscience* 2(4): 364–369.

Mehta, A. D., Ulbert, I., and Schroeder, C. E. (2000a). Intermodal selective attention in monkeys. I: Distribution and timing of effects across visual areas. *Cerebral Cortex* 10(4): 343–358.

Mehta, A. D., Ulbert, I., and Schroeder, C. E. (2000b). Intermodal selective attention in monkeys. II: Physiological mechanisms of modulation. *Cerebral Cortex* 10(4): 359–370.

Mesulam, M. M. (1981). A cortical network for directed attention and unilateral neglect. *Annals of Neurology* 10(4): 309–325.

Mesulam, M. M. (1999). Spatial attention and neglect: Parietal, frontal and cingulate contributions to the mental representation and attentional targeting of salient extrapersonal events. *Philosophical Transactions of the Royal Society B: Biological Sciences* 354(1387): 1325–1346.

Miller, E. K., Gochin, P. M., and Gross, C. G. (1993). Suppression of visual responses of neurons in inferior temporal cortex of the awake macaque by addition of a second stimulus. *Brain Research* 616(1–2): 25–29.

Moore, T. and Armstrong, K. M. (2003). Selective gating of visual signals by microstimulation of frontal cortex. *Nature* 421(6921): 370–373.

Moran, J. and Desimone, R. (1985). Selective attention gates visual processing in the extrastriate cortex. *Science* 229(4715): 782–784.

Mort, D. J., Malhotra, P., Mannan, S. K., Rorden, C., Pambakian, A., Kennard, C., and Husain, M. (2003). The anatomy of visual neglect. *Brain* 126(9): 1986–1997.

Motter, B. C. (1993). Focal attention produces spatially selective processing in visual cortical areas V1, V2, and V4 in the presence of competing stimuli. *Journal of Neurophysiology* 70(3): 909–919.

Muller, N. G., Bartelt, O. A., Donner, T. H., Villringer, A., and Brandt, S. A. (2003). A physiological correlate of the 'Zoom Lens' of visual attention. *Journal of Neuroscience* 23(9): 3561–3565.

Murray, S. O. (2008). The effects of spatial attention in early human visual cortex are stimulus independent. *Journal of Vision* 8(10): 2.1–11.

Murray, S. O. and He, S. (2006). Contrast invariance in the human lateral occipital complex depends on attention. *Current Biology* 16(6): 606–611.

Nobre, A. C., Sebestyen, G. N., Gitelman, D. R., Mesulam, M. M., Frackowiak, R. S., and Frith, C. D. (1997). Functional localization of the system for visuospatial attention using positron emission tomography. *Brain* 120(3): 515–533.

Norman, D. A. (1968). Toward a theory of memory and attention. *Psychological Review* 75(6): 522–536.

Nothdurft, H. C., Gallant, J. L., and Van Essen, D. C. (1999). Response modulation by texture surround in primate area V1: Correlates of 'popout' under anesthesia. *Visual Neuroscience* 16(1): 15–34.

O'Connor, D. H., Fukui, M. M., Pinsk, M. A., and Kastner, S. (2002). Attention modulates responses in the human lateral geniculate nucleus. *Nature Neuroscience* 5(11): 1203–1209.

Palmer, S. E. (1992). Common region: A new principle of perceptual grouping. *Cognitive Psychology* 24(3): 436–447.

Palmer, S. and Rock, I. (1994). Rethinking perceptual organization: The role of uniform connectedness. *Psychonomic Bulletin & Review* 1(1): 29–55.

Parks, N. A., Beck, D. M., et al. (submitted). The distribution of enhancement and suppression in the visual field under perceptual load.

Parks, N. A., Hilimire, M. R., and Corballis, P. M. (2010). Steady-state signatures of visual perceptual load, multimodal distractor filtering, and neural competition. *Journal of Cognitive Neuroscience* 23(5): 1113–1124.

Petersen, S. E., Robinson, D. L., and Keys, W. (1985). Pulvinar nuclei of the behaving rhesus monkey: Visual responses and their modulation. *Journal of Neurophysiology* 54(4): 867–886.

Pinsk, M. A., Doniger, G. M., and Kastner, S. (2004). Push-pull mechanism of selective attention in human extrastriate cortex. *Journal of Neurophysiology* 92(1): 622–629.

Polat, U., Mizobe, K., Pettet, M. W., Kasamatsu, T., and Norcia, A. M. (1998). Collinear stimuli regulate visual responses depending on cell's contrast threshold. *Nature* 391(6667): 580–584.

Posner, M. I., Nissen, N. J., and Ogden, W. C. (1978). Attended and unattended processing modes: The role of set for spatial location. In H. L. Picks and I. J. Saltzman (eds.), *Modes of Perceiving and Processing Information* (pp. 137–157). Hillsdale, N.J.: Erlbaum.

Posner, M. I., Snyder, C. R., and Davidson, B. J. (1980). Attention and the detection of signals. *Journal of Experimental Psychology* 109(2): 160–174.

Potter, M. C. (1976). Short-term conceptual memory for pictures. *Journal of Experimental Psychology: Human Learning and Memory* 2(5): 509–522.

Qiu, F. T., Sugihara, T., and von der Haydt, R. (2007). Figure-ground mechanisms provide structure for selective attention. *Nature Neuroscience* 10(11): 1492–1499.

Rafal, R. and Robertson, L. C. (1995). The neurology of visual attention. In M. Gazzaniga (ed.), *Handbook of Cognitive Neuroscience* (pp. 625–648). Cambridge, Mass.: MIT Press.

Recanzone, G. H. and Wurtz, R. H. (2000). Effects of attention on MT and MST neuronal activity during pursuit initiation. *Journal of Neurophysiology* 83(2): 777–790.

Recanzone, G. H., Wurtz, R. H., and Schwarz, U. (1997). Responses of MT and MST neurons to one and two moving objects in the receptive field. *Journal of Neurophysiology* 78(6): 2904–2915.

Reddy, L., Kanwisher, N. G., and VanRullen, R. (2009). Attention and biased competition in multi-voxel object representations. *Proceedings of the National Academy of Sciences USA* 106(50): 21447–21452.

Rees, G., Frith, C. D., and Lavie, N. (1997). Modulating irrelevant motion perception by varying attentional load in an unrelated task. *Science* 278(5343): 1616–1619.

Reynolds, J. H. and Chelazzi, L. (2004). Attentional modulation of visual processing. *Annual Review of Neuroscience* 27: 611–647.

Reynolds, J. H., Chelazzi, L., and Desimone, R. (1999). Competitive mechanisms subserve attention in macaque areas V2 and V4. *Journal of Neuroscience* 19(5): 1736–1753.

Reynolds, J. H. and Desimone, R. (2003). Interacting roles of attention and visual salience in V4. *Neuron* 37(5): 853–863.

Reynolds, J. H. and Heeger, D. J. (2009). The normalization model of attention. *Neuron* 61(2): 168–185.

Reynolds, J. H., Pasternak, T., and Desimone, R. (2000). Attention increases sensitivity of V4 neurons. *Neuron* 26(3): 703–714.

Robinson, D. L. and Kertzman, C. (1995). Covert orienting of attention in macaques. III: Contributions of the superior colliculus. *Journal of Neurophysiology* 74(2): 713–721.

Rubin, E. (1915). *Visuell wahrgenommene Figuren*. Copenhagen: Glydenalske.

Ruff, C. C., Bestmann, S., Blankenburg, F., et al. (2008). Distinct causal influences of parietal versus frontal areas on human visual cortex: Evidence from concurrent TMS-fMRI. *Cerebral Cortex* 18(4): 817–827.

Ruff, C. C., Blankenburg, F., Bjoertomt, O., et al. (2006). Concurrent TMS-fMRI and psychophysics reveal frontal influences on human retinotopic visual cortex. *Current Biology* 16(15): 1479–1488.

Saalmann, Y. B. and Kastner, S. (2009). Gain control in the visual thalamus during perception and cognition. *Current Opinion in Neurobiology* 19(4): 408–414.

Saalmann, Y. B. and Kastner, S. (2011). Cognitive and perceptual functions of the visual thalamus. *Neuron* 71(2): 209–223.

Saalmann, Y. B., Pinsk, M. A., Wang, L., Li, X., and Kastner, S. (2012). The pulvinar regulates information transmission between cortical areas based on attention demands. *Science* 337(6095): 753–756.

Saenz, M., Buracas, G. T., and Boynton, G. M. (2002). Global effects of feature-based attention in human visual cortex. *Nature Neuroscience* 5(7): 631–632.

Scalf, P. E., Basak, C., and Beck, D. M. (2011). Attention does more than modulate suppressive interactions: attending to multiple items. *Experimental Brain Research* 212(2): 293–304.

Scalf, P. E. and Beck, D. M. (2010). Competition in visual cortex impedes attention to multiple items. *Journal of Neuroscience* 30(1): 161–169.

Schluppeck, D., Glimcher, P., and Heeger, D. J. (2005). Topographic organization for delayed saccades in human posterior parietal cortex. *Journal of Neurophysiology* 94(2): 1372–1384.

Schneider, K. A. (2011). Subcortical mechanisms of feature-based attention. *Journal of Neuroscience* 31(23): 8643–8653.

Schneider, K. A. and Kastner, S. (2009). Effects of sustained spatial attention in the human lateral geniculate nucleus and superior colliculus. *Journal of Neuroscience* 29(6): 1784–1795.

Schwartz, S., Vuilleumier, P., Hutton, C., Maravita, A., Dolan, R. J., and Driver, J. (2005). Attentional load and sensory competition in human vision: Modulation of fMRI responses by load at fixation during task-irrelevant stimulation in the peripheral visual field. *Cerebral Cortex* 15(6): 770–786.

Serences, J. T. and Boynton, G. M. (2007). Feature-based attentional modulations in the absence of direct visual stimulation. *Neuron* 55(2): 301–312.

Sereno, M. I., Dale, A. M., Reppas, J. B., et al. (1995). Borders of multiple visual areas in humans revealed by functional magnetic resonance imaging. *Science* 268(5212): 889–893.

Sereno, M. I., Pitzalis, S., and Martinez, A. (2001). Mapping of contralateral space in retinotopic coordinates by a parietal cortical area in humans. *Science* 294(5545): 1350–1354.

Shipp, S. (2003). The functional logic of cortico-pulvinar connections. *Philosophical Transactions of the Royal Society B: Biological Sciences* 358(1438): 1605–1624.

Shiu, L. P. and Pashler, H. (1995). Spatial attention and vernier acuity. *Vision Research* 35(3): 337–343.

Shulman, G. L., Astafiev, S. V., McAvoy, M. P., d'Avossa, G., and Corbetta, M. (2007). Right TPJ deactivation during visual search: functional significance and support for a filter hypothesis. *Cerebral Cortex* 17(11): 2625–2633.

Sillito, A. M., Grieve, K. L., Jones, H. E., Cudeiro, J., and Davis, J. (1995). Visual cortical mechanisms detecting focal orientation discontinuities. *Nature* 378(6556): 492–496.

Silver, M. A., Ress, D., and Heeger, D. J. (2005). Topographic maps of visual spatial attention in human parietal cortex. *Journal of Neurophysiology* 94(2): 1358–1371.

Smania, N., Martini, M. C., Gambina, G., Tomelleri, G., Palamara, A., Natale, E., and Marzi, C. A. (1998). The spatial distribution of visual attention in hemineglect and extinction patients. *Brain* 121(9): 1759–1770.

Smith, A. T., Cotton, P. L., Bruno, A., and Moutsiana, C. (2009). Dissociating vision and visual attention in the human pulvinar. *Journal of Neurophysiology* 101(2): 917–925.

Snowden, R. J., Treue, S., Erickson, R. G., and Andersen, R. A. (1991). The response of area MT and V1 neurons to transparent motion. *Journal of Neuroscience* 11(9): 2768–2785.

Somers, D. C., Dale, A. M., Seiffert, A. E., and Tootell, R. B. H. (1999). Functional MRI reveals spatially specific attentional modulation in human primary visual cortex. *Proceedings of the National Academy of Sciences USA* 96(4): 1663–1668.

Sprague, J. M. (1966). Interaction of cortex and superior colliculus in mediation of visually guided behavior in the cat. *Science* 153(3743): 1544–15447.

Swisher, J. D., Halko, M. A., Merabet, L. B., McMains, S. A., and Somers, D. C. (2007). Visual topography of human intraparietal sulcus. *Journal of Neuroscience* 27(20): 5326–5337.

Sylvester, R., Josephs, O., Driver, J., and Rees, G. (2007). Visual FMRI responses in human superior colliculus show a temporal-nasal asymmetry that is absent in lateral geniculate and visual cortex. *Journal of Neurophysiology* 97(2): 1495–1502.

Szczepanski, S. M., Konen, C. S., and Kastner, S. (2010). Mechanisms of spatial attention control in frontal and parietal cortex. *Journal of Neuroscience* 30(1): 148–160.

Taylor, P. C., Nobre, A. C., and Rushworth, M. F. (2007). FEF TMS affects visual cortical activity. *Cerebral Cortex* 17(2): 391–399.

Thiele, A., Pooresmaeili, A., Delicato, L. S., Herrero, J. L., and Roelfsema, P. R. (2009). Additive effects of attention and stimulus contrast in primary visual cortex. *Cerebral Cortex* 19(12): 2970–2981.

Tootell, R. B., Hadjikhani, N., Hall, E. K., Marrett, S., Vanduffel, W., Vaughan, J. T., and Dale, A. M. (1998). The retinotopy of visual spatial attention. *Neuron* 21(6): 1409–1422.

Torralbo, A. and Beck, D. M. (2008). Perceptual-load-induced selection as a result of local competitive interactions in visual cortex. *Psychological Science* 19(10): 1045–1050.

Treisman, A. M. (1969). Strategies and models of selective attention. *Psychological Review* 76(3): 282–299.

Treisman, A. M. and Gelade, G. (1980). A feature-integration theory of attention. *Cognitive Psychology* 12(1): 97–136.

Treue, S. and Martinez Trujillo, J. C. (1999). Feature-based attention influences motion processing gain in macaque visual cortex. *Nature* 399(6736): 575–579.

Vallar, G. (1993). The anatomical basis of spatial neglect in humans. In I. H. Robertson and J. C. Marshall (eds.), *Unilateral Neglect: Clinical and Experimental Studies* (pp. 27–62). Hillsdale, N.J.: Erlbaum.

Vallar, G. and Perani, D. (1987). The anatomy of unilateral neglect after right-hemisphere stroke lesions: A clinical/CT-scan correlation study in man. *Neuropsychologia* 24: 609–622.

Vanduffel, W., Tootell, R. B., and Orban, G. A. (2000). Attention-dependent suppression of metabolic activity in the early stages of the macaque visual system. *Cerebral Cortex* 10(2): 109–126.

Watanabe, T., Harner, A. M., Miyauchi, S., Sasaki, Y., Nielsen, M., Palomo, D., and Mukai, I. (1998). Task-dependent influences of attention on the activation of human primary visual cortex. *Proceedings of the National Academy of Sciences USA* 95(19): 11489–11492.

Wertheimer, M. (1923). Untersuchungen zur Lehre von der Gestalt II. Psychologische Forschung 4: 301–350. Translation in W. D. Ellis (ed.), *A Sourcebook of Gestalt Psychology* (pp. 71–88). London: Routledge & Kegan Paul.

White, A. L. and Carrasco, M. (2011). Feature-based attention involuntarily and simultaneously improves visual performance across locations. *Journal of Vision* 11(6): Article 15.

Williford, T. and Maunsell, J. H. (2006). Effects of spatial attention on contrast response functions in macaque area V4. *Journal of Neurophysiology* 96(1): 40–54.

Yantis, S., Schwarzbach, J., Serences, J. T., Carlson, R. A., Steinmetz, M. A., Pekar, J. J., and Courtney, S. M. (2002). Transient neural activity in human parietal cortex during spatial attention shifts. *Nature Neuroscience* 5(10): 995–1002.

Yeshurun, Y. and Carrasco, M. (1998). Attention improves or impairs visual performance by enhancing spatial resolution. *Nature* 396(6706): 72–75.

Zhou, H., Friedman, H. S., and von der Heydt, R. (2000). Coding of border ownership in monkey visual cortex. *Journal of Neuroscience* 20(17): 6594–6611.

CHAPTER 10

THE TIME COURSE OF SPATIAL ATTENTION: INSIGHTS FROM EVENT-RELATED BRAIN POTENTIALS

MARTIN EIMER

INTRODUCTION

FOR many years, human perception, cognition, and action, and the role of attentional mechanisms in these domains, have been studied primarily with behavioural measures. The ability to measure neural correlates of these processes is a relatively recent achievement, and event-related potential (ERP) research was at the forefront of this development. Although electroencephalographic (EEG) recordings of human brain activity date back to the 1920s, the method of averaging stimulus-locked EEG activity, and using the resulting ERP waveforms to study cognitive processes, started in a systematic fashion only in the late 1960s. ERPs reflect the synchronized postsynaptic activity of a large number of cortical neurons that is time-locked to specific external or internal events. Typical ERP waveforms consist of a series of successive positive and negative deflections or peaks that are often referred to as ERP components. The ERP technique is attractive to cognitive neuroscientists because of its excellent temporal resolution: ERPs can trace electrical brain activity on a millisecond-by-millisecond basis, and the effects of an experimental manipulation on a distinct ERP component at a specific post-stimulus latency can be helpful to develop models of the temporal organization of human cognitive abilities. But due to the properties of electrical volume conduction inside the head and across the skull, and because of complex interactions between several simultaneously active neural generator processes, ERP scalp recordings provide only limited information about the localization of underlying brain processes. Although several methods of reconstructing sources of electrical activity in the brain on the basis of scalp recordings are available, their precision and spatial resolution are not comparable to those of other neuroimaging methods such as fMRI. For this reason, this chapter will focus primarily on research that has used ERP measures to study specific questions about the time course of attentional processing.

The central theoretical issues addressed by attention researchers have changed considerably in the past 40 years, and so have the questions that have been investigated with ERP measures during this period. Traditional models of selective attention have postulated a fundamental distinction between early, capacity-unlimited, and parallel processing stages, and late, capacity-limited, and serial stages. This view, which was most influentially expressed in Donald Broadbent's Filter Theory of Attention (1958), characterizes selective attention as the mechanism that gates the access of perceptual information to late capacity-limited processes. If attention acts as a filter that controls the transition between early parallel and late serial processing stages, it is important to identify where and when in the information processing hierarchy the transition point between early pre-attentive and late attentive mechanisms is located. Because of their excellent temporal resolution, ERP measures have played a prominent role in this quest to specify the locus of attentional selection, and this role will be reviewed in the second section of this chapter.

In the past twenty years, attention research has moved beyond the traditional debate about early versus late selection. Attempts to develop general models of attentional selectivity have been replaced by investigations of more specific theoretical issues, and this change in emphasis is also reflected by contemporary ERP research on selective attention. As will be described in the third section, it has now become clear that the mechanisms of spatial attention do not operate in a strict modality-specific fashion, but that there are instead strong crossmodal links in spatially selective attentional processing between vision, audition, and touch. In addition, an important distinction has been proposed between control processes in modality-unspecific fronto-parietal regions (the 'source' of top-down attentional control) and attentional modulations of processing in modality-specific sensory areas (the 'sites' where top-down control signals produce their selective effects).

Another major focus of contemporary attention research is the study of competitive interactions between relevant stimuli and distractors in situations where multiple stimuli are simultaneously present. Biased competition accounts of selective attention (e.g. Desimone and Duncan 1995; Beck and Kastner 2009) describe attentional phenomena as the consequence of such competitions for neural and cognitive representation. This competition takes place at different levels of processing, and its outcome is controlled both by top-down selection intentions and bottom-up salience. Visual search paradigms have been particularly useful to study competitive mechanisms in attention, and ERP measures of attentional selectivity have become important tools to investigate the temporal dynamics of competitive interactions in multi-stimulus visual scenes. In the fourth section of this chapter, the N2pc component is introduced as an important ERP correlate of the attentional selection of targets among non-targets. The final section presents ERP research that has used the N2pc component to address two critical questions about the temporal organization of stimulus selection in visual search. First, do all stimuli in a multi-stimulus array compete in parallel for attentional selection, or is attention allocated sequentially to specific stimulus locations in the visual field? And second, is the selection of perceptually distinct visual events determined by top-down search intentions, or driven by their bottom-up salience?

The Locus of Attentional Selectivity: Early Versus Late Selection

The historically most influential conceptualization of selective attention in modern times is undoubtedly the filter model proposed by Donald Broadbent (1958). According to this model, basic physical attributes of incoming sensory information are initially analysed in parallel, and the results of this parallel processing stage are stored in an unlimited-capacity short-term buffer. Because subsequent processing stages such as semantic analysis and response selection operate in a serial and capacity-limited fashion, only a fraction of the content stored in the short-term buffer can gain access to these stages. Selective attention acts as a gatekeeper that controls which stimuli are permitted to make the transition from parallel to serial processing. In the filter model, attentional selection is 'early', because it operates on the basis of low-level physical stimulus features that are represented in the short-term buffer, and precedes the semantic analysis of selected stimuli. This early selection hypothesis has not gone unchallenged. Others (e.g. Deutsch and Deutsch 1963) have proposed that selective attention operates at a 'late' stage that follows the semantic analysis of attended as well as unattended stimuli.

The debate whether attentional selection is 'early' or 'late' has dominated mainstream attention research for decades. The critical assumption was that there is a fundamental division in human information processing between early, unlimited-capacity, parallel, and pre-attentive stages, and late, limited-capacity, serial, and attentive stages. If this basic dichotomy does in fact exist, it is important to determine exactly where and when the transition from pre-attentive to attentive processing occurs. It has proved to be remarkably difficult to find a decisive answer to this critical question on the basis of behavioural measures, and this is one reason why the early-versus-late selection controversy has remained an active concern for attention researchers over many years. Because this locus-of-selection debate is essentially a disagreement about the temporal organization of functionally defined stages of information processing, the ability of ERPs to provide high temporal resolution measures of cognitive processing has come to play an important role in this debate.

In early ERP studies of auditory and visual selective attention (e.g. Hillyard et al. 1973; Van Voorhis and Hillyard 1977), ERPs were recorded to physically identical stimuli in two different conditions where attention was either directed to the location of these stimuli, or was focused at a different location. Results demonstrated that ERP differences between these two conditions emerged remarkably early after stimulus onset: In audition, selective attention resulted in amplitude modulations of the auditory Nl component that started around 80 ms after stimulus onset (Hillyard et al. 1973). In vision, the earliest attentional modulations were observed for the Pl component, which also has a typical post-stimulus onset latency of 80–90 ms (Van Voorhis and Hillyard 1977). In these pioneering ERP investigations of selective spatial attention, participants were usually instructed at the start of each block to direct their attention to one specific location and to keep it focused at this location for an entire experimental block. Later studies have demonstrated that very similar attentional ERP modulations at short post-stimulus latencies are also triggered when the focus of spatial attention is not sustained for an extended period, but is instead manipulated in a trial-by-trial fashion by pre-cues such as left-pointing or right-pointing arrows (e.g. Mangun and Hillyard 1991; Eimer 1994).

Figure 10.1 illustrates the typical pattern of spatial attention effects on visual ERPs observed in an experiment where the focus of spatial attention was manipulated on a trial-by-trial basis (Eimer and Schröger 1998). On each trial, a single stimulus was presented to the left or right of fixation, and was preceded by an arrow cue. Participants had to direct their attention to the side indicated by the cue, in order to detect and respond to infrequent visual target stimuli on that side, while ignoring all stimuli on the opposite uncued side. The ERPs in Fig. 10.1 were recorded from occipital electrodes over the hemisphere contralateral to the side of a visual stimulus, separately for stimuli that appeared on the attended side, and stimuli that were presented on the uncued/unattended side. The earliest attentional modulation was an increase in the amplitude of the Pl component for attended stimuli. This effect started approximately 80 ms after stimulus onset, and was followed by an attentional enhancement of the Nl component, and then by a sustained 'processing negativity' for attended visual stimuli that emerged after more than 200 ms following stimulus onset. The ERP effects shown in Fig. 10.1 have been observed in many ERP studies of visual-spatial attention. Attentional enhancements on Pl amplitudes are often interpreted as the effect of sensory gain control mechanisms that are activated during preparatory shifts of attention towards likely target location. Nl amplitude modulations have been linked to the active engagement of attention at a specific location (e.g. Mangun and Hillyard 1991; Mangun 1995). Attention-induced ERP modulations at post-stimulus latencies of 200 ms and beyond are usually linked to subsequent post-perceptual processing stages (e.g. stimulus identification and/or classification of response-relevant features; e.g. Mangun and Hillyard 1991; Eimer 1996a).

The consistent finding that ERP effects of sustained or transient spatial attention emerge at post-stimulus latencies of 100 ms or even earlier is often interpreted as evidence in support of early selection accounts. At latencies where the visual Pl or auditory Nl components are generated, sensory signals are still processed in modality-specific visual or auditory cortical areas. In the first 100 ms after stimulus onset, sensory

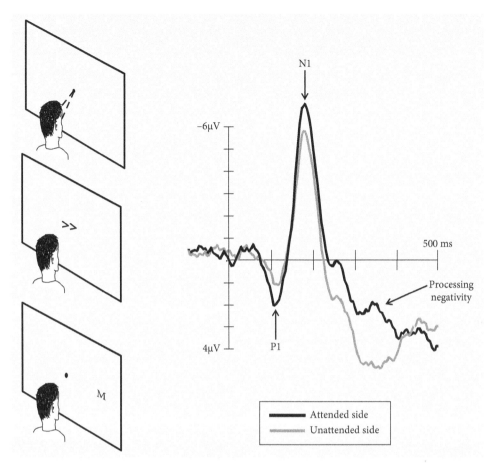

FIGURE 10.1 ERPs triggered in response to laterally presented visual stimuli in an experiment where these stimuli were preceded by arrow pre-cues that signalled the to-be-attended location for a visual target/non-target discrimination on that trial. ERP waveforms were measured at lateral occipital electrodes contralateral to the side where the stimulus was presented, and are shown separately for visual stimuli on the cued/attended side and on the uncued/unattended side. Cued visual-spatial attention produces amplitude enhancements of visual Pl and Nl components and a later sustained processing negativity. Data from Eimer and Schröger (1998), E. ERP effects of intermodal attention and cross-modal links in spatial attention. *Psychophysiology* 35, pp. 313–327, 1998.

processing is assumed to proceed in a feedforward fashion, prior to any effects of recurrent modulatory input from higher-level control areas on activity in lower-level cortical regions (Lamme and Roelfsema 2000). Source localization studies (e.g. Di Russo et al. 2003) have indeed suggested that the neural generators responsible for the visual Pl component are located in relatively early extrastriate cortical regions in middle and ventral occipital cortex, which correspond to visual areas V3 and V4. These observations suggest a direct link between attentional effects on the amplitudes of early sensory-specific ERP components and spatially selective attentional modulations of early stages of sensory-perceptual processing, which is consistent with early selection models of attention. Importantly, there is other ERP evidence which strongly suggests that the initial activation of primary visual cortex (VI) by incoming sensory events is not affected by attention. The arrival of visual input in VI is reflected by the Cl component, which is triggered approximately 60 ms after stimulus onset, and shows a retinotopic pattern of polarity inversion for stimuli in the upper versus lower visual field (Clark et al. 1995) that strongly points to the calcarine sulcus (which contains area VI) as its origin. In marked contrast to Pl and Nl components, Cl amplitudes remain unaffected by manipulations of spatial attention (e.g. Martínez et al. 1999). The attention-independence of the Cl component and the strong attention-sensitivity of subsequent Pl and Nl components provide temporally precise evidence for the earliest locus of spatial selectivity in the visual processing hierarchy: The initial activation of primary visual cortex that is triggered within 50 or 60 ms after stimulus onset by afferent signals in the geniculostriate pathway can be regarded as genuinely pre-attentive, because it is not modulated by the current focus of spatial attention. In contrast, neural activity in adjacent extrastriate visual cortical areas that is elicited only 20–30 ms after the initial VI activation is selectively enhanced for visual events that originate from attended locations, and thus marks the transition from pre-attentive to attention-sensitive visual processing.

The observation that spatial attention affects the amplitudes of visual and auditory ERP components which originate in sensory-specific cortical areas and are triggered at post-stimulus latencies of less than 100 ms demonstrates beyond reasonable doubt that brain activity during these early stages of sensory processing is subject to attentional modulations. But documenting early attention-induced effects on activation levels in visual or auditory cortex does not by itself provide conclusive evidence for the veracity of the early selection theories of attention such as Broadbent's filter model. It is problematic to directly link the concept of 'attentional selection', as defined in cognitive-psychological debates about the locus of selectivity, and attention-induced amplitude modulations of visual Pl or Nl components. What such ERP effects demonstrate is that the level of neural activation triggered in modality-specific cortical areas is selectively affected by the location of a sensory stimulus within or outside the current focus of spatial attention. But this does not represent selective attentional processing in the sense that is invoked by models which describe the function of attention as allowing specific stimuli access to limited-capacity serial processing stages, and preventing access by other stimuli. Additional arguments are clearly required before attentional effects on the amplitudes of early ERP components (i.e. short-latency modulations of cortical processing) can be interpreted as directly reflecting the transition of sensory information from parallel pre-attentive to serial capacity-limited processing stages.

Another caveat against an uncritical interpretation of spatial attention effects on visual Pl and auditory Nl components as directly demonstrating the early locus of selection comes from the fact that the presence of such effects does by no means preclude the existence of additional attention-induced ERP modulations at later post-stimulus latencies. In fact, many studies have reported effects of selective attention on ERP components that are elicited between 200 ms and 800 ms after stimulus onset and often do not show a sensory-specific scalp topography. These effects are likely to be generated at processing stages that follow the sensory-perceptual analysis of incoming stimuli. Figure 10.1 shows one example for a late effect of spatial attention—the sustained 'processing negativity' that is frequently triggered by potentially task-relevant visual stimuli at attended locations and emerges beyond 200 ms post-stimulus. This enhanced posterior negativity for stimuli at attended versus unattended locations has been linked to stimulus identification and categorization, which often involves their comparison to stored representations of target-defining visual features (e.g. Eimer 1994, 1996a).

ERP evidence for an even later locus of attentional selectivity has come from experiments that employed the attentional blink (AB) paradigm. In AB experiments, two targets are embedded in a rapidly presented sequential stream of distractors. Detection of the second target (T2) is greatly impaired when it is presented in close temporal proximity to the first target (Tl), indicating attentional suppression of T2 processing while Tl is still being analysed (Raymond et al. 1992). To locate the stage at which this suppression takes place, Luck et al. (1996) recorded ERPs in response to T2 stimuli (words) when these were presented during the critical attentional blink interval. Interestingly, there was no attenuation of visual Pl and Nl components, suggesting that perceptual processes were unaffected by attentional suppression. Even more surprisingly, a later ERP component that is associated with semantic processing of words (the N400 component) also remained present during the attentional blink, indicating that in spite of their attentional inhibition, T2 words were still semantically analysed. The one ERP component that was suppressed during the attentional blink interval was the P3, which is often linked to the updating of working memory. These results are clearly inconsistent with the hypothesis that the locus of attentional selectivity is invariably early, because they show that the attentional blink is a post-perceptual effect which is produced at a late stage of information processing which follows semantic identification (e.g. Vogel et al. 1998).

In summary, many ERP studies investigating the locus of attentional selectivity have found evidence for attention-induced modulations of early sensory-perceptual stages of stimulus processing, while others have demonstrated that attention can also affect later stages of processing. These findings suggest that the traditional question whether selective attention is early or late represents a false dichotomy, because attention can operate at different processing stages, and within different cognitive subsystems and cortical areas. This insight is one of the reasons why the search for the locus of selection is no longer regarded as the single most important task for attention researchers. Another reason is that the general theoretical background that motivated this search has now been called into question. This includes the idea that human information processing is organized in a strict serial sequence of processing stages, and that the locus of the attentional bottleneck can be uniquely identified within this sequence (see Allport 1993, for an early incisive critique of these assumptions). The new consensus is that the locus of attentional selectivity can be shifted flexibly and rapidly between stages and subsystems, in accordance with a variety of factors that include stimulus parameters, current task demands, and top-down selection intentions. But ERP measures of attention-induced processing modulations remain valuable, because they allow researchers to track variable loci of attentional selectivity across a wide variety of task contexts.

CROSSMODAL LINKS IN SPATIAL ATTENTION

Information about external objects and events is often conveyed simultaneously and independently by different sensory systems. However, this information is initially represented within modality-specific coordinate systems (retinotopic in vision, somatotopic in touch, tonotopic in audition), and this makes its integration and the attentional selection of objects that are specified by multisensory signals a non-trivial problem. Spatially selective processing can help to solve this problem, as visual, auditory, or tactile information about the same object originates from the same location in external space. If attentional selectivity is integrated across perceptual modalities, this should be reflected by spatial synergies in the processing of sensory events across vision, audition, and touch. Behavioural studies of crossmodal links in voluntary (endogenous) spatial attention between vision and audition (e.g. Spence and Driver 1996) or vision and touch (e.g. Spence et al. 2000) have indeed demonstrated the existence of such synergies (see Robbins (chapter 18), this volume, for a detailed discussion). In these experiments, attention was directed to the expected location of target stimuli within one primary modality. Stimuli in the other (secondary) modality were presented only infrequently, and were equally likely (or even more likely) to appear on the side that was unattended in the primary modality. In spite of these contingencies, performance in response to secondary modality targets was superior when they appeared on the side that was attended in the primary modality. These results demonstrate that the locus of endogenous attention within one modality (that is, a spatial expectancy that is specific for that modality) affects the processing of information in other modalities. Similarly, rapid shifts of involuntary (exogenous) spatial attention triggered by salient but irrelevant stimuli in one modality modulate performance to subsequently presented stimuli in another modality, demonstrating the existence of crossmodal spatial links in exogenous attention (e.g. McDonald et al. 2000).

   While such behavioural observations demonstrate the existence of crossmodal links in spatial attention, they cannot provide direct insight into the locus of such spatial synergies at perceptual and/or post-perceptual processing stages. Because they provide temporally precise markers of attentional effects, ERP measures have been used in many studies to find out when and how crossmodal spatial synergies in endogenous or exogenous attention affect the processing of visual, auditory, and tactile stimuli. In a typical ERP experiment of crossmodal links between vision and touch (Eimer and Driver 2000), visual stimuli were delivered via light-emitting diodes (LEDs), and tactile stimuli by punctators attached to the left and right index finger, close to the location of the LED on the same side (Fig. 10.2, top panel). Participants directed attention to the left or right side, in order to detect and to respond to infrequent targets in one primary modality on the attended side, while ignoring stimuli in the other secondary modality on that side,

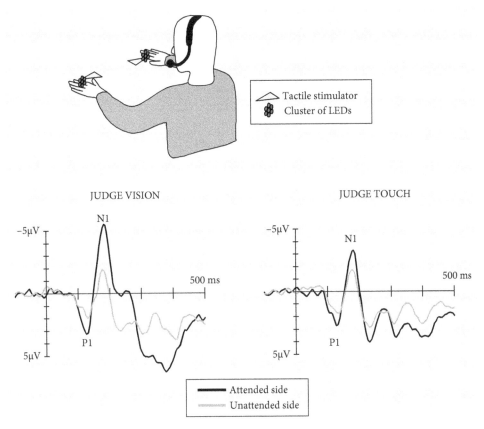

FIGURE 10.2 ERPs triggered in an experiment on crossmodal attention where observers directed attention to the left or right side for a visual or tactile task. Visual stimuli were delivered via LEDs, tactile events via punctators. ERPs were recorded in response to laterally presented visual stimuli at contralateral posterior electrodes. In the 'Judge Vision' task, visual stimuli on the attended side triggered larger Pl and Nl amplitudes relative to visual stimuli on the opposite unattended side. In the 'Judge Touch' task where visual stimuli could be entirely ignored, visual ERP components were generally reduced in amplitude, but attentional modulations of Pl and Nl components were still present. Data from Eimer and Driver (2000). Data from Eimer, M. and Driver, J., An event-related brain potential study of cross-modal links in spatial attention between vision and touch. *Psychophysiology* 37, pp. 697–705, 2000.

as well as stimuli in either modality on the unattended side. Attentional modulations of visual and somatosensory ERPs were measured separately for blocks where vision was the attended modality ('Judge Vision'), and for blocks where touch was task-relevant and therefore attended ('Judge Touch').

Figure 10.2 (bottom panels) shows ERPs measured at occipital electrodes contralateral to the visual field of stimulus presentation in response to visual stimuli on the currently attended side or on the opposite unattended side. As expected, attended visual stimuli triggered enhanced Pl and Nl components in 'Judge Vision' blocks where vision was the task-relevant modality, thus confirming that visual-spatial attention modulates activity in early visual areas (see the second section above). In 'Judge Touch' blocks, Pl and Nl components in response to visual stimuli were generally smaller than in 'Judge Vision' blocks, demonstrating that when attention is directed away from vision towards a different task-relevant sensory modality, activation of visual cortical areas is reduced. But even more importantly, early spatially selective modulations of visual ERPs were still reliably present in 'Judge Touch' blocks: Visual stimuli presented next to tactually attended locations elicited larger Pl and Nl components than visual stimuli close to the opposite unattended hand, in spite of the fact that participants focused spatial attention solely on the relevant location of tactile events and visual stimuli could be entirely ignored. The observation that attentional modulations of visual ERPs in 'Judge Touch' blocks started within 100 ms after stimulus onset not only provides strong evidence for the existence of crossmodal links in spatial attention, but also demonstrates that links from touch to vision affect early perceptual stages of visual processing. Analogous results were obtained in the same study for ERP components in response to tactile events that were measured over somatosensory cortex: Tactile stimuli at attended locations triggered enhanced sensory-specific N140 components, and this was the case not only in blocks where touch was the task-relevant modality, but also in blocks where vision was primary. Other studies (e.g. Eimer and Schröger 1998; Teder-Sälejärvi et al. 1999) found similar ERP evidence for the existence of symmetrical crossmodal spatial synergies between vision and audition, and have demonstrated that such audiovisual attentional links modulate early perceptual stages of visual and auditory processing.

While these results demonstrate the existence of crossmodal links for endogenous shifts of spatial attention, other ERP studies have studied spatial synergies in involuntary (exogenous) spatial attention. McDonald and Ward (2000) measured ERPs to visual target stimuli that were preceded by spatially uninformative but salient auditory events at the same or at a different location. Responses to visual stimuli were faster on same-location as compared to different-location trials. Critically, this behavioural benefit was accompanied by an enhancement of occipital ERP components for visual stimuli that appeared at the same location as a preceding auditory event, suggesting that crossmodal links in exogenous spatial attention modulate early perceptual stages of visual processing. Along similar lines, salient but irrelevant tactile events improve discrimination performance and trigger enhanced early ERP components in response to subsequent visual stimuli that are presented at the same location (Kennett et al. 2001). Overall, these findings demonstrate that spatial synergies across sensory modalities exist for both endogenous and exogenous attention, and that these synergies modulate the sensory-perceptual processing of visual, auditory, or tactile stimuli at short post-stimulus latencies.

The question remains whether such spatial synergies across sensory modalities, as reflected by ERP effects of crossmodal spatial attention, are due to fixed and possibly hard-wired links between modalities, or instead just reflect a default preference for shifting attention simultaneously to the same locations in different modalities when this does not impair task performance. To answer this question, an experiment was conducted where participants had to detect infrequently presented single visual or auditory targets in the left or right hemifield (Eimer 1999). In Same-Side blocks, attention was directed to the same location in both modalities, because response-relevant visual or auditory targets always appeared at the same location. In Opposite-Side blocks, attention had to be directed to opposite sides in vision and audition, as visual targets had to be detected on the left, and auditory targets on the right, or vice versa. ERP results in Same-Side blocks were as expected (Fig. 10.3, left side): Relative to stimuli on the unattended side, attended visual stimuli elicited enhanced Pl and Nl components and a later sustained processing negativity. A very different pattern of results was observed in Opposite-Side blocks (Fig. 10.3, right side): There were no enhancements of visual Pl and Nl components in response to stimuli on the visually attended side when auditory attention had to be simultaneously directed to the opposite side. Under these conditions, spatially selective ERP effects only emerged at about 200 ms post-stimulus in the form of a sustained processing negativity. Analogous results were observed for auditory ERPs (not shown in Fig. 10.3): In Same-Side blocks, attended auditory stimuli triggered an enhanced negativity that started around 100 ms after stimulus onset and overlapped with the auditory Nl component. In Opposite-Side blocks, this early effect was eliminated. Overall, these findings strongly suggest that spatial synergies between sensory modalities observed in behavioural and ERP studies of crossmodal attention do not just

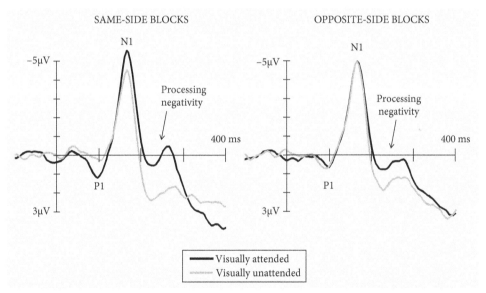

FIGURE 10.3 ERPs triggered in response to laterally presented visual stimuli at contralateral posterior electrodes in an audiovisual experiment. In Same-Side blocks, participants directed their visual and auditory attention to the same side in order to detect infrequent visual or auditory targets on that side. Here, larger Pl and Nl amplitudes and a sustained processing negativity were elicited by visual stimuli on the attended side relative to stimuli on the opposite unattended side. In Opposite-Side blocks, where visual and auditory attention were directed to opposite sides, attentional Pl and Nl modulations were completely eliminated and only the late processing negativity remained present. Data from Eimer (1999). Data from Eimer, M., Can attention be directed to opposite locations in different modalities? An ERP study. *Clinical Neurophysiology* 110, pp. 1252–1259, 1999.

reflect optional attentional allocation strategies, but more permanent, and perhaps even hard-wired links in spatially selective processing across different sensory systems.

While the existence of crossmodal spatial synergies in attentional processing is an important phenomenon in its own right, it may also provide valuable clues about how attentional control mechanisms that initiate and guide shifts of attention are organized. For example, it has been suggested that the control of spatial orienting in different sensory modalities is implemented by a single supramodal system (e.g. Farah et al. 1989). If attentional control was indeed supramodal, strong crossmodal links in spatial attention between vision, audition, and touch would be an obvious consequence. While control processes involved in directing visual-spatial attention have been studied most prominently with fMRI measures (e.g. Corbetta and Shulman 2002; Beck and Kastner 2009; see also chapters 4, 5, and 9, this volume), important insights into the temporal organization of these processes have been obtained in ERP studies. In these studies, ERPs were recorded in response to symbolic central cues that directed attention to the left or right side, during the interval prior to the arrival of a subsequent imperative stimulus. Activity unrelated to spatial attention shifts, such as sensory responses to the cue, or ERP correlates of temporal attention, was eliminated by subtracting ERP waveforms obtained during rightward attentional shifts from ERPs during shifts of attention to the left side. It is important to note that this procedure also removes ERP correlates of top-down attentional control that do differ during the orienting of attention to the left versus right side.

In a pioneering study by Harter et al. (1989), an early negative deflection at posterior electrodes contralateral to the direction of an attentional shift ('Early Directing Attention Negativity'; EDAN) emerged around 200 ms after cue onset, and was followed at about 500 ms post-stimulus by a posterior contralateral positivity ('Late Directing Attention Positivity'; LDAP). Later studies (e.g. Nobre et al. 2000) have also observed an enhanced negativity at frontal electrodes contralateral to the direction of attentional shifts ('Anterior Directing Attention Negativity'; ADAN) with an onset latency of 300–400 ms after cue onset. The earliest of these components (EDAN) may not be a genuine reflection of covert attentional control, but instead a lateralized visual response to non-symmetrical visual cues such as left-pointing and right-pointing arrows (Van Velzen and Eimer 2003). The ADAN is assumed to reflect the activation of dorsolateral frontal control processes that are involved in programming and initiating shifts of attention (Nobre et al. 2000). In line with this hypothesis, source localization studies have placed the neural generators of the ADAN component in lateral premotor cortex (e.g. Praamstra et al. 2005). The LDAP has been linked to preparatory changes in the excitability of ventral occipitotemporal visual areas in anticipation of an expected visual stimulus at a specific location (Harter et al. 1989).

While most research on ERP correlates of preparatory spatial orienting has investigated shifts of visual attention, other studies have demonstrated that ADAN and LDAP components are also triggered in tasks where attention is directed towards the cued location of auditory or tactile events (e.g. Eimer et al. 2002; Green et al. 2005). This is illustrated in Fig. 10.4, which shows ERPs elicited during rightward and leftward

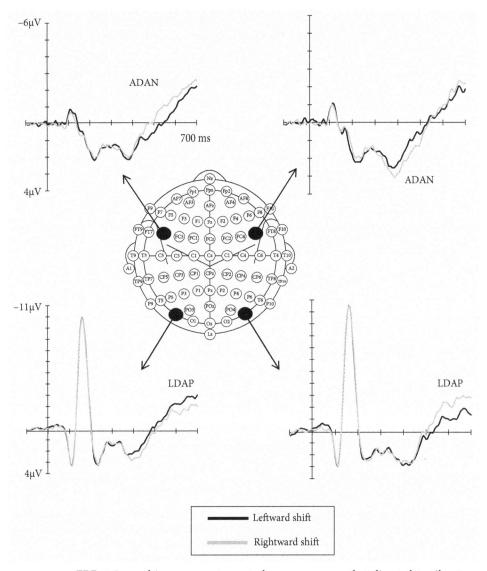

FIGURE 10.4 ERPs triggered in response to central arrow pre-cues that directed tactile attention to the left or right side in an experiment where participants had to detect infrequent tactile targets that were delivered to the hand on the cued side. The top panel shows ERPs from the fronto-central electrode pair FC5/6, where the anterior directing attention negativity (ADAN) was elicited at electrodes contralateral to the side of a cued attentional shift. The bottom panel shows ERPs from the posterior electrode pair PO7/8, where the late directing attention positivity (LDAP) emerged contralateral to the side of the attentional shift. Data from Eimer, M., Van Velzen, J., and Driver, J., Crossmodal interactions between audition, touch and vision in endogenous spatial attention: ERP evidence on preparatory states and sensory modulations. *Journal of Cognitive Neuroscience* 14, pp. 254–271, 2002.

shifts of tactile attention in the 700 ms interval following the onset of a central spatial pre-cue, and prior to the presentation of an imperative stimulus on the left or right side. Observers were instructed by the cue to direct their attention to their left or right hand, in order to discriminate tactile targets and non-targets that were delivered to the index finger of the cued hand. The top panels in Fig. 10.4 show ERPs recorded at a lateral fronto-central electrode pair (FC5 and FC6), the bottom panels show ERPs recorded at a lateral posterior electrode pair (PO7 and PO8). Shifts of tactile attention were accompanied by an enhanced contralateral negativity at anterior fronto-central electrodes (ADAN) that emerged at about 350 ms after cue onset, and a contralateral positivity at posterior electrodes (LDAP) with a post-cue onset latency of approximately 500 ms. Critically, these lateralized components were very similar to ERP effects previously observed during shifts of visual-spatial attention. In addition, virtually identical ADAN and LDAP components were observed in the same study (Eimer et al. 2002) in another task where observers were cued to direct their attention to the location of task-relevant auditory events.

The presence and similarity of ADAN and LDAP components during shifts of visual, tactile, and auditory attention seems to provide strong support for the hypothesis that spatial orienting is controlled by a single multimodal system (Farah et al. 1989). However, alternative interpretations remain viable. It is possible that even when auditory or tactile stimuli are task-relevant, shifts of spatial attention towards these stimuli are always controlled by visual-spatial information, because vision provides superior spatial acuity relative to hearing or touch, and therefore allows a more precise tuning of focal attention. If this was correct, lateralized ERP components that are measured during attentional shifts towards anticipated tactile or auditory events would primarily reflect shifts of attention within visual space. This hypothesis was tested by measuring ERP correlates of attentional orienting in congenitally blind people. Due to the absence of any visual input, the congenitally blind cannot develop a visually defined spatial frame of reference that could guide preparatory shifts of attention towards auditory or tactile events. In a study with congenitally blind participants that measured ERPs during cued attention shifts towards task-relevant tactile stimuli (Van Velzen et al. 2006), the ADAN component was clearly present, indicating that this component reflects attentional control processes that do not rely on visually coded representations of external space. In contrast, the posterior LDAP component was absent in the congenitally blind, which suggests that the preparatory attentional mechanisms associated with this component are strongly dependent upon visually defined spatial reference frames. This dissociation suggests that ADAN and LDAP components may be linked to functionally separable control mechanisms that mediate the control of attentional shifts within vision-independent egocentric/somatotopic and visually mediated allocentric/external frames of reference, respectively.

In summary, the ERP research reviewed in this section has demonstrated the existence of strong spatial synergies in endogenous and exogenous spatial attention between vision, audition, and touch. It has shown that these synergies modulate perceptual processing in modality-specific sensory cortices, that they reflect permanent links rather than optional strategies, and that there are remarkable similarities in ERP correlates of top-down attentional control across modalities. Such observations are in line with two interpretations, which are not necessarily mutually exclusive. Some aspects of attentional control may be genuinely supramodal, while others may be dominated by visually coded spatial representations, irrespective of whether attention is directed in vision, audition, or touch.

THE N2PC COMPONENT AND ATTENTIONAL TARGET SELECTION IN VISUAL SEARCH

Most of the ERP studies discussed so far have employed experimental designs where attention is directed in advance to a particular location, and a single stimulus is then presented at this attended location or at a different unattended position in the visual field. This research has demonstrated that spatial attention can modulate sensory activity generated at early stages of perceptual processing, and that shifts of spatial attention and their effects on sensory modulations show remarkable spatial synergies across vision, audition, and touch. However, other important aspects of attentional processing cannot be directly assessed with such experimental designs. In many situations, multiple simultaneous stimuli compete for the control of perception and action, and no advance spatial information is available to guide selective attention towards the location of anticipated task-relevant events. Under such circumstances, a critical function of attention is to resolve the competition between different stimuli in favour of those that are relevant to current task goals, and to filter out others that are not (Desimone and Duncan 1995). To identify mechanisms that operate when there is competition for attentional selection, procedures where single stimuli are presented in an otherwise empty field are insufficient, and multi-stimulus paradigms such as visual search tasks need to be employed.

In visual search experiments, observers are presented with visual arrays that can contain numerous items. Their task is to report the presence or absence of a predefined target among distractors. The detection of targets is fast and efficient when they can be distinguished from distractors on the basis of a unique feature, and less efficient when they are defined by a conjunction of features (Treisman and Gelade 1980). An important electrophysiological marker of attentional target selection in visual search is the N2pc component. This component, which was first described by Luck and colleagues (Luck et al. 1993; Luck and Hillyard 1994a, 1994b), represents an enhanced negativity at posterior electrodes contralateral to the target's visual field, and usually emerges around 200 ms after search array onset. This is illustrated in Fig. 10.5, which shows N2pc components measured in response to search arrays that contained a uniquely coloured diamond target (Mazza et al. 2007). In different blocks, observers either had the relatively easy task of localizing these targets in the left versus right hemifield, or the more difficult

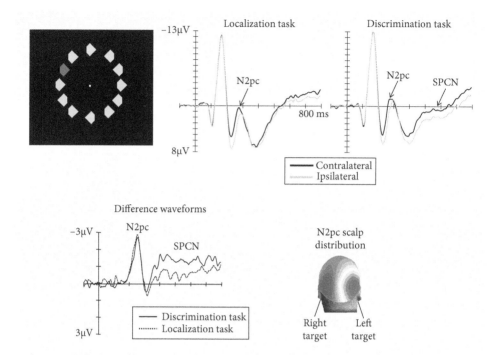

FIGURE 10.5 ERPs triggered at posterior electrodes PO7/8 contralateral and ipsilateral to the target side in response to visual search arrays that contained a colour singleton target diamond. Results are shown separately for an easy target localization task and a more difficult target discrimination task. The bottom panels show difference waveforms obtained by subtracting ipsilateral from contralateral ERPs, and a topographic scalp distribution map (back-of-the-head view) of the N2pc component. N2pc components did not differ between the two tasks, but the subsequent sustained posterior contralateral negativity (SPCN) was larger in the discrimination task. Data from Mazza, V., Turatto, M., Umiltà, C., and Eimer, M., Attentional selection and identification of visual objects are reflected by distinct electrophysiological responses. *Experimental Brain Research* 181, pp. 531–536, 2007.

task of discriminating on which side the target diamond had a cut. Very similar N2pc components were triggered in both tasks (Fig. 10.5, top panels). Difference waveforms obtained by subtracting ipsilateral from contralateral ERP waveforms (Fig. 10.5, bottom left) show that N2pc amplitudes and onset latencies were virtually identical in both tasks, even though the discrimination task was much more difficult. This result suggests that the N2pc component is generated during the initial attentional selection of targets among distractors that precedes the subsequent detailed analysis of specific target features. In contrast, a sustained posterior contralateral negativity (SPCN) that followed the N2pc and emerged around 350 ms after search array onset was much larger during the discrimination task. This SPCN component has also been observed during the retention period of working memory tasks and has been associated with the spatially selective activation of visual working memory (e.g. Vogel and Machizawa 2004).

The results shown in Fig. 10.5 demonstrate that N2pc components are triggered by singleton targets that can be discriminated from distractors on the basis of a unique feature (see also Luck and Hillyard 1994a). Other studies have observed an N2pc in response to targets that are defined by a feature conjunction (e.g. Luck et al. 1997). N2pc components are triggered not just by target items, but also by non-targets that possess target-defining features (Luck and Hillyard 1994b). In contrast, even highly salient stimuli such as orientation singletons do not elicit an N2pc when they are task-irrelevant (Luck and Hillyard 1994a). This latter observation underlines that the N2pc component is a genuine marker of spatially selective attentional processing, and not an artefact of asymmetric hemispheric activations that are caused by low-level physical differences between visual fields. Its distinct occipitotemporal focus and its sensitivity to the retinal location of target stimuli (Luck et al. 1997) strongly suggests that the N2pc is generated in retinotopically organized sensory-perceptual regions of visual cortex. Brain source localization analyses based on magnetoencephalographic (MEG) recordings have identified extrastriate occipitotemporal cortex as the main generator region of the N2pc, although activity in posterior parietal areas may also contribute to the early phase of this component (Hopf et al. 2000).

With respect to the functional interpretation of the N2pc, the first thing to note is that this component emerges about 100 ms later than the earliest effects of visual-spatial attention on the Pl component that were discussed in the second section above. Attentional Pl modulations are found in experiments where relevant locations are known in advance, and preparatory shifts of spatial attention can take place prior to target onset. The observation that Pl enhancements for visual events at attended locations are elicited for targets as well as for non-target stimuli (e.g. Mangun and Hillyard 1987), demonstrates that the underlying spatially specific modulations of visual processing precede the discrimination between targets and distractors. In contrast, the N2pc component is observed in visual search tasks where target locations are not cued in advance, and is triggered only by candidate target events, but not by events that lack target-defining features. These differences demonstrate that attention-induced Pl amplitude enhancements and N2pc components reflect qualitatively distinct attentional effects. The Pl component is triggered during the initial parallel feedforward sweep of visual processing (Lamme and Roelfsema 2000) and its attentional modulation reflects a pre-existing spatial bias that is the result of preparatory shifts of spatial attention prior to stimulus onset. In contrast, the N2pc component is triggered only after evidence for the presence of a task-relevant visual stimulus has been obtained in the course of the initial feedforward analysis of the visual field. If such evidence is present, control signals from higher-level attentional centres in posterior parietal cortex are sent to lower-level extrastriate visual cortex, where they induce spatially selective processing biases, which are reflected by the N2pc (Luckand Hillyard 1994b).

It is important to note that the N2pc indexes the selection of distinct visual objects, and not purely space-based selectivity: N2pc components are triggered when observers select the location of an anticipated target stimulus and this location is marked by a placeholder object, whereas no N2pc is triggered under otherwise identical circumstances in the absence of such placeholders (Woodman et al. 2009). Along similar lines, a study that combined spatial cueing procedures and a visual search paradigm (Kiss et al. 2008) has demonstrated that the N2pc is not associated with shifts of attention in visual space towards the location of anticipated target locations, but instead reflects the subsequent spatial selection of visual target stimuli.

The question whether the N2pc reflects target selection or distractor inhibition has been a matter of considerable debate. Results from early N2pc experiments have suggested that this component might be primarily associated with the inhibition of non-target stimuli. For example, N2pc components were observed for target stimuli that were surrounded by task-irrelevant distractors, but not when targets were presented in isolation (Luck and Hillyard 1994b). Furthermore, increasing the number of distractors, and thus the need for distractor inhibition, results in larger N2pc amplitudes (Mazza et al. 2009; see also Luck et al. 1997). Such observations have led to the suggestion that the N2pc component is an index for spatially selective distractor inhibition ('spatial filtering') that is activated when distractors and targets compete for attentional selection (Luck and Hillyard 1994b; Luck et al. 1997). Because distractor inhibition should be maximal when target and distractor items are presented in close proximity and thus are strong competitors (Desimone and Duncan 1995), the spatial filtering account implies that the N2pc should be sensitive to the relative spatial locations of targets and distractors. However, this prediction has not been supported by experimental results. An early study (Eimer 1996b) demonstrated that N2pc components are triggered by target stimuli that are presented in isolation in one visual hemifield, and are accompanied by a single distractor stimulus in the opposite hemifield. Under such conditions, target selection should require little if any distractor inhibition. Along similar lines, Mazza et al. (2009) have shown that N2pc amplitudes are unaffected by manipulations of the spatial proximity of targets and distractors, which is inconsistent with the inhibitory spatial filtering account. Such results suggest that the N2pc is primarily associated with the spatially selective attentional enhancement of target processing, rather than the selective inhibition of distractor items.

However, more recent findings suggest that the N2pc may reflect target enhancement as well as distractor suppression. Several ERP studies (Eimer and Kiss 2008; Hickey et al. 2009; Sawaki and Luck 2010) have reported a lateralized posterior ERP component in response to distractors that is similar to the N2pc in terms of its latency and topography, but shows an inverse polarity (i.e. a contralateral positivity rather than a contralateral negativity). For example, Hickey et al. (2009) found this distractor positivity (Pd) in response to lateral colour distractors in a task where observers had to discriminate the orientation of luminance targets that were located on the vertical meridian, and thus did not elicit any lateralized posterior ERP activity. They interpreted the Pd component as a marker of active distractor inhibition. Interestingly, no Pd was triggered by the same stimuli in a task that required only target detection, suggesting that distractors are only suppressed when the demands on attentional target processing are high. Similar results were reported by Sawaki and Luck (2010), who found a Pd component to salient colour distractors when observers searched for non-salient target letters. These authors concluded that attentional capture by salient but task-irrelevant stimuli can be prevented by active top-down suppression, and that the Pd reflects this inhibitory process. In line with this interpretation, a Pd component was also observed in a spatial cueing study (Eimer and Kiss 2008; see Fig. 10.7) in response to salient colour singleton cues in a task where participants searched for size-defined targets, and colour was therefore task-irrelevant. Overall, these recent findings suggest that N2pc components that are triggered in response to search arrays where a target appears among distractor items may be composed of two temporally overlapping subcomponents—a negativity contralateral to targets that reflects the attentional enhancement of target processing, and a positivity contralateral to distractors that is associated with their active inhibition. One important task for future ERP investigations into the mechanisms of selective attention in multi-stimulus arrays will be to verify the existence of a distinct Pd component and its relationship to distractor inhibition, and to provide a more detailed account of the relative roles of target enhancement and distractor suppression for the attentional selection of targets among non-targets in visual search.

ATTENTIONAL SELECTIVITY IN MULTI-STIMULUS ARRAYS: PARALLEL OR SERIAL AND BOTTOM-UP OR TOP-DOWN?

The question about the early versus late locus of selection (see the second section above) is not the only important debate among attention researchers that is focused on the time course of attentional selectivity. This final section discusses two other controversies that have arisen about the operation of selective attention in multi-stimulus arrays. Both controversies are based on disagreements about the time course of attentional processes, and both have been addressed with ERP measures of attentional target selection such as the N2pc component. The first debate to be discussed concerns the question whether the allocation of attention to candidate targets operates in a serial or parallel fashion. The other debate addresses the relative roles of top-down intentional control and bottom-up stimulus salience for attentional target selection.

In many visual search tasks, target detection time increases as the number of distractor items (set size) increases. This increase typically occurs when search targets share some features with non-targets, and when non-target items are perceptually heterogeneous (Duncan and Humphreys 1989), and has often been attributed to the necessity of serial visual search. For example, Feature Integration Theory (e.g. Treisman 1988) postulates that in difficult visual search tasks, attention has to be directed on one stimulus at a time and that the focus of attention switches between different objects in a serial fashion. The speed with which attention switches between individual objects has been calculated by measuring the increase in search time when set size is increased, which is typically between 20 and 80 ms per item. Others (e.g. Duncan et al. 1994; Ward et al. 1996) have argued that this procedure seriously underestimates the time demands of focal attentional processing, and that the correct 'attentional dwell time' is in the order of several hundreds of milliseconds. This is much longer than would be plausible for any strictly serial model of visual search, and therefore suggests an alternative parallel search scenario which does not involve a rapid serial focusing and re-allocation of spatial attention to individual stimuli. Instead, all visual objects compete in parallel for attentional processing, with target detection the result of a gradually evolving resolution of this competition (e.g. Desimone and Duncan 1995).

In a series of ERP studies, Woodman and Luck (1999, 2003) have used the N2pc component as a temporal marker of attentional target selection in perceptually demanding visual search tasks in order to discriminate between serial and parallel models. Observers had to perform a difficult gap localization task in response to infrequent targets, which were squares with a gap at a particular location (Fig. 10.6, left panel). In one experiment (Woodman and Luck 1999), search arrays contained four differently coloured objects among black background items, and one of these objects was likely to be the target. To control the order in which candidate target objects were selected, participants were informed that targets would have one colour (e.g. red) on 75% of all target trials, and another colour (e.g. blue) on 25% of these trials. If visual search was serial, this manipulation should ensure that red objects would be selected first, followed by blue objects. Fig. 10.6 (right) shows ERPs from target-absent trials where the objects in the two possible target colours were presented in opposite visual fields. An N2pc component initially emerged over the hemisphere contralateral to the object in the more likely target colour (C_{75}), and then shifted to the hemisphere contralateral to the object in the other less likely colour (C_{25}). This pattern of results supports serial models of

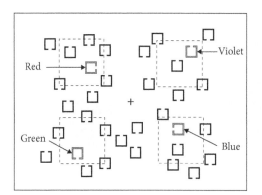 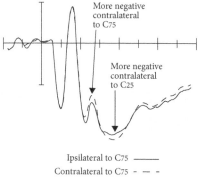

FIGURE 10.6 The left panel shows the visual search task employed by Woodman and Luck (1999). Search arrays contained four different colour singletons among black background items. Observers had to detect a target square defined by a specific gap location. 75% of all targets had one specific colour (C_{75}), and 25% had another colour (C_{25}). ERPs shown in the right panel are from non-target trials where the C_{75} and C_{25} items appeared on opposite sides, and were obtained at posterior electrodes contralateral and ipsilateral to the C_{75} item. The N2pc was triggered first contralateral to the C_{75} item, and then contralateral to the C_{25} stimulus. Reproduced with permission from Woodman and Luck (2003). Adapted from *Journal of Experimental Psychology: Human Perception and Performance*, 29(1), Woodman, G. F., and Luck, S. J., Serial deployment of attention during visual search pp. 121–38. Copyright © 2003 by the American Psychological Association.

visual search, because it suggests that attention was shifted within about 100 ms between the two candidate target objects. Parallel models of visual search should predict a sustained N2pc contralateral to the more likely target colour, indicative of a top-down task set for this colour that biases attentional competition in a spatially specific fashion. In a second experiment, Woodman and Luck (1999) controlled search order by presenting one candidate target object near fixation and another at a greater eccentricity, as observers tend to examine near objects prior to far objects. Here, the N2pc emerged initially contralateral to the near object, and shifted after about 100 ms to the far object, which again supports serial models of visual search.

There is, however, an important methodological problem for the interpretation of these N2pc polarity reversals in terms of serial search. Because the N2pc component is quantified as the difference between occipital ERP amplitudes at contralateral versus ipsilateral electrodes, it is not an absolute measure of attentional allocation to one specific object in a multi-stimulus search array, but instead reflects the difference in the degree to which attention is focused on a stimulus in the left versus right visual field. Because of this fact, the N2pc results observed by Woodman and Luck (1999) may still be consistent with models that assume that attention was allocated in parallel to both candidate target objects, and that only the relative bias in favour of one versus the other object changed slightly across time. To meet this challenge, Woodman and Luck (2003) employed search arrays where one candidate target object was located on the vertical meridian and the other on the horizontal meridian. The contralateral nature of this component implies that visual stimuli on the vertical midline will elicit no N2pc, and that an N2pc measured on such trials can be exclusively interpreted as reflecting the attentional selection of the other candidate target object on the left or right side. Search order was again manipulated via stimulus eccentricity. Results were straightforward: The N2pc emerged about 150 ms earlier in search arrays with near horizontal targets than in arrays with far horizontal targets, and there was very little temporal overlap between the N2pc components elicited by these two search array types. These findings suggest that attention was not allocated in parallel to both possible targets, but was first shifted to near targets, and then reoriented to far targets. Overall, the N2pc results reported by Woodman and Luck (1999, 2003) provide novel insights into the time course of attentional allocation in visual search, and demonstrate the power of ERP measures as temporal markers of selective attention. Their findings provide strong evidence for the sequential nature of attentional processing in demanding visual search tasks, and thus support serial models of visual search such as Feature Integration Theory (Treisman 1988) or Guided Search (Wolfe 1994), but are more difficult to reconcile with parallel models of visual search (e.g. Ward et al. 1996).

It is important to underline that the detection of target items in visual search does not always require the serial allocation of spatial attention. When there is one stimulus with a distinct feature in a context of perceptually uniform stimuli (e.g. one red apple on a plate of green apples), it will usually 'pop out' and rapidly capture attention. In contrast to targets that are defined by feature conjunctions, the speed of detecting such feature singleton targets is unaffected by the number of distractor items in a visual search array (Treisman and Gelade 1980). It is natural to assume that such feature singletons capture attention in an automatic bottom-up fashion that is determined exclusively by their perceptual salience, and is independent of current top-down search goals (see also Theeuwes (chapter 8), this volume). In fact, the relative roles of bottom-up and top-down factors in the control of attentional capture by feature singletons remain controversial, and ERP measures such as the N2pc component have recently played an important role in this debate.

In several models of attentional selectivity, stimulus salience is represented in a topographical map that combines local contrast signals from different dimension- and feature-specific maps (e.g. Koch and Ullman 1985; Itti and Koch 2000). Attention will normally be directed towards the location with the highest combined salience value, but the controversial question is whether and to what degree this salience-driven attentional capture can be modulated or even prevented by top-down control processes (e.g. Fecteau and Munoz 2006). Behavioural studies that have investigated the relative roles of top-down task sets and bottom-up salience for attentional capture by feature singleton stimuli in visual search tasks have yielded apparently inconsistent results. When observers search for a shape singleton (e.g. a unique diamond target presented among distractor circles) the presence of an additional salient but task-irrelevant stimulus (e.g. a colour singleton; Theeuwes 1991) slows down reaction times relative to trials where no irrelevant singleton is present. This observation appears to suggest that salient singleton stimuli capture attention in a bottom-up fashion that is unaffected by current selection goals (Theeuwes 2010). In contrast, experiments by Folk and colleagues (Folk et al. 1992, 1994; Folk and Remington 1998) have demonstrated that attentional capture by salient but irrelevant visual singletons is determined by top-down task sets. In their experiments, spatially non-predictive singleton cues were presented prior to the onset of a target search display. Responses were faster for targets at cued as compared to uncued locations, indicating that the cues captured attention. Critically, these spatial cueing effects were only present when cue features matched the current task set. For example, when observers searched for a colour-defined target, cueing effects were found for colour singleton cues that matched the current target colour, but not for cues in a different colour, or for singletons defined in a different dimension (e.g. abrupt onset items). These findings strongly suggest that attentional capture by visual singletons is not a bottom-up phenomenon driven by salience, but is instead determined by whether or not these objects match task-relevant attributes as defined by an active task set.

The controversy whether attentional capture by salient visual feature singletons is determined by current top-down task sets or is triggered in a purely bottom-up fashion has continued for two decades. On both sides of this debate, specific assumptions about the time course of attentional capture have been invoked, and these have proved to be difficult to confirm or reject on the basis of behavioural performance data. The observation that target detection is delayed when visual search arrays contain an additional task-irrelevant salient singleton item has been attributed to the increased visual complexity of such search arrays, which extends pre-attentive processing and thus delays attention shits towards targets (Folk and Remington 1998). On the other side, the observation that spatial cueing effects are eliminated for salient singleton cues that do not match current target-defining features has been explained by assuming that such cues do initially capture attention in a bottom-up fashion, but that attention is then rapidly disengaged, thereby preventing the emergence of spatial cueing effects in response to subsequently presented target stimuli (e.g. Theeuwes et al. 2000).

Again, ERP markers of attentional target selection such as the N2pc component allow more precise insights into the time course of the attentional selection processes that are elicited by visual arrays that contain salient feature singletons, and thus offer the possibility to decide between competing top-down and bottom-up accounts of attentional capture. Hickey et al. (2006) measured the N2pc during visual search for shape singleton targets that were accompanied by salient but task-irrelevant colour singleton distractors on some trials. Critically, an N2pc component was triggered by laterally presented colour singleton distractors on trials where shape targets were located on the vertical meridian, and thus did not elicit any N2pc activity. This observation appears to provide strong evidence for the bottom-up capture of attention by salient distractors. Further support for this bottom-up account comes from the finding that in trials where a shape target and a colour distractor appeared in opposite hemifields, a small N2pc to distractors preceded the N2pc to targets, suggesting that attention was initially drawn to the distractor before it was re-allocated to the target.

While the N2pc results reported by Hickey et al. (2006) appear to provide clear ERP evidence for the bottom-up nature of attentional capture, findings from other N2pc studies that used spatial cueing procedures strongly support the view that capture is always contingent on top-down task set. Fig. 10.7 (left) shows the setup of an experiment where spatially uninformative colour singleton cues preceded target search arrays (Eimer and Kiss 2008). In different blocks, observers either searched for red targets among grey distractors (Colour Task), or for a small target bar among larger distractor bars (Size Task). In the Colour Task, colour singleton cues elicited a large N2pc indicative of attentional capture (Fig. 10.7, right side). In contrast, no N2pc was triggered by physically identical colour singleton cues in the Size Task where colour was task-irrelevant. In fact, Fig. 10.7 shows that under these task instructions, these cues triggered an enhanced contralateral positivity. As mentioned earlier, this Pd component is thought to reflect active top-down inhibition (e.g. Hickey et al., 2009). The observation that an N2pc was elicited by perceptually salient colour singleton cues only when colour was task-relevant strongly suggests that attentional capture depends on top-down task sets, and is not driven in a bottom-up fashion by stimulus salience (see also Lien et al. 2008; Eimer et al. 2009, for additional N2pc evidence for top-down control of capture). The absence of any early-onset N2pc component to colour singleton cues that did not match the current top-down task set also casts doubt on the hypothesis that these cues trigger rapid salience-driven attentional capture which is later followed by rapid disengagement (see also Ansorge et al. 2011, for more direct N2pc evidence against this rapid disengagement account).

There is an obvious conflict between N2pc studies which employed the additional singleton paradigm and found evidence for the bottom-up salience-driven nature of attentional capture (e.g. Hickey et al. 2006), and N2pc results from spatial cueing experiments which seem to demonstrate that capture is fully controlled by top-down task sets (e.g. Eimer and Kiss 2008). However, this apparent discrepancy might be linked to the

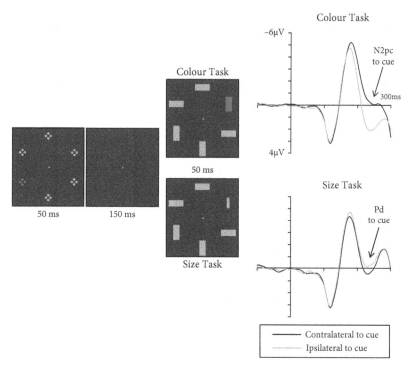

FIGURE 10.7 ERPs triggered in response to spatially uninformative cue arrays that contained a red colour singleton, measured in a task where participants searched for red target singletons, and a task where they searched for size singletons. An N2pc was triggered by colour singleton cues in the Colour Task, whereas a contralateral positivity (Pd) was elicited by the same cues in the Size Task. Data from Eimer and Kiss (2008).

time demands that are imposed on attentional selectivity in these two different paradigms. In additional singleton experiments, search displays usually remain visible until a response is executed, and observers therefore have sufficient time to select and identify targets even if attention is initially drawn to a more salient distractor. In spatial cueing experiments, search array durations are typically much shorter, which imposes stricter temporal demands on target selection, as attentional capture by distractors will likely result in targets being missed. To investigate the impact of temporal task demands on the top-down versus bottom-up control of attentional capture by feature singletons, a recent ERP study (Kiss et al. 2012) measured lateralized posterior ERP components in response to search arrays that contained a shape singleton target and a colour singleton distractor. The critical factor was display duration, as search arrays remained visible until response execution for one group of participants, but were presented for only 200 ms for another group. Figure 10.8 shows lateralized ERP components measured for both groups at posterior electrodes. In the long duration group, salient colour distractors triggered an N2pc, confirming earlier observations by Hickey et al. (2006), and demonstrating these distractors did capture attention even though they were known to be task-irrelevant. But in the short

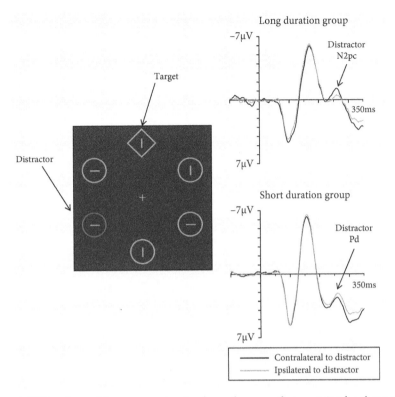

FIGURE 10.8 ERPs triggered in response to visual search arrays that contained a shape target on the vertical meridian and a lateral task-irrelevant colour singleton. For participants in the long duration group, arrays remained visible until response execution. In the short duration group, they disappeared after 200 ms. In the long duration group, colour distractors triggered an N2pc indicative of attentional capture. In the short duration group, the same distractors elicited a Pd component, indicating that they were subject to active inhibition. Data from Kiss et al. (2012).

duration group, the same colour distractors elicited no N2pc, but instead a contralateral positivity (Pd). Because this Pd component is believed to mark the top-down inhibition of salient distractors, its presence under conditions of high temporal task demands suggests that attentional capture by salient distractors can be prevented by active inhibition when it would otherwise disrupt task performance. These ERP findings point towards a resolution of the dispute between bottom-up and top-down accounts of attentional capture. Salience-driven capture may represent a default mode of attentional selectivity, such that salient distractors will capture attention when the time demands on target selection are relatively relaxed. However, salience-driven capture is not strongly automatic, because it can be prevented by top-down inhibitory control when this is necessitated by the demands of a specific task context.

In summary, the results discussed in this section have illustrated the special role that ERP measures can play in investigations of attentional processes that govern the selection of targets in multi-stimulus arrays. As temporally precise markers of attentional processes, ERP components such as the N2pc have been particularly useful to shed new light on controversial issues about the functional and temporal organization of the mechanisms that are responsible for spatially selective stimulus processing.

References

Allport, A. (1993). Attention and control: Have we been asking the wrong questions? A critical review of twenty-five years. In D. E. Meyer and S. Kornblum (eds.), *Attention and Performance* (vol. 14, pp. 183–218). Cambridge, Mass.: MIT Press.

Ansorge, U., Kiss, M., Worschech, F., and Eimer, M. (2011). The initial stage of visual selection is controlled by top-down task set: New ERP evidence. *Attention, Perception, & Psychophysics* 73: 113–122.

Beck, D. M. and Kastner, S. (2009). Top-down and bottom-up mechanisms in biasing competition in the human brain. *Vision Research* 49: 1154–1165.

Broadbent, D. E. (1958). *Perception and Communication*. New York: Elsevier.

Clark, V. P., Fan, S., and Hillyard, S. A. (1995). Identification of early visually evoked potential generators by retinotopic and topographic analysis. *Human Brain Mapping* 2: 170–187.

Corbetta, M. and Shulman, G. L. (2002). Control of goal-directed and stimulus-driven attention in the brain. *Nature Reviews Neuroscience* 3: 215–229.

Desimone, R. and Duncan, J. (1995). Neural mechanisms of selective visual attention. *Annual Review of Neuroscience* 18: 193–222.

Deutsch, J. A. and Deutsch, D. (1963). Attention: Some theoretical considerations. *Psychological Review* 70: 80–90.

Di Russo, F., Martínez, A., and Hillyard, S. A. (2003). Source analysis of event-related cortical activity during visuo-spatial attention. *Cerebral Cortex* 13: 486–499.

Duncan, J. and Humphreys, G. W. (1989). Visual search and stimulus similarity. *Psychological Review* 96: 433–458.

Duncan, J., Ward, R., and Shapiro, K. L. (1994). Direct measurement of attentional dwell time in human vision. *Nature* 369: 313–315.

Eimer, M. (1994). 'Sensory gating' as a mechanism for visuo-spatial orienting: Electro-physiological evidence from trial-by-trial cueing experiments. *Perception & Psychophysics* 55: 667–675.

Eimer, M. (1996a). ERP modulations indicate the selective processing of visual stimuli as a result of transient and sustained spatial attention. *Psychophysiology* 33: 13–21.

Eimer, M. (1996b). The N2pc component as an indicator of attentional selectivity. *Electroencephalography and Clinical Neurophysiology* 99: 225–234.

Eimer, M. (1999). Can attention be directed to opposite locations in different modalities? An ERP study. *Clinical Neurophysiology* 110: 1252–1259.

Eimer, M. and Driver, J. (2000). An event-related brain potential study of cross-modal links in spatial attention between vision and touch. *Psychophysiology* 37: 697–705.

Eimer, M. and Kiss, M. (2008). Involuntary attentional capture is determined by task set: Evidence from event-related brain potentials. *Journal of Cognitive Neuroscience* 20: 1423–1433.

Eimer, M., Kiss, M., Press, C., and Sauter, D. (2009). The roles of feature-specific task set and bottom-up salience in attentional capture: An ERP study. *Journal of Experimental Psychology: Human Perception and Performance* 35: 1316–1328.

Eimer, M. and Schröger, E. (1998). ERP effects of intermodal attention and cross-modal links in spatial attention. *Psychophysiology* 35: 313–327.

Eimer, M., Van Velzen, J., and Driver, J. (2002). Crossmodal interactions between audition, touch and vision in endogenous spatial attention: ERP evidence on preparatory states and sensory modulations. *Journal of Cognitive Neuroscience 14*: 254–271.

Farah, M. J., Wong, A. B., Monheit, M. A., and Morrow, L. A. (1989). Parietal lobe mechanisms of spatial attention: Modality-specific or supramodal? *Neuropsychologia 27*: 461–470.

Fecteau, J. H. and Munoz, D. P. (2006). Salience, relevance, and firing: a priority map for target selection. *Trends in Cognitive Sciences 10*: 382–390.

Folk, C. L. and Remington, R. W. (1998). Selectivity in distraction by irrelevant featural singletons: Evidence for two forms of attentional capture. *Journal of Experimental Psychology: Human Perception and Performance 24*: 847–858.

Folk, C. L., Remington, R. W., and Johnston, J. C. (1992). Involuntary covert orienting is contingent on attentional control settings. *Journal of Experimental Psychology: Human Perception and Performance 18*: 1030–1044.

Folk, C. L., Remington, R. W., and Wright, J. H. (1994). The structure of attentional control: Contingent attentional capture by apparent motion, abrupt onset, and colour. *Journal of Experimental Psychology: Human Perception and Performance 20*: 317–329.

Green, J. J., Teder-Sälerjärvi, W. A., and McDonald, J. J. (2005). Control mechanisms mediating shifts of attention in auditory and visual space: A spatio-temporal ERP analysis. *Experimental Brain Research 166*: 358–369.

Harter, M. R., Miller, S. L, Price, N. J., LaLonde, M. E., and Keyes, A. L. (1989). Neural processes involved in directing attention. *Journal of Cognitive Neuroscience 1*: 223–237.

Hickey, C., Di Lollo, V., and McDonald, J. J. (2009). Electrophysiological indices of target and distractor processing in visual search. *Journal of Cognitive Neuroscience 21*: 760–775.

Hickey, C., McDonald, J. J., and Theeuwes, J. (2006). Electrophysiological evidence of the capture of visual attention. *Journal of Cognitive Neuroscience 18*: 604–613.

Hillyard, S. A., Hink, R. F., Schwent, V. L., and Picton, T. W. (1973). Electrical signs of selective attention in the human brain. *Science 182*: 177–180.

Hopf, J.-M., Luck, S. J., Girelli, M., Hagner, T., Mangun, G. R., Scheich, H., and Heinze, H. J. (2000). Neural sources of focused attention in visual search. *Cerebral Cortex 10*: 1233–1241.

Itti, L. and Koch, C. (2000). A saliency-based search mechanism for overt and covert shifts of visual attention. *Vision Research 40*: 1489–1506.

Kennett, S., Eimer, M., Spence, C., and Driver, J. (2001). Tactile–visual links in exogenous spatial attention under different postures: Convergent evidence from psychophysics and ERPs. *Journal of Cognitive Neuroscience 13*: 462–478.

Kiss, M., Grubert, A., Petersen, A., and Eimer, M. (2012). Attentional capture by salient distractors during visual search is determined by temporal task demands. *Journal of Cognitive Neuroscience 24*: 749–759.

Kiss, M., Van Velzen, J., and Eimer, M. (2008). The N2pc component and its links to attention shifts and spatially selective visual processing. *Psychophysiology 45*: 240–249.

Koch, C. and Ullman, S. (1985). Shifts in selective visual attention: towards the underlying neural circuitry. *Human Neurobiology 4*: 219–227.

Lamme, V. A. F. and Roelfsema, P. R. (2000). The distinct modes of vision offered by feedforward and recurrent processing. *Trends in Neuroscience 23*: 571–579.

Lien, M.-C., Ruthruff, E., Goodin, Z., and Remington, R. W. (2008). Contingent attentional capture by top-down control settings: Converging evidence from event-related potentials. *Journal of Experimental Psychology: Human Perception and Performance 34*: 509–530.

Luck, S. J., Fan, S., and Hillyard, S. A. (1993). Attention-related modulation of sensory-evoked brain activity in a visual search task. *Journal of Cognitive Neuroscience 5*: 188–195.

Luck, S. J., Girelli, M., McDermott, M. T., and Ford, M. A. (1997). Bridging the gap between monkey neurophysiology and human perception: An ambiguity resolution theory of visual selective attention. *Cognitive Psychology* 33: 64–87.

Luck, S. J. and Hillyard, S. A. (1994a). Electrophysiological correlates of feature analysis during visual search. *Psychophysiology* 31: 291–308.

Luck, S. J. and Hillyard, S. A. (1994b). Spatial filtering during visual search: Evidence from human electrophysiology. *Journal of Experimental Psychology: Human Perception and Performance* 20: 1000–1014.

Luck, S. J., Vogel, E. K., and Shapiro, K. L. (1996). Word meanings are accessed but cannot be reported during the attentional blink. *Nature* 383: 616–618.

McDonald, J. J., Teder-Sälejärvi, W. A., and Hillyard, S. A. (2000). Involuntary orienting to sound improves visual perception. *Nature* 407: 906–908.

McDonald, J. J. and Ward, L. M. (2000). Involuntary listening aids seeing: Evidence from human electrophysiology. *Psychological Science* 11: 167–171.

Mangun, G. R. (1995). Neural mechanisms of visual selective attention. *Psychophysiology* 32: 4–18.

Mangun, G. R. and Hillyard, S. A. (1987). The spatial allocation of visual attention as indexed by event-related brain potentials. *Human Factors* 29: 195–211.

Mangun, G. R. and Hillyard, S. A. (1991). Modulation of sensory-evoked brain potentials provide evidence for changes in perceptual processing during visual-spatial priming. *Journal of Experimental Psychology: Human Perception and Performance* 17: 1057–1074.

Martínez, A. Anllo-Vento, L., Sereno, M. I., Frank, L. R., Buxton, R. B., Dubowitz, D. J., Wong, E. C., Hinrichs, H., Heinze, H. J., and Hillyard, S. A. (1999). Involvement of striate and extrastriate visual cortical areas in spatial attention. *Nature Neuroscience* 2: 364–369.

Mazza, V., Turatto, M., and Caramazza, A. (2009). Attention selection, distractor suppression, and N2pc. *Cortex* 45: 879–890.

Mazza, V., Turatto, M., Umiltà, C., and Eimer, M. (2007). Attentional selection and identification of visual objects are reflected by distinct electrophysiological responses. *Experimental Brain Research* 181: 531–536.

Nobre A. C., Sebestyen, G. N., and Miniussi, C. (2000). The dynamics of shifting visuospatial attention revealed by event-related brain potentials. *Neuropsychologia* 38: 964–974.

Praamstra, P., Boutsen, L., and Humphreys, G. W. (2005). Frontoparietal control of spatial attention and motor intention in human EEG. *Journal of Neurophysiology* 94: 764–774.

Raymond, J. E., Shapiro, K. L., and Arnell, K. M. (1992). Temporary suppression of visual processing in an RSVP task: An attentional blink? *Journal of Experimental Psychology: Human Perception and Performance* 18: 849–860.

Sawaki, R. and Luck, S. (2010). Capture versus suppression of attention by salient singletons: Electrophysiological evidence for an automatic attend-to-me signal. *Attention, Perception, & Psychophysics* 72: 1455–1470.

Spence, C. and Driver, J. (1996). Audiovisual links in endogenous covert spatial attention. *Journal of Experimental Psychology: Human Perception and Performance* 22: 1005–1030.

Spence, C., Pavani, F., and Driver, J. (2000). Crossmodal links between vision and touch in covert endogenous spatial attention. *Journal of Experimental Psychology: Human Perception and Performance* 26: 1298–1319.

Teder-Sälejärvi, W. A., Münte, T. F., Sperlich, F. J., and Hillyard, S. A. (1999). Intra-modal and cross-modal spatial attention to auditory and visual stimuli: An event-related brain potential (ERP) study. *Cognitive Brain Research* 8: 327–343.

Theeuwes, J. (1991). Cross-dimensional perceptual selectivity. *Perception & Psychophysics* 50: 184–193.

Theeuwes, J. (2010). Top-down and bottom-up control of visual selection. *Acta Psychologica* 135: 77–99.

Theeuwes, J., Atchley, P., and Kramer, A. F. (2000). On the time course of top-down and bottom-up control of visual attention. In S. Monsell and J. Driver (eds.), *Attention and Performance* (vol. 18, pp. 105–124). Cambridge, Mass.: MIT Press.

Treisman, A. (1988). Features and objects: The Fourteenth Bartlett Memorial Lecture. *Quarterly Journal of Experimental Psychology* 40A: 201–237.

Treisman, A. and Gelade, G. (1980). A feature integration theory of attention. *Cognitive Psychology* 12: 97–136.

Van Velzen, J., Eardley, A., Forster, B., and Eimer M. (2006). Shifts of attention in the early blind: An ERP study of attentional control processes in the absence of visual spatial information. *Neuropsychologia* 44: 2533–2546.

Van Velzen, J. and Eimer, M. (2003). Early posterior ERP components do not reflect the control of attentional shifts towards expected peripheral events. *Psychophysiology* 40: 827–831.

Van Voorhis, S. and Hillyard, S. (1977). Visual evoked potentials and selective attention to points in space. *Perception & Psychophysics* 22: 54–62.

Vogel, E. K., Luck, S. J., and Shapiro, K. L. (1998). Electrophysiological evidence for a post-perceptual locus of suppression during the attentional blink. *Journal of Experimental Psychology: Human Perception and Performance* 24: 1656–1674.

Vogel, E. K. and Machizawa, M. G. (2004). Neural activity predicts individual differences in visual working memory capacity. *Nature* 428: 748–751.

Ward, R., Duncan, J., and Shapiro, K. L. (1996). The slow time-course of visual attention. *Cognitive Psychology* 30: 79–109.

Wolfe, J. M. (1994). Guided search 2.0: A revised model of visual search. *Psychonomic Bulletin & Review* 1: 202–238.

Woodman, G. F., Arita, J. T., and Luck, S. J. (2009). A cuing study of the N2pc component: An index of attentional deployment to objects rather than spatial locations. *Brain Research* 1297: 110–121.

Woodman, G. F. and Luck, S. J. (1999). Electrophysiological measurement of rapid shifts of attention during visual search. *Nature* 400: 867–869.

Woodman, G. F. and Luck, S. J. (2003). Serial deployment of attention during visual search. *Journal of Experimental Psychology: Human Perception and Performance* 29: 121–138.

CHAPTER 11

....

NEURONAL MECHANISMS OF SPATIAL ATTENTION IN VISUAL CEREBRAL CORTEX

....

MARLENE R. COHEN AND
JOHN H. R. MAUNSELL

Introduction

It is well established that the responses of individual visual neurons are modulated when subjects shift their attention from one location in visual space to another (reviewed by Olson 2001; Bisley and Goldberg 2010; Reynolds and Chelazzi 2004; Carrasco 2011; Gilbert and Sigman 2007; Maunsell and Cook 2002; Braun et al. 2001). Most neurons respond more strongly when the subject attends to a stimulus within their receptive fields relative to when attention is directed to a distant location. Shifts in spatial attention have been associated with changes in the responses of individual neurons in every visual cortical area that has been examined, including primary visual cortex (V1; Roelfsema et al. 1998; Thiele et al. 2009; McAdams and Maunsell 1999; Motter 1993).

More recently, electrophysiological studies have begun to elucidate the mechanisms underlying attention-related changes in the responses of sensory neurons and to establish a link between the modulation of sensory neurons and improvements in performance on psychophysical tasks. Progress in three areas has been particularly notable. First, while it has long been understood that a bottom-up sensory processing mechanism known as normalization can explain some aspects of modulation with attention (Lee et al. 1999; Reynolds et al. 1999; Carandini and Heeger 2012), recent results have underscored that normalization is critical for interpreting many aspects of the way that sensory responses change with attention. This insight has led to a refined understanding of the range of attention-related effects that are seen under different stimulus conditions. Second, studies that have recorded simultaneously from many neurons during attention tasks have found that attention has striking effects on correlations between the responses of nearby neurons. Such changes in the way that populations of neurons encode sensory signals cannot be seen when recording from one neuron at a time, but they might prove critical to the behavioural advantages associated with attention. Third, simultaneous recordings from a few dozen neurons have provided the statistical power needed to link attention-related modulation of sensory neurons with improvements in performance on a trial-by-trial basis. This discovery allows for temporally precise measures of attentional state (milliseconds), compared with the traditional approach of averaging over many trials (minutes).

These conceptual advances, combined with the advent of new recording technologies that have made identifying neurons and recording simultaneously from groups of neurons experimentally tractable, have improved our understanding of how spatial attention is linked to neuronal responses and have opened new avenues for future research. Here, we review these recent findings, focusing on experiments that have recorded the responses of individual neurons (recorded one at a time or simultaneously) in the visual cortex of trained, behaving monkeys. Although our subject is spatial attention, we will also refer to results from feature attention when they bear directly on the interpretation of the data. A comprehensive treatment of feature attention can be found elsewhere in this volume (see Wolfe, chapter 2; Scholari, Esther, and Serences, chapter 20; and Treue, chapter 21). We also discuss the potential of these ideas for extending our knowledge of how the responses of sensory neurons in different states of attention can affect perceptual performance.

Single Unit Measures: Modulations and Normalization

Sensory response modulation

Scaling of tuning curves

Attention to a visual stimulus is typically associated with increases in the responses of cortical neurons that represent that stimulus. Early attempts to understand the mechanism underlying this attentional modulation focused on the link between attention and the selectivity of neurons to different stimulus attributes. Neurons in visual cortex respond selectively to stimulus properties such as colour, orientation, and direction of motion. This selectivity is captured in plots of neuronal response as a function of the value of a given stimulus attribute (tuning curves; see Fig. 11.1). Although some early observations suggested that tuning curves for orientation in area V4 might be sharper when subjects attended to the stimuli (Haenny and Schiller 1988; Spitzer et al. 1988), it has subsequently been shown that in many situations responses to all stimuli are enhanced more or less proportionally, resulting in an overall multiplicative scaling of tuning curves.

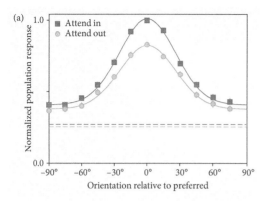

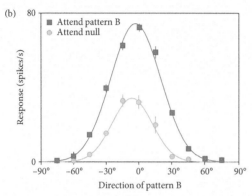

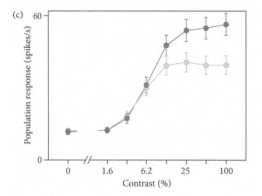

FIGURE 11.1 Attention is associated with the multiplicative scaling of responses of neurons in visual cortex. (a) The tuning curves of V4 neurons tend to be scaled upward when attention is directed to a stimulus inside the neurons' receptive fields (red line) compared to when attention is directed to a stimulus outside the receptive field (blue line). The dashed lines are average spontaneous activities. Reproduced from *Journal of Neuroscience*, 19 (1) McAdams, C. J. and Maunsell, J. H. R. Effects of attention on orientation-tuning functions of single neurons in macaque cortical area v4. pp. 431–441. Fig. 4 © 1999, The Society for Neuroscience. (b) Feature attention is also associated with the multiplicative scaling of tuning curves. Two stimuli were present in the receptive field: one patch of dots that always moved in each neuron's non-preferred (null) direction and one patch that moved in different directions for different measurements (pattern). Direction tuning curves of MT neurons are scaled when monkeys pay attention to motions close to the preferred direction, and are scaled down when monkeys pay attention to motion in the null direction. Reprinted by permission from Macmillan Publishers Ltd: *Nature* 399 (6736), Stefan Treue and Julio C. Martinez Trujillo, Feature-based attention influences motion processing gain in macaque visual cortex, pp. 575–579, copyright, 1999, Nature Publishing Group. (c) Spatial attention is often associated with an upward scaling of contrast response functions. Error bars in each panel are SEM. Adapted from *Journal of Neurophysiology*, 104 (2), Joonyeol Lee and John H. R. Maunsell, Feature-based attention influences motion processing gain in macaque visual cortex, pp. 960–971 © 2010, The American Physiological Society.

A scaling of tuning functions with attention has been seen for responses to many stimulus dimensions by neurons in several visual areas. In area V4, responses to all orientations increase by approximately the same proportion when attention is directed toward the stimulus. Fig. 11.1a shows average orientation tuning curves for single neuron responses when attention was directed to or away from the visual stimulus in the neuron's receptive field (McAdams and Maunsell 1999). In the middle temporal area (MT), attention to a stimulus is similarly associated with a scaling of average direction tuning curves (Fig. 11.1b, Treue and Martinez-Trujillo 1999b). Spatial attention can also be associated with scaling of contrast response functions for neurons in MT (Fig. 11.1c, Lee and Maunsell 2010b) and V4 (Williford and Maunsell 2006). Measurements of the temporal integration function used by MT neurons show that attention is associated with a scaling of the function with no shift in time or change in direction selectivity (Cook and Maunsell 2004). In area V4, receptive field profiles scale when attention is directed to different points around the receptive field (Connor et al. 1996, 1997), and in inferotemporal cortex (IT) behavioural differences between reward-contingent stimuli and other stimuli are coupled to scaling of orientation-tuning curves (Vogels and Orban 1994).

Like visual responses, spontaneous activity also changes with attention. Spontaneous activity in cortex typically amounts to only a few spikes per second, and modulation of such modest rates can be difficult to detect. Nevertheless, reliable changes in spontaneous activity have been reported in many visual areas (Luck et al. 1997; Reynolds et al. 2000; Williford and Maunsell 2006; Li and Basso 2008). Relatively indiscriminate scaling of both spontaneous activity and visual responses suggests that attention is associated with an increase in the overall sensitivity of neurons to all their inputs.

While an increase in sensitivity might be the primary signature of attention in sensory neurons, responses are affected in other ways. In particular, as we describe in the following section, shifting attention between preferred and non-preferred stimuli inside a neuron's receptive field can be associated with more complex effects. Even with a single stimulus in the receptive field, changes that are inconsistent with a simple scaling of sensitivity can occur with shifts in attention. For example, although contrast response functions are often scaled upward during attention to a stimulus (Fig. 11.1c), in some cases contrast response functions can instead shift to the left (Reynolds et al. 2000; Martinez-Trujillo and Treue 2002). Additive offsets of tuning curves have also been described (Williford and Maunsell 2006; Thiele et al. 2009). Moreover, attention to stimulus motion has been associated with changes in the way that MT neurons sum motion in space and time that differ from what would be expected from a simple scaling of responses (Ghose and Bearl 2010). Attention to stimulus features has been linked to shifts in the orientation and spatial frequency tuning of neurons in V4 (David et al. 2008).

Results like these show that there is considerable diversity in attention-related changes in the selectivity of individual visual neurons. While a range of effects on the selectivity of sensory neurons has been observed, the relative potency of each effect remains to be established. Currently it seems that a simple scaling of responses is the most common and strongest effect associated with attention, while other effects might require careful measurement or specific circumstances.

Modulation with multiple stimuli in the receptive field

Typically, the neuronal correlates of attention are studied by shifting attention between a single stimulus inside a neuron's receptive field and a distant stimulus. This manipulation usually produces a modest modulation, in the range of 5–20% of the rate of firing. However, it has long been known that shifting attention between two stimuli inside a neuron's receptive field can yield much stronger changes in response. Moran and Desimone (1985) were the first to show this effect. They trained monkeys to shift attention between a preferred stimulus that strongly drove the neuron being recorded and a non-preferred stimulus that produced little or no response when presented alone, both of which were placed inside the neuron's receptive field. When the animal attended to the preferred stimulus, responses of the neurons they recorded in V4 and IT were greatly enhanced compared to when the animal attended to the non-preferred stimulus. Strong response modulation from shifting attention between preferred and non-preferred stimuli has since been shown many times (Moran and Desimone 1985; Treue and Maunsell 1996; Luck et al. 1997; Reynolds et al. 1999; Ghose and Maunsell 2008; Ghose 2009).

A direct comparison of modulation with one versus two stimuli in a neuron's receptive field has been difficult to obtain. Attending to one of two closely spaced stimuli in a receptive field is more demanding than attending to a single stimulus, and differences in the effort of the subject could account for much of the stronger modulation with two stimuli in the receptive field (Spitzer et al. 1988; Boudreau et al. 2006; Chen et al. 2008). This problem has been addressed by randomly interleaving brief presentations of either one or two receptive field stimuli that are too fleeting to allow the animal to alter its attentional effort. Such brief presentations facilitate comparisons of the modulations of the responses of MT neurons under equivalent attention conditions (Lee and Maunsell 2010a). Shifting attention from outside a cell's receptive field to a single, preferred stimulus in the receptive field was associated with a 9% increase in response (Fig. 11.2a). However, shifting attention from outside the field to a preferred stimulus paired with a non-preferred stimulus inside the receptive field yielded a 28% enhancement (Fig. 11.2b; red vs black). Responses increased by 59% when attention was shifted from a non-preferred stimulus in the receptive field to a preferred stimulus in the receptive field (Fig. 11.2b; red vs blue). These measurements show that stimulus configurations greatly affect how much neuronal responses vary when spatial attention is shifted.

Normalization and attention

As described above, attention to a single stimulus inside a neuron's receptive field is generally associated with an increase in that neuron's response, as if attention was related to an overall increase in the sensitivity of the neuron. With two stimuli, however, attention can be associated with either an increase or a decrease in a neuron's response, depending

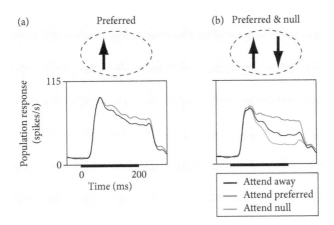

FIGURE 11.2 Attention is associated with greater modulation when there are multiple stimuli in a neuron's receptive field. (a) Peristimulus time histograms for the average of many MT neurons when attention is directed toward a single stimulus in its receptive field (red line) or a stimulus in the opposite hemifield (black line). (b) Same, for multiple stimuli within the receptive field. Attention is associated with increased modulation when it is directed to either a preferred (red line) or a null (blue line) stimulus within the receptive field, compared with the condition with a single stimulus in the receptive field. The thick line on the x-axis marks the period when the stimulus was present. Reproduced from Lee, J. and Maunsell , J. Attentional modulation of MT neurons with single or multiple stimuli in their receptive fields, *Journal of Neuroscience*, 30, pp. 3058–3066, (c) 2010, The Society for Neuroscience.

on whether a preferred or non-preferred stimulus lies at the focus of attention. This effect on cells' responses cannot be accounted for by an overall increase in sensitivity. Recently, it has become widely recognized that the attention-related changes seen with either one or two stimuli in a neuron's receptive field can be explained by a mechanism called response normalization.

Normalization describes the way that neurons respond when presented with more than one stimulus at the same time in their receptive fields. It was first introduced to explain failures of linear summation when sensory neurons are presented with multiple stimuli (Albrecht and Geisler 1991; Heeger 1992, 1993). In particular, normalization explains why adding a weakly excitatory stimulus to a receptive field containing a strongly excitatory stimulus will reduce, rather than increase, the response of a neuron (see Carandini and Heeger 2012). Normalization accurately explains responses to a broad range of stimulus conditions for neurons in V1 and extrastriate cortex, both for single units (Heeger et al. 1996; Carandini et al. 1997) and for populations of neurons (Busse et al. 2009). In the absence of attention, normalization causes a neuron's response to reflect the similarity between the entire set of stimuli in its receptive field and its preferred stimulus. Therefore, the response to the combination of a preferred and non-preferred stimulus is more similar to the average than the sum of the responses to each stimulus alone.

Neurophysiological support for a role of normalization in spatial attention

Several reports have shown how normalization models can account for many aspects of the way that the activity of sensory neurons varies with attention (Boynton 2009; Ghose 2009; Lee and Maunsell 2009; Reynolds and Heeger 2009). Normalization readily explains why shifting attention between a stimulus in a neuron's receptive field and a distant stimulus produces relatively little modulation compared to shifting attention between two different stimuli that both lie within the receptive field (Fig. 11.2). This difference occurs because normalization mechanisms have relatively little influence when only one stimulus is present, but come into play strongly when multiple stimuli are present. Normalization can also explain how shifts in attention can scale the tuning response function and why neuronal modulations differ when shifting attention between stimuli that have either the same contrast or different contrast (Khayat et al. 2010). Some normalization models can produce leftward shifts of contrast response functions (contrast gain; Ghose 2009; Reynolds and Heeger 2009; Boynton 2009). More elaborate normalization models allow attention to be distributed narrowly or broadly in space (Reynolds and Heeger 2009; Ghose and Bearl 2010), thereby capturing a characteristic of attention that is well established in behavioural studies (LaBerge 1983; Eriksen and Yeh 1985) and seen in some single-unit experiments (Boudreau et al. 2006; Ghose 2009). When spatial attention is misaligned with the receptive field of a neuron, these models account for how attention can shift receptive fields (Connor et al. 1997; Womelsdorf et al. 2006). The ability of normalization to robustly accommodate a wide range of effects from attention suggests that it is an important mechanism for changing sensory responses when attention is directed to different stimuli.

While many neurophysiological results can be explained by normalization, few studies have provided evidence for a direct relationship between normalization and attention in the responses of neurons. Reynolds and colleagues (1999) measured the responses of neurons in V2 and V4 to two stimuli when they were presented alone or together. As in other studies, when the two stimuli were presented together, attention to the preferred stimulus was associated with an increase in the neuron's response, while attention to the non-preferred stimulus was associated with a lower response. Because each neuron was tested with many stimulus pairs, some pairs included stimuli that were equally preferred by a cell. Normalization models of attention predict that there should be no modulation from shifting attention between two such stimuli, and that was what these investigators found. In MT, shifting attention between two identical stimuli is also associated with little response modulation compared to shifting attention between two differently preferred stimuli (Lee and Maunsell 2010a). Similarly, Chelazzi and colleagues (1998) showed that two stimuli placed within the receptive field of an inferotemporal neuron showed more modulation from shifting attention when both stimuli were placed on the same side of the vertical meridian, a configuration that associated with stronger stimulus interactions.

A cell-by-cell correlation between normalization and attention-related modulation was observed in an experiment that examined responses in MT (Lee and Maunsell 2009). Each cell was tested with a pair of stimuli within the receptive field that included

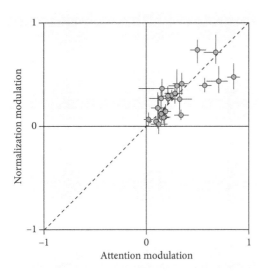

FIGURE 11.3 Across a population of MT neurons, the amount of modulation associated with sensory normalization (y-axis) is highly correlated with the amount of modulation that occurs when attention is shifted between preferred and non-preferred stimuli within the receptive field (x-axis; r = 0.76). Adapted from *PLoS ONE*, 4, Lee, J. and Maunsell, J. H. R., A normalization model of attentional modulation of single unit responses, e4651 © 2009, Creative Commons License.

a preferred stimulus and a non-preferred stimulus. With this pairing, cells are expected to show pronounced modulation when attention is shifted from one stimulus to the other. Normalization should also cause the addition of the non-preferred stimulus to reduce a cell's response to a preferred stimulus. That was the case for many, but not all cells. MT neurons that showed little evidence of normalization also showed little modulation when attention was shifted between the stimuli. This strong correlation between the strength of normalization and the strength of modulation with attention was apparent in the population of MT neurons (Fig. 11.3). The modulation associated with attention approached zero when normalization approached zero. These results suggest that normalization and modulation by attention are tightly coupled in sensory neurons.

Implications of normalization for attentional modulation

Sensory normalization has long provided an important framework for understanding stimulus interactions in the generation of neuronal response. Recent work also shows that normalization provides insight into many aspects of the modulation of sensory responses associated with shifts in spatial attention. However, important questions remain unanswered. In particular, the precise relationship between normalization and attention remains to be established. It has been suggested that attention shifts are associated with changes in the potency of normalization (Lee and Maunsell 2009), which would imply that normalization mechanisms are critical for attention-related modulations in sensory cortex. However, the relationship might be less direct. Attention might primarily be associated with a scaling of the visual signals that provide input to a downstream neuron. Following this scaling, inputs might be combined according to normalization rules that are constant over different attention conditions, as in input gain models (Ghose 2009). In that case, normalization might amplify attention-related modulations but have no special relationship to attention. It will be important to determine whether any essential relationship exists between attention and normalization.

Another important question is whether normalization will have as prominent a role for feature attention as it does for spatial attention (Boynton 2009; Reynolds and Heeger 2009). Normalization models are generally conceptualized with each stimulus driving a separate population of neurons that spans a range of stimulus preferences, with shifts in attention differentially modulating these separate populations (Boynton 2009; Ghose 2009; Lee and Maunsell 2009; Reynolds and Heeger 2009). It is easy to envision two populations of neurons when two stimuli are spatially offset, as in experiments on spatial attention. However, the effects of feature attention span the visual field (Treue and Martinez-Trujillo 1999a, 1999b; Maunsell and Treue 2006). While it is possible that normalization can work with populations of neurons that are intermixed in cortex, it remains to be seen whether normalization is closely related to feature attention when it involves this more challenging configuration.

Normalization might also explain differences in the strength of attention-related modulation observed both within (Fig. 11.3) and between cortical visual areas. One possibility is that this variance is optimized for enhancing behaviour. For example, it might be beneficial for neurons to be modulated differently depending on how well their responses distinguish targets from distractors (Navalpakkam and Itti 2007; Scolari and Serences 2009; Scolari et al. 2012). However, if attention-related modulation depends on the strength of normalization, its variance might have little to do with behavioural strategies. Instead, variance in attention-related modulation might be simply incidental to the variance in normalization mechanisms (due to inherent differences in normalization between cells or details of how experimental stimuli are configured relative to a cell's receptive field). The data in Fig. 11.3 suggest that at least half of the variance in attention-related modulation across neurons in MT reflects variance in normalization. Similarly, the larger attention-related modulations seen in later stages of visual cortex (see Maunsell and Cook 2002; O'Connor et al. 2002) might depend more on changes related to sensory normalization, such as differences in receptive field size or the need to remove redundancy in sensory coding (Schwartz and Simoncelli 2001), than on differences in the strength of inputs from higher cortical centres.

POPULATION MEASURES: CORRELATIONS AND FLUCTUATIONS IN ATTENTION

Most of our knowledge of how the responses of visual neurons change with attention comes from single-neuron studies such as those described in the previous sections. Typically, the average response of a neuron across many trials is compared between attention conditions. In general, attention is associated with improvements in the sensitivity of single neurons that arise from increased mean responses and, sometimes, decreased trial-to-trial variability (Mitchell et al. 2007). The resulting improvement in neuronal sensitivity is consistent with the hypothesis that the attention-related modulations of visual responses are responsible for the associated improvement in perception, although the improvement in the sensitivity of any individual neuron is typically small (McAdams and Maunsell 1999).

Rather than averaging the responses of single neurons over many stimulus presentations, however, animals must act on the sensory information encoded in populations of neurons over a short period. Single-neuron studies cannot measure several critical aspects of the way changes in attention are linked to changes in cortical circuits, interactions between neurons, or the relationship between specific subpopulations of cells and behaviour. The average responses of single neurons provide only limited access to the relationship between attention and changes in the underlying circuit, in part because in most studies the cell type or laminar location of the recorded studies is unknown. Furthermore, because so many neurons respond to any visual stimulus, it seems unlikely that the small changes in the signal-to-noise ratio of individual neurons underlie the dramatic perceptual improvement associated with attention. Theoretical studies suggest that interactions between neurons profoundly affect the amount of information encoded by a population of neurons (Shadlen and Newsome 1996; Abbott and Dayan 1999; Averbeck et al. 2006), so it is critical to consider how such interactions might change between states of attention. Finally, the activity of single neurons is only weakly related to an animal's perceptual decisions (Parker and Newsome 1998; Nienborg and Cumming 2010). Analysing the activity of large groups of neurons circumvents this problem and provides the statistical power necessary to determine subtleties in the relationship between attention-related modulation of particular groups of neurons and perception (Cohen and Maunsell 2010, 2011b; Nienborg et al. 2012).

Recent advances in multi-neuron recording technologies such as multielectrode arrays, laminar probes, and two-photon imaging have made recording from populations of neurons in behaving animals more tractable and more popular. Here, we review studies of attention-related changes in populations of visual neurons and discuss possibilities for using population metrics to uncover the mechanisms underlying attention.

Attention and correlations between the activity of pairs of neurons

Beyond properties of single neurons, the simplest higher-order measures of attention-related changes in visual neurons concern interactions between pairs of neurons. Cortical neurons respond variably to identical presentations of a sensory stimulus (Tolhurst et al. 1983). The extent to which this response variability is shared across a population of neurons can in principle affect two of the hypothesized functions of attention: the efficacy of spikes in driving downstream cells and the amount of information available in the population.

The most straightforward way of assessing the shared variability in a neuronal population is to measure correlations in the trial-to-trial fluctuations in the responses of a pair of neurons. The word correlation can refer to a relationship between responses over timescales that range from millisecond-level precision (synchrony) to the timescale of sensory stimuli or behavioural responses (typically hundreds of milliseconds). Correlations on these longer timescales (called spike count correlations, noise correlations, or r_{SC}) are typically quantified as the Pearson's correlation coefficient between spike count responses from two neurons measured over trials with identical stimulus and task conditions (for review, see Kohn et al. 2009; Cohen and Kohn 2011).

Neuronal correlations can vary depending on a variety of factors. Both synchrony and spike count correlations depend on the sensory stimulus (Espinosa and Gerstein 1988; Aertsen et al. 1989; Ahissar et al. 1992; Kohn and Smith 2005), learning (Ahissar et al. 1992; Gutnisky and Dragoi 2008; Komiyama et al. 2010; Gu et al. 2011), and behavioural context (Vaadia et al. 1995; Cohen and Newsome 2008; Poulet and Petersen 2008; Cohen and Maunsell 2009; Mitchell et al. 2009), as well as on cognitive factors including attention. Synchrony on short timescales is thought to improve the ability of cortical neurons to drive downstream cells, and increasing synchrony has been hypothesized as a mechanism by which signal efficacy might be improved when attention is directed to a stimulus (for review, see Womelsdorf and Fries 2007). Synchrony between cortical areas has also been suggested as a mechanism by which inter-area communication might be enhanced in some attention conditions (Buschman and Miller 2007; Saalmann et al. 2007; Fries 2009; Gregoriou et al. 2009). Because synchrony between pairs of cells in visual cortex is typically weak and requires large amounts of data to measure, most studies of attention and synchrony have focused on coherence measures based on spiking or local field potential responses (for review, see Fries 2009). The two studies that have measured neuronal correlates of attention on short-timescale synchrony between spiking responses have found either very weak (Roy et al. 2007) or no (Roelfsema et al. 2004) differences between attention conditions (Steinmetz et al. 2000).

Recent studies have shown profound attention-related changes in spike count correlations (r_{SC}) measured over hundreds of milliseconds. In two different tasks that modulated spatial attention, spike count correlations between pairs of neurons in V4 with overlapping receptive fields decreased by approximately 40% when the animals attended to locations inside the joint receptive fields of the neurons under study (Cohen and Maunsell 2009; Mitchell et al. 2009). This reduction in spike count correlation was substantially larger than the effects of attention on firing rates (<20%) and the variability of the individual neurons' responses (quantified as a ratio of the variance of the spike counts to the mean, or Fano factor; <10%) in the same studies.

Implications for population coding

Pairwise correlations can profoundly affect the amount of information encoded by a population of neurons, so any process that modulates correlations will affect the sensory information available to guide behaviour. Attending to a location or feature improves perception of the attended stimulus, and recent evidence suggests that the associated large reduction in correlated activity might account for these perceptual improvements.

Correlations affect the information in neuronal populations because they affect the extent to which coding is improved by incorporating the responses of multiple neurons. If the fluctuations between neurons are independent, the amount of information available in a neuronal population grows with the square root of the population size (Zohary et al. 1994; Shadlen and Newsome 1996, 1998; Abbott and Dayan 1999). Intuitively, increasing the population size improves accuracy because independent noise can simply be averaged away.

The effect of correlations on population coding depends on how sensory information is read out by downstream cells, but it is almost always dramatic (Zohary et al. 1994; Shadlen and Newsome 1998; Abbott and Dayan 1999; Nirenberg and Latham 2003; Averbeck et al. 2006; Berens et al. 2011). For example, if a downstream cell were to average the responses of neurons with similar tuning properties, correlations would limit the benefit of having multiple cells. In this case, correlated fluctuations could never be averaged out, leading to a more variable (and less accurate) estimate of the mean rate. However, if a downstream cell responded to the difference between the responses of two neurons (for example, comparing the responses of cells with opposite tuning properties as in a discrimination task), a higher proportion of correlated noise would be beneficial as these shared fluctuations would be subtracted away.

Under most conditions, the amount and structure of correlated variability has a greater effect on the coding capacity of the population than do the signalling capabilities of single neurons. Many neurons will respond to any given sensory stimulus, so variability in the responses of single neurons can be compensated for by simply considering the responses of large groups of neurons. Correlations, however, can limit or enhance the benefit of reading out sensory information from multiple neurons.

Two recent studies in area V4 suggest that the reduction in correlation associated with spatial attention can account for the vast majority of the observed behavioural improvements (Cohen and Maunsell 2009; Mitchell et al. 2009). In these studies, pairs (Mitchell et al. 2009) or groups of neurons (Cohen and Maunsell 2009) were recorded simultaneously, the attention-related improvement in the stimulus sensitivity of these neuronal populations was quantified (Cohen and Maunsell 2009) or modelled, and the relative importance of different physiological changes for this improvement was measured. There was a strong link between the improvement in the sensitivity of the population and the monkey's behavioural improvement due to attention (Fig. 11.4a), suggesting that the physiological factors that account for the improvement in sensitivity may also play a role in improving perception.

Increased attention was associated with at least three effects on populations of sensory neurons. Consistent with results from single-unit studies, firing rates increased and the variability of individual neurons decreased (quantified as the Fano factor; Mitchell et al. 2009). Additionally, spike count correlations decreased substantially. While each of these physiological changes could have contributed to the improvement in population sensitivity, the decrease in pairwise correlations was by far the most important factor in

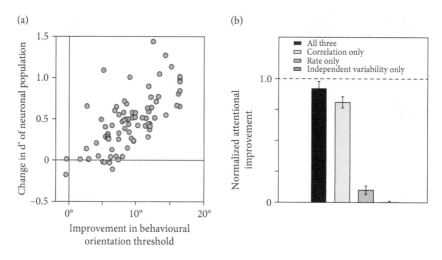

FIGURE 11.4 Changes in spike count correlations can account for most of the improvement in performance associated with spatial attention. (a) Each point represents attention-related changes in neuronal and behavioural responses during one recording session. Across experimental sessions, the improvement in the sensitivity of a population of a few dozen simultaneously recorded V4 neurons (quantified as d′ between population responses to two stimuli) associated with shifting attention toward the stimuli is correlated with the corresponding improvement in the subject's performance on a change detection task (quantified as improvement in psychophysical threshold in an orientation change detection task). (b) Proportion of the observed improvement in population sensitivity that can be accounted for by the modulation in correlation (green), firing rate (blue), within-neuron variability (red, quantified as the Fano factor), or all three factors (black). The modulation in spike count correlation accounts for over 80% of the observed improvement in population sensitivity. Adapted by permission from Macmillan Publishers Ltd: *Nature Neuroscience* 12 (12) Cohen, M. and Maunsell, J. H. R., Attention improves performance primarily by reducing interneuronal correlations, pp. 1594–1600 copyright, 2009, Nature Publishing Group.

explaining the improvement in population sensitivity, accounting for over 80% of the observed improvement (Fig. 11.b). Importantly, the ideal way for a downstream brain region to combine the responses of V4 neurons to solve the detection task in the study that measured behavioural improvement was similar to averaging (Cohen and Maunsell 2009), so decreasing correlations is beneficial to coding efficiency. It remains to be seen whether increased attention can be associated with increased correlations or no change in correlations in situations in which that would be beneficial.

The effects of correlations on the representation of stimulus information in populations of neurons in general and the way this representation changes with attention are complicated and only beginning to be understood. These results suggest, however, that studies of the average responses of single neurons miss interactions between neurons that can have critical effects on behaviour. Consequently, the future of studying population coding must rely on multielectrode or imaging technologies that allow glimpses of population activity on the timescale of a single behavioural decision.

Implications for the neuronal mechanisms underlying attention

Studying correlations is also useful because it can provide insights about the neuronal mechanisms underlying attention that are inaccessible from the responses of single neurons. For example, correlations can shed light on the question of whether attention is associated with modulations of all aspects of neuronal responses or a particular communication channel in a specific frequency range (for review, see Womelsdorf and Fries 2007). A study by Mitchell and colleagues (2009) showed that attention is predominantly associated with changes in correlations on the timescale of tens to hundreds of milliseconds rather than precise synchrony that occurs over shorter periods. The authors trained monkeys to do a stimulus tracking task and recorded from pairs of V4 neurons during 1000 ms periods in which the attended object paused in the joint receptive field of the recorded neurons. They computed the spike-to-spike coherence as a function of frequency (which is monotonically related to correlation with sufficient amounts of data) and spike count correlation as a function of counting window. Consistent with other studies in visual cortex (Bair et al. 2001; Kohn and Smith 2005), the correlations they measured were dominated by co-fluctuations on the timescale of tens to hundreds of milliseconds (Fig. 11.5). Attention appears to be linked to substantial decreases in correlations at longer timescales, but only barely measurable effects on

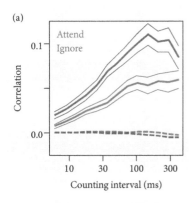

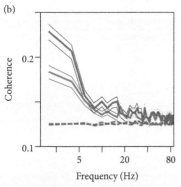

FIGURE   11.5 The   modulation   of   correlation and coherence associated with attention is not restricted to a specific range of temporal frequencies. (a) Correlation as a function of the period over which spikes were counted when attention was directed to a stimulus either inside (red line) or outside (blue line) the joint receptive field of a pair of V4 neurons. (b) Spike–spike coherence as a function of temporal frequency. The greatest modulation was seen in the low frequencies, where coherence is greatest. Reprinted from *Neuron*, 63 (6), Jude F. Mitchell, Kristy A. Sundberg, and John H. Reynolds, Spatial Attention Decorrelates Intrinsic Activity Fluctuations in Macaque Area V4, pp. 879–88, Copyright (2009), with permission from Elsevier.

the already weak high-frequency synchrony. These results suggest that attention-related modulation of correlations is not frequency-specific, but instead affects the same mechanisms that cause these correlations in the first place.

Changes in correlations may also provide clues about attention-related changes in the underlying functional circuitry. Spike count correlations are thought to reflect the balance between the activity of common same-sign (excitatory or inhibitory) direct or indirect inputs and common opposite-sign inputs (e.g. mutual inhibition) to the two neurons (Zohary et al. 1994; Bair et al. 2001; Kohn and Smith 2005; Smith and Kohn 2008). Changes in correlations may therefore indicate changes in either the connection in the underlying circuit or in the relative activity levels of different inputs.

Recent evidence suggests that the modulations of rates and correlations associated with spatial attention are linked: the pairs of neurons that show large increases in rate show large decreases in correlations, and pairs with very little rate change show little correlation change (Cohen and Maunsell 2011a; Fig. 11.6, black line). A similar relationship was observed for a form of feature attention in which the same monkeys were trained to detect, in alternating blocks of trials, a change in either the orientation or spatial frequency of a stimulus. Like other forms of feature attention (for review, see Maunsell and Treue 2006), the stimulus feature that the animals expected to change either increased or decreased firing rates depending on the similarity of the neuron's tuning to the attended feature (Cohen and Maunsell 2011a). Like spatial attention, the rate changes associated with feature attention were accompanied by changes in correlations, and large increases in firing rate were associated with large decreases in correlation (Fig. 11.6, right side of the grey line). The opposite relationship held as well: pairs of neurons whose rates decreased with feature attention showed increases in correlation (Fig. 11.6, left side of the grey line). The relationship between rate and correlation changes therefore appears to be similar for the two types of attention.

The results reviewed here show that studying correlations can provide new insights into both the mechanisms underlying attention and the impact of attention-related modulation of sensory neurons on the amount of information those neurons encode. These early results open several avenues for future research. Characterizing the conditions under which correlations change will be a first step towards understanding the way neural circuits reflect shifts in attention. For example, knowing whether shifts in attention are selectively associated with changes in correlations between neurons of different subtypes or in different cortical layers can provide clues about how the responses of populations of sensory neurons change with attention. Similarly, understanding whether there is always a fixed relationship between rate and correlation changes places limits on the mechanisms underlying modulation by attention or other cognitive, sensory, or motor factors. If the link between gain and correlation changes holds for simple processes such as normalization, the underlying mechanisms could be studied using genetic tools in rodents or other species without training complex attentional tasks. Finally, the role of correlations in population coding could be further investigated using tasks in which information coding would be improved by a different relationship between rate and correlation changes.

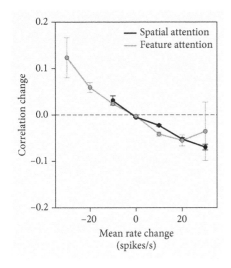

FIGURE 11.6 For both spatial (black line) and feature attention (grey line), attention-related increases in firing rate (x-axis) are associated with decreases in correlation. Conversely, decreases in rate are associated with increases in correlation. The relationship between rate and correlation modulation is similar for the two types of attention. Reprinted from *Neuron*, 70 (6), Marlene R. Cohen and John H.R. Maunsell, Using Neuronal Populations to Study the Mechanisms Underlying Spatial and Feature Attention, pp. 1192–1204, Copyright (2011), with permission from Elsevier.

Using fluctuations in attention to study its neuronal basis

Changes in perception or sensory representations with attention are typically studied by comparing psychophysical performance or neural responses between sets of trials that differ in their instructions to the subject. Analyses that compare mean perceptual performance or mean neuronal responses implicitly assume that subjects follow task instructions reliably, making every trial within an attention condition identical. Despite the best efforts of experimenters and subjects, however, a subject's attentional state will vary, even within the same task condition. Such uncontrolled fluctuations in attention can have important consequences for both perception and neuronal responses. The dynamics and cortical extent of these fluctuations and the extent to which fluctuations in different types of attention are coordinated can also provide new insight into the mechanisms underlying attention.

Measuring uncued attentional fluctuations requires an estimate of the subject's attentional state on each trial, which has been impractical using either behavioural or neuronal responses. A single trial typically yields a single behavioural response, which is not easily decomposed into contributions from the subject's behavioural state and perceptual capacity. The responses of individual sensory neurons are so variable that they have been similarly difficult to use to determine a subject's attentional state. While many previous studies have found a relationship between single-neuron responses and behavioural choice (e.g., choice probability), the relationship between any one neuron and behaviour is typically weak (Parker and Newsome 1998; Nienborg and Cumming 2010). A neuron's response on a single trial therefore cannot provide useful information about behavioural state.

The resolution lies in combining the responses of many neurons. Fluctuations in signals from scalp recordings (Thut et al. 2006; Bollimunta et al. 2008) and the BOLD signal from fMRI studies (Ress et al. 2000; Grill-Spector et al. 2004; Sapir et al. 2005; Fox et al. 2007; Leber 2010), which presumably reflect the activity of a large number of cells, are related to behavioural outcome. As with the responses of single neurons, however, fluctuations in these signals are only weakly correlated with behaviour and EEG and imaging methods do not allow flexibility in the way the responses of different neurons are combined for analysis.

Recent work shows that basing a single trial measure of attention on the responses of a few dozen simultaneously recorded neurons provides the power to accurately predict behaviour on a trial-by-trial basis (Cohen and Maunsell 2011a, 2011b). In the next section, we discuss this method for measuring attention at a single moment, some insights into attentional mechanisms, and avenues for future work.

Measuring attention on a single trial

A set of recent studies showed that a single-trial measure of attention can be based on the responses of a few dozen simultaneously recorded neurons in each hemisphere of visual area V4. These neurons can be used to identify fluctuations in attention in the context of a task involving either spatial attention alone (Cohen and Maunsell 2010) or spatial and feature attention simultaneously (Cohen and Maunsell 2011a). Just as traditional measures of attention compare mean responses in two attention conditions, the population analysis assessed the monkey's attentional state on each trial in a similar way: by using a linear discriminator to quantify the similarity of the population response at a given moment to the average in each of the attention conditions.

A putative 'attention axis' was defined as the line connecting mean responses before correct detections in each of two cued attention conditions (Cohen and Maunsell 2010, 2011a, 2011b). The population responses for each trial, which form a high dimensional space (where each neuron represents one dimension) are projected onto this axis (Fig. 11.7a). The attention axis was constructed based only on data from correct trials, so missed trials provided an important test of whether position on the attention axis correlates with behavioural performance. On average, projections for trials in which the animal missed the orientation change had smaller values than for correct detections, meaning that attention was shifted toward the mean of the opposite attention condition (Cohen and Maunsell 2010).

The population projection provides a metric of attention that strongly correlates with the animal's performance (Fig. 11.7b). On trials in which the animal's attention was putatively directed to the stimulus on the left, the monkey did well detecting stimulus changes on the left (Fig. 11.7b, grey line) and poorly detecting changes on the right (Fig. 11.7b, black line). Conversely, on trials in which the population response was more similar to the mean for correct attend-right trials, the monkey correctly detected most changes on the right but few on the left. This metric, which was based on the responses of a few dozen visual neurons over just 200 ms, therefore provides a glimpse into the animal's attentional state at a given moment, and the results in Fig. 11.7 show that fluctuations in attention are associated with changes in perception.

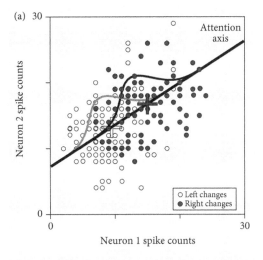

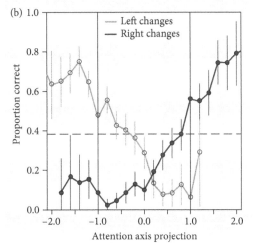

FIGURE 11.7 Fluctuations in attention are associated with large changes in psychophysical performance on a difficult change detection task. (a) Construction of a putative attention axis. The responses of each simultaneously recorded neuron are plotted in an n-dimensional space, where n is the number of neurons (shown here for a two-neuron example). These responses are projected onto the line connecting the mean responses on correct trials in each cued attention condition to give two distributions of projections onto the attention axis. On this axis a value of 1 corresponds to the average response across all trials when the animal was instructed to pay attention to the stimulus on the right, and a value of −1 corresponds to the average response across all trials when the animal was instructed to pay attention to the stimulus on the left. (b) The animal's ability to detect changes in the left (grey line) or right visual field (black line) was strongly correlated with projection on the attention axis. When the neurons indicated strong attention to the left, the animal was able to detect changes in that location more than half of the time and was almost never able to detect changes in the opposite hemifield. The dashed line represents the average proportion correct across all conditions. Adapted from Cohen, M. and Maunsell, J., A neuronal population measure of attention predicts behavioral performance on individual trials, *Journal of Neuroscience*, 30, pp. 15241–15253 © 2010, The Society for Neuroscience.

Insights from fluctuations in attention

Beyond establishing a relationship between attentional fluctuations and psychophysical performance, examining these fluctuations can provide insights about the mechanisms underlying attention that are inaccessible from firing rates and pairwise correlations. For example, comparing fluctuations in feature and spatial attention provides a new way to address long-standing questions about whether these two forms of attention share underlying mechanisms (Cohen and Maunsell 2011a). Such insights illustrate the importance of studying fluctuations in attention and other cognitive processes in the future.

A recent study compared feature and spatial attention by recording from populations of V4 neurons in both hemispheres of monkeys that performed a mixed spatial and feature attention task (Cohen and Maunsell 2011a). On each trial, four estimates of attention were obtained: one for spatial and one for feature attention calculated from the responses of the subset of neurons recorded in each hemisphere. With these measures, it was possible to ask whether spatial and feature attention are co-modulated by calculating the correlation coefficient between projections onto the feature and spatial attention axes both within (Fig. 11.8b) and across hemispheres (Fig. 11.8a). In both cases, the mean correlation coefficient was statistically indistinguishable from zero. Therefore, although feature and spatial attention are associated with similar changes in the rates and correlation of nearby neurons (Fig. 11.7), and likely mediated by similar mechanisms, these mechanisms nevertheless appear to function independently.

Calculating the correlation coefficient between projections onto attention axes defined separately for neurons recorded from the two hemispheres can also provide insight into the cortical extent of modulation by spatial and feature attention. The correlation between projections on the spatial attention axes for the two cerebral hemispheres was indistinguishable from zero (Fig. 11.8a). This lack of correlation was not a result of insufficient statistical power: when neurons recorded within each hemisphere were randomly divided into two equal-sized groups, a positive correlation between projections onto spatial attention axes calculated from each subgroup was easily detected. These data indicate that fluctuations in the amount of spatial attention allocated to the two stimuli arise from fluctuations in groups of neurons within a hemisphere, rather than because the animal attends to the wrong stimulus.

The cortical extent of neuronal changes related to feature attention is qualitatively different. The statistical power for detecting correlations along the feature attention axes was similar for feature and spatial attention (Fig. 11.8b). However, in contrast to spatial attention, projections on the two feature attention axes were positively correlated across hemispheres (Fig. 11.8a, grey bar).

These results are consistent with the idea that spatial attention involves coordination among local groups of neurons, and that the amount of attention allocated to locations in opposite hemifields is independent. In contrast, attention to features appears to involve coordination across neurons representing the entire visual field, selectively

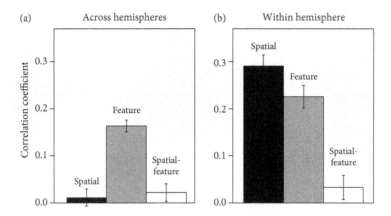

FIGURE 11.8 Fluctuations in feature, but not spatial attention are coordinated across the two cerebral hemispheres. (a) Mean correlation coefficient between projections onto the attention axes constructed using simultaneously recorded neurons in the two hemispheres. The mean correlation coefficient was statistically greater than zero for feature attention and indistinguishable from zero for spatial attention or the correlation between spatial and feature attention. (b) Same, for randomly chosen subsets of neurons within a hemisphere. The correlation coefficients were statistically greater than zero for both spatial and feature attention and indistinguishable from zero for the correlation between the two types of attention. Reprinted from *Neuron*, 70 (6), Marlene R. Cohen and John H. R. Maunsell, Using Neuronal Populations to Study the Mechanisms Underlying Spatial and Feature Attention, pp. 1192–1204, Copyright (2011), with permission from Elsevier.

co-modulating neurons located far apart, even across hemispheres. The idea that spatial and feature attention operate on different spatial scales is supported by psychophysical evidence. A subject's ability to attend to an object in one hemifield is unaffected by attention to objects in the other hemifield (Alvarez and Cavanagh 2005). Conversely, feature attention can affect visual processing independent of stimulus location (Motter 1994; Saenz et al. 2002, 2003; Liu and Mance 2011). Together, these results are consistent with the idea that feature and spatial attention are mediated by a unified attentional mechanism that can modulate the responses of arbitrary subgroups of neurons. More generally, they suggest that studying populations of neurons can provide ways of distinguishing between mechanisms underlying different cognitive processes.

Future directions

Attention and the dynamics of neuronal modulations

As the studies of attentional fluctuations show, attention varies over short intervals. These fluctuations can occur even within a trial. When subjects scan a visual scene, they shift their eyes every few hundred milliseconds (DiCarlo and Maunsell 2000), and each shift is associated with a change in spatial attention (Zhou and Desimone 2011). Studies that have examined shifts in attention have found that changes in neuronal responses can be correspondingly rapid. When distracting stimuli appear unexpectedly, the responses of neurons in the lateral parietal area (LIP) to distractors rise and fall quickly and closely match the dynamics of behavioural distraction (Bisley and Goldberg 2003, 2006). When monkeys are given a signal to shift their attention from one target to another, neurons in V4 reflect the change in attention within 100–200 ms (Motter 1994). Corresponding experiments that compared latencies for attentional modulation in LIP and MT found similarly rapid shifts, but with modulation in LIP responses ~60 ms earlier than those in MT, consistent with a top-down flow of attention-related signals in visual cortex (Herrington and Assad 2009).

Subjects can also shift their attention during trials without any external cue or instruction. Monkeys that are familiar with the dynamics of a task will shift their attention to different spatial locations at appropriate times to maximize their chance of getting a reward. When the probability of receiving a reward varies predictably within trials, neurons in V4 (Ghose and Maunsell 2002) and LIP (Janssen and Shadlen 2005) are more strongly modulated with attention during periods of greater reward probability, with the strength of modulation varying over periods of no more than a few hundred milliseconds.

The dynamic aspects of attention pose a challenge for studies that aim to compare differences in neuronal activity across different tasks and conditions. When direct quantitative comparisons must be made, not only the stimulus conditions but also task difficulty and reward expectations must be carefully balanced. When considering the neuronal correlates of spatial attention, quantitative comparisons from different studies are problematic because neuronal modulations are greatly affected by the difficulty of the behavioural task. Subjects adjust the amount of attention that is allocated to different stimuli in response to task demands (Lavie and Tsal 1994; Urbach and Spitzer 1995; Lee et al. 1999), and this is reflected in neuronal activity. When subjects are faced with more difficult tasks, neuronal responses to given stimuli are stronger (Spitzer et al. 1988; Spitzer and Richmond 1991) and the modulation of neuronal responses associated with shifting attention between two stimuli is larger (Spitzer et al. 1988; Spitzer and Richmond 1991; Boudreau et al. 2006). Because task difficulty and attentional effort will vary between studies, precise quantitative comparisons of neurophysiological results from different laboratories are not practical. Studies that wish to quantitatively compare neuronal modulation linked to attention and other cognitive factors across stimuli and brain areas must therefore carefully control for task difficulty and reward expectation.

The ability to detect fluctuations in attention using populations of neurons provides a new avenue for studying the dynamics of switches in attention and other cognitive factors. The ability to estimate attention at a given moment will allow much more detailed studies of the dynamics of attention switching and the extent to which they depend on the demands of the behavioural task.

Attention and cortical cell classes

There is growing interest in whether attention is preferentially associated with modulation of the responses of specific cell classes in cortex. Extracellular recordings can distinguish two classes of neurons on the basis of spike duration. 'Narrow' spikes are thought to arise from inhibitory interneurons, while 'broad' spikes are thought to arise from pyramidal neurons, whose axons carry signals to other brain regions (McCormick et al. 1985; Connors and Gutnick 1990; Contreras and Palmer 2003). In prefrontal cortex, attention has been shown to be associated with changes in the selectivity of visually responsive neurons. When monkeys switch from a direction discrimination task to a speed discrimination task, the direction selectivity of narrow-spiking neurons in prefrontal cortex is reduced more than that of broad-spiking neurons (Hussar and Pasternak 2009). In V4, however, the responses of narrow-spiking and broad-spiking neurons scale by the same factor when spatial attention varies (Mitchell et al. 2007). Equivalent effects on both classes of neurons are consistent with the organization of the anatomical projection from prefrontal cortex to V4, which does not preferentially target inhibitory interneurons (Anderson et al. 2011a).

While both narrow- and broad-spiking V4 neurons change their mean rates proportionally when attention varies, they show differential effects on the variance of their responses across repeated presentations of the same stimulus. Mitchell and colleagues (2007) found that the variance of the broad-spiking neurons did not change with attention, and was the same as the variance of the narrow-spiking neurons when attention was directed toward their receptive fields. However, when attention was directed away from the receptive field, the narrow-spiking neurons increased their variance. Another difference in the effect of attention on narrow- and broad-spiking V4 neurons is the relationship between attention-related modulation and burstiness of firing. Among broad-spiking neurons, attention-related modulation is strongest among those broad-spiking neurons that have bursty patterns of firing (Anderson et al. 2011b), a relationship that is not found among the narrow-spiking neurons. Future studies of the circuits underlying attention might help explain why attention is associated with different effects for different cell classes in cortex.

Concluding remarks

Although one could imagine designing a nervous system in which cognitive factors do not affect basic sensory representations, it is clear that attention is associated with modulation of the responses of neurons throughout visual cortex. The studies described here have made promising strides toward understanding the neuronal mechanisms underlying this modulation and establishing a link between the modulation of sensory responses and changes in perception. Recent improvements in technology for recording from, identifying, and manipulating populations of neurons suggest that the field is well positioned to build on these insights to improve our understanding of how the changes observed in visual cortex improve observers' perceptual abilities.

References

Abbott, L. F. and Dayan, P. (1999). The effect of correlated variability on the accuracy of a population code. *Neural Computation* 11: 91–101.

Aertsen, A. M. H. J., Gerstein, G. L., Habib, M. K., and Palm, G. (1989). Dynamics of neurons firing correlation: Modulation of 'effective connectivity'. *Journal of Neurophysiology* 61: 900–917.

Ahissar, E., Vaadia, E., Ahissar, M., Bergman, H., Arieli, A., and Abeles, M. (1992). Dependence of cortical plasticity on correlated activity of single neurons and on behavioral context. *Science* 257: 1412–1415.

Albrecht, D. G. and Geisler, W. S. (1991). Motion selectivity and the contrast-response function of simple cells in the visual cortex. *Visual Neuroscience* 7: 531–546.

Alvarez, G. and Cavanagh, P. (2005). Independent resources for attentional tracking in the left and right visual hemifields. *Psychological Science* 16: 637–643.

Anderson, J., Kennedy, H., and Martin, K. (2011a). Pathways of attention: Synaptic relationships of frontal eye field to v4, lateral intraparietal cortex, and area 46 in macaque monkey. *Journal of Neuroscience* 31: 10872–10881.

Anderson, E., Mitchell, J., and Reynolds, J. (2011b). Attentional modulation of firing rate varies with burstiness across putative pyramidal neurons in macaque visual area v4. *Journal of Neuroscience* 31: 10983–10992.

Averbeck, B., Latham, P., and Pouget, A. (2006). Neural correlations, population coding and computation. *Nature Reviews Neuroscience* 7: 358–366.

Bair, W., Zohary, E., and Newsome, W. T. (2001). Correlated firing in macaque visual area MT: Time scales and relationship to behavior. *Journal of Neuroscience* 21: 1676–1697.

Berens, P., Ecker, A., Gerwinn, S., Tolias, A., and Bethge, M. (2011). Reassessing optimal neural population codes with neurometric functions. *Proceedings of the National Academy of Sciences of the USA* 108: 4423–4428.

Bisley, J. and Goldberg, M. (2003). Neuronal activity in the lateral intraparietal area and spatial attention. *Science* 299: 81–86.

Bisley, J. and Goldberg, M. (2006). Neural correlates of attention and distractibility in the lateral intraparietal area. *Journal of Neurophysiology* 95: 1696–1717.

Bisley, J. and Goldberg, M. (2010). Attention, intention, and priority in the parietal lobe. *Annual Review of Neuroscience* 33: 1–21.

Bollimunta, A., Chen, Y., Schroeder, C., and Ding, M. (2008). Neuronal mechanisms of cortical alpha oscillations in awake-behaving macaques. *Journal of Neuroscience* 28: 9976–9988.

Boudreau, C., Williford, T., and Maunsell, J. H. R. (2006). Effects of task difficulty and target likelihood in area v4 of macaque monkeys. *Journal of Neurophysiology* 96: 2377–2387.

Boynton, G. (2009). A framework for describing the effects of attention on visual responses. *Vision Research* 49: 1129–1143.

Braun, J., Koch, C., and Davis, J. L. (2001). *Visual Attention and Cortical Circuits* (p. 313). Cambridge, Mass.: MIT Press.

Buschman, T. and Miller, E. (2007). Top-down versus bottom-up control of attention in the prefrontal and posterior parietal cortices. *Science* 315: 1860–1862.

Busse, L., Wade, A. R., and Carandini, M. (2009). Representation of concurrent stimuli by population activity in visual cortex. *Neuron* 64: 931–942.

Carandini, M., Heeger, D. J., and Movshon, J. A. (1997). Linearity and normalization in simple cells of the macaque primary visual cortex. *Journal of Neuroscience* 17: 8621–8644.

Carandini, M. and Heeger, D. J. (2012). Normalization as a canonical neural computation. *Nature Reviews Neuroscience* 13: 51–62.

Carrasco, M. (2011). Visual attention: The past 25 years. *Vision Research* 51: 1484–1525.

Chelazzi, L., Duncan, J., Miller, E. K., and Desimone, R. (1998). Responses of neurons in inferotemporal cortex during memory-guided visual search. *Journal of Neurophysiology* 80: 2918–2940.

Chen, Y., Martinez-Conde, S., Macknik, S., Bereshpolova, Y., Swadlow, H., and Alonso, J. (2008). Task difficulty modulates the activity of specific neuronal populations in primary visual cortex. *Nature Neuroscience* 11: 974–982.

Cohen, M. and Newsome, W. (2008). Context-dependent changes in functional circuitry in visual area MT. *Neuron* 60: 162–173.

Cohen, M. and Maunsell, J. H. R. (2009). Attention improves performance primarily by reducing interneuronal correlations. *Nature Neuroscience* 12: 1594–1600.

Cohen, M. R. and Maunsell, J. H. R. (2010). A neuronal population measure of attention predicts behavioral performance on individual trials. *Journal of Neuroscience* 30: 15241–15253.

Cohen, M. R. and Kohn, A. (2011). Measuring and interpreting neuronal correlations. *Nature Neuroscience* 14: 811–819.

Cohen, M. R. and Maunsell, J. H. R. (2011a). Using neuronal populations to study the mechanisms underlying spatial and feature attention. *Neuron* 70: 1192–1204.

Cohen, M. R. and Maunsell, J. H. R. (2011b). When attention wanders: How uncontrolled fluctuations in attention affect performance. *Journal of Neuroscience* 31: 15802–15806.

Connor, C. E., Gallant, J. L., Preddie, D. C., and Van Essen, D. C. (1996). Responses in area v4 depend on the spatial relationship between stimulus and attention. *Journal of Neurophysiology* 75: 1306–1308.

Connor, C. E., Preddie, D. C., Gallant, J. L., and Van Essen, D. C. (1997). Spatial attention effects in macaque area v4. *Journal of Neuroscience* 17: 3201–3214.

Connors, B. and Gutnick, M. (1990). Intrinsic firing patterns of diverse neocortical neurons. *Trends in Neurosciences* 13: 99–104.

Contreras, D. and Palmer, L. A. (2003). Response to contrast of electrophysiologically defined cell classes in primary visual cortex. *Journal of Neuroscience* 23: 6936–6945.

Cook, E. P. and Maunsell, J. H. R. (2004). Attentional modulation of motion integration of individual neurons in the middle temporal visual area (MT). *Journal of Neuroscience* 24: 7964–7977.

David, S., Hayden, B., Mazer, J., and Gallant, J. (2008). Attention to stimulus features shifts spectral tuning of v4 neurons during natural vision. *Neuron* 59: 509–521.

Dicarlo, J. J. and Maunsell, J. H. R. (2000). Form representation in monkey inferotemporal cortex is virtually unaltered by free viewing. *Nature Neuroscience* 3: 814–821.

Eriksen, C. and Yeh, Y. (1985). Allocation of attention in the visual field. *Journal of Experimental Psychology: Human Perception and Performance* 11: 583–597.

Espinosa, I. and Gerstein, G. (1988). Cortical auditory neuron interactions during presentation of 3-tone sequences: Effective connectivity. *Brain Research* 450: 39–50.

Fox, M., Snyder, A., Vincent, J., and Raichle, M. (2007). Intrinsic fluctuations within cortical systems account for intertrial variability in human behavior. *Neuron* 56: 171–184.

Fries, P. (2009). Neuronal gamma-band synchronization as a fundamental process in cortical computation. *Annual Review of Neuroscience* 32: 209–224.

Ghose, G. M. and Maunsell, J. H. R. (2002). Attentional modulation in visual cortex depends on task timing. *Nature* 419: 616–620.

Ghose, G. M. and Maunsell, J. H. R. (2008). Spatial summation can explain the attentional modulation of neuronal responses to multiple stimuli in area v4. *Journal of Neuroscience 28*: 5115–5126.

Ghose, G. M. (2009). Attentional modulation of visual responses by flexible input gain. *Journal of Neurophysiology 101*: 2089–2106.

Ghose, G. M. and Bearl, D. (2010). Attention directed by expectations enhances receptive fields in cortical area MT. *Vision Research 50*: 441–451.

Gilbert, C. and Sigman, M. (2007). Brain states: Top-down influences in sensory processing. *Neuron 54*: 677–696.

Gregoriou, G., Gotts, S., Zhou, H., and Desimone, R. (2009). High-frequency, long-range coupling between prefrontal and visual cortex during attention. *Science 324*: 1207–1210.

Grill-Spector, K., Knouf, N., and Kanwisher, N. (2004). The fusiform face area subserves face perception, not generic within-category identification. *Nature Neuroscience 7*: 555–562.

Gu, Y., Liu, S., Fetsch, C., et al. (2011). Perceptual learning reduces interneuronal correlations in macaque visual cortex. *Neuron 71*: 750–761.

Gutnisky, D. and Dragoi, V. (2008). Adaptive coding of visual information in neural populations. *Nature 452*: 220–224.

Haenny, P. E. and Schiller, P. H. (1988). State-dependent activity in monkey visual cortex, I: Single cell activity in v1 and v4 on visual tasks. *Experimental Brain Research 69*: 225–244.

Heeger, D. J. (1992). Normalization of cell responses in cat striate cortex. *Visual Neuroscience 9*: 181–197.

Heeger, D. J. (1993). Modeling simple-cell direction selectivity with normalized, half-squared, linear operators. *Journal of Neurophysiology 70*: 1885–1898.

Heeger, D. J., Simoncelli, E. P., and Movshon, J. A. (1996). Computational models of cortical visual processing. *Proceedings of the National Academy of Science (USA) 93*: 623–627.

Herrington, T. and Assad, J. (2009). Neural activity in the middle temporal area and lateral intraparietal area during endogenously cued shifts of attention. *Journal of Neuroscience 29*: 14160–14176.

Hussar, C. and Pasternak, T. (2009). Flexibility of sensory representations in prefrontal cortex depends on cell type. *Neuron 64*: 730–743.

Janssen, P. and Shadlen, M. N. (2005). A representation of hazard rate of elapsed time in macaque area lip. *Nature Neuroscience 8*: 234–241.

Khayat, P., Niebergall, R., and Martinez-Trujillo, J. C. (2010). Attention differentially modulates similar neuronal responses evoked by varying contrast and direction stimuli in area MT. *Journal of Neuroscience 30*: 2188–2197.

Kohn, A. and Smith, M. (2005). Stimulus dependence of neuronal correlation in primary visual cortex of the macaque. *Journal of Neuroscience 25*: 3661–3673.

Kohn, A., Zandvakili, A., and Smith, M. (2009). Correlations and brain states: From electrophysiology to functional imaging. *Current Opinion in Neurobiology 19*: 434–438.

Komiyama, T., Sato, T., O'Connor, D. H., et al. (2010). Learning-related fine-scale specificity imaged in motor cortex circuits of behaving mice. *Nature 464*: 1182–1186.

Laberge, D. (1983). Spatial extent of attention to letters and words. *Journal of Experimental Psychology: Human Perception and Performance 9*: 371–379.

Lavie, N. and Tsal, Y. (1994). Perceptual load as a major determinant of the locus of selection in visual attention. *Perception & Psychophysics 56*: 183–197.

Leber, A. (2010). Neural predictors of within-subject fluctuations in attentional control. *Journal of Neuroscience 30*: 11458–11465.

Lee, D. K., Itti, L., Koch, C., and Braun, J. (1999). Attention activates winner-take-all competition among visual filters. *Nature Neuroscience 2*: 375–381.

Lee, J. and Maunsell, J. H. R. (2009). A normalization model of attentional modulation of single unit responses. *PLoS One 4*: e4651.

Lee, J. and Maunsell, J. H. R. (2010a). Attentional modulation of MT neurons with single or multiple stimuli in their receptive fields. *Journal of Neuroscience 30*: 3058–3066.

Lee, J. and Maunsell, J. H. R. (2010b). The effect of attention on neuronal responses to high and low contrast stimuli. *Journal of Neurophysiology 104*: 960–971.

Li, X. and Basso, M. (2008). Preparing to move increases the sensitivity of superior colliculus neurons. *Journal of Neuroscience 28*: 4561–4577.

Liu, T. and Mance, I. (2011). Constant spread of feature-based attention across the visual field. *Vision Research 51*: 26–33.

Luck, S. J., Chelazzi, L., Hillyard, S. A., and Desimone, R. (1997). Neural mechanisms of spatial selective attention in areas v1, v2, and v4 of macaque visual cortex. *Journal of Neurophysiology 77*: 24–42.

Martinez-Trujillo, J. C. and Treue, S. (2002). Attentional modulation strength in cortical area MT depends on stimulus contrast. *Neuron 35*: 365–370.

Maunsell, J. H. R. and Cook, E. P. (2002). The role of attention in visual processing. *Philosophical Transactions of the Royal Society of London B 357*: 1063–1072.

Maunsell, J. H. R. and Treue, S. (2006). Feature-based attention in visual cortex. *Trends in Neurosciences 29*: 317–322.

McAdams, C. J. and Maunsell, J. H. R. (1999). Effects of attention on orientation-tuning functions of single neurons in macaque cortical area v4. *Journal of Neuroscience 19*: 431–441.

McCormick, D., Connors, B., Lighthall, J., and Prince, D. (1985). Comparative electrophysiology of pyramidal and sparsely spiny stellate neurons of the neocortex. *Journal of Neurophysiology 54*: 782–806.

Mitchell, J. F., Sundberg, K., and Reynolds, J. H. (2007). Differential attention-dependent response modulation across cell classes in macaque visual area v4. *Neuron 55*: 131–141.

Mitchell, J. F., Sundberg, K., and Reynolds, J. H. (2009). Spatial attention decorrelates intrinsic activity fluctuations in macaque area v4. *Neuron 63*: 879–888.

Moran, J. and Desimone, R. (1985). Selective attention gates visual processing in the extrastriate cortex. *Science 229*: 782–784.

Motter, B. C. (1993). Focal attention produces spatially selective processing in visual cortical areas v1, v2, and v4 in the presence of competing stimuli. *Journal of Neurophysiology 70*: 909–919.

Motter, B. C. (1994). Neural correlates of feature selective memory and pop-out in extrastriate area v4. *Journal of Neuroscience 14*: 2190–2199.

Navalpakkam, V. and Itti, L. (2007). Search goal tunes visual features optimally. *Neuron 53*: 605–617.

Nienborg, H. and Cumming, B. (2010). Correlations between the activity of sensory neurons and behavior: How much do they tell us about a neuron's causality? *Current Opinion in Neurobiology 20*: 376–381.

Nienborg, H., Cohen, M., and Cumming, B. (2012). Decision-related activity in sensory neurons: Correlations among neurons and with behavior. *Annual Review of Neuroscience 35*: 463–483.

Nirenberg, S. and Latham, P. (2003). Decoding neuronal spike trains: How important are correlations? *Proceedings of the National Academy of Sciences of the USA 100*: 7348–7353.

O'Connor, D. H., Fukui, M. M., Pinsk, M. A., and Kastner, S. (2002). Attention modulates responses in the human lateral geniculate nucleus. *Nature Neuroscience* 5: 1203–1209.

Olson, C. R. (2001). Object-based vision and attention in primates. *Current Opinion in Neurobiology* 11: 171–179.

Parker, A. J. and Newsome, W. T. (1998). Sense and the single neuron: Probing the physiology of perception. *Annual Review of Neuroscience* 21: 227–277.

Poulet, J. and Petersen, C. (2008). Internal brain state regulates membrane potential synchrony in barrel cortex of behaving mice. *Nature* 454: 881–885.

Ress, D., Backus, B. T., and Heeger, D. J. (2000). Activity in primary visual cortex predicts performance in a visual detection task. *Nature Neuroscience* 3: 940–945.

Reynolds, J. H., Chelazzi, L., and Desimone, R. (1999). Competitive mechanisms subserve attention in macaque areas v2 and v4. *Journal of Neuroscience* 19: 1736–1753.

Reynolds, J. H., Pasternak, T., and Desimone, R. (2000). Attention increases sensitivity of v4 neurons. *Neuron* 26: 703–714.

Reynolds, J. H. and Chelazzi, L. (2004). Attentional modulation of visual processing. *Annual Review of Neuroscience* 27: 611–647.

Reynolds, J. H. and Heeger, D. (2009). The normalization model of attention. *Neuron* 61: 168–185.

Roelfsema, P. R., Lamme, V. A. F., and Spekreijse, H. (1998). Object-based attention in the primary visual cortex of the macaque monkey. *Nature* 395: 376–381.

Roelfsema, P. R., Lamme, V., and Spekreijse, H. (2004). Synchrony and covariation of firing rates in the primary visual cortex during contour grouping. *Nature Neuroscience* 7: 982–991.

Roy, A., Steinmetz, P., Hsiao, S., Johnson, K., and Niebur, E. (2007). Synchrony: A neural correlate of somatosensory attention. *Journal of Neurophysiology* 98: 1645–1661.

Saalmann, Y., Pigarev, I., and Vidyasagar, T. (2007). Neural mechanisms of visual attention: How top-down feedback highlights relevant locations. *Science* 316: 1612–1615.

Saenz, M., Buracas, G. T., and Boynton, G. M. (2002). Global effects of feature-based attention in human visual cortex. *Nature Neuroscience* 5: 631–632.

Saenz, M., Buracas, G. T., and Boynton, G. M. (2003). Global feature-based attention for motion and color. *Vision Research* 43: 629–637.

Sapir, A., D'Avossa, G., McAvoy, M., Shulman, G., and Corbetta, M. (2005). Brain signals for spatial attention predict performance in a motion discrimination task. *Proceedings of the National Academy of Sciences of the USA* 102: 17810–17815.

Schwartz, O. and Simoncelli, E. P. (2001). Natural signal statistics and sensory gain control. *Nature Neuroscience* 4: 819–825.

Scolari, M. and Serences, J. (2009). Adaptive allocation of attentional gain. *Journal of Neuroscience* 29: 11933–11942.

Scolari, M., Byers, A., and Serences, J. (2012). Optimal deployment of attentional gain during fine discriminations. *Journal of Neuroscience* 32: 7723–7733.

Shadlen, M. N. and Newsome, W. T. (1996). Motion perception: Seeing and deciding. *Proceedings of the National Academy of Sciences USA* 93: 628–633.

Shadlen, M. N. and Newsome, W. T. (1998). The variable discharge of cortical neurons: Implications for connectivity, computation, and information coding. *Journal of Neuroscience* 18: 3870–3896.

Smith, M. and Kohn, A. (2008). Spatial and temporal scales of neuronal correlation in primary visual cortex. *Journal of Neuroscience* 28: 12591–12603.

Spitzer, H., Desimone, R., and Moran, J. (1988). Increased attention enhances both behavioral and neuronal performance. *Science* 240: 338–340.

Spitzer, H. and Richmond, B. J. (1991). Task difficulty: Ignoring, attending to, and discriminating a visual stimulus yield progressively more activity in inferior temporal neurons. *Experimental Brain Research 83*: 340–348.

Steinmetz, P. N., Roy, A., Fitzgerald, P. J., Hsiao, S. S., Johnson, K. O., and Niebur, E. (2000). Attention modulates synchronized firing in primate somatosensory cortex. *Nature 404*: 187–190.

Thiele, A., Pooresmaeili, A., Delicato, L., Herrero, J., and Roelfsema, P. (2009). Additive effects of attention and stimulus contrast in primary visual cortex. *Cerebral Cortex 19*: 2970–2981.

Thut, G., Nietzel, A., Brandt, S., and Pascual-Leone, A. (2006). Alpha-band electroencephalographic activity over occipital cortex indexes visuospatial attention bias and predicts visual target detection. *Journal of Neuroscience 26*: 9494–9502.

Tolhurst, D. J., Movshon, J. A., and Dean, A. F. (1983). The statistical reliability of signals in single neurons in cat and monkey visual cortex. *Vision Research 23*: 775–785.

Treue, S. and Maunsell, J. H. R. (1996). Attentional modulation of visual motion processing in cortical areas MT and MST. *Nature 382*: 539–541.

Treue, S. and Martinez-Trujillo, J. C. (1999a). Reshaping neuronal representations of visual scenes through attention. *Current Psychology of Cognition 18*: 951–972.

Treue, S. and Martinez-Trujillo, J. C. (1999b). Feature-based attention influences motion processing gain in macaque visual cortex. *Nature 399*: 575–579.

Urbach, D. and Spitzer, H. (1995). Attentional effort modulated by task difficulty. *Vision Research 35*: 2169–2177.

Vaadia, E., Haalman, I., Abeles, M., et al. (1995). Dynamics of neuronal interactions in monkey cortex in relation to behavioural events. *Nature 373*: 515–518.

Vogels, R. and Orban, G. A. (1994). Activity of inferior temporal neurons during orientation discrimination with successively presented gratings. *Journal of Neurophysiology 71*: 1428–1451.

Williford, T. and Maunsell, J. H. R. (2006). Effects of spatial attention on contrast response functions in macaque area v4. *Journal of Neurophysiology 96*: 40–54.

Womelsdorf, T., Anton-Erxleben, K., Pieper, F., and Treue, S. (2006). Dynamic shifts of visual receptive fields in cortical area MT by spatial attention. *Nature Neuroscience 9*: 1156–1160.

Womelsdorf, T. and Fries, P. (2007). The role of neuronal synchronization in selective attention. *Current Opinion in Neurobiology 17*: 154–160.

Zhou, H. and Desimone, R. (2011). Feature-based attention in the frontal eye field and area v4 during visual search. *Neuron 70*: 1205–1217.

Zohary, E., Celebrini, S., Britten, K. H., and Newsome, W. T. (1994). Neuronal plasticity that underlies improvement in perceptual performance. *Science 263*: 1289–1292.

....

CHAPTER 12

NEURONAL MECHANISMS OF ATTENTIONAL CONTROL: PARIETAL CORTEX

....

JACQUELINE GOTTLIEB

INTRODUCTION

....

SINCE the nineteenth century, neuropsychological evidence has suggested that the parietal cortex is important in spatial attention. Patients with damage to the parietal lobe can develop the syndrome of *neglect*, a specific inability to notice sensory stimuli in the contralateral space. A milder form of the disease is that of *extinction* or *perceptual rivalry*, where patients can perceive a contralateral object when it is presented alone but, if presented with two objects simultaneously tend to choose the ipsilateral one. Accompanying their attentional deficits, patients with parietal lesions can also have *optic ataxia*, difficulty looking at or reaching contralateral targets. These syndromes suggest that the parietal lobes are important for linking perception and action, and specifically in assigning importance (or 'interest') to the contralateral space (see also Vallar and Bolognini, chapter 33, this volume).

This view of the parietal lobe emerging from neurological studies is upheld in neurophysiological work in monkeys. Based on anatomical and physiological evidence, the monkey parietal lobe has been subdivided into two broad sectors that lie dorsal and ventral to the intraparietal sulcus (IPS) and are called the superior and inferior parietal lobes (SPL and IPL) (Fig. 1). Areas within the SPL are responsive primarily to touch (somatosensation) and skeletal (limb) movements and represent the near peripersonal space (Colby and Goldberg 1999), while areas in the IPL respond to visual inputs and movements of the eyes and head and represent the farther visual space (Colby and Goldberg 1999).

The IPL, which has been most intensively studied in relation to attention, is further subdivided into three areas. Area VIP (the ventral intraparietal area) lies in the fundus

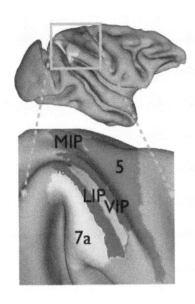

FIGURE 12.1 The parietal lobe in the monkey. Lateral view of the rhesus monkey brain indicating the approximate location of individual parietal areas. The IPL is located ventral and posterior to the intraparietal sulcus and includes areas 7a, LIP (the lateral intraparietal area, ventral and dorsal divisions) and VIP (ventral intraparietal area). The SPL is located dorsal and medial to the sulcus and includes area 5 and the medial intraparietal area (MIP). Reprinted from *Current Opinion in Neurobiology*, 20 (6), Jacqueline Gottlieb and Lawrence H. Snyder, Spatial and non-spatial functions of the parietal cortex, pp. 731–40, Copyright (2010), with permission from Elsevier.

of the IPS and is a transitional area that responds to both visual and somatosensory stimulation. VIP neurons have bimodal receptive fields (RF) on the upper body and face (Colby et al. 1993). Area 7a is a visual area that covers the cortical convexity lateral to the IPL and conveys information about full-field visual motion, visual salience, and eye position (Constantinidis and Steinmetz 2005; Raffi and Siegel 2005). Finally the lateral intraparietal area (LIP) is a small area in the lateral bank of the intraparietal sulcus that has strong ties to the oculomotor system.

As will become clear in this chapter, area LIP has been intensively investigated and is believed to reflect internal processes related to attention, learning, and decision formation. LIP receives visual inputs from the lateral pulvinar thalamic nucleus and from cortical areas in the dorsal and ventral visual streams, and has strong anatomical connections to two oculomotor areas—the frontal eye fields (FEF) and the superior colliculus (SC) (Blatt et al. 1990; Lewis and Van Essen 2000). LIP neurons have visual RF located mostly in the contralateral hemifield and respond to small stimuli that drive attention and shifts of gaze (Blatt et al. 1990). This chapter will focus on physiological studies that explore the function of this area with respect to attention and eye movement control.

ADAPTIVE SPATIAL REPRESENTATION

Although LIP contains several types of cells, the vast majority of studies have focused on neurons that have visual receptive fields (RF)—i.e. respond to visual inputs in a limited range of retinal locations. In terms of its layout in the IPS the retinotopic map in LIP has only a coarse organization, and adjacent neurons can respond to disparate retinal locations (Ben Hamed and Duhamel 2002; Ben Hamed et al. 2002). Nevertheless, by virtue of their RF the neurons convey spatial information, encoding the location of objects in the external world.

The spatiotopic map in LIP is distinguished from maps in earlier visual areas by several characteristics. First, LIP neurons encode not the mere presence of a visual input but are strongly modulated by the salience or behavioural significance of that input. Second, even though the RF of LIP neurons are retinotopic (meaning that they move relative to the external world each time the eye moves) neurons maintain an accurate memory of salient locations across shifts of gaze. And third, the visual responses that are encoded in LIP can be quite complex and are modulated by a variety of behavioural ('extraretinal') factors.

A good illustration of the sensitivity of LIP neurons to salience and behavioural significance comes from an experiment that trained monkeys to make eye movements across a stable visual scene (Gottlieb et al. 1998). A circular array containing several objects remained stable on the screen (Fig. 2, top cartoon). On each trial the monkey looked at (fixated) a peripheral location (FP1) where no array stimulus was in a neuron's RF (labelled RF1 in the cartoon) and then made a saccade to a central location (FP2) that brought the RF onto a portion of the stable array (RF2). This mode of presentation emulates natural viewing conditions, where stimuli are stable and inconspicuous in their environment but move on the retina by virtue of the observer's motion.

In one variant of this task, all eight stimuli remained stable and unchanging for a long block of trials, and one of these stimuli entered the RF by virtue of the monkeys' saccade. In a second variant, the visual stimulation to the neurons' RF was identical, except that the stimulus entering the RF was rendered salient by abruptly appearing and disappearing on each trial.

Even though the visual stimulation to their RF was identical in both cases LIP neurons distinguished between the stable and recent-onset contexts. Neurons had barely any response when a stable stimulus entered their RF (Fig. 2, left) but responded exuberantly if the same object had recently flashed on (Fig. 2, right). Note that this visual response arose even though the stimulus onset had occurred before the saccade and outside of the neuron's RF; thus, the neuron responded after the saccade as if it had 'remembered' the salient event that occurred before the saccade. Thus LIP neurons have a remarkable ability to filter out most objects in rich visual scenes and selectively respond to salient locations, and they track these locations across shifts of gaze.

To see if neurons also encode top-down, deliberate selection, a modified version of the stable array task was used, in which the RF stimulus was inconspicuous and stable but on some trials, could become relevant for the task (Fig. 3). After achieving fixation on a given trial, monkeys saw a cue that matched one of the stable stimuli and instructed the monkey to make a saccade to it. The cue was flashed at the centre of gaze outside the neurons' RF, so that it did not activate the cell. However, LIP neurons responded selectively if the stable stimulus in their RF became the designated target . This is illustrated for the cell in Fig. 12.3, which responded if the designated target was in its RF (i.e. upward saccade in the left column) but remained quiescent if another stimulus

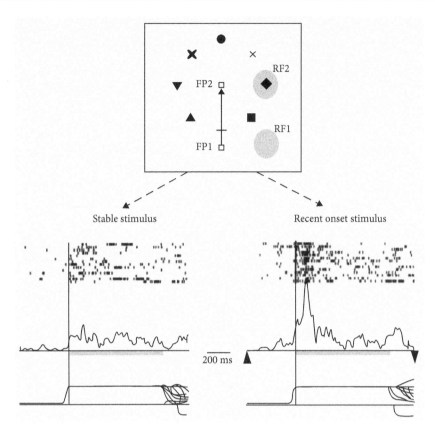

FIGURE 12.2 LIP neurons respond selectively to salient events. The top cartoon shows the experiment design. A circular object array was continuously present on the screen. The monkey began each trial by looking at an initial fixation point (FP1), chosen so that the RF of the neuron under study was on a blank visual location (RF1). The fixation point then jumped to the centre of the array (FP2) and the monkey made a saccade to it (arrow). This saccade brought the neuron's RF onto one of the array objects (RF2). The bottom panels show the activity of one LIP neuron. Raster plots show the times of individual action potentials relative to the saccade that brings the stimulus in the RF (marked by the vertical bar). Traces underneath the rasters show average firing rate across trials. Bottom traces show the horizontal and vertical eye position, superimposed for multiple trials. The neuron had only weak activation if the stimulus entering its RF was stable for a long period of time (left). In contrast the neuron responded strongly if the same stimulus had been rendered salient by virtue of an abrupt onset (right). Adapted by permission from Macmillan Publishers Ltd: *Nature* 391 (6666) Gottlieb, J. P., Kusunoki, M., and Goldberg, M. E., The representation of visual salience in monkey parietal cortex, pp. 481–4 copyright, 1998, Nature Publishing Group.

was selected for the saccade (i.e. all other saccade directions). In a separate condition the cue itself appeared in the RF (Fig. 3, right column). In this condition neurons had two responses—the first to the flashed visual cue and the second to the selected target (which could be at any location in the array). While these responses occurred respectively, early and late during the delay, they overlapped in time in the neural population

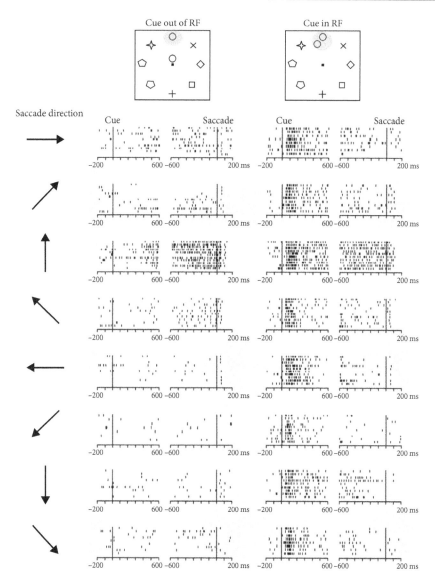

FIGURE 12.3 LIP neurons respond selectively to relevant targets. The top panels show the task design. Monkeys viewed a circular array containing eight peripheral saccade targets, of which one was constantly in the neuron's RF (shaded oval). On each trial a cue was flashed for 200 ms and, after a 600–800 ms delay, monkeys were rewarded for making a saccade to the target matching the cue. The rasters show responses of a representative neuron sorted according to the direction of the saccade. If the cue was out of the RF (left column), the neuron had no response to the cue; however, gradually during the delay period it developed a response to target selection—e.g. became active only if the designated target was in its RF (upward saccades). If the cue was in the RF (right column) the neuron responded first to the cue and later encoded saccade direction. Reproduced from Gottlieb, J., Kusunoki, M., and Goldberg, M. E., Simultaneous representation of saccade targets and visual onsets in monkey lateral intraparietal area, *Cerebral Cortex*, 15 (8), pp. 1198–206 (c) 2005, Oxford University Press.

(Gottlieb et al. 1998, 2005). In other words, while some LIP cells were still responding to the cue location, others were beginning to select the target for the forthcoming saccade.

These findings show that LIP neurons encode a very selective visual representation that integrates information about visual conspicuity and task demands, and tracks salient locations across shifts of gaze. As mentioned above, the spatial accuracy of the LIP response can be best appreciated in Fig. 12.2, where neurons responded to a visual event (abrupt onset) whose location entered their RF, even though the event itself occurred at a separate retinal location (before the shift of gaze). This spatially accurate remapping is thought to reflect the integration of retinotopic visual information with extraretinal responses, about eye position and corollary discharge signals specifying the direction of the upcoming saccade (Bisley and Goldberg 2010). Such retinal–extraretinal integration may be the basis of spatial encoding in different reference frames (Pouget et al. 2002). It may also account for the fact that spatial deficits in neglect can occur in multiple reference frames, as patients ignore stimuli that are contralateral with respect to the centre of gaze, with respect to their head or body or with respect to external landmarks (Behrmann and Geng 2002).

Neurons Encode Visual Selection

As described above, LIP neurons respond selectively to salient or relevant information and can signal a vector, or pointer, from the centre of gaze to the selected location. Such a retinotopic vector is in principle suitable for both influencing visual processing and guiding shifts of gaze. For the visual system this vector could act as a top-down bias facilitating sensory processing at the selected locations. For the oculomotor system it could act as a motor command, specifying the direction and amplitude of a desired saccade. Indeed, if the same signal were broadcast simultaneously to the visual and oculomotor systems this could explain the close natural coordination between attention and gaze.

Psychophysical studies, however, show that despite their close relationship, eye movements and attention are not identical and show important dissociations. On one hand, when an overt saccade is made there does seem to be an obligatory link, since perceptual performance is by default improved at the saccade goal (Kowler et al. 1995). The converse association, however, is not absolute: attention (defined as an improvement in perceptual discrimination) can be allocated without shifts of gaze, as if by an internal—'covert'— movement of the mind's eye (Carrasco and Yeshurun 2009). Covert shifts of attention contribute to efficient visual analysis before a shift of gaze, and are also beneficial in social situations. For example, it is often desirable to attend to a dominant individual without shifting gaze, as direct eye contact can signify a threat. In more general terms, the capacity for covert attention points to the brain's capacity to generate mental processes and flexibly determine how (or even whether) to translate these processes into action.

From the point of view of neural processing this flexibility implies that the brain must have partially dissociable mechanisms of visual and oculomotor selection. Multiple studies have addressed the question of which process is more closely encoded in LIP, and the bulk of the evidence from these studies favours an interpretation in terms of visual selection.

Perhaps the simplest and strongest evidence in this direction is the fact that LIP neurons respond strongly to salient stimuli even when these do not evoke saccades. This can be appreciated in the experiment shown in Fig. 12.2, where monkeys were not rewarded for making saccades to the salient object or to the briefly flashed cue. And yet in this study (and many like it) LIP neurons emit some of their strongest responses to salient stimuli even as monkeys deliberately fix their gaze (Gottlieb et al. 2005; Powell and Goldberg 2000).

A follow-up experiment expanded on this observation by asking how neurons respond in a condition of visuomotor conflict—when monkeys make saccades *away* from a salient cue (Gottlieb and Goldberg 1999). On each trial in the task monkeys were first shown a cue that flashed briefly at one of two possible locations—either inside or opposite to the neurons' RF. Depending on the colour of the fixation point, monkeys had to make a saccade toward the cue (an easy or habitual 'pro-saccade') or a saccade to an unmarked location opposite the cue (a more difficult, controlled 'anti-saccade'). By randomly interleaving the two cue locations and two mapping rules, the task achieved a full dissociation, such that on any given trial the cue, the saccade goal, neither or both could be in the RF.

As expected from the earlier results, LIP neurons had strong transient responses when the cue flashed in their RF, and these responses were highly consistent regardless of whether the cue instructed a pro- or an anti-saccade. Also consistent with prior studies, the neural responses continued until the saccade; however, this presaccadic response was inconsistent and dependent on visual stimulation. Fig. 12.4a shows the responses of a representative neuron while the monkey executed saccades toward its RF, sorted according to whether the saccade had been preceded by a flash at the same location (top row and solid traces, 'pro-saccades') or by a flash at the opposite location, outside the RF (bottom row and dotted traces, 'anti-saccades'). On pro-saccade trials the neuron had strong responses before the saccade (top row) and, if a delay was imposed between the cue and the saccade, it had an initial response to the cue followed by a dip in activity and a re-activation just before the movement itself (top right). However, *all* of the cell's responses (including the re-activation just before the saccade) vanished in the anti-saccade condition, when the saccades were identical but there had been no RF visual stimulation. Thus, the neuron's responses, even immediately before the saccade, were strongly dependent on visual stimulation. This visual dependence was the rule for most cells, with most neurons responding much more weakly before anti-saccades relative to pro-saccades (Fig. 4b), and limited the neurons' ability to encode the saccade goal. An information analysis that included all stimulus configurations showed that neurons conveyed reliable information about cue location (responding strongly if the cue appeared in their RF), but transmitted hardly any information about saccade direction even as monkeys were making that saccade (Fig. 4c). Thus, LIP neurons have robust responses to visual stimuli and visually guided saccades, but only weak responses for internally generated movements that are not congruent with a visual cue.

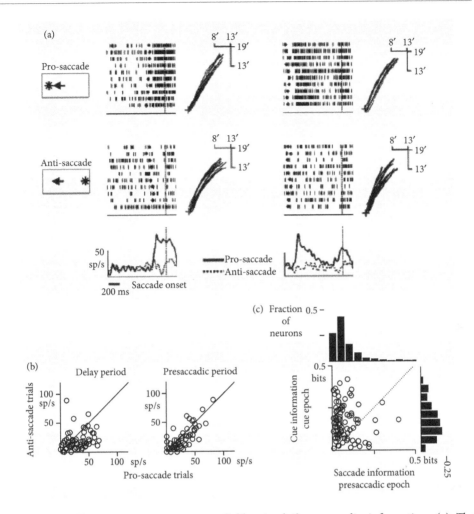

FIGURE 12.4 LIP neurons convey more reliable visual than saccadic information. (a) The responses of a representative neuron on trials in which the monkey made a pro-saccade (top) or an anti-saccade (bottom) toward its RF. The raster plots show action potentials aligned on saccade onset, and the time of cue onset is indicated by a dot. The left column shows no-delay trials, in which the saccade was made immediately upon cue onset, and the right column shows delay trials in which a variable delay was imposed after cue presentation. The bottom panels show average firing rates for pro- and anti-saccades. The traces next to each raster show the two-dimensional trajectory (horizontal and vertical position) for the corresponding saccades, even though the eye movements were equivalent in both cases. (b) The vast majority of cells showed stronger responses on delayed pro-saccades relative to anti-saccade trials, both during the delay period and immediately before the saccade. (c) The vast majority of cells transmitted more information about the location of the cue in their visual response than about the location of the saccade goal in their pre-saccadic response. Each dot shows the information transmitted by one cell, and the histograms show the marginal distributions of cue and saccade direction information. Adapted by permission from Macmillan Publishers Ltd: *Nature Neuroscience* 2 (10) Gottlieb, J. and Goldberg, M. E., Activity of neurons in the lateral intraparietal area of the monkey during an antisaccade task, pp. 906–12, copyright, 1999, Nature Publishing Group.

What do these findings imply about the relation between LIP activity and the ocu-lomotor system? Converging evidence shows that saccade production depends on a gradual visuomotor transformation that is implemented in neural populations distrib-uted throughout LIP, FEF, and the SC. Many neurons in the FEF and SC are similar to those in LIP in that they have spatially tuned visual and pre-saccadic responses (Schall et al. 2011). However, in contrast with LIP, the FEF and SC also contain a distinct popu-lation of 'movement' neurons that are scarce or absent in LIP, and which very consist-ently encode an impending saccade. In contrast with the LIP neurons described so far, movement cells in the FEF and SC do not respond to visual stimulation but respond consistently before an actual saccade and, in FEF, these movement cells seem to reach a fixed threshold at the time of the eye movement onset (Hanes and Schall 1996). These cells therefore are reliable reporters of an actual saccade plan and of the integration of evidence toward such a plan (Schall et al. 2011; Stanford et al. 2010).

Given their anatomical connections, it is likely that LIP neurons influence, directly or indirectly, the movement mechanisms in the FEF and SC. Clearly, however. the integra-tion of the LIP visual selection signal into a motor plan is not automatic but is gated in task-dependent fashion depending on what the subjects want to do about the visual cue. One gating mechanism is thought to involve inhibition of movement neurons by the substantia nigra and collicular 'fixation cells' (Lo and Wang 2006; Pouget et al. 2011), which are tonically active during sustained fixation and may prevent an automatic sac-cade if a movement has to be withheld (e.g. as in Fig. 2). To generate more complex behaviours such as an anti-saccade, the brain also requires additional mechanisms that generate an alternative action, and these mechanisms are not strongly encoded in LIP. Thus, LIP neurons can contribute to visual selection and suggest a possible saccade plan but, to reach a final action decision, their activity must be supplemented by additional mechanisms that proceed in parallel or in downstream structures.

A final noteworthy point is that rather than reflecting a feedforward motor effect, much of the saccade-related response in LIP may reflect *feedback* from downstream motor mechanisms. Information about saccade direction continues to accumulate in LIP after the saccade itself (Powell and Goldberg 2000) and for anti-saccades, seems to arise at delays longer than the natural latency of the saccade (Zhang and Barash 2004). It is therefore possible that the saccade response reflects, at least in part, corollary infor-mation about a saccade plan that is computed in downstream structures (for example, the FEF or the SC) and is fed back to LIP where it modulates a visual response (Sommer and Wurtz 2002). This hypothesis can explain both the presence of saccade activity in LIP and its dependence on visual stimulation.

LIP ACTIVITY AND VISUAL ATTENTION

As described above, the selective visual responses in LIP seem to have a direct corre-spondence with visual attention. Neurons respond selectively to salient or behaviourally relevant items, and emit these responses independently of a shift of gaze. Unlike neurons in earlier visual areas, LIP neurons are not feature-selective and do not describe the sensory world. Rather they convey a more abstract measure of 'target selection' that signals the attention-worthiness of an object or location.

According to an influential 'biased competition' hypothesis of attention, selective responses such as the one encoded in LIP can modulate perception through top-down feedback to earlier sensory representations (Desimone and Duncan 1995) that selectively increases the gain of neurons tuned to the selected features or locations (Reynolds et al. 2000; Reynolds and Chelazzi 2004; Reynolds and Heeger 2009). In addition, top-down signals can enhance competitive weight, allowing the selected item to suppress competition from irrelevant distractors (Reynolds et al. 1999; Reynolds and Heeger 2009). To see whether LIP neurons are indeed a possible source of attentional bias, several studies have tested the relation between LIP responses and perceptual selection as assessed by psychophysical measures of contrast sensitivity and visual search.

Bisley and Goldberg used a dual-task design that measured the monkeys' locus of attention based on contrast thresholds on a visual discrimination task (Bisley and Goldberg 2003). Monkeys were first shown a saccade target whose location they had to memorize throughout a memory (delay) period (Fig. 5a). On some trials a distractor was flashed during this period, which monkeys were instructed to ignore. While engaged in this task, monkeys received a secondary task designed to test covert attention. At some point after target presentation the monkeys were shown a visual cue—a C-like stimulus that could have two possible orientations. The cue's orientation instructed the monkey whether to proceed with the planned saccade or to cancel it and maintain fixation. By presenting this cue very briefly at several randomized locations and levels of contrast, experimenters could measure the monkeys' contrast sensitivity at these different locations. This in turn allowed the estimation of the monkey's attentional focus: the locus of attention was defined as the location that showed the lowest contrast threshold for cue discrimination.

Using this approach, Bisley and Goldberg showed that while holding stable fixation, monkeys shifted their attention from the target to the distractor and back again, and these shifts correlated with the balance of LIP activity, between the target and distractor locations. As shown in Fig. 12.5b, LIP neurons responded to the target with a transient response followed by a lower-level sustained activation (blue trace), and also had a strong response to the distractor (red trace). This dual responsiveness confirms the earlier finding that, although selective, the population of LIP neurons can encode more than one stimulus at a time (Gottlieb et al. 2005). In contrast with this dual response, however, perceptual attention (the locus of lowered thresholds) was only found at a single location at a time—namely, the location that elicited the higher response in LIP. Attention was allocated to the distractor for as long as the distractor response exceeded that to the target, but shifted back to the target location when the balance of activity reversed in LIP.

These findings suggest that, just as LIP plays an indirect role in driving saccades, it may have an indirect role in controlling attention. Given a complex visual scene, the priority map in LIP may select several locations as candidates for enhanced discrimination; however, enhanced discrimination may only materialize at one of these locations, possibly due

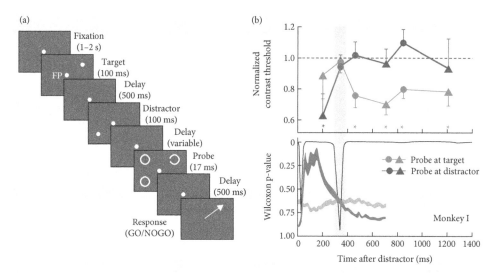

FIGURE 12.5 LIP activity predicts the locus of attention. (a) The task design showing the parameters of target and distractor presentation, followed by the presentation of the no-go instruction (the Landoldt-C) that also served as an attentional probe. (b) Data from monkey I. The top panel shows normalized contrast thresholds for discriminating the probe when it appeared at the target versus distractor locations. Thresholds are normalized to a value of 1 that represents the threshold at the remaining two locations that contained neither the target nor the distractor. Stars indicate thresholds that are significantly lower than the reference value. The bottom panel shows the population response of LIP neurons to the target and distractor in their RF. The black trace shows the p-value from a moving window paired test, showing that these responses were reliably different for most of the delay period. The brief window of ambiguity when the two responses were equivalent (shaded window, downward deflection in the p-value trace) corresponds to times when attention shifted from the distractor to the target location. Adapted from Bisley, JW and Goldberg, ME, Attention, intention, and priority in the parietal lobe, *Annual Review of Neuroscience*, 33, pp. 1–21 © 2010, Annual Reviews.

to a winner-take-all mechanism that operates downstream of LIP. This additional selection may be implemented in a discrete stage subsequent to LIP, or simply reflect the properties of sensory processing itself. It is important to note that the experiment of Bisley and Goldberg used very brief (16 ms) masked visual presentations and shows that attention has a unitary locus on these very brief time scales. It remains possible that attention rapidly shifts between locations, being effectively distributed across multiple locations on longer time scales.

While Bisley and Goldberg focused on saccade-related and bottom-up attention, a second set of studies focused on visual search tasks, where monkeys have to find targets that are embedded in distractor arrays. These studies capitalized on the classic observation that if the target is inconspicuous, the time required to find it increases as a function of the number of distractors, a set-size effect that is indicative of inefficient or attentionally demanding search (Haslam et al. 2001). An involvement of LIP in difficult search was suggested by two experiments using reversible inactivation with the GABA agonist muscimol. These studies showed that inactivation impairs visual selection during difficult search, whether the search occurs covertly or in conjunction with overt saccades (Wardak et al. 2002, 2004).

To determine the neural responses underlying this function, Balan et al. (Balan et al. 2008) trained monkeys to discriminate a visual cue—an E-like shape—that appeared in the visual periphery in an array of distractors (Fig. 6a). Monkeys were required to maintain central fixation and suppress saccades to stimuli in the search array. They were rewarded for reporting the cue orientation by releasing a bar held in the right or the left

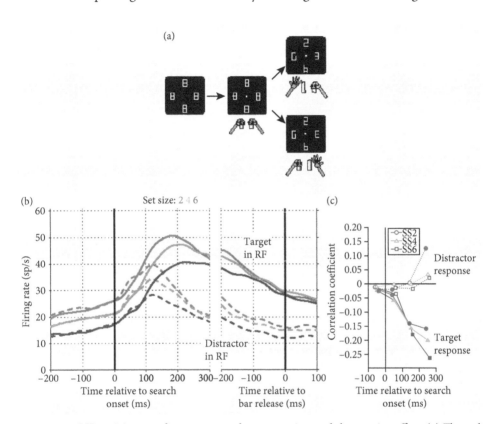

FIGURE 12.6 LIP activity encodes covert top-down attention and the set-size effect. (a) The task design. An array of figure-8 placeholders remained stably on the screen. In interleaved blocks of trials the array contained two, four, or six placeholders. Each trial began when the monkey achieved fixation, bringing a placeholder into the RF. Two line segments were then removed from each placeholder, revealing a display with one target and several distractors. The target (a right or left facing letter 'E') appeared at a random location. Without shifting gaze, monkeys had to find the target and report its orientation by releasing a bar. (b) During the time between search onset (stimulus presentation) and the manual release LIP neurons encoded target location, responding more strongly when the 'E' relative to a distractor appeared in their RF. These responses declined as a function of set size. The set-size effect was evident even before search onset, when a different number of placeholders were present on the screen. (c) Correlation coefficients between neuronal firing rates and reaction times for trials in which the target (solid lines) or a distractor (dotted lines) were in the RF. Significant correlations (filled symbols) were found for the target response, showing that the larger this response the shorter the reaction time. In contrast, the distractor response was more weakly related to performance. Adapted from *PLoS Biol*, 6 (7), Balan, P. F., et al., Neuronal correlates of the set-size effect in monkey lateral intraparietal area, e158 © 2008, Creative Commons License.

paw. Performance showed a set-size effect in both reaction time and accuracy, indicating effortful, attentionally demanding search.

LIP neurons had robust responses encoding the cue location, responding more strongly if the cue rather than a distractor was in their RF (Fig. 6b). Consistent with the behavioural set-size effect, these responses diminished as a function of the number of distractors. The set-size related decline in activity was seen in the fixation period, when the monkeys viewed a variable number of placeholders but could not yet begin their search (Fig. 6b— 200 to 0 ms). Behavioural testing showed that monkeys were insensitive to changes in location probability per se, suggesting that the set-size effect was not due to changes in the monkeys' estimate of the probability that a target will appear at a given location. A simple explanation is that this neural set-size effect reflected competitive visual interactions triggered by surrounding distractors (Falkner et al. 2006), suggesting that these interactions explain capacity limitations during visual search.

The robust responses that the cells had on this task underscore the fact that LIP encodes visual selection independently of a specific action, i.e. for guiding saccades or limb motor actions. Notably, however, while in saccade tasks neural responses typically increase up to the time of a saccade (e.g. Fig. 4a), in this task activity peaked in the middle of the reaction time and declined well before the motor response. This suggests that LIP accumulates visual information, and then passes control to skeletomotor mechanisms.

The results also provided data regarding the specific behavioural correlates of the response. If a distractor was in the RF, neurons showed an enduring set-size effect that persisted until the bar release (Fig. 6b, dashed traces). By contrast, if the target was in the RF, the set-size effect diminished gradually over time, so that the response reached a comparable *peak* level at all set-sizes (solid traces). These findings are consistent with a biased competition account whereby the influence of distractors is filtered through top-down control. In addition, the monkeys' reaction times were better correlated with the target than with the distractor response (Fig. 6c), suggesting that the top-down signal may primarily influence performance through its actions on target representations.

In sum, the studies described in this section establish correlations between LIP activity and perceptually defined attention, whether attention is driven in bottom-up or top-down fashion, and whether it guides ocular or skeletal actions.

Combining Bottom-up and Top-Down Information

Psychophysical studies show that the effects of salient distractors are not immutable but depend strongly on task context and the observers' search set (Burnham 2007). Given that LIP neurons integrate the influences of bottom-up and top-down factors, they are possible candidates for mediating interactions between these forms of control.

To address this question, Balan and Gottlieb (Balan and Gottlieb 2006) used the E-search task described in Fig. 12.6 but, in addition to the target, introduced a salient visual perturbation. On each trial the appearance of the search display containing a target and multiple distractors was preceded by a 50 ms visual perturbation—which could be a brief change in the position, luminance, or colour of a stable placeholder, or the brief appearance of a frame around a placeholder. The significance of the perturbation was varied in interleaved trial blocks. In some blocks the perturbation appeared at the same location as the search target—and was thus a valid cue to the target location. In other blocks the perturbation appeared at a different, unrelated location and was irrelevant to the search. These statistical associations remained constant during a block, and monkeys could exploit them to adjust their attentional strategy. Indeed, in SAME location blocks the monkey's reaction time was shorter than in OPPOSITE blocks, showing that the animals learned to use the perturbation as a valid cue or block its distracting effects, according to the context.

LIP neurons reflected these contextual adjustments, emitting enhanced responses to the perturbation in the relevant relative to the irrelevant context. Moreover, the relative size of their responses to the perturbation correlated with the behavioural effect. In the perturbation-relevant block, perturbation responses were higher overall (Fig. 7a), and an increase in the visual response correlated with a decrease in reaction time (Fig. 7b), consistent with the hypothesis that the perturbation facilitated target selection. In the perturbation-irrelevant block, by contrast, perturbation responses were lower (Fig. 7b) and a higher response was correlated with *longer* search reaction times, indicating that the perturbation had a distracting effect. Interestingly, the increment in the perturbation response in the relevant context was accompanied by an increase in the neurons' baseline activity even before the perturbation occurred, and the fractional increase in baseline activity was not different from the fractional increase in the visual response, suggesting a multiplicative gain (Fig. 7a). Multiplicative gain was shown previously to enhance responses to weak stimuli when these are the focus of attention (McAdams and Maunsell 1999; Williford and Maunsell 2006). In this task, however, response gain increased in a non-spatial fashion, before the animal could direct attention to a specific location. Thus, abstract knowledge of task context can produce multiplicative effects on baseline firing rates that influence sensitivity to subsequent sensory stimulation.

A task-dependent encoding of salient stimuli was also shown in a visual search task in which a pop-out (colour-contrasting) distractor was present along with an inconspicuous target (Ipata et al. 2006). Neurons showed variable responses to this distractor, which correlated with the monkeys' ability to suppress saccades to it, supporting the idea that LIP is a possible substrate for integrating top-down and bottom-up information.

Determinants of visual selection I: Semantic associations

The studies described above show that the selective response in LIP can be a source of top-down bias that selectively guides visual processing. However, this raises an

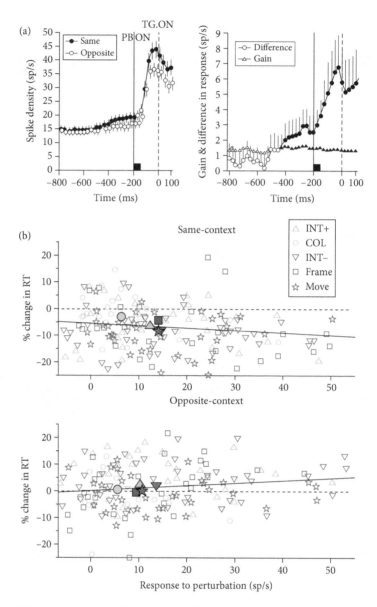

FIGURE 12.7 LIP neurons integrate bottom-up and top-down information. (a) Left panel shows the population responses on trials in which a salient perturbation was relevant ('Same') or irrelevant ('Opposite') for the location of the search target. Responses are aligned on the time of the perturbation (PB ON) and truncated after the appearance of the target (TG ON). An enhancement is seen in the relevant blocks starting 200–300 ms before onset of the perturbation. The right panel shows the difference and ratio (gain) between firing rates in the two conditions. While the difference increases sharply at the time of the visual response the gain remains constant throughout the trial. (b) The perturbation response in LIP correlates with the effect of the perturbation on search reaction times. In the Same context a larger perturbation response is associated with a large fractional decrease in reaction time, while in the Opposite context a larger response produces a larger increase in reaction time. Each point shows the data from one neuron and one perturbation type (increase or decrease in luminance, INT+ and INT–, isoluminant colour change (COL), appearance of a frame (FRAME) or movement of a placeholder (MOVE)). Adapted from Cohen, M. and Maunsell, J., Functional significance of nonspatial information in monkey lateral intraparietal area, *Journal of Neuroscience*, 29 (25), pp. 8166–76 © 2009, The Society for Neuroscience.

important question. How do LIP neurons know the 'relevance' of a visual cue and how do they know which target to select?

Psychophysical studies show that the significance of visual cues is established by multiple factors, which include the learned contextual and action associations of the cues, the usefulness of a cue in providing information, and the Pavlovian (reward) associations of the cues. The following sections discuss the role of these factors in modulating the LIP response and their possible contribution to a relevance computation.

A fundamental step in computing relevance is learning the associations between stimuli and the broader task, including the context, actions, or goals of that task. Imagine, for example, that you want to drive to a remote location. By virtue of information stored in long-term memory, you have learned to associate the task of driving with the category of a 'car'. This can in turn activate a visual template (of a 'big object with wheels') which can produce an attentional bias and ultimately allow you to focus on a car (Huang and Grossberg 2010; Navalpakkam and Itti 2005). The idea of associative top-down control is consistent with psychophysical evidence that attention can be guided by context or gist (Oppermann et al. 2012) or by the motor associations (affordances) of a visual cue (Roberts and Humphreys 2011a, 2011b).

Consistent with the importance of associative learning in behaviour, neurophysiological studies have shown that the target selection response in LIP is not stereotyped but is shaped by the motor, visual, and categorical associations of visual cues. Evidence regarding motor associations comes from the covert visual search task that was described in Fig. 12.6 (Oristaglio et al. 2006). As described above, in that task monkeys were required to find a visual cue while maintaining central fixation, and report its orientation with a manual release. Specifically, monkeys learned to release a bar held in the right paw if the cue was a right-facing 'E' but to release a bar held in the left paw if the cue was a left-facing 'E' (a '3'). This manual response occurred outside the monkeys' field of view and it was non-targeting—i.e. independent of the location of the cue. Nevertheless, each motor response had a non-spatial (semantic) association with a cue, and this association was encoded in LIP.

In about half of the cells encoding target location, the cue-evoked response was not constant but depended on the manual release. Of these cells, some had stronger responses if the cue appeared in the RF and instructed a left bar release (Fig. 8a, left column, red vs. blue). Other cells had the complementary preference, responding best for the cue signalling right release. Control experiments showed that the effect was not linked to the cue's orientation or to the location of the limb. Thus, when monkeys were trained to indicate the orientation of a new set of cues (an upright or inverted U-like shape) a majority of neurons showed the same limb preference as they did for the E-like cues. Similarly, when monkeys were trained to perform the same task with their limbs crossed across the body midline, limb effects remained unchanged: neurons that preferred the right or left limb in the standard arm position continued to have the same preference in the crossed position (Fig. 8b), showing that the modulatory effects were linked to a specific limb regardless of its position in space.

An important aspect of these limb effects is that, while they occurred reliably in over half the cells, they were not the neurons' primary response. Rather they *modulated* a

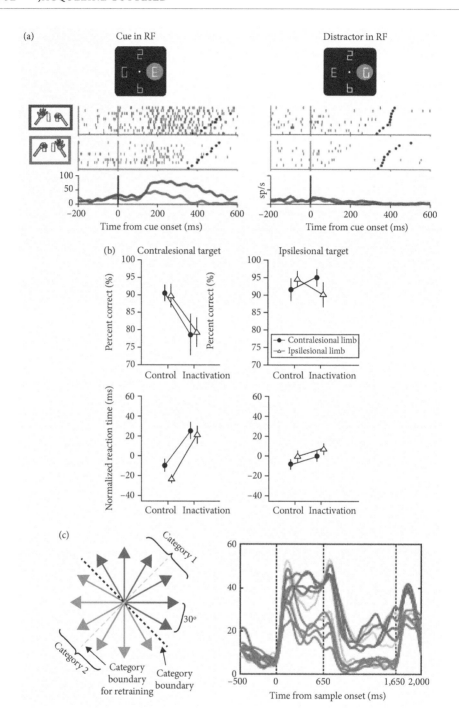

FIGURE 12.8 LIP neurons encode motor and categorical associations. (a) Modulation by manual release. Responses of a representative neuron in the 'E' search task shown in Fig. 6. Monkeys were rewarded for maintaining fixation and reporting the orientation of the 'E'— right or left facing—by releasing a bar held, respectively, in the right or left paw. The bars themselves were outside of the field of view. Rightward-facing cues could appear on the left and vice

primary response to visual selection. The cell in Fig. 12.8a, for example, had robust limb selectivity if the cue appeared in its RF. However, the neuron remained silent if a distractor was in the RF even though the monkeys performed the same manual action (right column). The primacy of the visual response was confirmed by a further experiment that used reversible inactivation, which showed that inactivation impaired only visual but not motor selection (Balan and Gottlieb 2009). Infusion of muscimol into LIP in one hemisphere impaired performance in spatially selective manner—i.e. if the cue was contralateral but not if it was ipsilateral to the inactivation site (Fig. 8b). However, inactivation caused no deficits in the manual release—neither a global impairment in the manual action nor a limb-specific deficit. These findings suggest that the limb responses in LIP do not indicate a primary involvement of this area in the execution or release of a grasp. Rather they are effects of a visuo-manual association on the target selection response.

Other experiments have shown that LIP neurons can also reflect more abstract properties such as the categorical membership or visuo-visual associations of an instructive cue (Freedman and Assad 2011). In a task where monkeys were trained to report the

---

versa, so the laterality of the motor response was independent of the laterality of the visual cue. The neuron responded only if the 'E' appeared in the RF but was silent if a distractor did (left vs. right column). In addition, when an 'E' appeared in its RF, the cell was more active if the monkey released the left bar than the right bar (blue vs. red traces). Raster plots in the top panels show individual trials. Each dot represents the time of an action potential aligned on cue onset, and the black dots show the time of manual release. Trials are sorted offline in order of manual reaction time. The bottom panel shows the corresponding averaged spike density histograms (smoothed with a Gaussian kernel, sigma 10 ms). Adapted from Oristaglio, J., et al., Integration of visuospatial and effector information during symbolically cued limb movements in monkey lateral intraparietal area, *Journal of Neuroscience*, 26 (32), pp. 8310–9 © 2006, The Society for Neuroscience. (b) Muscimol inactivation impairs visual but not motor selection. Performance of the 'E' search task in control conditions and after muscimol inactivation of LIP in one hemisphere. The top row shows discrimination accuracy and the bottom row, reaction times. Symbols show average and standard errors. Data are segregated according to the hemifield of the target and the side of the active limb (contralateral or ipsilateral to the inactivation site). Adapted from Balan, P. F. and Gottlieb, J., Functional significance of nonspatial information in monkey lateral intraparietal area', *Journal of Neuroscience*, 29 (25), pp. 8166–76 © 2009, The Society for Neuroscience. (c) Modulation by stimulus category. The left panel illustrates the behavioural task. Monkeys viewed a sample stimulus containing random dot motion in one of eight possible directions. After a delay period (650 to 1650 ms) a test motion stimulus appeared and monkeys had to release a bar if the test stimulus matched the category of motion of the sample, but continue to hold the bar otherwise. Monkeys were initially trained to categorize directions according to one category boundary (black dotted line) and then retrained to use a different boundary (green dashed line). Top right panel shows a representative LIP neuron that had visual and delay period activity following presentation of a sample inside its RF as well as sensitivity to sample category. Firing rates were much more strongly modulated by changes in direction across, relative to within a category boundary, dissociating this modulation from simple selectivity for motion direction. Reprinted by permission from Macmillan Publishers Ltd: *Nature*, 443 (7107), David J. Freedman and John A. Assad, Experience-dependent representation of visual categories in parietal cortex, copyright (2006), Nature Publishing Group.

category of a motion stimulus using a delayed match to sample task, neural responses to the stimulus were category selective, with different neurons responding more for one or the other category (Freedman and Assad 2006). Similar differentiation was found in different tasks testing visuo-visual associations (Fitzgerald et al. 2011) or visual search based on feature conjunctions. Although using very different tasks, these studies converge on a similar conclusion—that LIP neurons reflect not only the location but the learned visual, action, and semantic associations of task-relevant cues.

These findings were proposed to contribute to abstract decisions based on the semantic associations of visual cues (Freedman and Assad 2011) and, given the role of LIP in visual selection they may also contribute to the learning of relevance and top-down control. This hypothesis raises new questions about this control. In the traditional view of attention, top-down signals for features or locations are thought to arise from different neurons and recruit different attentional mechanisms (Desimone and Duncan 1995; Maunsell and Treue 2006). The multifaceted nature of the LIP response, however, suggests that top-down signals may be selective for both space and high-level features (Gottlieb and Snyder 2010). For example, if neurons such as the limb-selective cells in Fig. 7a provide the top-down bias, this implies that a different populations of neurons provide the bias for cues signalling right—or left—release. In other words, directing attention to a given location may be accomplished by different neuronal populations depending on the significance of the attended object. While counterintuitive at first glance, such a differentiated (combinatorial) signal may provide an efficient interface with visual and motor mechanisms, which are themselves selective for feature and/or categories. An alternative possibility is that neurons with dual spatial/non-spatial selectivity represent only the hidden layer in a network computing relevance, and the output of the network (the attentional bias itself) may be conveyed by the neurons that lack associative effects. Future experiments are needed to clarify this question.

A second set of questions concerns the mechanism generating associative effects. One possibility is that the effects reflect online feedback from structures that accumulate evidence regarding categories or actions. Alternatively, however, it is possible that through prolonged training, visual associations produce plasticity in visual areas themselves or in the connections between these areas and LIP. Such plasticity can be produced in simple reinforcement models (Ferrera and Grinband 2006) and is consistent with the presence of semantic/categorical effects in earlier visual areas such as V4 (Mirabella et al. 2007).

Determinants of visual selection II: Utility and information

While semantic associations are necessary for determining relevance, to efficiently guide attention the brain must also estimate the *usefulness* of a visual cue. To appreciate this distinction, consider the pattern of eye movements made by a subject during natural behaviour—a simple task such as filling a kettle for making tea (Fig. 9a). Consistent with the seminal work of Yarbus in the early twentieth century, the vast majority of eye movements made in such conditions are directed to task-relevant cues. However, these movements do not target *all* the stimuli that have task associations, which in the tea-making example would include the kitchen walls, cabinets, and floor. Instead, they are highly selective for stimuli that bring new information for the subject's immediate actions. This suggests that additional mechanisms must operate within the set of task-associated cues, to further select those stimuli that inform—and thus increase the likelihood of success of—a future action.

Consistent with this idea, multiple studies have shown that oculomotor decisions are sensitive to expected reward and have proposed that the target selection response in LIP (and possibly other areas) encodes the value of alternative options (Kable and Glimcher 2009; Sugrue et al. 2004, 2005). Monkeys are easily trained to direct gaze for liquid rewards, and human subjects make optimal tradeoffs between expected gain and salience during visual search (Navalpakkam et al. 2010). Reward effects have been described in multiple structures including the FEF (Ding and Hikosaka 2006), and SC (Ikeda and Hikosaka 2003). Multiple studies have shown that in LIP the target selection response increases monotonically with the desirability of a specific reward, whether desirability is manipulated through the magnitude, probability or timing of the eventual reward, and whether animals perform instructed or free-choice tasks (Dorris and Glimcher 2004; Louie and Glimcher 2010; Louie et al. 2011; Platt and Glimcher 1999; Sugrue et al. 2004). These findings suggest the powerful hypothesis that the target selection response in LIP encodes a common currency of visual utility, with utility being computed based on a variety of factors (Kable and Glimcher 2009; Sugrue et al. 2005).

An important question, however, is if neurons encode expected reward per se or the specific form of utility that is important for attention—the utility of information, which depends on the observer's uncertainty at a point in time (Sprague and Ballard 2005; Tatler et al. 2011). Consider again the eye movements of the subject in Fig. 12.9a. To complete her task the subject is simultaneously manipulating the kettle and walking from the stove to the sink. Both her hand and leg actions have high *value* and are necessary for the task. However, our subject guides her eye movements exclusively to the targets of the hand actions, since these have higher uncertainty and have more to gain from new information.

While the specific utility of information has not been examined in the oculomotor domain, insights into this question come from reinforcement learning studies of attention in humans and rats (Pearce and Mackintosh 2010). A central idea in these studies is that attentional weight is assigned not based on expected reward but based on the *prediction errors* associated with a cue. A prediction error is a measure of the difference between the agent's expectations and the actual experienced outcome. Outcomes that are better or worse than expected generate respectively, positive and negative errors, and these errors drive learning in iterative algorithms. Reinforcement learning theories of attention postulate that the 'informativeness' of a sensory signal can be estimated through the absolute value of the prediction errors associated with that signal. Cues that are reliable predictors will reduce uncertainty and have low associated errors, while cues that make uncertain predictions will have higher prediction errors.

(a)

(b)

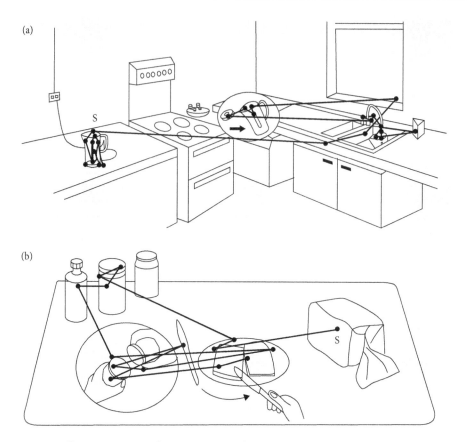

FIGURE 12.9 Eye movements during active tasks. (a) Eye movements of a subject filling water in a tea-kettle. (b) Eye movements of a subject preparing a sandwich. Reproduced from *Visual Neuroscience*, 26 (1), Land, M. F. Vision, eye movements, and natural behavior, pp. 51–62 © 2009, Cambridge University Press.

Consistent with this framework, psychophysical studies show that human attention is guided by the predictive qualities of visual cues (Hogarth et al. 2010). Furthermore, studies in rats suggest that this guidance may involve two distinct mechanisms (Pearce and Mackintosh 2010). One mechanism, dubbed 'attention for action', is thought to depend on the frontal lobe and assigns priority to stimuli that have low prediction errors—i.e. reliable predictors that can guide future actions (e.g. the tap or sink in Fig. 9a). A second mechanism, dubbed 'attention for learning', involves the amygdala and parietal lobe and assigns value to novel or uncertain cues in order to learn *about* such cues.

So far little is known about the importance of prediction errors in the visual and ocu-lomotor system, as most studies have focused on the role of expected reward. A key question for future work therefore is to integrate this work with a reinforcement learn-ing framework and understand how parietal and frontal neurons assign priority based on predictive or informational properties of visual cues.

Determinants of attention III: Pavlovian (emotional) associations

A central assumption of reinforcement theories of attention is that attention is guided by the *absolute* magnitude of prediction errors regardless of their sign. In this way attention is guided by the information value of a stimulus independent of whether the stimulus brings 'good' or 'bad' news. This seems to correspond to our intuition that attention should proceed in a 'rational', 'value neutral' fashion: while seeing a tiger on your hiking trail is an unpleasant prospect, there should not be a problem in attending to confirm that there is, in fact, a tiger in the bush. Put differently, reliable information is valuable whether it brings good or bad news.

In contrast with this purely informational view, however, converging psychophysical evidence shows that attention does have strong emotional components and is sensitive to the social or affective valence of external cues (Vuilleumier 2005). Stimuli that are initially neutral but gain positive reward associations can automatically attract attention even when they are irrelevant to a task (Anderson et al. 2011; Libera and Chelazzi 2009) while stimuli with negative associations can repel gaze and reduce fixation time at their locations (Hogarth et al. 2010). Unlike the goal-directed attention discussed above, these effects produce task-independent attentional biases. Affective biases in attention are strong in psychiatric disease (Williams et al. 1996). For example, patients with drug addiction have automatic biases toward drug-related cues that may reinstate drug craving and cause relapse even after periods of abstinence (Flagel et al. 2009).

Despite the possible importance of emotional attention, little is known about its neural mechanisms. However, a recent experiment shows that conditioned cues produce valence-specific biases in spatial attention and in the neural responses in LIP (Peck et al. 2009).

In the experiment, the monkeys performed a probabilistic reward task where each trial had a 50% prior probability of ending in a reward or no-reward. At the outset of a trial monkeys viewed a peripheral conditioned stimulus (CS) that provided full information about the trial's reward. Some cues brought 'good news', signalling that the trial will end in a reward (CS+); others brought 'bad news', signalling that, even if correctly completed, the trial will end in no reward (CS–). If attention depends solely on predictive validity it should be directed in a similar fashion to the positive and negative cues, as both conveyed reliable information. By contrast, if attention depends on reward associations, it may be differently allocated to the positive and negative cues.

Consistent with the latter possibility, attentional biases differed according to affective value—such that 'good news' cues (CS+) attracted attention, while 'bad news' (CS–) cues repelled attention from their location. As shown in Fig. 12.10a, upon presentation of a CS, LIP neurons had a fast transient visual response followed by sustained activity that lasted after disappearance of the cue. The sustained response that followed a CS+ was excitatory, resulting in a higher response when the cue appeared in the RF relative to when it appeared at the opposite location (Fig. 10b, top, black vs. grey traces). By contrast, the response evoked by a CS– was suppressive, producing lower activity at the cue location relative to the opposite location (Fig. 10b, bottom).

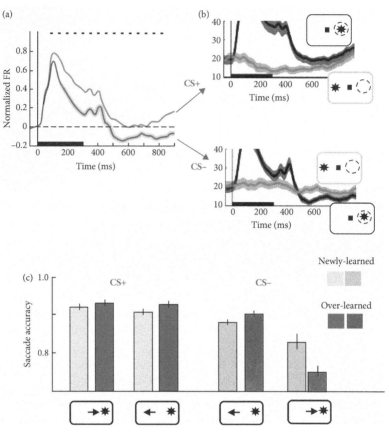

FIGURE 12.10 Pavlovian cues bias attention and LIP activity. (a) Population responses to Pavlovian cues. A cue flashes in the RF for 300 ms (dark bar) and is followed by a delay period during which monkeys maintain fixation. LIP neurons have transient and sustained responses that are selective for cue value, being stronger for a positive cue predicting a reward (CS+, blue) relative to a negative cue predicting no reward (CS–, red). The stars show time bins with a significant difference between the two conditions. The bottom dashed line shows the pre-cue level of activity. Shading shows the standard error of the mean. (b) Cue-evoked biases are spatially specific. The dark traces in each panel are the same as, respectively, the blue and red traces in panel A, but shown on an expanded vertical axis. The grey traces show responses when the cues appeared opposite the RF. Responses evoked by an RF cue are higher than (CS+) or lower than (CS–) those evoked by a cue at the opposite location. (c) Attentional biases are spatially specific. Panels show mean and SEM for saccade accuracy across all sessions. Opaque colours show trials with over-learned CS, which had consistent reward associations for tens of thousands of trials. Pale colours show trials with novel CS, which were introduced and trained within a single session. Measurement of anticipatory licking showed that monkeys learned the value of the novel CS within the first 5–10 trials. Data collection began after this learning was complete. On CS– trials (red) accuracy is somewhat lower than on CS+ trials, indicating a modest effect of motivation. The strongest effect, however, is on CS– congruent trials, when the saccade is directed toward the CS– location (rightmost bars). Moreover, the accuracy on these trials decreases further with training, being lower after over-learned relative to newly learned cues. Adapted from Peck, C. J., Jangraw, D. C., et al., Reward modulates attention independently of action value in posterior parietal cortex, *Journal of Neuroscience*, 29 (36), pp. 11182–91 © 2009, The Society for Neuroscience.

To see whether these neural biases had behavioural correlates, monkeys were trained to maintain fixation for a brief delay period then make a saccade to a second target that appeared unpredictably either at the opposite or same location as the cue. By comparing saccades that were directed toward versus opposite the CS location, investigators could detect whether the CS had attractive or repulsive effects.

Consistent with the neural biases in LIP, saccades were slightly facilitated if they were directed toward a CS+ location but strongly impaired if directed toward a CS– location (Fig. 10c). Performance on a CS– trial was much better if the saccade was directed away from the CS–, showing that the impairment was spatially specific and distinct from a global decrease in motivation on unrewarded trials (Fig. 10c, rightmost two bars). Moreover, the impairment on CS– congruent trials affected both reaction times and accuracy. The dysmetria (inaccuracy) produced by a CS– is particularly important because it distinguishes this repulsion from inhibition of return, which has only been reported to prolong latency (Fecteau and Munoz 2006). In addition, by reducing accuracy, the CS– produced many targeting errors and lowered the monkeys' rate of reward, showing that the CS– repulsion interfered with the monkeys' task. Nevertheless, despite its detrimental consequences, this repulsion *increased* rather than decreasing with training, becoming stronger for over-learned relative to newly learned cues (Fig. 10c, solid vs. pale colours).

These effects therefore seem to be neuronal correlates of the emotional biases documented in human subjects. Like these biases, the effects produced by the CS depended on the valence of the cue, arose automatically, and persisted despite their maladaptive effects.

Taken together with the previous discussion, these findings indicate the need to distinguish between two classes of reward-based attention mechanisms. One is a goal-directed mechanism that estimates the operant value of a cue in informing future actions. This mechanism requires knowledge of the task demands and may involve cortical areas that can plan a series of actions (Gershman and Niv 2010). A second mechanism, however, seems independent of action relevance and may be guided solely by conditioned Pavlovian associations, such as those encoded, for example, by dopamine (DA) neurons of the midbrain (Flagel et al. 2011). As described above, affective biases operate automatically and can produce maladaptive effects. However, because they are computationally simpler and quickly learnt, they may be useful in detecting biologically relevant information.

CONCLUSIONS

Converging evidence from anatomical, single-neuron recordings and inactivation studies implicates area LIP in the allocation of visual attention. Neurons in this area encode a sparse visual representation that selects candidate stimuli for shifts of attention and gaze, and integrates sensory and behavioural information.

The complex behavioural influences in LIP raise important questions about the nature of top-down control. Understanding these influences requires that we consider the multiple mechanisms by which the brain assigns relevance, including the task associations, information content, and emotional value of cues. Thus a critical goal for future research will be to integrate evidence from behavioural and computational research toward a better understanding of the neurophysiological mechanisms.

Acknowledgements

This research was supported by the National Alliance for Research on Schizophrenia and Depression, the Gatsby Charitable Foundation, and the National Eye Institute.

Disclosure Statement

The authors declare that they have no conflict of interest.

References

Anderson, B. A., Laurent, P.A., and Yantis, S. (2011). Value-driven attentional capture. *Proceedings of the National Academy of Sciences USA 108*(25): 10367–10371.

Balan, P. F. and Gottlieb, J. (2006). Integration of exogenous input into a dynamic salience map revealed by perturbing attention. *Journal of Neuroscience 26*(36): 9239–9249.

Balan, P. F. and Gottlieb, J. (2009). Functional significance of nonspatial information in monkey lateral intraparietal area. *Journal of Neuroscience 29*(25): 8166–8176.

Balan, P. F., Oristaglio, J., Schneider, D. M., and Gottlieb, J. (2008). Neuronal correlates of the set-size effect in monkey lateral intraparietal area. *PLoS Biology 6*(7): e158.

Behrmann, M. and Geng, J. J. (2002). What is 'left' when all is said and done? Spatial coding in hemispatial neglect. In H. O. Karnath, D. Milner, and G. Vallar (eds.), *The Cognitive and Neural Basis of Spatial Neglect* (pp. 85–100). Oxford: Oxford University Press.

Ben Hamed, S. and Duhamel, J. R. (2002). Ocular fixation and visual activity in the monkey lateral intraparietal area. *Experimental Brain Research 142*(4): 512–528.

Ben Hamed, Duhamel, J. R., Bremmer, F., and Graf, W. (2002). Visual receptive field modulation in the lateral intraparietal area during attentive fixation and free gaze. *Cerebral Cortex 12*(3): 234–245.

Bisley, J. W. and Goldberg, M. E. (2003). Neuronal activity in the lateral intraparietal area and spatial attention. *Science 299*(5603): 81–86.

Bisley, J. W. and Goldberg, M. E. (2010). Attention, intention, and priority in the parietal lobe. *Annual Review of Neuroscience 33*: 1–21.

Blatt, G. J., Andersen, R. A., and Stoner, G. R. (1990). Visual receptive field organization and cortico-cortical connections of the lateral intraparietal area (area LIP) in the macaque. *Journal of Computational Neurology 299*(4): 421–445.

Burnham, B. R. (2007). Displaywide visual features associated with a search display's appearance can mediate attentional capture. *Psychonomic Bulletin & Review 14*(3): 392–422.

Carrasco, M. and Yeshurun, Y. (2009). Covert attention effects on spatial resolution. *Progress in Brain Research 176*: 65–86.

Colby, C. L., Duhamel, J.-R., and Goldberg, M. E. (1993). Ventral intraparietal area of the macaque: Anatomic location and visual response properties. *Journal of Neurophysiology 69*(3): 902–914.

Colby, C. L. and Goldberg, M. E. (1999). Space and attention in parietal cortex. *Annual Review of Neuroscience 23*: 319–349.

Constantinidis, C. and Steinmetz, M. A. (2005). Posterior parietal cortex automatically encodes the location of salient stimuli. *Journal of Neuroscience 25*(1): 233–238.

Desimone, R. and Duncan, J. (1995). Neural mechanisms of selective visual attention. *Annual Review of Neuroscience 18*: 183–222.

Ding, L. and Hikosaka, O. (2006). Comparison of reward modulation in the frontal eye field and caudate of the macaque. *Journal of Neuroscience 26*(25): 6695–6703.

Dorris, M. C. and Glimcher, P. W. (2004). Activity in posterior parietal cortex is correlated with the relative subjective desirability of action. *Neuron 44*(2): 365–378.

Falkner, A. L., Krisha, B. S., and Goldberg, M. E. (2006). Lateral inhibitory interactions in the lateral intraparietal area (LIP) of the monkey. *Abstracts of the Society for Neuroscience 37*: 606.8.

Fecteau, J. H. and Munoz, D. P. (2006). Salience, relevance, and firing: A priority map for target selection. *Trends in Cognitive Neurosciences 10*(8): 382–390.

Ferrera, V. P. and Grinband, J. (2006). Walk the line: Parietal neurons respect category boundaries. *Nature Neuroscience 9*(10): 1207–1208.

Fitzgerald, J. K., Freedman, D. J., and Assad, J. A. (2011). Generalized associative representations in parietal cortex. *Nature Neuroscience 14*(8): 1075–1079.

Flagel, S. B., Akil, H., and Robinson, T. E. (2009). Individual differences in the attribution of incentive salience to reward-related cues: Implications for addiction. *Neuropharmacology 56* Suppl. 1: 139–148.

Flagel, S. B., Clark, J. J., Robinson, T. E., Mayo, L., Czuj, A., et al. (2011). A selective role for dopamine in stimulus-reward learning. *Nature 469*(7328): 53–57.

Freedman, D. J. and Assad, J. A. (2006). Experience-dependent representation of visual categories in parietal cortex. *Nature 443*(7107): 85–88.

Freedman, D. J. and Assad, J. A. (2011). A proposed common neural mechanism for categorization and perceptual decisions. *Nature Neuroscience 14*(2): 143–146.

Gershman, S. J. and Niv, Y. (2010). Learning latent structure: Carving nature at its joints. *Current Opinion in Neurobiology 20*(2): 251–256.

Gottlieb, J. and Goldberg, M. E. (1999). Activity of neurons in the lateral intraparietal area of the monkey during an antisaccade task. *Nature Neuroscience 2*(10): 906–912.

Gottlieb, J., Kusunoki, M., and Goldberg, M. E. (1998). The representation of visual salience in monkey parietal cortex. *Nature 391*(6666): 481–484.

Gottlieb, J., Kusunoki, M., and Goldberg, M. E. (2005). Simultaneous representation of saccade targets and visual onsets in monkey lateral intraparietal area. *Cerebral Cortex 15*(8): 1198–1206.

Gottlieb, J. and Snyder, L. H. (2010). Spatial and non-spatial functions of the parietal cortex. *Current Opinion in Neurobiology 20*(6): 731–740.

Hanes, D. P. and Schall, J. D. (1996). Neural control of voluntary movement initiation. *Science 274*(5286): 427–430.

Haslam, N., Porter, M., and Rothschild, L. (2001). Visual search: Efficiency continuum or distinct processes? *Psychonomic Bulletin & Review 8*(4): 742–746.

Hogarth, L., Dickinson, A., and Duka, T. (2010). Selective attention to conditioned stimuli in human discrimination learning: Untangling the effects of outcome prediction, valence, arousal and uncertainty. In C. Mitchell and M. Le Pelley (eds.), *Attention and Associative Learning* (pp. 71–98). New York and Oxford: Oxford University Press.

Huang, T. R. and Grossberg, S. (2010). Cortical dynamics of contextually cued attentive visual learning and search: Spatial and object evidence accumulation. *Psychological Review* 117(4): 1080–1112.

Ikeda, T. and Hikosaka, O. (2003). Reward-dependent gain and bias of visual responses in primate superior colliculus. *Neuron* 39(4): 693–700.

Ipata, A. E., Gee, A. L., Gottlieb, J., Bisley, J. W., and Goldberg, M. E. (2006). LIP responses to a popout stimulus are reduced if it is overtly ignored. *Nature Neuroscience* 9(8): 1071–1076.

Kable, J. W. and Glimcher, P. W. (2009). The neurobiology of decision: Consensus and controversy. *Neuron* 63(6): 733–745.

Kowler, E., Anderson, E., Dosher, B., and Blaser, E. (1995). The role of attention in the programming of saccades. *Vision Research* 35(13): 1897–1916.

Land, M. F. (2009). Vision, eye movements, and natural behavior. *Visual Neuroscience* 26(1): 51–62.

Lewis, J. W. and Van Essen, D. C. (2000). Corticocortical connections of visual, sensorimotor, and multimodal processing areas in the parietal lobe of the macaque monkey. *Journal of Comparative Neurology* 428(1): 112–137.

Libera, C. D. and Chelazzi, L. (2009). Learning to attend and to ignore is a matter of gains and losses. *Psychological Science* 20(6): 778–784.

Lo, C. C. and Wang, X. J. (2006). Cortico-basal ganglia circuit mechanism for a decision threshold in reaction time tasks. *Nature Neuroscience* 9(7): 956–963.

Louie, K. and Glimcher, P. W. (2010). Separating value from choice: Delay discounting activity in the lateral parietal area. *Journal of Neuroscience* 30(16): 5498–5507.

Louie, K., Grattan, L. E., and Glimcher, P. W. (2011). Reward value-based gain control: Divisive normalization in parietal cortex. *Journal of Neuroscience* 31(29): 10627–10639.

McAdams, C. J. and Maunsell, J. H. R. (1999). Effects of attention on orientation-tuning functions of single neurons in macaque cortical area V4. *Journal of Neuroscience* 19(1): 431–441.

Maunsell, J. H. and Treue, S. (2006). Feature-based attention in visual cortex. *Trends in Neurosciences* 29(6): 317–322.

Mirabella, G., Bertini, G., Samengo, I., Kilavik, B. E., Della Libera, C., and Chelazzi, L. (2007). Neurons in area V4 of the macaque translate attended visual features into behaviorally relevant categories. *Neuron* 54(2): 303–318.

Navalpakkam, V. and Itti, L. (2005). Modeling the influence of task on attention. *Vision Research* 45(2): 205–231.

Navalpakkam, V., Koch, C., Rangel, A., and Perona, P. (2010). Optimal reward harvesting in complex perceptual environments. *Proceedings of the National Academy of Sciences USA* 107(11): 5232–5237.

Oppermann, F., Hassler, U., Jescheniak, J. D., and Gruber, T. (2012). The rapid extraction of gist-early neural correlates of high-level visual processing. *Journal of Cognitive Neuroscience* 24(2): 521–529.

Oristaglio, J., Schneider, D. M., Balan, P. F., and Gottlieb, J. (2006). Integration of visuospatial and effector information during symbolically cued limb movements in monkey lateral intraparietal area. *Journal of Neuroscience* 26(32): 8310–8319.

Pearce, J. M. and Mackintosh, N. J. (2010). Two theories of attention: A review and a possible integration. In C. J. Mitchell and M. E. Le Pelley (eds.), *Attention and Associative Learning* (pp. 11–40). New York and Oxford: Oxford University Press.

Peck, C. J., Jangraw, D. C., Suzuki, M., Efem, R., and Gottlieb, J. (2009). Reward modulates attention independently of action value in posterior parietal cortex. *Journal of Neuroscience* 29(36): 11182–11191.

Platt, M. L. and Glimcher, P. W. (1999). Neural correlates of decision variables in parietal cortex. *Nature* 400(6741): 233–238.

Pouget, A., Deneve, S., and Duhamel, J. R. (2002). A computational perspective on the neural basis of multisensory spatial representations. *Nature Reviews Neuroscience* 3(9): 741–747.

Pouget, P., Logan, G. D., Palmeri, T. J., Boucher, L., Paré, M., and Schall, J. D. (2011). Neural basis of adaptive response time adjustment during saccade countermanding. *Journal of Neuroscience* 31(35): 12604–12612.

Powell, K. D. and Goldberg, M. E. (2000). Response of neurons in the lateral intraparietal area to a distractor flashed during the delay period of a memory-guided saccade. *Journal of Neurophysiology* 84(1): 301–310.

Raffi, M. and Siegel, R. M. (2005). Functional architecture of spatial attention in the parietal cortex of the behaving monkey. *Journal of Neuroscience* 25(21): 5171–5186.

Reynolds, J. H. and Chelazzi, L. (2004). Attentional modulation of visual processing. *Annual Review of Neuroscience* 27: 611–647.

Reynolds, J. H., Chelazzi, L., and Desimone, R. (1999). Competitive mechanisms subserve attention in macaque areas V2 and V4. *Journal of Neuroscience* 19(5): 1736–1753.

Reynolds, J. H. and Heeger, D. J. (2009). The normalization model of attention. *Neuron* 61(2): 168–185.

Reynolds, J. H., Pasternak, T., and Desimone, R. (2000). Attention increases sensitivity of V4 neurons. *Neuron* 26(3): 703–714.

Roberts, K. L. and Humphreys, G. W. (2011a). Action relations facilitate the identification of briefly-presented objects. *Attention, Perception, & Psychophysics* 73(2): 597–612.

Roberts, K. L. and Humphreys, G. W. (2011b). Action-related objects influence the distribution of visuospatial attention. *Quarterly Journal of Experimental Psychology (Hove)* 64(4): 669–688.

Schall, J. D., Purcell, B. A., Heitz, R. P., Logan, G. D., and Palmeri, T. J. (2011). Neural mechanisms of saccade target selection: Gated accumulator model of the visual-motor cascade. *European Journal of Neuroscience* 33(11): 1991–2002.

Sommer, M. A. and Wurtz, R. H. (2002). A pathway in primate brain for internal monitoring of movements. *Science* 296(5572): 1480–1482.

Sprague, N. and Ballard, D. H. (2005). Modeling embodied visual behaviors. *ACM Transactions on Applied Perception* 1(1): 1–26.

Stanford, T. R., Shankar, S., Massoglia, D. P., Costello, M. G., and Salinas, E. (2010). Perceptual decision making in less than 30 milliseconds. *Nature Neuroscience* 13(3): 379–385.

Sugrue, L. P., Corrado, G. S., and Newsome, W. T. (2004). Matching behavior and the representation of value in the parietal cortex. *Science* 304(5678): 1782–1787.

Sugrue, L. P., Corrado, G. S., and Newsome, W. T. (2005). Choosing the greater of two goods: Neural currencies for valuation and decision making. *Nature Reviews Neuroscience* 6(5): 363–375.

Tatler, B. W., Hayhoe, M. M., Land, M. F., and Ballard, D. H. (2011). Eye guidance in natural vision: reinterpreting salience. *Journal of Vision* 11(5): 5–25.

Vuilleumier, P. (2005). How brains beware: Neural mechanisms of emotional attention. *Trends in Cognitive Neurosciences* 9(12): 585–594.

Wardak, C., Olivier, E., and Duhamel, J. R. (2002). Saccadic target selection deficits after lateral intraparietal area inactivation in monkeys. *Journal of Neuroscience* 22(22): 9877–9884.

Wardak, C., Olivier, E., and Duhamel, J. R. (2004). A deficit in covert attention after parietal cortex inactivation in the monkey. *Neuron* 42(3): 501–508.

Williams, J. M., Mathews, A., and MacLeod, C. (1996). The emotional Stroop task and psychopathology. *Psychological Bulletin* 120(1): 3–24.

Williford, T. and Maunsell, J. H. (2006). Effects of spatial attention on contrast response functions in macaque area V4. *Journal of Neurophysiology* 96(1): 40–54.

Zhang, M. and Barash, S. (2004). Persistent LIP activity in memory antisaccades: Working memory for a sensorimotor transformation. *Journal of Neurophysiology* 91(3): 1424–1441.

CHAPTER 13

··

NEURONAL MECHANISMS OF ATTENTIONAL CONTROL: FRONTAL CORTEX

··

KELSEY L. CLARK, BEHRAD NOUDOOST,
ROBERT J. SCHAFER, AND TIRIN MOORE

THE ACTIVITY OF FRONTAL EYE FIELD (FEF) NEURONS DURING ENDOGENOUS SPATIAL ATTENTION

··

IT is now well established that the responses of neurons within visual cortex to a stimulus are enhanced when a subject pays attention to that stimulus, compared to when the stimulus is ignored. In a typical neurophysiological experiment, the subject (e.g. a monkey) is trained to pay attention to different stimuli appearing at peripheral locations while maintaining central fixation. In other words, the subject *covertly* attends to the different peripheral stimuli. The responses of visual cortical neurons to physically identical stimuli presented to their receptive fields (RFs) are then compared between the different conditions. During covert attention, the visual response of neurons to the RF stimulus is enhanced when the animal pays attention to that stimulus, compared to when the animal attends elsewhere (e.g. Motter 1993). Moreover, this enhancement leads to changes in orientation tuning, direction of motion tuning, contrast sensitivity, colour tuning, and the representations of multiple, competing RF stimuli (Reynolds and Chelazzi 2004). It is assumed that the perceptual benefits of covert attention are supported by these correlative changes in neuronal sensitivity within visual cortex. If this assumption is correct, then the crucial question to be addressed is: what mechanisms give rise to these correlates of attention? What neural circuits modulate the 'gain' of visual signals when particular stimuli are selected by covert attention? In this chapter, we discuss evidence that implicates the FEF as one of the structures causally involved in that control.

The FEF is an area of prefrontal cortex (PFC) with a well-known role in the control of saccadic eye movements (Schall 1995). That is, this area is involved in the *overt* shifting of attention, via shifts of gaze, from one stimulus to another. In recent years, however, single-neuron recordings in behaving monkeys have yielded much data supporting a role of the FEF in the control of *covert* attention as well. Firing rates of FEF neurons are enhanced when the animal pays attention to a stimulus within an FEF neuron's receptive field (RF), similar to what is observed in posterior visual areas. The firing rates of FEF neurons thus signal the location of spatial attention, even in the absence of eye movements, and they've been shown to do so in a variety of covert attention tasks. For example, such modulation occurs during change blindness tasks (Armstrong et al. 2009), change detection tasks (Gregoriou et al. 2009; Kodaka et al. 1997), and during covert visual search (Monosov and Thompson 2009; Thompson et al. 2005a, 2005b; Buschman and Miller 2009). Simultaneous recordings from visual area V4 and the FEF during the deployment of covert attention have revealed that modulation of neuronal firing rates arises earlier in the FEF (Gregoriou et al. 2009). Critically, in this task the target stimuli appeared well before the cue directing attention to a particular location, allowing the onset of attentional modulation to be measured independently of the visual latency of the neurons and without being obscured by visual onset transients. Within the FEF itself, spiking activity reflects target selection earlier than the local field potential (LFP), which suggests that the attentional signal may emerge from within the circuitry of the FEF (Monosov et al. 2008).

In addition to facilitating comparisons of the latency of attentional signals between areas, simultaneous recordings from frontal and extrastriate regions also provide insight into the interaction of these reciprocally connected areas during the deployment of spatial attention. Onset of a spatial cue toward the RF is followed by a rise in firing rates in both FEF and V4, and an increase in gamma-band LFP power in both areas (Gregoriou et al. 2009). Changes in FEF firing rate precede the increase in gamma power in both areas, which in turn precede significant increases in V4 firing rates. Synchrony between the spike times and LFP phases, as measured by the spike-field coherence, also increases in the gamma band, both within and between areas. If this synchrony were the product of a common driving input to the two areas, then the difference in phase between the activity across areas would be expected to be zero; instead, both spike-field and field-field coherence showed that V4 activity lagged FEF activity by approximately half a gamma cycle (8–13 ms). Granger causality analysis of the gamma power in LFPs of the two areas suggests that this synchrony is initiated by the FEF: although within 200 ms of the spatial cue there is significant Granger causality both from FEF to V4 and from V4 to FEF (as might be expected given that each receives projections from the other), the cue-evoked rise in Granger values occurs significantly sooner in the FEF to V4 direction than the reverse (100 ms vs 160 ms after cue onset, respectively). This work begins to bridge the gap between the bodies of research previously focused on characterizing the effects of attention in each area independently. Neurophysiological studies of this type seem to complement a variety of observations in the human literature. For example, attentional state has been found to modify propagation of TMS-induced activity from frontal to posterior visual areas (Morishima et al. 2009). In fMRI studies, measures of frontal activity and frontal-extrastriate connectivity have proven effective predictors of both attentional modulation of visual cortical responses and task performance (Bressler et al. 2008; Gazzaley et al. 2007; Zanto et al. 2010).

EXOGENOUS ATTENTION

The above-mentioned evidence primarily addresses the involvement of the FEF in *endogenous* spatial attention, that is, attention that is directed to a location by virtue of internal goals. This type of attention is also referred to as *top-down, voluntary*, or *goal-directed* attention. Less clear is the role of the FEF in *exogenous* attention. Unlike endogenous attention, which is deployed according to the goal or task relevance of particular stimuli, *exogenous* attention is governed primarily by the physical salience of sensory stimuli. This type of attention is also referred to as *bottom-up, involuntary*, or *stimulus-driven* attention. One major question of recent interest is the relative contribution of frontal and parietal regions to exogenous attention, particularly the FEF and the lateral intraparietal area (LIP), respectively. Both the FEF and the LIP have been proposed to contain 'salience maps', combining task goals and stimulus salience into a priority map of space for directing gaze and attention (Bisley and Goldberg 2010; Thompson and Bichot 2005; Moore and Fallah 2001). One such exogenous form of attention is 'pop-out', in which a stimulus with unique features is easily distinguished from among any number of dissimilar distractors (Treisman and Gelade 1980). Neurons in both LIP (Ipata et al. 2006) and FEF (Bichot et al. 2001) have been found to respond more strongly to pop-out stimuli than to stimuli that share features with the distractors. Buschman and Miller sought to clarify the contributions of parietal and frontal regions to exogenous and endogenous attention by simultaneously recording from areas LIP, FEF, and lateral prefrontal cortex (LPFC) during both pop-out search and an attentionally demanding covert visual search (Buschman and Miller 2007). All three areas showed target selectivity under both pop-out and covert search conditions, but the relative timing of the emergence of these effects in the different areas was markedly different in the two tasks. In pop-out, target selectivity appeared first in the responses of LIP neurons, followed by LPFC and finally FEF neurons. In all three areas a significant subpopulation of neurons showed target selectivity before the animal's behavioural response. In the search task, selectivity arose in the FEF and LPFC significantly earlier than in LIP, which didn't select target location until after the monkey's saccade. These results suggest that while the FEF and LPFC may exert control over target selection in top-down, covert search, this function might be performed first in LIP during stimulus-driven, pop-out search.

Given the apparent overlap in the set of areas representing exogenous and endogenous attentional signals, a natural question to ask is how the two types of attentional modulation interact. Burrows and Moore recently examined the effect of saccade plan-ning, and the accompanying attentional deployment toward the saccade target, on the representation of bottom-up, pop-out salience in area V4 responses (Burrows and Moore 2009). Monkeys passively viewed pop-out arrays either while fixating or just prior to directing a saccade to a target located away from the array. During fixation the V4 neurons showed an enhanced response to pop-out stimuli. The same neurons that exhibited this pop-out selectivity during fixation showed no selectivity just prior to a saccade away from the pop-out array, suggesting that this exogenous attentional sig-nal is limited by the availability of endogenous resources. A model of exogenous sali-ence by Soltani and Koch suggests that although feedforward and lateral connectivity within extrastriate cortex are sufficient to generate pop-out selectivity, such signals can be either disrupted or enhanced by incorporating top-down feedback with or without a saccade preparation signal, respectively (Soltani and Koch 2010). These results suggest a role for oculomotor or attentional feedback signals, perhaps from LIP or FEF, in main-taining pop-out selectivity in extrastriate cortex, in addition to mediating the behav-ioural consequences of such salient stimulus properties.

FEF MICROSTIMULATION

Although a relationship between attention and gaze control has been noted for some time (e.g. Ferrier 1890; Ribot 1890), only in the last twenty years or so has this rela-tionship been thoroughly examined psychophysically and neurophysiologically. Gaze shifts, which are most often achieved by saccadic eye movements (saccades) seem to occur in conjunction with shifts in attention, as shown by the decrement in target detection thresholds observed near the endpoints of upcoming saccades (Hoffman and Subramaniam 1995; Peterson et al. 2004). Conversely, covert attention has been shown to alter the metrics of saccades, impacting latencies (Rizzolatti et al. 1987) and trajec-tories of both cue-driven and electrically evoked saccades, with the magnitude of the deviation increasing with difficulty of the attention task (Sheliga et al. 1995; Kustov and Robinson 1996). Additionally, if the eyes are maximally rotated in their orbits, spatial cues in the visual hemifield toward which no further movement is possible no longer produce their typical reaction time benefits, suggesting a functional coupling between eye movements and attention (Craighero et al. 2004).

Prompted by the psychophysical evidence of a link between saccades and attention, Moore and Fallah (2001, 2004) examined whether manipulating neural activity within the FEF could affect the deployment of spatial attention. Neurons in the FEF exhibit both visual and motor properties, responding to stimuli positioned at particular loca-tions and/or prior to saccades toward those locations; in other words, FEF neurons can have receptive fields (RFs) or movement fields (MFs) or both (Bruce and Goldberg 1985). Microstimulation of the FEF at sufficiently high currents evokes saccades of an amplitude and direction such that gaze shifts to the location of the RFs/MFs of neurons near the electrode tip (Bruce et al. 1985; Robinson and Fuchs 1969). Moore and Fallah stimulated FEF sites using currents too low to evoke eye movements (subthreshold currents) while monkeys monitored a target stimulus among distractors for a small change in luminance (Fig. 13.1a). On trials in which microstimulation occurred, monkeys were able to detect smaller luminance changes than on control trials. This effect was spatially and temporally specific—an increase in sensitivity was observed only if the target location matched the endpoint of saccades evoked from the microstimulation site, and was strongest when onset of microstimulation immediately preceded and temporally overlapped the luminance change (Fig. 13.1b). The magnitude of the change in sensitivity produced by microstimulation was comparable to removing the distractors altogether.

In addition to producing perceptual benefits, voluntary deployment of covert attention is known to modulate visual responses of neurons in visual cortex (Treue and Maunsell 1999; Desimone and Duncan 1995). Armstrong and colleagues investigated whether subthreshold microstimulation of the FEF could alter responses in area V4 of visual cortex in a manner similar to that observed during spatial attention. Microstimulation of the FEF enhanced responses of V4 neurons to visual stimuli (Fig. 13.1c). This modulation was stronger in the presence of distractors (Moore and Armstrong 2003), and was critically dependent upon an overlap in the RF of the V4 neuron and the endpoint of saccades evoked from the microstimulation site (Fig. 13.1d). The enhancement also depended upon the placement of the visual stimulus precisely at the endpoint of evoked saccades and not merely anywhere within the larger V4 receptive field (Fig. 13.1f; Armstrong et al. 2006). This enhancement was larger for the V4 neuron's preferred stimulus than a non-preferred stimulus, resulting in an increase in the ability of a V4 cell to discriminate between a preferred and non-preferred orientation (Fig. 13.1e; Armstrong and Moore 2007). Placing both a preferred and non-preferred stimulus within a V4 neuron's RF produces a response that is intermediate in magnitude between its response to either stimulus alone (Reynolds et al. 1999). The responses of V4 neurons to such competing RF stimuli could be biased toward one stimuli or the other with FEF microstimulation, depending on which stimulus was aligned with the stimulated FEF vector (Fig. 13.1g). These effects of FEF microstimulation mirror those of voluntary covert spatial attention on V4 responses (Reynolds et al. 1999; Reynolds and Chelazzi 2004).

Ekstrom and colleagues also examined the influence of FEF microstimulation on visual cortical activity, but did so using functional magnetic resonance imaging (fMRI), thus allowing them to see effects in all visual areas. They evaluated blood-oxygen-level-dependent (BOLD) responses throughout the visual cortical hierarchy following visual stimulation alone, subthreshold FEF microstimulation, or microstimulation combined with visual stimuli of varying contrast (Ekstrom et al. 2009). The impact of microstimulation depended upon the presence of distractors, and was more effective for low-contrast stimuli, consistent with electrophysiological studies of attentional modulation of visual cortical responses (Reynolds et al. 2000). Analogous effects have also been observed in humans, where TMS of the FEF increases extrastriate cortical sensitivity, as assessed by the ability of TMS to evoke visual percepts (Silvanto et al.

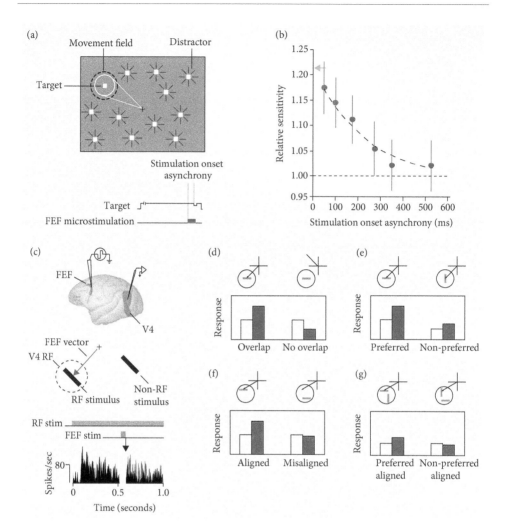

FIGURE 13.1 Effects of subthreshold FEF microstimulation on covert spatial attention and on the responses of neurons within posterior visual cortex. (a) Change detection task used to test the effect of FEF microstimulation on attention. Monkeys were trained to maintain central fixation and to pay attention (spotlight icon) to a peripheral target while ignoring flashing distractors. The target was transiently dimmed at random times and the monkey had to indicate it with a manual response. The event plot at the bottom shows the temporal relationship between the timing of the target dimming and the train of FEF microstimulation, the *stimulation onset asynchrony*, which was varied across experiments. (b) FEF microstimulation increased the monkeys' sensitivity to the target dimming depending on the stimulation onset asynchrony. Relative sensitivity values denote performance relative to control trials and are given as ratios, unity being equal performance and greater values indicating improvement. The black arrow shows the improvement that results from removing the distractors in control trials. (c) Modulation of visually driven responses of area V4 neurons with microstimulation of the FEF. Sites within the FEF were electrically stimulated while recording from neurons in area V4. Cartoon shows a side view of the macaque brain. Top: the locations of the FEF in the anterior bank of the arcuate sulcus and of area V4 in the prelunate

2006) or by the size of event-related potentials (Taylor et al. 2007) or BOLD signals (Ruff et al. 2006) evoked by visual stimuli. Lastly, similar results have even been obtained in the owl brain, where microstimulation of a forebrain gaze control area homologous with the primate FEF, the archopallial gaze field (AGF), modulates the gain of tectal visual and auditory responses (Winkowski and Knudsen 2008).

One early concern with the experiments linking microstimulation of the FEF to attention was the possibility that microstimulation did not directly manipulate the brain's attentional circuitry, but simply produced a localized visual percept (a 'phosphene') that in turn drew the animal's attention. Humans report perceiving brief flashes of light during microstimulation of V1 and a variety of other cortical and subcortical areas (Brindley and Lewin 1968; Nashold 1970), and behavioural studies in monkeys are consistent with the animal experiencing a similar phenomenon (Bartlett and Doty 1980). However, humans do not report visual percepts during microstimulation of the FEF, despite experiencing involuntary eye movements (Blanke et al. 2000; Penfield and Rasmussen 1950). Attempts to introduce an 'artificial phosphene' in the form of a veridical visual cue have had either no or negative effects on an animal's attentional performance and neural discriminability in visual cortex (Armstrong and Moore 2007; Cavanaugh et al. 2006; Müller et al. 2005), suggesting that the attention-like effects of FEF microstimulation are not simply due to a visual percept. A more recent study provides further support that FEF microstimulation directly drives attentional deployment and does so in conjunction with the preparation of saccades (Schafer and Moore 2007). In this study, the authors exploited the fact that visual motion can distort the position of objects (Devalois and Devalois 1991) such that the endpoints of saccades to a drifting grating tend to be biased in the direction of motion (Schafer and Moore 2007). Subthreshold microstimulation of the FEF not only increased the tendency of monkeys to choose targets aligned with the stimulated representation, but it also enhanced the

---

←

gyrus and below the inferior occipital sulcus are shown (both shaded). Monkeys performed a fixation task while oriented bar stimuli were presented inside the recorded V4 neuron's RF (dotted circle) and at another location outside the RF. The stimulation and recording sites in the FEF and area V4, respectively, could be chosen such that the FEF saccade vector (arrow) and the area V4 neuron's RF overlapped spatially. Bottom: mean response of a V4 neuron during control trials (black) and on trials in which a 50 ms microstimulation train (FEF stim) was applied to the FEF site (red). (d) Dependence of V4 modulation on the spatial overlap of stimulated FEF representation (black arrow) and the V4 RF (black circle). 'Response' schematically depicts the V4 activity during control (open) and stimulation (red) trials. (e) Dependence of V4 modulation on the efficacy of the RF stimulus. (f) Dependence of the V4 modulation on the alignment of the RF stimulus with the stimulated FEF vector *within* the V4 RF. (g) Effect of FEF microstimulation on the responses of V4 neurons to competing (preferred and non-preferred) RF stimuli. Effects depicted in (d–g) mirror the modulations observed during covert spatial attention. Data from *Journal of Neurophysics* 91, Moore T and Fallah M. Microstimulation of the frontal eye field and its effects on covert spatial attention, pp. 152–62 © 2004, American Physiological Society and Nature 421, Moore T, Armstrong KM., Selective gating of visual signals by microstimulation of frontal cortex, pp. 370–373 © 2003, Nature Publishing Group.

motion-induced bias (MIB) of saccadic endpoints made to the targets. The latter stimulation effect was unambiguously perceptual rather than motor, since introduction of a
fixed saccadic vector would have reduced, not enhanced, the MIB. This effect is also
inconsistent with a microstimulation-induced visual percept, as such a percept should
also be expected to reduce, not enhance, the MIB.

Even in the absence of an evoked visual percept, any localized perception of the microstimulation itself could serve as a cue which the animal uses to guide attention, rather
than directly driving attentional deployment. To address this potential confound, in the
form of either a phosphene or more abstract sensation, a recent study directly probed the
ability of animals to detect microstimulation of the FEF (Murphey and Maunsell 2008). It
was found that monkeys could indeed detect when stimulation occurred, and could do so
at currents below the threshold for producing eye movements. The mean value for detecting microstimulation was approximately 66% of the threshold for evoking saccades (Fig.
13.2b). Interestingly, the previously reported attentional benefits of FEF microstimulation were found to decrease as the current approached the saccade threshold, disappearing when the current reached ~75% of the saccade threshold (Moore and Fallah 2004,
Fig. 13.2a). This observation served as the basis for subsequently fixing all 'subthreshold' currents to 50% of the saccadic threshold in this and further studies (e.g. Moore and
Armstrong 2003). Thus, the results by Murphey and Maunsell (2008) suggest that the
currents at which microstimulation can be detected (relative to saccadic threshold) do
not appear to overlap with the currents at which microstimulation produces attentional
benefits. More recent work by Corneil and colleagues suggests a possible mechanism
for both the detection of microstimulation and the negative effects of increasing microstimulation current on behavioural performance. In natural vision, saccades are often
accompanied by head movements. Recording muscle activity from head-restrained and
head-unrestrained monkeys, they found that FEF microstimulation evoked neck muscle contraction, even for small saccades in head-restrained monkeys (Corneil et al. 2010;
Elsley et al. 2007). Furthermore, the current required to evoke muscle activity was found
to be lower than that required to evoke saccades, averaging ~70% of the saccade threshold (Fig. 13.2c). These results suggest that the basis of monkeys' ability to detect FEF
microstimulation might be neck muscle proprioception, rather than visual phosphenes.
Moreover, these results suggest that the attention-related enhancement observed with
lower currents (relative to saccadic threshold) were not accompanied by such effects.

In spite of the above, a remaining limitation with any microstimulation result is that
effects cannot be definitively attributed to the neurons near the electrode tip, as microstimulation is known to activate areas projecting to or receiving input from the stimulated
site (via orthodromic or antidromic potentials), and could even activate cells in remote
regions whose axons pass in proximity to the electrode tip (see Clark et al. 2011 for
review). Indeed, it is known that microstimulation of the SC, to which the FEF projects,
produces attention-like behavioural benefits similar to those seen with FEF microstimulation (Cavanaugh and Wurtz 2004; Müller et al. 2005). With only these experiments to go
by, either set of results could in fact be entirely dependent on activation of neurons in the
other brain area. Different methods of manipulating neural activity are therefore desirable in the search for causal attribution of attentional deployment to a specific brain area.

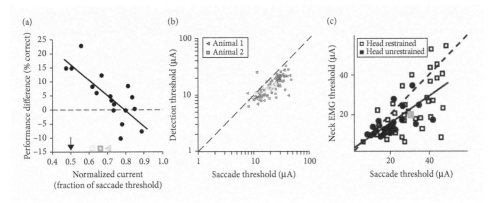

FIGURE 13.2 Relationship of attention effects of FEF microstimulation and the detection of microstimulation itself to the current threshold to evoke a saccade. (a) Performance improvement with microstimulation (positive values) as a function of current magnitude, expressed as a fraction of threshold current for evoking saccades (normalized current). Arrow denotes the normalized current value (50%) used in studies of the effects of FEF microstimulation on attention and visual cortex (e.g. Moore and Armstrong 2003) (adapted from Moore and Fallah 2004). Green triangle and blue square show the mean normalized current at which two monkeys detected FEF microstimulation (Murphey and Maunsell 2008). Orange square shows mean normalized current at which stimulation-evoked neck EMG becomes measurable. Adapted from *Journal of Neurophysiology*, 91 (1), Tirin Moore and Mazyar Fallah, Microstimulation of the Frontal Eye Field and Its Effects on Covert Spatial Attention, pp. 152–62 © 2004, The American Physiological Society. (b) Current detection threshold across FEF sites as a function of threshold for evoking saccades. Detection thresholds are consistently lower than saccade thresholds. Green triangle and blue square show the means for two monkeys. Adapted from Murphey D. K., Maunsell J. H. R., Electrical microstimulation thresholds for behavioral detection and saccades in monkey frontal eye fields, *Proceedings of the National Academy of Sciences of the United States of America*, 105, pp. 7315–20 © 2008, The National Academy of Sciences. C. Threshold for neck muscle EMG across FEF sites as a function of saccadic threshold, for head-restrained (open squares) and head-unrestrained (filled circles) monkeys. Orange square shows mean head-restrained value. Adapted from Corneil B. D., Elsley J. K., Nagy B., Cushing S. L., Motor output evoked by subsaccadic stimulation of primate frontal eye fields, *Proceedings of the National Academy of Sciences of the United States of America*, 107, pp. 6070–5 © 2010, The National Academy of Sciences. Dotted diagonal lines in b and c denote the line of unity.

DOPAMINE-MEDIATED FEF CONTROL OF VISUAL CORTICAL SIGNALS

In spite of a wealth of evidence for a role of PFC dopamine in attention (Robbins and Arnsten 2009) and good evidence that attentional control is achieved in part by the PFC's modulation of signals within sensory cortices (Barcelo et al. 2000; Moore 2006), these two lines of evidence have remained largely separate. However, recent neurophysiological work suggests that the PFC's control of signals within visual cortex may rely on PFC dopamine receptors (Noudoost and Moore 2011a). Dopaminergic innervation of the PFC originates from neurons within the ventral tegmental area making up the mesocortical pathway. As elsewhere in the brain, within the PFC dopamine receptors are classified into two classes, D1 and D2 (Missale et al. 1998). Compared to other subtypes, D1 receptors (D1Rs) are more abundant in PFC, suggesting a more prominent role in regulating cognitive functions (Lidow et al. 1991; Lidow et al. 1998; Goldman-Rakic et al. 1992). Within the PFC, D1Rs exhibit a bilaminar pattern of expression, while D2 receptors (D2Rs) are less abundant and appear to be expressed primarily within infragranular layers (Farde et al. 1987; Gaspar et al. 1995; Santana et al. 2009). As dopamine is a neuromodulator, evidence from a variety of experimental approaches suggests that when acting via D1Rs, dopamine's effects on PFC neurons are complex. However, these effects appear to have two general properties. First, dopamine can alter the strength and reliability of converging excitatory (glutamatergic) synapses (Seamans and Yang 2004). Second, dopamine's modulatory influence can exhibit an inverted-U-shaped property wherein a positive effect on PFC activity is observed at 'low' dopamine levels, but a negative effect is observed at 'high' levels (Vijayraghavan et al. 2007).

Noudoost and Moore (2011a) studied the impact of manipulating D1R-mediated activity within the FEF on saccadic target selection and on visual responses of extrastriate area V4 neurons (Fig. 13.3). With respect to the latter, since the FEF appears to be the part of the PFC from which modulation of visual cortical signals originates during spatially directed attention, we might expect that if dopamine plays a role in visuospatial attention, then changes in dopaminergic activity within the FEF should alter signals within visual cortex. Manipulation of D1R-mediated FEF activity was achieved via volume injections of a D1 antagonist (SCH23390) into sites within the FEF where neurons represented the same part of visual space as simultaneously recorded area V4 neurons. As mentioned above, modulation of PFC activity via D1Rs is complex and thus infusing a D1 antagonist can be expected to increase (at relatively low concentrations) or decrease (at relatively high concentrations) local FEF activity (Williams and Goldman-Rakic 1995; Vijayraghavan et al. 2007). Thus, the manipulation of D1R-mediated FEF activity might be expected to either increase or decrease target selection and visual cortical responses. In this particular case, it was the former. Following the D1R manipulation, visual targets presented within the affected part of space were more likely to be chosen by monkeys as targets for saccades than during control trials. Thus, the D1R manipulation increased saccadic target selection (Fig. 13.3b). In addition, the responses of area V4 neurons with RFs within the part of space affected by the D1R manipulation were measured. It was found that during passive fixation those responses were altered in three ways (Fig. 13.3c). First, there was an enhancement in the magnitude of responses to visual stimulation. Second, the visual responses became more selective to stimulus orientation. And third, the visual responses became less variable across trials. Importantly, all three changes in V4 visual activity have also been observed in monkeys trained to covertly attend to RF stimuli (Motter 1993; McAdams and Maunsell 1999; Mitchell et al. 2007). Thus, manipulation of D1R-mediated FEF activity not only increased

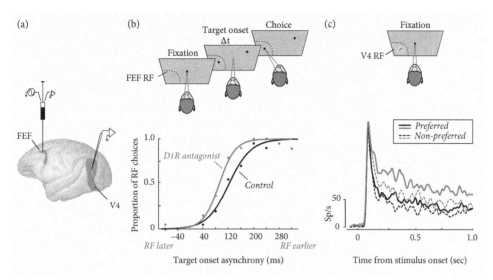

FIGURE 13.3 Dopamine-mediated FEF control of saccadic target selection and visual cortical processing. (a) Local manipulation of dopamine D1 receptor (D1R)-mediated activity within the FEF during single-neuron electrophysiology in area V4. Lateral view of the macaque brain depicts the location of a recording microinjectrode within the FEF and of recording sites within area V4. (b) Free-choice saccade task used to measure the monkey's tendency to make saccades to a target within the FEF RF vs one at an opposite location. In the task, two targets appear at varying temporal onset asynchronies. The RF target can appear earlier or later than a target outside of the RF. The monkey's bias toward either target is measured as the asynchrony at which the monkey chooses the target with equal probability. The bottom plot shows the leftward shift in the asynchrony curve, indicating more RF choices, following manipulation of D1R-mediated FEF activity. (c) Visual responses of a V4 neuron with an RF that overlapped the FEF RF measured during passive fixation. The plot shows mean visual responses over time to bar stimuli presented at the preferred (solid) or non-preferred (dotted) orientation both before (black) and after (red) the FEF D1R manipulation. Reprinted by permission from Macmillan Publishers Ltd: *Nature*, 474, Noudoost, B. and Moore T. Assad, Control of visual cortical signals by prefrontal dopamine, copyright (2011), Nature Publishing Group.

saccadic target selection but it also increased the magnitude, selectivity, and reliability of V4 visual responses within the corresponding part of space. The manipulation effectively elicited correlates of covert attention within extrastriate cortex in the absence of a behavioural task. Interestingly, infusion of a D2 agonist into FEF sites resulted in equivalent target selection increases as the D1 antagonist. However, only the D1 antagonist produced attention-like effects within area V4. Thus, in addition to being dissociable at the level of functional subclasses of FEF neurons (Thompson et al. 2005b), the control of attention and target selection appear to be dissociable at the level of dopamine receptors as well.

The effect of manipulating D1R-mediated FEF activity on V4 neurons shows that changes in FEF neuronal activity are sufficient to exert a long-range influence on representations within visual cortex, an influence suggested, but not demonstrated, by previous studies (Moore and Armstrong 2003; Gregoriou et al. 2009). In addition, these studies demonstrate that dopamine, acting via D1Rs, is involved in the FEF's influence on visual cortical signals as well as on saccadic preparation. As there is a wealth of evidence implicating D1Rs in the neural mechanisms of spatial working memory, specifically in regulating the persistent activity of neurons within dorsolateral prefrontal cortex (dlPFC) (Williams and Goldman-Rakic 1995; Vijayraghavan et al. 2007), the above results suggest that D1Rs may be a part of a common mechanism underlying spatial attention and spatial working memory (Noudoost and Moore 2011a, b). Like dlPFC neurons, FEF neurons also exhibit persistent, delay-period activity, even in tasks not involving saccades (Armstrong et al. 2009). Persistent activity within the PFC is thought to be generated by recurrent glutamatergic connections between prefrontal pyramidal neurons (Goldman-Rakic 1995). Dopaminergic modulation of persistent activity within the PFC appears to be achieved by the influence of D1Rs on these recurrent connections (Gao et al. 2001). The above results suggest a model in which D1Rs contribute to signatures of attention within visual cortex by a mechanism similar to their influence on persistent activity, namely by modulating long-range, recurrent connections between the FEF and visual cortex (Fig. 13.4). Consistent with this idea is the finding that FEF neurons exhibiting persistent activity tend to exhibit greater attentional modulation than those without (Armstrong et al. 2009). In the model, attention (and/or saccadic preparation) is directed toward particular locations according to the pattern of activity across the map of visual space within the FEF, similar to what has been proposed for parietal area LIP (Bisley et al. 2011). Cortical columns with greater activity would correspond to locations of greater attentional deployment (and/or saccadic preparation) and consequently higher 'gain' of spatially overlapping visual cortical signals, compared to non-overlapping signals. A possible role of dopamine would be to control the extent of the FEF gain modulation, effectively setting its dynamic range. Thus, optimum dopamine levels would translate into larger differences between attended and unattended stimuli while suboptimal dopamine would result in small differences and perhaps a less stable attentional focus. At least superficially, such a role of dopamine in attentional deployment would be consistent with the perceptual deficits characteristic of ADHD patients, patients who generally exhibit prefrontal dopaminergic abnormality (Ernst et al. 1998).

OPERANT CONDITIONING OF FEF ACTIVITY

Previous studies have demonstrated the ability of humans and monkeys to voluntarily manipulate activity within motor cortical areas via operant conditioning, even when actual movements are withheld (Fetz and Finocchio 1975; Fetz 1969). Recently Schafer and Moore employed a similar operant training paradigm to examine the extent to which FEF neurons could be controlled voluntarily (Schafer and Moore 2011). Monkeys were provided with real-time auditory feedback based on the firing rate of FEF neurons, and rewarded for either increasing or decreasing that activity to some threshold (in

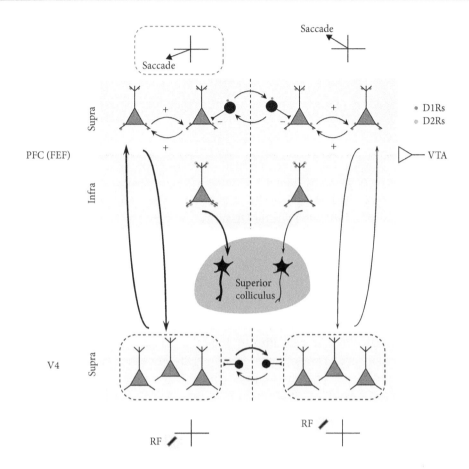

FIGURE 13.4 Possible influence of dopamine receptors on recurrent networks within the PFC (specifically FEF) and between the PFC and V4. The diagram depicts two adjacent FEF or V4 columns representing different but adjacent locations in saccadic or visual space, respectively. The columns are assumed to interact competitively (black inhibitory neurons). Positive arrows between FEF neurons within the same column depict the recurrent excitatory connections thought to underlie the persistence of spatial signals while remembering saccades or locations. Recurrence between the FEF and V4 is proposed to underlie the influence of the FEF on the gain of visual inputs within V4. Dopaminergic input from the ventral tegmental area (VTA, input at right) to the PFC may modulate recurrence both within the FEF and between FEF and V4 through D1Rs and to influence competition between spatial representations. For example, increases in recurrence in a particular column while remembering or attending to a corresponding location (thicker arrows at left) can be modulated by the level of dopamine. Biases in competitive interactions between columns within visual cortex can also be achieved by experimental manipulation of D1R-mediated FEF activity. Also shown are the projections from infragranular FEF neurons to the superior colliculus (SC). Other anatomical details are omitted for simplicity. Red circles represent D1Rs and blue circles D2Rs. Note the localization of D2Rs primarily in infragranular, SC-projecting layers which is consistent with the observation that changes in D2R-mediated FEF activity only affect target selection, and not visual cortical activity. Adapted from *Trends in Cognitive Sciences*, 15 (12), Behrad Noudoost and Tirin Moore, The role of neuromodulators in selective attention, pp. 585–91, Copyright (2011), with permission from Elsevier.

alternating Up and Down blocks of trials) while remaining fixated (Fig. 13.5a). Overall, monkeys were able to alter the average firing rate of FEF neurons in Up vs Down operant control trials and maintained that firing rate for several seconds. Interestingly, the magnitude of voluntary modulation was uncorrelated with the visual or oculomotor properties of the recorded neurons; neurons exhibiting little or no saccade-related activity were equally likely to be controlled as those solely modulated by saccades, but not visual stimuli. Thus, the degree of voluntary control appeared to be equal across functionally defined classes of FEF neurons. Furthermore, voluntary control of FEF firing rates was associated with a frequency-specific modulation of power in the local field potentials (LFPs) at the recording site. Despite the fact that the neurofeedback and rewards were not contingent upon the LFPs, power in the beta (13–30 Hz) and gamma (30–70 Hz) frequency bands were increased during Up trials, compared to Down. LFP and EEG power in both of these frequency bands is believed to be a signature of visual attention (Benchenane et al. 2011; Womelsdorf and Fries 2007; Wróbel 2000).

In addition to demonstrating that FEF neuronal activity could be modulated via endogenous means, Schafer and Moore also probed the consequences of that control on behaviour. The particular behavioural (or cognitive) strategy employed by the monkeys to achieve control of FEF activity could be unrelated to the saccadic or attentional functions attributed to this area, and instead simply be an effective strategy for modulating neuronal activity across any number of brain areas. For example, neuronal control might be achieved merely by non-specific changes in arousal or vigilance. Thus, it is important to probe for specific effects of the neuronal control strategy on the monkeys' behaviour or neurophysiology, and determine the degree to which the monkeys converged upon the same strategy. Schafer and Moore therefore introduced probe trials during the voluntary control paradigm to assess the consequences of voluntary control. In these probe trials, which occurred randomly on 29% of trials, the auditory feedback ceased abruptly and a visual search task was suddenly initiated. In this task, an array of visual shapes appeared on the screen and the monkey was rewarded for making a saccade to an oriented bar target if it was present in the array, or for withholding the saccade if the target was absent (Fig. 13.5b). If the monkey's strategy for altering FEF firing rates was one of general vigilance or arousal, any effects of neuronal control on visual search performance should be independent of task conditions, and in particular, independent of target location. Instead, the behavioural effects of neuronal control were limited to trials in which the target appeared within the RF of the controlled FEF neurons. When the target appeared within the RF, failures to detect the target ('misses') were more frequent on the Down trials than the Up trials, while the frequency of such errors for targets appearing outside the RF was unaffected by voluntary control. In contrast to the effects of voluntary control on visual search performance, Schafer and Moore failed to find any clear effects of control on the metrics of saccades. The probability of a saccade being directed toward stimuli within the FEF RF, across all visual search conditions, was equal for Up and Down conditions, as was the reaction time for saccades to RF targets. In addition, the saccadic main sequence, the trade-off between saccadic amplitude and saccadic velocity (Bahill 1975; Boghen et al. 1974), also appeared to be identical between movements made during Up and Down trials.

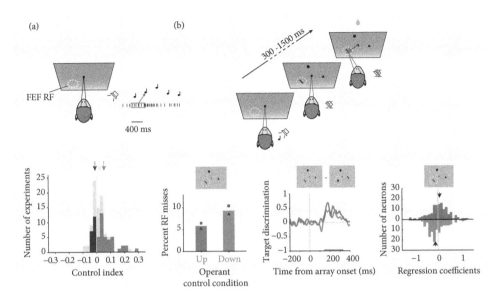

FIGURE 13.5 Operant control of FEF neurons and its effects on selective attention measured behaviourally and neurophysiologically. (a) Operant control task in which the monkey fixated a central spot on an otherwise blank video display and was rewarded for increasing or decreasing the firing rate of FEF neurons. Dotted circle shows the FEF RF; speaker icon and musical notes depict auditory feedback of FEF neuronal activity (spike train) during a sliding 500 ms window (open rectangle). Bottom: population histogram of control indices across a population of FEF neurons. The control index measures the change in FEF firing rate in the rewarded direction (Up or Down); positive values denote correct control. Light grey histogram shows all experiments, purple histogram shows experiments with individually significant positive control, and dark grey histogram shows experiments with significant negative control. (b) Behavioural and neurophysiological consequences of operant FEF control. Top: visual-search probe trials, in which a search array appeared, the auditory feedback ceased ('x' on speaker icon), and the monkey was rewarded (blue droplet) for directing a saccade toward an oriented bar target. Bottom left: mean proportion of target misses opposite the RF was increased during downward operant control of FEF activity in both monkeys (square and triangle symbols). Bottom middle: target discrimination by FEF neurons, defined as the difference in FEF responses between 'Target in RF' and 'Target opposite' trials, was increased during upward operant control relative to downward. Bottom right: correlation of spontaneous activity with FEF responses to the target array. Population histogram shows the regression coefficients describing the relationship between spontaneous activity and responses to targets during upward (red) and downward (blue) operant control. The direction of operant control determined the sign of the relationship between pre-target (baseline) and target-driven FEF activity.

Previous work by Schall and colleagues has established that neurons in the FEF signal the identification of target stimuli during visual search tasks (e.g. Thompson et al. 1996). Schafer and Moore took advantage of this property of FEF neurons and measured the neurons' ability to identify targets in the probe search trials during Up vs Down neuronal control. They found that target discrimination was greater during Up trials than

Down trials, reflecting both a larger response to the target during Up trials and smaller response to the distractor in Down trials. Importantly, the change in target discrimination by FEF neurons was dependent on the direction of neuronal control, rather than simply their spontaneous firing rate just prior to the visual search probe trial. Pooling across Up and Down conditions, there was no correlation between spontaneous firing rate and subsequent target-driven responses. However, dividing Up and Down trials revealed a positive correlation between spontaneous firing rate and target-driven responses during Up trials, but a negative correlation during Down trials. Distractor responses were not correlated with spontaneous activity for Up or Down trials. These results therefore show that the strategy employed by monkeys to exert voluntary control on FEF neuronal activity qualitatively altered how exogenous visual signals interacted with endogenous neural activity.

Spatial Attention and Working Memory

Long before their role in attention was made apparent, FEF neurons were known to display spatially selective persistent activity during the delay period of a memory-guided saccade task (Bruce and Goldberg 1985), as do neurons in nearby dlPFC (Goldman-Rakic 1995). Evidence suggests that maintaining a location in working memory may automatically direct attention to that location: when subjects remember a location, visual processing at that location is enhanced compared to elsewhere in space, as measured by visual discrimination (Awh et al. 1998), visually evoked ERPs in visual cortex (Awh et al. 2000; Jha 2002), or visually evoked BOLD responses in visual cortex (Postle et al. 2004). Performing an attentionally demanding task removed from a memorized location impairs memory performance (Awh et al. 1998; Smyth 1996). The known role of the FEF in both working memory and attention, in combination with demonstrated links between these two processes on a behavioural level, naturally raises the question of whether signals representing attention vs memory are distinguishable within the FEF on the cellular level.

To investigate the relationship between attentional modulation and sustained memory activity within the FEF, Armstrong and colleagues recorded FEF activity during a change blindness task. In change blindness tasks, observers have difficulty detecting localized changes between two visual scenes when they are flashed in quick succession (Cavanaugh and Wurtz 2004; Rensink 2002). Directing spatial attention to a particular location can greatly increase the ability of observers to correctly detect changes (Rensink 2002). Monkeys were cued to one of six possible locations; after a variable delay, oriented grating stimuli appeared at all six locations, followed by a brief blank interval, after which the oriented grating stimuli reappeared, with or without a change in the orientation of the grating at the cued location (Fig. 13.6a). Animals indicated a change in grating orientation by

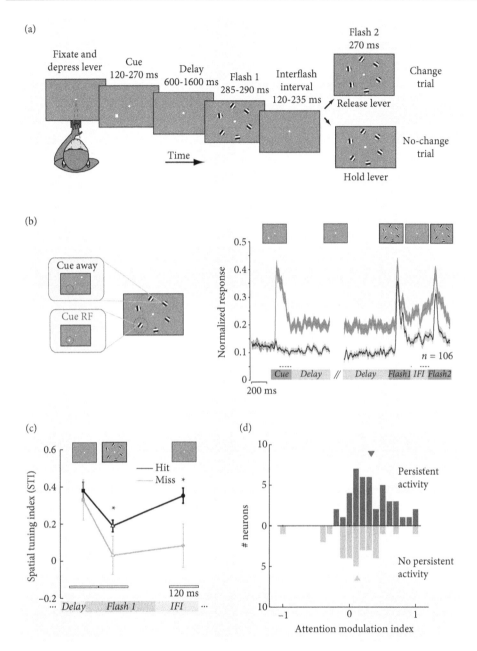

FIGURE 13.6 (a) Change detection task used to measure the selection and maintenance of spatial information by FEF neurons. In the task, the monkey maintained fixation throughout the duration of the trial. To initiate a trial, the monkey manually depressed a lever, and after a few hundred milliseconds, a peripheral cue was presented briefly, indicating the target location. Following a fixed delay period, an array of six oriented gratings was flashed twice. On trials in which the target stimulus changed orientation across flashes (change trial), the monkey was rewarded for releasing the lever. On trials where the target stimulus did not change (no-change trial), the monkey was rewarded for continuing to hold the lever.

releasing a bar to receive juice. The activity of FEF neurons with RFs at the cued location was enhanced during the delay immediately following the cue, during the presentation of the visual stimuli themselves, and in the interval between the two flashed grating stimulus arrays (Fig. 13.6b). FEF thus showed persistent activity maintaining memory of the cue location, and enhanced activity during visual stimulation which could direct attention to the target grating. FEF neurons with RFs at the cued location had greater activity during the interval between the two visual stimuli on correct detection trials (hits) than on incorrect non-responses (misses), such that FEF activity during this period could reliably predict the monkey's subsequent detection performance (Fig. 13.6c). Most interestingly, those neurons which showed persistent activity during the delay period were also those with the greatest enhancement of activity during the presentation of the visual stimuli (Fig. 13.6d), suggesting mechanistic overlap between the maintenance of location information and the deployment of visual attention.

To uncover any potential difference between the representation of location memory vs the locus of attention, one might wish to dissociate the remembered location from that of targets requiring attentional deployment. To date no FEF recordings have been made during a task requiring both spatial memory and attention to a separate location, but this type of experiment has recently been conducted in dlPFC. The dlPFC is reciprocally connected with the FEF (Stanton et al. 1993), and while most of the dlPFC electrophysiology has focused on working memory rather than spatial attention tasks (Funahashi et al. 1989; Rainer et al. 1998), it also exhibits an enhanced target response during covert visual search (Buschman and Miller 2007). Lebedev and colleagues trained monkeys to remember one location while attending to a second, visually cued location, which was monitored for a change in target luminance (Lebedev et al. 2004). The remembered and attended locations could be varied independently from trial to trial, allowing construction of tuning curves for each. A majority of neurons in the dlPFC showed spatially selective activity reflecting the remembered location, the attended location, or both. Significantly more neurons represented the attended location than the remembered location, but nearly a third of those showing any selectivity were modulated

---

(b) Trials in which the monkey was cued to attend to the opposite array location are labelled 'Cue away', while trials in which the monkey was cued to attend to the FEF RF are labelled 'Cue RF'. Histograms show the average response of the population of FEF neurons (n = 106) on correct trials in which the monkey was cued to attend to the RF location (red) and cued to attend away (grey). Panels along the top show a schematic diagram of the display seen by the monkey during the task and the trial epochs are also indicated at the bottom. (c) FEF neuronal responses distinguished between Cue RF and Cue away trials (spatial tuning index) across the flash1 and inter-flash-interval (IFI) epochs more effectively on correct (hit) trials than on incorrect (miss) trials. (d) Dark and light histograms show the distribution of attention modulation indices for neurons that had persistent delay period activity and for neurons that lacked persistent activity, respectively. Adapted from Armstrong K. M, Chang M. H., Moore T., Selection and maintenance of spatial information by frontal eye field neurons, *Journal of Neuroscience*, 29 (50), pp. 15621–9 © 2009, The Society for Neuroscience.

by both the remembered and the attended location, referred to as multitasking neurons. Interestingly, it was found that within cells signalling both location memory and locus of attention, spatial tuning curves usually differed for the remembered vs attended location, often even favouring diametrically opposite positions (Messinger et al. 2009). This dissociation in mnemonic vs attentional tuning, as well as generally stronger tuning, makes multitasking neurons more informative than specialized neurons in extracting the remembered or attended location from neural activity. To what extent this differential tuning in PFC arises through the training of an explicit and perhaps unnatural dissociation of the locus of attention from working memory, and whether a similar dissociation in mnemonic and attentional tuning could arise in the more topographically organized FEF under similar behavioural conditions, is not yet known.

Future Directions

Thus far there has been only limited success in correlating the functional properties of FEF neurons between saccadic and cognitive tasks. For example, delay activity in memory-guided saccade tasks appears to be equally frequent across neurons with varying visual and motor properties (Sommer and Wurtz 2000). In addition, neurons that exhibit covert attentional modulation are likewise distributed among neurons with or without motor properties (Zhou and Thompson 2009), and only purely motor neurons appear to be exempt from that modulation (Thompson et al. 2005b). An important goal of future research will be to determine which types of neurons send feedback to visual cortical areas and influence visual representations during the selection or maintenance of relevant information.

References

Armstrong, K. M., Fitzgerald, J. K., and Moore, T. (2006). Changes in visual receptive fields with microstimulation of frontal cortex. *Neuron* 50: 791–798.

Armstrong, K. M. and Moore, T. (2007). Rapid enhancement of visual cortical response discriminability by microstimulation of the frontal eye field. *Proceedings of the National Academy of Sciences USA* 104: 9499–9504.

Armstrong, K. M., Chang, M. H., and Moore, T. (2009). Selection and maintenance of spatial information by frontal eye field neurons. *Journal of Neuroscience* 29: 15621–15629.

Awh, E., Jonides, J., and Reuter-Lorenz, P. A. (1998). Rehearsal in spatial working memory. *Journal of Experimental Psychology: Human Perception and Performance* 24: 790–780.

Awh, E., Anllo-Vento, L., and Hillyard, S. A. (2000). The role of spatial selective attention in working memory for locations: Evidence from event-related potentials. *Journal of Cognitive Neuroscience* 12: 840–847.

Bahill, A. (1975). The main sequence, a tool for studying human eye movements. *Mathematical Biosciences* 24: 191–204.

Barcelo, F., Suwazono, S., and Knight, R. T. (2000). Prefrontal modulation of visual processing in humans. *Nature Neuroscience* 3: 399–403.

Bartlett, J. R. and Doty, R. W. (1980). An exploration of the ability of macaques to detect microstimulation of striate cortex. *Acta Neurobiologica Experimentalis* 40: 713–727.

Benchenane, K., Tiesinga, P. H., and Battaglia, F. P. (2011). Oscillations in the prefrontal cortex: A gateway to memory and attention. *Current Opinion in Neurobiology* 21: 475–485.

Bichot, N. P., Rao, S. C., and Schall, J. D. (2001). Continuous processing in macaque frontal cortex during visual search. *Neuropsychologia* 39: 972–982.

Bisley, J. W. and Goldberg, M. E. (2010). Attention, intention, and priority in the parietal lobe. *Annual Review of Neuroscience* 33: 1–21.

Bisley, J. W., Mirpour, K., Arcizet, F., and Ong, W. S. (2011). The role of the lateral intraparietal area in orienting attention and its implications for visual search. *European Journal of Neuroscience* 33: 1982–1990.

Blanke, O., Spinelli, L., Thut, G., Michel, C. M., Perrig, S., Landis, T., and Seeck, M. (2000). Location of the human frontal eye field as defined by electrical cortical stimulation: Anatomical, functional and electrophysiological characteristics. *NeuroReport* 11: 1907–1913.

Boghen, D., Troost, B. T., Daroff, R. B., Dell'Osso, L. F., and Birkett, J. E. (1974). Velocity characteristics of normal human saccades. *Investigations in Ophthalmology* 13: 619–623.

Bressler, S. L., Tang, W., Sylvester, C. M., Shulman, G. L., and Corbetta, M. (2008). Top-down control of human visual cortex by frontal and parietal cortex in anticipatory visual spatial attention. *Journal of Neuroscience* 28: 10056–10061.

Brindley, G. S. and Lewin, W. S. (1968). The sensations produced by electrical stimulation of the visual cortex. *Journal of Physiology* 196: 479–493.

Bruce, C. J. and Goldberg, M. E. (1985). Primate frontal eye fields, I: Single neurons discharging before saccades. *Journal of Neurophysiology* 53: 603–635.

Bruce, C. J., Goldberg, M. E., Bushnell, M. C., and Stanton, G. B. (1985). Primate frontal eye fields, II: Physiological and anatomical correlates of electrically evoked eye movements. *Journal of Neurophysiology* 54: 714–734.

Burrows, B. E. and Moore, T. (2009). Influence and limitations of popout in the selection of salient visual stimuli by area V4 neurons. *Journal of Neuroscience* 29: 15169–15177.

Buschman, T. J. and Miller, E. K. (2007). Top-down versus bottom-up control of attention in the prefrontal and posterior parietal cortices. *Science* 315: 1860–1862.

Buschman, T. J. and Miller, E. K. (2009). Serial, covert shifts of attention during visual search are reflected by the frontal eye fields and correlated with population oscillations. *Neuron* 63: 386–396.

Cavanaugh, J. and Wurtz, R. H. (2004). Subcortical modulation of attention counters change blindness. *Journal of Neuroscience* 24: 11236–11243.

Cavanaugh, J., Alvarez, B. D., and Wurtz, R. H. (2006). Enhanced performance with brain stimulation: Attentional shift or visual cue? *Journal of Neuroscience* 26: 11347–11358.

Corneil, B. D., Elsley, J. K., Nagy, B., and Cushing, S. L. (2010). Motor output evoked by subsaccadic stimulation of primate frontal eye fields. *Proceedings of the National Academy of Sciences of the USA* 107: 6070–6075.

Clark, K. L., Armstrong, K. M., and Moore T. (2011). Probing neural circuitry and function with electrical microstimulation. *Proceedings of the Royal Society B: Biological Sciences* 278: 1121–1130.

Craighero, L., Nascimben, M., and Fadiga, L. (2004). Eye position affects orienting of visuospatial attention. *Current Biology* 14: 331–333.

Desimone, R. and Duncan, J. (1995). Neural mechanisms of selective visual attention. *Annual Review of Neuroscience 18*: 193–222.

Devalois, R. L. and Devalois, K. K. (1991). Vernier acuity with stationary moving Gabors. *Vision Research 31*: 1619–1626.

Ekstrom, L. B., Roelfsema, P. R., Arsenault, J. T., Kolster, H., and Vanduffel, W. (2009). Modulation of the contrast response function by electrical microstimulation of the macaque frontal eye field. *Journal of Neuroscience 29*: 10683–10694.

Elsley, J. K., Nagy, B., Cushing, S. L., and Corneil, B. D. (2007). Widespread presaccadic recruitment of neck muscles by stimulation of the primate frontal eye fields. *Journal of Neurophysiology 98*: 1333–1354.

Ernst, M., Zametkin, A. J., Matochik, J. A., Jons, P. H., and Cohen, R. M. (1998). DOPA decarboxylase activity in attention deficit hyperactivity disorder adults: A [fluorine-18]fluorodopa positron emission tomographic study. *Journal of Neuroscience 18*: 5901–5907.

Farde, L., Halldin, C., Stoneelander, S., and Sedvall, G. (1987). Pet analysis of human dopamine receptor subtypes using C-11 Sch 23390 and C-11 Raclopride. *Psychopharmacology 92*: 278–284.

Ferrier, D. (1890). *Cerebral Localisation*. London: Smith, Elder and Co.

Fetz, E. E. (1969). Operant conditioning of cortical unit activity. *Science 163*: 955–958.

Fetz, E. E. and Finocchio, D. V. (1975). Correlations between activity of motor cortex cells and arm muscles during operantly conditioned response patterns. *Experimental Brain Research 23*: 217–240.

Funahashi, S., Bruce, C. J., and Goldman-Rakic, P. S. (1989). Mnemonic coding of visual space in the monkey's dorsolateral prefrontal cortex. *Journal of Neurophysiology 61*: 331–349.

Gao, W. J., Krimer, L. S., and Goldman-Rakic, P. S. (2001). Presynaptic regulation of recurrent excitation by D1 receptors in prefrontal circuits. *Proceedings of the National Academy of Sciences of the USA 98*: 295–300.

Gaspar, P., Bloch, B., and Lemoine, C. (1995). D1 and D2 receptor gene expression in the rat frontal cortex: Cellular localization in different classes of efferent neurons. *European Journal of Neuroscience 7*: 1050–1063.

Gazzaley, A., Rissman, J., Cooney, J., Rutman, A., Seibert, T., Clapp, W., and D'Esposito, M. (2007). Functional interactions between prefrontal and visual association cortex contribute to top-down modulation of visual processing. *Cerebral Cortex 17*: i125–i135.

Goldman-Rakic, P. S., Lidow, M. S., Smiley, J. F., and Williams, M. S. (1992). The anatomy of dopamine in monkey and human prefrontal cortex. *Journal of Neural Transmission 36*: 163–177.

Goldman-Rakic, P. S. (1995). Cellular basis of working memory. *Neuron 14*: 477–485.

Gregoriou, G. G., Gotts, S. J., Zhou, H. H., and Desimone, R. (2009). High-frequency, long-range coupling between prefrontal and visual cortex during attention. *Science 324*: 1207–1210.

Hoffman, J. E. and Subramaniam, B. (1995). The role of visual attention in saccadic eye movements. *Perception & Psychophysics 57*: 787–795.

Ipata, A. E., Gee, A. L., Gottlieb, J., Bisley, J. W., and Goldberg, M. E. (2006). LIP responses to a popout stimulus are reduced if it is overtly ignored. *Nature Neuroscience 9*: 1071–1076.

Jha, A. P. (2002). Tracking the time-course of attentional involvement in spatial working memory: An event-related potential investigation. *Brain Research 15*: 61–69.

Kodaka, Y., Mikami, A., and Kubota, K. (1997). Neuronal activity in the frontal eye field of the monkey is modulated while attention is focused on to a stimulus in the peripheral visual field, irrespective of eye movement. *Neuroscience Research 28*: 291–298.

Kustov, A. A. and Robinson, D. L. (1996). Shared neural control of attentional shifts and eye movements. *Nature 384*: 74–77.

Lebedev, M. A., Messinger, A., Kralik, J. D., and Wise, S. P. (2004). Representation of attended versus remembered locations in prefrontal cortex. *PLoS Biology 2*: e365.

Lidow, M. S., Goldman-Rakic, P. S., Gallager, D. W., and Rakic, P. (1991). Distribution of dopaminergic receptors in the primate cerebral cortex: Quantitative autoradiographic analysis using [H-3] Raclopride, [H-3] Spiperone and [H-3] Sch23390. *Neuroscience 40*: 657–671.

Lidow, M. S., Wang, F., Cao, Y., Goldman-Rakic, P. S. (1998). Layer V neurons bear the majority of mRNAs encoding the five distinct dopamine receptor subtypes in the primate prefrontal cortex. *Synapse 28*: 10–20.

McAdams, C. J. and Maunsell, J. H. R. (1999). Effects of attention on orientation-tuning functions of single neurons in macaque cortical area V4. *Journal of Neuroscience 19*: 431–441.

Messinger, A., Lebedev, M. A., Kralik, J. D., and Wise, S. P. (2009). Multitasking of attention and memory functions in the primate prefrontal cortex. *Journal of Neuroscience 29*: 5640–5653.

Missale, C., Nash, S. R., Robinson, S. W., Jaber, M., and Caron, M. G. (1998). Dopamine receptors: From structure to function. *Physiological Review 78*: 189–225.

Mitchell, J. F., Sundberg, K. A., and Reynolds, J. H. (2007). Differential attention-dependent response modulation across cell classes in macaque visual area V4. *Neuron 55*: 131–141.

Monosov, I. E., Trageser, J. C., and Thompson, K. G. (2008). Measurements of simultaneously recorded spiking activity and local field potentials suggest that spatial selection emerges in the frontal eye field. *Neuron 57*: 614–625.

Monosov, I. E. and Thompson, K. G. (2009). Frontal eye field activity enhances object identification during covert visual search. *Journal of Neurophysics 102*: 3656–3672.

Moore, T. and Fallah, M. (2001). Control of eye movements and spatial attention. *Proceedings of the National Academy of Sciences of the USA 98*: 1273–1276.

Moore, T. and Armstrong, K. M. (2003). Selective gating of visual signals by microstimulation of frontal cortex. *Nature 421*: 370–373.

Moore, T. and Fallah, M. (2004). Microstimulation of the frontal eye field and its effects on covert spatial attention. *Journal of Neurophysics 91*: 152–162.

Moore, T. (2006). The neurobiology of visual attention: Finding sources. *Current Opinion in Neurobiology 16*: 159–165.

Morishima, Y., Akaishi, R., Yamada, Y., Okuda, J., Toma, K., and Sakai, K. (2009). Task-specific signal transmission from prefrontal cortex in visual selective attention. *Nature Neuroscience 12*: 85–91.

Motter, B. C. (1993). Focal attention produces spatially selective processing in visual cortical areas V1, V2, and V4 in the presence of competing stimuli. *Journal of Neurophysics 70*: 909–919.

Müller, J. R., Philiastides, M. G., and Newsome, W. T. (2005). Microstimulation of the superior colliculus focuses attention without moving the eyes. *Proceedings of the National Academy of Sciences of the USA 102*: 524–529.

Murphey, D. K. and Maunsell, J. H. R. (2008). Electrical microstimulation thresholds for behavioral detection and saccades in monkey frontal eye fields. *Proceedings of the National Academy of Sciences of the USA 105*: 7315–7320.

Nashold, B. S. (1970). Phosphenes resulting from stimulation of the midbrain in man. *Archives of Opthalmology 84*: 433–435.

Noudoost, B. and Moore, T. (2011a). Control of visual cortical signals by prefrontal dopamine. *Nature 474*: 372–375.

Noudoost, B. and Moore, T. (2011b). The role of neuromodulators in selective attention. *Trends in Cognitive Sciences* 15: 585–591.

Penfield, W. and Rasmussen, T. (1950). *The Cerebral Cortex of Man: A Clinical Study of Localization of Function*. New York: Macmillan.

Peterson, M. S., Kramer, A. F., and Irwin, D. E. (2004). Covert shifts of attention precede involuntary eye movements. *Perception & Psychophysics* 66: 398–405.

Postle, B. R., Awh, E., Jonides, J., Smith, E. E., and D'Esposito, M. (2004). The where and how of attention-based rehearsal in spatial working memory. *Brain Research* 20: 194–205.

Rainer, G., Asaad, W. F., Miller, and E. K. (1998). Memory fields of neurons in the primate prefrontal cortex. *Proceedings of the National Academy of Sciences of the USA* 95: 15008–15013.

Rensink, R. A. (2002). Change detection. *Annual Review of Psychology* 53: 245–277.

Reynolds, J. H., Chelazzi, L., and Desimone, R. (1999). Competitive mechanisms subserve attention in macaque areas V2 and V4. *Journal of Neuroscience* 19: 1736–1753.

Reynolds, J. H., Pasternak, T., and Desimone, R. (2000). Attention increases sensitivity of V4 neurons. *Neuron* 26: 703–714.

Reynolds, J. H. and Chelazzi, L. (2004). Attentional modulation of visual processing. *Annual Review of Neuroscience* 27: 611–647.

Ribot, T. (1890). *The Psychology of Attention*. Chicago: Open Court Publishing.

Rizzolatti, G., Riggio, L., Dascola, I., and Umiltá, C. (1987). Reorienting attention across the horizontal and vertical meridians: Evidence in favor of a premotor theory of attention. *Neuropsychologia* 25: 31–40.

Robbins, T. W. and Arnsten, A. F. T. (2009). The neuropsychopharmacology of fronto-executive function: Monoaminergic modulation. *Annual Review of Neuroscience* 32: 267–287.

Robinson, D. A. and Fuchs, A. F. (1969). Eye movements evoked by stimulation of frontal eye fields. *Journal of Neurophysics* 32: 637–648.

Ruff, C. C., Blankenburg, F., Bjoertomt, O., Bestmann, S., Freeman, E., Haynes, J. D., Rees, G., Josephs, O., Deichmann, R., and Driver, J. (2006). Concurrent TMS-fMRI and psychophysics reveal frontal influences on human retinotopic visual cortex. *Current Biology* 16: 1479–1488.

Santana, N., Mengod, G., and Artigas, F. (2009). Quantitative analysis of the expression of dopamine D(1) and D(2) receptors in pyramidal and GABAergic neurons of the rat prefrontal cortex. *Cerebral Cortex* 19: 849–860.

Schafer, R. J. and Moore, T. (2007). Attention governs action in the primate frontal eye field. *Neuron* 56: 541–551.

Schafer, R. J. and Moore, T. (2011). Selective attention from voluntary control of neurons in prefrontal cortex. *Science* 332: 1568–1571.

Schall, J. D. (1995). Neural basis of saccade target selection. *Review of Neuroscience* 6: 63–85.

Seamans, J. K. and Yang, C. R. (2004). The principal features and mechanisms of dopamine modulation in the prefrontal cortex. *Progress in Neurobiology* 74: 1–57.

Sheliga, B. M., Riggio, L., Craighero, L., and Rizzolatti, G. (1995). Spatial attention-determined modifications in saccade trajectories. *NeuroReport* 6: 585–588.

Silvanto, J., Lavie, N., and Walsh, V. (2006). Stimulation of the human frontal eye fields modulates sensitivity of extrastriate visual cortex. *Journal of Neurophysics* 96: 941–945.

Smyth, M. M. (1996). Interference with rehearsal in spatial working memory in the absence of eye movements. *Human Experimental Psychology* 49: 940–949.

Soltani, A. and Koch, C. (2010). Visual saliency computations: Mechanisms, constraints, and the effect of feedback. *Journal of Neuroscience* 30: 12831–12843.

Sommer, M. A. and Wurtz, R. H. (2000). Composition and topographic organization of signals sent from the frontal eye field to the superior colliculus. *Journal of Neurophysics 83*: 1979–2001.

Stanton, G. B., Bruce, C. J., and Goldberg, M. E. (1993). Topography of projections to the frontal lobe from the macaque frontal eye fields. *Journal of Comparative Neurology 330*: 286–301.

Taylor, P. C. J., Nobre, A. C., and Rushworth, M. F. S. (2007). FEF TMS affects visual cortical activity. *Cerebral Cortex 17*: 391–399.

Thompson, K. G., Hanes, D. P., Bichot, N. P., and Schall, J. D. (1996). Perceptual and motor processing stages identified in the activity of macaque frontal eye field neurons during visual search. *Journal of Neurophysics 76*: 4040–4055.

Thompson, K. G. and Bichot, N. P. (2005). A visual salience map in the primate frontal eye field. *Progress in Brain Research 147*: 251–262.

Thompson, K. G., Bichot, N. P., and Sato, T. R. (2005a). Frontal eye field activity before visual search errors reveals the integration of bottom-up and top-down salience. *Journal of Neurophysics 93*: 337–351.

Thompson, K. G., Biscoe, K. L., and Sato, T. R. (2005b). Neuronal basis of covert spatial attention in the frontal eye field. *Journal of Neuroscience 25*: 9479–9487.

Treisman, A. M. and Gelade, G. (1980). Feature-integration theory of attention. *Cognitive Psychology 12*: 97–136.

Treue, S. and Maunsell, J. H. R. (1999). Effects of attention on the processing of motion in macaque middle temporal and medial superior temporal visual cortical areas. *Journal of Neuroscience 19*: 7591–7602.

Vijayraghavan, S., Wang, M., Birnbaum, S. G., Williams, G. V., and Arnsten, A. F. T. (2007). Inverted-U dopamine D1 receptor actions on prefrontal neurons engaged in working memory. *Nature Neuroscience 10*: 376–384.

Williams, G. V. and Goldman-Rakic, P. S. (1995). Modulation of memory fields by dopamine D1 receptors in prefrontal cortex. *Nature 376*: 572–575.

Winkowski, D. E. and Knudsen, E. I. (2008). Distinct mechanisms for top-down control of neural gain and sensitivity in the owl optic tectum. *Neuron 60*: 698–708.

Womelsdorf, T. and Fries, P. (2007). The role of neuronal synchronization in selective attention. *Current Opinion in Neurobiology 17*: 154–160.

Wróbel, A. (2000). Beta activity: A carrier for visual attention. *Acta Neurobiologica Experimentalis 60*: 247–260.

Zanto, T. P., Rubens, M. T., Bollinger J., and Gazzaley, A. (2010). Top-down modulation of visual feature processing: The role of the inferior frontal junction. *NeuroImage 53*: 736–745.

Zhou, H. H. and Thompson, K. G. (2009). Cognitively directed spatial selection in the frontal eye field in anticipation of visual stimuli to be discriminated. *Vision Research 49*: 1205–1215.

CHAPTER 14

NEURAL MECHANISMS OF SPATIAL ATTENTION IN THE VISUAL THALAMUS

YURI B. SAALMANN AND SABINE KASTNER

INTRODUCTION

THE thalamus has been extensively studied in terms of its anatomical organization, efferent and afferent connectivity patterns, basic neural response properties, and synaptic, biochemical, and molecular characteristics (Jones 2007; Sherman and Guillery 2006). However, its role in cognitive processes such as spatial attention has remained poorly understood. Studies in awake, behaving monkeys during the last decades have focused almost exclusively on defining the roles of cortical areas in cognition. Similarly, human neuroimaging studies have heavily emphasized the functions of cortical rather than subcortical networks, partially due to technical limitations in terms of spatial resolution. The emphasis on studying cortical function ultimately led to a concept assuming a major, if not exclusive role for cortical networks in cognition. This notion has begun to be revised during the last few years due to the development of functional magnetic resonance imaging (fMRI) at high resolution that permitted for the first time the study of the human thalamus in some detail (reviewed in Saalmann and Kastner 2009, 2011), followed by a renewed interest of physiologists in thalamic function in awake, behaving monkeys (e.g. McAlonan et al. 2006, 2008). In this chapter, we will focus on the visual thalamus as a model system to exemplify the changing views of the thalamus's role in cognition and particularly in spatial attention, which have begun to emerge from these studies.

The visual thalamus consists of three main nuclei, the lateral geniculate nucleus (LGN), the thalamic reticular nucleus (TRN), and the pulvinar. These three structures are characterized by differences in their efferent and afferent connectivity patterns

(Jones 2007; Sherman and Guillery 2006). The LGN is considered a first-order thalamic nucleus because it transmits peripheral signals to the cortex along the retino-cortical pathway. In addition to retinal afferents that form only a minority of the input to the LGN, it receives projections from multiple sources including primary visual cortex (V1), the TRN, and brainstem. Thus, the LGN represents the first stage in the visual pathway at which modulatory influences from other sources could affect information processing. The TRN forms a thin shell of neurons that covers the lateral and anterior surface of the dorsal thalamus, and it receives input from branches of both thalamo-cortical and cortico-thalamic fibers. The TRN in turn sends its output exclusively to the thalamus and is positioned to provide inhibitory control over thalamo-cortical transmission. The pulvinar is the largest nucleus in the primate thalamus and is considered a higher-order thalamic nucleus because it forms input-output loops almost exclusively with the cortex. The extensive and reciprocal connectivity with the cortex suggests that the pulvinar serves in aiding cortico-cortical transmission through thalamic loops. Thus, from an anatomical perspective, the visual thalamus is ideally positioned to regulate the transmission of information to the cortex and between cortical areas, as was originally proposed more than twenty years ago (Crick 1984; Sherman and Koch 1986; Singer 1977). Based on its anatomical connectivity the thalamus may be able to strongly influence cortical networks involved with cognitive processing. The experimental evidence in favour of such a functional role will be reviewed in the following sections that are organized by thalamic nucleus.

LGN: Early Modulation of Visual Information

LGN topography and the response properties of LGN neurons have been extensively studied in anaesthetized non-human primates (e.g. Connolly and Van Essen 1984; Kaas et al. 1972; Malpeli and Baker 1975). The LGN is typically organized into six main layers, and each layer receives input from either the contra- or ipsilateral eye. The four dorsal layers contain small (parvocellular) neurons that are characterized by sustained discharge patterns and low contrast sensitivity, largely processing form and colour information. The two ventral layers contain large (magnocellular) neurons that are characterized by transient discharge patterns and high contrast sensitivity, largely processing motion and depth information (Creutzfeldt et al. 1979; Derrington and Lennie 1984; Dreher et al. 1976; Merigan and Maunsell 1993; Shapley et al. 1981; Wiesel and Hubel 1966). In addition, there are six thin LGN layers, located ventral to each of the parvo- and magnocellular layers, that contain very small (koniocellular) neurons, some of which carry signals from short-wavelength-sensitive (blue) cones (Hendry and Reid 2000; Martin et al. 1997; Roy et al. 2009; Xu et al. 2001). These three LGN cell classes target different cortical layers (Fig. 14.1a). Parvocellular and magnocellular neurons

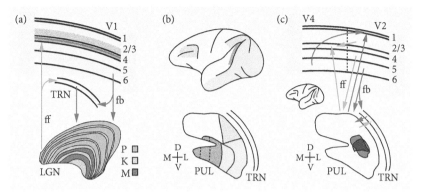

FIGURE 14.1 Thalamo-cortical connectivity. (a) Feedforward (ff) projections from parvo-, konio-, and magnocellular (P, K, M) neurons in the LGN target specific layers in V1 (colour-coded). Layer 6 feedback (fb) from V1 respectively targets P, K, and M layers of the LGN. (b) Fronto-parietal (yellow), medio-temporal (violet), infero-temporal and occipital (green) cortical regions preferentially connect with different divisions of the pulvinar (PUL). The ventro-lateral and ventro-central divisions shown in green are retinotopically organized. Note that there are alternative parcellation schemes of the pulvinar based on neurochemical criteria (Gutierrez et al. 1995; Stepniewska and Kaas 1997; Adams et al. 2000); however, there is reasonable agreement on subdivisions of the ventro-medial pulvinar (dotted lines). (c) Direct cortico-cortical connections (top) and indirect cortico-pulvino-cortical loops exemplified by V2-pulvino-V4 circuitry. Tracer injections into V2 (blue) and V4 (pink; inset) showed overlapping (purple) projection zones in the pulvinar (bottom). (c) Adapted from *Journal of Comparative Neurology*, 419 (3), Michelle M. Adams, Patrick R. Hof, Ricardo Gattass, Maree J. Webster, and Leslie G. Ungerleider, Visual cortical projections and chemo-architecture of macaque monkey pulvinar, pp. 377–93, figure 8 © 2000, Wiley-Liss, Inc.

project to layer 4 and to a lesser extent to layer 6, while koniocellular cells project to layers 1 and 3 of area V1 and to extrastriate areas as well (reviewed in Callaway 2005).

In addition to retinal afferents, the LGN receives modulatory input from multiple sources. Cortico-thalamic feedback projections from V1 comprise about 30% of the input to the LGN, and inhibitory input from the TRN and local interneurons contributes another 30% of LGN input (Sherman and Guillery 2006). Both V1 and TRN represent visual information in retinotopically organized maps and can thereby influence LGN responses in spatially specific ways. Moreover, V1 feedback arises from three classes of neurons, each selectively targeting parvo-, magno-, or koniocellular LGN neurons (Briggs and Usrey 2009). This finding suggests that cortico-thalamic feedback may differentially modulate information processing in parvo-, magno-, and koniocellular afferent pathways, and thus be more selective than the TRN input to LGN. A third major modulatory influence that represents another 30% of input to the LGN arises from brainstem nuclei, that is, the pedunculopontine tegmentum and the parabigeminal nucleus. These cholinergic projections are more diffusely organized than the V1 and TRN projections (Bickford et al. 2000; Erisir et al. 1997) and, consequently, are likely to influence LGN responses with less spatial specificity. Due to the multiple modulatory inputs, the LGN is well positioned for early regulation of visual information transmission.

Attentional response modulation

Human fMRI studies provided the first compelling evidence of cognitive tasks that modulated LGN responses. In a series of attention experiments, O'Connor et al. (2002) showed that selective attention affects visual processing in at least three different ways, similar to the modulatory effects observed in visual cortex: by enhancing responses to attended relative to ignored stimuli, by suppressing responses evoked by unattended stimuli, and by increasing baseline activity in the absence of visual stimulation and in anticipation of an upcoming stimulus (see Beck and Kastner, chapter 9, this volume). The finding of attentional modulation in the human LGN has been corroborated by a subsequent single-cell recording study in the macaque LGN that provided a more

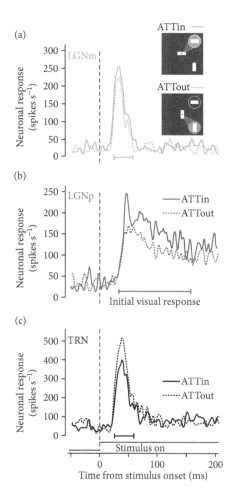

FIGURE 14.2 Attention effects on macaque LGN and TRN neurons. (Inset) Monkeys were cued to direct their attention to a visual stimulus inside (ATTin) or outside (ATTout) the receptive field (circle). Selective attention increased spike rates of (a) magno- and (b) parvocellular LGN neurons, but reduced spike rates of (C) TRN neurons. Reprinted by permission from Macmillan Publishers Ltd: *Nature*, 456 (7220), Kerry McAlonan, James Cavanaugh and Robert H. Wurtz, Guarding the gateway to cortex with attention in visual thalamus, pp. 391–394, figure 1, copyright (2008), Nature Publishing Group.

space- and time-resolved view of the attention effects (McAlonan et al. 2008). The spike rate of LGN neurons increased for attended stimuli relative to unattended stimuli, with slightly stronger effects on magnocellular neurons (11% enhancement) than parvocellular neurons (9%; Fig. 14.2a and b) across the population. Selective attention also influenced magnocellular neurons earlier than parvocellular neurons (the influence of attention on koniocellular neurons is not known). The attention effects varied over time, as evidenced by an early period of attentional modulation within the first 100 ms after stimulus onset, and a later period of modulation starting around 200 ms, possibly reflecting different sources of modulatory input. Based on the response patterns of TRN and V1 neurons, it is possible that the early period of attentional effects in the LGN is attributable to TRN influences, whereas the late period may reflect feedback from V1 (Fig. 14.1a).

Burst and tonic response modes

Modulating the response magnitude of LGN neurons is one mechanism by which information transmitted to the cortex can be influenced depending on behavioural context. Switching the response mode of LGN neurons potentially represents another important mechanism to regulate thalamo-cortical transmission. Thalamic neurons respond in one of two modes, tonic or burst firing mode, depending on a calcium current (I_T) through a low threshold calcium channel (T channel). The calcium channel is inactivated when the neuron is depolarized and de-inactivated when the neuron is hyperpolarized for at least 50 ms. When the calcium current is inactivated, the neuron responds linearly to its input, with a relatively steady train of action potentials (tonic mode). When the calcium current is activated, the neuron responds to its input in a less linear fashion, with a burst of action potentials (burst mode); that is, I_T activates a Ca^{2+}-dependent spike, activating a burst of Na^+ spikes (Huguenard 1996). For example, suppressive stimuli may cause sufficiently prolonged hyperpolarization of an LGN neuron to de-inactivate low-threshold calcium channels. A subsequent depolarizing input is then more likely to induce the LGN neuron to burst fire (Alitto et al. 2005; Denning and Reinagel 2005; Lesica and Stanley 2004). Because bursts are more efficacious in activating thalamo-cortical synapses than tonic spikes (Swadlow and Gusev 2001), burst firing mode may be useful for initially detecting stimuli (Fanselow et al. 2001). After stimulus detection, a switch to tonic firing mode would allow thalamic neurons to be more faithful to their retinal input, reliably transmitting information from retinal afferents to the cortex, for more detailed information processing. Such switching of firing modes has been shown in the cat LGN, in which most bursting occurred during early responses to a visual stimulus, followed by tonic firing (Guido and Weyand 1995). The degree of vigilance also appears to influence the firing mode of thalamo-cortical neurons. LGN neurons tended to burst more when rabbits were in a low vigilance state than in an alert state; and this switch in firing mode occurred within one second of the EEG-defined state transition (Bezdudnaya et al. 2006). The increased bursting may allow the detection of stimuli that are relevant for ongoing behaviour even when in an inattentive state. Importantly, both cortical feedback as well as cholinergic brainstem influences have been shown to depolarize LGN neurons (Scharfman et al. 1990) and thus are able to switch their firing mode from burst to tonic (Lu et al. 1993; McCormick and von Krosigk 1992; Varela and Sherman 2007). However, little is known about the way in which selective attention and other cognitive processes may impact the firing mode of thalamic neurons.

Neural synchrony and oscillations

Thus far, we have considered influences on response magnitude and firing mode as mechanisms to modulate the efficacy of thalamic drive to the cortex. Synchronizing thalamic output represents yet a third relevant mechanism, which may be particularly effective in light of the reported low efficacy of thalamo-cortical synapses (Bruno and Sakmann 2006). Accordingly, simultaneous recordings from the LGN and V1 in anaesthetized cats have found that correlated spiking of LGN neurons increased their efficacy in driving cortical neurons (Alonso et al. 1996). Neurons with greater overlap of their RFs showed greater synchrony. A recent modelling study estimated that as few as five to ten synchronized LGN cells may be sufficient to drive a cortical neuron (Wang et al. 2010). Thus, modulating the synchrony of a group of thalamic neurons may be a potent mechanism to regulate information transmission to cortex.

Synchronizing the activity of two groups of neurons can also increase their information exchange (Gregoriou et al. 2009; Saalmann et al. 2007; Tiesinga and Sejnowski 2009; Womelsdorf et al. 2007). Spikes are more likely to be relayed if those from presynaptic neurons arrive during periods of reduced inhibition of postsynaptic neurons. This spike-timing relationship can be achieved by synchronizing oscillatory activity of pre- and postsynaptic neurons with an appropriate phase lag. Consequently, synchrony between thalamic and cortical neurons, with LGN leading, may increase the efficacy of thalamic input to cortex. Consistent with such a gain control mechanism, it has been found that attentive viewing synchronizes beta frequency oscillations of LFPs in cat LGN and V1 (Bekisz and Wrobel 1993; Wrobel et al. 1994). Such synchrony largely seems to occur between interconnected groups of neurons in each area (Briggs and Usrey 2007; Steriade et al. 1996), offering the possibility of spatially specific control of information transmission.

LGN synchrony and oscillations are controlled by the areas that provide modulatory inputs to the LGN, that is, V1, TRN, and cholinergic brainstem nuclei. Importantly, these sources may differentially influence different oscillation frequencies (the TRN input is discussed in its own section below). For example, evidence suggests that the cholinergic input to the thalamus regulates alpha oscillations in the LGN, as evidenced by activation of muscarinic cholinergic receptors that induce alpha oscillations of LFPs in the LGN (Lorincz et al. 2008). Thalamo-cortical cell firing appears to be correlated with these alpha oscillations, with different groups of LGN neurons firing at distinct phases of the alpha oscillation (Lorincz et al. 2009). Thus, cholinergic inputs to the LGN may influence thalamo-cortical transmission by changing the synchrony of LGN neurons (Hughes and Crunelli 2005; Steriade 2004). Because cholinergic tone increases with vigilance (Datta and Siwek 2002), cholinergic influence on thalamo-cortical transmission may be modulated by behavioural context. Moreover, the thalamus is critically involved in generating cortical alpha rhythms (Hughes and Crunelli 2005), which are linked to spatial attention bias and stimulus visibility (Mathewson et al. 2009; Romei et al. 2010; Thut et al. 2006). In comparison, feedback from V1 may influence alpha oscillations in the LGN to a lesser degree (Lorincz et al. 2009). However, feedback from V1 appears to play an important role at higher frequencies. For instance, inter-areal synchrony in the beta frequency range can help route information during selective attention (Buschman and Miller 2007; Saalmann et al. 2007). Accordingly, feedback from V1 has been reported to modulate beta oscillatory activity in the LGN according to attentional demands (Bekisz and Wrobel 1993).

In summary, there is growing evidence from human fMRI and macaque physiology studies that the response magnitude of LGN neurons is influenced by attentive processing. Thus, the LGN may regulate information transmission from the retina to visual cortex according to behavioural context. Although the spike timing of LGN neurons is important in influencing thalamo-cortical transmission, modulation of spike timing by selective attention in the LGN of awake, behaving primates has been largely unexplored.

PULVINAR: MODULATION OF INFORMATION TRANSMISSION BETWEEN CORTICAL AREAS

Traditionally, the pulvinar has been divided into medial, lateral, inferior, and anterior areas. However, these cytoarchitectonically defined divisions do not correspond well with divisions based on connectivity, neurochemistry, or electrophysiological properties (Adams et al. 2000; Gutierrez et al. 1995; Stepniewska and Kaas 1997). Based on retinotopic organization and cortical connections, at least four visual areas of the pulvinar have been differentiated. There are two areas with clearly organized retinotopic maps in the lateral and inferior parts of the pulvinar, which connect with ventral visual cortex. The other two pulvinar areas do not show clear retinotopy: an inferomedial area that connects with dorsal visual cortex (areas MT, MST, and FST); and a dorsal area that connects with the posterior parietal cortex (PPC) and frontal eye fields (Fig. 14.1b). The RF size of pulvinar neurons appears to roughly correspond to that of cortical neurons to which they connect (Bender 1982; Petersen et al. 1985). The majority of pulvinar neurons respond phasically to the onset of visual stimuli, although a number of pulvinar neurons show more tonic responses (Petersen et al. 1985). Pulvinar neurons have been reported to show broad orientation tuning and weak directional preference for moving stimuli;

and a subset of neurons show colour-sensitivity, including colour-opponent responses (Bender 1982; Felsten et al. 1983; Petersen et al. 1985).

The pulvinar is heavily connected to the cortex and forms cortico-thalamo-cortical pathways. As a general principle, directly connected cortical areas will be indirectly connected via the pulvinar (Fig. 14.1c; Sherman and Guillery 2006; Shipp 2003). Cortical areas project to restricted zones within the pulvinar, and directly connected cortical areas have overlapping projection zones in the pulvinar. Originally investigated using anatomical tracers, the cortical projection zones in the pulvinar can now be visualized *in vivo* using diffusion tensor imaging (DTI). For example, Saalmann and colleagues (2012) performed probabilistic tractography on DTI data to map probable connections between the pulvinar and the directly connected cortical areas V4 and TEO. Figure 14.3a and b show pulvinar zones connected with V4 (yellow) and TEO (red), as well as the region of overlap (green) through which the V4-pulvinar-TEO pathway likely traverses. V4 and TEO predominantly connect with the ventral pulvinar, and there is substantial overlap between V4 and TEO projection zones in the pulvinar, with the TEO projection zone extending more caudally. These probabilistic tractography results are broadly consistent with previous anatomical tracer work (Baleydier and Morel 1992; Shipp 2003). However, the probabilistic tractography data has the advantage of delineating projection zones specific to individual monkeys, which cannot be precisely ascribed based on tracer data from the literature.

The direct cortico-cortical feedforward connections originate in layer 3 and terminate in layer 4 in a higher cortical area (Felleman and Van Essen 1991). In parallel, the putative feedforward pathways through the pulvinar originate in cortical layer 5 and terminate in layer 4 of the higher cortical area as well. There are also direct and indirect

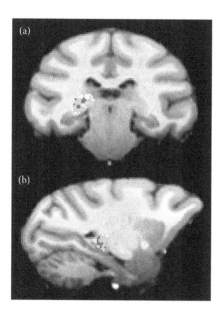

FIGURE 14.3 Pulvino-cortical networks defined using DTI. (a) Coronal and (b) sagittal slices containing pulvinar voxels with high probability of connection with V4 (yellow), TEO (red), or both (green). Broadly consistent with published anatomical tracer results (Baleydier and Morel 1992), the probabilistic tractography on the DTI data had the advantage of showing projection zones in the pulvinar specific to the individual monkeys participating in our study. This allowed us to target electrodes to interconnected pulvino-cortical network sites, improving the precision of the simultaneous multi-site electrophysiological recordings. From *Science*, 337 (6095), Yuri B. Saalmann, Mark A. Pinsk, Liang Wang, Xin Li, and Sabine Kastner, The Pulvinar Regulates Information Transmission Between Cortical Areas Based on Attention Demands, pp. 753–6, figure 1 (c) 2012, AAAS. Reprinted with permission from AAAS.

feedback pathways between cortical areas. The direct cortico-cortical feedback connections commonly project from layer 6 to layer 1 of the lower cortical area. Cortical layer 6 also provides feedback to the pulvinar, which itself projects to cortical layer 1 (Benevento and Rezak 1976; Lund et al. 1975; Shipp 2003). The fact that the direct and indirect pathways terminate in similar cortical layers presents an opportunity for the two pathways to interact. Due to the overall connectivity pattern, the pulvinar is positioned to regulate cortico-cortical transmission according to behavioural context.

Effects of pulvinar lesions

Arguably the most compelling evidence for the pulvinar playing an important role in visual perception and behaviour comes from lesion studies in humans and monkeys. Cortical lesions involving the posterior parietal cortex (PPC) may lead to profound attentional deficits such as visuospatial hemineglect, a syndrome associated with a failure to direct attention to contralesional space (see Vallar and Bolognini, chapter 33, this volume). Neglect is not only associated with cortical lesions, but can also occur after thalamic lesions that include the pulvinar (Karnath et al. 2002; Petersen et al. 1987). More specifically, the PPC is interconnected with the dorsal pulvinar and, accordingly, inactivation of the dorsal pulvinar in monkeys leads to deficits in directing attention to contralateral space (Wilke et al. 2010). Even though thalamic neglect in humans is rare and severe attentional deficits that occur as a consequence of pulvinar lesions typically do not persist, a milder deficit that may be a residual form of thalamic neglect has been observed as a slowing of orienting responses to contralesional space (Danziger et al. 2001; Rafal and Posner 1987).

More generally, patients with pulvinar lesions present with deficits in coding spatial information in the contralesional visual field. They have difficulty localizing stimuli in the affected visual space and these difficulties extend to the binding of visual features based on spatial information (Ward et al. 2002), which is one of the most fundamental operations that the visual system has to perform in order to integrate visual information across various feature dimensions. For example, these patients may have difficulties binding the appropriate colour to each of multiple shapes that are presented simultaneously: a red square and a blue circle may be mistaken to be a blue square or red circle. Such errors in binding information from different feature dimensions that require accurate spatial coding are classically associated with PPC lesions (Friedman-Hill et al. 1995), but appear to be associated with pulvinar lesions as well (Arend et al. 2008; Ward et al. 2002). Interestingly, the spatial coding deficits have been observed in different spatial reference frames (e.g. retinotopic or object-based), thus underlining the close functional relationship between the (dorsal) pulvinar and PPC (Ward and Arend 2007).

In accordance with its role in visual attention, patients with pulvinar lesions also show deficits in filtering distractor information. While these patients have no difficulty discriminating target stimuli when shown alone, discrimination performance is impaired when salient distractors are present that compete with the target for attentional resources, consistent with a difficulty in filtering out the unwanted information present in the visual display (Danziger et al. 2004; Snow et al. 2009). Similar filtering deficits have been observed after PPC lesions in humans (Friedman-Hill et al. 2003) and after extrastriate cortex lesions that include area V4 in humans (Gallant et al. 2000) and monkeys (De Weerd et al. 1999), suggesting that the pulvinar is part of a distributed network of brain areas that subserves visuospatial attention.

Taken together, lesion studies point to the critical involvement of the pulvinar, not only in selective attention, but in a number of fundamental cognitive functions, including orienting responses and the exploration of visual space, and the spatial coding of visual information necessary for feature binding. These studies indicate that the pulvinar is an integral subcortical part of multiple large-scale networks that regulate behaviour.

Behavioural response modulation

The findings from lesion studies are corroborated by physiology studies showing that neural responses in the pulvinar reflect the behavioural relevance of stimuli. It has been demonstrated that spatial attention modulates the response magnitude of neurons in dorsal, lateral, and inferior parts of the pulvinar. Evoked neural responses typically increased by up to 25% or more and, in some cases, spontaneous activity was also affected (Bender and Youakim 2001; Petersen et al. 1985). When attention was maintained in the absence of visual stimuli, many pulvinar neurons showed a small but significant elevation in spiking activity (Fig. 14.4a and b; Saalmann et al. 2012). In addition to response magnitude, the timing and variability of pulvinar responses is likely to influence

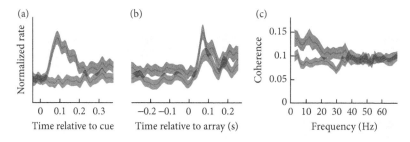

FIGURE 14.4 Spatial attention modulated the spike rate of pulvinar neurons and their synchrony. Population activity (± standard error) aligned to (a) cue and (b) target onset. Mean of 51 pulvinar cells. The monkey's attention was drawn to the location of the spatial cue and maintained there until target presentation. In (b), the preferred stimulus appeared at the RF, flanked by congruent distractors. (c) Population average of the transformed spike-field coherence in the pulvinar, calculated in the 300 ms window prior to target onset. Red, attention at RF; blue, attention away from RF. From Science, 337 (6095), Yuri B. Saalmann, Mark A. Pinsk, Liang Wang, Xin Li, and Sabine Kastner, The Pulvinar Regulates Information Transmission Between Cortical Areas Based on Attention Demands, pp. 753–6, figure 2 (c) 2012, AAAS. Reprinted with permission from AAAS.

information transmission to the cortex. Accordingly, pulvinar neurons show reduced response variability during peripheral attention and saccade tasks (Petersen et al. 1985). During spatial attention, increased synchrony between pulvinar neurons may increase the efficacy of pulvinar influence on the cortex (Fig. 14.4c; Saalmann et al. 2012).

Like other thalamic cells, pulvinar neurons are able to respond in burst or tonic firing modes. Because the activity of the low-threshold calcium channel depends on cell membrane potential, modulatory inputs to the pulvinar may influence the firing mode. Cholinergic inputs will likely depolarize most pulvinar neurons, switching their firing from burst to tonic mode (Varela and Sherman 2007). However, unlike the LGN, muscarinic activation hyperpolarized about one fifth of rat pulvinar neurons, suggesting that cholinergic inputs can induce bursting in these neurons (Varela and Sherman 2007). In addition, inhibitory input to the pulvinar from sources such as the TRN, anterior pretectal nucleus, and the zona incerta (Bokor et al. 2005; Power et al. 1999) may sufficiently hyperpolarize pulvinar neurons, to enable burst firing. Although data on the relationship between pulvinar burst firing mode and behaviour is lacking, it has been shown that pulvinar neurons are more frequently in burst firing mode than LGN neurons (Ramcharan et al. 2005), and thus burst firing may play a larger role in cortico-cortical transmission than retino-cortical transmission.

Regulation of cortico-cortical transmission

The direct cortico-cortical pathways are commonly thought to be the major routes for the transmission of visual information between cortical areas (but see, e.g., Sherman and Guillery 2006). Given that these direct pathways are paralleled by indirect pathways through the pulvinar, it is important to ask what function these cortico-thalamo-cortical pathways may serve. *In vitro* studies have shown that microstimulation of the indirect pathways strongly activated cortical areas (Theyel et al. 2010). Moreover, inactivation of the thalamic projection zone that two interconnected cortical areas share led to a failure of cortico-cortical communication, raising the possibility that all cortico-cortical information transmission may strongly depend on thalamic loops (Theyel et al. 2010).

How does pulvinar output influence cortical activity? Simultaneous recordings from the lateral posterior-pulvinar complex and visual cortex of cats performing a spatial discrimination task have demonstrated inter-areal synchrony of beta-band oscillations when the animal anticipated the visual target (Wrobel et al. 2007). Similarly, simultaneous recordings from the pulvinar and visual cortex of macaques performing a spatial attention task have shown synchrony in a pulvino-cortical network predominantly in the alpha frequency range (Saalmann et al. 2012). In anaesthetized cats, deactivating the pulvinar has been reported to disrupt oscillatory activity in visual cortex (Molotchnikoff and Shumikhina 1996; Shumikhina and Molotchnikoff 1999). Together, these results suggest that the pulvinar may facilitate oscillatory activity in visual cortical areas.

What may be the functional role of such oscillatory activity in cortico-thalamo-cortical communication? Simultaneous recordings from two cortical areas suggest that the selective routing of behaviourally relevant information across the cortex depends on the degree of synchrony between cortical areas (Buschman and Miller 2007; Gregoriou et al. 2009; Saalmann et al. 2007). Saalmann and colleagues tested whether the pulvinar synchronized oscillations between interconnected cortical areas according to attentional demands, thereby modulating the efficacy of cortico-cortical information transfer. To do this, simultaneous recordings were obtained from two interconnected cortical areas along the ventral visual pathway, V4 and TEO, as well as from the corresponding projection zone in the pulvinar of macaques performing a spatial attention task (Saalmann et al. 2012). Recording electrodes targeted pulvinar sites interconnected with the cortical areas, as determined by probabilistic tractography on DTI data (Fig. 14.3a and b). While monkeys maintained spatial attention, cortical areas V4 and TEO synchronized in the alpha frequency range and to a smaller extent in the gamma frequency range. At the same time, the pulvinar causally influenced oscillatory activity in both V4 and TEO predominantly in the alpha frequency range (Fig. 14.5a and b), suggesting that the pulvinar controlled the alpha frequency synchrony between cortical areas. Pulvinar influence on the cortex may also extend to gamma frequencies through a cross-frequency coupling mechanism. Pulvinar-controlled alpha oscillations in the cortex modulated gamma frequency activity in both V4 and TEO, likely contributing to the

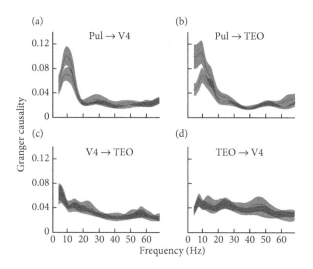

FIGURE 14.5 Strong pulvino-cortical influences and weak cortico-cortical influences during the maintenance of attention in the absence of visual stimuli. Population average of the conditional Granger causality for (a) pulvinar influence on V4, (b) pulvinar influence on TEO, (c) V4 influence on TEO, and (d) TEO influence on V4, calculated in the 200 ms window before target onset. The pulvinar influenced both V4 and TEO oscillatory activity predominantly in the alpha frequency range. Because V4 and TEO activity synchronized in the same frequency range, these results suggest that the pulvinar regulates neural synchrony between cortical areas according to the locus of attention. Red, attend in; Blue, attend out. From Science, 337 (6095), Yuri B. Saalmann, Mark A. Pinsk, Liang Wang, Xin Li, and Sabine Kastner, The Pulvinar Regulates Information Transmission Between Cortical Areas Based on Attention Demands, pp. 753–6, figure 4 (c) 2012, AAAS. Reprinted with permission from AAAS.

synchrony observed between these cortical areas in the gamma frequency range. Thus, the pulvinar may be able to regulate information transfer between cortical areas based on attentional demands. Because direct and indirect feedforward pathways project to cortical layer 4 and direct and indirect feedback pathways project to cortical layer 1 (Fig. 14.1c), the pulvinar is well positioned to regulate both feedforward and feedback cortical pathways.

Together, these results provide evidence for an important role of the pulvinar in regulating cortico-cortical information transmission through the modulation of inter-areal synchrony during cognitive tasks. The prevailing view that information about our visual environment is transmitted through a network of cortical areas for detailed processing needs to be revised by considering extensive pulvino-cortical loops that regulate the information transmitted between each cortical stage of visual processing. Because of common cellular mechanisms and thalamo-cortical connectivity principles across sensorimotor domains, a general function of higher-order thalamic nuclei may be regulation of cortical synchrony to selectively route information across cortex.

Pulvinar control of cortical processing challenges the common conceptualizing of cognitive functions as being restricted to cortex. During maintained spatial attention in the delay period between a cue and subsequent target, pulvino-cortical influences were strong, predominantly in the alpha frequency range (Fig. 14.5a and b), whereas direct cortico-cortical influences were weak (Fig. 14.5c and d). This suggests that internal processes such as maintenance of attention in expectation of visual stimuli and short-term memory rely heavily on pulvino-cortical interactions. Pulvinar regulation of alpha activity is consistent with the important role ascribed to alpha oscillations in these internal processes (Palva and Palva 2011; von Stein et al 2000).

In summary, lesion studies have shown that the pulvinar is critically involved in visual perception, attention, and visually guided behaviour. Electrophysiology evidence suggests that the neural mechanisms supporting these visual functions involve the pulvinar synchronizing distributed groups of cortical neurons, to selectively transmit behaviourally relevant information across the cortex. How the different subdivisions of the pulvinar contribute to cognitive processing remains to be clarified.

TRN: Modulator and Pacemaker of Thalamo-cortical Signals?

The TRN is subdivided into sectors, each associated with a different thalamo-cortical pathway. The visual sector of the TRN receives cortical input from layer 6 as well as thalamic input from the LGN and pulvinar in the form of collaterals from descending or ascending fibers. However, the TRN only projects to the thalamus, providing inhibitory input to the LGN and pulvinar. The TRN contains topographically organized representations of the visual field, with the RF size of many TRN neurons comparable to that of LGN neurons (McAlonan et al. 2006). The TRN input to the LGN is retinotopically organized (Crabtree and Killackey 1989; Montero et al. 1977), suggesting that the TRN can influence thalamic processing at specific locations in the visual field. However, the TRN is unlikely to selectively modulate magno-, parvo-, or koniocellular pathways, because an individual TRN axon projects to multiple LGN layers (Uhlrich et al. 2003). In contrast with the high spatial specificity of the TRN's input to the LGN, the TRN input to the pulvinar appears to be only roughly topographically organized (Fitzgibbon et al. 1995). Tracer studies have shown that there are reciprocal connections between the TRN and the LGN or pulvinar, forming closed loops. Nonetheless, incomplete overlap in thalamic labelling after the injection of retrograde and anterograde tracers into the TRN suggests that a number of TRN neurons synapse on thalamo-cortical neurons which do not project back to the same TRN neurons, consequently forming open loops (Fitzgibbon et al. 1995; Pinault and Deschenes 1998). Such open and closed loops offer lateral and feedback inhibition, respectively. In addition to these loops formed between the TRN and an individual thalamic nucleus, there are pathways between different thalamic nuclei via the TRN. These disynaptic, intrathalamic pathways can connect first-order and higher-order thalamic nuclei within the same modality, or connect two nuclei of different modalities. These pathways inhibit the target nucleus, thereby providing a means to facilitate information transmission through one thalamic nucleus, while suppressing another one (Crabtree et al. 1998; Crabtree and Isaac 2002).

TRN neurons respond transiently and with short latency to visual stimuli (McAlonan et al. 2006), suggesting that the TRN can influence early evoked responses of LGN and pulvinar neurons. TRN neurons also have high spontaneous activity (McAlonan et al. 2006), consistent with a tonic inhibition of thalamic nuclei. There is growing evidence for modulation of TRN responses depending on stimulus context. For example, in anaesthetized rats, TRN neurons have been reported to habituate to repetitive stimuli (Yu et al. 2009a) and to increase their response to deviant stimuli in an oddball paradigm (Yu et al. 2009b). The TRN receives input from the prefrontal cortex, visual cortex, superior colliculus, and cholinergic brainstem nuclei (Kolmac and Mitrofanis 1998; Montero 2000; Zikopoulos and Barbas 2006), which may enable the TRN to integrate information from various processing levels and to modulate its output according to behavioural needs.

Attentional modulation

The TRN has been implicated in playing an important role in selective attention by regulating thalamo-cortical information transmission (e.g. Crick 1984; Guillery et al. 1998; Yingling and Skinner 1976). The effects of TRN lesions are consistent with such a role. For example, like in humans, the reaction times of rats to visual targets that are cued are faster than those to targets that are not. However, a unilateral TRN lesion has been shown to abolish this behavioural advantage for the cued stimulus, suggesting that the TRN normally contributes to directing attention to a cued location (Weese et al. 1999).

Rat TRN lesions have also been reported to impair orienting responses and, more generally, to reduce exploratory behaviour (Friedberg and Ross 1993).

There is converging evidence from metabolic mapping and electrophysiology studies that selective attention modulates the activity of TRN neurons. Increased activity, as gauged by the number of Fos-labelled cells, has been observed in the visual sector of the rat TRN for attended visual stimuli relative to unattended stimuli (McAlonan et al. 2000). Moreover, increased deoxyglucose uptake has been demonstrated in the TRN of macaques performing a feature-based attention task (Vanduffel et al. 2000). Single-neuron recordings in macaques using cues to guide their attention directly show specific modulatory effects of attention on TRN neuronal responses. When visual and auditory stimuli were simultaneously presented, the spike rate of neurons in the visual sector of the TRN increased when monkeys directed attention to the visual stimulus relative to when they attended to the auditory stimulus (McAlonan et al. 2006). When a monkey attended to one of two visual stimuli presented simultaneously, the spike rate of TRN neurons decreased relative to that evoked by the same stimulus when unattended (Fig. 14.3c; McAlonan et al. 2008). Although magnocellular LGN neurons tended to have a slightly shorter response latency to the visual stimuli, the attentional modulation started in the TRN before LGN, suggesting that the TRN contributed to the attention effects on the LGN. Interestingly, the attentional modulation of TRN responses in the intra-modal attention task differed in sign relative to that found in the cross-modal attention task. The implications of these modulatory effects on thalamo-cortical neurons will be further discussed below.

Response modes and oscillatory activity

Like LGN and pulvinar neurons, TRN neurons fire in burst or tonic modes depending on the level of vigilance. Importantly, the firing mode can significantly influence the TRN response to sensory stimulation. TRN neurons reach their peak response rate more rapidly for sensory stimulation during tonic mode relative to burst mode. Considering the corresponding time courses of inhibition exerted on thalamo-cortical neurons, tonic mode may thereby facilitate rapid changes in thalamo-cortical signalling, while burst mode may permit an initially strong evoked response from thalamo-cortical neurons (Hartings et al. 2003).

TRN neurons are critically involved in initiating and sustaining thalamo-cortical oscillations. For example, a deafferented TRN is able to self-generate oscillations in the 7–15 Hz range (spindles; Steriade et al. 1987). Moreover, interactions between TRN and thalamo-cortical neurons sustain oscillations, that is, TRN neurons inhibit thalamo-cortical neurons, which rebound fire to excite TRN neurons, thereby initiating another oscillatory cycle (Steriade et al. 1993). In addition to its prominent role in spindle generation, the TRN has been shown to oscillate at lower (Amzica et al. 1992) and higher frequencies, including the beta/gamma frequency range (Pinault and Deschenes 1992). These different oscillation frequencies manifest during different behavioural contexts. Spindles and lower frequencies commonly occur during states of low vigilance, while beta/gamma frequencies are more associated with increased vigilance (Steriade et al. 1993). It appears that spindle oscillations may contribute to reduced efficacy of information transfer across retino-thalamic synapses, by decorrelating retinal input from thalamic output (Le Masson et al. 2002). A more specific role of response modes and oscillatory TRN activity in selective attention remains to be defined.

Influences on thalamo-cortical transmission

TRN neurons may influence thalamo-cortical neurons of the LGN and pulvinar in a number of ways. First, TRN neurons reduce the spike rate of thalamo-cortical neurons through direct inhibition. For example, the responses of TRN neurons evoked by stimuli at unattended locations were shown to increase, while the responses of LGN neurons decreased (McAlonan et al. 2008), thus suppressing thalamo-cortical transmission of information at unattended locations. In the case of an attended visual stimulus, the converse response pattern was found. That is, responses of LGN neurons increased, while the responses of TRN neurons decreased, thus facilitating the transmission of information at attended locations. Such an inverse correlation has also been reported in anaesthetized cats between simultaneously recorded neurons in the LGN and the perigeniculate nucleus, the equivalent of the TRN's visual sector in the cat (Funke and Eysel 1998).

Second, it is possible that TRN neurons increase the responses of thalamo-cortical neurons through disinhibition. Disinhibition of thalamo-cortical neurons has been shown to arise from TRN neurons inhibiting other TRN cells via dendrodendritic synapses (Pinault et al. 1997) or from TRN neurons synapsing on local inhibitory thalamic neurons, which constitutes about 10% of the synapses formed by TRN neurons projecting to the dorsal thalamus of the cat (Liu et al. 1995; Steriade et al. 1986). Such disinhibitory mechanisms may facilitate the thalamo-cortical transmission of relevant information (Steriade 1999).

Third, TRN neurons may contribute to switching the firing mode of thalamo-cortical neurons. Direct TRN input hyperpolarizes thalamo-cortical cells, which typically invokes burst firing (Huguenard 1996). Consequently, modulation of TRN activity may change the firing mode of thalamo-cortical neurons and the way information is transmitted to cortex (Yu et al. 2009b).

Finally, the TRN may impact the synchrony and oscillatory patterns of thalamic neurons. TRN inhibitory input to LGN and pulvinar neurons may constrain their spike times to time windows following periods of inhibition, thereby helping to synchronize thalamic output (Steriade et al. 1996). Furthermore, it has been argued that the TRN might function as a pacemaker of thalamo-cortical oscillations (Fuentealba and Steriade 2005). For thalamo-cortical synchrony at spindle frequencies, cortical feedback appears to drive TRN-mediated inhibition and rebound firing of thalamic neurons. Thus, these neurons are recruited into thalamo-cortical spindle oscillations during states of low vigilance (Destexhe et al. 1998). In contrast, thalamo-cortical synchrony at higher frequencies, in the beta/gamma band, may rely more on direct cortical feedback providing excitatory input to thalamo-cortical neurons. In this case, the role of the TRN neurons may be to influence thalamo-cortical beta/gamma oscillations by resetting their phase (Pedroarena and Llinas 1997). Such a phase reset may help to synchronize localized beta/gamma oscillations between the thalamus and cortex, thereby increasing information exchange during states of increased vigilance. This is consistent with the localized enhancement of gamma oscillations in sensory cortex that has been reported after electrical stimulation of the TRN (Macdonald et al. 1998). Such an account is also supported by a recent computational model showing that the TRN, via other thalamic nuclei, is well positioned to help synchronize areas of the cortex (Drover et al. 2010). However, a functional role of such TRN influences on thalamo-cortical synchrony and oscillations in perception and cognition remains to be determined.

In summary, the TRN forms cortico-reticular-thalamic loops that allow the TRN to influence both the LGN and pulvinar, and this may include playing the role of a pacemaker coordinating the visual thalamus. Although the empirical evidence is sparse, the TRN has a rich mechanistic infrastructure to flexibly control both thalamo-cortical and cortico-thalamic signal transmission according to behavioural context.

CONCLUSION

The overall evidence that has emerged during recent years suggests that the visual thalamus serves a fundamental function in regulating information transmission to the cortex and between cortical areas according to behavioural context. Selective attention has been shown to modulate LGN activity, thus indicating that the LGN filters visual information before it reaches the cortex. Behavioural context appears to even more strongly modulate pulvinar activity and, due to its connectivity, the pulvinar is well positioned to influence feedforward and feedback information transmission between cortical areas. Because the TRN provides strong inhibitory input to both the LGN and pulvinar, the TRN may control and coordinate the information transmitted along both retino-cortical and cortico-cortical pathways.

Although the experimental evidence in support of some of these notions is still sparse and there are many unanswered questions about the role of the thalamus in cognitive processing, converging evidence from neuroimaging, physiological, anatomical, and computational studies suggests that the classical view of cognitive functions exclusively depending on the cortex needs to be thoroughly revised. Only with detailed knowledge of thalamic processing and thalamo-cortical interactions will it be possible to fully understand cognition.

ACKNOWLEDGEMENTS

This chapter builds upon and extends a recent review of the authors (Saalmann and Kastner 2011). We thank the National Institutes of Health and National Science Foundation for grant support of our research.

References

Adams, M. M., Hof, P. R., Gattass, R., Webster, M. J., and Ungerleider, L. G. (2000). Visual corti-cal projections and chemoarchitecture of macaque monkey pulvinar. *Journal of Comparative Neurology* 419: 377–393.

Alitto, H. J., Weyand, T. G., and Usrey, W. M. (2005). Distinct properties of stimulus-evoked bursts in the lateral geniculate nucleus. *Journal of Neuroscience* 25: 514–523.

Alonso, J. M., Usrey, W. M., and Reid, R. C. (1996). Precisely correlated firing in cells of the lat-eral geniculate nucleus. *Nature* 383: 815–819.

Amzica, F., Nuñez, A., and Steriade, M. (1992). Delta frequency (1–4 Hz) oscillations of peri-geniculate thalamic neurons and their modulation by light. *Neuroscience* 51: 285–294.

Arend, I., Rafal, R., and Ward, R. (2008). Spatial and temporal deficits are regionally dissociable in patients with pulvinar lesions. *Brain* 131: 2140–2152.

Baleydier, C. and Morel, A. (1992). Segregated thalamocortical pathways to inferior parietal and inferotemporal cortex in macaque monkey. *Visual Neuroscience* 8: 391–405.

Beck, D. M. and Kastner, S. (forthcoming). Neural systems for spatial attention in the human brain: Evidence from neuroimaging in the framework of biased competition. In S. Kastner and K. Nobre (eds.), *The Oxford Handbook of Attention*. Oxford: Oxford University Press.

Bekisz, M. and Wrobel, A. (1993). 20 Hz rhythm of activity in visual system of perceiving cat. *Acta Neurobiologiae Experimentalis (Wars)* 53: 175–182.

Bender, D. B. (1982). Receptive-field properties of neurons in the macaque inferior pulvinar. *Journal of Neurophysiology* 48: 1–17.

Bender, D. B. and Youakim, M. (2001). Effect of attentive fixation in macaque thalamus and cortex. *Journal of Neurophysiology* 85: 219–234.

Benevento, L. A. and Rezak, M. (1976). The cortical projections of the inferior pulvinar and adjacent lateral pulvinar in the rhesus monkey (Macaca mulatta): An autoradiographic study. *Brain Research* 108: 1–24.

Bezdudnaya, T., Cano, M., Bereshpolova, Y., Stoelzel, C. R., Alonso, J. M., and Swadlow, H. A. (2006). Thalamic burst mode and inattention in the awake LGNd. *Neuron* 49: 421–432.

Bickford, M. E., Ramcharan, E., Godwin, D. W., Erisir, A., Gnadt, J., and Sherman, S. M. (2000). Neurotransmitters contained in the subcortical extraretinal inputs to the monkey lateral geniculate nucleus. *Journal of Comparative Neurology* 424: 701–717.

Bokor, H., Frere, S. G., Eyre, M. D., Slezia, A., Ulbert, I., Luthi, A., and Acsady, L. (2005). Selective GABAergic control of higher-order thalamic relays. *Neuron* 45: 929–940.

Briggs, F. and Usrey, W. M. (2007). Cortical activity influences geniculocortical spike efficacy in the macaque monkey. *Frontiers in Integrative Neuroscience* 1: 3.

Briggs, F. and Usrey, W. M. (2009). Parallel processing in the corticogeniculate pathway of the macaque monkey. *Neuron* 62: 135–146.

Bruno, R. M. and Sakmann, B. (2006). Cortex is driven by weak but synchronously active thalamocortical synapses. *Science* 312: 1622–1627.

Buschman, T. J. and Miller, E. K. (2007). Top-down versus bottom-up control of attention in the prefrontal and posterior parietal cortices. *Science* 315: 1860–1862.

Callaway, E. M. (2005). Structure and function of parallel pathways in the primate early visual system. *Journal of Physiology* 566: 13–19.

Connolly, M. and Van Essen, D. (1984). The representation of the visual field in parvicellular and magnocellular layers of the lateral geniculate nucleus in the macaque monkey. *Journal of Comparative Neurology* 226: 544–564.

Crabtree, J. W. and Killackey, H. P. (1989). The topographic organization and axis of projection within the visual sector of the rabbit's thalamic reticular nucleus. *European Journal of Neuroscience* 1: 94–109.

Crabtree, J. W., Collingridge, G. L., and Isaac, J. T. (1998). A new intrathalamic pathway linking modality-related nuclei in the dorsal thalamus. *Nature Neuroscience* 1: 389–394.

Crabtree, J. W. and Isaac, J. T. (2002). New intrathalamic pathways allowing modality-related and cross-modality switching in the dorsal thalamus. *Journal of Neuroscience* 22: 8754–8761.

Creutzfeldt, O. D., Lee, B. B., and Elepfandt, A. (1979). A quantitative study of chromatic organisation and receptive fields of cells in the lateral geniculate body of the rhesus monkey. *Experimental Brain Research* 35: 527–545.

Crick, F. (1984). Function of the thalamic reticular complex: The searchlight hypothesis. *Proceedings of the National Academy of Sciences USA* 81: 4586–4590.

Danziger, S., Ward, R., Owen, V., and Rafal, R. (2001). The effects of unilateral pulvinar damage in humans on reflexive orienting and filtering of irrelevant information. *Behavioural Neurology* 13: 95–104.

Danziger, S., Ward, R., Owen, V., and Rafal, R. (2004). Contributions of the human pulvinar to linking vision and action. *Cognitive, Affective, & Behavioral Neuroscience* 4: 89–99.

Datta, S. and Siwek, D. F. (2002). Single cell activity patterns of pedunculopontine tegmentum neurons across the sleep-wake cycle in the freely moving rats. *Journal of Neuroscience Research* 70: 611–621.

De Weerd, P., Peralta, M. R., III, Desimone, R., and Ungerleider, L. G. (1999). Loss of attentional stimulus selection after extrastriate cortical lesions in macaques. *Nature Neuroscience* 2: 753–758.

Denning, K. S. and Reinagel, P. (2005). Visual control of burst priming in the anesthetized lateral geniculate nucleus. *Journal of Neuroscience* 25: 3531–3538.

Derrington, A. M. and Lennie, P. (1984). Spatial and temporal contrast sensitivities of neurones in lateral geniculate nucleus of macaque. *Journal of Physiology* 357: 219–240.

Destexhe, A., Contreras, D., and Steriade, M. (1998). Mechanisms underlying the synchronizing action of corticothalamic feedback through inhibition of thalamic relay cells. *Journal of Neurophysiology* 79: 999–1016.

Dreher, B., Fukada, Y., and Rodieck, R. W. (1976). Identification, classification and anatomical segregation of cells with X-like and Y-like properties in the lateral geniculate nucleus of old-world primates. *Journal of Physiology* 258: 433–452.

Drover, J. D., Schiff, N. D., and Victor, J. D. (2010). Dynamics of coupled thalamocortical modules. *Journal of Computational Neuroscience* 28: 605–616.

Erisir, A., Van Horn, S. C., Bickford, M. E., and Sherman, S. M. (1997). Immunocytochemistry and distribution of parabrachial terminals in the lateral geniculate nucleus of the cat: A comparison with corticogeniculate terminals. *Journal of Comparative Neurology* 377: 535–549.

Fanselow, E. E., Sameshima, K., Baccala, L. A., and Nicolelis, M. A. (2001). Thalamic bursting in rats during different awake behavioral states. *Proceedings of the National Academy of Sciences USA* 98: 15330–15335.

Felleman, D. J. and Van Essen, D. C. (1991). Distributed hierarchical processing in the primate cerebral cortex. *Cerebral Cortex* 1: 1–47.

Felsten, G., Benevento, L. A., and Burman, D. (1983). Opponent-color responses in macaque extrageniculate visual pathways: The lateral pulvinar. *Brain Research* 288: 363–367.

Fitzgibbon, T., Tevah, L. V., and Sefton, A. J. (1995). Connections between the reticular nucleus of the thalamus and pulvinar-lateralis posterior complex: A WGA-HRP study. *Journal of Comparative Neurology* 363: 489–504.

Friedberg, E. B. and Ross, D. T. (1993). Degeneration of rat thalamic reticular neurons following intrathalamic domoic acid injection. *Neuroscience Letters 151*: 115–119.

Friedman-Hill, S. R., Robertson, L. C., and Treisman, A. (1995). Parietal contributions to visual feature binding: Evidence from a patient with bilateral lesions. *Science 269*: 853–855.

Friedman-Hill, S. R., Robertson, L. C., Desimone, R., and Ungerleider, L. G. (2003). Posterior parietal cortex and the filtering of distractors. *Proceedings of the National Academy of Sciences USA 100*: 4263–4268.

Fuentealba, P. and Steriade, M. (2005). The reticular nucleus revisited: Intrinsic and network properties of a thalamic pacemaker. *Progress in Neurobiology 75*: 125–141.

Funke, K. and Eysel, U. T. (1998). Inverse correlation of firing patterns of single topographically matched perigeniculate neurons and cat dorsal lateral geniculate relay cells. *Visual Neuroscience 15*: 711–729.

Gallant, J. L., Shoup, R. E., and Mazer, J. A. (2000). A human extrastriate area functionally homologous to macaque V4. *Neuron 27*: 227–235.

Gregoriou, G. G., Gotts, S. J., Zhou, H., and Desimone, R. (2009). High-frequency, long-range coupling between prefrontal and visual cortex during attention. *Science 324*: 1207–1210.

Guido, W. and Weyand, T. (1995). Burst responses in thalamic relay cells of the awake behaving cat. *Journal of Neurophysiology 74*: 1782–1786.

Guillery, R. W., Feig, S. L., and Lozsadi, D. A. (1998). Paying attention to the thalamic reticular nucleus. *Trends in Neurosciences 21*: 28–32.

Gutierrez, C., Yaun, A., and Cusick, C. G. (1995). Neurochemical subdivisions of the inferior pulvinar in macaque monkeys. *Journal of Comparative Neurology 363*: 545–562.

Hartings, J. A., Temereanca, S., and Simons, D. J. (2003). State-dependent processing of sensory stimuli by thalamic reticular neurons. *Journal of Neuroscience 23*: 5264–5271.

Hendry, S. H. and Reid, R. C. (2000). The koniocellular pathway in primate vision. *Annual Review of Neuroscience 23*: 127–153.

Hughes, S. W. and Crunelli, V. (2005). Thalamic mechanisms of EEG alpha rhythms and their pathological implications. *Neuroscientist 11*: 357–372.

Huguenard, J. R. (1996). Low-threshold calcium currents in central nervous system neurons. *Annual Review of Physiology 58*: 329–348.

Jones, E. G. (2007). *The Thalamus*, 2nd edn. New York: Cambridge University Press.

Kaas, J. H., Guillery, R. W., and Allman, J. M. (1972). Some principles of organization in the dorsal lateral geniculate nucleus. *Brain, Behavior and Evolution 6*: 253–299.

Karnath, H. O., Himmelbach, M., and Rorden, C. (2002). The subcortical anatomy of human spatial neglect: Putamen, caudate nucleus and pulvinar. *Brain 125*: 350–360.

Kolmac, C. I. and Mitrofanis, J. (1998). Patterns of brainstem projection to the thalamic reticular nucleus. *Journal of Comparative Neurology 396*: 531–543.

Le Masson, G., Renaud-Le Masson, S., Debay, D., and Bal, T. (2002). Feedback inhibition controls spike transfer in hybrid thalamic circuits. *Nature 417*: 854–858.

Lesica, N. A. and Stanley, G. B. (2004). Encoding of natural scene movies by tonic and burst spikes in the lateral geniculate nucleus. *Journal of Neuroscience 24*: 10731–10740.

Liu, X. B., Warren, R. A., and Jones, E. G. (1995). Synaptic distribution of afferents from reticular nucleus in ventroposterior nucleus of cat thalamus. *Journal of Comparative Neurology 352*: 187–202.

Lorincz, M. L., Crunelli, V., and Hughes, S. W. (2008). Cellular dynamics of cholinergically induced alpha (8–13 Hz) rhythms in sensory thalamic nuclei in vitro. *Journal of Neuroscience 28*: 660–671.

Lorincz, M. L., Kekesi, K. A., Juhasz, G., Crunelli, V., and Hughes, S. W. (2009). Temporal framing of thalamic relay-mode firing by phasic inhibition during the alpha rhythm. *Neuron 63*:
683–696.

Lu, S. M., Guido, W., and Sherman, S. M. (1993). The brain-stem parabrachial region controls
mode of response to visual stimulation of neurons in the cat's lateral geniculate nucleus.
Visual Neuroscience 10: 631–642.

Lund, J. S., Lund, R. D., Hendrickson, A. E., Bunt, A. H., and Fuchs, A. F. (1975). The origin of
efferent pathways from the primary visual cortex, area 17, of the macaque monkey as shown
by retrograde transport of horseradish peroxidase. *Journal of Comparative Neurology 164*:
287–303.

Macdonald, K. D., Fifkova, E., Jones, M. S., and Barth, D. S. (1998). Focal stimulation of the
thalamic reticular nucleus induces focal gamma waves in cortex. *Journal of Neurophysiology*
79: 474–477.

Malpeli, J. G. and Baker, F. H. (1975). The representation of the visual field in the lateral geniculate nucleus of Macaca mulatta. *Journal of Comparative Neurology 161*: 569–594.

Martin, P. R., White, A. J., Goodchild, A. K., Wilder, H. D., and Sefton, A. E. (1997). Evidence
that blue-on cells are part of the third geniculocortical pathway in primates. *European Journal*
of Neuroscience 9: 1536–1541.

Mathewson, K. E., Gratton, G., Fabiani, M., Beck, D. M., and Ro, T. (2009). To see or not to
see: Prestimulus alpha phase predicts visual awareness. *Journal of Neuroscience 29*: 2725–2732.

McAlonan, K., Brown, V. J., and Bowman, E. M. (2000). Thalamic reticular nucleus activation reflects attentional gating during classical conditioning. *Journal of Neuroscience 20*:
8897–8901.

McAlonan, K., Cavanaugh, J., and Wurtz, R. H. (2006). Attentional modulation of thalamic
reticular neurons. *Journal of Neuroscience 26*: 4444–4450.

McAlonan, K., Cavanaugh, J., and Wurtz, R. H. (2008). Guarding the gateway to cortex with
attention in visual thalamus. *Nature 456*: 391–394.

McCormick, D. A. and von Krosigk, M. (1992). Corticothalamic activation modulates thalamic
firing through glutamate 'metabotropic' receptors. *Proceedings of the National Academy of*
Sciences USA 89: 2774–2778.

Merigan, W. H. and Maunsell, J. H. (1993). How parallel are the primate visual pathways? *Annual*
Review of Neuroscience 16: 369–402.

Molotchnikoff, S. and Shumikhina, S. (1996). The lateral posterior-pulvinar complex modulation of stimulus-dependent oscillations in the cat visual cortex. *Vision Research 36*: 2037–2046.

Montero, V. M., Guillery, R. W., and Woolsey, C. N. (1977). Retinotopic organization within
the thalamic reticular nucleus demonstrated by a double label autoradiographic technique.
Brain Research 138: 407–421.

Montero, V. M. (2000). Attentional activation of the visual thalamic reticular nucleus depends
on 'top-down' inputs from the primary visual cortex via corticogeniculate pathways. *Brain*
Research 864: 95–104.

O'Connor, D. H., Fukui, M. M., Pinsk, M. A., and Kastner, S. (2002). Attention modulates
responses in the human lateral geniculate nucleus. *Nature Neuroscience 5*: 1203–1209.

Palva, S. and Palva, J. M. (2011). Functional roles of alpha-band phase synchronization in local
and large-scale cortical networks. *Frontiers in Psychology 2*: 204.

Pedroarena, C. and Llinas, R. (1997). Dendritic calcium conductances generate high-frequency
oscillation in thalamocortical neurons. *Proceedings of the National Academy of Sciences USA*
94: 724–728.

Petersen, S. E., Robinson, D. L., and Keys, W. (1985). Pulvinar nuclei of the behaving rhesus monkey: Visual responses and their modulation. *Journal of Neurophysiology 54*: 867–886.

Petersen, S. E., Robinson, D. L., and Morris, J. D. (1987). Contributions of the pulvinar to visual spatial attention. *Neuropsychologia 25*: 97–105.

Pinault, D. and Deschenes, M. (1992). Voltage-dependent 40-Hz oscillations in rat reticular thalamic neurons in vivo. *Neuroscience 51*: 245–258.

Pinault, D., Smith, Y., and Deschenes, M. (1997). Dendrodendritic and axoaxonic synapses in the thalamic reticular nucleus of the adult rat. *Journal of Neuroscience 17*: 3215–3233.

Pinault, D. and Deschenes, M. (1998). Anatomical evidence for a mechanism of lateral inhibition in the rat thalamus. *European Journal of Neuroscience 10*: 3462–3469.

Power, B. D., Kolmac, C. I., and Mitrofanis, J. (1999). Evidence for a large projection from the zona incerta to the dorsal thalamus. *Journal of Comparative Neurology 404*: 554–565.

Rafal, R. D. and Posner, M. I. (1987). Deficits in human visual spatial attention following thalamic lesions. *Proceedings of the National Academy of Sciences USA 84*: 7349–7353.

Ramcharan, E. J., Gnadt, J. W., and Sherman, S. M. (2005). Higher-order thalamic relays burst more than first-order relays. *Proceedings of the National Academy of Sciences USA 102*: 12236–12241.

Romei, V., Gross, J., and Thut, G. (2010). On the role of prestimulus alpha rhythms over occipito-parietal areas in visual input regulation: Correlation or causation? *Journal of Neuroscience 30*: 8692–8697.

Roy, S., Jayakumar, J., Martin, P. R., Dreher, B., Saalmann, Y. B., Hu, D., and Vidyasagar, T. R. (2009). Segregation of short-wavelength-sensitive (S) cone signals in the macaque dorsal lateral geniculate nucleus. *European Journal of Neuroscience 30*: 1517–1526.

Saalmann, Y. B., Pigarev, I. N., and Vidyasagar, T. R. (2007). Neural mechanisms of visual attention: How top-down feedback highlights relevant locations. *Science 316*: 1612–1615.

Saalmann, Y. B. and Kastner, S. (2009). Gain control in the visual thalamus during perception and cognition. *Current Opinions in Neurobiology 19*: 408–414.

Saalmann, Y. B. and Kastner, S. (2011) Cognitive and perceptual functions of the visual thalamus. *Neuron 71*: 209–223.

Saalmann, Y. B., Pinsk, M. A., Wang, L., Li, X., and Kastner, S. (2012). The pulvinar regulates information transmission between cortical areas based on attention demands. *Science 337*: 753–6.

Scharfman, H. E., Lu, S. M., Guido, W., Adams, P. R., and Sherman, S. M. (1990). N-methyl-D-aspartate receptors contribute to excitatory postsynaptic potentials of cat lateral geniculate neurons recorded in thalamic slices. *Proceedings of the National Academy of Sciences USA 87*: 4548–4552.

Shapley, R., Kaplan, E., and Soodak, R. (1981). Spatial summation and contrast sensitivity of X and Y cells in the lateral geniculate nucleus of the macaque. *Nature 292*: 543–545.

Sherman, S. M. and Koch, C. (1986). The control of retinogeniculate transmission in the mammalian lateral geniculate nucleus. *Experimental Brain Research 63*: 1–20.

Sherman, S. M. and Guillery, R. W. (2006). *Exploring the Thalamus and its Role in Cortical Function*, 2nd edn. Cambridge, Mass.: MIT Press.

Shipp, S. (2003). The functional logic of cortico-pulvinar connections. *Philosophical Transactions of the Royal Society of London B: Biological Sciences 358*: 1605–1624.

Shumikhina, S. and Molotchnikoff, S. (1999). Pulvinar participates in synchronizing neural assemblies in the visual cortex, in cats. *Neuroscience Letters 272*: 135–139.

Singer, W. (1977). Control of thalamic transmission by corticofugal and ascending reticular pathways in the visual system. *Physiological Reviews* 57: 386–420.

Snow, J. C., Allen, H. A., Rafal, R. D., and Humphreys, G. W. (2009). Impaired attentional selection following lesions to human pulvinar: Evidence for homology between human and monkey. *Proceedings of the National Academy of Sciences USA* 106: 4054–4059.

Stepniewska, I. and Kaas, J. H. (1997). Architectonic subdivisions of the inferior pulvinar in New World and Old World monkeys. *Visual Neuroscience* 14: 1043–1060.

Steriade, M., Domich, L., and Oakson, G. (1986). Reticularis thalami neurons revisited: Activity changes during shifts in states of vigilance. *Journal of Neuroscience* 6: 68–81.

Steriade, M., Domich, L., Oakson, G., and Deschenes, M. (1987). The deafferented reticular thalamic nucleus generates spindle rhythmicity. *Journal of Neurophysiology* 57: 260–273.

Steriade, M., McCormick, D. A., and Sejnowski, T. J. (1993). Thalamocortical oscillations in the sleeping and aroused brain. *Science* 262: 679–685.

Steriade, M., Contreras, D., Amzica, F., and Timofeev, I. (1996). Synchronization of fast (30–40 Hz) spontaneous oscillations in intrathalamic and thalamocortical networks. *Journal of Neuroscience* 16: 2788–2808.

Steriade, M. (1999). Coherent oscillations and short-term plasticity in corticothalamic networks. *Trends in Neuroscience* 22: 337–345.

Steriade, M. (2004). Acetylcholine systems and rhythmic activities during the waking–sleep cycle. *Progress in Brain Research* 145: 179–196.

Swadlow, H. A. and Gusev, A. G. (2001). The impact of 'bursting' thalamic impulses at a neocortical synapse. *Nature Neuroscience* 4: 402–408.

Theyel, B. B., Llano, D. A., and Sherman, S. M. (2010). The corticothalamocortical circuit drives higher-order cortex in the mouse. *Nature Neuroscience* 13: 84–88.

Thut, G., Nietzel, A., Brandt, S. A., and Pascual-Leone, A. (2006). Alpha-band electroencephalographic activity over occipital cortex indexes visuospatial attention bias and predicts visual target detection. *Journal of Neuroscience* 26: 9494–9502.

Tiesinga, P. and Sejnowski, T. J. (2009). Cortical enlightenment: Are attentional gamma oscillations driven by ING or PING? *Neuron* 63: 727–732.

Uhlrich, D. J., Manning, K. A., and Feig, S. L. (2003). Laminar and cellular targets of individual thalamic reticular nucleus axons in the lateral geniculate nucleus in the prosimian primate Galago. *Journal of Comparative Neurology* 458: 128–143.

Vanduffel, W., Tootell, R. B., and Orban, G. A. (2000). Attention-dependent suppression of metabolic activity in the early stages of the macaque visual system. *Cerebral Cortex* 10: 109–126.

Varela, C. and Sherman, S. M. (2007). Differences in response to muscarinic activation between first- and higher-order thalamic relays. *Journal of Neurophysiology* 98: 3538–3547.

von Stein, A., Chiang, C., and Konig, P. (2000). Top-down processing mediated by interareal synchronization. *Proceedings of the National Academy of Sciences USA* 97: 14748–14753.

Wang, H. P., Spencer, D., Fellous, J. M., and Sejnowski, T. J. (2010). Synchrony of thalamocortical inputs maximizes cortical reliability. *Science* 328: 106–109.

Ward, R., Danziger, S., Owen, V., and Rafal, R. (2002). Deficits in spatial coding and feature binding following damage to spatiotopic maps in the human pulvinar. *Nature Neuroscience* 5: 99–100.

Ward, R. and Arend, I. (2007). An object-based frame of reference within the human pulvinar. *Brain* 130: 2462–2469.

Weese, G. D., Phillips, J. M., and Brown, V. J. (1999). Attentional orienting is impaired by unilateral lesions of the thalamic reticular nucleus in the rat. *Journal of Neuroscience* 19: 10135–10139.

Wiesel, T. N. and Hubel, D. H. (1966). Spatial and chromatic interactions in the lateral geniculate body of the rhesus monkey. *Journal of Neurophysiology 29*: 1115–1156.

Wilke, M., Turchi, J., Smith, K., Mishkin, M., and Leopold, D. A. (2010). Pulvinar inactivation
disrupts selection of movement plans. *Journal of Neuroscience 30*: 8650–8659.

Womelsdorf, T., Schoffelen, J. M., Oostenveld, R., Singer, W., Desimone, R., Engel, A. K., and
Fries, P. (2007). Modulation of neuronal interactions through neuronal synchronization.
Science 316: 1609–1612.

Wrobel, A., Bekisz, M., Kublik, E., and Waleszczyk, W. (1994). 20 Hz bursting beta activity in
the cortico-thalamic system of visually attending cats. *Acta Neurobiologiae Experimentalis
(Wars) 54*: 95–107.

Wrobel, A., Ghazaryan, A., Bekisz, M., Bogdan, W., and Kaminski, J. (2007). Two streams of
attention-dependent beta activity in the striate recipient zone of cat's lateral posterior-pulvinar
complex. *Journal of Neuroscience 27*: 2230–2240.

Xu, X., Ichida, J. M., Allison, J. D., Boyd, J. D., Bonds, A. B., and Casagrande, V. A. (2001). A
comparison of koniocellular, magnocellular and parvocellular receptive field properties in
the lateral geniculate nucleus of the owl monkey (Aotus trivirgatus). *Journal of Physiology
531*: 203–218.

Yingling, C. D. and Skinner, J. E. (1976). Selective regulation of thalamic sensory relay nuclei
by nucleus reticularis thalami. *Electroencephalography and Clinical Neurophysiology 41*:
476–482.

Yu, X. J., Xu, X. X., Chen, X., He, S., and He, J. (2009a). Slow recovery from excitation of thalamic reticular nucleus neurons. *Journal of Neurophysiology 101*: 980–987.

Yu, X. J., Xu, X. X., He, S., and He, J. (2009b). Change detection by thalamic reticular neurons.
Nature Neuroscience 12: 1165–1170.

Zikopoulos, B. and Barbas, H. (2006). Prefrontal projections to the thalamic reticular nucleus
form a unique circuit for attentional mechanisms. *Journal of Neuroscience 26*: 7348–7361.

CHAPTER 15

ATTENTIONAL FUNCTIONS OF THE SUPERIOR COLLICULUS

RICHARD J. KRAUZLIS

INTRODUCTION

The superior colliculus (SC) is an evolutionarily conserved structure in the vertebrate brainstem that plays a major role in sensory-motor integration in a wide range of species. Here we focus on the primate SC, which is best known for its role in the control of orienting movements of the eyes and head. As might be expected from the linkage between shifts of attention and orienting of the body, the primate SC plays an important role in attention. However, we now understand that this role extends beyond executing motor commands based on attention effects accomplished elsewhere, and includes the process of selecting targets for orienting movements, and the control of covert attention for perceptual judgements, even in the absence of orienting movements. We begin by summarizing how the primate SC contributes to the control of orienting movements, and then describe how successive studies have advanced our understanding of the role of the SC in attention.

MOTOR CONTROL OF SACCADES

The SC is a major component of the motor circuits that control how we orient our eyes and head in space. In fact, the primate SC was one of the first structures to be thoroughly investigated using the techniques of single-neuron electrophysiology in awake and behaving primates, and our knowledge of the role played by the SC in the control of orienting movements has continuously advanced over the past several decades. A full review of the role of the SC in the motor control of orienting movements is beyond the scope of this chapter, and several excellent reviews can be found elsewhere (Gandhi and Katnani 2011; Sparks 1999; Wurtz and Albano 1980). However, to provide an appropriate context for describing the role of the SC in attention, a few key facts should be summarized.

First, the SC is a multi-layered structure that contains neurons with different properties in its different layers. In the primate, these are usually divided broadly into superficial, intermediate, and deep layers. The superficial layers receive direct projections from retinal ganglion cells and contain 'visual' neurons with brisk responses to visual stimulus onsets, offsets, and motion, but without clear preferences for complex stimulus features or the direction of motion. The intermediate and deep layers contain neurons with activity related to orienting movements as well as responses to sensory stimuli. 'Burst' neurons in these SC layers show phasic increases in spiking activity that are time-locked to the occurrence of saccadic eye movements that have a particular direction and amplitude (Munoz and Wurtz 1995; Schiller and Koerner 1971; Sparks 1975; Wurtz and Goldberg 1971). 'Prelude' or 'build-up' neurons also show activity for particular saccades, but they also exhibit increases in tonic activity over the several hundreds of milliseconds that precede the onset of the movement (Glimcher and Sparks 1992; Mohler and Wurtz 1976; Munoz and Wurtz 1995). These neurons are described as possessing 'response fields', reflecting the observation that their activity is not purely sensory. As we will explore in more detail below, both visual and build-up neurons show activity related to attention.

Second, the SC forms a topographic map of visual space that is organized in retinotopic (or alternately, oculocentric) coordinates. This feature of SC organization was first suggested by recording the activity of single neurons and finding that the receptive fields of visual neurons and the movement fields of movement-related neurons varied systematically across the SC (Schiller and Koerner 1971; Wurtz and Goldberg 1971). However, the best-known description of the SC's retinotopic map comes from applying electrical microstimulation to artificially activate SC neurons (Robinson 1972). Microstimulation in the intermediate and deep layers of the SC evoked saccadic eye movements at short latencies (~20 ms), and the direction and amplitude of the evoked saccade depends on the stimulation site; when the stimulating electrode is relocated to another site, the evoked saccades have a different direction and amplitude. The resulting map of evoked saccades provides the iconic image of the saccade motor map in the SC (Fig. 1). If the amount of current is dialled down to levels that no longer directly evoke eye movements, it is still possible to influence behaviour and, as we describe below, this approach has been used to explore the role of the SC in the control of attention.

Third, the read-out mechanism for controlling saccades by the SC involves a population code. The direction and amplitude of the saccades is based on the weighted average of the entire population of active saccade-related neurons, and thus involves activity spread over a large extent of the intermediate and deep layers of the SC. This property was first identified by reversibly inactivating neuronal activity in the SC by injecting small amounts of lidocaine, which interrupts neuronal transmission by blocking sodium channels (Lee, Rohrer, and Sparks, 1988). During such inactivation, it is still possible to make saccades to the epicentre of the affected retinotopic region, albeit at

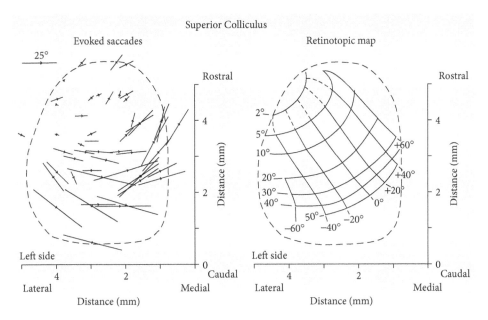

FIGURE 15.1 The retinotopic map of the superior colliculus. Electrical microstimulation in the superior colliculus causes eye movements whose direction and amplitude depends on the location (left). Each arrow corresponds to a stimulation site in the left superior colliculus, and the length and direction of the arrow indicate the metrics of the evoked saccade. As in the visual cortex, the SC represents the opposite side of the visual field; accordingly, the evoked saccades are directed rightward. Also as in the visual cortex, the representation of the centre of the visual field is amplified. Sites toward the front (rostral) are associated with smaller movements than those toward the back (caudal), and medial sites are associated with upward movements whereas lateral sites are associated with downward movements. On the right, the retinotopic map in the SC is summarized, based on the results from the micro-stimulation experiments. Reprinted from *Vision Research*, 12 (11), D. A. Robinson, Eye movements evoked by collicular stimulation in the alert monkey, pp. 1795–1808, Copyright (1972), with permission from Elsevier.

slightly slower speeds, because the halo of intact neurons surrounding the inactivated site continues to provide signals for making the saccade. Saccades directed nearby the epicentre are systematically deviated away from the affected region, reflecting the operation of a mechanism that averages across the population of active neurons. Similar manipulations have subsequently been used to test how the population of SC neurons may contribute to the selection of targets during overt shifts of attention, and to the formation of perceptual decisions during covert attention tasks.

In summary, the primate SC is well known to contain a retinotopically organized motor map for the control of saccades. The same classic trio of physiology methods (single-neuron recording, electrical microstimulation, pharmacologic manipulation) that have been used to understand the role of the SC in the motor execution of saccadic eye movements have also been used to investigate how it contributes to the control of overt and covert attention.

SELECTION FOR SACCADES

When we attend to an object, we typically look directly at it. Because the SC plays a central role in the motor control of orienting movements, it might be expected to play some role in implementing the shifts of attention during overt orienting. However, in addition to this expected role as part of the motor read-out for attention shifts, the SC also plays a central role in the preceding step of identifying where to shift overt attention—namely, selecting which saccade should be made and, more generally, selecting the targets of orienting movements.

Neurons in the superficial layers of the SC respond to visual stimuli, including those that will be the target of a saccadic eye movement. In fact, this observation provided one of the earliest known neuronal correlates of visual spatial attention in the primate brain (Goldberg and Wurtz 1972). Approximately one-half of the visual neurons in the superficial layers of the SC show markedly enhanced responses when the visual stimulus in the neuron's receptive field will be the target of a saccadic eye movement. This enhancement was observed during a straightforward task—the monkey was simply required to make a saccade to a spot stimulus presented in the visual field. When the saccade was directed outside the neuron's receptive field, the neuron did not show enhanced responses, showing that the effect was spatially specific and not due to general arousal.

Subsequent studies have explored how neuronal activity in the intermediate and deep layers participates in the winner-take-all selection for saccades—how to choose where to redirect the eyes when the visual environment presents two or more competing alternatives. This question has most often been studied using some form of visual search. One experimental strategy is to place one visual stimulus in the receptive field or response field of the neuron, together with other stimuli outside the neuron's response field, and then use a cue to instruct the animal which one should be chosen as the endpoint of the saccade. Another strategy is to use visual 'pop out', rather than cues, to indicate where the saccade should go; in this case, the task is to saccade to the one odd-coloured stimulus presented with several same-coloured distractors. Both of these approaches have the advantage of keeping the visual conditions constant while varying the behavioural relevance—the same stimulus in the neuron's response field can be either a cued target or an irrelevant distractor.

Single-neuron recordings using these types of visual search tasks demonstrate that neuronal activity in the intermediate and deeper layers of the SC is related to saccade selection (Glimcher and Sparks 1992; Krauzlis and Dill 2002; McPeek and Keller 2002). Neurons show enhanced activity for a visual stimulus when it is selected as the endpoint of a saccadic eye movement, compared to when it will be ignored, and this preference typically emerges over a time course (~150–250 ms after stimulus onset) that precedes and predicts the saccade choice. However, not all neurons show the same type of modulation. Neurons with some form of saccade-related activity tend to discriminate targets from distractors before saccade onset, but neurons with only visual activity do not (McPeek and Keller 2002). Moreover, for some neurons the discrimination is time-locked to the onset of the visual stimuli, whereas for other neurons it is time-locked to the onset of the saccadic eye movement. These differences presumably reflect the distinct roles played by these neurons in the sequence of steps linking visual selection to the motor control of the saccade that ensues, but the detailed circuitry is not yet understood.

The variety of neuronal signals in the SC correlated with saccade selection is also illustrated by another experimental strategy that involves perceptual discrimination, rather than visual search. In this task design, the animal is presented with random-dot motion displays, in which the fraction of dots that move together coherently in one particular direction is varied, and usually kept near the threshold level that is necessary for correctly discriminating the direction of motion (Britten, Shadlen, Newsome, and Movshon 1992). Unlike visual search, in which the peripheral stimuli immediately provide all the necessary information required to select the correct saccade, in this task the motion signals must be integrated over time in order to determine the correct direction. Also unlike visual search, which involves making a saccade directly to the same stimulus that was used for the discrimination, the motion task involves making a saccade to another peripheral stimulus, usually a spot, based on the direction identified in the motion patch. This makes it possible to introduce a distinction between the direction of motion identified in the motion patch and the direction of motion of the selected saccade, because the peripheral stimuli used as choice targets can be placed at arbitrary locations in the display. For example, the animal might identify the direction for a motion patch presented at the centre of display as 'rightward', and then be asked to indicate his choice by making a saccade to the right-hand member of a pair of dots placed in the top of the display; this would require the animal to make an upward saccade to indicate his 'rightward' choice.

Single-neuron recordings in the intermediate layers of the SC during this type of discrimination task reveal that neurons with prelude or build-up activity fall into two distinct types (Horwitz and Newsome 1999, 2001; Horwitz, Batista, and Newsome 2004). The first type of neuron shows activity that predicts which of the peripheral stimuli will be chosen as the saccade target. This type of modulation appears to be similar to the elevated activity that predicts saccade choice during visual search tasks. However, the second type of neuron shows activity that predicts the direction of motion that will be identified, but not necessarily the direction of saccade that will be made. For example, the neuron might show elevated activity for 'rightward' choices, even if this choice required an upward saccade. Notably, these neurons generally prefer motion that was directed toward the location of their movement fields. Consequently, one interpretation of their activity is that it represents a type of 'motor mnemonic', an intermediate stage of saccade selection that helps bias the animal toward the correct choice once the actual saccade is prepared and executed. This intermediate stage of processing might also be related to the population of neurons mentioned before whose saccade selection is time-locked to the stimulus rather than to the movement itself (McPeek and Keller 2002), but this has not been directly tested.

Activity in the SC is not only correlated with the selection of the saccade, but also plays a causal role. Performance in the pop-out visual search tasks described above is dramatically altered when activity in the intermediate layers of the SC is reversibly blocked by injection of pharmacological agents like lidocaine (McPeek and Keller 2004). When the pop-out target was presented in the part of the visual field affected by the SC inactivation, saccades were often directed to one of the distractor stimuli rather than to the target. Importantly, when no choice was required and the subject was simply asked to make saccades to single stimuli, the saccades were only mildly impaired, ruling out the possibility that the problem with saccade selection was due to a motor deficit. Moreover, the degree of impairment depended on the level of difficulty in discriminating the target stimulus from the distractors, again consistent with a problem with saccade selection rather than saccade execution.

Artificially increasing neuronal activity in the SC by electrical microstimulation, rather than suppressing it by chemical inactivation, has provided complementary evidence for a causal role in saccade selection. In visual search tasks, stimulation biases saccade selection in favour of the stimulus location matching the activated SC site (Carello and Krauzlis 2004; Dorris, Olivier, and Munoz 2007), providing additional support for the idea that the SC plays a causal role in the process of selecting where to orient, and is not just involved in implementing a motor command for a decision accomplished elsewhere.

SACCADES AND SPATIAL ATTENTION

It has been known for some time that there is functional overlap between the role of the SC in the control of saccades and the mechanisms for spatial attention. One of the earliest demonstrations of this overlap was achieved by evoking saccades by microstimulation of the SC, and showing that the endpoints of the evoked saccades could be shifted by manipulations known to affect spatial attention (Kustov and Robinson 1996). In these experiments, animals were trained to report the onset of a target on either the left or right side of the visual display, and were presented cues during fixation as they awaited the appearance of the target (Fig. 15.2). The cues consisted of either a peripheral flash indicating the likely spatial location of the upcoming target, or a central cue whose colour likewise indicated the likely target location, albeit indirectly. As expected, if the appearance of the cues caused a shift of attention, valid cues reduced reaction times and invalid cues increased reaction times. The novel finding was that the endpoints of saccades evoked by SC microstimulation were systematically deviated in the direction of the cue, supporting the idea that the shifts of attention caused by the cues automatically led to the preparation of saccades. Moreover, the time course of these deviations provided nice corroboration of the attention shifts—peripheral cues led to deviations at short delays, consistent with a stimulus-driven effect, whereas central cues led to deviations at longer delays, consistent with a top-down effect.

Activity in the intermediate layers of the SC also shows striking correlates of the interaction between top-down and bottom-up influences on attention during the programming of saccades. This has been studied by flashing a peripheral visual stimulus briefly

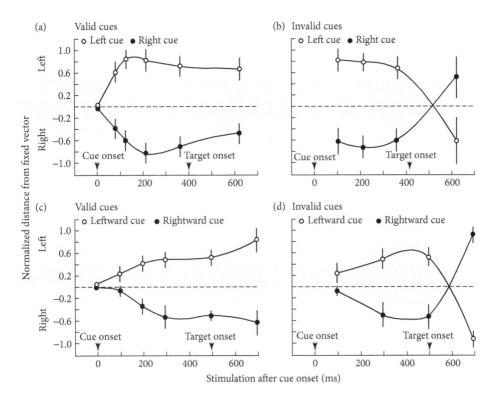

FIGURE 15.2 The effects of attention cues on the saccades evoked by SC microstimulation. The y-axis in these plots is the normalized distance between the saccade vectors evoked by SC microstimulation under control conditions and those evoked under experimental conditions when either peripheral (a, b) or symbolic (c, d) attention cues were presented to the animal. The x-axis is the time of SC microstimulation relative to the onset of the cue. The cues were valid on 80% of the trials, and led to systematic deviations in the saccade vectors evoked by SC microstimulation. The effects for peripheral cues showed a faster time course than the effects for symbolic cues. Reprinted by permission from Macmillan Publishers Ltd: *Nature*, 384 (6604), Kustov, A. and Robinson, D. Shared neural control of attentional shifts and eye movements, pp. 74–7, copyright (1996), Nature Publishing Group.

on one side of the visual display, and after a variable delay, presenting the target on either the same or opposite side; the task of the animal is simply to make a saccade to the target after it is presented. By manipulating the timing of when the flashed stimulus appears with respect to the target stimulus, and by making the flashed stimulus either predictive or not predictive of the target location, it is possible to document both behavioural and neuronal correlates of spatial attention during saccade preparation (Bell, Fecteau, and Munoz 2004; Fecteau, Bell, and Munoz 2004).

Some effects on saccades and SC activity can be explained by the capture of attention. When the flashed peripheral stimulus appears just before the appearance of the target (e.g. 50 ms prior), it reduces saccade latency if it is flashed on the same side of the visual display. Similarly, the activity evoked by the appearance of the target in the neuron's response field is facilitated if a stimulus was just flashed at the same location. These effects are time-locked to the onset of the stimulus, suggesting that they are automatic consequences driven by sensory, bottom-up processing. However, when the flashed stimulus is predictive of the target location, these effects are larger and more prolonged than when the flashed stimulus is not predictive, indicating an additional influence of top-down factors. Thus, the behavioural consequences of attention capture, at least for saccades, can be partly explained by changes in the activity of SC neurons evoked by the stimulus onsets.

Other effects on saccades and SC activity appear to be related to the inhibition of return—the tendency to avoid coming back to a previously explored location (Klein 2000). When the flashed stimulus appears 100 milliseconds or longer before the appearance of the target, it increases the latency of saccades if it was flashed on the same side of the display, and decreases the latency of saccades if it was flashed on the opposite side. Similarly, the activity of SC neurons evoked by the target is suppressed if a stimulus was flashed at the same location longer than 100 milliseconds ago. These effects support the idea that the SC is part of the mechanism that mediates inhibition of return, which acts to automatically bias orienting toward new locations in space. However, just as with attention capture, inhibition of return can also be modulated by top-down factors. When the flashed stimulus is predictive of the target location—in which case the tendency to avoid previously explored locations is counter-productive—the size of inhibition of return is reduced for both saccade latency and SC activity.

Together, these results support the view of the SC as a priority map for saccade target selection (Fecteau and Munoz 2006). The term 'priority map' is meant to draw a distinction with other terms that emphasize the role of bottom-up or top-down processes. 'Salience map' has been used in several ways, but it typically refers to the physical distinctiveness of a sensory stimulus, and therefore connotes a function tightly linked to bottom-up processes. 'Relevance' is a term that is often used to describe the behavioural significance of a visual object, regardless of its physical properties, and therefore connotes functions linked to top-down processes. As described above, the selection of saccades and the activity of neurons in the SC involve a combination of both bottom-up and top-down processes. The term 'priority map' has therefore been proposed, and largely adopted, to recognize that the map in the superior colliculus contains a representation of visual space that combines both physical salience and behavioural relevance.

MICROSACCADES AND SPATIAL ATTENTION

Modulation of SC neuronal activity with shifts of spatial attention helps explain an interesting phenomenon that occurs during fixation. When subjects are required to maintain fixation of a central stimulus, and also asked to covertly attend to a peripheral stimulus, they tend to make very small saccades—microsaccades—in the direction of the attention shift. This effect of covert attention on microsaccades can be explained by the combination of neuronal events taking place in the intermediate layers of the SC.

First, as might be expected from the description of the SC as a priority map, neurons in the rostral part of the SC, which represent the central visual field, are modulated by the behavioural relevance and physical salience of foveal goals (Hafed and Krauzlis 2008). In addition to contributing to the control of fixation, these neurons also play a causal role in the generation of microsaccades (Hafed, Goffart, and Krauzlis 2009). In fact, rostral SC neurons show build-up and bursts for microsaccades that are nearly identical to the behaviour of SC neurons elsewhere in the map, except that the saccadic eye movements themselves are about an order of magnitude smaller in amplitude (Hafed et al. 2009; Hafed and Krauzlis 2012).

Second, the trigger for saccades appears to coincide with the occurrence of an imbalance in activity across the SC (Hafed, Goffart, and Krauzlis 2008). Typically, this imbalance arises when a peripheral target appears and the subject is allowed to look directly at it. In this scenario, activity in the central part of the SC map drops, and the movement is guided by the activity of SC neurons at the peripheral site. If the subject is required to ignore the peripheral stimulus and maintain fixation, activity in the central part of the SC map is maintained, and activity at the peripheral site is suppressed, preventing the generation of an inappropriate saccade that would take the eye outside of the fixation window. However, the transient change in activity caused by the appearance of the peripheral stimulus can create an imbalance in activity sufficient to trigger a saccade, whose amplitude is then determined by the population average of activity present across the SC map. This model has not been directly tested, but it provides a plausible explanation for the link between microsaccades and covert shifts of attention (Hafed et al. 2009).

TARGET SELECTION FOR SMOOTH PURSUIT

The results from various saccade selection tasks share an ambiguity. Because the motor response consists of a saccade to the selected target, it is possible that the importance of the SC depends on the preparation of the saccade, rather than the selection of the target. The single-neuron recordings provide evidence that some SC activity is indeed linked to the process of selecting between sensory stimuli, and that SC activity provides correlates of spatial attention linked to saccades. However, because these are correlates, it is unclear whether these signals are necessary for target selection or the control of spatial attention. Manipulations like chemical inactivation and electrical stimulation can test for causality, but their effects are not limited to these particular neuronal signals. Consequently, it is ambiguous from the saccade selection tasks whether SC activity is involved in target selection or spatial attention per se or is instead only necessary for controlling the saccade that follows.

One approach for disambiguating these possibilities is to use smooth pursuit eye movements, rather than saccades. Smooth pursuit is another voluntary eye movement, well developed in primates, that makes it possible to smoothly track an object of interest as it moves through the visual environment, even in the presence of other moving or stationary distractors (Krauzlis 2005; Lisberger 2010). The function of smooth pursuit is to keep the retinal images of objects of interest relatively stable on the retina so that they can be seen clearly. One of the classic results in the eye movement literature was the demonstration by Rashbass (1961) that smooth pursuit moves the eye in the direction of the target motion, even if this moves the target's image further from the centre of the fovea. The best-known scenario introduced by Rashbass is referred to as the 'step-ramp'—this involves stepping the target slightly to one side, while at the same time moving the target smoothly back toward the centre. In this scenario, smooth pursuit gradually follows the motion of the target after a short latency (e.g. about 100 ms), directing the eyes away from the starting position of the target and, if the step size and target speed are chosen appropriately, the eye intercepts the target as it moves through the centre of the display with no need for a saccade. For our purposes, the important feature of this manipulation is that the target initially appears on one side of the display, while the eye movement is directed to the opposite side. This difference is useful for the purposes of investigating target selection—it makes it possible to dissociate the location of the target from the direction of the eye movement, a distinction that cannot be made in saccade visual search tasks.

Single-neuron recordings in the intermediate layers of the SC have used Rashbass' technique of step-ramp target motions to identify modulations in firing rate during smooth pursuit eye movements, even in the absence of saccades (Krauzlis 2003; Krauzlis, Basso, and Wurtz 1997, 2000). SC neurons discharge during smooth pursuit in a manner that is consistent with the location of their response fields—they increase their discharge when the retinal location of the pursuit stimulus falls inside their response field, and decrease their discharge otherwise.

More relevant to our discussion of overt attention, SC neurons have also been studied during a pursuit version of a visual search task. As in some studies of saccade visual search, the task involves presenting two differently coloured stimuli and providing a cue that identifies one as the target, and the other as a distractor. However, to evoke saccade-free smooth pursuit, both stimuli are initially located off to the side of the fixated central spot, and then move toward and through the centre of the display in classic Rashbass style. The subject can track either of the two stimuli without the need to make a targeting saccade, but only gets rewarded for tracking the cued stimulus. As in the saccade versions of this task, neurons show enhanced activity for a visual stimulus when it is selected as the target of a pursuit eye movement, compared to when it will be ignored. Indeed, when SC neurons are examined in both saccade and pursuit versions of the task, they show selectivity for targets regardless of the type of eye movement used to acquire the target (Krauzlis and Dill 2002). However, in the pursuit version of the task, the neurons show enhanced responses for the target, even though the eye movement is directed away from the starting position of the target. This distinction supports the idea that the neuronal activity is related to the selection of the target, rather than to the direction of the eye movement.

One caveat to this interpretation is that the elevated activity during pursuit could possibly be related to the planning of saccades, rather than to the selection of the target. The task is designed so that the animal does not make saccades to acquire the target, but with single-neuron recording data it is hard to rule out the possibility that the animal plans a saccade that is subsequently cancelled.

Clear evidence for a role in target selection per se comes from causal manipulations of SC activity using electrical microstimulation or chemical inactivation. When weak microstimulation is applied to the intermediate layers of the SC (i.e. microstimulation at levels below the threshold for evoking saccades), the animal shows a bias in favour of the stimulus placed at the corresponding location in the visual field (Carello and Krauzlis 2004). For saccades, this target location is the same as the saccade endpoint, so selection of the target is confounded with saccade selection. For pursuit, however, this initial location is opposite the direction of target motion, so selection of the target can be dissociated from selecting the direction of the eye movement, and the results show that the behavioural deficit is based on the location of the target.

These effects on target selection can by explained by a 'race model' in which signals representing the possible choices rise toward a threshold, and the behavioural choice is determined by which signal reaches the threshold first (Logan, Cowan, and Davis 1984). In this formulation, stimulation of the SC raises the level of activity of one of the possible choices closer to the threshold, increasing the probability that it will be selected as the target. This shift in activity level predicts that, in addition to changing the probability of choosing one stimulus over the other, there should also be changes in reaction times, because the raised level of activity should take less time to reach the threshold. Indeed, microstimulation does change the latencies of pursuit and saccades, as well as the choices, as predicted by this simple model (Carello and Krauzlis 2004)—reaction times are decreased for stimuli at locations matching the stimulated site and increased for stimuli at other locations.

A complementary pattern of results is found when neuronal activity in the intermediate layers of the SC is focally inactivated (Fig. 3). Using the same types of visual search tasks, chemical inactivation causes a bias in target choice away from the stimulus placed inside the affected part of the visual field (Nummela and Krauzlis 2010). Deficits in target selection are observed for both pursuit and saccadic eye movements, and once again, the deficits for pursuit are based on the location of the stimulus rather than the direction of movement required to acquire it. SC inactivation also affects the reaction times of target choices, and the results again are in agreement with predictions from the race model— latencies are increased for stimuli placed inside the affected region, consistent with the interpretation that the level of SC was lowered further away from the decision threshold. Activity in the SC therefore appears to be crucial for selecting the target for eye movements, in addition to its role in the selection, preparation, and execution of saccades.

The results from these types of experiments show that activity in the SC is important for the winner-take-all selection of a single visual target in the presence of distractors. However, there is also evidence that SC activity contributes to the integration of

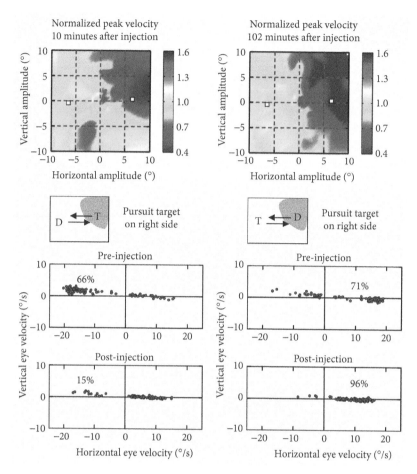

FIGURE 15.3 Effects of SC inactivation on target selection for pursuit eye movements. The extent of SC inactivation is estimated by measuring the change in peak velocity of saccades to visual targets either shortly after the injection (a) or toward the end of the experimental session (b). The region of the visual field with slower saccades indicates the portion of the SC affected by the chemical inactivation. The distributions of target choices are illustrated by plotting the mean horizontal eye velocity against mean vertical eye velocity over the first 100 milliseconds of the pursuit eye movement response. When the pursuit target initially appeared in the affected part of the visual field, correct pursuit choices dropped from 66% correct to 15% correct (c). Conversely, when the distractor appeared in the affected part of the visual field, correct pursuit choices improved from 71% correct to 96% correct. Thus, SC inactivation biased choices in favour of the stimulus appearing outside the affected region, even though these required movements to the opposite side. Adapted from *Journal of Neurophysiology*, 104 (3), Nummela, S. U., and Krauzlis, R. J., Inactivation of primate superior colliculus biases target choice for smooth pursuit, saccades, and button press responses, pp. 1538–48 © 2010, The American Physiological Society.

visual signals before a single winner is selected. This evidence come from a task called 'vector-averaging'. In this task, there are again two moving stimuli for pursuit, but they are arranged to move orthogonal to one another, rather than in opposite directions. The behavioural outcome from this scenario is that the initial smooth pursuit eye movements do not strictly follow either of the two motions, but instead move in a direction that is based on a weighted average of the two individual stimulus motions (Case and Ferrera 2007; Lisberger and Ferrera 1997). The particular weights applied to the two motion signals can vary from trial to trial, and can be influenced by instructions to the subject, but the initial response almost always includes a contribution from both stimulus motions. On an individual trial, the weights change over time and typically evolve toward a winner-take-all outcome in favour of one of the two stimuli, followed by a targeting saccade to the winning stimulus.

Activity in the SC plays a causal role in establishing these weights (Nummela and Krauzlis 2011). When activity in the SC is suppressed by chemical inactivation, the contribution of the moving stimulus placed in the affected part of the visual field is reduced. Conversely, the contribution of the moving stimulus placed outside the affected field tends to be increased. These results show that SC activity helps determine how visual signals are combined during the earliest phases of orienting eye movements, in addition to the role that it plays in the winner-take-all selection of the target.

TARGET SELECTION FOR HAND MOVEMENTS

A few studies have investigated target selection and SC activity using manual responses, such as pressing a button to indicate the choice, instead of asking the animal to make an eye movement. For example, in a visual search task, rather than asking the animal to make a saccade to the target stimulus, the animal is asked to press one of two buttons on a response pad that he can reach with his hands but cannot see. When SC activity is suppressed by chemical inactivation, the animal's choices are biased away from the stimulus placed in the affected part of the visual field, qualitatively similar to the effects seen on saccade and pursuit tasks (Nummela and Krauzlis 2010). However, in these experiments, the effects on target selection for manual responses were notably smaller than the effects on target selection for eye movements measured at the same time. This difference could be due to the extra time that was necessarily allowed for the manual responses compared to eye movements, or the fact that the buttons for the manual response were at a different spatial location from the visual stimuli.

Larger effects on target selection have been found when animals are asked to directly reach to the visual targets (Song, Rafal, and McPeek 2011). In these experiments, the target and distractor stimuli were presented sequentially, and the animal was rewarded for making a reaching movement to the stimulus that had appeared first. The difficulty of the task was varied by changing the delay between the appearance of the target and the appearance of the distractor. Before SC inactivation, animals correctly selected the reach target on most trials if the target appeared only about 50 milliseconds before the distractor; after SC inactivation, the target needed to precede the distractor by about 100 milliseconds to achieve the same level of performance, when the target appeared in the affected part of the visual field. Activity in the SC is therefore important to target selection for reach movements, as well as eye movements.

Overall, the results from the pursuit and hand movement tasks are important for a couple of reasons. First, they show that the role of the SC in visual selection is not limited to a specific type of movement, because inactivation of the SC does not only affect saccades, but also affects smooth pursuit eye movements and movements of the hand. This supports the idea that activity in the SC is not just involved in selecting the goal for saccades, but is part of a more general mechanism that selects targets for a range of actions and effector systems. Second, these results imply a remote site of action. The directional motion signals needed for pursuit are not contained within the SC, but are found elsewhere—for example, in extrastriate cortex (Newsome and Pare 1988; Newsome, Wurtz, and Komatsu 1988; Priebe and Lisberger 2004). Similarly, although there are some neurons in the SC active during reaching movements (Stuphorn, Bauswein, and Hoffmann 2000; Werner, Dannenberg, and Hoffmann 1997), the control of button presses and reaching movements involves signals processed in motor cortex (Graziano 2006; Kalaska 2009; Kalaska and Crammond 1992).

These findings therefore represent a dramatic departure from the view of the SC as a motor map for saccades. When viewed as a motor map, it is possible to explain the role of the SC in terms of local interactions within the SC that could mediate the winner-take-all selection of the final saccade endpoint. Instead, the results from pursuit target selection and manual responses support the view of the SC as a general-purpose priority map that is important for selecting the target for a range of orienting movements, and the mechanisms involved include multiple brain regions outside the SC. Viewing the SC as a priority map raises questions about how the SC interacts with other brain regions, and what range of functions are mediated by these interactions. As we shall see, several lines of evidence show that these functions include the control of attention even in the absence of orienting movements.

ORIENTING OF COVERT ATTENTION

Work on saccade and target selection can claim some of the credit for developing the idea that the SC is not just a saccade motor map, but also acts as a priority map with links to attention. However, some models of attention have outlined a role for the SC in the orienting of attention that predates this work on target selection. These older models are based largely on clinical observations, and distinguished three operations in the control of attention: disengaging attention from the currently attended object, shift attention to the new target, and engaging attention on the new target (Posner and Petersen 1990; Posner, Walker, Friedrich, and Rafal 1984). These three different operations have been linked to different brain regions. Patients with damage to the parietal lobe of cortex have abnormally long reaction times following invalid cues presented in the unaffected visual field, consistent with a deficit in the ability to disengage attention from visual stimuli (Posner et al. 1984). In contrast, patients with progressive supranuclear palsy (PSP), which affects midbrain structures including the SC, require more time after valid cues to show the expected decreases in reaction times, suggesting that they shift attention more slowly than normal (Posner, Cohen, and Rafal 1982; Rafal, Posner, Friedman, Inhoff, and Bernstein 1988). Finally, patients with damage to nuclei in the thalamus show improvements in reaction time after valid cues, but their overall reaction times are slower, suggesting a problem with engaging attention (Rafal and Posner 1987).

These clinical studies provide intriguing evidence that the SC plays a specific role in the control of attention. It is also noteworthy that, because many of these studies involved manual responses, such as button-presses in the absence of targeting saccades, they suggest that the role of the SC extends to the control of covert attention, in addition to its role in overt orienting. Unfortunately, clinical cases do not provide a level of anatomical specificity to unequivocally demonstrate whether or how the SC contributes to the control of attention. To clearly test the role of the SC in attention, we look once again at the results from primate animal models.

Single-neuron recordings in the intermediate layers have provided strong evidence that SC activity is correlated with the allocation of attention, even in the absence of orienting movements (Ignashchenkova, Dicke, Haarmeier, and Thier 2004). In these tasks, animals were trained to discriminate the orientation of the letter 'C', presented at some peripheral location, and the size of the gap was varied to adjust the difficulty of the task and to measure the animal's acuity. On some trials, the onset of the 'C' was preceded by a spatial cue indicating where the letter would subsequently be presented; this type of spatial cueing led to significant improvements in discrimination performance. In a separate experiment, the onset of the 'C' was preceded by a symbolic cue—a dot presented to the side of the fixation spot—again indicating where the letter would appear; once again, cueing improved performance.

Both visual neurons and visual-motor neurons in the SC show effects related to attention in these tasks, but with interesting differences (Fig. 4). Visual neurons respond to the appearance of the 'C' in their receptive field, and this evoked activity is higher when the location was previously cued, regardless of whether the cue was spatial or symbolic; this enhanced activity with cues is a neuronal correlate of covert attention. In contrast, visual-motor neurons also respond to the appearance of the 'C' in their response fields, and show higher activity when the location was previously cued; however this enhancement only occurs for spatial cues and not for symbolic cues. In addition, visual-motor neurons also show elevated activity during the time period after the cue but before the appearance of the 'C', and again this only occurs for spatial cues. This time period after the cue presumably is when attention is shifted, showing that visual-motor neurons in the SC show correlates of this attention shift, but only for spatially precise cues. These results suggest that visual-motor neurons in the SC may be especially important for stimulus-driven shifts of attention.

As with other single-neuron studies, a limitation of these studies is that they provide correlative evidence of a role in covert attention, but do not provide a test of causality. It

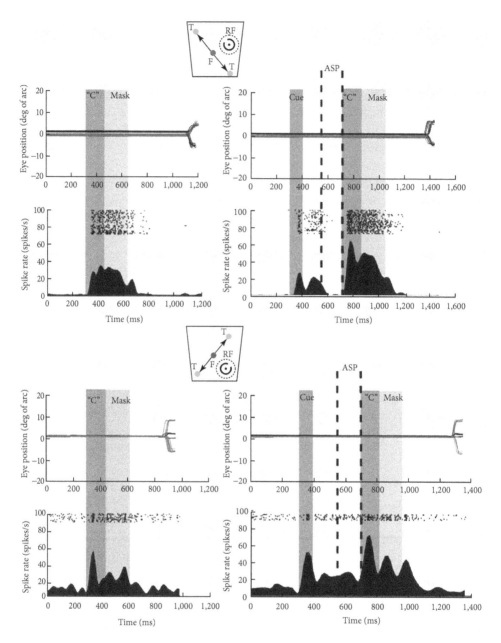

FIGURE 15.4 Examples of enhanced activity in the SC with covert shifts of attention, for a sample visual neuron (top row) and visual-motor neuron (bottom row). The left column shows activity on trials when no cue was presented; the right column shows activity on trials when a spatially precise cue was presented. Both the visual and visual-motor neurons respond to the presentation of the 'C', but this activity is higher when the location of the 'C' was cued than when it was not cued. Also, the visual-motor neuron shows activity during the time epoch before the presentation of the 'C' (attention shift period, ASP), but the visual neuron does not. Reprinted by permission from Macmillan Publishers Ltd: *Nature Neuroscience*, 7(1), Alla Ignashchenkova, Peter W. Dicke, Thomas Haarmeier, and Peter Their, Neuron-specific contribution of the superior colliculus to overt and covert shifts of attention, copyright (2004), Nature Publishing Group.

remains possible that the observed modulations in SC activity are related to the preparation of saccades, even if the animal refrains from making those saccades during the covert attention task. However, several causal tests have now been performed, and they confirm that the SC does play a causal role in the control of covert attention, and is in fact necessary for the normal control of attention.

One of these studies involved applying microstimulation in the SC during a test of change-blindness (Cavanaugh and Wurtz 2004). Change-blindness describes the inability to detect even large changes in a visual scene when those changes are accompanied by a full-field transient, such as a blank screen or the blurred visual input during saccades (Rensink 2002). In this task, animals fixated a central spot and were shown three patches of random-dot motion arranged across the visual display; after about one second, a blank screen replaced the patches briefly, and then the three patches reappeared. However, upon their reappearance, one of the three patches may have changed its direction of motion. The task of the animal was to detect the change, if it occurred, and make a saccade to that patch; if no change was detected, they should remain fixated on the central spot.

In the control experiments, the animals were first given a visual cue on half of the trials indicating which motion patch might change its direction, and as evident from the improvement in the animal's detection performance and their reduced reaction times, they were able to use this visual cue to covertly orient attention to the cued location. In the SC microstimulation trials, instead of providing the animal with a visual cue, the SC was stimulated at a location corresponding to one of the three motion patches, while the animal maintained fixation; the stimulation was applied at levels that were below the threshold for eliciting saccadic eye movements. The striking finding was that the SC microstimulation caused effects similar to those observed with visual cues— the animal's detection performance improved and their reaction times were reduced. Additional experiments showed that these effects on performance cannot be explained by SC stimulation generating a visual phosphene that only indirectly affects spatial attention (Cavanaugh, Alvarez, and Wurtz 2006). Together, these results provide support for the premotor theory of attention—the proposal that the same mechanisms involved in preparing overt movements are also involved in the covert shifting of attention (Sheliga, Riggio, and Rizzolatti 1994).

Microstimulation of the SC also alters performance during a visual-motion discrimination task that requires covert spatial attention (Müller, Philiastides, and Newsome 2005). In this task, animals were asked to judge the direction of motion in a patch containing random-dot motion, which was surrounded by flickering distractor dots elsewhere in the display. By varying the fraction of dots that moved coherently in the motion patch, it was possible to construct a psychometric curve that describes how the animal's performance varied as a function of the strength of the visual motion signal. When subthreshold microstimulation was applied to the SC, the animal's performance improved, so that less motion was required for the animal to achieve a certain level of performance. This improvement in performance was only observed if the motion patch and the site of SC stimulation were at spatially coincident locations. These results provide additional evidence that the SC plays a causal role in the control of covert spatial attention, perhaps as part of an extended network of structures including the frontal eye fields and the lateral intraparietal areas in cerebral cortex.

The results from these microstimulation studies provide clear evidence that the SC is part of the neuronal circuitry for controlling covert attention. However, they leave open the possibility that the SC is not crucial for the normal control of covert attention, but is instead simply updated about covert processes that primarily take place elsewhere. To test whether the SC is necessary for covert attention, the performance of animals has been tested before and after reversible chemical inactivation that targeted activity in the intermediate layers of the SC (Lovejoy and Krauzlis 2010). In these experiments, animals were again asked to discriminate the direction of motion in a random-dot motion patch that appeared at a previously cued location in the visual display. However, to ensure that spatial attention was involved in the task, the display included a 'foil' patch that contained an equivalent motion, but was placed at an uncued location and was therefore irrelevant to the performance of the task. Thus, in addition to discriminating the direction of motion at the cued motion patch, the animals also had to ignore the motion signals presented at the irrelevant foil patch.

Reversible inactivation of the SC caused a profound impairment in the performance of this discrimination task, and was selective for stimuli placed in the part of the visual field affected by the SC chemical inactivation. When the cued stimulus was placed in the affected part of the visual field, performance was severely impaired, but the animal did not make random errors; instead, he tended to base his choices on the irrelevant foil stimulus placed outside the affected region (Fig. 5). This shows that the animal still followed the rules of the task lawfully after SC inactivation, but erroneously based his choices on the stimulus at the wrong spatial location. Importantly, when only a single motion patch was presented in the affected part of the visual field, the animal had only a minor impairment in performance, showing that the processing of visual motion signals per se was largely unaffected. Instead, the primary deficit caused by SC inactivation appears to be an inability to filter out distracting or misleading sensory information. These results demonstrate that SC activity is necessary for the normal operation of spatial attention, even when the response involves a perceptual judgement rather than an orienting movement.

CONCLUSIONS AND OPEN QUESTIONS

It is now well established that the primate SC is involved in the control of both overt and covert shifts of attention. However, several lines of questions remain unanswered about the specific role played by the SC and how this role is implemented through neuronal mechanisms.

Is the SC important for both endogenous and exogenous attention? Single-neuron recording studies have provided seemingly conflicting results, with some studies suggesting the role of the SC is limited to the availability of spatially specific cues, whereas other studies support the conclusion that the SC is involved with voluntary attention as well.

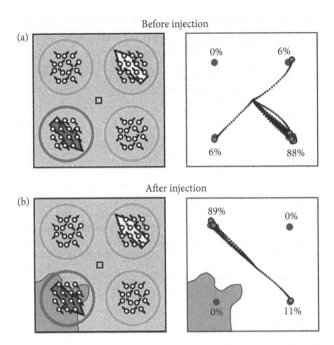

FIGURE 15.5 Impairments in covert selection of signals for perceptual judgements after SC inactivation. The figure shows data from one stimulus condition from one experimental session. The top-left panel shows the stimulus configuration, with the cued motion stimulus located in the lower left quadrant, and the foil stimulus in the upper right quadrant. The top-right panel shows the choices made by the animal in this condition before injection of muscimol into the SC. Almost all of his choices were correctly directed based on the motion in the cued patch. The bottom-left panel shows the stimulus configuration again, with the region affected by the SC inactivation highlighted in blue. After SC inactivation, most of the animal's choices are incorrectly directed based on the motion in the irrelevant foil patch. Thus, the animal no longer correctly allocated spatial attention during the task. Reprinted by permission from Macmillan Publishers Ltd: *Nature Neuroscience*, 13(2), Lovejoy, L. P., & Krauzlis, R. J. Inactivation of primate superior colliculus impairs covert selection of signals for perceptual judgments, copyright (2010), Nature Publishing Group.

Does the SC play a special role in attention to visual motion? Studies of the SC and visual attention have used random dot motion stimuli, so it is presently unclear whether the role of the SC in attention extends generally across visual features, such as orientation and colour. Neurons in the SC are particularly responsive to visual motion stimuli, so it is possible that visual motion occupies a privileged status in the SC's contribution to attention.

Which SC neurons are especially important for attention, and do they play specialized roles? Several classes of SC neurons have been found to show attention-related modulation, with a current emphasis on visual-motor neurons in the intermediate layers. However, it is unknown which types of neurons mediate the causal effects of electrical microstimulation and chemical inactivation, or whether different classes of neurons might be involved in different aspects of attention.

Which neuronal circuits are involved in the SC's control of attention? By analogy with the results from studies of the frontal eye fields and attention (Moore and Armstrong 2003; Moore and Fallah 2004; Tirin Moore 2001), current models emphasize the role of ascending projections from the SC through thalamus to cortical visual areas, or possibly to other cortical areas implicated in attention, such as the frontal eye fields or the lateral intraparietal area (Moore 2006). The actual circuits involved in controlling attention are not known, and the anatomical connections of the SC raise several other possibilities, including the basal ganglia, cerebellum, and other nuclei in the brainstem (Wurtz and Albano 1980).

REFERENCES

Bell, A. H., Fecteau, J. H., and Munoz, D. P. (2004). Using auditory and visual stimuli to investigate the behavioral and neuronal consequences of reflexive covert orienting. *Journal of Neurophysiology* 91(5): 2172–2184. doi: 10.1152/jn.01080.2003.

Britten, K., Shadlen, M., Newsome, W., and Movshon, J. (1992). The analysis of visual motion: A comparison of neuronal and psychophyscial performance. *Journal of Neuroscience* 12(12): 4745–4765.

Carello, C. D. and Krauzlis, R. J. (2004). Manipulating intent: Evidence for a causal role of the superior colliculus in target selection. *Neuron* 43(4): 575–583. doi: 10.1016/j.neuron.2004.07.026.

Case, G. R. and Ferrera, V. P. (2007). Coordination of smooth pursuit and saccade target selection in monkeys. *Journal of Neurophysiology* 98(4): 2206–2214. doi: 10.1152/jn.00021.2007.

Cavanaugh, J., Alvarez, B., and Wurtz, R. (2006). Enhanced performance with brain stimulation: Attentional shift or visual cue. *Journal of Neuroscience* 26(44): 11347–11358.

Cavanaugh, J. and Wurtz, R. (2004). Subcortical modulation of attention counters change blindness. *Journal of Neuroscience* 24(50): 11236–11243.

Dorris, M., Olivier, E., and Munoz, D. (2007). Competitive integration of visual and preparatory signals in the superior colliculus during saccadic programming. *Journal of Neuroscience* 27(19): 5053–5062.

Fecteau, J. H., Bell, A. H., and Munoz, D. P. (2004). Neural correlates of the automatic and goal-driven biases in orienting spatial attention. *Journal of Neurophysiology* 92(3): 1728–1737. doi: 10.1152/jn.00184.2004.

Fecteau, J. H. and Munoz, D. P. (2006). Salience, relevance, and firing: A priority map for target selection. *Trends in Cognitive Sciences* 10(8): 382–390. doi: 10.1016/j.tics.2006.06.011.

Gandhi, N. J. and Katnani, H. A. (2011). Motor functions of the superior colliculus. *Annual Review of Neuroscience* 34: 205–231. doi: 10.1146/annurev-neuro-061010-113728.

Glimcher, P. W. and Sparks, D. L. (1992). Movement selection in advance of action in the superior colliculus. *Nature* 355(6360): 542–545. doi: 10.1038/355542a0.

Goldberg, M. E. and Wurtz, R. H. (1972). Activity of superior colliculus in behaving monkey. II: Effect of attention on neuronal responses. *Journal of Neurophysiology* 35(4): 560–574.

Graziano, M. (2006). The organization of behavioral repertoire in motor cortex. *Annual Review of Neuroscience* 29: 105–134. doi: 10.1146/annurev.neuro.29.051605.112924.

Hafed, Z. M., Goffart, L., and Krauzlis, R. J. (2008). Superior colliculus inactivation causes stable offsets in eye position during tracking. *Journal of Neuroscience* 28(32): 8124–8137. doi: 10.1523/JNEUROSCI.1317-08.2008.

Hafed, Z. M., Goffart, L., and Krauzlis, R. J. (2009). A neural mechanism for microsaccade generation in the primate superior colliculus. *Science* 323(5916): 940–943. doi: 10.1126/science.1166112.

Hafed, Z. M. and Krauzlis, R. J. (2008). Goal representations dominate superior colliculus activity during extrafoveal tracking. *Journal of Neuroscience* 28(38): 9426–9439. doi: 10.1523/JNEUROSCI.1313-08.2008.

Hafed, Z. M. and Krauzlis, R. J. (2012). Similarity of superior colliculus involvement in microsaccade and saccade generation. *Journal of Neurophysiology* 107(7): 1904–1916. doi: 10.1152/jn.01125.2011.

Horwitz, G. D., Batista, A. P., and Newsome, W. T. (2004). Representation of an abstract perceptual decision in macaque superior colliculus. *Journal of Neurophysiology* 91(5): 2281–2296. doi: 10.1152/jn.00872.2003.

Horwitz, G. D. and Newsome, W. T. (1999). Separate signals for target selection and movement specification in the superior colliculus. *Science* 284(5417): 1158–1161.

Horwitz, G. D. and Newsome, W. T. (2001). Target selection for saccadic eye movements: Prelude activity in the superior colliculus during a direction-discrimination task. *Journal of Neurophysiology* 86(5): 2543–2558.

Ignashchenkova, A., Dicke, P. W., Haarmeier, T., and Thier, P. (2004). Neuron-specific contribution of the superior colliculus to overt and covert shifts of attention. *Nature Neuroscience* 7(1): 56–64. doi: 10.1038/nn1169.

Kalaska, J. F. (2009). From intention to action: Motor cortex and the control of reaching movements. *Advances in Experimental Medicine and Biology* 629: 139–178. doi: 10.1007/978-0-387-77064-2_8.

Kalaska, J. F. and Crammond, D. (1992). Cerebral cortical mechanisms of reaching movements. *Science* 255(5051): 1517–1523.

Klein, R. (2000). Inhibition of return. *Trends in Cognitive Sciences* 4(4): 138–147.

Krauzlis, R. J. (2003). Neuronal activity in the rostral superior colliculus related to the initiation of pursuit and saccadic eye movements. *Journal of Neuroscience* 23(10): 4333–4344.

Krauzlis, R. J. (2005). The control of voluntary eye movements: New perspectives. *Neuroscientist* 11(2): 124–137. doi: 10.1177/1073858404271196.

Krauzlis, R. J., Basso, M. A., and Wurtz, R. H. (1997). Shared motor error for multiple eye movements. *Science* 276(5319): 1693–1695.

Krauzlis, R. J., Basso, M. A., and Wurtz, R. H. (2000). Discharge properties of neurons in the rostral superior colliculus of the monkey during smooth-pursuit eye movements. *Journal of Neurophysiology* 84(2): 876–891.

Krauzlis, R. and Dill, N. (2002). Neural correlates of target choice for pursuit and saccades in the primate superior colliculus. *Neuron* 35(2): 355–363.

Kustov, A. and Robinson, D. (1996). Shared neural control of attentional shifts and eye movements. *Nature* 384(6604): 74–77.

Lee, C., Rohrer, W. H., and Sparks, D. L. (1988). Population coding of saccadic eye movements by neurons in the superior colliculus. *Nature* 332(6162): 357–360. doi: 10.1038/332357a0.

Lisberger, S. G. (2010). Visual guidance of smooth-pursuit eye movements: Sensation, action, and what happens in between. *Neuron* 66(4): 477–491. doi: 10.1016/j.neuron.2010.03.027.

Lisberger, S. G. and Ferrera, V. (1997). Vector averaging for smooth pursuit eye movements initiated by two moving targets in monkeys. *Journal of Neuroscience* 17(19): 7490–7502.

Logan, G., Cowan, W., and Davis, K. (1984). On the ability to inhibit simple and choice reaction time responses: A model and a method. *Journal of Experimental Psychology: Human Perception and Performance* 10(2): 276–291.

Lovejoy, L. P. and Krauzlis, R. J. (2010). Inactivation of primate superior colliculus impairs covert selection of signals for perceptual judgments. *Nature Neuroscience* 13(2): 261–266. doi: 10.1038/nn.2470.

McPeek, R. M. and Keller, E. L. (2002). Saccade target selection in the superior colliculus during a visual search task. *Journal of Neurophysiology* 88(4): 2019–2034.

McPeek, R. M. and Keller, E. L. (2004). Deficits in saccade target selection after inactivation of superior colliculus. *Nature Neuroscience* 7(7): 757–763. doi: 10.1038/nn1269.

Mohler, C. W. and Wurtz, R. H. (1976). Organization of monkey superior colliculus: Intermediate layer cells discharging before eye movements. *Journal of Neurophysiology* 39(4): 722–744.

Moore, T. (2006). The neurobiology of visual attention: Finding sources. *Current Opinion in Neurobiology* 16(2): 159–165. doi: 10.1016/j.conb.2006.03.009.

Moore, T. and Armstrong, K. M. (2003). Selective gating of visual signals by microstimulation of frontal cortex. *Nature* 421(6921): 370–373. doi: 10.1038/nature01341.

Moore, T. and Fallah, M. (2004). Microstimulation of the frontal eye field and its effects on covert spatial attention. *Journal of Neurophysiology* 91(1): 152–162.

Müller, J. R., Philiastides, M. G., and Newsome, W. T. (2005). Microstimulation of the superior colliculus focuses attention without moving the eyes. *Proceedings of the National Academy of Sciences USA* 102(3): 524–529. doi: 10.1073/pnas.0408311101.

Munoz, D. P. and Wurtz, R. H. (1995). Saccade-related activity in monkey superior colliculus. I: Characteristics of burst and buildup cells. *Journal of Neurophysiology* 73(6): 2313–2333.

Newsome, W. and Pare, E. (1988). A selective impairment of motion perception following lesions of the middle temporal visual area (MT). *Journal of Neuroscience* 8(6): 2201–2211.

Newsome, W., Wurtz, R., and Komatsu, H. (1988). Relation of cortical areas MT and MST to pursuit eye movements. II: Differentiation of retinal from extraretinal inputs. *Journal of Neurophysiology* 60(2): 604–620.

Nummela, S. U. and Krauzlis, R. J. (2010). Inactivation of primate superior colliculus biases target choice for smooth pursuit, saccades, and button press responses. *Journal of Neurophysiology* 104(3): 1538–1548. doi: 10.1152/jn.00406.2010.

Nummela, S. U. and Krauzlis, R. J. (2011). Superior colliculus inactivation alters the weighted integration of visual stimuli. *Journal of Neuroscience* 31(22): 8059–8066. doi: 10.1523/JNEUROSCI.5480-10.2011.

Posner, M., Cohen, Y., and Rafal, R. (1982). Neural systems control of spatial orienting. *Philosophical Transactions of the Royal Society B: Biological Sciences* 298(1089): 187–198.

Posner, M. I. and Petersen, S. E. (1990). The attention system of the human brain. *Annual Review of Neuroscience* 13: 25–42. doi: 10.1146/annurev.ne.13.030190.000325.

Posner, M. I., Walker, J. A., Friedrich, F. J., and Rafal, R. D. (1984). Effects of parietal injury on covert orienting of attention. *Journal of Neuroscience* 4(7): 1863–1874.

Priebe, N. and Lisberger, S. (2004). Estimating target speed from the population response in visual area MT. *Journal of Neuroscience* 24(8): 1907–1916.

Rafal, R. D. and Posner, M. I. (1987). Deficits in human visual spatial attention following thalamic lesions. *Proceedings of the National Academy of Sciences USA* 84(20): 7349–7353.

Rafal, R. D., Posner, M. I., Friedman, J. H., Inhoff, A. W., and Bernstein, E. (1988). Orienting of visual attention in progressive supranuclear palsy. *Brain* 111(2): 267–280.

Rashbass, C. (1961). The relationship between saccadic and smooth tracking eye movements. *Journal of Physiology* 159(2): 326–338.

Rensink, R. A. (2002). Change detection. *Annual Review of Psychology* 53: 245–277. doi: 10.1146/annurev.psych.53.100901.135125.

Robinson, D. A. (1972). Eye movements evoked by collicular stimulation in the alert monkey. *Vision Research* 12(11): 1795–1808.

Schiller, P. H. and Koerner, F. (1971). Discharge characteristics of single units in superior colliculus of the alert rhesus monkey. *Journal of Neurophysiology* 34(5): 920–936.

Sheliga, B. M., Riggio, L., and Rizzolatti, G. (1994). Orienting of attention and eye movements. *Experimental Brain Research* 98(3): 507–522.

Song, J.-H., Rafal, R. D., and McPeek, R. M. (2011). Deficits in reach target selection during inactivation of the midbrain superior colliculus. *Proceedings of the National Academy of Sciences USA* 108(51): E1433–1440. doi: 10.1073/pnas.1109656108.

Sparks, D. L. (1975). Response properties of eye movement-related neurons in the monkey superior colliculus. *Brain Research* 90(1): 147–152.

Sparks, D. L. (1999). Conceptual issues related to the role of the superior colliculus in the control of gaze. *Current Opinion in Neurobiology* 9(6): 698–707.

Stuphorn, V., Bauswein, E., and Hoffmann, K.-P. (2000). Neurons in the primate superior colliculus coding for arm movements in gaze-related coordinates. *Journal of Neurophysiology* 83(3): 1283–1299.

Tirin Moore, M. F. (2001). Control of eye movements and spatial attention. *Proceedings of the National Academy of Sciences USA* 98(3): 1273–1276.

Werner, W., Dannenberg, S., and Hoffmann, K.-P. (1997). Arm-movement-related neurons in the primate superior colliculus and underlying reticular formation: Comparison of neuronal activity with EMGs of muscles of the shoulder, arm and trunk during reaching. *Experimental Brain Research* 115(2): 191–205.

Wurtz, R. and Albano, J. (1980). Visual-motor function of the primate superior colliculus. *Annual Review of Neuroscience* 3: 189–226.

Wurtz, R. and Goldberg, M. (1971). Superior colliculus cell responses related to eye movements in awake monkeys. *Science* 171(966): 82–84.

CHAPTER 16

ORIENTING ATTENTION: A CROSSMODAL PERSPECTIVE

CHARLES SPENCE

INTRODUCTION: OVERT AND COVERT ORIENTING

ATTENTION can be oriented either overtly or covertly. So, for example, we make overt eye movements in order to fixate objects and events of interest in the environment. On occasion, we might also turn our head in order to hear better what someone else is saying at a noisy cocktail party, and we overtly palpate hand-held objects in order to discern their material properties. Sniffing, meanwhile, can be thought of as a form of overt olfactory orienting, and putting a foodstuff in our mouth allows us to attend to its gustatory qualities. These forms of overt orienting primarily facilitate the perception of stimuli in the modality associated with the receptors that have been moved (or oriented).

It is important to note that planning, or executing, an eye movement may also facilitate the processing of both auditory and tactile stimuli that happen to be presented at, or from close to, the endpoint of that saccade (see Rorden and Driver 1999; Rorden, Greene, Sasine, and Baylis 2002). This can be considered as a crossmodal form of overt orienting. Similarly, the processing of visual stimuli that just so happen to be presented from close to a body-part also tend to be enhanced (or prioritized). That said, most of the research in this area has tended to focus on the perception of visual stimuli presented from close to, or far from, an observer's hands (e.g. Abrams, Davoli, Du, Knapp, and Paull 2008; Dufour and Touzalin 2008; Hari and Jousmäki 1996; Reed, Grubb, and Steele 2006; Spence, Pavani, Maravita, and Holmes 2008), or even from close to a rubber (or virtual) hand that may have been incorporated into the observer's body image (Hartcher-O'Brien, Levitan, and Spence 2010). As such, it is currently somewhat unclear to what extent such facilitatory effects also occur for visual stimuli presented to other body parts (cf. Makin, Holmes, and Ehrsson 2008). And while there will not be space to cover the limited literature on attentional orienting (either overt or covert) as it impacts on the processing of chemosensory signals (see Ashkenazi and Marks 2004), the fact that salivation that can be triggered by sniffing certain foodstuffs will also likely impact on the information processing of gustatory signals (see Spence 2011a, for a review).

In summary, then, there are extensive crossmodal links in attention that result from the *overt* orienting of the sensory receptors (e.g. the eyes, ears, hands, etc.). The majority of the cognitive neuroscience research that has been conducted over the last 50 years or so has tended to focus on the consequences of the *covert* orienting of attention for the processing of auditory, visual, and tactile stimuli (see Posner 1978; Spence and Driver 2004; Wright and Ward 2008), and it is on this rapidly growing body of research that the present review will focus. While there is now a reasonably large body of neuropsychological data relevant to the topic of crossmodal attention and multisensory integration[1] (e.g. see Farah, Wong, Monheit, and Morrow 1989; Inhoff, Rafal, and Posner 1992; Sarri, Blankenburg, and Driver 2006; Valenza Murray, Ptak, and Vuilleumier 2004; Van Vleet and Robertson 2006, for representative examples), the focus of this review will instead primarily be on human psychophysics and neuroimaging data.

ATTENDING TO A SENSORY MODALITY

One of the simplest ways in which an individual can orient their attention in a crossmodal manner is by endogenously choosing to focus their attention on a sensory modality. So, for example, numerous studies have now demonstrated that voluntarily (or endogenously) choosing to do this often allows an individual to respond more rapidly and/or more accurately than they would otherwise have done if their attentional resources were to have been divided between several senses simultaneously, or else focused on a different sensory modality instead (see Spence, Nicholls, and Driver 2001a, for a review). That said, carefully controlled psychophysical studies involving participants making unspeeded discrimination responses have not always found much evidence of a benefit associated with participants focusing their attention on a specific modality (either audition or vision) as compared to when attention is divided between two modalities (that is, when the modality of the target on the upcoming trial, either auditory or visual, is uncertain; Alais, Morrone, and Burr 2006; Shiffrin and Grantham 1974; see also Larsen, McIlhagga, Baert, and Bundesen 2003).

There are a number of ways in which this seemingly inconsistent pattern of behavioural results can potentially be explained. It may simply be that the costs of endogenously focusing attention on the wrong sensory modality are larger than the benefits of focusing attention on the correct target modality (see Spence et al. 2001a). Alternatively, however, there is also evidence to suggest that people find it somewhat more difficult (or time-consuming) to shift their attention to or from the tactile modality than to shift their attention between the auditory and visual modalities (Spence et al. 2001a; Spence, Shore, and Klein, 2001b). However, another way in which to reconcile these seemingly inconsistent results is to suggest that endogenous attention to a sensory modality may speed up the relative time of arrival of stimuli in the attended modality without necessarily enhancing the perceptual representations of those stimuli that happen to be attended (though see Prinzmetal, McCool, and Park 2005; Prinzmetal, Park, and Garrett 2005, for contradictory evidence).

There is robust psychophysical and event-related potential (ERP) evidence demonstrating the 'prior entry' of target stimuli presented in a modality that is attended endogenously as compared to the same events when a participant's attention is divided between multiple sensory modalities, or when it is endogenously directed to another modality instead (Spence et al. 2001b; Vibell, Klinge, Zampini, Spence, and Nobre 2007; Zampini, Shore, and Spence 2005; see Spence and Parise 2010, for a review). For example, Vibell et al. (2007) reported a study in which their participants' attention was endogenously directed either to the visual or tactile modality on a block-by-block basis. The participants had to determine on which side the first stimulus had been presented. A significant (38 ms) prior-entry effect was demonstrated behaviourally. Importantly, latency shifts of the early visual evoked potentials were also observed: in particular, the latencies of the early visual P1, N1, N2 components all peaked significantly earlier in time over contralateral (than over ipsilateral) cortex when the visual stimulus was attended as compared to when attention was directed to the tactile modality instead. The P1 and N1 components were temporally shifted by 3–4 ms, while the latency of the late P300 potential was shifted by 14 ms. What is more, the mean amplitude of the P1 and N1 components for the attended visual stimuli were also increased over selected scalp sites, hence suggesting that the subjective perception of temporal order may result from some as yet unknown combination of neural latency and amplitude-modulation effects. The presentation of a task-irrelevant and non-informative auditory, visual, or tactile stimulus has also been shown to elicit a short-lasting exogenous shift of attention to the modality of the cue (see Miles, Brown, and Poliakoff 2011; Turatto, Benso, Galfano, Gamberini, and Umilta 2002; Turatto, Galfano, Bridgeman, and Umiltà, 2004).

A number of neuroimaging studies conducted over the last decade or so have converged on the conclusion that attending to a particular sensory modality typically results in enhanced neural processing of the attended stimuli in the relevant early cortical areas (e.g. occipital areas when attending to vision, somatosensory areas when attending to touch, and so on) while neural activity tends to be suppressed in those cortical areas that are associated with those modalities that are in some sense 'unattended'. So, for example, when a participant's attention is drawn away from the processing of an auditory event by the presentation of a visual stimulus, and particularly when their attention is directed to vision by their performing a visual task (as compared with a non-competitive baseline condition), auditory cortex, especially secondary auditory cortical areas, exhibits decreased activity in response to auditory stimuli (Johnson and Zatorre 2005; Kawashima, O'Sullivan, and Roland 1995; Laurienti, Burdette, Wallace,

Yen, Field, and Stein 2002; Shomstein and Yantis 2004; see also Just, Kellar, and Cynkar 2008). The available evidence suggests that the extent of this suppression may well depend upon the difficulty of the participant's task (e.g. Hairston, Hodges, Casanova, Hayasaka, Kraft, Maldjian, and Burdette 2008; see also Otten, Alain, and Picton 2000; Rees, Frith, and Lavie 2001).

By analysing the functional connectivity between the auditory and visual cortical areas in participants performing auditory and visual tasks, Johnson and Zatorre (2005, 2006) were able to highlight a reciprocal inverse relationship with decreasing visual activation correlating with increased auditory activation and vice versa. Furthermore, it turns out that temporarily lesioning cortical areas such as dorsolateral prefrontal cortex using transcranial magnetic stimulation (TMS) impairs an individual's ability to simultaneously divide attention between two sensory modalities (Johnson, Strafella, and Zatorre 2007).

Crossmodal Exogenous Spatial Orienting

Attention may be directed to a spatial location following the presentation of an auditory, visual, or tactile cue. The presentation of such peripheral cues, even though they may be entirely task-irrelevant (that is, they provide no information concerning the likely location of the upcoming target) has been shown to give rise to a short-lasting facilitation of information-processing at the cued location (see Fig. 16.1; e.g. Ferris and Sarter 2008; Gray, Mohebbi, and Tan 2009; see Spence, McDonald, and Driver 2004; Wright and Ward 2008, for reviews). The extent of the spread of attention appears to be related to the localizability of the cue stimulus, with visual cues typically giving rise to a more tightly focused spotlight of attentional enhancement than either auditory or tactile cues. In fact, the failure to present the cue and target stimuli from a similar enough position on 'validly' (or ipsilaterally) cued trials has now been shown to be responsible for the failure to demonstrate certain crossmodal links in spatial attention (see Prime, McDonald, Green, and Ward 2008; Spence et al. 2004).

This short-lasting attentional facilitation (which normally lasts for a few hundred milliseconds after the onset of the cue stimulus) is then followed by a much longer period of inhibition, known as inhibition-of-return (IOR) (see Klein 2000, for a review). IOR has now been demonstrated to occur between all possible pairings of successively presented auditory, visual, and tactile stimuli (Spence, Lloyd, McGlone, Nicholls, and Driver, 2000a). To date, such crossmodal inhibitory effects, which may last for several seconds after cue onset, have primarily been reported in those studies in which the participants were required to make a speeded detection (rather than discrimination) response to the target stimulus. That said, the intramodal visual cuing literature would certainly appear to suggest that crossmodal IOR ought to be observed at longer SOAs in speeded discrimination tasks as well (see Lupiáñez, Milán, Tornay, Madrid, and Tudela 1998).

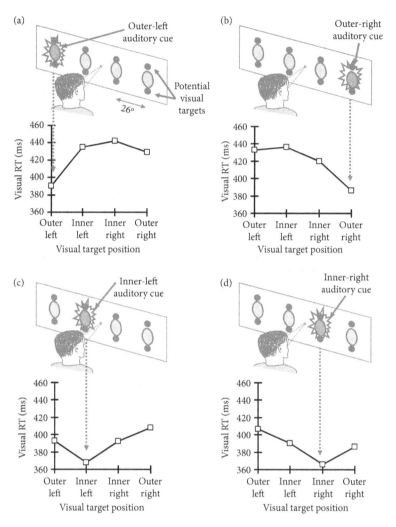

FIGURE 16.1 (a–d) Schematic experimental set-up, plus results, from a study designed to investigate the spatial specificity of auditory cuing effects on visual elevation discrimination responses (Driver and Spence 1998). On each trial, a spatially non-predictive auditory cue was presented randomly from one of the four loudspeaker cones sketched at the top of each panel (these loudspeakers were evenly spaced with 26° between neighbouring columns). A visual target, defined as the offset of any one of the 8 LEDs situated immediately above and below each loudspeaker, was presented 100–150 ms later (requiring an elevation discrimination response of 15° vertically). The auditory cue did not predict the location of the subsequent visual target on each trial. The four graphs illustrate the results (reaction times in the visual up/down task) after: (a) an outer-left auditory cue; (b) an outer-right auditory cue; (c) an inner-left auditory cue; and (d) an inner-right auditory cue. Despite the fact that audition was completely irrelevant to the participant's visual task, visual performance was nevertheless faster (and tended to be more accurate) when the immediately preceding sound came from the same lateral location as the visual target within its hemifield (see dotted arrow pointing to the visual eccentricity with best performance in each graph). Reproduced from Spence, C., McDonald, J., and Driver, J. Exogenous spatial cuing studies of human crossmodal attention and multisensory integration. In C. Spence and J. Driver (Eds.), Crossmodal Space and Crossmodal Attention, pp. 277–320, figure 11.2 © 2004, Oxford University Press with permission.

Perhaps the best-studied example of exogenous crossmodal spatial attentional orient-ing relates to the consequences of presenting task-irrelevant peripheral auditory cues (normally presented from the left or right of fixation) on visual perception. Crossmodal spatial attentional cuing effects can influence visual processing in a number of ways (McDonald, Teder-Sälejärvi, and Hillyard 2000; Spence and Driver 1997). Peripheral auditory cues, for example, have been shown to enhance the apparent contrast of visual targets, with changes in perceived contrast correlating positively with enlargements of the contralateral neural response (P1 and N1) starting within 100 ms of stimulus onset (Störmer, McDonald, and Hillyard 2009). Crossmodal spatial attentional cuing can also speed up the neural processing of visual target stimuli (this is the prior entry effect; see Spence and Parise 2010, for a review; though see also McDonald, Teder-Sälejärvi, Di Russo, and Hillyard 2005; Schneider and Bavelier 2003). That said, there is quite some debate about whether such crossmodal effects are best conceptualized in terms of exogenous spatial attention or in terms of multisensory integration (see Bolognini, Frassinetti, Serino, and Làdavas 2005; Macaluso, Frith, and Driver 2000a; McDonald, Teder-Sälejärvi, and Ward 2001).

It may well be that both accounts provide appropriate explanations for the data that have been collected by various researchers at different SOAs and using somewhat differ-ent experimental paradigms. For example, those studies that have documented maximal crossmodal exogenous spatial cuing effects when the onset of the cue precedes that of the target by several hundred milliseconds would appear more consistent with the pres-entation of the cue triggering a shift of spatial attention that facilitates the participant's perception of the subsequently presented target. By contrast, those studies in which the maximal cuing effects appear to occur when the cue and target stimuli are presented near simultaneously would appear more consistent with an explanation in terms of mul-tisensory integration instead (Lu, Tse, Dosher, Lesmes, Posner, and Chu 2009; Spence et al. 2004). We will return later to the long-standing and thorny issue of whether spatial attention modulates multisensory integration and/or whether instead shifts of spatial attention may themselves be directed to specific locations as a result of the multisensory integration of unimodal signals.

It has frequently been argued in the literature that crossmodal exogenous spatial ori-enting occurs automatically. Now, while different researchers often appear to mean quite different things by the term 'automatic' (e.g. see Santangelo and Spence 2008: Section 2), with some using the term to refer to phenomena that are unaffected by the performance of another task and others using the term to refer to phenomena that are not under vol-untary control, what is clear is that when a participant's attentional resources are engaged with a demanding central task (such as monitoring a rapid serial presentation stream for a target), then the peripheral presentation of an auditory, visual, or tactile cue fails to exogenously capture spatial attention. That said, if a spatially congruent multisensory cue is presented, it will capture a participant's attention no matter what the central task hap-pens to be (see Spence 2010a, for a review). This seems to be true for audiovisual, visuo-tactile, and audiotactile cue combinations (see also Van der Burg, Olivers, Bronkhorst, and Theeuwes 2008a). It appears as though multisensory spatial coincidence is capable of capturing a person's attention in a way that unisensory cues (or even spatially misaligned multisensory cues) simply cannot (see Ho, Santangelo, and Spence 2009).

However, that said, under those conditions in which a participant's task involves searching for a visual target in a complex (and potentially densely crowded) visual search display, precisely co-locating an auditory or tactile cue with a visual target turns out not to be absolutely necessary. In fact, several studies have demonstrated that presenting a temporally synchronous auditory cue will facilitate a participant's performance in a variety of different visual search tasks, even when the cue and target stimuli happen to be presented from very different spatial positions (e.g. Ngo, Pierce, and Spence 2012; Van der Burg, Olivers, Bronkhorst, and Theeuwes 2008b, 2009; Van der Burg, Talsma, Olivers, Hickey, and Theeuwes 2011; see also Matusz and Eimer 2011). There is, however, an interesting dissociation here: when the auditory stimuli are potentially task-relevant it appears as though spatial coincidence (of the auditory and visual stimuli) is not such an important factor in terms of modulating participants' behavioural performance (see Ngo and Spence 2010a, 2010b). Determining why exactly it is that exact co-location turns out to be critical in certain studies/tasks but not in others will certainly be an interesting area for future research (Spence 2013): one possibly important factor here is whether the participant (or the participant's brain) happens to treat the component unimodal stimuli as relating to each other (as in the visual search studies) versus treats them as referring to separate unisensory events (as possibly the case in crossmodal spatial attentional cuing studies, when the location of the cue is independent of that of the target, and the cue and target presented as some variable asynchrony with respect to one another).

Researchers have used TMS in order to investigate the neural substrates underlying the crossmodal links in exogenous spatial attention that have been documented behaviourally (Chambers, Payne, and Mattingley 2007). The participants in Chambers et al.'s study were presented with a spatially non-predictive lateralized tactile or visual cue shortly before a tactile or visual target requiring the participants to make an elevation discrimination response. When TMS was delivered over the right supramarginal gyrus and over the angular gyrus, synchronously with the tactile (but not visual) cue, the magnitude of the exogenous spatial cuing effects for targets presented in both sensory modalities was significantly reduced. Such results (i.e. the fact that both intramodal and crossmodal spatial orienting were interfered with by TMS over a single site) have been taken to suggest that the right inferior parietal cortex controls exogenous shifts (both crossmodal and intramodal) of covert spatial attention.

CROSSMODAL LINKS IN ENDOGENOUS SPATIAL ORIENTING

Crossmodal links have also been demonstrated in the case of endogenous attentional orienting. So, for example, several studies have shown that people find it easier to endogenously direct their auditory, visual, and tactile spatial attention to the same side than to try and attend to one side in one sensory modality, but to the opposite side in the other modality (Spence and Driver 1996; Spence et al. 2000a; see Driver and Spence 2004, for a review). Several putative accounts for such behavioural effects have been put forward including the suggestion that there may be a supramodal attentional spotlight, or some kind of 'separable-but-linked' attentional mechanism (see Fig. 16.2). What is more, it has also been demonstrated that when a participant attempts to focus his/her spatial attention endogenously on a specific location (or side of space) in anticipation of a target being presented on that side in a particular modality (say, vision), their spatial attention is normally focused on (or oriented toward) the same side in the other modalities (e.g. touch and audition) too. This is true even when targets in the other modalities actually happen to be more likely on the opposite side of fixation (see Fig. 16.3; see Spence and Driver 1996; Spence, Pavani, and Driver 2000b). Such results are consistent with their being crossmodal links in *endogenous* spatial attention.

Importantly, however, the shifts of endogenous spatial attention that have been documented in the secondary modality generally tend to be weaker than those seen in the primary modality. Such results are entirely consistent with the hypothesis that attention is controlled by a separable-but-linked mechanism. That said, there are at least two possible reasons as to why the attentional shifts documented in the secondary modality might end up being smaller than those observed in the primary modality. First, the spatial focus of attention in the secondary modality might only have shifted part of the way (from central fixation) toward the location attended in the primary modality. Alternatively, however, the focus of attention in the secondary modality might be focused on exactly the same spatial location as that in the primary modality, but there

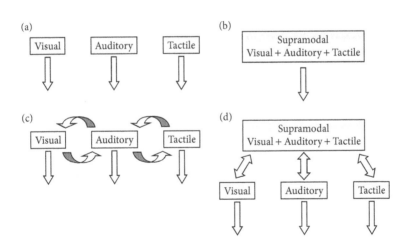

FIGURE 16.2 Schematic illustration of four different ways in which scientists have conceptualized how crossmodal attentional resources might be configured across the 'spatial' modalities of audition, vision, and touch: (a) Independent modality-specific attentional resources (Hancock, Oron-Gilad, and Szalma 2007; Wickens 1992, 2008); (b) Single supramodal attention system (Eimer and van Velzen 2002; Farah et al. 1989); (c) Separable-but-linked attentional systems (Ferlazzo et al. 2002; Spence and Driver 1996); and (d) Hierarchical supramodal plus modality-specific attentional systems (Posner 1990). Reproduced from *Scholarpedia*, 5 (5), Spence, C., Crossmodal Attention, pp. 6309 © 2010, Creative Commons License.

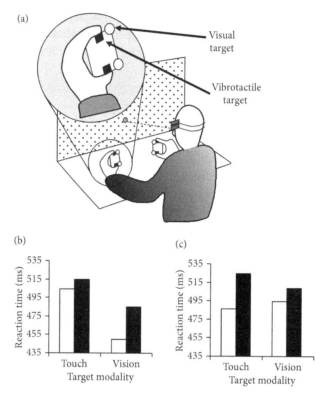

(a)

Visual
target

Vibrotactile
target

(b)

Reaction time (ms)

535
515
495
475
455
435

Touch   Vision
Target modality

(c)

Reaction time (ms)

535
515
495
475
455
435

Touch   Vision
Target modality

FIGURE 16.3 Schematic illustration of the experimental set-up, plus results, from Spence et al.'s (2000) studies probing the nature of the crossmodal links in endogenous spatial attentional orienting between touch and vision. (a) Participants fixated straight-ahead throughout each block of trials while a visual or tactile target could be presented at either an upper or lower location (see blown-up inset) near one or the other hand on each trial. In one experiment, tactile targets were much more common (thus serving as the 'primary' modality), with vision serving as the secondary modality; while in another experiment these roles were reversed. Participants reported whether each target came from an upper or lower location, regardless of its side or modality. The likely side for targets in the primary modality on each trial was manipulated on a block-by-block basis. (b and c) The results showed faster judgements (and better or equivalent accuracy) for targets in the primary modality (i.e. vision in B, and touch in C) when appearing on the cued side (empty bars), where they were most likely, than on the uncued side (filled bars). Critically, this advantage for the cued side was also found for targets in the secondary modality (i.e. vision in b, and touch in c), even though such targets were themselves more likely to appear on the *uncued* side. This again implies that a strong spatial expectancy for one (primary) modality can lead to spatially corresponding attention effects in another (secondary) modality, now extending this to the case of vision and touch; see main text for more details. Reproduced from Driver, J. and Spence, C., Crossmodal spatial attention: Evidence from human performance. In C. Spence and J. Driver (Eds.), *Crossmodal Space and Crossmodal Attention*, pp. 179–220, figure 8.6 © 2004, Oxford University Press with permission.

might be some kind of gating mechanism at play that simply attenuates spatial attention effects in the secondary modality. Elegant psychophysical research conducted by Martin Eimer and his colleagues in London has provided some support for the latter account (Eimer and Van Velzen 2005; Eimer, Van Velzen, and Driver 2004).

It is by no means easy to distinguish between the various accounts of the crossmodal links in endogenous spatial attention that have been proposed to date on the basis of behavioural/psychophysical data alone (see Driver and Spence 2004, for a review). However, the last decade or so has seen a number of studies attempting to investigate the neural substrates underlying such behavioural effects (see Spence and Driver 2004). In one influential positron emission tomography (PET) study reported by Macaluso, Frith, and Driver (2000b), participants were presented bilaterally with a stream of tactile or visual stimuli. Attending endogenously (that is, in a sustained manner) to one side or the other had consequences that were both multisensory and modality-specific. In particular, unimodal spatial attentional effects were observed in modality-specific brain areas, such as the superior occipital gyrus (for vision) and the superior postcentral gyrus (for touch). Meanwhile, multisensory spatial effects—that is, patterns of neural activation that were observed regardless of the particular modality that the participant happened to be attending to—were demonstrated in the intraparietal sulcus (a polysensory association area) and in the occipitotemporal junction. Sustained attention to one side versus the other (regardless of the sensory modality being attended) has also been shown to modulate neural activity in contralateral visual cortical areas, with such effects being somewhat more pronounced when it was the participant's visual attention that was being endogenously oriented (Macaluso, Frith, and Driver 2002b).

In another study, Kida, Inui, Wasaka, Akatsuka, Tanaka, and Kakigi (2007) looked at the magnetoencephalography (MEG) response to electrocutaneous stimuli, when their participants endogenously directed their attention to the tactile or visual stimuli presented randomly on either the left or right of fixation. The results demonstrated that neural responses close to the Sylvian fissures (bilaterally) were significantly enhanced by spatial attention 85–100 ms after stimulus onset, regardless of the modality (vision or touch) that was attended. These responses were traced to a generator in the secondary somatosensory cortex (see also Sterr, Shen, Zaman, Roberts, and Szameitat 2007).

While the authors of a number of the early neuroimaging studies in this area jumped to the conclusion that crossmodal links in endogenous spatial attention must be underpinned by some kind of supramodal attentional orienting mechanism (e.g. see Eimer and Van Velzen 2002; Macaluso et al. 2002b; Spence 2010a), the TMS research that has been published subsequently has tended to support the separable-but-linked account instead (see Fig. 16.2). So, for example, in one study, Chambers, Stokes, and Mattingley (2004) demonstrated that temporarily lesioning the supramarginal gyrus of the right inferior parietal lobe using TMS selectively reduced the magnitude of endogenous spatial cuing effects for *visual* targets, while leaving such spatial cuing effects intact when probed via the presentation of *tactile* targets. Such results, suggesting the ability to temporarily interfere with the endogenous spatial orienting of attention in a modality-specific manner, are clearly inconsistent with the supramodal account (see also Chambers et al. 2007, for evidence regarding exogenous spatial orienting). Instead, they are more consistent with the 'separable-but-linked' hypothesis (as originally suggested by Spence and Driver 1996; see also Spence, 2010b).

POSTURE CHANGE AND CROSSMODAL SPATIAL ATTENTIONAL ORIENTING

At the start of this article, evidence concerning the crossmodal consequences of the *overt* orienting of attention was reviewed. Since then, the focus has been primarily on the *covert* (i.e. in the absence of any movement of the receptors) orienting of attention instead. It is, however, important to note that the overt orienting of the eyes with respect to the head, and/or the head or hands with respect to the torso, will all likely result in a misalignment of the various sensory receptors. The obvious question to ask here, then, is whether such receptor misalignment has any consequences for the crossmodal orienting of covert spatial attention (see Pöppel 1973; Spence et al. 2004). Here, it is worth highlighting the fact that the vast majority of laboratory studies of crossmodal spatial attentional orienting have been conducted under conditions where participants were instructed *not* to move their eyes or head away from the straight-ahead position. To date, there has only been a handful of studies in which the participants have been instructed to divert their gaze, to either the left or right, while keeping their head pointing straight-ahead (see Spence et al. 2004; see also Ferlazzo, Couyoumdjian, Padovani, and Belardinelli 2002), or else to cross the hands over the midline, while keeping the eyes and head pointing forward (Spence et al. 2000b, 2008). That said, the results of the studies that have been published demonstrate that the crossmodal spatial orienting of attention that follows the presentation of a spatially non-predictive auditory, visual, or tactile cue appears to be directed to more or less the correct external location (meaning that information processing is facilitated for stimuli presented at the appropriate environmental location of the cue, regardless of the modality of the target or the posture adopted; see Fig. 16.4; Eimer, Cockburn, Smedley, and Driver 2001; Kennett, Eimer, Spence, and Driver 2001; Kennett, Spence, and Driver 2002; Macaluso, Frith, and Driver 2002a).

TEMPORAL ORIENTING OF CROSSMODAL ATTENTION

The last few years have seen growing research interest in the temporal orienting (or allocation) of crossmodal attention, both when participants are presented with relatively simple stimulus displays (Lippert, Logothetis, and Kayser 2007) and when they have to

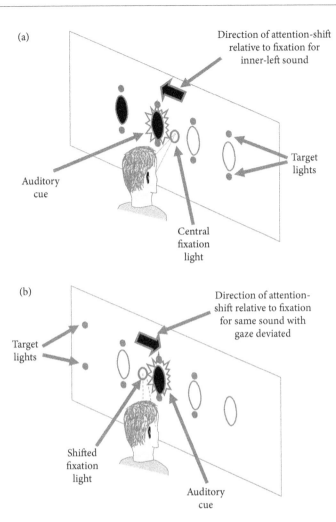

FIGURE 16.4 Illustration of Driver and Spence's (1998) manipulation of gaze-direction in their audiovisual cuing study. (a) With the eyes and head in alignment (i.e. both pointing straight-ahead, as in the majority of audiovisual spatial cuing studies, and as for Fig. 16.1 here), an auditory cue positioned to the left of the participant's head (at an inner-left location here) produces a crossmodal spatial cuing effect with most efficient visual performance at inner-left retinal locations (cf. Fig. 16.1c). But when the eyes are deviated 26° to the left of straight-ahead (as in b here) exactly the same auditory cue (still to the *left* of the participant's head) now benefits visual targets to the *right* of current fixation (i.e. in the *opposite* retinotopic direction; see white arrows). This indicates that current gaze-posture is taken into account by auditory-upon-visual exogenous spatial cuing effects. Reproduced from Spence, C., McDonald, J., and Driver, J. Exogenous spatial cuing studies of human crossmodal attention and multisensory integration. In C. Spence and J. Driver (Eds.), *Crossmodal Space and Crossmodal Attention*, pp. 277–320, figure 11.3 © 2004, Oxford University Press with permission.

search for a target in a more crowded temporal array such as in a rapid serial visual presentation stream (RSVP; e.g. Chen and Yeh 2008, 2009; Olivers and Van der Burg 2008; Vroomen and de Gelder 2000). There is, in fact, evidence to suggest that the facilitatory crossmodal effect resulting from the presentation of a task-irrelevant auditory cue when it happens to coincide temporally with the presentation of the visual target may exert its influence either by capturing a participant's attention exogenously in the temporal domain (Dalton and Spence 2007) or by providing a temporal cue that facilitates endogenous temporal orienting (see Spence and Ngo 2012, for a recent review). There is also a large, if somewhat hard to interpret, literature on the crossmodal attentional blink that is relevant here. However, I would argue that it is difficult to draw any straightforward conclusions from the published data, given the very mixed results that have been reported to date. Indeed, while some researchers have documented reliable crossmodal attentional blinks (e.g. Jolicoeur 1999; Soto-Faraco, Spence, Fairbank, Kingstone, Hillstrom, and Shapiro 2002), others have failed to document any such effect (Duncan, Martens, and Ward 1997; Soto-Faraco and Spence 2002).

ATTENTION AND MULTISENSORY INTEGRATION

One of the most hotly debated areas in multisensory research on auditory–visual interactions in recent years concerns the role of attention in multisensory integration (e.g. see Koelewijn, Bronkhorst, and Theeuwes 2010; Navarra, Alsius, Soto-Faraco, and Spence 2009, for reviews). The available behavioural evidence suggests that performance on certain tasks, such as the ventriloquism effect observed in spatial localization tasks with discrepant auditory and visual stimuli, is relatively immune to manipulations of a participant's attention, either to a sensory modality or to a spatial location (e.g. Bertelson, Vroomen, de Gelder, and Driver 2000; Vroomen, Bertelson, and de Gelder 2001; see Spence 2012). By contrast, performance in a variety of other tasks is modulated by attentional manipulations (e.g. Alsius, Navarra, Campbell, and Soto-Faraco 2005; Alsius, Navarra, and Soto-Faraco 2007; Mozolic, Hugenschmidt, Peiffer, and Laurienti 2008; Spence 2010a). So, for example, Salvador Soto-Faraco and his colleagues have demonstrated that the magnitude of audiovisual integration (as indexed by the McGurk effect; McGurk and MacDonald 1976) is modulated by the perceptual load of the visual or tactile task that the participant happens to be performing at the same time. Apparent differences in the patterns of results observed in these various studies may turn out to relate to the differing ways in which attention was manipulated (e.g. via instruction or by manipulating the perceptual load of a participant's task; see Lavie 2005; Spence 2010a). Of course, it may turn out that multisensory integration occurs more automatically for certain types (or combinations) of stimuli than for others. Indeed, audiovisual integration (e.g. for speech stimuli) has been shown to occur even when it is detrimental to a participant's performance (e.g. see Driver 1996; though note that several research groups have found it very difficult, if not impossible, to replicate this particular effect). Here, it would be interesting to determine whether the spatial (or for that matter, temporal) ventriloquism effects are modulated by variations in perceptual load.

Currently, neuroscientists are using the various techniques at their disposal to try to figure out exactly what the relation between multisensory integration and attention really is (e.g. Busse, Roberts, Crist, Weissman, and Woldorff 2005; Driver and Noesselt 2008; Fairhall and Macaluso 2009; Senkowski, Schneider, Foxe, and Engel 2008; Talsma, Doty, and Woldorff 2007; see Talsma, Senkowski, Soto-Faraco, and Woldorff 2010, for a review). The lack of a commonly agreed-upon definition of what attention is (Spence 2010b; see also Stein, Burr, Costantinides, Laurienti, Meredith, Perrault, et al. 2010) makes such a task all the more difficult. That said, research conducted using functional magnetic resonance imaging (fMRI) by Fairhall and Macaluso has suggested that spatial attention can modulate multisensory integration at multiple cortical and subcortical sites. In their study, a central auditory speech stream was presented together with two visual streams, one presented on either side of central fixation. The participants were instructed to attend to the visual stream that could either be congruent or incongruent with the auditory stream. The results revealed that attention to the congruent audiovisual speech stimuli gave rise to increased activation in multisensory association areas (the superior temporal sulcus), in early modality-specific visual cortex (striate and extrastriate retinotopic visual areas), and in subcortical structures (the superior colliculus). However, one might question whether such results should be taken to support the claim that attention drives multisensory integration or whether instead multisensory integration guides attention? It seems likely that this debate will rumble on for some years to come.

CROSSMODAL FACILITATION VERSUS CROSSMODAL COMPETITION

It is important to note that when multiple sensory stimuli compete for a person's behavioural response then crossmodal competition may ensue (Hein, Alink, Kleinschmidt, and Müller 2007a). Under certain conditions, such crossmodal competition has even been shown to lead to the *extinction* of one of the competing stimuli. While such effects have constituted a popular topic of study amongst neuroscientists interested in the consequences of brain damage for crossmodal attentional control and multisensory perception (e.g. Inhoff et al. 1992; Rapp and Hendel 2003; Sarri et al. 2006), perhaps the best-known example of crossmodal competition in neurologically normal participants comes from research on the Colavita visual dominance task (see Colavita 1974).

In a typical study of the Colavita effect, participants are presented with a random sequence of unimodal auditory and visual target stimuli. They are required to make a speeded modality-discrimination response, pressing one key in response to auditory targets and another key in response to visual targets. Occasionally, though, the auditory and visual targets are presented at the same time. On such trials, the participant is either instructed to press both response keys, or else to press a third response key (to indicate the presence of a bimodal target). The results of numerous studies using this paradigm conducted over the last 35 years or so have demonstrated that people sometimes fail to respond to the auditory target on the bimodal target trials, despite the fact that they respond near-perfectly to all of the unimodal target stimuli (see Spence, Parise, and Chen 2011, for a review). By contrast, participants never seem to miss the visual target, suggesting, once again, a kind of visual dominance.

This kind of crossmodal competition has now been documented between all pairings of auditory, visual, and tactile stimuli (Hartcher-O'Brien, Gallace, Krings, Koppen, and Spence 2008; Hecht and Reiner 2009; Occelli, Hartcher-O'Brien, Spence, and Zampini 2010). What is more, it can result in a lowering of perceptual sensitivity to stimuli in the sensory modality that ends up being extinguished (Koppen, Levitan, and Spence 2009). Perhaps surprisingly, though, it turns out that the semantic congruency between the auditory and visual target stimuli presented on the bimodal target trials does not seem to modulate the size of the Colavita visual dominance effect (see Koppen, Alsius, and Spence 2008). What is more, while directing a participant's attention toward the auditory modality reduces (and possibly even eliminates) this particular example of visual sensory dominance, it does not appear capable of reversing it (e.g. Koppen and Spence 2007; Sinnett, Spence, and Soto-Faraco 2007).

Intriguingly, one can move from a situation in which crossmodal facilitation is observed to a situation in which crossmodal competition is found simply by changing the demands of the participant's task (e.g. from the facilitation of speeded target detection in a redundant targets effect type of paradigm through to competition when the participant's task involves discriminating between the modalities of the targets that have been presented; see Sinnett, Soto-Faraco, and Spence 2008). Diaconescu, Alain, and McIntosh (2011) recently utilized MEG in order to investigate the neural circuitry underlying these differing behavioural effects. Their research highlighted a key role for early posterior parietal activity in multisensory facilitation effects (i.e. for those facilitatory effects taking place within 100 ms of stimulus onset). By contrast, multisensory conflict (elicited by presenting semantically matched stimuli—such as the sound of a barking dog being paired with a black and white line drawing of a dog—from different sides) resulted in the activation of the cingulate, temporal, and prefrontal cortices instead. It would be intriguing in future research to determine whether such crossmodal competition could be reduced, or perhaps even eliminated, simply by applying TMS to the latter sites (cf. Bien, ten Oever, Goebel, and Sack 2012).

CONCLUSIONS

The large body of research that has been published in recent years on the topic of crossmodal orienting has documented the existence of extensive crossmodal links in both overt and covert attentional orienting. *Endogenous* shifts of covert attention (either to a sensory modality or to a spatial location) speed up the relative time of arrival of attended (relative to unattended) stimuli while only having a modest impact on the salience/perceptual sensitivity of attended stimuli. By contrast, *exogenous* spatial attentional orienting enhances the perceptibility (perceived contrast) of stimuli presented at the attended location (McDonald et al. 2000; Spence and Driver 1997; Störmer et al. 2009), while at the same time giving rise to a prior entry effect (Spence and Parise 2010; though see McDonald et al. 2005). Researchers have, for many years, tended to study crossmodal links in endogenous and exogenous spatial orienting separately (sometimes coming to somewhat different conclusions regarding the nature of the underlying neural mechanisms; see Chambers et al. 2004, 2007; Spence 2010b). That said, a number of researchers have now started to investigate how these two forms of attentional orienting interact (e.g. Chica, Sanabria, Lupiáñez, and Spence 2007; Koelewijn, Bronkhorst, and Theeuwes 2009a, 2009b; Santangelo, Olivetti Belardinelli, Spence, and Macaluso 2009), as they surely must in everyday life. In the past, researchers have also tended to focus on the crossmodal orienting in the space directly in front of a participant. Interestingly though, similar links have now been demonstrated over a much wider range of spatial locations (Perrott, Cisneros, McKinley, and D'Angelo 1996; Perrott, Sadralodabai, Saberi, and Strybel 1991). Particularly interesting here is research showing the differences in the representation of space and multisensory integration of auditory and tactile signals in the region just behind the back of the head (e.g. Ho and Spence 2009; Zampini, Torresan, Spence, and Murray 2007).

One area of growing research interest relates to the question of how attention spreads across the various modality-specific features of an object (Turatto, Mazza, and Umiltà 2005) or event as a function of the semantic relationship (or crossmodal correspondence) between the component parts (Spence 2011b). It has recently been suggested, for example, that people may find it harder to attend to (and prioritize) the stimulus presented in one modality if it happens to be meaningfully related to any stimuli that are simultaneously presented in the other modalities (see Spence and Parise 2010). Certainly, the available research currently suggests that the spread of attention across pairs of simultaneously presented auditory and visual stimuli is significantly affected by their prior history of being co-presented (or paired; e.g. Baier, Kleinschmidt, and Müller 2006; Busse et al. 2005; Fiebelkorn, Foxe, and Molholm 2010; see also Hein, Doehrmann, Müller, Kaiser, Muckli, and Naumer 2007b; Zangenehpour and Zatorre 2010). It may also depend on the observer's assumption concerning whether the stimuli belong together or not—the so-called unity assumption (see Sato, Toyoizumi, and Aihara 2007; Vatakis and Spence 2007). What such results appear to demonstrate is that the crossmodal orienting of a person's attention may depend on the meaningfulness (not to mention relevance) of the stimuli that happen to be presented to them.

With this thought in mind, it is noticeable how abstract and ecologically invalid many of the stimuli used in previous crossmodal orienting studies have been (see also de Gelder and Bertelson 2003, on this point). In fact, it is surprising to see how little spatial coincidence actually matters to multisensory integration when people respond to meaningful combinations of auditory, visual, and tactile stimuli (Spence 2012). It certainly appears as though crossmodal spatial orienting effects have a more pronounced influence on people's perception and performance when space is somehow relevant to their task (see Spence 2012). Here it will also be interesting in future research to pursue the question of how crossmodal orienting effects change as a function of the ecological relevance/salience of the cue stimuli that happen to be presented (e.g. in a spatial cuing study; Ho and Spence 2008; Poliakoff, Miles, Li, and Blanchette 2007; Van Damme, Gallace, Spence, Crombez, and Moseley 2009; see also Van Damme, Crombez, and Spence 2009).

Given that the majority of studies of crossmodal orienting have been conducted in neurologically normal young adults, another area of growing research interest for the coming years will be to investigate how crossmodal orienting develops in childhood, and how (if at all) it declines in old age (see Hugenschmidt, Peiffer, McCoy, Hayasaka, and Laurienti 2009; Poliakoff, Ashworth, Lowe, and Spence 2006). Similarly, there is also widespread interest in the results of neurophysiological studies of those patients suffering from selective spatial difficulties in information processing, such as those suffering from neglect or extinction (Farah et al. 1989; Inhoff et al. 1992; Sarri et al. 2006).

In terms of the neural substrates, and consequences, of crossmodal attentional orienting, it is, by now, well established that the early neural processing of attended auditory, visual, and tactile stimuli is enhanced, while the processing of unattended distractor stimuli is simultaneously suppressed (Hairston et al. 2008). This appears to be true no matter whether attention is directed exogenously or endogenously and either when attention is directed to a sensory modality or to a specific spatial location (or hemifield). Control circuits for the strategic control of attention to stimuli in one sensory modality versus another appear to include areas such as the dorsolateral prefrontal cortex (Johnson et al. 2007). Parietal areas also appear to be engaged in the integration of auditory and visual stimuli that, for whatever reason, have fallen out of spatiotemporal alignment but which the brain appears to want to integrate/bind (e.g. Bien et al. 2012; Meienbrock, Naumer, Doehrmann, Singer, and Muckli 2007). Certainly, TMS over inferior parietal areas has been shown to interfere with multisensory perception/integration (Bien et al. 2012), while TMS over other cortical sites has been shown to interfere with attentional selection/orientation instead (e.g. Chambers et al. 2004, 2007). As this chapter has hopefully made clear, the latest techniques to emerge in the field of cognitive neuroscience are increasingly being used to further understand the networks of neural structures that determine how attention is distributed crossmodally, across space, time, and sensory modality.

NOTE

1. Note that the term 'multisensory integration' grew out of the neurophysiological research conducted at the single-cell level, and typically in the anaesthetized preparation, often in the superior colliculus, a subcortical orienting structure (see Spence 2012). This kind of research has been popularized by the work of Barry Stein and his colleagues (see Stein

and Meredith 1993; Stein et al. 2010). In recent years, many cognitive neuroscientists have attempted to determine whether the rules of multisensory integration documented at the single-cell level in the animal model can also be used to help to explain the interactions between stimuli presented in different sensory modalities that have been observed in awake humans (see Bolognini et al. 2005; Macaluso et al. 2000a, 2001; McDonald et al. 2001; Spence et al. 2004).

References

Abrams, R., Davoli, F., Du, C., Knapp, W., and Paull, D. (2008). Altered vision near the hands. *Cognition* 107: 1035–1047.

Alais, D., Morrone, C., and Burr, D. (2006). Separate attentional resources for vision and audition. *Philosophical Transactions of the Royal Society B: Biological Sciences* 273: 1339–1345.

Alsius, A., Navarra, J., Campbell, R., and Soto-Faraco, S. (2005). Audiovisual integration of speech falters under high attention demands. *Current Biology* 15: 1–5.

Alsius, A., Navarra, J., and Soto-Faraco, S. (2007). Attention to touch weakens audiovisual speech integration. *Experimental Brain Research* 183: 399–404.

Ashkenazi, A. and Marks, L. E. (2004). Effect of endogenous attention on detection of weak gustatory and olfactory flavors. *Perception & Psychophysics* 66: 596–608.

Baier, B., Kleinschmidt, A., and Müller, N. (2006). Cross-modal processing in early visual and auditory cortices depends on the statistical relation of multisensory information. *Journal of Neuroscience* 26: 12260–12265.

Bertelson, P., Vroomen, J., de Gelder, B., and Driver, J. (2000). The ventriloquist effect does not depend on the direction of deliberate visual attention. *Perception & Psychophysics* 62: 321–332.

Bien, N., ten Oever, S., Goebel, R., and Sack, A. T. (2012). The sound of size: Crossmodal binding in pitch-size synesthesia: A combined TMS, EEG, and psychophysics study. *NeuroImage* 59: 663–672.

Bolognini, N., Frassinetti, F., Serino, A., and Làdavas, E. (2005). 'Acoustical vision' of below threshold stimuli: Interaction among spatially converging audiovisual inputs. *Experimental Brain Research* 160: 273–282.

Busse, L., Roberts, K. C., Crist, R. E., Weissman, D. H., and Woldorff, M. G. (2005). The spread of attention across modalities and space in a multisensory object. *Proceedings of the National Academy of Sciences USA* 102: 18751–18756.

Chambers, C. D., Payne, J. M., and Mattingley, J. B. (2007). Parietal disruption impairs reflexive spatial attention within and between sensory modalities. *Neuropsychologia* 45: 1715–1724.

Chambers, C. D., Stokes, M. G., and Mattingley, J. B. (2004). Modality-specific control of strategic spatial attention in parietal cortex. *Neuron* 44: 925–930.

Chen, Y. C. and Yeh, S. L. (2008). Visual events modulated by sound in repetition blindness. *Psychonomic Bulletin & Review* 15: 404–408.

Chen, Y.-C. and Yeh, S.-L. (2009). Catch the moment: Multisensory enhancement of rapid visual events by sound. *Experimental Brain Research* 198: 209–219.

Chica, A., Sanabria, D., Lupiáñez, J., and Spence, C. (2007). Comparing intramodal and crossmodal cuing in the endogenous orienting of spatial attention. *Experimental Brain Research* 179: 353–364, 531.

Colavita, F. B. (1974). Human sensory dominance. *Perception & Psychophysics* 16: 409–412.

Dalton, P. and Spence, C. (2007). Attentional capture in serial audiovisual search tasks. *Perception & Psychophysics 69*: 422–438.

De Gelder, B. and Bertelson, P. (2003). Multisensory integration, perception and ecological validity. *Trends in Cognitive Sciences 7*: 460–467.

Diaconescu, A. O., Alain, C., and McIntosh, A. R. (2011). The co-occurrence of multisensory facilitation and cross-modal conflict in the human brain. *Journal of Neurophysiology 106*: 2896–2909.

Driver, J. (1996). Enhancement of selective listening by illusory mislocation of speech sounds due to lip-reading. *Nature 381*: 66–68.

Driver, J. and Noesselt, T. (2008). Multisensory interplay reveals crossmodal influences on 'sensory-specific' brain regions, neural responses, and judgments. *Neuron 57*: 11–23.

Driver, J. and Spence, C. (1998). Attention and the crossmodal construction of space. *Trends in Cognitive Sciences 2*: 254–262.

Driver, J. and Spence, C. (2004). Crossmodal spatial attention: Evidence from human performance. In C. Spence and J. Driver (eds.), *Crossmodal Space and Crossmodal Attention* (pp. 179–220). Oxford: Oxford University Press.

Dufour, A. and Touzalin, P. (2008). Improved sensitivity in the perihand space. *Experimental Brain Research 190*: 91–98.

Duncan, J., Martens, S., and Ward, R. (1997). Restricted attentional capacity within but not between sensory modalities. *Nature 387*: 808–810.

Eimer, M., Cockburn, D., Smedley, B., and Driver, J. (2001). Cross-modal links in endogenous spatial attention are mediated by common external locations: Evidence from event-related brain potentials. *Experimental Brain Research 139*: 398–411.

Eimer, M. and Van Velzen, J. (2002). Crossmodal links in spatial attention are mediated by supramodal control processes: Evidence from event-related potentials. *Psychophysiology 39*: 437–449.

Eimer, M. and Van Velzen, J. (2005). Spatial tuning of tactile attention modulates visual processing within hemifields: An ERP investigation of crossmodal attention. *Experimental Brain Research 166*: 402–410.

Eimer, M., Van Velzen, J., and Driver, J. (2004). ERP evidence for cross-modal audiovisual effects of endogenous spatial attention within hemifields. *Journal of Cognitive Neuroscience 16*: 272–288.

Fairhall, S. L. and Macaluso, E. (2009). Spatial attention can modulate audiovisual integration at multiple cortical and subcortical sites. *European Journal of Neuroscience 29*: 1247–1257.

Farah, M. J., Wong, A. B., Monheit, M. A., and Morrow, L. A. (1989). Parietal lobe mechanisms of spatial attention: Modality-specific or supramodal? *Neuropsychologia 27*: 461–470.

Ferlazzo, F., Couyoumdjian, A., Padovani, T., and Belardinelli, M. O. (2002). Head-centered meridian effect on auditory spatial attention orienting. *Quarterly Journal of Experimental Psychology (A) 55*: 937–963.

Ferris, T. K. and Sarter, N. B. (2008). Cross-modal links among vision, audition, and touch in complex environments. *Human Factors 50*: 17–26.

Fiebelkorn, I. C., Foxe, J. J., and Molholm, S. (2010). Dual mechanisms for the cross-sensory spread of attention: How much do learned associations matter? *Cerebral Cortex 20*: 109–120.

Gray, R., Mohebbi, R., and Tan, H. Z. (2009). The spatial resolution of crossmodal attention: Implications for the design of multimodal interfaces. *ACM Transactions on Applied Perception 6*: 1–14.

Hairston, W. D., Hodges, D. A., Casanova, R., Hayasaka, S., Kraft, R., Maldjian, J. A., and Burdette, J. H. (2008). Closing the mind's eye: Deactivation of visual cortex related to auditory task difficulty. *NeuroReport 19*: 151–154.

Hancock, P. A., Oron-Gilad, T., and Szalma, J. L. (2007). Elaborations of the multiple-resource theory of attention. In A. F. Kramer, D. A. Wiegmann, and A. Kirlik (eds.), *Attention: From Theory to Practice* (pp. 45–56). Oxford: Oxford University Press.

Hari, R. and Jousmäki, V. (1996). Preference of personal to extrapersonal space in a visuomotor task. *Journal of Cognitive Neuroscience 8*: 305–307.

Hartcher-O'Brien, J., Gallace, A., Krings, B., Koppen, C., and Spence, C. (2008). When vision 'extinguishes' touch in neurologically-normal people: Extending the Colavita visual dominance effect. *Experimental Brain Research 186*: 643–658.

Hartcher-O'Brien, J., Levitan, C., and Spence, C. (2010). Out-of-touch: Does vision dominate over touch when it occurs off the body? *Brain Research 1362*: 48–55.

Hecht, D. and Reiner, M. (2009). Sensory dominance in combinations of audio, visual and haptic stimuli. *Experimental Brain Research 193*: 307–314.

Hein, G., Alink, A., Kleinschmidt, A., and Müller, N. G. (2007a). Competing neural responses for auditory and visual decisions. *PLoS One 3*: e320.

Hein, G., Doehrmann, O., Müller, N. G., Kaiser, J., Muckli, L., and Naumer, M. J. (2007b). Object familiarity and semantic congruency modulate responses in cortical audiovisual integration areas. *Journal of Neuroscience 27*: 7881–7887.

Ho, C., Santangelo, V., and Spence, C. (2009). Multisensory warning signals: When spatial correspondence matters. *Experimental Brain Research 195*: 261–272.

Ho, C. and Spence, C. (2008). *The Multisensory Driver: Implications for Ergonomic Car Interface Design*. Aldershot: Ashgate Publishing.

Ho, C. and Spence, C. (2009). Using peripersonal warning signals to orient a driver's gaze. *Human Factors 51*: 539–556.

Hugenschmidt, C. E., Peiffer, A. M., McCoy, T. P., Hayasaka, S., and Laurienti, P. J. (2009). Preservation of crossmodal selective attention in healthy aging. *Experimental Brain Research 198*: 273–285.

Inhoff, A. W., Rafal, R. D., and Posner, M. I. (1992). Bimodal extinction without cross-modal extinction. *Journal of Neurology, Neurosurgery, & Psychiatry 55*: 36–39.

Johnson, J. A., Strafella, A. P., and Zatorre, R. J. (2007). The role of the dorsolateral prefrontal cortex in bimodal divided attention: Two transcranial magnetic stimulation studies. *Journal of Cognitive Neuroscience 19*: 907–920.

Johnson, J. A. and Zatorre, R. J. (2005). Attention to simultaneous unrelated auditory and visual events: Behavioral and neural correlates. *Cerebral Cortex 15*: 1609–1620.

Johnson, J. A. and Zatorre, R. J. (2006). Neural substrates for dividing and focusing attention between simultaneous auditory and visual events. *NeuroImage 31*: 1673–1681.

Jolicoeur, P. (1999). Restricted attentional capacity between sensory modalities. *Psychonomic Bulletin & Review 6*: 87–92.

Just, M. A., Kellar, T. A., and Cynkar, J. (2008). A decrease in brain activation associated with driving when listening to someone speak. *Brain Research 1205*: 70–80.

Kawashima, R., O'Sullivan, B. T., and Roland, P. E. (1995). Positron-emission tomography studies of cross-modality inhibition in selective attentional tasks: Closing the 'mind's eye'. *Proceedings of the National Academy of Sciences USA 92*: 5969–5972.

Kennett, S., Eimer, M., Spence, C., and Driver, J. (2001). Tactile–visual links in exogenous spatial attention under different postures: Convergent evidence from psychophysics and ERPs. *Journal of Cognitive Neuroscience 13*: 462–478.

Kennett, S., Spence, C., and Driver, J. (2002). Visuo-tactile links in covert exogenous spatial attention remap across changes in unseen hand posture. *Perception & Psychophysics 64*: 1083–1094.

Kida, T., Inui, K., Wasaka, T., Akatsuka, K., Tanaka, E., and Kakigi, R. (2007). Time-varying cortical activations related to visual–tactile cross-modal links in spatial selective attention. *Journal of Neurophysiology* 97: 3585–3596.

Klein, R. (2000). Inhibition of return. *Trends in Cognitive Sciences* 4: 138–147.

Koelewijn, T., Bronkhorst, A., and Theeuwes, J. (2009a). Competition between auditory and visual spatial cues during visual task performance. *Experimental Brain Research* 195: 593–602.

Koelewijn, T., Bronkhorst, A., and Theeuwes, J. (2009b). Auditory and visual capture during focused visual attention. *Journal of Experimental Psychology: Human Perception and Performance* 35: 1303–1315.

Koelewijn, T., Bronkhorst, A., and Theeuwes, J. (2010). Attention and the multiple stages of multisensory integration: A review of audiovisual studies. *Acta Psychologica* 134: 372–384.

Koppen, C., Alsius, A., and Spence, C. (2008). Semantic congruency and the Colavita visual dominance effect. *Experimental Brain Research* 184: 533–546.

Koppen, C., Levitan, C., and Spence, C. (2009). A signal detection study of the Colavita effect. *Experimental Brain Research* 196: 353–360.

Koppen, C. and Spence, C. (2007). Assessing the role of stimulus probability on the Colavita visual dominance effect. *Neuroscience Letters* 418: 266–271.

Larsen, A., McIlhagga, W., Baert, J., and Bundesen, C. (2003). Seeing or hearing? Perceptual independence, modality confusions, and crossmodal congruity effects with focused and divided attention. *Perception & Psychophysics* 65: 568–574.

Laurienti, P. J., Burdette, J. H., Wallace, M. T., Yen, Y.-F., Field, A. S., and Stein, B. E. (2002). Deactivation of sensory-specific cortex by cross-modal stimuli. *Journal of Cognitive Neuroscience* 14: 1–10.

Lavie, N. (2005). Distracted and confused? Selective attention under load. *Trends in Cognitive Sciences* 9: 75–82.

Lippert, M., Logothetis, N. K., and Kayser, C. (2007). Improvement of visual contrast detection by a simultaneous sound. *Brain Research* 1173: 102–109.

Lu, Z. L., Tse, H. C., Dosher, B. A., Lesmes, L. A., Posner, C., and Chu, W. (2009). Intra- and crossmodal cuing of spatial attention: Time courses and mechanisms. *Vision Research* 49: 1081–1096.

Lupiáñez, J., Milán, E. G., Tornay, F. J., Madrid, E., and Tudela, P. (1998). Does IOR occur in discrimination tasks? Yes, it does, but later. *Perception & Psychophysics* 59: 1241–1254.

Macaluso, E., Frith, C., and Driver, J. (2000a). Modulation of human visual cortex by cross-modal spatial attention. *Science* 289: 1206–1208.

Macaluso, E., Frith, C., and Driver, J. (2000b). Selective spatial attention in vision and touch: Unimodal and multimodal mechanisms revealed by PET. *Journal of Neurophysiology* 83: 3062–3075.

Macaluso, E., Frith, C. D., and Driver, J. (2001). A reply to J. J. McDonald, W. A. Teder-Sälejärvi, and L. M. Ward, Multisensory integration and crossmodal attention effects in the human brain. *Science* 292: 1791.

Macaluso, E., Frith, C. D., and Driver, J. (2002a). Crossmodal spatial influences of touch on extrastriate visual areas take current gaze direction into account. *Neuron* 34: 647–658.

Macaluso, E., Frith, C. D., and Driver, J. (2002b). Supramodal effects of covert spatial orienting triggered by visual or tactile events. *Journal of Cognitive Neuroscience* 14: 389–401.

McDonald, J. J., Teder-Sälejärvi, W. A., Di Russo, F., and Hillyard, S. A. (2005). Neural basis of auditory-induced shifts in visual time-order perception. *Nature Neuroscience* 8: 1197–1202.

McDonald, J. J., Teder-Sälejärvi, W. A., and Hillyard, S. A. (2000). Involuntary orienting to sound improves visual perception. *Nature 407*: 906–908.

McDonald, J. J., Teder-Sälejärvi, W. A., and Ward, L. M. (2001). Multisensory integration and crossmodal attention effects in the human brain. *Science 292*: 1791.

McGurk, H. and MacDonald, J. (1976). Hearing lips and seeing voices. *Nature 264*: 746–748.

Makin, T. R., Holmes, N. P., and Ehrsson, H. H. (2008). On the other hand: Dummy hands and peripersonal space. *Behavioural Brain Research 191*: 1–10.

Matusz, P. J. and Eimer, M. (2011). Multisensory enhancement of attentional capture in visual search. *Psychonomic Bulletin & Review 18*: 904–909.

Meienbrock, A., Naumer, M. J., Doehrmann, O., Singer, W., and Muckli, L. (2007). Retinotopic effects during spatial audio-visual integration. *Neuropsychologia 45*: 531–539.

Miles, E., Brown, R. J., and Poliakoff, E. (2011). Investigating the nature and time-course of the modality shift effect between vision and touch. *Quarterly Journal of Experimental Psychology 64*: 871–888.

Mozolic, J. L., Hugenschmidt, C. E., Peiffer, A. M., and Laurienti, P. J. (2008). Modality-specific selective attention attenuates multisensory integration. *Experimental Brain Research 184*: 39–52.

Navarra, J., Alsius, A., Soto-Faraco, S., and Spence, C. (2009). Assessing the role of attention in the audiovisual integration of speech. *Information Fusion 11*: 4–11.

Ngo, M. K. and Spence, C. (2010a). Auditory, tactile, and multisensory cues facilitate search for dynamic visual stimuli. *Attention, Perception, & Psychophysics 72*: 1654–1665.

Ngo, M. and Spence, C. (2010b). Crossmodal facilitation of masked visual target identification. *Attention, Perception, & Psychophysics 72*: 1938–1947.

Ngo, M. K., Pierce, R., and Spence, C. (2012). Utilizing multisensory cues to facilitate air traffic management. *Human Factors 54*: 1093–1103.

Occelli, V., Hartcher O'Brien, J., Spence, C., and Zampini, M. (2010). Assessing the audiotactile Colavita effect in near and rear space. *Experimental Brain Research 203*: 517–532.

Olivers, C. N. L. and Van der Burg, E. (2008). Bleeping you out of the blink: Sound saves vision from oblivion. *Brain Research 1242*: 191–199.

Otten, L. J., Alain, C., and Picton, T. W. (2000). Effects of visual attentional load on auditory processing. *NeuroReport 11*: 875–880.

Perrott, D. R., Cisneros, J., McKinley, R. L., and D'Angelo, W. (1996). Aurally aided visual search under virtual and free-field listening conditions. *Human Factors 38*: 702–715.

Perrott, D. R., Saberi, K., Brown, K., and Strybel, T. Z. (1990). Auditory psychomotor coordination and visual search performance. *Perception & Psychophysics 48*: 214–226.

Perrott, D. R., Sadralodabai, T., Saberi, K., and Strybel, T. Z. (1991). Aurally aided visual search in the central visual field: Effects of visual load and visual enhancement of the target. *Human Factors: The Journal of the Human Factors and Ergonomics Society 33*: 389–400.

Poliakoff, E., Ashworth, S., Lowe, C., and Spence, C. (2006). Vision and touch in ageing: Crossmodal selective attention and visuotactile spatial interactions. *Neuropsychologia 44*: 507–517.

Poliakoff, E., Miles, E., Li, X., and Blanchette, I. (2007). The effect of visual threat on spatial attention to touch. *Cognition 102*: 405–414.

Pöppel, E. (1973). Comments on 'Visual system's view of acoustic space'. *Nature 243*: 231.

Posner, M. I. (1978). *Chronometric Explorations of Mind*. Hillsdale, N.J.: Erlbaum.

Posner, M. I. (1990). Hierarchical distributed networks in the neuropsychology of selective attention. In A. Caramazza (ed.), *Cognitive Neuropsychology and Neurolinguistics: Advances in Models of Cognitive Function and Impairment* (pp. 187–210). Hillsdale, N.J.: Erlbaum.

Prime, D. J., McDonald, J. J., Green, J., and Ward, L. M. (2008). When crossmodal attention fails: A controversy resolved? *Canadian Journal of Experimental Psychology* 62: 192–197.

Prinzmetal, W., McCool, C., and Park, S. (2005). Attention: Reaction time and accuracy reveal different mechanisms. *Journal of Experimental Psychology: General* 134: 73–92.

Prinzmetal, W., Park, S., and Garrett, R. (2005). Involuntary attention and identification accuracy. *Perception & Psychophysics* 67: 1344–1353.

Rapp, B. and Hendel, S. K. (2003). Principles of cross-modal competition: Evidence from deficits of attention. *Psychonomic Bulletin & Review* 10: 210–219.

Reed, C. L., Grubb, J. D., and Steele, C. (2006). Hands up: Attentional prioritization of space near the hand. *Journal of Experimental Psychology: Human Perception and Performance* 32: 166–177.

Rees, G., Frith, C., and Lavie, N. (2001). Processing of irrelevant visual motion during performance of an auditory attention task. *Neuropsychologia* 39: 937–949.

Rorden, C. and Driver, J. (1999). Does auditory attention shift in the direction of an upcoming saccade? *Neuropsychologia* 37: 357–377.

Rorden, C., Greene, K., Sasine, G. M., and Baylis, G. C. (2002). Enhanced tactile performance at the destination of an upcoming saccade. *Current Biology* 12: 1–6.

Santangelo, V., Olivetti Belardinelli, M., Spence, C., and Macaluso, E. (2009). Multisensory interactions between voluntary and stimulus-driven spatial attention mechanisms across sensory modalities. *Journal of Cognitive Neuroscience* 21: 2384–2397.

Santangelo, V. and Spence, C. (2008). Is the exogenous orienting of spatial attention truly automatic? Evidence from unimodal and multisensory studies. *Consciousness and Cognition* 17: 989–1015.

Sarri, M., Blankenburg, F., and Driver, J. (2006). Neural correlates of crossmodal visual-tactile extinction and of tactile awareness revealed by fMRI in a right-hemisphere stroke patient. *Neuropsychologia* 44: 2398–2410.

Sato, Y., Toyoizumi, T., and Aihara, K. (2007). Bayesian inference explains perception of unity and ventriloquism aftereffect: Identification of common sources of audiovisual stimuli. *Neural Computation* 19: 3335–3355.

Schneider, K. A. and Bavelier, D. (2003). Components of visual prior entry. *Cognitive Psychology* 47: 333–366.

Senkowski, D., Schneider, T. R., Foxe, J. J., and Engel, A. K. (2008). Crossmodal binding through neural coherence: Implications for multisensory processing. *Trends in Neurosciences* 31: 401–409.

Shiffrin, R. M. and Grantham, D. W. (1974). Can attention be allocated to sensory modalities? *Perception & Psychophysics* 15: 460–474.

Shomstein, S. and Yantis, S. (2004). Control of attention shifts between vision and audition in human cortex. *Journal of Neuroscience* 24: 10702–10706.

Sinnett, S., Soto-Faraco, S., and Spence, C. (2008). The co-occurrence of multisensory competition and facilitation. *Acta Psychologica* 128: 153–161.

Sinnett, S., Spence, C., and Soto-Faraco, S. (2007). Visual dominance and attention: The Colavita effect revisited. *Perception & Psychophysics* 69: 673–686.

Soto-Faraco, S. and Spence, C. (2002). Modality-specific auditory and visual temporal processing deficits. *Quarterly Journal of Experimental Psychology (A)* 55: 23–40.

Soto-Faraco, S., Spence, C., Fairbank, K., Kingstone, A., Hillstrom, A. P., and Shapiro, K. (2002). A crossmodal attentional blink between vision and touch. *Psychonomic Bulletin & Review* 9: 731–738.

Spence, C. (2010a). Crossmodal spatial attention. *Annals of the New York Academy of Science (The Year in Cognitive Neuroscience)* 1191: 182–200.

Spence, C. (2010b). Crossmodal attention. *Scholarpedia* 5(5): 6309. doi: 10.4249/scholarpedia.6309.

Spence, C. (2011a). Mouth-watering: The influence of environmental and cognitive factors on salivation and gustatory/flavour perception. *Journal of Texture Studies* 42: 157–171.

Spence, C. (2011b). Crossmodal correspondences: A tutorial review. *Attention, Perception, & Psychophysics* 73: 971–995.

Spence, C. (2012). Multisensory perception, cognition, and behavior: Evaluating the factors modulating multisensory integration. In B. E. Stein (ed.), *The New Handbook of Multisensory Processing* (pp. 241–264). Cambridge, Mass.: MIT Press.

Spence, C. (2013). Just how important is spatial coincidence to multisensory integration? Evaluating the spatial rule. *Annals of the New York Academy of Sciences* 1296: 31–49.

Spence, C. and Driver, J. (1996). Audiovisual links in endogenous covert spatial attention. *Journal of Experimental Psychology: Human Perception and Performance* 22: 1005–1030.

Spence, C. and Driver, J. (1997). Audiovisual links in exogenous covert spatial orienting. *Perception & Psychophysics* 59: 1–22.

Spence, C. and Driver, J. (eds.) (2004). *Crossmodal Space and Crossmodal Attention*. Oxford: Oxford University Press.

Spence, C., Lloyd, D., McGlone, F., Nicholls, M. E. R., and Driver, J. (2000a). Inhibition of return is supramodal: A demonstration between all possible pairings of vision, touch and audition. *Experimental Brain Research* 134: 42–48.

Spence, C., McDonald, J., and Driver, J. (2004). Exogenous spatial cuing studies of human crossmodal attention and multisensory integration. In C. Spence and J. Driver (eds.), *Crossmodal Space and Crossmodal Attention* (pp. 277–320). Oxford: Oxford University Press.

Spence, C. and Ngo, M. K. (2012). Does attention or multisensory integration explain the crossmodal facilitation of masked visual target identification? In B. E. Stein (ed.), *The New Handbook of Multisensory Processing* (pp. 345–358). Cambridge, Mass.: MIT Press.

Spence, C., Nicholls, M. E. R., and Driver, J. (2001a). The cost of expecting events in the wrong sensory modality. *Perception & Psychophysics* 63: 330–336.

Spence, C. and Parise, C. (2010). Prior entry. *Consciousness and Cognition* 19: 364–379.

Spence, C., Parise, C., and Chen, Y.-C. (2011). The Colavita visual dominance effect. In M. M. Murray and M. Wallace (eds.), *Frontiers in the Neural Bases of Multisensory Processes* (pp. 523–550). Boca Raton, Fla.: CRC Press.

Spence, C., Pavani, F., and Driver, J. (2000b). Crossmodal links between vision and touch in covert endogenous spatial attention. *Journal of Experimental Psychology: Human Perception and Performance* 26: 1298–1319.

Spence, C., Pavani, F., Maravita, A., and Holmes, N. P. (2008). Multi-sensory interactions. In M. C. Lin and M. A. Otaduy (eds.), *Haptic Rendering: Foundations, Algorithms, and Applications* (pp. 21–52). Wellesley, Mass.: A K Peters.

Spence, C., Shore, D. I., and Klein, R. M. (2001b). Multimodal prior entry. *Journal of Experimental Psychology: General* 130: 799–832.

Stein, B. E., Burr, D., Costantinides, C., Laurienti, P. J., Meredith, A. M., Perrault, T. J., et al. (2010). Semantic confusion regarding the development of multisensory integration: A practical solution. *European Journal of Neuroscience* 31: 1713–1720.

Stein, B. E. and Meredith, M. A. (1993). *The Merging of the Senses.* Cambridge, Mass.: MIT Press.

Sterr, A., Shen, S., Zaman, A., Roberts, N., and Szameitat, A. (2007). Activation of SI is modulated by attention: A random effects fMRI study using mechanical stimuli. *NeuroReport* 18: 607–611.

Störmer, V. S., McDonald, J. J., and Hillyard, S. A. (2009). Cross-modal cueing of attention alters appearance and early cortical processing of visual stimuli. *Proceedings of the National Academy of Sciences USA* 106: 22456–22461.

Talsma, D., Doty, T. J., and Woldorff, M. G. (2007). Selective attention and audiovisual integration: Is attending to both modalities a prerequisite for early integration? *Cerebral Cortex* 17: 691–701.

Talsma, D., Senkowski, D., Soto-Faraco, S., and Woldorff, M. G. (2010). The multifaceted interplay between attention and multisensory integration. *Trends in Cognitive Sciences* 14: 400–410.

Turatto, M., Benso, F., Galfano, G., Gamberini, L., and Umilta, C. (2002). Non-spatial attentional shifts between audition and vision. *Journal of Experimental Psychology: Human Perception and Performance* 28: 628–639.

Turatto, M., Galfano, G., Bridgeman, B., and Umiltà, C. (2004). Space-independent modality-driven attentional capture in auditory, tactile and visual systems. *Experimental Brain Research* 155: 301–310.

Turatto, M., Mazza, V., and Umiltà, C. (2005). Crossmodal object-based attention: Auditory objects affect visual processing. *Cognition* 96: B55–B64.

Valenza, N., Murray, M. M., Ptak, R., and Vuilleumier, P. (2004). The space of senses: Impaired crossmodal interactions in a patient with Balint syndrome after bilateral parietal damage. *Neuropsychologia* 42: 1737–1748.

Van Damme, S., Crombez, G., and Spence, C. (2009). Is the visual dominance effect modulated by the threat value of visual and auditory stimuli? *Experimental Brain Research* 193: 197–204.

Van Damme, S., Gallace, A., Spence, C., Crombez, G., and Moseley, G. L. (2009). Does the sight of physical threat induce a tactile processing bias? Modality-specific attentional facilitation induced by viewing threatening pictures. *Brain Research* 1253: 100–106.

Van der Burg, E., Olivers, C. N. L., Bronkhorst, A. W., and Theeuwes, J. (2008a). Audiovisual events capture attention: Evidence from temporal order judgments. *Journal of Vision* 8(5): 2.1–10.

Van der Burg, E., Olivers, C. N. L., Bronkhorst, A. W., and Theeuwes, J. (2008b). Non-spatial auditory signals improve spatial visual search. *Journal of Experimental Psychology: Human Perception and Performance* 34: 1053–1065.

Van der Burg, E., Olivers, C. N. L., Bronkhorst, A. W., and Theeuwes, J. (2009). Poke and pop: Tactile-visual synchrony increases visual saliency. *Neuroscience Letters* 450: 60–64.

Van der Burg, E., Talsma, D., Olivers, C. N. L., Hickey, C., and Theeuwes, J. (2011). Early multisensory interactions affect the competition among multiple visual objects. *NeuroImage* 55: 1208–1218.

Van Vleet, T. M. and Robertson, L. C. (2006). Cross-modal interactions in time and space: Auditory influences on visual attention in patients with hemispatial neglect. *Journal of Cognitive Neuroscience* 18: 1368–1379.

Vatakis, A. and Spence, C. (2007). Crossmodal binding: Evaluating the 'unity assumption' using audiovisual speech stimuli. *Perception & Psychophysics* 69: 744–756.

Vibell, J., Klinge, C., Zampini, M., Spence, C., and Nobre, A. C. (2007). Temporal order is coded temporally in the brain: Early ERP latency shifts underlying prior entry in a crossmodal temporal order judgment task. *Journal of Cognitive Neuroscience* 19: 109–120.

Vroomen, J., Bertelson, P., and de Gelder, B. (2001). The ventriloquist effect does not depend on the direction of automatic visual attention. *Perception & Psychophysics 63*: 651–659.

Vroomen, J. and de Gelder, B. (2000). Sound enhances visual perception: Cross-modal effects of auditory organization on vision. *Journal of Experimental Psychology: Human Perception and Performance 26*: 1583–1590.

Wickens, C. D. (1992). *Engineering Psychology and Human Performance*, 2nd edn. New York: HarperCollins.

Wickens, C. D. (2008). Multiple resources and mental workload. *Human Factors 50*: 449–454.

Wright, R. D. and Ward, L. M. (2008). *Orienting of Attention*. Oxford: Oxford University Press.

Zampini, M., Shore, D. I., and Spence, C. (2005). Audiovisual prior entry. *Neuroscience Letters 381*: 217–222.

Zampini, M., Torresan, D., Spence, C., and Murray, M. M. (2007). Audiotactile multisensory interactions in front and rear space. *Neuropsychologia 45*: 1869–1877.

Zangenehpour, S. and Zatorre, R. J. (2010). Cross-modal recruitment of primary visual cortex following brief exposure to bimodal audiovisual stimuli. *Neuropsychologia 48*: 591–600.

CHAPTER 17

NEURONAL DYNAMICS AND THE MECHANISTIC BASES OF SELECTIVE ATTENTION

CHARLES E. SCHROEDER, JOSE L. HERRERO, AND SASKIA HAEGENS

INTRODUCTION

In traditional models, sensory processing begins when a stimulus initiates activity in peripheral sensory receptors. Over a population of receptors, activation results in a volley of activity that penetrates the brain along multiple parallel neuronal pathways that course through subcortical relays and then through a hierarchy of cortical regions. The initial encoding of a stimulus by different classes of receptors provides a virtual 'riot' of input signals, which in general are carried centrally by dedicated neuronal pathways, such as the parvocellular (P) and magnocellular (M) divisions of the primary visual pathways (Ungerleider and Mishkin 1982). The patterns of feedforward and feedback connections between neurons which bridge each ascending step in a pathway produce convergence and/or divergence of these signals during their transit through the synaptic stages of the ascending systems (Felleman and Van Essen 1991). The result is progressive transformation or 'processing' of the original sensory input. Studies in the visual, auditory, and somatosensory systems of macaque monkeys have outlined many basic selectivities of sensory receptor populations, as well as subsequent signal transformations, that provide passive mechanisms for sensory processing.

Selective attention's crucial role in such an information processing scheme is obvious when we consider the magnitude of sensory input volleys set in complex natural settings. There are, for example, more than 1,000,000 output lines (axons) in each optic nerve, and more than 30,000 axons in each auditory nerve. Thus, a moderately salient stimulus that impinges on these two senses could send several million signals per second into the brain, creating an overwhelming processing bottleneck. Selective attention attacks this problem, by modulating sensory-evoked neuronal responses so as to enhance the processing of task-relevant stimuli while suppressing that of irrelevant stimuli (Desimone and Duncan 1995; Harter and Aine 1984). This 'active control' processing is essential to normal perception and cognition because it enables information processing to adapt to the immediate goals of the observer.

Early electrophysiological studies in humans clearly recognized several varieties of selective attention, most notably spatial and feature attention (Harter et al. 1982; Parasuraman and Davies 1984), and these were later explored in detail by seminal studies using single-unit recordings in monkeys (Moran and Desimone 1985; Motter 1993; Treue and Maunsell 1996). Early studies in humans also recognized the conceptual necessity of distinguishing selective attention from non-specific arousal (Naatanen and Michie 1979), as well as that of separating the key components of attention (Posner 1980). These distinctions became guiding principles in the rapidly expanding study of attention, and helped shape the exploration of mechanistic issues such as top-down control, and local modulatory control of specific ascending circuits (Desimone and Duncan 1995; Maunsell 1995; Schroeder et al. 2001); they are expanded in several of the accompanying chapters in this volume.

This chapter will focus on recent conceptual and empirical developments in four areas that we think have significantly advanced the discussion and debate on the mechanistic underpinnings of selective attention: (1) the role of neuronal oscillations, (2) the distinctions between differing modes of dynamic operation, (3) potentially unique roles of specific oscillatory frequencies, and (4) the neurochemistry of attention.

NEURONAL OSCILLATIONS AS INSTRUMENTS OF BRAIN OPERATION

Based on recordings in rabbit optic tract over 75 years ago, Bishop (1933) proposed that neuroelectric oscillations reflect rhythmic shifting of excitability in ensembles of neurons, and this fundamental proposition stands: *Neuroelectric oscillations in general reflect rhythmic fluctuations of neuronal ensembles between high and low excitability states* (Fig. 17.1). Over the ensuing decades, seminal studies by Llinas, Singer, Buzsaki, and others (Buzsaki and Draguhn 2004; Llinas 1988; Singer et al. 1990) explored the idea that *neuronal oscillations are instrumental rather than incidental to brain operations* (for recent in-depth reviews see Buzsaki 2010a; Schroeder and Lakatos 2009;Wang 2010). The question of exactly what causes neurons to oscillate and to synchronize dynamically (e.g. Kopell et al. 2011; Roopun et al. 2008b; Roopun et al. 2008a) is of fundamental importance, but beyond the scope of this discussion. However, even if only as a noise source, these excitability fluctuations have an undeniable impact on sensory processing, and mounting evidence points to their potential causal relationships with cognitive operations. While much of the focus in this arena is on the functional role of

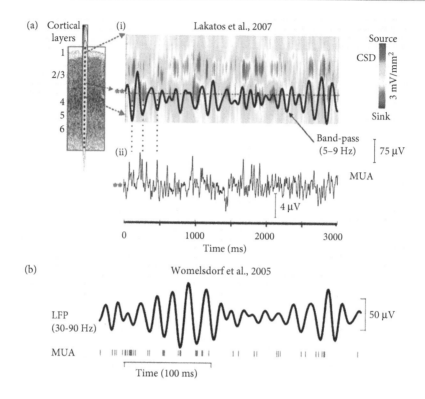

FIGURE 17.1 Coupling of excitability and oscillatory phase: (a) (i) Theta-band (5–9 Hz band pass) oscillatory activity from a lower supragranular site in primary auditory cortex (asterisks at left) superimposed on the underlying current source density (CSD) profile for the supragranular layers. Net outward transmembrane current flow generates net extracellular current sources (blue), whereas net inward current flow generates current sinks (red). The theta oscillation at this site represents the 'underside' of the superficial current dipole so that negative deflections correspond to current sinks and positive deflections reflect current sources, alternating at a theta rhythm. (ii) Multiunit activity (MUA) simultaneously recorded from the same site. Drop lines are provided to show the relationship between the initial three negative deflections/sinks at this site and MUA correlates. Note that current sinks and sources correspond to MUA peaks and troughs, indicating alternations in local neuronal excitability. Reprinted from *Neuron*, 53 (2), Peter Lakatos, Chi-Ming Chen, Monica N. O'Connell, Aimee Mills, and Charles E. Schroeder, Neuronal Oscillations and Multisensory Interaction in Primary Auditory Cortex, pp. 279–92, Copyright (2007), with permission from Elsevier. (b) Relation between gamma-band (30–90 Hz) oscillatory phase and neuronal firing (MUA) from a recording in macaque visual area V4. Vertical lines at the bottom represent occurrence of action potentials. Reprinted by permission from Macmillan Publishers Ltd: *Nature*, 439 (7077), Thilo Womelsdorf, Pascal Fries, Partha P. Mitra and Robert Desimone, Gamma-band synchronization in visual cortex predicts speed of change detection, pp. 733–736, copyright 2006).

high frequency 'gamma' oscillations (Fries et al. 2008), and this is not without controversy (e.g. Ray and Maunsell 2010), we focus on the idea that *selective attention uses low frequency neuronal oscillations in primary sensory cortices as 'instruments' for parsing complex input streams, for selecting task-relevant inputs and for amplifying their representation across processing stages* (Schroeder and Lakatos 2009). Several lines of evidence support this proposition.

Discontinuities in perception

One of the obvious reasons to think that neuronal oscillations are used in sensory processing is the long-standing impression that visual perception is 'quantized' into temporal chunks that are on the order of the period of low-frequency oscillations (Harter 1967; Harter and White 1968; Dehaene 1993). A decade ago, VanRullen and Koch (2003) suggested specifically that cortical or thalamocortical oscillations may provide a neuronal basis for these effects. More recently, VanRullen and colleagues have shown that even with a single target, visual attention appears to operate at a sampling rate of about 7 Hz (VanRullen and Koch 2003; VanRullen et al. 2007), which corresponds to the frequency of theta/alpha oscillations. In line with this idea, several studies report that the phase of ongoing oscillations predicts perceptual and attentional variability on a trial-by-trial basis. Ongoing phase, for example, has been shown to influence the neuronal response, perceptual detection, reaction times, and transcranial magnetic stimulation (TMS)-induced phosphenes (reviewed by VanRullen et al. 2011). Various low-frequency oscillations have been implicated in this, including alpha, which is thought to function as a filter to phasically suppress task-irrelevant stimuli (see below), while still letting through salient input (Jensen et al. 2012).

Rhythm in natural stimulation

Complementing the idea of 'discrete' (quantized) perception are the indications that most of the stimulation our brains receive under natural conditions is itself rhythmic. Indeed, our motor behaviour is patterned by numerous oscillatory (rhythmic) influences in the 1–4 Hz (delta), 5–8 Hz (theta), 9–12 Hz (alpha/mu), and higher (beta, etc.) ranges (review by Schroeder et al. 2010), which means that even the most static, inert objects that we 'sample' with our hands and our eyes are presented to the brain as rhythmic input. This also means that, independent of our sensory sampling routines, stimuli produced by other animals will be generally rhythmic. Vocal communication is our best-developed illustration of this point. Prosody, a key organizing element in speech perception, is conveyed at rates of 1–3 Hz (Munhall et al. 2004). Perceptually salient envelope frequencies in normal human speech are focused at the 4–8 Hz range, and many transitions within the envelope occur over 20–30 ms periods (Drullman 1995; Luo and Poeppel 2007). Strikingly, humans and other primates emit these rhythmic vocalizations while in view of their conspecifics, thus bringing vision into play, and allowing visual stimulus rhythms to predict auditory stimulus rhythms (Fig. 17.2). This has important implications for our understanding of how the brain allocates attention in time during audiovisual speech processing (Schroeder et al. 2008). All of these observations converge to suggest that sensory rhythms are likely to have a strong influence on the neural substrates of perceptual operations under normal conditions (Schroeder and Lakatos 2009).

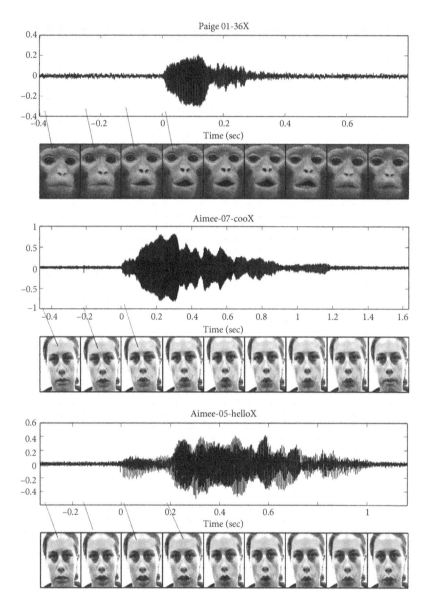

FIGURE 17.2 Visuo-auditory integration: In order for visual inputs to *predictively* modulate primary auditory processing, the ideal arrangement would be for visual inputs to arrive there before the time of auditory response onset. One factor that allows this to occur is the typical delay between visual articulatory gestures and the accompanying vocalizations (Chandrasekaran et al. 2009) . Examples of this V-A offset are illustrated here, using a monkey making an affiliative 'coo' call (top), a human imitating this monkey coo (middle), and a human making a human affiliative vocalization ('hello'—bottom). In each case, the auditory amplitude envelope of the call (sampled at 44.1 kHz) is displayed above a series of simultaneous video frames; these were acquired at 30 Hz (33.3 ms/frame), but only a key subset of the frames are shown, linked by arrows to the appropriate point in the auditory time line. The lag between the first detectable opening of the mouth and the onset of the auditory envelope function is displayed for each case (arrows and corresponding values in sec).

Mirroring of event rhythms by brain rhythms

It merits emphasis that there is a remarkable a priori match between the rhythmic structures of many behaviourally relevant events, and those of brain oscillations. The temporal structures of the three speech parameters discussed above correspond to those of delta, theta, and gamma oscillations, respectively, which are the three most prominent ambient rhythms in primary auditory cortex (Lakatos et al. 2005). Also, because of the temporal structure of vocalizations, formant and other high-frequency transitions are 'nested' within the lower frequency envelope, which is in turn nested within prosodic rate (see Schroeder et al. 2008). Significantly, this matches the hierarchical coupling pattern observed in A1, in which higher frequency amplitude is coupled to ('nested within') lower frequency phase (Lakatos et al. 2005). These parallels make brain rhythms an ideal instrument for parsing and selecting stimuli that occur in natural rhythmic event streams like natural speech. On the larger stage, dynamic cross-frequency coupling appears common to most brain regions (Bragin et al. 1995; Canolty et al. 2006; Lakatos et al. 2005), and coupling is modulated by attention (Canolty and Knight 2010; Lakatos et al. 2008), suggesting that it may represent a general computational strategy implemented by the brain to solve a range of sensory and motor problems (Burgess et al. 2007; Buzsaki and Draguhn 2004; Maurer and McNaughten 2007; Schroeder et al. 2008).

DIFFERING MODES OF OSCILLATORY OPERATION IN ATTENTIONAL SELECTION

The findings reviewed above provide reasonable, albeit indirect support for the hypothesis that oscillations are instruments of sensory selection. A central question for this hypothesis is how task demands influence the brain's oscillatory dynamics—which oscillatory tools are selected and how are they combined and applied. We have proposed (Schroeder and Lakatos 2009) that there are two modes of processing, *rhythmic* and *random/continuous* (Fig. 17.3), that these modes are implemented based on task demands, and that they determine how oscillations are used in sensory processing. Below we elaborate three key predictions of this hypothesis, and considerations that help to frame them.

Prediction 1: Entrainment promotes input amplification/suppression in rhythmic mode: When events occur in rhythmic streams (Fig. 17.3a(bottom)), low frequency oscillations entrain or phase-lock to the temporal structure of attended (Lakatos et al. 2008), or otherwise salient, 'attention-grabbing' (Lakatos et al. 2007) input. Entrainment shifts the high excitability phases of local delta oscillations, aligning them with attended events, causing amplification. At the same time, there is suppression of inputs that are 'out-of-phase' with attended events (i.e. those that occur outside of rhythmically occurring high excitability phases). These effects are illustrated in Fig. 17.4. The first point

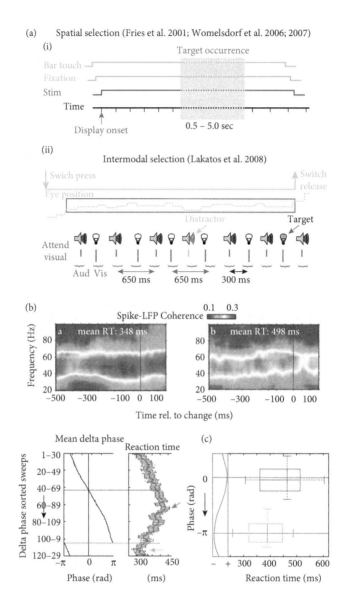

FIGURE 17.3 Random and rhythmic modes of attending: Two distinctive forms of task demand that have characteristic effects on oscillatory dynamics and behaviour. At the top is a depiction of a vigilance paradigm (i) (Fries et al. 2001b; Moran and Desimone 1985; Womelsdorf et al. 2006), and a rhythmic stream paradigm (ii) (Jones and Boltz 1989; Lakatos et al. 2008, 2009; Large and Jones 1999). In both cases the subjects make manual responses to target stimuli. The key difference is that stimuli occur randomly in the first case but are arranged in a rhythmic stream in the second. The former suppresses low-frequency oscillatory entrainment, whereas the latter facilitates it. (b) Behavioural correlates of oscillatory modulation by attention in the same two studies. Reaction time is predicted by gamma-band amplitude in the former (upper) and by delta-band phase in the latter (lower). (c) Variations in stimulus discriminability (d′) in a tone discrimination, depending on whether targets occurred in (middle) or out of phase (left and right) with an attended rhythm. Adapted from Mari Riess Jones, Heather Moynihan, Noah MacKenzie, and Jennifer Puente, *Psychological Science*, 4 (7), Temporal Aspects of Stimulus-Driven Attending in Dynamic Arrays pp. 313–19, copyright © 2002 by SAGE Publications. Reprinted by Permission of SAGE Publications.

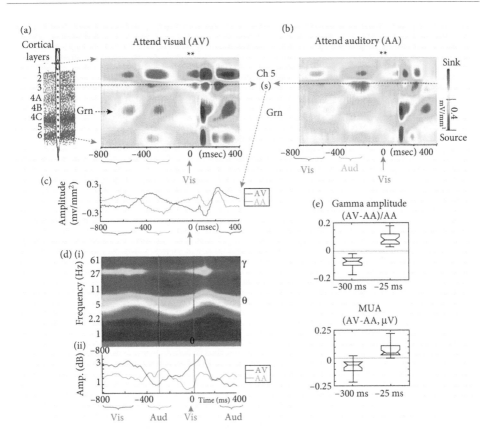

FIGURE 17.4 Attentional modulation of delta phase and its related cascade of effects. (a, b) Colour maps show average CSD profiles related to standard visual (Vis) stimuli in the attend visual (AV) and attend auditory (AA) conditions for the −800 to +400 ms time frame from a representative experiment. Red arrow indicates the visual event used as a trigger (0 ms). Blue and red brackets indicate the time frame where adjoining auditory (Aud) and visual events occur; because stimuli are jittered the responses to prior stimuli are somewhat 'smeared' over time. (c) Overlay of CSD waveforms from supragranular site (S) in the AV and AA conditions. (d) (i) Time–frequency plot of the average oscillatory amplitude of the wavelet transformed single trials from the supragranular site in (a); note variations in theta (~6 Hz) and gamma (~40 Hz) amplitudes are coupled to stimulus-entrained delta phase. (ii) An overlay of the variations in time course of averaged (37–57 Hz) gamma amplitude in the AV and AA conditions. (e) Pooled (n = 24) normalized gamma amplitude and MUA differences between AV and AA conditions ([AV−AA]/AA) for the −325 to −275 and −50 to 0 ms time frames. Notches in the boxes depict a 95% confidence interval about the median of each distribution.

to note is that low frequency fluctuations of excitability entrain to the structure of the task in both attended (Fig. 17.4a) and ignored (attend auditory—Fig. 17.4b) conditions. Importantly, those in the extragranular layers entrain in opposite phases (best seen in superimposed waveforms Fig. 17.4c) depending on which of the streams (i.e. favouring either the auditory or visual input pattern) the subjects attend to; the granular (thalamic input layers) are entrained to the visual input stream regardless of the attention condition. Another noteworthy observation is the coupling of mid (theta band) and high frequency (gamma band) oscillatory power, as well as the coupling of neuronal firing as measured by multiunit activity (MUA) to the phase of the lower frequency activity, which as mentioned first, is entrained to the tempo of the attended stream (Fig. 17.4d, e). In our framework, rhythmic mode would be the 'preferred' state of the system, in part because of its efficiency; i.e. after the high excitability phase is aligned to attended events, inputs that are out-of-phase with the attended stream (i.e. irrelevant ones) are automatically suppressed. Also, gamma band activity appears to be more metabolically demanding than low frequency oscillations (Mukamel et al. 2005; Niessing et al. 2005), and in rhythmic mode, due to hierarchical coupling (Canolty et al. 2006; Lakatos et al. 2005; review by Canolty and Knight, 2010), gamma activity is 'rationed', or selectively enhanced at time points when high excitability is most useful. At a mechanistic level, neuronal oscillations appear to provide a way for *modulatory inputs* to control the processing of *driving* inputs (using Sherman's terminology: Sherman and Guillery 2002). That is, a modulatory input by itself does not cause a response (e.g. it produces no change in action potentials), but it can reset local oscillations to a high excitability phase so that accompanying sensory (driving) inputs are amplified (Lakatos et al. 2007, 2009). It is worth noting that an oscillation can also be reset to its low excitability phase (Lakatos et al. 2007). In theory, this would have the immediate effect of suppressing a coincident driving input, but could also produce anticipatory increase in excitability for events that are predicted to occur at a later time point. Unfortunately, while rhythmic entrainment effects are widespread, they are generally not analysed. In monkey selective attention studies, lower frequencies are usually ignored. However, when the paradigm entails predictable rhythmic stimulation, their influence can still be detected as a slow variation of gamma amplitude/synchrony and/or neuronal firing, entrained to stimulation. For example, Fig. 17.2a vs. 2b of Ghose and Maunsell (2002) shows attentional enhancement of the coupling of firing rate to a 4 Hz contrast alternation in the stimuli. Similarly, Fig. 17.4 of Taylor et al. (2005) shows coupling of high-gamma power to an underlying 0.7 Hz task rhythm. Finally, Fig. 17.3 of Saalmann et al. (2007a) shows coupling of gamma coherence to a 1 Hz task structure. The reason these effects are obvious is that attentive processing increases the ambient coupling of both gamma amplitude and unit firing rates with the phase of an underlying lower (theta, delta, or sub-delta) frequency (Canolty and Knight 2010). In human psychophysical and electrophysiological studies, attentional entrainment to an anticipated rhythm affects d' measures for targets that are 'on' versus 'off' rhythm (Jones and Boltz 1989; Large and Jones 1999; Large and Snyder 2009; Stefanics et al. 2010); an effect of this sort was shown above (Fig. 17.3). Prior studies in primary sensory cortices (above) already provide strong support for Prediction 1; however, if selection via entrained oscillations is a general strategy in sensory processing it should be reflected at additional levels of the system. While this notion already has some indirect support (Buffalo et al. 2011), it clearly will require further investigation.

Prediction 2: Random, non-rhythmic operation entails low frequency suppression. It is at first paradoxical that selective attention appears to both suppress delta oscillations

(Fries et al. 2001), and to use them as an instrument of response amplification (above). However, as proposed recently (Schroeder and Lakatos 2009), it is likely that low frequency suppression in Fries et al. (2001) is due simply to the use of a 'vigilance' paradigm, in which the occurrence of target stimuli is completely unpredictable. When there is no task-relevant rhythm to entrain them, low frequency oscillations are actually detrimental to processing, as by definition, they entail relatively long periods of low excitability during which detection of a subtle random stimulus would be less likely. Under these conditions, a continuous (vigilance) mode of operation is implemented, low frequency oscillations are suppressed, and the system is pushed as well as possible into a continuous state of high excitability. Brain–behaviour relationships support the differentiation of the continuous and rhythmic processing modes. In continuous/vigilance mode (delta suppression), variations in gamma power/synchrony predict reaction time variations (Womelsdorf et al. 2006), while in rhythmic mode, where attentional modulation harnesses low frequency rhythmic entrainment, variations of delta phase predict reaction time variations, as well as gamma amplitude modulation (Lakatos et al. 2008). These behavioural and neural effects are shown in Figs. 17.3 and 17.4, respectively. It is worth pointing out that even in its most intense form, continuous mode processing may entail only a relative suppression of low frequency oscillatory rhythms (Schroeder and Lakatos 2009); this 'residual' low frequency modulation can be seen in a subtle variation (rolling) over time in gamma band amplitude and centre frequency (Fig. 17.3b). We think that is because the rhythmic oscillatory mode is the preferred mode of the system, and thus has to be actively, and often incompletely, suppressed. Consistent with this idea, it is predicted that during continuous mode operation, there will be periodic spontaneous lapses into rhythmic mode, evidenced by lapses in behavioural responding and phasic increase in low frequency power.

Prediction 3: Characteristics of inter-ensemble communication vary with rhythmicity. Specifically, the functional coupling of neuronal ensemble activity across cortical layers, and across cortical areas (reflecting the strength of a sensory representation) should differ significantly between rhythmic and continuous modes. A notable feature of attention-induced oscillatory entrainment in V1 is that it is biased to the extragranular, particularly the supragranular layers (Lakatos et al. 2008; i.e. Layers 2/3 [red lines in Fig. 17.4a, b; overlay in c] entrain to attended stimuli, and thus are in phase opposition across conditions [Fig. 17.4c], while Layer 4 ['Grn' in Fig. 17.4a, b] remains phase-locked to visual stimulation, regardless of attention condition). In other words, attention is in a position to control transmission from Layer 4 to 2/3 using phase coherence and opposition. While it may be that gamma band oscillations have a special role in cross-areal communication, as embodied in the 'Communication through Coherence' model (Fries 2005), there is good evidence that cross-areal phase coherence at different frequencies reflects differing aspects and scales of brain operation (Leopold et al. 2003; Singer 1999; Von Stein and Sarntheim 2000). For example, different parts of the gamma/beta bands could be specialized for top-down and bottom-up communications between frontal and parietal cortices (Buschman and Miller 2007); at least during random mode operations. In Saalmann et al. (2007b), the electrophysiological measurement that appears coupled to the low frequency rhythm is cross-areal coherence, and it clearly extends down to sub-gamma frequencies, though the delta band was not analysed. Thus, we predict that in rhythmic processing, delta band cross-layer and cross-areal coherence will increase with attention, facilitating transient coherence increase in coupled higher frequency bands, and multiunit activity. In continuous mode, the strength of cross-laminar and cross-areal interactions will be more constant, with random decreases related to lapses of attention.

Unique Roles for Specific Oscillatory Frequencies: The Question of Alpha

An important question that arises here is whether specific oscillatory frequencies have unique roles in brain operations. The foregoing discussion carries the obvious implication that delta and theta band dynamics may be special when it comes to parsing natural event streams, and there is strong evidence for this proposition (Besle et al. 2011; Lakatos et al. 2008, 2009, 2013; Zion-Golumbic et al. 2013; Stefanics et al. 2010). Several recent reviews have addressed the question of whether gamma and beta oscillations are prime mediators of feedforward and feedback processes respectively (Engel and Fries 2010; Fries 2005; Siegel et al. 2012). The question remains highly controversial, particularly since it is clear that the overall dynamics of oscillatory activity are themselves likely to be *dynamic*, if, as we discuss above, the oscillatory frequencies and constraints that the brain implements depend on the rhythms and predictabilities inherent in the task at hand. We focus here on another controversy in the field, the idea that alpha oscillations may play a special role in attentional suppression of task-irrelevant sensory input. The somatosensory or rolandic alpha is traditionally known as the mu rhythm, which is sometimes defined as a combination of the alpha and beta bands. As here we are specifically referring to the 10 Hz rhythm being a general mechanism throughout the brain, we will use the term 'alpha' for all sensory systems.

The prominent occipital alpha rhythm was first recorded by Hans Berger (1929) and long considered to reflect cortical idling (Adrian and Matthews 1934; Pfurtscheller et al. 1996). More recent evidence has suggested that alpha oscillations actually play an important and active role in cognitive processing (Cooper et al. 2003; Jensen and Mazaheri 2010; Klimesch et al. 2007). In particular, alpha activity is proposed to reflect a mechanism of (phasic) attentional inhibition (Jensen et al. 2012; Mathewson et al. 2011), which serves to suppress irrelevant and distracting stimuli. In this view, alpha activity decreases to facilitate processing in task-relevant (attended) regions, whereas it increases to actively inhibit interference from task-irrelevant (unattended) regions.

Both alpha power and phase are relevant in this regard. The phasic (or pulsed) inhibition hypothesis of alpha proposes that alpha suppresses neuronal processing at its peaks, while still providing windows of opportunity at its troughs during which processing can occur (Mathewson et al. 2011). These windows represent the 'duty cycle', and their length depends on the alpha amplitude (Jensen et al. 2012). Thus, alpha works as a

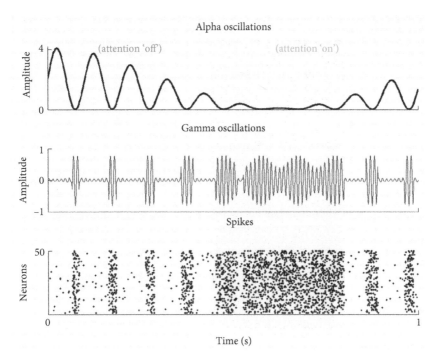

FIGURE 17.5 Phasic inhibition. Alpha band oscillations fluctuate over time (upper panel; simulated data), thereby modulating neuronal processing as reflected by gamma band activity (middle panel) and spikes (lower panel). Neuronal processing is strong when alpha amplitude is low, and during a certain phase of the alpha cycle. The green time window reflects a period of strong attention and thus low alpha activity, whereas the yellow time window shows a non-attended period with strong alpha activity.

kind of 'windscreen wiper', with the amount of wiping dependent upon the amplitude. With low alpha amplitude, processing (in terms of spikes or gamma oscillations) can occur throughout most of the cycle, whereas with a higher alpha amplitude, processing is limited to a short duty cycle in the trough of the oscillation and only salient activity survives. This provides a flexible gating mechanism that can be applied in a gradual way, adapting the amount of (unattended) information that is allowed through (Fig. 17.5). Via top-down control of both alpha power and phase, one would have an effective mechanism for sampling and filtering sensory inputs.

The role of alpha activity in sensory processing has been studied in two main ways: by looking at the influence of spontaneous fluctuations in ongoing alpha activity on sensory detection, or by employing a cued-attention paradigm and studying the top-down modulation of alpha and its consequences. Evidence from various paradigms and sensory modalities will be discussed below.

Alpha power

The study of spontaneous fluctuations in ongoing oscillatory activity starts from the premise that these oscillations reflect the internal state of the sensory systems prior to perception and are relevant for subsequent processing of external information. In this view, ongoing (intrinsic) alpha reflects the current state of arousal or vigilance. Several studies have shown that spontaneous fluctuations in ongoing alpha activity predict detection of near-threshold visual (Ergenoglu et al. 2004; Hanslmayr et al. 2007, 2011; Van Dijk et al. 2008) and tactile stimuli (Linkenkaer-Hansen et al. 2004; Zhang and Ding 2010), with lower (or intermediate) alpha levels related to better perceptual performance. These results support the notion that the alpha rhythm reflects the state of the brain in terms of arousal level, and influences processing ability.

In cued-attention paradigms, one aims to influence alpha levels by instructing the subject what/where to attend. In this view, alpha reflects a more specific anticipatory attention. Traditionally, most of the studies on alpha have focused on visual spatial attention, showing that alpha oscillations in visual cortex reflect the focus of attention (Worden et al. 2000). Anticipatory alpha activity decreases contralateral to the attended location (Sauseng et al. 2005; Thut et al. 2006) and increases contralateral to the ignored location (Fu et al. 2001; Kelly et al. 2006; Rihs et al. 2007, 2009; Worden et al. 2000). The latter effect is often (but not exclusively) observed in demanding paradigms that include distractors on the ipsilateral side. Importantly, lateralized alpha activity correlates with visual detection performance (Gould et al. 2011; Thut et al. 2006), suggesting it has behaviourally relevant consequences.

Recently, it was reported that this functionality of alpha can be generalized to the somatosensory system (Anderson and Ding 2011; Haegens et al. 2011a, 2012; Jones et al. 2010; Van Ede et al. 2011). Thus, also in tactile spatial attention, alpha lateralizes to reflect the focus of attention and influences detection performance. Indeed, the alpha lateralization exceeds a mere left vs. right pattern: Jones et al. (2010) looked at attention towards hand vs. foot, and previous studies have suggested a 'centre–surround' pattern of alpha modulation for directing focal attention (Pfurtscheller and Lopes da Silva 1999; Suffczynski et al. 2001). A recent study using an auditory spatial attention paradigm suggests that a similar alpha modulation pattern may occur in the auditory modality (Banerjee et al. 2011). Furthermore, alpha does not only reflect spatial attention, but can also be modulated by temporal expectations, such that alpha modulation peaks right before the anticipated stimulus (Rohenkohl and Nobre 2011; Van Ede et al. 2011). The temporal specificity seems to be in the order of a couple of alpha cycles. Additionally, alpha modulation was observed in a feature-based attention paradigm (Snyder and Foxe 2010). Thus, the inhibitory role of alpha seems to generally apply to attentional modulation evidences shown here are mainly in the random mode in the sensory systems, with increased alpha power reflecting active suppression and reduced alpha power reflecting engagement of the respective region, with subsequent consequences for sensory processing.

Alpha phase

Not only alpha power, also alpha phase modulates neuronal processing. It was shown that the phase of ongoing alpha oscillations predicts visual perception (Busch et al. 2009; Mathewson et al. 2009). These studies looked at the (random) phase of the alpha cycle at which the stimulus happened to be presented. By post-hoc sorting of trials based on stimulus detection, they showed that when a stimulus was presented in the alpha trough, it was more likely to be detected than when it happened to coincide with the alpha peak. In another study, it was shown that alpha phase can be entrained by rhythmic visual stimulation, and that presentation of a target in the (induced) optimal phase improves detection performance compared to suboptimal phase (Mathewson et al. 2010). These results confirm the hypotheses on phasic inhibition by alpha (Jensen et al. 2012; Klimesch et al. 2007; Mathewson et al. 2011). Another implication of these ideas would be that, when stimuli are presented in a temporally predictable fashion (i.e. not jittered), alpha-phase reset could be utilized by the brain to optimize the alpha phase in which the stimulus is going to fall, i.e. trough for a target and peak for a distractor. Indeed, Bonnefond and Jensen (2012) find that in anticipation of a strong distractor, alpha phase is adjusted in order to protect working memory maintenance.

In addition to these studies linking detection performance to alpha phase upon stimulus presentation, there are several studies looking at alpha phase and neuronal processing. Indeed, if alpha phase is relevant for performance, it should be so via modulation of the actual neuronal processing underlying that detection performance. Recordings in monkeys provide direct evidence for the phasic modulation of task-related neuronal activity by alpha oscillations (Bollimunta et al. 2008; Buffalo et al. 2011; Haegens et al. 2011b; Bollimunta et al. 2011; Mo et al. 2011). It was shown that, in addition to a negative correlation between alpha power and spike firing rates, firing is modulated by the phase of the alpha rhythm, with the lowest firing rate at the alpha peak (Haegens et al. 2011b; Bollimunta et al. 2011). Furthermore, combined EEG–fMRI studies show a relationship between alpha phase and the blood oxygen level-dependent (BOLD) response (Scheeringa et al. 2011). Visual stimuli presented at the peak of the alpha cycle yielded a lower BOLD response in early visual cortex than stimuli arriving at the alpha trough. Overall, these findings indicate that alpha oscillations reflect cyclical fluctuations in local neuronal excitability and that alpha phase has a crucial impact on the temporal patterning of excitation and inhibition in neuronal processing of information.

Alpha generation and modulation

Surprisingly, the physiological mechanisms underlying the alpha rhythm remain poorly understood. While most previous work on alpha oscillations has focused on functional aspects—correlating alpha oscillations with cognitive functions and performance— relatively few studies have been devoted to the physiological mechanisms generating the alpha rhythm. Traditionally, alpha was thought to be a purely thalamocortical rhythm. However, this view was contested by studies showing independent local cortical alpha generators (Bollimunta et al. 2008, 2011; Lopes da Silva et al. 1973, 1980; Mo et al. 2011). It is likely that both thalamic and cortical generators interact to produce cortical alpha oscillations. Indeed, thalamus generates alpha oscillations which have been linked to cortical alpha activity (Lopes da Silva et al. 1980; Lorincz et al. 2009; Saalmann and Kastner 2011; Saalmann et al. 2012). Investigation of the laminar distribution of alpha oscillations in cortical areas V1, V2, V4, and inferotemporal (IT) cortex generally shows current generators grouped in the supragranular, granular, and infragranular layers (Bollimunta et al. 2008, 2011; Mo et al. 2011). However, there may be some disagreement on this point, as a report by another group suggests a weighting of spike-field in the lower frequencies, including alpha band, toward the infragranular layers (Buffalo et al. 2011). In any case, the general patterns of inter-laminar interactions in the alpha band using Granger causality analyses (Bollimunta et al. 2008, 2011; Mo et al. 2011) point to both cortico–cortical and thalamic driving of cortical alpha oscillations. It is clear from these studies that attention modulates the impact of alpha oscillations on cortical excitability, but it remains unknown what the respective contribution is of thalamic vs. cortical alpha generators in the context of attention, and how exactly these two interact.

In addition to the question of the location of alpha generators, there is the question of which specific neuronal networks drive alpha. Early work suggested Layer 5 pyramidal cells as cortical pacemakers for alpha (Steriade et al. 1990). These excitatory cells receive inhibitory feedback from GABA-ergic interneurons, and computational modelling shows this interaction can, in principle, produce alpha oscillations (Jones et al. 2000; Roopun et al. 2010). As similar networks have also been implicated in the generation of gamma (Jones et al. 2000; Roopun et al. 2010; Whittington et al. 2000), additional research will be necessary to resolve their overlap and differences, e.g. which neuronal properties lead to one rhythm rather than another, and whether these networks employ different types of interneurons.

As to the driving of cortical alpha oscillations, it was recently shown that thalamocortical interactions, involving the pulvinar, modulate alpha coherence in visual cortex depending on attentional demands (Saalmann et al. 2012). Based on this work, pulvinar joins the non-specific thalamic projections (matrix) as an important player in regulation of cortical synchrony (Schroeder and Lakatos 2009), and perhaps for regulation of cortical alpha synchrony in particular.

Regarding cortico–cortical modulation, it is suggested that (pre-) frontal control regions exert a top-down influence on alpha activity in sensory regions (Ungerleider and Kastner 2000). Indeed, Capotosto and colleagues (Capotosto et al. 2009) showed that TMS interference with preparatory activity in frontoparietal cortex (FEF and IPS) disrupted anticipatory occipital alpha lateralization and impaired behavioural performance in a visual spatial attention task. Interestingly, even this influence may be at least partially mediated through thalamic circuits (Zikopoulos and Barbas 2006; Zikopoulos and Barbas 2007b).

Remaining questions include, what are the underlying physiological mechanisms involved in this modulation? It is conceivable that synchronization or (cross-frequency) oscillatory coupling between the regions involved could function as a top-down control mechanism. What is the role of phasic vs. tonic neuromodulation in this context? Further, if alpha phase is indeed an important way to modulate processing and suppress irrelevant input, it will be important to define the mechanism causing alpha phase reset.

To conclude, there is substantial evidence supporting alpha's role as a mechanism of attentional suppression of task-irrelevant sensory input. Future work should focus on the physiological mechanisms underlying the generation and modulation of the alpha rhythm, and its interaction with other oscillations and spikes. An important question is how general this mechanism is throughout the brain, and how it relates to other low frequency attentional mechanisms.

Neurochemistry of
Attention: Cholinergic Modulation
of Glutamatergic Processes

Clearly, there are numerous neurotransmitters that likely play a role in attention, most notably glutamate, gamma amino butyric acid (GABA), noradrenaline (NE), and acetylcholine (ACh). We focus on the ACh system as it is a reasonably well-developed theme in attention research.

Recent findings support the idea that cortical cholinergic inputs mediate essential aspects of attentional modulation of information processing (Everitt and Robbins 1997; Hasselmo and McGaughy 2004; Parikh and Sarter 2008; Yu and Dayan 2002). In tasks that do not explicitly tax attentional processes, removal of forebrain cholinergic neurons does not have strong effects on the performance of animals. Examples are the only small impairments found in the matching-to-place task in the Morris water maze (Baxter et al. 1995), in the ability to learn this task (Frick et al. 2004), in the radial arm maze (Galani et al. 2002), in the T-maze alternation task (Galani et al. 2002; Pang and Nocera 1999), and visual scene learning (Browning et al. 2010). On the other hand, strong impairments are found in tasks that explicitly tax attentional processes (Dalley et al. 2001; Kozak et al. 2006; Passetti et al. 2000; Sarter et al. 2006; Botly and De 2009). Several microdialysis studies indicate that levels of cortical ACh release in attentional task-performing animals vary as a function of the task load (Dalley et al. 2001; Kozak et al. 2006; Passetti et al. 2000; Sarter et al. 2006). Animals performing behavioural procedures that controlled for non-cognitive performance variables, such as lever pressing and reward rates, or the presentation of stimuli and distractors in contexts that do not require attention, do not find concomitant increases in cortical ACh release (Arnold et al. 2003; Himmelheber et al. 1997).

A recent microdialysis study using enzyme-coated electrodes (Parikh et al. 2007) indicates changes in cholinergic modulation on a timescale of seconds. On a sustained attention task in rats, the authors found cue-evoked cholinergic transients in prefrontal cortex in trials yielding hits (ITI is 9 seconds on average). It is important to note that the sustained attention task may correspond reasonably to the random or vigilance mode of attending discussed above. In this task, there was a steep increase in cholinergic activity that lagged the onset of the cue by 2–3 seconds, and it was not observed in (1) missed trials, (2) trials with reward but no cue, and (3) before the cue–reward contingency was learned. However, these changes triggered by sensory cues do not occur in hit trials that are followed by another hit trial (see also Howe et al. 2010; Parikh et al. 2007). The authors explained the effect by a lack of *reorienting*, attributing cholinergic transients to the need for reorienting attentional resources (towards a new target port) rather than non-specific *alerting* mechanisms. The noradrenergic system has been proposed to contribute to alerting (Posner 1980; Witte and Marrocco 1997). However, interactions between the different neuromodulatory systems likely occur. In addition, alerting and reorienting are not independent functions, suggesting that a tonic component of cholinergic neurotransmission may be necessary for both (Briand et al. 2007; Dalley et al. 2001).

In line with this idea, a recent *in vitro* study (Unal et al. 2012) reported two distinct types of cholinergic neurons, one with fast spiking and adaption properties more suitable for phasic changes in cortical ACh release associated with reorienting, and another with slow firing and poor adaption dynamics which could support general arousal by maintaining tonic ACh levels. It is possible that the second type of neurons (slow firing) may be differentially important in Random Mode Tasks requiring sustained attention to unpredictably occurring stimuli (Unal et al. 2012; Womelsdorf et al. 2006), and the first type (faster firing) may be more involved in more rhythmic tasks where subjects attend to more predictable rhythmic streams of stimuli (Lakatos et al. 2008). The ideal neuromodulatory strategy in the latter would be that ACh transients are entrained at the pace of the task so that excitability is modulated 'predictively' in a way that anticipates the occurrence of the events in the task-relevant stream (both standards and targets). A key question is whether the phasic cholinergic system can modulate on the tempo required for reasonably fast (0.5–4 Hz) rhythmic entrainment. Given the rapid destruction of ACh by AChE, ACh release may be capable of fluctuating at the pace of fast stimulation rates (e.g. 5 Hz), but whether the system as a whole can modulate at that rate is unclear. Another question is whether the ACh system might be controlled such that the two types of cholinergic neurons are engaged optimally based on task demand. Addressing these questions could provide insight into the temporal resolution of cortical ACh release and its role in selective attention.

Role of ACh in Response Gain and Attention

One important question is whether the attentional modulation observed in sensory areas (e.g. increased firing rates of neurons in V1) is mediated by ACh, and which receptor types contribute to it. One study (Herrero et al. 2008) addressed this question in V1 of the macaque, and found that the amount of attentional modulation was augmented when the cholinergic system was pharmacologically enhanced. This enhancement occurred mainly through the activation of muscarinic receptors (mAChRs).

Fig. 17.6 illustrates the effect showing how cholinergic modulation of glutamatergic transmission may contribute to control of response gain (A) and attentional modulation (B) of sensory responses in V1 neurons. Note that many receptors, neurons (e.g. inhibitory interneurons), and connections are excluded for simplicity. A basic sequence of steps and some relevant details and caveats are as follows:

(1) Depolarization of thalamocortical (TC) terminals leads to glutamate release from vesicles on the presynaptic side, activating AMPA and NMDA receptors in the postsynaptic density of the cortical neuron (Fig. 17.6a).

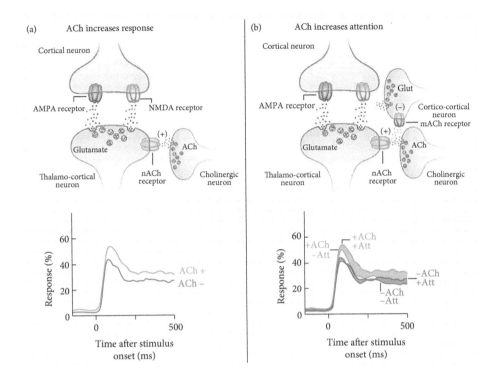

FIGURE 17.6 Mechanisms of action of ACh on response gain and attentional modulation in V1. (a) ACh increases neuronal gain. Glutamate (Glu) release from presynaptic TC terminals is modulated by ACh. ACh activates presynaptic nAChRs increasing Glu release from TC terminals (see + sign), likely contributing to larger firing rates as shown in the histograms (bottom). ACh can also activate postsynaptic mAChRs (not drawn for simplicity), likewise increasing neuronal excitability. (b) ACh increases attentional modulation (coloured shaded area shows strength of attention effect). In addition to activating presynaptic nAChRs at TC terminals, ACh can also activate presynaptic mAChRs at IC terminals. Activation of these receptors can in some cases decrease the excitability of p2/3 cells (e.g. Mrzljak et al. 1996). Thus less Glu is released from IC terminals (reducing their efficacy), while more Glu is released from TC terminals (increasing their efficacy).

(2) ACh contributes to glutamatergic transmission in a modulatory role. Depolarization of cholinergic neurons (from the NBM) leads to ACh release and activation of nAChRs located presynaptically at TC terminals. This results in further glutamate release (e.g. ACh increases $Ca+2$ influx through nAChRs and glutamate-induced depolarization); i.e. ACh modulates rather than triggers the release of glutamate. This is shown by the firing histograms (Fig. 17.6a, bottom) where application of ACh in the extracellular space of V1 neurons resulted in increased firing rates.

(3) When ACh levels are high due to the rapid activation of nAChRs, more glutamate is released, and the conductances controlled by AMPA and NMDA
receptors in the postsynaptic cortical neuron are larger. The resulting increase
in excitation of the postsynaptic cortical neuron increases its probability of firing action potentials, triggering neurotransmitter release onto downstream
neurons. This represents one mechanism by which neuronal responsiveness is
increased with visual stimulation. Additionally, this mechanism could underlie gain enhancement (Fig. 17.6b), due to increased synaptic efficacy of TC
connections (e.g. increased response reliability and signal-to-noise ratio). The
location of nAChRs, mainly in the thalamic input layers (Gil et al. 1997; Vidal
and Changeux 1993; Wonnacott 1997), makes them ideally suited for this role
(Hasselmo 2010). A number of studies suggest that selective nicotinic agonists
enhance attentional performance (Wilens et al. 1999). Herrero and colleagues
(Herrero et al. 2008) found that blockade of nAChRs reduced the overall gain
of V1 neurons but did not reduce attentional modulation, unlike blockade of
mAChRs (Fig. 17.6b, bottom).

(4) These are not necessarily opposing effects, but rather, may mean that nicotinic
and muscarinic receptors act synergistically to mediate attention effects (Ellis
et al. 2006). As shown (Fig. 17.6b), ACh boosts attention most efficiently
when two requirements are met: the synaptic efficacy of TC connections
is increased and at the same time, the synaptic efficacy of IC connections
is reduced. IC influence could be minimized by ACh acting on presynaptic mAChRs (Gil et al. 1997; Kimura 2000; Oldford and Castro-Alamancos
2003; Vidal and Changeux 1993). These studies showed that at least within
superficial cortical layers, ACh reduces glutamate release at IC synapses via
mAChRs receptors. Less glutamate release could mean less spread of excitation; however, the rapid degradation of ACh (due to ACHE action) may
prevent this effect. In any case, such ACh–Glu interactions suggest that ACh
is capable of shifting the dynamics of the cortical networks into a state where
afferent influence predominates over intracortical influence (Hasselmo and
Bower 1992; Kimura, 2000).

(5) In addition to presynaptic mAChRs, there are also postsynaptic mAChRs (not
drawn; McCormick and Prince 1986a). Activation of these channels within
supragranular layers increases neuronal excitability through blockade of several
K+ currents. This effect may contribute to the increase in firing rates observed
by Herrero and colleagues (Herrero et al. 2008) (see histograms in Fig. 17.6a),
as most recordings were from supragranular pyramidal neurons. Activation of
mAChRs on these neurons causes cell depolarization, increased excitability, and
reduced spike frequency adaptation (Herrero et al. 2008; McCormick and Prince
1986b; Mrzljak et al. 1996). The effect of ACh can be indirect however, as ACh
applied to Layer 1 interneurons can inhibit Layer 2/3 basket cells (b2/3), which
in turn would increase the excitability of pyramidal cells (p2/3) (Christophe
et al. 2002). ACh can also have opposed effects. For example, activation of

postsynaptic mAChRs on Layer 4 cells can decrease the excitability of Layer 4 neurons (Mrzljak et al. 1996), possibly reducing the excitatory feedforward drive to p2/3 cells. Additionally, a simultaneous activation of mAChRs located on interneurons would counteract the depolarization of the pyramidal cells, due to increased GABA-ergic inhibition (McCormick and Prince 1985; but note that hyperpolarization of interneurons can also occur: Xiang et al. 1998).

Synergy between cholinergic and other systems

Additional neuromodulatory systems may interact with the cholinergic system to mediate attention. Recent amperiometric studies have found that the amplitude of the cholinergic transients is determined by glutamatergic stimulation of ionotropic glutamate receptors (Howe and Purves 2005; Parikh and Sarter 2008). Projections from the thalamic mediodorsal (MD) nucleus to the PFC are mostly glutamatergic, but because there are AMPA and NMDA receptors on cholinergic terminals in PFC, glutamate is capable of modulating ACh release. In turn, ACh modulates further glutamate release through specific presynaptic ACh receptors located on MD glutamatergic terminals. These Glu–ACh interactions determine amplitude changes in ACh transients but they do not seem to play an important role in the duration and rate of ACh release (Hasselmo and Sarter 2011); these temporal parameters are sensitive to stimulation of nicotinic receptors. Parik and colleagues (Parikh et al. 2008) showed that stimulation of $\alpha 4\beta 2$ nAChR with ABT-089 results in more potent amplitude enhancement and faster signal rise time and decay rate as compared to nicotine. These results suggest that glutamatergic mechanisms mediate the cholinergic effects of nAChR agonists but that the effects tightly depend on the specific receptor type and on its kinetics. This latter point leads to the question of the experimental paradigm used. For example, when visual stimuli are presented at low frequency rates (<0.1Hz), there is no detectable increase in extracellular ACh levels in V1 (Kang and Vaucher 2009). In contrast, high frequency visual and auditory stimulation (9Hz) contributes to sensory-LTP in visual and auditory cortices (Clapp et al. 2005, 2006a), possibly through cholinergic-induced glutamatergic action. Interestingly, in the latter case there is event-related desynchronization of ongoing alpha oscillations (Clapp et al. 2006b). These results suggest different neurobiological mechanisms involved in high and low sensory stimulation, and predict interesting interactions with behaviour. One prediction is that attention in the oddball task with higher frequency stimulation rates could be enhanced by stimulation of $\alpha 4\beta 2$ nAChR but not $\alpha 7$ nAChR.

A recent study in macaque V1 (Self et al. 2012) has shown the contribution of the glutamatergic system to figure–ground segregation, a task known to recruit both feedforward and feedback projections. It was shown that blockade of AMPA receptors with CNQX strongly reduced the main stimulus-driven response of V1 neurons but it had little effect on the figure–ground modulation. In contrast, blocking NMDA receptors with APV reduced the figure–ground modulation but had little effect on the stimulus-induced activity. The authors discussed that feedback connections target synapses especially rich in NMDA receptors, whereas feedforward connections target synapses rich in AMPA receptors. The importance of NMDA receptors is not limited to figure–ground segregation, but applies to other tasks demanding feedback processing such as the antisaccade task (Skoblenick and Everling 2012). A previous paper (Herrero et al. 2008) reported that muscarinic, rather than NMDA, receptors play a role in processes involving feedback mechanisms. These are not opposed effects, rather, a synergistic role for cholinergic and NMDA mechanisms in attention is likely (Herrero et al. 2013). Recent modelling suggests that feedback targets NMDA-rich synapses and that ACh adjusts the network properties to increase the probability of this happening (Deco and Thiele 2011). Increased amounts of ACh elevate the excitability of V1 neurons, which may then allow spatially specific glutamatergic feedback to enhance specific incoming information. The PFC can exert a profound influence over the basal forebrain. The PFC projects back to the BF both directly and indirectly through the NAcc. Activation of NBM cholinergic neurons could increase tonic levels of ACh in V1, and allow spatially specific glutamatergic feedback to enhance specific incoming information. Alternatively, phasic and spatially specific releases of ACh (on top of any tonic ACh level) could also account for more rapid attention effects (Sarter et al. 2009a), and possibly also for relatively fast rhythmic modulation of excitability oscillations (Lakatos et al. 2008). According to Sarter (Sarter et al. 2009b), these phasic releases of ACh are controlled by the PFC: the glutamatergic input from the PFC would modulate the release of ACh in cholinergic terminals from the NBM. Future pharmacological studies of attentional modulation should further address these alternative possibilities, as well as studying the role of the recently described cholinergic cortical interneurons (Von et al. 2007).

Role of ACh in Neuronal Oscillations and Attention

Changes in cholinergic function produce characteristic alterations of cortical activity at the network level. Administration of cholinergic antagonists or excitotoxic lesions of cholinergic neurons in the BF increase slow-wave power and decrease high-frequency power (Buzsaki et al. 1988; Buzsaki and Gage 1989; Holschneider et al. 1998; Vanderwolf et al. 1993). They also diminish theta synchronization (Holschneider et al. 1998). Cholinergic agonists reduce slow-wave power and increase high-frequency power (Vanderwolf et al. 1993). Indirect cholinergic agonists (e.g. physostigmine, eserine) enhance the synchronization of theta activity. Cholinergic deafferentation has also been shown to impair intrahemispheric coherence in the 4–8 Hz band, consistent with the largely ipsilateral projections of cholinergic nerve fibres (Holschneider et al. 1999). Studies using electrical stimulation of the mesenphalic reticular formation (MRF) in conjunction with light stimuli found enhanced gamma oscillations and response synchronization in V1 (Herculano-Houzel et al. 1999). Another study (Rodriguez et al. 2004), used intracortical application of cholinergic drugs in V1, and showed that the MRF-induced gamma oscillations and response synchronization are reduced after blocking muscarinic receptors. Similarly, the visually induced gamma oscillations and response synchronization itself were also reduced by muscarinic blockade. The amplitude power in the gamma band was also reduced. This is contrary to a study (Kimura et al. 1999) that found systematic increases in power with muscarinic blockade, and thus contrary to the hypothesis that ACh reduces the spread of membrane voltage fluctuations (Kimura et al. 1999) and the spread of BOLD activation (Silver et al. 2008). According to the latter studies, blockade of muscarinic receptors would increase the spread of excitation, leading to an increase in LFP power. A recent *in vitro* study (Lucas-Meunier et al. 2009) found complex interactions between different types of nicotinic receptors and between deep and superficial layers in V1. One such finding was that endogenous ACh enhances inhibition by acting directly on GABA-ergic interneurons presynaptic to the recorded cell. Under such a scenario, blockade of specific nicotinic receptors would release the recorded cell from a bath of inhibition, possibly leading to increased oscillatory activity. Another study in V1 of the awake behaving monkey (Chalk et al. 2010), found that directing attention to the RF of the recorded neurons reduced the stimulus-induced LFP power and spike-field coherence in a broad range of frequency bands. This attention-induced reduction of power was counteracted by blocking muscarinic receptors: scopolamine reduced the influence of attention on LFP power (unpublished data).

CONCLUSIONS AND OPEN QUESTIONS FOR FUTURE STUDIES

Despite the fact that neuronal oscillations were first described over 80 years ago, the concerted investigation of their mechanistic role in brain operations is still a relatively young field, plagued by pitfall and uncertainty, with many more questions than answers. Going forward, several key questions are immediately obvious. Many of these, though requiring further experimentation, already have partial answers.

(1) *Do attentional entrainment effects in primary cortices generalize to higher cortical areas and to other attentional varieties?* The fact that, as discussed above, evidence of rhythmic entrainment can be seen in findings related to feature attention in V4 (Taylor et al. 2005), spatial attention in parietal areas (Saalmann et al. 2007b), and even feature discrimination nested within spatial attention in V4 (Ghose and Maunsell, 2002), indicates that generalization across higher cortical areas and varieties of attention likely does occur. The attention sensitivity of entrainment per se is supported by the observation that attention strengthens entrainment in steady-state VEP studies (Ding et al. 2006; Kim et al. 2007; Morgan et al. 1996). Most importantly, recent reports from event-related potential (ERP) studies (e.g. Stefanics et al. 2010a), and direct recordings from the cortical surface in surgical epilepsy patients (Besle et al. 2011; Zion-Golumbic et al. 2013) confirm that entrainment occurs with different varieties of attention

and on a 'network level', involving a large number of cortical (and probably subcortical) areas.

(2) *Do neuronal oscillations utilize unique cellular circuits?* The answer to this question will turn out to be nuanced. On one hand, the laminar current source and sink profiles generating field potential oscillations across most frequencies are coextensive with those generating evoked responses (Lakatos et al. 2005, 2009; Shah et al. 2004), meaning that largely the same supragranular, granular, and infragranular cell ensembles generate both phenomena. On the other hand the laminar current flow profiles of ambient oscillations and evoked responses differ in amplitude weighting due to the large flux of added power in Layer 4 in the latter (evoked) case (Shah et al. 2004). Thus, it seems that while ambient oscillations and evoked responses use that same cellular architecture, the way the local circuit is accessed and utilized is different. This idea is consistent with the observation that spontaneous activity in the auditory cortices has underlying structure that mirrors the local functional (tonotopic) organization and areal boundaries (Fukushima et al. 2012; Schroeder and Lakatos, 2012).

(3) *Can oscillatory phase reset be distinguished from an evoked response?* Again an answer to this question must be nuanced. First of all, the fact that the extragranular layers of V1 can entrain flexibly to either an auditory or a visual input stream depending on which is attended, while Layer 4 remains enslaved to visual input regardless of attention (Fig. 17.4), coupled with the fact that evoked responses to auditory stimuli have never been documented in *normal* V1, indicates that attention-related phase opposition in the extragranular layers occurs via phase-reset. Second, isolation of the initial effects of *phase-resetting*, heteromodal inputs to the uppermost layers in primary cortices (e.g. somatosensory input into auditory cortices; Lakatos et al. 2007) indicates that these inputs: (a) are not carried by the specific thalamocortical system that terminates most densely in Layer 4, but rather by non-specific, or 'matrix' thalamic projections that terminate in superficial layers (Jones 2001), and (b) reflect *modulatory* rather than *driving* inputs; i.e. they do not drive action potentials directly, but by resetting the phase of ambient oscillations, they modulate the excitability of the local neuronal ensembles in a way that modulates the probability that an appropriate, preferred sensory input will drive action potentials (Schroeder and Lakatos 2009).

(4) *Do different frequencies have distinctive laminar distributions and functions?* Based on quantification of oscillatory power/amplitude profiles for spontaneous delta, theta, alpha, beta, and gamma band activity (Lakatos et al. 2005, 2009; Rajkai et al. 2008; Shah et al. 2004; Bollimunta et al. 2008, 2011; Mo et al. 2011), this does not appear to be the case. However, a recent report indicated that higher beta and gamma frequencies may be differentially engaged in feedback versus feedforward modulation respectively (Buschman and Miller 2007), and given that feedforward and feedback terminations do have different laminar weighting patterns, differential laminar distributions of gamma and beta oscillations would be predicted. So in a sense, the question becomes: *'do different brain*

operations such as top-down and bottom-up processes operate in different frequencies?' In line with the above discussion of a special role for alpha oscillations in information processing, another recent report weighed in on the positive side of this question with the observation that *spike-field coherence* in the gamma band (putative feedforward activity) is weighted toward supragranular laminae, while that in lower frequencies (putative feedback activity) is weighted toward infragranular layers (Buffalo et al. 2011). Given these divergent sets of findings, and some obvious differences between spike-field coherence versus oscillatory power/amplitude measures, this question will require further investigation. In particular, it will be important to pay close attention to the specific mode in which attentional operations are engaged (i.e. *random* versus *rhythmic*), as mode will undoubtedly impact the utilization of the available dynamics.

(5) *How important are cortico–subcortical interactions?* Traditional models of alpha-band modulation have often considered the rhythm to be *essentially* thalamocortical (Lopes da Silva et al. 1973, 1980; Pfurtscheller et al. 1996). This idea is strongly seconded by the recent proposition that pulvinar gates cortico–cortical communication by promoting oscillatory synchrony between regions (Saalmann et al. 2012), and it fits in at least a general sense with the thalamic gating model of cortical sensory processing of Sherman and Guillery (2002). Similarly, based on findings of attentional modulation of synchrony at both intra-cortical/inter-laminar (Lakatos et al. 2008) and inter-areal scales (Besle et al. 2011), it seems likely that attentional modulation of synchrony between the LGN and V1 will prove critical in selective processing rhythmic input streams, though clear evidence on this point is thus far slim (Bollimunta et al. 2011). Finally, it is noteworthy that even top-down prefrontal control in the operation of attention may be executed through the use of thalamic circuitry, in particular the reticular nucleus of the thalamus, and the non-specific thalamic projection system (Zikopoulos and Barbas 2006, 2007a, 2007b), discussed above in the context of modulatory input to superficial layers of cortex.

(6) *Role of motor cortex in covert attentional operations?* According to the 'Premotor Theory of Attention' (Rizzolatti et al. 1987), covert orienting to space, and by implication to features and to timing/rhythm, utilizes the same circuits as those involved in overt motoric orienting. In both cases, predictive top-down modulation is used to improve the quality of sensory processing, and effectively, deployment of attention amounts to a suppressed motor response. *Active sensing* is a related perspective in cognitive neuroscience, which holds that sensory input that is given precedence in information processing is that which is actively acquired by an overt motoric or covert attentional sampling routine (Schroeder et al. 2010). An important feature of the active sensing view is that it explicitly incorporates neuronal oscillations as an implementation of the brain's predictions; i.e. top-down signals use reset of ongoing neuronal oscillations as instruments in modulation of sensory processing. One important implication of this perspective that is yet to be fully explored is that ambient neuronal oscillatory

rhythms in sensory and association regions are likely patterned by rhythms present in the motor cortical system and its subcortical components.

(7) *Do neuronal oscillations help to connect different brain areas into 'cell assemblies' and 'networks'?* Refinements of the influential idea that gamma oscillations bind cell assemblies together to enable dynamic control of brain operations (Gray and Singer 1989) that have been put forward by Kopell and colleagues (Kopell and LeMasson 1994; Kopell et al. 2000, 2010) emphasize the qualities of gamma rhythms, in particular the interactions of co-located excitatory and inhibitory neuron populations, in forming cell assemblies that are useful for computing purposes. Parallel propositions have been put forward using theta oscillations in hippocampus and entorhinal cortex (Buzsaki and Chrobak 1995; Buzsaki 2010; O'Keefe and Burgess 1999, 2005), and delta oscillations in the neocortex (Besle et al. 2011; Lakatos et al. 2009a; Stefanics et al. 2010b). Most recently, several propositions have been advanced for use of cross-frequency coupling of neuronal oscillations as a framework for parsing, selection, and representation of complex natural input patterns (Canolty and Knight 2010; Fujisawa and Buzsaki 2011; Schroeder et al. 2008). Interestingly, a recent study provided evidence that when multiple values of visual stimulus contrast are present within a scene, the precise frequency of local oscillations within the gamma band is regulated by stimulus contrast (Ray and Maunsell 2010). The pattern of results in this study is consistent with both the encoding of contrast information by oscillatory frequency, and with the idea that ensembles encoding different contrasts in the stimulus may be linked by common oscillatory frequency with counterpart neuronal ensembles in downstream areas. This would amount to multiplexing of information about contrast variation in a scene through different oscillatory channels. There thus seems to be a wealth of propositions, some with excellent empirical support. The biggest challenge in the immediate future for this area will be to build the findings and hypotheses into a unified framework for guiding future investigations.

(8) *Do cholinergic systems underpin attentional modulation through changes in functional connectivity across cortical layers and across brain areas?* Given the differential receptor distribution across cortical areas and laminae (Gil et al. 1997; Kimura and Baughman 1997), it would be interesting to record laminar activity profiles with linear array multielectrodes together with glutamatergic and cholinergic receptor manipulations. One earlier study (Kimura et al. 1999) used optical recording to examine the laminar selectivity of cholinergic suppression in cortical slices of rat visual cortex. They found that ACh suppressed the initial synaptic component in all cortical layers, with the strongest suppressive effect in the SG and IG layers and the weakest in the middle layer. One prediction is that high levels of ACh in Layers 2/3 results in increased amount of attentional modulation, whereas high levels in Layer 4 mostly increase the gain (to all stimuli) but not the attentional modulation (e.g. increased gain to target stimuli). High ACh levels in Layers 2/3 may shift the flow of cortical processing in favour of relevant feedforward signals, such that incoming target stimuli are processed preferentially.

At the network level, the entrainment hypothesis (Lakatos et al. 2008) may predict high ACh levels in Layers 2/3 to improve phase alignment of delta-band oscillations to rhythmic stimuli, promoting increased response gain for task-relevant events and faster reaction times. It is also possible ACh effects improve phase alignment (coherence) across layers, such as between Layer 4 and supragranular output layers and across areas, such as between the supragranular layers of V1 or A1 and the granular layers of the next higher order target region (V2 or belt cortices). This would both enhance transmission of inputs through the system, and amplify the representation of task-relevant inputs in higher order neurons.

(9) *Do cholinergic systems contribute to attentional modulation of response specificity (tuning)?* The effects of ACh in stimulus selectivity (Sato et al. 1987) are controversial. Some studies reported that raised ACh levels sharpen sensory tuning curves (Sillito and Kemp 1983; Murphy and Sillito 1991), enhance stimulus detectability through improved signal-to-noise ratio (Sato et al. 1987) or reduced influence of spatial context (Roberts al. 2005). However, others (Sato et al. 1987; Zinke et al. 2006) observed that raised ACh levels broaden sensory tuning curves, or have no effect (Thiele et al. 2012). The discrepancy possibly arises from the type of neurons sample and other factors (e.g. experimental paradigm, animal species). It seems sensible to ask whether a more detailed approach using laminar electrodes could shed light on the effects of ACh on sensory processing. Optimal frequency (OF) stimuli would result in stronger input drive to Layer 4 neurons compared to non-optimal stimuli. Thalamocortical (TC) terminals depolarized by OF stimuli release large amounts of glutamate from vesicles in the presynaptic side, increasing the conductance through AMPA and NMDA receptors in the postsynaptic membrane. The resulting larger excitation of the postsynaptic cortical neuron causes it to more likely fire action potentials. An underlying current sink (net inward transmembrane current flow) supports this with concomitant increase in neuronal firing in Layer 4, followed by later responses in extragranular layers. This sequence of activation is coupled with a *source over sink* in the supragranular layers, and it is typical of an excitatory 'feedforward' type activation profile. However, this profile is reversed for non-OF stimulation in the SG layers with a *sink over source* (O'Connell et al. 2011). Future research should question whether ACh contributes to the reversal and whether attention leads to similar effects. For example, pairing ACh release in SG layers with non-OF stimuli could result in *source over sink*. Seemingly, directing attention to non-OF stimuli would yield to a similar effect. This could be a mechanism by which ACh shifts the dynamics in cortical network (Kimura 2000; Hasselmo 2010), modulating neuronal responsiveness to optimal or attended stimulus features.

REFERENCES

Adrian, E. D. and Matthews B. H. C. (1934). The Berger rhythm: Potential changes from the occipital lobes in man. *Brain 57*: 355–385.

Anderson, K. L. and Ding M (2011). Attentional modulation of the somatosensory mu rhythm. *Neuroscience 180*: 165–180.

Arnold, H. M., Nelson, C. L., Sarter, M., and Bruno, J. P. (2003). Sensitization of cortical acetylcholine release by repeated administration of nicotine in rats. *Psychopharmacology (Berlin) 165*: 346–358.

Banerjee, S., Snyder, A. C., Molholm, S., and Foxe, J. J. (2011). Oscillatory alpha-band mechanisms and the deployment of spatial attention to anticipated auditory and visual target locations: Supramodal or sensory-specific control mechanisms? *Journal of Neuroscience 31*: 9923–9932.

Baxter, M. G., Bucci, D. J., Gorman, L. K., Wiley, R. G., and Gallagher, M. (1995). Selective immunotoxic lesions of basal forebrain cholinergic cells: Effects on learning and memory in rats. *Behavioral Neuroscience 109*: 714–722.

Berger, H. (1929). Über das elektrenkephalogramm des Menschen [On the electroencephalogram of humans]. *Archiv für Psychiatrie und Nervenkrankeheiten 87*: 527–570.

Besle, J., Schevon, C. A., Mehta, A. D., Lakatos, P., Goodman, R. R., McKhann, G. M., Emerson, R. G., and Schroeder, C. E. (2011). Tuning of the human neocortex to the temporal dynamics of attended events. *Journal of Neuroscience 31*: 3176–3185.

Bishop, G. (1933). Cyclical changes in excitability of the optic pathway of the rabbit. *American Journal of Physiology 103*: 213–224.

Bollimunta, A., Chen, Y., Schroeder, C. E., and Ding, M. (2008). Neuronal mechanisms of cortical alpha oscillations in awake-behaving macaques. *Journal of Neuroscience 28*: 9976–9988.

Bollimunta, A., Mo, J., Schroeder, C. E., and Ding, M. (2011). Neuronal mechanisms and attentional modulation of corticothalamic alpha oscillations. *Journal of Neuroscience 31*: 4935–4943.

Bonnefond, M. and Jensen, O. (2012). Alpha oscillations serve to protect working memory maintenance against anticipated distractors. *Current Biology 22*: 1969–1974.

Botly, L. C. and De, R. E. (2009). The nucleus basalis magnocellularis contributes to feature binding in the rat. *Physiology & Behavior 97*: 313–320.

Bragin, A., Jando, G., Nadasdy, Z., Hetke, J., Wise, K., and Buzsaki, G. (1995). Gamma (40–100Hz) oscillation in the hippocampus of the behaving rat. *Journal of Neuroscience 15*: 47–60.

Browning, P. G., Gaffan, D., Croxson, P. L., and Baxter, M. G. (2010). Severe scene learning impairment, but intact recognition memory, after cholinergic depletion of inferotemporal cortex followed by fornix transection. *Cerebral Cortex 20*: 282–293.

Buffalo, E. A., Fries, P., Landman, R., Buschman, T. J., and Desimone, R. (2011). Laminar differences in gamma and alpha coherence in the ventral stream. *Proceedings of the National Academy of Sciences USA 108*: 11262–11267.

Burgess, N., Barry, C., and O'Keefe, J. (2007). An oscillatory interference model of grid cell firing. *Hippocampus 17*: 801–812.

Busch, N. A., Dubois, J., and VanRullen, R. (2009). The phase of ongoing EEG oscillations predicts visual perception. *Journal of Neuroscience 29*: 7869–7876.

Buschman, T. J. and Miller, E. K. (2007). Top-down versus bottom-up control of attention in the prefrontal and posterior parietal cortices. *Science 315*: 1860–1862.

Buzsaki, G. (2010). Neural syntax: Cell assemblies, synapsembles, and readers. *Neuron 68*: 362–385.

Buzsaki, G., Bickford, R. G., Ponomareff, G., Thal, L. J., Mandel, R., and Gage, F. H. (1988). Nucleus basalis and thalamic control of neocortical activity in the freely moving rat. *Journal of Neuroscience 8*: 4007–4026.

Buzsaki, G. and Chrobak, J. J. (1995). Temporal structure in spatially organized neuronal ensembles: A role for interneuronal networks. *Current Opinion in Neurobiology 5*: 504–510.

Buzsaki, G. and Draguhn A (2004). Neuronal oscillations in cortical networks. *Science 304*: 1926–1929.

Buzsaki, G. and Gage, F. H. (1989). The cholinergic nucleus basalis: A key structure in neocortical arousal. *EXS 57*: 159–171.

Canolty, R. T., Edwards, E., Dalal, S. S., Soltani, M., Nagarajan, S. S., Kirsch, H. E., Berger, M. S., Barbaro, N. M., and Knight, R. T. (2006). High gamma power is phase-locked to theta oscillations in human neocortex. *Science 313*: 1626–1629.

Canolty, R. T. and Knight, R. T. (2010). The functional role of cross-frequency coupling. *Trends in Cognitive Sciences 14*: 506–515.

Capotosto, P., Babiloni, C., Romani, G. L., and Corbetta, M. (2009). Frontoparietal cortex controls spatial attention through modulation of anticipatory alpha rhythms. *Journal of Neuroscience 29*: 5863–5872.

Chandrasekaran, C., Trubanova, A., Stillittano, S., Caplier, A., and Ghazanfar, A. A. (2009). The natural statistics of audiovisual speech. *PLoS Computational Biology 5*: e1000436.

Christophe, E., Roebuck, A., Staiger, J. F., Lavery, D. J., Charpak, S., and Audinat, E. (2002). Two types of nicotinic receptors mediate an excitation of neocortical layer I interneurons. *Journal of Neurophysiology 88*: 1318–1327.

Clapp, W. C., Eckert, M. J., Teyler, T. J., and Abraham, W. C. (2006a). Rapid visual stimulation induces N-methyl-D-aspartate receptor-dependent sensory long-term potentiation in the rat cortex. *NeuroReport 17*: 511–515.

Clapp, W. C., Muthukumaraswamy, S. D., Hamm, J. P., Teyler, T. J., and Kirk, I. J. (2006b). Long-term enhanced desynchronization of the alpha rhythm following tetanic stimulation of human visual cortex. *Neuroscience Letters 398*: 220–223.

Clapp, W. C., Zaehle, T., Lutz, K., Marcar, V. L., Kirk, I. J., Hamm, J. P., Teyler, T. J., Corballis, M. C., and Jancke, L. (2005). Effects of long-term potentiation in the human visual cortex: A functional magnetic resonance imaging study. *NeuroReport 16*: 1977–1980.

Cooper, N. R., Croft, R. J., Dominey, S. J. J., Burgess, A. P., and Gruzelier, J. H. (2003). Paradox lost? Exploring the role of alpha oscillations during externally vs. internally directed attention and the implications for idling and inhibition hypotheses. *International Journal of Psychophysiology 47*: 65–74.

Dalley, J. W., McGaughy, J., O'Connell, M. T., Cardinal, R. N., Levita, L., and Robbins, T. W. (2001). Distinct changes in cortical acetylcholine and noradrenaline efflux during contingent and noncontingent performance of a visual attentional task. *Journal of Neuroscience 21*: 4908–4914.

Deco, G. and Thiele, A. (2011). Cholinergic control of cortical network interactions enables feedback-mediated attentional modulation. *European Journal of Neuroscience 34*: 146–157.

Dehaene, S. (1993). Temporal oscillations in human perception. *Psychological Science 4*: 264–270.

Desimone, R. and Duncan, J. (1995). Neural mechanisms of selective visual attention. *Annual Review of Neuroscience 18*: 193–222.

Ding, J., Sperling, G., and Srinivasan, R. (2006). Attentional modulation of SSVEP power depends on the network tagged by the flicker frequency. *Cerebral Cortex 16*: 1016–1029.

Drullman, R. (1995). Temporal envelope and fine structure cues for speech intelligibility. *Journal of the Acoustical Society of America 97*: 585–592.

Ellis, J. R., Ellis, K. A., Bartholomeusz, C. F., Harrison, B. J., Wesnes, K. A., Erskine, F. F., Vitetta, L., and Nathan, P. J. (2006). Muscarinic and nicotinic receptors synergistically modulate working memory and attention in humans. *International Journal of Neuropsychopharmacology* 9: 175–189.

Engel, A. K. and Fries, P. (2010). Beta-band oscillations—signalling the status quo? *Current Opinion in Neurobiology* 20: 156–165.

Ergenoglu, T., Demiralp, T., Bayraktaroglu, Z., Ergen, M., Beydagi, H., and Uresin, Y. (2004). Alpha rhythm of the EEG modulates visual detection performance in humans. *Brain Research: Cognitive Brain Research* 20: 376–383.

Everitt, B. J. and Robbins, T. W. (1997). Central cholinergic systems and cognition. *Annual Review of Psychology* 48: 649–684.

Felleman, D. J. and Van Essen, D. C. (1991). Distributed hierarchical processing in the primate cerebral cortex. *Cerebral Cortex* 1: 1–47.

Frick, K. M., Kim, J. J., and Baxter, M. G. (2004). Effects of complete immunotoxin lesions of the cholinergic basal forebrain on fear conditioning and spatial learning. *Hippocampus* 14: 244–254.

Fries, P. (2005). A mechanism for cognitive dynamics: Neuronal communication through neuronal coherence. *Trends in Cognitive Sciences* 9: 474–480.

Fries, P., Reynolds, J. H., Rorie, A. E., and Desimone, R. (2001). Modulation of oscillatory neuronal synchronization by selective visual attention. *Science* 291: 1560–1563.

Fries, P., Womelsdorf, T., Oostenveld, R., and Desimone, R. (2008). The effects of visual stimulation and selective visual attention on rhythmic neuronal synchronization in macaque area V4. *Journal of Neuroscience* 28: 4823–4835.

Fu, K. M., Foxe, J. J., Murray, M. M., Higgins, B. A., Javitt, D. C., and Schroeder, C. E. (2001). Attention-dependent suppression of distractor visual input can be cross-modally cued as indexed by anticipatory parieto-occipital alpha-band oscillations. *Brain Research: Cognitive Brain Research* 12: 145–152.

Fujisawa, S. and Buzsaki, G. (2011). A 4 Hz oscillation adaptively synchronizes prefrontal, VTA, and hippocampal activities. *Neuron* 72: 153–165.

Fukushima, M., Saunders, R. C., Leopold, D. A., Mishkin, M., and Averbeck, B. B. (2012). Spontaneous high-gamma band activity reflects functional organization of auditory cortex in the awake macaque. *Neuron* 74: 899–910.

Galani, R., Lehmann, O., Bolmont, T., Aloy, E., Bertrand, F., Lazarus, C., Jeltsch, H., and Cassel, J. C. (2002). Selective immunolesions of CH4 cholinergic neurons do not disrupt spatial memory in rats. *Physiology & Behavior* 76: 75–90.

Ghose, G. M. and Maunsell, J. H. (2002). Attentional modulation in visual cortex depends on task timing. *Nature* 419: 616–620.

Gil, Z., Connors, B. W., and Amitai, Y. (1997). Differential regulation of neocortical synapses by neuromodulators and activity. *Neuron* 19: 679–686.

Gould, I. C., Rushworth, M. F., and Nobre, A. C. (2011). Indexing the graded allocation of visuospatial attention using anticipatory alpha oscillations. *Journal of Neurophysiology* 105: 1318–1326.

Gray, C. M. and Singer, W. (1989). Stimulus-specific neuronal oscillations in orientation columns of cat visual cortex. *Proceedings of the National Academy of Sciences USA* 86: 1698–1702.

Haegens, S., Handel, B. F., and Jensen, O. (2011a). Top-down controlled alpha band activity in somatosensory areas determines behavioral performance in a discrimination task. *Journal of Neuroscience* 31: 5197–5204.

Haegens, S., Luther, L., and Jensen, O. (2012). Somatosensory anticipatory alpha activity increases to suppress distracting input. *Journal of Cognitive Neuroscience* 24: 677–685.

Haegens, S., Nácher, V., Luna, R., Romo, R., and Jensen, O. (2011b). α-oscillations in the monkey sensorimotor network influence discrimination performance by rhythmical inhibition of neuronal spiking. *Proceedings of the National Academy of Sciences USA 108*: 19377–19382.

Hanslmayr, S., Aslan, A., Staudigl, T., Klimesch, W., Herrmann, C. S., and Bäuml, K. H. (2007). Prestimulus oscillations predict visual perception performance between and within subjects. *NeuroImage 37*: 1465–1473.

Hanslmayr, S., Gross, J., Klimesch, W., and Shapiro, K. L. (2011). The role of alpha oscillations in temporal attention. *Brain Research Reviews 67*: 331–343.

Harter, M. R. (1967). Excitability cycles and cortical scanning: a review of two hypotheses of central intermittency in perception. *Psychological Bulletin 68*: 47–58.

Harter, R. and Aine, C. J. (1984). Brain mechanisms of visual selective attention. In R. Parasuraman and D. R. Davies (eds.), *Varieties of Attention* (pp. 293–321). London: Academic Press.

Harter, M. R., Aine, C., and Schroeder, C. E. (1982). Hemispheric differences in the neural processing of stimulus location and type: Effects of selective attention on visual evoked potentials. *Neuropsychologia 20*: 421–438.

Harter, M. R. and White, C. T. (1968). Periodicity within reaction time distributions and electromyograms. *Quarterly Journal of Experimental Psychology 20*: 157–166.

Hasselmo, M. E. and Bower, J. M. (1992). Cholinergic suppression specific to intrinsic not afferent fiber synapses in rat piriform (olfactory) cortex. *Journal of Neurophysiology 67*: 1222–1229.

Hasselmo, M. E. and McGaughy, J. (2004). High acetylcholine levels set circuit dynamics for attention and encoding and low acetylcholine levels set dynamics for consolidation. *Progress in Brain Research 145*: 207–231.

Hasselmo, M. E. and Sarter, M. (2011). Modes and models of forebrain cholinergic neuromodulation of cognition. *Neuropsychopharmacology 36*: 52–73.

Herculano-Houzel, S., Munk, M. H., Neuenschwander, S., and Singer, W. (1999). Precisely synchronized oscillatory firing patterns require electroencephalographic activation. *Journal of Neuroscience 19*: 3992–4010.

Herrero, J. L., Roberts, M. J., Delicato, L. S., Gieselmann, M. A., Dayan, P., and Thiele, A. (2008). Acetylcholine contributes through muscarinic receptors to attentional modulation in V1. *Nature 454*: 1110–1114.

Herrero, J. L., Gieselmann, M. A., sanavai, M., and Thiele, A. (2013). Attention-induced variance and noise correlation reduction in macaque V1 is mediated by NMDA receptors. *Neuron 78* (4): 729–739.

Himmelheber, A. M., Sarter, M., and Bruno, J. P. (1997). Operant performance and cortical acetylcholine release: Role of response rate, reward density, and non-contingent stimuli. *Brain Research: Cognitive Brain Research 6*: 23–36.

Holschneider, D. P., Leuchter, A. F., Scremin, O. U., Treiman, D. M., and Walton, N. Y. (1998). Effects of cholinergic deafferentation and NGF on brain electrical coherence. *Brain Research Bulletin 45*: 531–541.

Holschneider, D. P., Scremin, O. U., Chen, K., and Shih, J. C. (1999). Lack of protection of monoamine oxidase B-deficient mice from age-related spatial learning deficits in the Morris water maze. *Life Sciences 65*: 1757–1763.

Howe, C. Q. and Purves, D. (2005). Natural-scene geometry predicts the perception of angles and line orientation. *Proceedings of the National Academy of Sciences USA 102*: 1228–1233.

Howe, W. M., Ji, J., Parikh, V., Williams, S., Mocaer, E., Trocme-Thibierge, C., and Sarter, M. (2010). Enhancement of attentional performance by selective stimulation of alpha4beta2(*) nAChRs: Underlying cholinergic mechanisms. *Neuropsychopharmacology 35*: 1391–1401.

Jensen, O., Bonnefond, M., and VanRullen, R. (2012). An oscillatory mechanism for prioritizing salient unattended stimuli. *Trends in Cognitive Sciences 16*: 200–206.

Jensen, O. and Mazaheri, A. (2010). Shaping functional architecture by oscillatory alpha activity: Gating by inhibition. *Frontiers in Human Neuroscience 4*: 186.

Jones, E. G. (2001). The thalamic matrix and thalamocortical synchrony. *Trends in Neurosciences 24*: 595–601.

Jones, M. R. and Boltz, M. (1989). Dynamic attending and responses to time. *Psychological Review 96*: 459–491.

Jones, M. R., Moynihan, H., Mackenzie, N., and Puente, J. (2002). Temporal aspects of stimulus-driven attending in dynamic arrays. *Psychological Science 13*: 313–319.

Jones, S. R., Kerr, C. E., Wan, Q., Pritchett, D. L., Hamalainen, M., and Moore, C. I. (2010). Cued spatial attention drives functionally relevant modulation of the mu rhythm in primary somatosensory cortex. *Journal of Neuroscience 30*: 13760–13765.

Jones, S. R., Pinto, D. J., Kaper, T. J., and Kopell, N. (2000). Alpha-frequency rhythms desynchronize over long cortical distances: A modeling study. *Journal of Computational Neuroscience 9*: 271–291.

Kang, J. I. and Vaucher, E. (2009). Cholinergic pairing with visual activation results in long-term enhancement of visual evoked potentials. *PLoS One 4*: e5995.

Kelly, S. P., Lalor, E. C., Reilly, R. B., and Foxe, J. J. (2006). Increases in alpha oscillatory power reflect an active retinotopic mechanism for distractor suppression during sustained visuospatial attention. *Journal of Neurophysiology 95*: 3844–3851.

Kim, Y. J., Grabowecky, M., Paller, K. A., Muthu, K., and Suzuki, S. (2007). Attention induces synchronization-based response gain in steady-state visual evoked potentials. *Nature Neuroscience 10*: 117–125.

Kimura, F. (2000). Cholinergic modulation of cortical function: A hypothetical role in shifting the dynamics in cortical network. *Neuroscience Research 38*: 19–26.

Kimura, F. and Baughman, R. W. (1997). Distinct muscarinic receptor subtypes suppress excitatory and inhibitory synaptic responses in cortical neurons. *Journal of Neurophysiology 77*: 709–716.

Klimesch W., Sauseng P., Hanslmayr S. (2007). EEG alpha oscillations: The inhibition-timing hypothesis. *Brain Research Reviews 53*: 63–88.

Kopell, N., Ermentrout, G. B., Whittington, M. A., and Traub, R. D. (2000). Gamma rhythms and beta rhythms have different synchronization properties. *Proceedings of the National Academy of Sciences USA 97*: 1867–1872.

Kopell, N., Kramer, M. A., Malerba, P., and Whittington, M. A. (2010). Are different rhythms good for different functions? *Frontiers in Human Neuroscience 4*: 187.

Kopell, N. and LeMasson, G. (1994). Rhythmogenesis, amplitude modulation, and multiplexing in a cortical architecture. *Proceedings of the National Academy of Sciences USA 91*: 10586–10590.

Kopell, N., Whittington, M. A., and Kramer, M. A. (2011). Neuronal assembly dynamics in the beta1 frequency range permits short-term memory. *Proceedings of the National Academy of Sciences USA 108*: 3779–3784.

Kozak, R., Bruno, J. P., and Sarter, M. (2006). Augmented prefrontal acetylcholine release during challenged attentional performance. *Cerebral Cortex 16*: 9–17.

Lakatos, P., Chen, C. M., O'Connell, M. N., Mills, A., and Schroeder, C. E. (2007). Neuronal oscillations and multisensory interaction in primary auditory cortex. *Neuron 53*: 1–14.

Lakatos, P., Karmos, G., Mehta, A. D., Ulbert, I., and Schroeder, C. E. (2008). Entrainment of neuronal oscillations as a mechanism of attentional selection. *Science 320*: 110–113.

Lakatos, P., Musacchia, G. E., O'Connell, M. N., Falchier, A. Y. Javitt, D. C., and Schroeder, C. E. (2013). The spectrotemporal filter mechanism of auditory selective attention. *Neuron 77*: 750–761.

Lakatos, P., O'Connell, M. N., Barczak, A., Mills, A., Javitt, D. C., and Schroeder, C. E. (2009). The leading sense: Supramodal control of neurophysiological context by attention. *Neuron* 64: 419–430.

Lakatos, P., Shah, A. S., Knuth, K. H., Ulbert, I., Karmos, G., and Schroeder, C. E. (2005). An oscillatory hierarchy controlling neuronal excitability and stimulus processing in the auditory cortex. *Journal of Neurophysiology* 94: 1904–1911.

Large, E. W. and Jones, M. R. (1999). The dynamics of attending: How we track time-varying events. *Psychological Review* 106: 119–159.

Large, E. W. and Snyder, J. S. (2009). Pulse and meter as neural resonance. *Annals of the New York Academy of Sciences* 1169: 46–57.

Leopold, D., Murayama, Y., and Logothetis, N. (2003). Very slow activity fluctuations in monkey visual cortex: Implications for functional brain imaging. *Cerebral Cortex* 12: 422–433.

Linkenkaer-Hansen, K., Nikulin, V. V., Palva, S., Ilmoniemi, R. J., and Palva, J. M. (2004). Prestimulus oscillations enhance psychophysical performance in humans. *Journal of Neuroscience* 24: 10186–10190.

Llinas, R. R. (1988). The intrinsic electrophysiological properties of mammalian neurons: Insights into central nervous system function. *Science* 242: 1654–1664.

Lopes da Silva, F. H., van Lierop, T. H. M. T., Schrijer, C. F., and Storm van Leeuwen, W. (1973). Organization of thalamic and cortical alpha rhythms: Spectra and coherences. *Electroencephalography and Clinical Neurophysiology* 35: 627–639.

Lopes da Silva, F. H., Vos, J. E., Mooibroek, J., and van Rotterdam, A. (1980). Relative contributions of intracortical and thalamo-cortical processes in the generation of alpha rhythms, revealed by partial coherence analysis. *Electroencephalography and Clinical Neurophysiology* 50: 449–456.

Lőrincz M. L., Kékesi K. A., Juhász G., Crunelli V., and Hughes S. W. (2009). Temporal framing of thalamic relay-mode firing by phasic inhibition during the alpha rhythm. *Neuron* 63: 683–696.

Luo, H. and Poeppel, D. (2007). Phase patterns of neuronal responses reliably discriminate speech in auditory cortex. *Neuron* 54: 1001–1010.

McCormick, D. A. and Prince, D. A. (1985). Two types of muscarinic response to acetylcholine in mammalian cortical neurons. *Proceedings of the National Academy of Sciences USA* 82: 6344–6348.

McCormick, D. A. and Prince, D. A. (1986a). Acetylcholine induces burst firing in thalamic reticular neurones by activating a potassium conductance. *Nature* 319: 402–405.

McCormick, D. A. and Prince, D. A. (1986b). Mechanisms of action of acetylcholine in the guinea-pig cerebral cortex in vitro. *Journal of Physiology* 375: 169–194.

Mathewson, K. E., Fabiani, M., Gratton, G., Beck, D. M., and Lleras, A. (2010). Rescuing stimuli from invisibility: Inducing a momentary release from visual masking with pre-target entrainment. *Cognition* 115: 186–191.

Mathewson, K. E., Gratton, G., Fabiani, M., Beck, D. M., and Ro, T. (2009). To see or not to see: Prestimulus alpha phase predicts visual awareness. *Journal of Neuroscience* 29: 2725–2732.

Mathewson, K. E., Lleras, A., Beck, D. M., Fabiani, M., Ro, T., and Gratton, G. (2011). Pulsed out of awareness: EEG alpha oscillations represent a pulsed inhibition of ongoing cortical processing. *Frontiers in Psychology* 2: 99.

Maunsell, J. H. R. (1995). The brain's visual world: Representation of visual targets in cerebral cortex. *Science* 270: 764–769.

Maurer, A. P. and McNaughton, B. L. (2007). Network and intrinsic cellular mechanisms underlying theta phase precession of hippocampal neurons. *Trends in Neurosciences* 30: 325–333.

Mo, J., Schroeder, C. E., and Ding, M. (2011). Attentional modulation of alpha oscillations in macaque inferotemporal cortex. *Journal of Neuroscience 31*: 878–882.

Moran, J. and Desimone, R. (1985). Selective attention gates visual information processing in extrastriate cortex. *Science 229*: 782–784.

Morgan, S. T., Hansen, J. C., and Hillyard, S. A. (1996). Selective attention to stimulus location modulates the steady-state visual evoked potential. *Proceedings of the National Academy of Sciences USA 93*: 4770–4774.

Motter, B. C. (1993). Focal attention produces spatially selective processing in visual cortical areas V1, V2, and V4 in the presence of competing stimuli. *Journal of Neurophysiology 70*: 909–919.

Mrzljak, L., Levey, A. I., and Rakic, P. (1996). Selective expression of m2 muscarinic receptor in the parvocellular channel of the primate visual cortex. *Proceedings of the National Academy of Sciences USA 93*: 7337–7340.

Mukamel, R., Gelbard, H., Arieli, A., Hasson, U., Fried, I., and Malach, R. (2005). Coupling between neuronal firing, field potentials, and FMRI in human auditory cortex. *Science 309*: 951–954.

Munhall, K. G., Jones, J. A., Callan, D. E., Kuratate, T., and Vatikiotis-Bateson, E. (2004). Visual prosody and speech intelligibility: Head movement improves auditory perception. *Psychological Science 15*: 133–137.

Naatanen, R. and Michie, P. T. (1979). Early selective-attention effects on the evoked potential: A critical review and reinterpretation. *Biological Psychology 8*: 81–136.

Niessing, J., Ebisch, B., Schmidt, K. E., Niessing, M., Singer, W., and Galuske, R. A. (2005). Hemodynamic signals correlate tightly with synchronized gamma oscillations. *Science 309*: 948–951.

O'Keefe, J. and Burgess, N. (1999). Theta activity, virtual navigation and the human hippocampus. *Trends in Cognitive Sciences 3*: 403–406.

O'Keefe, J. and Burgess, N. (2005). Dual phase and rate coding in hippocampal place cells: Theoretical significance and relationship to entorhinal grid cells. *Hippocampus 15*: 853–866.

Oldford, E. and Castro-Alamancos, M. A. (2003). Input-specific effects of acetylcholine on sensory and intracortical evoked responses in the 'barrel cortex' in vivo. *Neuroscience 117*: 769–778.

Pang, K. C. and Nocera, R. (1999). Interactions between 192-IgG saporin and intraseptal cholinergic and GABAergic drugs: Role of cholinergic medial septal neurons in spatial working memory. *Behavioral Neuroscience 113*: 265–275.

Parasuraman, R. and Davies, D. R. (eds.) (1984). *Varieties of Attention*. London: Academic Press.

Parikh, V., Kozak, R., Martinez, V., and Sarter, M. (2007). Prefrontal acetylcholine release controls cue detection on multiple timescales. *Neuron 56*: 141–154.

Parikh, V., Man, K., Decker, M. W., and Sarter, M. (2008). Glutamatergic contributions to nicotinic acetylcholine receptor agonist-evoked cholinergic transients in the prefrontal cortex. *Journal of Neuroscience 28*: 3769–3780.

Parikh, V. and Sarter, M. (2008). Cholinergic mediation of attention: Contributions of phasic and tonic increases in prefrontal cholinergic activity. *Annals of the New York Academy of Sciences 1129*: 225–235.

Passetti, F., Dalley, J. W., O'Connell, M. T., Everitt, B. J., and Robbins, T. W. (2000). Increased acetylcholine release in the rat medial prefrontal cortex during performance of a visual attentional task. *European Journal of Neuroscience 12*: 3051–3058.

Pfurtscheller, G. and Lopes da Silva, F. H. (1999). Event-related EEG/MEG synchronization and desynchronization: Basic principles. *Clinical Neurophysiology 110*: 1842–1857.

Pfurtscheller, G., Stancak, A., and Neuper, C. (1996). Event-related synchronization (ERS) in the alpha band: An electrophysiological correlate of cortical idling—a review. *Journal of Psychophysiology* 24: 39–46.

Posner, M. (1980). Orienting of attention. *Quarterly Journal of Experimental Psychology* 32: 3–25.

Rajkai, C., Lakatos, P., Chen, C. M., Pincze, Z., Karmos, G., and Schroeder, C. E. (2008). Transient cortical excitation at the onset of visual fixation. *Cerebral Cortex* 18: 200–209.

Ray, S. and Maunsell, J. H. (2010). Differences in gamma frequencies across visual cortex restrict their possible use in computation. *Neuron* 67: 885–896.

Rihs, T. A., Michel, C. M., and Thut, G. (2007). Mechanisms of selective inhibition in visual spatial attention are indexed by alpha-band EEG synchronization. *European Journal of Neuroscience* 25: 603–610.

Rihs, T. A., Michel, C. M., and Thut, G. (2009). A bias for posterior alpha-band power suppression versus enhancement during shifting versus maintenance of spatial attention. *NeuroImage* 44: 190–199.

Rizzolatti, G., Riggio, L., Dascola, I., and Umiltá, C. (1987). Reorienting attention across the horizontal and vertical meridians: Evidence in favor of a premotor theory of attention. *Neuropsychologia* 25: 31–40.

Rohenkohl, G. and Nobre, A. C. (2011). Alpha oscillations related to anticipatory attention follow temporal expectations. *Journal of Neuroscience* 31: 14076–14084.

Roopun, A. K., Kramer, M. A., Carracedo, L. M., Kaiser, M., Davies, C. H., Traub, R. D., Kopell, N. J., and Whittington, M. A. (2008a). Period concatenation underlies interactions between gamma and beta rhythms in neocortex. *Frontiers in Cellular Neuroscience* 2: 1.

Roopun, A. K., Kramer, M. A., Carracedo, L. M., Kaiser, M., Davies, C. H., Traub, R. D., Kopell, N. J., and Whittington, M. A. (2008b). Temporal interactions between cortical rhythms. *Frontiers in Neuroscience* 2: 145–154.

Roopun, A. K., Lebeau, F. E., Ramell, J., Cunningham, M. O., Traub, R. D., and Whittington, M. A. (2010). Cholinergic neuromodulation controls directed temporal communication in neocortex in vitro. *Frontiers in Neural Circuits* 4: 8.

Saalmann, Y. B. and Kastner, S. (2011). Cognitive and perceptual functions of the visual thalamus. *Neuron* 71: 209–223.

Saalmann, Y. B., Kirkcaldie, M. T., Waldron, S., and Calford, M. B. (2007a). Cellular distribution of the GABAA receptor-modulating 3alpha-hydroxy, 5alpha-reduced pregnane steroids in the adult rat brain. *Journal of Neuroendocrinology* 19: 272–284.

Saalmann, Y. B., Pigarev, I. N., and Vidyasagar, T. R. (2007b). Neural mechanisms of visual attention: How top-down feedback highlights relevant locations. *Science* 316: 1612–1615.

Saalmann, Y. B., Pinsk, M. A., Wang, L., Li, X., and Kastner, S. (2012). The pulvinar regulates information transmission between cortical areas based on attention demands. *Science* 337: 753–756.

Sarter, M., Gehring, W. J., and Kozak, R. (2006). More attention must be paid: The neurobiology of attentional effort. *Brain Research Reviews* 51: 145–160.

Sarter, M., Parikh, V., and Howe, W. M. (2009a). nAChR agonist-induced cognition enhancement: Integration of cognitive and neuronal mechanisms. *Biochemical Pharmacology* 78: 658–667.

Sarter, M., Parikh, V., and Howe, W. M. (2009b). Phasic acetylcholine release and the volume transmission hypothesis: Time to move on. *Nature Reviews Neuroscience* 10: 383–390.

Sauseng, P., Klimesch, W., Stadler, W., Schabus, M., Doppelmayr, M., Hanslmayr, S., Gruber, W. R., and Birbaumer, N. (2005). A shift of visual spatial attention is selectively associated with human EEG alpha activity. *European Journal of Neuroscience* 22: 2917–2926.

Scheeringa, R., Mazaheri, A., Bojak, I., Norris, D. G., and Kleinschmidt, A. (2011). Modulation of visually evoked cortical fMRI responses by phase of ongoing occipital alpha oscillations. *Journal of Neuroscience 31*: 3813–3820.

Schroeder, C. E. and Lakatos, P. (2009). Low-frequency neuronal oscillations as instruments of sensory selection. *Trends in Neurosciences 32*: 9–18.

Schroeder, C. E. and Lakatos, P. (2012). The signs of silence. *Neuron 74*: 770–772.

Schroeder, C. E., Lakatos, P., Kajikawa, Y., Partan, S., and Puce, A. (2008). Neuronal oscillations and visual amplification of speech. *Trends in Cognitive Sciences 12*: 106–113.

Schroeder, C. E., Mehta, A. D., and Foxe, J. J. (2001). Determinants and mechanisms of attentional modulation of neural processing. *Frontiers in Bioscience 6*: 672–84.

Schroeder, C. E., Wilson, D. A., Radman, T., Scharfman, H., and Lakatos, P. (2010). Dynamics of active sensing and perceptual selection. *Current Opinion in Neurobiology 20*: 172–176.

Self, M. W., Kooijmans, R. N., Super, H., Lamme, V. A., and Roelfsema, P. R. (2012). Different glutamate receptors convey feedforward and recurrent processing in macaque V1. *Proceedings of the National Academy of Sciences USA 109*: 11031–11036.

Shah, A. S., Bressler, S. L., Knuth, K. H., Ding, M., Mehta, A. D., and Schroeder, C. E. (2004). Neural dynamics and fundamental mechanisms of event-related potentials. *Cerebral Cortex 14*: 476–485.

Sherman, S. M. and Guillery, R. W. (2002). The role of the thalamus in the flow of information to the cortex. *Philosophical Transactions of the Royal Society of London B: Biological Sciences 357*: 1695–1708.

Siegel, M., Donner, T. H., and Engel, A. K. (2012). Spectral fingerprints of large-scale neuronal interactions. *Nature Reviews Neuroscience 13*: 121–134.

Singer, W. (1999). Neuronal synchrony: A versatile code for definition of relations? *Neuron 24*: 49–65.

Singer, W., Gray, C., Engel, A., Konig, P., Artola, A., and Brocher, S. (1990). Formation of cortical cell assemblies. *Cold Spring Harbor Symposia on Quantitative Biology 55*: 939–952.

Skoblenick, K. and Everling, S. (2012). NMDA antagonist ketamine reduces task selectivity in macaque dorsolateral prefrontal neurons and impairs performance of randomly interleaved prosaccades and antisaccades. *Journal of Neuroscience 32*: 12018–12027.

Snyder, A. C. and Foxe, J. J. (2010). Anticipatory attentional suppression of visual features indexed by oscillatory alpha-band power increases: A high-density electrical mapping study. *Journal of Neuroscience 30*: 4024–4032.

Stefanics, G., Hangya, B., Hernadi, I., Winkler, I., Lakatos, P., and Ulbert, I. (2010). Phase entrainment of human delta oscillations can mediate the effects of expectation on reaction speed. *Journal of Neuroscience 30*: 13578–13585.

Steriade, M., Gloor, P., Llinás, R. R., Lopes da Silva, F. H., and Mesulam, M. M. (1990). Basic mechanisms of cerebral rhythmic activities. *Electroencephalography and Clinical Neurophysiology 76*: 481–508.

Suffczynski, P., Kalitzin, S., Pfurtscheller, G., and Lopes da Silva, F. H. (2001). Computational model of thalamo-cortical networks: Dynamical control of alpha rhythms in relation to focal attention. *International Journal of Psychophysiology 43*: 25–40.

Taylor, K., Mandon, S., Freiwald, W., and Kreiter, A. (2005). Coherent oscillatory activity in monkey area V4 predicts successful allocation of attention. *Cerebral Cortex 15*: 1424–1437.

Thiele, A., Herrero, J. L., Distler, C., and Hoffmann, K. P. (2012). Contribution of cholinergic and GABAergic mechanisms to direction tuning, discriminability, response reliability, and neuronal rate correlations in macaque middle temporal area. *Journal of Neuroscience 32*: 16602–16615.

Thut, G., Nietzel, A., Brandt, S. A., and Pascual-Leone, A. (2006). Alpha-band electroencephalographic activity over occipital cortex indexes visuospatial attention bias and predicts visual target detection. *Journal of Neuroscience* 26: 9494–9502.

Treue, S. and Maunsell, J. H. (1996). Attentional modulation of visual motion processing in cortical areas MT and MST. *Nature* 382: 539–541.

Unal, C. T., Golowasch, J. P., and Zaborszky, L. (2012). Adult mouse basal forebrain harbors two distinct cholinergic populations defined by their electrophysiology. *Frontiers in Behavioral Neuroscience* 6: 21.

Ungerleider, L. G. and Kastner, S. (2000). Mechanisms of visual attention in the human cortex. *Annual Review of Neuroscience* 23: 315–341.

Ungerleider, L. G. and Mishkin, M. (1982). Two cortical visual systems. In D. J. Ingle, M. A. Goodale, and R. J. W. Mansfield (eds.), *Analysis of Visual Behavior* (pp. 549–586). Cambridge, Mass.: MIT Press.

Van Dijk, H., Schoffelen, J. M., Oostenveld, R., and Jensen, O. (2008). Prestimulus oscillatory activity in the alpha band predicts visual discrimination ability. *Journal of Neuroscience* 28: 1816–1823.

Van Ede, F., de Lange, F., Jensen, O., and Maris, E. (2011). Orienting attention to an upcoming tactile event involves a spatially and temporally specific modulation of sensorimotor alpha- and beta-band oscillations. *Journal of Neuroscience* 31: 2016–2024.

Vanderwolf, C. H., Raithby, A., Snider, M., Cristi, C., and Tanner, C. (1993). Effects of some cholinergic agonists on neocortical slow wave activity in rats with basal forebrain lesions. *Brain Research Bulletin* 31: 515–521.

VanRullen, R., Busch, N., Drewes, J., and Dubois, J. (2011). Ongoing EEG phase as a trial-by-trial predictor of perceptual and attentional variability. *Frontiers in Psychology* 2: 60.

VanRullen, R., Carlson, T., and Cavanagh, P. (2007). The blinking spotlight of attention. *Proceedings of the National Academy of Sciences USA* 104: 19204–19209.

VanRullen, R. and Koch, C. (2003). Is perception discrete or continuous? *Trends in Cognitive Sciences* 7: 207–213.

Vidal, C. and Changeux, J. P. (1993). Nicotinic and muscarinic modulations of excitatory synaptic transmission in the rat prefrontal cortex in vitro. *Neuroscience* 56: 23–32.

Von, E. J., Eliava, M., Meyer, A. H., Rozov, A., and Monyer, H. (2007). Functional characterization of intrinsic cholinergic interneurons in the cortex. *Journal of Neuroscience* 27: 5633–5642.

Von Stein, A. and Sarnthein, J. (2000). Different frequencies for different scales of cortical integration: From local gamma to long-range alpha/theta synchronization. *International Journal of Psychophysiology* 38: 301–313.

Wang, X. J. (2010). Neurophysiological and computational principles of cortical rhythms in cognition. *Physiological Reviews* 90: 1195–1268.

Whittington, M. A., Traub, R. D., Kopell, N., Ermentrout, B., and Buhl, E. H. (2000). Inhibition-based rhythms: Experimental and mathematical observations on network dynamics. *International Journal of Psychophysiology* 38: 315–336.

Wilens, T. E., Biederman, J., Spencer, T. J., Bostic, J., Prince, J., Monuteaux, M. C., Soriano, J., Fine, C., Abrams, A., Rater, M., and Polisner, D. (1999). A pilot controlled clinical trial of ABT-418, a cholinergic agonist, in the treatment of adults with attention deficit hyperactivity disorder. *American Journal of Psychiatry* 156: 1931–1937.

Witte, E. A. and Marrocco, R. T. (1997). Alteration of brain noradrenergic activity in rhesus monkeys affects the alerting component of covert orienting. *Psychopharmacology (Berlin)* 132: 315–323.

Womelsdorf, T., Fries, P., Mitra, P. P., and Desimone, R. (2006). Gamma-band synchronization in visual cortex predicts speed of change detection. *Nature 439*: 733–736.

Wonnacott, S. (1997). Presynaptic nicotinic ACh receptors. *Trends in Neurosciences 20*: 92–98.

Worden, M. S., Foxe, J. J., Wang, N., and Simpson, G. V. (2000). Anticipatory biasing of visuospatial attention indexed by retinotopically specific alpha-band electroencephalography increases over occipital cortex. *Journal of Neuroscience 20*: RC63.

Xiang, Z., Huguenard, J. R., and Prince, D. A. (1998). Cholinergic switching within neocortical inhibitory networks. *Science 281*: 985–988.

Yu, A. J. and Dayan, P. (2002). Acetylcholine in cortical inference. *Neural Networks 15*: 719–730.

Zhang, Y. and Ding, M. (2010). Detection of a weak somatosensory stimulus: Role of the prestimulus mu rhythm and its top-down modulation. *Journal of Cognitive Neuroscience 22*: 307–322.

Zikopoulos, B. and Barbas, H. (2006). Prefrontal projections to the thalamic reticular nucleus form a unique circuit for attentional modulation. *Journal of Neuroscience 26*: 7348–7361.

Zikopoulos, B. and Barbas, H. (2007a). Circuits for multisensory integration and attentional modulation through the prefrontal cortex and the thalamic reticular nucleus in primates. *Reviews in the Neurosciences 18*: 417–438.

Zikopoulos, B. and Barbas, H. (2007b). Parallel driving and modulatory pathways link the prefrontal cortex and thalamus. *PLoS One 2*: e848.

Zion-Golumbic, E., Ding, N., Bickel, S., Lakatos, P., Schevon, C. A., McKhann, G. M., Goodman, R. R., Emerson, R. G., Mehta, A. D., Simon, J. Z., Poeppel, D., and Schroeder, C. E. (2013). Mechanisms underlying selective neuronal tracking of attended speech at a 'cocktail party'. *Neuron 77*: 980–991.

CHAPTER 18

··

THE NEUROPSYCHO–
PHARMACOLOGY OF
ATTENTION

··

T. W. ROBBINS

INTRODUCTION

···

INVESTIGATING the neuropsychopharmacology of attention has several important goals, both theoretical and applied. Drugs generally have quite well-defined molecular actions and can produce specific effects on chemical neurotransmitter systems, sometimes in defined neurocircuits, which can be used to investigate the neurochemical basis of attention, as well as other aspects of cognition. Such investigations also enable the functions of these neurotransmitters to be defined, for example, in terms of characterizing specific states. Furthermore, there are important practical applications of studying drug effects on attention. First, some drugs are often used to improve vigilance or other aspects of attention in human operators performing certain tasks. Indeed, this is the mode of action of many so-called 'cognitive enhancers'. Second, some of the therapeutic effects of psychoactive drugs in psychiatric or neurological disorders may occur via actions on attention.

DRUGS, NEUROTRANSMITTERS,
AND NEURONAL NETWORKS

···

Drugs mainly affect chemical neurotransmitter function by interacting with receptors mediating components of synaptic processes, such as the synthesis, storage, release, reuptake, and catabolism of neurotransmitters, as well as the simulation or antagonism of their effects at pre- or post-synaptic receptors. Neurotransmitters may optimize transmission in neuronal networks via their signalling properties and their capacity to influence 'signal-to-noise' ratios in these networks. The functioning of neuronal networks in forebrain structures such as the cerebral cortex, hippocampus, and striatum is mediated by fast signalling excitatory (glutamate) or inhibitory (GABA-ergic) transmission. Hence they will almost certainly be implicated in several attentional mechanisms. Neuronal networks are also modulated by slow-acting, modulatory neurotransmitters such as the monoamines (dopamine (DA), noradrenaline (NA), serotonin or 5-hydroxytryptamine (5-HT), and histamine) and by acetylcholine (ACh), as well as by neuropeptides which may coexist as transmitters in the same neurons as, for example, DA (cholecystokinin), NA (neuropeptide Y), or ACh (vasoactive intestinal polypeptide or VIP) (see Table 18.1). These peptides also often function as hormones, and, both in the central nervous system and the periphery, may contribute importantly to state-changes, e.g. of stress, arousal, or motivation. Recently, novel neurotransmitters have been discovered in the hypothalamus, such as orexin and hypocretin, which may have especially important functions in sleep and arousal.

Commonly, a given neurotransmitter has multiple receptors, mediating different aspects of its functions, in complex ways that are difficult to unravel. Thus, acetylcholine has at least two main forms of receptor (muscarinic and nicotinic), DA has five main receptors (DA D1–5), serotonin (or 5-hydroxytryptamine, 5-HT) has at least 15, and glutamate has at least three main types (AMPA, NMDA, and kainate), the former being primarily responsible for the fast signalling functions of this transmitter and NMDA being linked to mechanisms of neural plasticity, including learning as well as shifts in attention and updating working memory (see Cooper et al. 2002).

Table 18.1 Major chemical neurotransmitters

Classical neurotransmitters	
'Fast signalling'	Receptors
Glutamate (excitatory) (GLU)	NMDA, AMPA, Kainate
Gamma-aminobutyric acid (inhibitory) (GABA)	GABA-a, GABA-b
'Slow modulatory'	
Acetylcholine (ACh)	Nicotinic, muscarinic
Dopamine (DA)	D1-D5
Noradrenaline (NA) (norepinephrine)	alpha1,2; beta 1,2
Serotonin (5-hydroxytryptamine, 5-HT)	At least 15, including 5-HT1a, 5-HT1b, 5HT2a, 5-HT1a, 5-HT1b, 5HT2a, 5-HT2c, 5-HT3, 5-HT6 etc
Neuropeptides	
Very slow modulators/co-transmitters	
Cholecystokinin (CCK)—co-transmitter for DA	
Neuropeptide Y—co-transmitter for NA	
Vasoactive intestinal polypeptide (VIP) —co-transmitter for ACh	
Orexin	
Oxytocin, vasopressin, etc.	

Strategies for investigating drug effects on attention have evolved in both human and non-human studies. In humans, one is limited in general to studying effects of drugs given systemically, which may thus also have peripheral effects (which have to be excluded when attributing central nervous system actions). Another limitation is that, of course, it is not possible to administer compounds to humans that have not been subjected to rigorous tests of safety (toxicity) to prevent adverse side-effects, and this often excludes experimental drugs with often more specific modes of action. The systemic route of administration in humans makes it difficult to localize effects of drugs in the brain, given that the relevant receptors are generally (though not always) widespread. This disadvantage can be partly offset by the combined use of drug treatments with such brain imaging methods as functional magnetic resonance imaging (fMRI). Some of these limitations can be overcome by animal studies, where it is possible to administer drugs centrally via implanted cannulae. However, the main difficulty is in translating findings obtained with animals to human, especially clinical, applications. Addressing this problem depends on using test methods in animals that can be clearly related to human paradigms, in terms of the underlying psychological processes and homologous mediating neural structures. Fortunately, this is not such a barrier to translation as would be provided by other aspects of cognition, most obviously, language.

Paradigms of Attention and Their Neural Basis

Most commentators agree that there are several distinct aspects of attention: selective, divided, and sustained attention, including vigilance (Parasuraman 1998; see also chapters 19 and 26, this volume). Attention also overlaps with the concept of executive function (that set of loosely defined processes which serve to optimize performance), notably in the domain of rule generation and selection (including set-shifting). This distinction is somewhat analogous to the distinction that is often made in cognitive neuroscience between anterior and posterior attentional networks (Posner and Petersen 1990; see also Posner, chapter 1, this volume). This distinction may perhaps be made in terms of 'input' attention versus 'controlled attention', the latter often assumed to be mediated by the prefrontal cortex and the former often involving involuntary processes. Another way of conceptualizing this distinction is in terms of 'posterior', involuntary, exogenous, 'bottom-up' versus 'anterior', voluntary, endogenous, 'top-down' processes, respectively (Noudoost and Moore 2011). A particularly influential 'biased competition' model of attention derives from single unit studies in the macaque monkey, in which the relative activity of cells towards external stimuli in visual regions such as V4 is influenced by attention paid to cues that predict food (Desimone and Duncan, 1995; see chapters 4 and 5, this volume). This biasing operation hence represents a likely 'top-down' influence of the prefrontal cortex to counteract processing of sensory salience in posterior cortical functioning. The paradigm may have implications for understanding selective attention in humans. Similar mechanisms may be inferred in humans from increased blood oxygenation level dependent activity (BOLD response) sensed using fMRI and also the occurrence of correlated waves or oscillations of neuronal activity such as gamma oscillations, which depend, for example, on interneurons using the inhibitory neurotransmitter GABA, as well as glutamate receptors, particularly of the NMDA sub-type (Bartos et al. 2007; Deco and Thiele 2009). To the extent that functioning of the neural networks depends on interactions in and among canonical cortical columnar micro-circuitry, comprising mainly pyramidal cells and interneurons, it can be inferred that attentional function will depend on glutamatergic and GABA-ergic neurotransmission, modulated by ascending neurotransmitter systems of subcortical origin, including the monoamines and acetylcholine.

Several questions can be addressed about the functions of these neurotransmitter systems in attention, and correspondingly, whether these can be discerned in the effects of drugs on cognitive performance. One issue is whether any effects on attention are essentially secondary to effects on overall arousal level, affected for example by circadian factors, stress, motivation, novelty, and fatigue. A second is whether discrete functions in attention can be discerned for these neurotransmitter systems arising from their unique neuronal actions to modulate signal-to-noise processing. Related to this issue is whether some chemical neurotransmitter systems are uniquely dedicated to different forms of attention (e.g. selective versus sustained; or top-down versus bottom-up). Thirdly, and most challenging, is how they might interact to influence attentional function.

Neuroscientists are beginning to discover the nature of glutamatergic and GABA-ergic mechanisms underlying network function and attention, and there are documented effects of drugs such as the benzodiazepines (indirect GABA agonists) and the NMDA receptor antagonist ketamine on human attention (see below). However, considerable research (as well as clinical practice in the case of treatment of attention deficit/hyperactivity disorder (ADHD) with stimulant drugs such as methylphenidate) has implicated the catecholamines, DA and NA, in modulatory, possibly complementary aspects of attention. Possibly the most investigated system, at all levels of analysis, is that using acetylcholine, especially in view of suggestions that the cholinergic deficit in dementia leads to attentional lapses that can be treated with anti-cholinesterases (Perry et al. 1999).

Acetylcholine and Attention

Research over the past 50 years or so, in both basic and human neuroscience, has strongly implicated acetylcholine in attention. Warburton was among the first to use signal detection theory in vigilance scenarios in rodents (Warburton and Brown 1971, 1972). Thus, for example, the anti-cholinesterase physostigmine dose-dependently enhanced d' in a visual target detection procedure in rats, whereas scopolamine reduced it. With Wesnes, he also showed that nicotine (in non-smokers) enhanced a test of sustained attention in humans requiring detection of rapidly presented (100/min), specified sequences of digits at a single location (the rapid visual information processing (RVIP) task) (Wesnes and Warburton 1984). Converging evidence from studies of the effects of the anti-muscarinic receptor antagonist scopolamine on cognition also implicated possible effects of the drug on cholinergically mediated attentional processes (e.g. Broks et al. 1988).

Soon after the early behavioural demonstrations of ACh involvement in attention, electrophysiological work on the V1 area of cat showed apparent effects of ACh to enhance signal processing in receptive fields of visual cortical neurons (Sillito and Kemp 1983), although some subsequent work has failed to confirm this (Zinke et al. 2006).

Research was also directed at the role of the major origin of the cholinergic projections to the neocortex, the nucleus basalis of Meynert (nbM; or nucleus basalis magnocellularis in rodents). Among the more consistent effects of excitotoxic lesions of this nucleus, which typically produced substantial loss of cholinergic terminals in the frontal cortex, was the disruption of performance by rats of a serial 5-choice serial reaction time task (5CSRTT—see Fig. 18.1), modelled on a similar continuous performance type task in humans (Robbins et al. 1989; Muir et al. 1994; Robbins 2002). Of particular importance was the impairment of detection of brief visual events presented randomly at one of five locations; this effect was later shown to be especially evident with longer test sessions where there was an apparent late decrement in accuracy, and when employing the more selective cholinergic immunotoxin 192-IgG-saporin (McGaughy et al. 2002; Dalley et al. 2004). Impaired discrimination performance could be remediated by systemic administration of optimal doses of physostigmine or nicotine, as well as by cholinergically enriched neural transplants into the rodent cortex (Muir et al. 1992, 1995). Further experiments using intracerebral monitoring of ACh with *in vivo* microdialysis showed the neurotransmitter to be released in the PFC when attentional demands were increased (Passetti et al. 2000; Dalley et al. 2001; Kozak et al. 2006). These results were paralleled by qualitatively similar findings for effects of 192-IgG-saporin-induced lesions of the nbM using a different sustained attention task in which rats were trained to detect the presence or absence of a visual cue (McGaughy et al. 1996), and also for another task measuring crossmodal divided attention between visual and auditory cues (Turchi and Sarter 1997). Careful analysis of performance on the former task suggested that ACh was especially important on cue detection trials in contrast to the 'blank' trials in which no stimuli were presented (McGaughy et al. 1996). Overall, the evidence implicating selective effects of ACh in attentional performance in rodents is perhaps more convincing than for any of the other major neurotransmitters.

The possible relevance of these findings to human disorders was demonstrated by the fact that the anti-cholinesterase tacrine improved performance of patients with probable Alzheimer's disease on the same 5-choice serial reaction-time tasks as used in rodents, with concomitant improvements in clinical rating scales of attention 'alerting' (Sahakian et al. 1993). Subsequent clinical experience has shown that such medications (e.g. rivastigmine) are also effective in the treatment of the fluctuating attentional capacities of

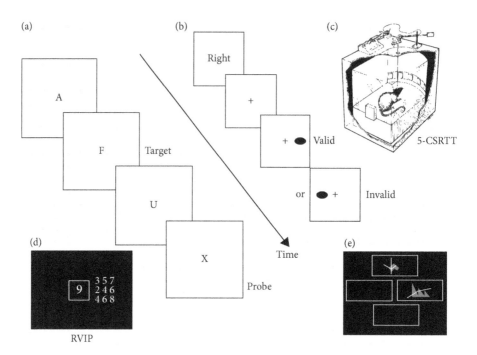

FIGURE 18.1 Paradigms for measuring attention in humans and other animals. (a) The 'attentional blink' task. In this paradigm the second of two rapidly presented targets (i.e. the probe) is detected with significantly lower accuracy if the rapid presentations exceed a certain rate in time (i.e. if the time-lag between target and probe is relatively short). (b) Posner's 'covert orienting' paradigm for spatial attention; invalid spatial cueing to where a visual target is expected significantly slows reaction time, whereas valid cueing has the opposite effect. (c) The rodent 5-choice serial reaction time task (5-CSRTT). The rat has to detect a brief visual target presented randomly at 1 of 5 locations in space. Reproduced from *Neuropharmacology of Attention*, Robbins, T.W., Milstein, J. & Dalley, J.W., In Attention (M Posner, Ed) 2004. Copyright Guilford Press. Reprinted with permission of The Guilford Press. (d) The rapid visual information processing (RVIP) test for sustained attention. Subject is required to detect specified sequences of rapidly presented digits (100/min). © Copyright 2013, Cambridge Cognition Limited. All rights reserved. (e) The intra-dimensional/ extra-dimensional shift task from the CANTAB battery for humans and monkeys; a translational analogue of the Wisconsin Card-Sorting Test. See text for further details. © Copyright 2013, Cambridge Cognition Limited. All rights reserved. (d) and (e) © Copyright 2013, Cambridge Cognition Limited. All rights reserved.

patients with Lewy Body dementia, who tend to have even more profound reductions of cholinergic function than do patients with Alzheimer's disease (Emre et al. 2004).

Work on non-human primates also implicated basal forebrain cholinergic projections in attentional functions that are classically thought to be mediated by posterior cortical regions (Voytko et al. 1994). These authors thus found that rhesus monkeys with lesions of the nbM exhibited specific deficits in Posner's test of covert attentional orienting (see Fig. 18.1; thought to depend on posterior parietal cortex, Posner et al. 1984). This finding is consistent with evidence that nicotine enhances attentional orienting in both monkeys (Witte et al. 1997) and humans (Murphy and Klein 1998) and also with the observation that intra-parietal cortex infusion of scopolamine impairs it (Davidson and Marrocco 2000). Thiele and co-workers additionally found that there was augmentation of responses of V1 neurons in their receptive fields to attended stimuli, by iontophoretically applied ACh in monkeys (see Deco and Thiele 2009). This action, on visual sensory processing, however, was mediated by muscarinic and not nicotinic receptors (Herrero et al. 2008). Thus, it appears likely that muscarinic receptors contribute to 'bottom-up' modulation of visual sensory processing and that both muscarinic and nicotinic receptors contribute to attentional orienting in primates. Thus, cholinergic modulation of visual attention probably occurs at different stages of the visual processing stream, which may differentially depend on muscarinic and nicotinic receptors. This situation may help to explain why anti-cholinesterases such as physostigmine can modulate both visual sensory processing and attentional performance patients with Alzheimer's disease, in relation to its effects on BOLD activity in extrastriatal cortex and fronto-parietal cortex, respectively (Bentley et al. 2008).

These findings nevertheless leave it unclear to what extent ACh may also affect top-down attentional control. The early work in rodents showed a definite connection between cholinergic function in the prefrontal cortex and performance of sustained attention tasks, whereas the electrophysiological and lesion work with non-human primates has focused on posterior cortical functions, including the extrastriate and posterior parietal cortex.

Recent advances in the use of *in vivo* electrochemical measures of cholinergic activity in rodents have lent a new dimension to the interpretation of the rodent data. The use of enzyme-coated microelectrodes has allowed monitoring ACh release at a sub-second resolution, thus permitting measurement of changes in ACh release in association with specific task events or behavioural responses. Visual cues predicting food presentation evoked transient increases in cholinergic activity in the rat medial prefrontal cortex (Parikh et al. 2007—see Fig. 18.2). Such transients were not observed on trials in which cues were missed (and they were not observed in a control region, the motor cortex). Even if a cue was missed, reward was eventually delivered and retrieved, but no cholinergic activity was then detected, strongly suggesting that the cholinergic transients were related to attentional processes.

Sarter's current hypothesis is that the cue evokes immediate release of glutamate which additionally causes the cholinergic transient and associated neuronal spiking activity to enable effective orienting (from the 'default' mode assumed to be present on blank trials) and responding to the target (Sarter et al. 2005; Hasselmo and Sarter 2011). This glutamate release itself can be stimulated by nicotinic receptors, as shown by the beneficial effect of alpha-4/beta-2 subunit nicotinic agonists. These drugs stimulate receptors found on afferents to the prefrontal cortex from the dorsomedial nucleus of the thalamus. This is hypothesized to be the main mechanism by which enhancement of attentional performance occurs following treatment with such drugs in several rodent studies. By contrast, similar evidence for a role for alpha-7 subunit nicotinic agonists is much more conflicting, and indeed there is some evidence that they even oppose the attentional enhancing action of the alpha-4 beta-2 agents (Howe et al.

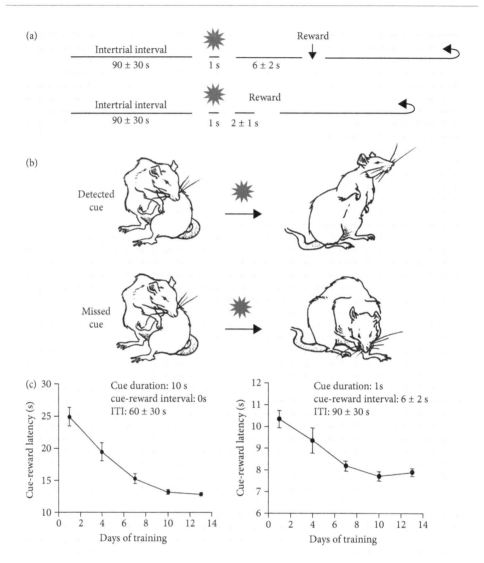

FIGURE 18.2 Task used for rodents in experiments on the role of cholinergic signalling in attention. (a) A cued appetitive task is used, in two versions, differing only in the interval between the cue offset and the delivery of food reward at one of two reward ports (randomly selected). (b) Trials on which cues were detected were monitored in terms of the rat's orienting behaviour (top), away from distracting activities such as grooming (bottom). (c) Demonstration of learning of the orientation response for cue detection over 14 days of training. Reprinted from *Neuron*, 56 (1), Vinay Parikh, Rouba Kozak, Vicente Martinez, and Martin Sarter, Prefrontal Acetylcholine Release Controls Cue Detection on Multiple Timescales, pp. 141–54, Copyright (2007), with permission from Elsevier.

2010). These data may help to explain the beneficial, though limited effects of nicotine itself on performance, and are also relevant to the potential use of such compounds in Alzheimer's disease and ADHD. They are also consistent with the findings of some fMRI studies in humans that demonstrate beneficial effects of nicotine in cue detection type tasks, associated with BOLD activity in the cingulate and fronto-parietal cortex (Vossel et al. 2008).

By contrast, there are as yet fewer data available to assess the likely efficacy of the newly developed selective muscarinic agonists on attentional performance, whether in rodents, infra-human primates, or humans, despite the fact that the muscarinic antagonist scopolamine is well known to produce attentional deficits. One intriguing observation is that stimulation of muscarinic receptors, presumably located on inhibitory interneurons, in the prefrontal cortex (as in V1) affects ACh release in posterior cortex (parietal cortex), presumably via feedback to the nbM which projects diffusely to the entire neocortex (Nelson et al. 2005). This would be an obvious example of top-down prefrontal control of attention mediated by cholinergic activity, possibly relevant to the regulation of biased competition and the capacity to ignore irrelevant, distracting stimuli. Thus it appears that cholinergic activity might simultaneously be affecting both 'bottom-up' and 'top-down' processing via different mechanisms. This illustrates the complexity of interpreting current drug effects on attention in humans, but also points to increasing selectivity of such effects with the emergence of more selective compounds.

ACh is also implicated, perhaps less convincingly, in memory functions, including working memory, recognition memory, and semantic retrieval, but it remains to be resolved whether its effects on attention contribute to these actions, as seems plausible, for example, for memory encoding, or persistence or resisting interference in working memory (Furey et al. 2000). It is, of course, possible that there are specific effects on memory-related processes, to those for attention, perhaps mediated by similar neuronal mechanisms, but in brain regions possibly more specialized for memory processing, such as the hippocampus.

NORADRENALINE AND ATTENTION

The catecholamines NA and DA also have important roles to play in attentional processes, although their precise contributions are complicated by their involvement in other functions that are sometimes difficult to unravel from attention. In the case of NA, it has also been linked with arousal, stress, anxiety, executive control, learning, and memory consolidation, probably as a consequence of its widely ramifying forebrain projections (most of which originate in the locus coeruleus of the pons). For example, an early theoretical suggestion was that the locus coeruleus functioned rather like the cognitive arm of a central sympathetic ganglion: 'Thus activation of the peripheral sympathetic nervous system prepares the animal physically for adaptive phasic responses to urgent stimuli, while parallel activation of the locus coeruleus increases attention and vigilance, preparing the animal cognitively for adaptive responses to such stimuli' (Amaral and Sinnamon 1977: 516). This notion remains at the heart of most of the theorizing about the functions of the coeruleo-cortical system in various forms.

For example, Posner has speculated that the system is implicated in 'alerting', mediated preferentially by modulation of his proposed attentional system, located predominantly in the right cerebral cortex, based on intriguing data suggesting an asymmetry of NA function in the rat thalamus (Oke et al. 1980). There is empirical evidence that a role for NA in mediating arousal or stress has indirect effects on attention or working memory. Arnsten and colleagues have shown how treatment with alpha-1 and alpha-2 agonists can affect spatial delayed response performance in rhesus monkeys according to a 'Yerkes–Dodson', inverted U-shaped function (Arnsten 1997, 2009). These effects can be interpreted in terms of effects of stress on working memory mediated by a neural network including the dorsolateral prefrontal cortex. However, possible relationships of working memory to 'working attention' are well known (see Chapter 28, this volume) and it may well be the case that the neuronal mechanisms by which NA affects performance on a working memory task may be identical to those affecting more globally, attentional performance.

Thus, based on microiontophoretic effects of applied NA, considerable evidence points to activity in the noradrenergic locus coeruleus producing alterations in signal-to-noise processing in terminal domains, such as the neocortex and hippocampus (review in Everitt et al. 1990; Foote et al. 1990; Segal and Bloom 1976). These alterations in signal-to-noise processing largely, but not completely, resulting from suppression of background neuronal activity ('noise') contrast with how ACh affects cortical neuronal activity. They result in an enhanced response of the terminal domain to another afferent input.

Another way in which a role for NA in mediating arousal or stress could affect attention can be derived from Easterbrook's hypothesis (Easterbrook 1959), which predicts that elevated levels of arousal narrow attentional focus. This concept has been applied specifically to the coeruleo-cortical NA system (Robbins 1984). One form of this hypothesis suggests a role for NA in attentional 'effort' (Cole and Robbins 1992; somewhat analogous to Sarter's hypothesis for ACh); that the NA system is 'recruited' or 'engaged' by top-down systems under arousing or stressful circumstances. This hypothesis gained some support from studies of effects of 6-hydroxydopamine-induced profound depletion of NA from the dorsal noradrenergic ascending bundle (DNAB, which provides the major NA-ergic innervation of the neocortex and hippocampus) in tests of spatial navigational learning and cue versus context aversive conditioning. Thus in the former case, learning was compared with the Morris water-maze with its conventional spatial cues around the pool in relation to a visual discrimination within the pool. In the latter case, a discrete CS and context were pitted against one another by a trace conditioning procedure. In brief, the results were that, under stressful circumstances, the rats with DNAB lesions showed greater attention to distal contextual and spatially diverse cues than to local cues (e.g. discrete visual stimuli). Thus, they appeared to have a broadened span of attention rather than exhibiting focused attention, suggestive of a loss of the focused attention occurring under high levels of arousal that is predicted by Easterbrook's hypothesis (Selden et al. 1990a, 1990b). More direct tests of the hypothesis employed the 5CSRTT. Rats with profound coeruleo-cortical NA depletion were impaired specifically under conditions when the visual targets were presented unpredictably in time, or when bursts of a white noise distractor were interpolated prior to the targets (Carli et al. 1983; Cole and Robbins 1992; Milstein et al. 2007).

Treatment of rodents or monkeys with adrenoceptor agonists at low doses can improve performance on similar tasks (Puumala et al. 1997; O'Neill et al. 2000). More recently, treatment with the relatively selective NA reuptake inhibitor atomoxetine has been shown to enhance accuracy of responding on the 5-choice serial reaction time task and also on a related multi-choice task under certain conditions (Jentsch et al. 2009; Robinson 2012). However, the main effect of the drug on performance of the 5CSRTT is to reduce premature ('impulsive') responding (Robinson et al. 2008). One problem of interpretation of such findings is that atomoxetine also up-regulates cortical dopamine levels as a consequence of the capacity of the cortical NA transporter also to control dopamine uptake (Bymaster et al. 2002).

Some evidence has accrued for the hypothesis that at least some of the modulatory effects of NA on attention are due to 'top-down' effects, resulting from its actions on prefrontal cortical mechanisms (e.g. Jentsch et al. 2009). Further evidence for this can be found from effects of noradrenergic manipulations on an attentional set-shifting paradigm for rodents, which is known to depend on the integrity of the medial prefrontal cortex. Dorsal noradrenergic bundle lesions selectively impaired extra-dimensional set-shifting (i.e. a shift in responding between tactile and olfactory stimuli) (Tait et al. 2007). This deficit was consistent with other evidence: (i) Chronic treatment with either idazoxan (alpha-2 receptor antagonist, Rowe et al. 1996) or desipramine (Lapiz et al. 2007) (which blocks NA reuptake) impaired and improved set-shifting performance, respectively. (ii) Enhancing NA-ergic function with atipamezole, an alpha-2 adrenergic autoreceptor antagonist (which increases activity in the dorsal noradrenergic bundle system via its actions at inhibitory autoreceptors located in the locus coeruleus) significantly improved attentional set-shifting (Lapiz and Morilak 2006). Moreover, this effect was blocked by infusions of a post-synaptic alpha-1 receptor antagonist infused into the medial prefrontal cortex (but not by β1 or β2 receptor antagonists) (Lapiz and Morilak 2006). (iii) This enhancement of shifting was also observed in rats with NA depletion treated with low doses of atomoxetine (Newman et al. 2008). Higher doses of atomoxetine administered to unoperated rats impaired attentional set-shifting performance. Overall, the evidence from rodent studies suggests that NA can play a role in remediating or modulating attentional function in a number of paradigms, and that the effects are not simply produced by changes in arousal level or states of stress, although they may interact with them.

A further dimension is provided by electrophysiological single unit recording from noradrenergic locus coeruleus cells during performance of a sustained attention task in which macaques had to detect rare targets presented in random intervals and inhibit responses to distractors (Aston-Jones et al. 1991; Usher et al. 1999; Rajkowski et al. 2004). The main findings were that optimal performance of the task

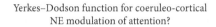

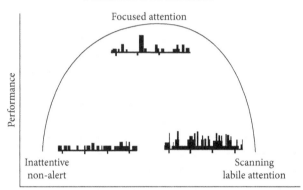

FIGURE 18.3 The inverted U-shaped 'Yerkes–Dodson' function, as applied to the relationship between efficient performance on a go/no-go visual discrimination, sustained attention task in monkeys and the balance between phasic/tonic activity of noradrenergic cells in the locus coeruleus. Reprinted from *Biological Psychiatry*, 46 (9), Gary Aston-Jones, Janusz Rajkowski, and Jonathan Cohen, Role of locus coeruleus in attention and behavioral flexibility, pp. 1309–20 Copyright (1999), with permission from Elsevier.

coincided with high phasic rates of coeruleal cell firing, whereas relatively poor performance corresponded to high tonic rates of firing, which were suggested to be associated with distractibility from the main task. This pattern of findings corresponds to an inverted-U shaped function relating locus coeruleus activity to optimal attentional performance, with the additional feature of the relative modes of phasic versus tonic firing (see Fig. 18.3). However, the tonic mode of locus coeruleus activity was not simply linked to impaired cognitive performance overall, as it was speculated that it represented a state that enabled task disengagement, in order to 'explore' other salient events in the environment of possible adaptive significance (Usher et al. 1999; Aston-Jones and Cohen 2005).

Peak phasic firing rates uniquely occurred approximately 100–150 msec post-target and 200 msec prior to the response—and were similar to the responses elicited by unexpected or intense salient stimuli. Other data indicate a direct relationship between firing rate of locus coeruleus cells and choice accuracy in a choice reaction time setting (Rajkowski et al. 2004).

Taking these non-human primate findings together with the rodent data, it would appear that optimal levels of noradrenergic activity are associated with superior performance in tests of sustained and selective attention, involving both 'top-down' and 'bottom-up' processes.

INVESTIGATION OF THE ROLE OF
NORADRENALINE IN HUMAN ATTENTION

Direct neuroimaging of human locus coeruleus activity is a challenging prospect because of the small size of the structure, which may possibly be approached using treatment with pharmacologically selective noradrenergic agents (or PET ligands) to highlight the nucleus. Some researchers have proposed that the cortical P-300 potential is controlled by locus coeruleus activity. The P-300 is certainly influenced by manipulation of central NA pharmacologically and lesions of the locus coeruleus in non-human primates selectively reduce it. There is evidence that the P-300 is closely related to the motivational salience of an event (somewhat like locus coeruleus activity), but it is still unclear precisely what this event potential reflects in information processing terms.

Nieuwenhuis et al. (2005) realized that a refractory period of firing of locus coeruleus cells approximately 250–450 msec after a phasic response to a stimulus coincides with the well-known 'attentional blink' phenomenon (the transient impairment in detecting the second of two signals if the second follows the first in rapid temporal proximity) and also absence of the P-300. De Martino et al. (2008) found that beta-adrenergic blockade using propanolol impaired attentional-blink performance, whereas an NA reuptake inhibitor (reboxetine) improved it (for emotionally salient stimuli). On the other hand, clonidine (an alpha-1/2 adrenoceptor agonist) has been reported to have no effect (Nieuwenhuis et al. 2007).

In general, studies with adrenergic agents on cognition in humans are complicated by possible effects on inhibitory autoreceptors. Thus, alpha-2 agonists such as clonidine and guanfacine will reduce firing of the locus coeruleus at low doses and thereby reduce NA release in terminal regions, though at the same time, at higher doses, acting as agonists at post-synaptic receptors. Therefore, effects on attention can be ambiguously interpreted sometimes as reflecting increasing or decreasing noradrenergic function. One way of addressing this difficulty is to use more than one dose of the agonist; a low dose targeting the autoreceptors, and a higher dose acting additionally at post-synaptic receptors. If the effects of the drug are in opposite directions at the low and high dose, this does aid interpretation. Unfortunately, however, relatively few studies have managed to achieve this ideal.

On the other hand, there is little doubt that low doses of clonidine impair attention, and are also sedative in some sense. For example, at a low dose, clonidine produces substantial deficits in performance on the RVIP test of sustained attention that were correlated with changes in heart rate variability (Middleton et al. 1994). Similarly, Coull et al. (1995) found impairments in RVIP at a low (but not at a higher) dose of clonidine, though with no interaction in terms of time on task. Importantly, the detrimental effect of clonidine was greatest in subjects who had been familiarized with the task, again suggesting that arousal factors induced by task novelty were important modulators of the effects of the drug. Coull (1998) notes that these effects of clonidine are directly comparable to those of patients with frontal lobe damage, suggesting a plausible location of the drug effects (and also consistent with beneficial effects of idazoxan on patients with frontal lobe dementia; Coull et al. 1996). Further evidence was provided by neuroimaging studies of performance of the RVIP task using PET, which were consistent with a fronto-parietal–anterior thalamic network for attention (Coull et al. 1997). Moreover, clonidine was found to reduce activity in the resting state rather than during performance of the attentional task, suggesting effects on arousal in networks determining activity in the 'default mode'.

Further evidence of a likely role of arousal in mediating effects of clonidine comes from the evidence that (i) clonidine impaired performance of a selective attention task more in quiet than in noisy conditions (Smith and Nutt 1996) and (ii) in rhesus monkeys spatial delayed response ('working memory') performance following clonidine was less impaired by distracting white noise in the delay intervals (Arnsten and Contant 1992). (iii) Clark et al. (1989) also found that clonidine impaired performance in a set of dichotic listening experiments that probed both selective and divided attention. They suggested that the drug reduced alertness or arousal. In contrast, a dopamine receptor blocker, whilst also impairing performance, reduced the readiness for action, leading to the authors' proposal that NA was concerned with the capacity for conscious registration of stimuli and DA with the capacity to respond to them.

One result that appears to contradict the hypothesis that clonidine's effects on arousal determine its actions on tasks of attention comes from Clark et al.'s use of Posner's test of attentional orienting. They found that a low dose of clonidine diminished the cost of invalid cueing while not affecting valid cueing or response speed. Moreover, idazoxan, an alpha-2 receptor antagonist, has been shown to enhance attention to the location of a previous cue (an impairment of 'inhibition of return') (Smith et al. 1992), which may possibly be construed as a complementary effect to that of clonidine. These findings are perhaps analogous to those in animals suggesting that NA depletion broadens the span of spatial attention.

However, the effects of clonidine on orienting of attention have to be reconsidered in the light of analogous studies in rhesus monkeys of effects of clonidine and another alpha-2 agent, guanfacine. In apparent contrast to the human studies, Witte et al. (1997) showed no effects on attentional orienting in rhesus monkeys, there being no significant effects of either drug on being invalidly cued to an incorrect target location. The drugs did, however, remove the benefit of advance cueing, suggesting selective effects of clonidine and guanfacine on arousal or alerting rather than attentional orienting. How best to reconcile the human and monkey data? First, Clark et al. (1989) did not index arousal in the same way as in the rhesus study. Second, they used a central cueing paradigm (see Fig. 18.1) in contrast to the peripheral cueing method employed by Witte and Marrocco, so the discrepancy may possibly be resolved by differential effects of clonidine on the 'anterior' (or 'top-down') and 'posterior' attentional orienting systems.

Overall, there is considerable evidence that the actions of NA on different aspects of attentional function are widespread (both in functional and neural terms), markedly dependent on level of baseline arousal or stress, and probably also upon the relative balance between fast phasic firing and tonic activity in the coeruleo-cortical system. The latter may also reflect to some degree the balance between top-down processing (affecting fast phasic activity of the locus coeruleus via descending projections from the cortex and other forebrain structures) and local mechanisms regulating NA levels within the synapse.

EFFECTS OF STIMULANT DRUGS ON ATTENTION

Stimulant drugs such as amphetamine and methylphenidate usually have facilitatory effects in humans on the performance of tests of sustained attention and vigilance, as well as upon other tasks (such as the Stroop or the continuous performance task) associated with different aspects of attention, both in healthy volunteers (Weiss and Laties 1962; Koelega 1993) and patients, notably those exhibiting ADHD (Swanson et al. 2011). Typically, the effects are dose-dependent, performance baseline-dependent, and arousal state-dependent in the sense that the largest drug effects are obtained when subjects are in sleep-deprived or fatigued conditions. However, their efficacy is not simply due to their capacity to combat fatigue or drowsiness. The effects are likely mediated by indirect actions to potentiate catecholamine (NA and DA) activity, through a number of actions (Cooper et al. 2002), including enhancement of neurotransmitter release, block of reuptake (transporter) mechanisms and monoamine oxidase inhibition, and likely at different neural locations. The dose-effect function is an inverted U-shaped curve, reminiscent of the Yerkes–Dodson principle relating to arousal, with optimal effects being shown at intermediate doses and even deficits relative to placebo being shown at the highest doses. This type of effect can be observed in paradigms such as the 5CSRTT in animal studies (where high doses often result in performance-disrupting impulsive behaviour), but has also been shown to be relevant in the treatment of juvenile or adult ADHD.

Stimulant drugs such as methylphenidate and amphetamine are routinely used to treat ADHD, but there is still considerable controversy about the core deficits in ADHD as well as which aspects of performance are affected (both acutely, and following chronic treatment) by stimulant drugs. Performance on tests of sustained attention (e.g. RVIP) and continuous performance is often impaired in ADHD, but ameliorated by stimulant drug treatment. A recent study has shown improved accuracy in a simultaneous matching-to-perceptual sample task (as well as with delay) (Coghill et al. 2007). There is consistent evidence that slowed stop-signal reaction times are improved (made faster) by stimulants (e.g. Tannock et al. 1989; Aron et al. 2003), although whether this reflects improvements in a response inhibitory process (thus reducing impulsivity) or attentional factors is not absolutely clear (Lijffijt et al. 2005). This is because Go reaction times (RT) are often also slowed or more variable in juvenile ADHD, with a positive skew in the RT distribution reflecting the occurrence of long RTs which may be associated with attentional lapses. Swanson et al. (2011) have suggested that this deficit reflects impairments in transitions between a task mode neural network and a default mode neural network, based largely on fMRI studies. However, precisely how drugs such as the stimulants or the chemical neurotransmitter pathways affect these transitions is not yet known. Nevertheless, a study by Epstein et al. (2006) using a sophisticated statistical analysis has shown that medication with stimulants may both slow Go RT and reduce RT variability, possibly reflecting both anti-impulsive and attention-enhancing effects, but also being reminiscent of rate-dependency effects seen in experimental animals (Robbins and Sahakian 1979). That the stimulants exert multiple effects on cognition including attention is plausible, given their actions on both catecholamines, NA and DA.

Dopamine and Attention

A fundamental possible confound in interpreting the role of dopamine in attention is its role in reinforcement, and additionally in putative motivational processes by which environmental stimuli gain 'incentive salience'. By definition, salience confers upon stimuli the capacity to compel or 'grab' attention. Efficient goal-directed behaviour requires a focusing of attention on the most salient stimuli predicting reward, and this may be achieved by 'attentional set', a component of 'top-down' executive functioning. Fast phasic firing of midbrain dopamine cells is correlated with the predictive properties of a conditioned stimulus (CS) for food reward; thus a discrepancy between an expected outcome and an actual outcome elicits such activity and corresponds to the beneficial effects of 'surprise' on learning (Schultz and Dickinson 2000). One phenomenon that has been linked to attentional function in the context of associative learning is latent inhibition, when learning about a conditioned CS is retarded if that stimulus has been pre-exposed uncorrelated with reinforcement. This retardation in rats is dramatically enhanced by exposure to a DA receptor antagonist drug such as haloperidol during the pre-exposure stage, suggesting that DA receptor blockade reduces the salience of the to-be-CS, possibly via an attentional-like process (Weiner and Feldon 1987).

Understanding the functions of dopamine at a systems level has to take into account the considerable evidence that the subcortical mesolimbic and mesostriatal DA systems may be functionally opposed to (or regulated by) the mesocortical DA system, which preferentially innervates the anterior cortex (including PFC) in rodents, although it also modulates more posterior cortical regions in the parietal and temporal lobes in humans. There is certainly evidence that manipulating PFC DA in experimental animals may up-regulate DA-dependent striatal functioning (Pycock et al. 1980; Roberts et al. 1994). The mesostriatal DA system also relates directly to motor functions, given its association with Parkinson's disease. This association also makes it sometimes difficult to measure attentional effects, which may be confounded for example by slowed response times.

One way in which this potential confound of sensory and motor effects has been manifested is in the analysis of an apparent 'neglect' syndrome following unilateral striatal dopamine depletion (Marshall and Teitelbaum 1977). Further studies have shown that such unilateral DA loss, when restricted to the dorsal striatum, impaired the capacity of rats to initiate a lateralized head movement into the hemispace contralateral to the side of the lesion rather than detect the stimulus in that space (Carli et al. 1985, 1989). If intact rats were required to make this response after unpredictable delays, such responding was 'primed' or speeded—an effect probably resulting from enhanced motor readiness (Brown and Robbins 1991). These authors found that lateralized dorsal striatal DA loss abolished the delay-dependent speeding effect, suggesting that striatal DA normally subserves lateralized motor readiness.

The neuronal mechanisms by which DA modulates the functioning of its terminal domains, like both ACh and NA, probably derives from its effects on signal-to-noise processing. Some aspects of this signalling are well understood, particularly for the dopamine D1-like receptor, which is in considerable preponderance in the PFC compared with the D2-like receptor. In the PFC, the signal-to-noise enhancing effect of DA at post-synaptic D1 receptors depends on several mechanisms, including the boosting of both glutamatergic NMDA receptor and GABA-ergic currents (Fig. 18.4—see

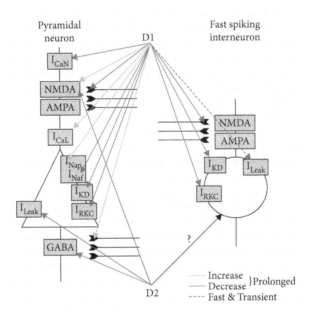

FIGURE 18.4 Complexities of signalling at the D1 and D2 dopamine receptors in the prefrontal cortex as discerned from *in vitro* studies. The D1 receptor affects a variety of ion channels and activity at GABA-ergic interneurons and NMDA-receptor bearing pyramidal cell and interneurons. Overall, the net effects of this activity are to (i) prolong activity initiated in pyramidal cells and (ii) prevent disruption of this activity from 'distracting' inputs. The net effect is to preserve neuronal activity in this prefrontal cortical 'module'. By contrast, via the mechanisms shown in the diagram, D2 receptors in the neocortex operate most effectively at different concentrations of extracellular DA and their activation opposes the optimal tuning provided by the D1 receptor to promote attentional lability and response flexibility. Reprinted from *Biological Psychiatry*, 64 (9), Tyrone D. Cannon, Robert Yolken, Stephen Buka, and E. Fuller Torrey, Decreased Neurotrophic Response to Birth Hypoxia in the Etiology of Schizophrenia, pp. 797–802, Copyright (2008), with permission from Elsevier.

Seamans and Yang 2004; Seamans and Robbins 2009). The former action may prolong neuronal activity in recurrently firing cell assemblies and the latter may prevent it from being interrupted by inputs from other neuronal assemblies. Durstewitz et al. (2000, Durstewitz and Seamans 2008) have modelled this action to predict several behavioural effects of manipulations of PFC DA on working memory and attention, according to a classic inverted U-shaped function (Yerkes and Dodson 1908; Arnsten 1997). Importantly, they also propose that the D2 receptors in the neocortex operate most effectively at different concentrations of extracellular DA and their activation opposes the optimal tuning provided by the D1 receptor, by promoting alternative modes of responding. This has led to the important concept of a 'balance' between selective attention to task-relevant representations and to shifting to alternative task sets. Analogous mechanisms may be operative in the striatum, where D1 and D2 receptors are, however, present in more or less equivalent densities.

Individual differences in PFC function may depend to some extent on genetic variation in the level of DA in this area. Remarkably, it appears that single nucleotide polymorphisms of the gene controlling the methylation of DA (catechol-O-methyltransferase, COMT) produce different levels of PFC DA by variation of a single allele (val 158met) (see Egan et al. 2001; Bilder et al. 2004). Thus, val/val homozygotes have efficient COMT and thus relatively low levels of PFC DA, whereas the opposite is true of met/met individuals. Within a population of individuals it appears that their performance on PFC-dependent tasks is in the form of an inverted-U shaped function with those subjects with val/val alleles (and hence putatively lower PFC DA) generally performing relatively worse. However, under certain circumstances, those with met/met alleles may perform worse (see Bilder et al. 2004), and this suggests a Yerkes–Dodson relationship by which different aspects of cognition are optimally performed at different levels of PFC DA functioning. This concept was originally applied to performance on working memory tasks but, as will be seen, may apply increasingly to aspects of attention along the lines suggested by the Durstewicz/Seamans model.

Individual differences may also affect response to DA receptor agents in both rodents and humans. Granon et al. (2000) divided rats into two groups, with low and high baseline levels of accuracy on the 5CSRTT and found that a partial D1 agonist (SKF-38393) enhanced performance only in the lower baseline group. By contrast, only higher performing rats were susceptible to the detrimental effects of an intra-PFC D1 receptor antagonist (Fig. 18.5). All rats were relatively unresponsive to sulpiride, a D2 receptor antagonist. These data parsimoniously indicate that the mesofrontal DA system is primarily engaged to optimize signal detection in this task. A follow-up study by Chudasama and Robbins (2004) used a combined attention and working memory (CAM) task in which rats had to commit the location of visual events they had successfully detected to working memory over a short delay. The full DA D1 receptor agonist SKF81297 produced dose-dependent effects on the attentional component, thereby replicating and expanding the findings of Granon et al. (2000). However, effects on the working memory component of the task were less obvious; improvements were evident when the stimulus duration was reduced, at certain doses and delays. At the highest dose, good memory at

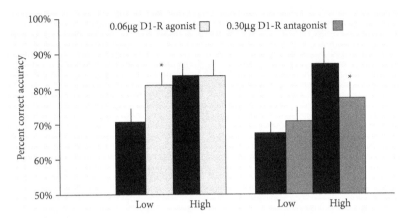

FIGURE 18.5 Comparative effects of a dopamine D1-R agonist and antagonist infused into the rat prefrontal cortex (PFC) on attentional performance in the 5-choice serial reaction time task for rats performing at relatively high and low baseline levels of accuracy. Note the baseline-dependency of the effects, which indicate a significant role for PFC D1 receptors in attentional function. Data redrawn from Granon, S., et al (2000) *Journal of Neuroscience*, 20, 1208–1215.

short delays was impaired whilst poor memory at longer delays was improved. Thus, D1 receptor stimulation sufficient to improve attentional accuracy could facilitate or disrupt working memory performance in a dose- and delay-dependent manner.

Depletion of PFC DA in the marmoset monkey produces impairments in the development of learning or attentional set, as shown in a series of repeated intra-dimensional shifts in discrimination learning by marmoset monkeys (Crofts et al. 2001), whereas distractibility is enhanced and the performance of extra-dimensional shifting can actually be improved by such PFC DA depletion (Roberts et al. 1994). This pattern is consistent with the hypothesis that DA modulates the stability of representation of response rules (Durstewitz et al. 2000).

A recent study of the 'lability of attentional set' using human variations of the intra-dimensional/extra-dimensional shift tasks has supported the hypothesis that low lateral PFC DA results in increased shifting or lability of attention, as compared with higher levels which are more important for a more stable mode of attentional set (as inferred by the comparison between val/val and met/met homozygotes, respectively; Fallon et al. 2013). The COMT inhibitor tolcapone (increasing PFC DA levels) has also been shown to specifically impair the establishment of attentional set (i.e. intra-dimensional set-shifting) in met/met individuals, whilst having the opposite effect on val/val homozygotes (Apud et al. 2007). This interpretation is also consistent with evidence that distraction during working memory tasks is particularly important for detecting deficits after prefrontal DA depletion (Roberts et al. 1994) and with the effects of systemic or intra-PFC agents on attention and working memory in rats (Granon et al. 2000; Chudasama and Robbins 2004). Overall, the data can be explained by assuming that task-irrelevant representations are suppressed at optimal levels of PFC

DA, allowing optimal attentional set, whereas low levels of PFC DA impair performance by allowing competing representations and high levels impair it by impairing all task representations either relevant or irrelevant.

Furthermore, the hypothesis that DA controls the optimal 'balance' between stability and flexibility of attentional set in the PFC is supported by evidence from human psychopharmacological studies where DA agents are (necessarily) administered systemically, though thereby affecting receptors in striatal as well as cortical sites. In general, progress has been limited by the unavailability of D1 agents for human use, and consequently, the predominant use of D2 agents. In general, the main paradigms employed have been those of working memory, but one study has compared examined effects of the D2 agonist bromocriptine on task-set switching and distractibility (Cools et al. 2007). These authors used a cued delayed matching-to-sample task in which healthy volunteers were required to retrieve either briefly presented faces or scenes, depending on the colour of the fixation cross. Distractors were also presented in the retention interval. Bromocriptine facilitated performance by reducing behavioural switch costs, but only in high-impulsive subjects. In contrast, low-impulsive subjects mainly had impaired performance. The drug-induced improvement was accompanied by a drug-induced modulation of activity in the putamen, whereas lateral PFC activity was unaltered during switching. However, although bromocriptine did not by itself affect behavioural performance during distraction, lateral frontal activity was nonetheless enhanced by bromocriptine during distraction, consistent with the prediction that D2 receptors mediate the impact of currently irrelevant distractors on prefrontal cortex function (Seamans and Yang 2004).

This study highlights several points other than generally supporting the hypothesis that PFC DA is implicated in attentional processes. First, D2 receptors exert effects on cognition in humans at striatal as well as prefrontal cortical sites. Second, brain imaging methodology (PET or fMRI) will probably be necessary for unravelling such effects in humans. Third, knowledge of individual differences (perhaps based on genetic polymorphisms and personality dimensions) will also be important for predicting effects of DA-ergic agents. High impulsivity has been related to reduced striatal DA receptor number (in rodents and humans) and impaired working memory; this can be predicted to place an individual on the left side of the putative 'inverted-U' relating DA function to performance.

Other evidence from both animal (e.g. Goto and Grace 2005; Pezze et al. 2007) and human studies indicates that attention-like processes are also probably mediated at striatal sites. Involuntary spatial attention is efficiently summoned by cues to targets presented after a short interval, but after a longer interval, target detection is slower because of inferred 'inhibition-of-return'. This inhibitory regulation of attention is impaired in Parkinson's disease (Filoteo et al. 1997) and is modulated by the D2 agonist bromocriptine, depending on a genetic marker of likely striatal DA activity. Bromocriptine did not affect involuntary spatial attention, but this DA D2 agonist enhanced inhibition of return in individuals with alleles predicting low striatal DA and abolished it in participants with alleles predicting high striatal DA (Colzato et al. 2009; Rokem et al. 2012).

Once again, the familiar inverted U-shaped curve relating performance to DA function can be invoked; and it is clear that this applies to attentional processes as well as to working memory function.

Overall, it is evident that DA influences forms of attentional function at both PFC and striatal sites, including both 'top-down' attentional processes such as task set, and also other modulations of spatial attention that can be regulated subcortically.

CONTROL OF ATTENTION BY ASCENDING MODULATORY CHEMICAL NEUROTRANSMITTER SYSTEMS: A SUMMARY

The evidence surveyed so far indicates important and potent, though complex, actions of the ascending cholinergic, noradrenergic, and dopaminergic neurotransmitter systems on aspects of attention. It is difficult to clearly differentiate functions of these systems because of incomplete information about how their manipulation might comparatively affect different types of attentional function, and these chemical systems ramify widely and can influence diverse forms of processing. However, certain themes are becoming apparent. The cholinergic system appears to be intimately implicated in target detection and sustained attention; the effects of NA on attention are intimately bound up with such factors as arousal and stress level, and dopamine is most obviously implicated in the regulation of the balance between attentional stability and flexibility, probably arising from the regulation of attentional set. As with NA, the effects of manipulating DA depend exquisitely on baseline states of performance and DA function, which might also be reflected in behavioural traits such as impulsivity.

NEW DIRECTIONS IN THE NEUROPSYCHOPHARMACOLOGY OF ATTENTION

New developments in understanding how attention may be modulated neuropharmacologically are coming from two directions. The first is a growing realization of how the complexity of subcortical neurotransmitter pathways may affect attention in a 'bottom-up' manner through actions on systems governing consciousness and sleep. The second comes from an appreciation of neural network theory born out of significant recent discoveries in neuroscience research such as gamma oscillations and the 'default mode network', often in the context of the need to find treatments for neuropsychiatric disorders. This concluding section considers some of the possible new directions arising from these developments.

One striking demonstration has been the finding that the 'wakefulness neuropeptide' hypocretin and nicotine excite the same thalamocortical pathways as shown by electrophysiological recordings at PFC synapses, and improve performance in a test of divided and sustained attention in rats following medial PFC infusion (Lambe et al. 2005). This observation is consonant with evidence that narcoleptic patients (who suffer from a deficiency in hypocretin) have deficits in aspects of attention even when awake (Rieger et al. 2003). It has long been speculated that the atypical stimulant modafinil, which has been shown to have some 'cognitive enhancing' actions (Turner et al. 2003; Minzenberg and Carter 2008), may also exert these effects through hypocretin receptors, although these is also evidence for actions on NA, DA, and indirectly, ACh (from actions on histamine).

The related neuropeptide orexin can also clearly modulate attention, though via its anatomical connections to the nucleus basalis and likely regulation of corticopetal cholinergic neurons (Fadel and Burk 2010). Thus, an orexin-1 receptor antagonist disrupted performance on a 2-choice sustained attention task when infused into the nucleus basalis of rats (Boschen et al. 2009). Histamine may similarly regulate cholinergic functioning and thereby mediate part of the interface between arousal and attention (Passani et al. 2000). Histamine-3 receptor antagonists and inverse agonists have been developed, partly with the aim of boosting attention in such disorders as ADHD (e.g. Iannone et al. 2010).

The other impetus for the neuropsychopharmacology of attention comes from an increasing interest in network properties of the cortex, as indexed by such phenomena as fast (30–90 Hz) gamma oscillations which probably bear specific relationships to cortical (including hippocampal) information processing, including memory and attention (Jensen et al. 2007). They are generated *in vivo* by fast-spiking parvalbumin-containing GABA interneurons and are evoked *in vitro* by metabotrophic glutamate and muscarinic ACh receptors (Bartos et al. 2007). One function that has been mooted for this activity is that of attentional binding of different elements of complex stimuli. Until recently, the relationship of gamma oscillations to the deactivation of the default mode network that normally accompanies task-related performance has been unclear. However, Ossandon et al. (2011) recently showed that all default mode regions displayed transient suppression of gamma activity during a visual search task in a manner correlated with task complexity and individual performance. Disruption of cortical gamma oscillatory activity has also been suggested to reflect cortical–cortical connectivity in schizophrenia, and given the postulated glutamatergic and GABA-ergic deficits in this disorder, this has refocused examination of drugs affecting glutamatergic and GABA-ergic function.

Ketamine, an anaesthetic drug with psychotogenic effects, which blocks NMDA receptors, also reduces subjective alertness and concentration, and impairs performance on sustained attention as measured by effects on continuous performance (e.g. Krystal et al. 1994). This drug reduces P-300 amplitudes, for example to oddball stimuli (Oranje et al. 2000) and also produces increased activity in the default mode network (Williamson 2007). A recent study (Knott et al. 2011) found that nicotine could antagonize some of the deficits on an RVIP task. The effects of ketamine on glutamate transmission are not entirely clear as, in common with other NMDA receptor antagonists, it can increase glutamate levels as a secondary effect of disinhibiting GABA-interneurons. A recent rodent study on sustained attentional performance of the 5CSRTT showed that infusion of an NMDA receptor antagonist into the rat medial PFC disrupted the accuracy of performance (Pozzi et al. 2011), similarly to the effects of ketamine on human sustained attention. But the disruptive effects in rodents were blocked by a drug reducing glutamatergic transmission, through its actions at glutamate metabotrophic 2/3 receptors. Intriguingly, this class of compounds has been shown to reduce psychotic symptoms in schizophrenia.

Parallel investigations of GABA receptor function in attention began with studies of effects of benzodiazepines such as triazolam, lorazepam, and diazepam. At higher doses, the effects of these drugs are sedating and sleep-inducing. However, greater specificity of effect is observed at lower doses; for example, diazepam was found to impair attentional set-shifting and learning at doses that did not impair RVIP performance (Coull et al. 1995). This effect on attentional set-shifting is consistent with some other observed effects, e.g. of triazolam which affected cue disengagement in a test of visual search (Johnson et al. 1995) although there is some inconsistency in findings with the Posner exogenous orienting paradigm (e.g. Carter et al. 1998). There is also evidence of a lengthening of the 'attentional blink' duration by benzodiazepines, an observation which has been incorporated into neocortical simulations of the attentional blink based on attractor networks, as a facilitation of GABA-A function (Silverstein and Lansner 2011).

Parvalbumin-positive GABA neurons implicated in schizophrenia regulate the synchronized oscillatory activity of cortical pyramidal neurons in the gamma band range (30–80 Hz) and frontal lobe gamma band oscillations have been shown to be reduced during a cognitive control task among individuals with schizophrenia. Therefore, it is possible that augmenting GABA transmission in interneurons, including chandelier cells, might restore both the oscillations and the impaired cognitive function. Lewis et al. (2008) tested this hypothesis in a group of patients with schizophrenia by administering a positive allosteric modulator of GABAA receptors containing the alpha-2 subunit (i.e. a drug which enhances chloride ion flow through GABAA receptors only when GABA itself is bound to the receptor). They showed some enhanced effects on frontal gamma activity and beneficial effects on working memory tasks, but also on the AX-CPT continuous performance task, which has a strong element of sustained attention. Further systematic analysis of such effects using other paradigms will greatly enhance our knowledge of the relationship between GABA-ergic function, gamma oscillations, and attention. However, this preliminary observation indicates the promise of this approach.

CONCLUSIONS

The recent advances illustrate the multidisciplinary neuroscientific endeavour that is now necessary to enhance our understanding of the neuropsychopharmacology of attention. As well as utilizing theoretically cogent methods for measuring different aspects of attentional function, it is necessary to combine these with functional brain imaging and human electrophysiological methodology, as well as translatable animal paradigms, in order to make significant progress. Attentional deficits are often central to different forms of psychopathology, ranging from Alzheimer's disease to ADHD and schizophrenia, and the recent progress in understanding promises ultimately to find more effective pharmacological treatments of these disorders.

REFERENCES

Amaral, D. G. and Sinnamon, H. M. (1977). The locus coeruleus: Neurobiology of a central noradrenergic nucleus. *Progress in Neurobiology* 9: 147–196.

Apud, J. A., Mattay, V., Chen, J. et al. (2007). Tolcapone improves cognition and cortical information processing in normal human subjects. *Neuropsychopharmacology* 32: 1011–1020.

Arnsten, A. F. T. (1997). Catecholamine modulation of prefrontal cortical function. *Trends in Cognitive Sciences* 2: 437–447.

Arnsten, A. F. T. (2009). Stress signalling pathways that impair prefrontal cortex structure and function. *Nature Reviews Neuroscience* 10: 410–422.

Arnsten, A. F. T. and Contant, T. A. (1992). Alpha-2 adrenergic agonists decrease distractibility in aged monkeys performing the delayed response task. *Psychopharmacology* 108: 159–169.

Aron, A. R., Dowson, J. H., Sahakian, B. J., and Robbins, T. W. (2003). Methylphenidate improves response inhibition in adults with attention-deficit/hyperactivity disorder. *Biological Psychiatry* 54: 1465–1468.

Aston-Jones, G., Chiang, G., and Alexinsky, T. (1991). Discharge of noradrenergic locus coeruleus neurons in behaving rats and monkeys suggest a role in vigilance. *Progress in Brain Research* 88: 501–520.

Aston-Jones, G. and Cohen, J. D. (2005). An integrative theory of locus coeruleus-norepinephrine function: Adaptive gain and optimal performance. *Annual Review of Neuroscience* 28: 403–450.

Aston-Jones, G., Rajkowski, J., and Cohen, J. D. (1999). The role of locus coeruleus in attention and behavioral flexibility. *Biological Psychiatry* 46: 1309–1320.

Bartos, M., Vida, I., and Jonas, P. (2007). Synaptic mechanisms of synchronized gamma oscillations in inhibitory interneuron networks. *Nature Reviews Neuroscience* 8: 45–56.

Bentley, P., Driver, J., and Dolan, R. J. (2008). Cholinesterase inhibition modulates visual and attentional brain responses in Alzheimer's disease and health. *Brain* 131(2): 409–424.

Bilder, R. M., Volavka, J., Lachman, H. M., and Grace, A. A. (2004). The catechol-O methyltransferase polymorphism: Relations to the tonic-phasic dopamine hypothesis and neuropsychiatric phenotypes. *Neuropsychopharmacology* 29: 1943–1961.

Boschen, K. E., Fadel, J. R., and Burk, J. A. (2009). Systemic and intrabasalis administration of the orexin-1 receptor antagonist, SN-334867, disrupts attentional performance in rats. *Psychopharmacology* 206: 205–213.

Broks, P., Preston, G. C., Traub, M., P.ppleton, P., Ward, C., and Stahl, S. M. (1988). Modelling dementia: Effects of scopolamine on memory and attention. *Neuropsychologia* 26: 685–700.

Brown, V. J. and Robbins, T. W. (1991). Simple and choice reaction time performance following unilateral striatal DA depletion in the rat. *Brain* 114: 513–525.

Bymaster, F. P., Katner, J. S., Nelson, D. L. et al. (2002). Atomoxetine increases extracellular levels of norepinephrine and dopamine in prefrontal cortex of rat: A potential mechanism for efficacy in attention deficit/hyperactivity disorder. *Neuropsychopharmacology* 27: 699–711.

Cannon, T. D., Yolken, R., Buka, B., and Torrey, E. F. (2008). Decreased neurotrophic response to birth hypoxia in the etiology of schizophrenia. *Biological Psychiatry* 64(9): 797–802.

Carli, M., Evenden, J. L., and Robbins, T. W. (1985). Depletion of unilateral striatal dopamine impairs initiation of contralateral actions and not sensory attention. *Nature* 313: 679–682.

Carli, M., Jones, G. H., and Robbins, T. W. (1989). Effects of unilateral dorsal and ventral striatal dopamine depletion on visual neglect in the rat: A neural and behavioural analysis. *Neuroscience* 29: 309–327.

Carli, M., Robbins, T. W., Evenden, J. L., and Everitt, B. J. (1983). Effects of lesions to ascending noradrenergic neurones on performance of a 5-choice serial reaction task in rats: Implications for theories of dorsal noradrenergic bundle function based on selective attention and arousal. *Behavioural Brain Research* 9: 361–380.

Carter, C. S., Maddock, R., Chaderjian, M., and Post, R. (1998). Attentional effects of single dose triazolam. *Progress in Neuropsychopharmacology & Biological Psychiatry* 22: 279–292.

Chudasama, Y. and Robbins, T. W. (2004). Dopaminergic modulation of visual attention and working memory in the rodent prefrontal cortex. *Neuropsychopharmacology* 29: 1628–1636.

Clark, C. R., Geffen, G. M., and Geffen, L. B. (1989). Catecholamines and the covert orientation of attention in humans. *Neuropsychologia* 27: 131–139.

Coghill, D. R., Rhodes, S. M., and Matthews, K. (2007). The neuropsychological effects of chronic methylphenidate on drug-naive boys with attention-deficit/hyperactivity disorder. *Biological Psychiatry* 62: 954–962.

Cole, B. J. and Robbins, T. W. (1992). Forebrain norepinephrine: Role in controlled information processing in the rat. *Neuropsychopharmacology* 7: 129–142.

Colzato, L. S., Pratt, J., and Hommel, B. (2009). Dopaminergic control of attentional flexibility: Inhibition of return is associated with the dopamine transporter gene (DAT1). *Frontiers in Human Neuroscience* 4: 53.

Cools, R., Sheridan, M., Jacobs, E., and D'Esposito, M. (2007). Impulsive personality predicts dopamine-dependent changes in frontostriatal activity during component processes of working memory. *Journal of Neuroscience* 27: 5506–5514.

Cooper, B., Bloom, F. E., and Roth, R. H. (2002). *The Biochemical Basis of Neuropharmacology*, 8th edn. New York: Oxford University Press.

Coull, J. T. (1998). Neural correlates of attention and arousal: Insights from electrophysiology, functional neuroimaging and psychopharmacology. *Progress in Neurobiology* 55: 343–361.

Coull, J. T., Frith, C. D., Dolan, R. J., Frackowiak, R. S. J., and Grasby, P. M. (1997). The neural correlates of the noradrenergic modulation of human attention, arousal and learning. *European Journal of Neuroscience* 9: 589–598.

Coull, J. T., Middleton, H. C., Robbins, T. W., and Sahakian, B. J. (1995a). Contrasting effects of clonidine and diazepam on tests of working memory and planning. *Psychopharmacology* 120: 311–321.

Coull, J. T., Middleton, H. C., Robbins, T. W., and Sahakian, B. J. (1995b). Clonidine and diazepam have differential effects on tests of attention and learning. *Psychopharmacology* 120: 322–332.

Coull, J. T., Sahakian, B. J., and Hodges, J. R. (1996). The alpha(2) antagonist idazoxan certain attentional and executive dysfunction in patients with dementia of frontal type. *Psychopharmacology* 123: 239–249.

Coull, J. T., Sahakian, B. J., Middleton, H. C. et al. (1995c). Differential effects of clonidine, halo-peridol, diazepam and tryptophan depletion on focused attention and attentional search. *Psychopharmacology* 121: 222–230.

Crofts, H. S., Dalley, J. W., Collins, P. et al. (2001). Differential effects of 6-OHDA lesions of the prefrontal cortex and caudate nucleus on the ability to acquire an attentional set. *Cerebral Cortex* 11: 1015–1026.

Dalley, J. W., McGaughy, J., O'Connell, M. T., Cardinal, R. N., Levita, L., and Robbins, T. W. (2001). Distinct changes in cortical acetylcholine and noradrenaline efflux during contin-gent and noncontingent performance of a visual attentional task. *Journal of Neuroscience* 21: 4908–4914.

Dalley, J. W., Theobald, D. E. H., Bouger, P., Chudasama, Y., Cardinal, R. N., and Robbins, T. W. (2004). Cortical cholinergic function and deficits in visual attentional performance in rats following 192 IgG-saporin-induced lesions of the medial prefrontal cortex. *Cerebral Cortex* 14: 922–932.

Davidson, M. C. and Marrocco, R. T. (2000). Local infusion of scololamine into intraparietal cortex slows covert orienting in rhesus monkeys. *Journal of Neurophysiology* 83: 1536–1549.

Deco, G. and Thiele, A. (2009). Attention: Oscillations and neuropharmacology. *European Journal of Neuroscience* 30: 247–354.

De Martino, B., Strange, B. A., and Dolan, R. J. (2008). Noradrenergic modulation of human attention for emotional neutral stimuli. *Psychopharmacology* 197: 127–136.

Desimone, R. and Duncan, J. (1995). Neural mechanisms of selective visual attention. *Annual Review of Neuroscience* 18: 193–222.

Durstewitz, D. and Seamans, J. K. (2008). The dual-state theory of prefrontal cortex dopamine function with relevance to catechol-o-methyltransferase genotypes and schizophrenia. *Biological Psychiatry* 64: 739–749.

Durstewitz, D., Seamans, J. K., and Sejnowski, T. (2000). Dopamine-mediated stabilization of delay-period activity in a network model of prefrontal cortex. *Journal of Neurophysiology* 19: 2807–2822.

Easterbrook, J. A. (1959). The effect of emotion on cue utilization and the organization of behav-ior. *Psychological Review* 66: 183–201.

Egan, F., Goldberg, T. E., Kolachana, B. S. et al. (2001). Effect of COMT Val108/158 Met genotype on frontal lobe function and risk for schizophrenia. *Proceedings of the National Academy of Sciences USA* 98: 6917–6922.

Emre, M., Aarsland, D., Albanese, A. et al. (2004). Rivastigmine for dementia associated with Parkinson's disease. *New England Journal of Medicine* 351: 2509–2518.

Epstein, J. N., Conners, C. K., Hervey, A. S. et al. (2006). Assessing medication effects in the MTA study using neuropsychological outcomes. *Journal of Child Psychology and Psychiatry* 47: 446–456.

Everitt, B. J., Robbins, T. W., and Selden, N. R. W. (1990). Functions of the locus coeruleus noradrenergic system: A neurobiological and behavioural synthesis. In S. A. Marsden and D. J. Heal (eds.), *The Pharmacology of Noradrenaline in the Central Nervous System* (pp. 349–378). New York: Oxford University Press,.

Fadel, J. and Burk, J. A. (2010). Orexin/hypocretin modulation of the basal forebrain choliner-gic system: Role in attention. *Brain Research* 1314: 112–123.

Fallon, S. J., Williams-Gray, C. H., Barker, R. A, Owen, A. M., and Hampshire, A. (2013). Prefrontal dopamine levels determine the balance between cognitive stability and flexibility. *Cerebral Cortex* 23: 361–369.

Filoteo, J. V., Delis, D. C., Salmon, D. P., Demadura, T., Roman, M. J., and Shults, C. W. (1997). An examination of the nature of attentional deficits in patients with Parkinson's disease: Evidence from a spatial orienting task. *Journal of the International Neuropsychological Society 3*: 337–347.

Foote, S. L., Bloom, F. E., and Aston-Jones, G. (1990). Nucleus locus ceruleus: New evidence of anatomical and physiological specificity. *Physiological Reviews 63*: 844–914.

Furey, M. L., P.etrini, P., and Haxby, J. V. (2000). Cholinergic enhancement and increased selectivity of perceptual processing during working memory. *Science 290*: 2315–2319.

Goto, Y. and Grace, A. A. (2005). Dopaminergic modulation of limbic and cortical drive of nucleus accumbens in goal-directed behavior. *Nature Neuroscience 8*: 805–812.

Granon, S., Passetti, F., Thomas, K. L., Dalley, J. W., Everitt, B. J., and Robbins, T. W. (2000). Enhanced and impaired attentional performance after infusion of D1 dopaminergic receptor agents into rat prefrontal cortex. *Journal of Neuroscience 20*: 1208–1215.

Hasselmo, M. E. and Sarter, M. (2011). Modes and models of forebrain cholinergic modulation of cognition. *Neuropsychopharmacology 36*: 52–73.

Herrero, J. L., Roberts, M. J., Delicato, L. S. et al. (2008). Acetylcholine contributes through muscarinic receptors to attentional modulation in V1. *Nature 454*: 1110–1114.

Howe, W. M., J., J., Parikh, V. et al. (2010). Enhanced attentional performance by selective stimulation of a4b2* nAChRs: Underlying cholinergic mechanisms. *Neuropsychopharmacology 35*: 1391–1401.

Iannone, R., Palcza, J., Renger, J. J. et al. (2010). Acute alertness-promoting effects of a novel histamine subtype in healthy sleep-deprived male volunteers. *Clinical Pharmacology and Therapeutics 88*: 831–839.

Jensen, O., Kaiser, J., and Lachaux, J,-P. (2007). Human gamma frequency oscillations associated with attention and memory. *Trends in Neurosciences 30*: 317–324.

Jentsch, J. D., Aarde, S. M., and Seu, E. (2009). Effects of atomoxetine and methylphenidate on performance of a lateralized reaction time task in rats. *Psychopharmacology (Berl) 202*: 497–504.

Johnson, D. N., Weingartner, H., Andreason, P., and George, D. T. (1995). An effect of triazolam on visual attention and information processing. *Psychopharmacology 121*: 145–149.

Knott, V. J., Millar, A. M., McIntosh, J. F. et al. (2011). Separate and combined effects of low dose ketamine and nicotine on behavioural and neural correlates of sustained attention. *Biological Psychology 68*: 83–93.

Koelega, H. S. (1993). Stimulant drugs and vigilance performance: A review. *Psychopharmacology (Berl) 111*: 1–16.

Kozak, R., Bruno, J. P., and Sarter, M. (2006). Augmented prefrontal acetylcholine release during challenged attentional performance. *Cerebral Cortex 16*: 9–17.

Krystal, J. H., Karper, L. P., Seibyl, J. P. et al. (1994). Subanesthetic effects of the noncompetitive NMDA antagonist, ketamine, in humans: Psychomimetic, perceptual, cognitive and neuroendocrine responses. *Archives of General Psychiatry 51*: 199–214.

Lambe, E. K., Olausson, P., Horst, N. K., and Taylor, J. R. (2005). Hypocretin and nicotine excite the same thalamocortical synapse with improved attention in the rat. *Journal of Neuroscience 25*: 5225–5229.

Lapiz, M. D., Bondi, C. O., and Morilak, D. A. (2007). Chronic treatment with desipramine improves cognitive performance of rats in an attentional set-shifting test. *Neuropsychopharmacology 32*: 1000–1010.

Lapiz, M. D. and Morilak, D. A. (2006). Noradrenergic modulation of cognitive function in rat medial prefrontal cortex as measured by attentional set shifting capability. *Neuroscience* 137: 1039–1049.

Lewis, D. A., Cho, R. Y., Carter, C. S. et al. (2008). Sub-unit-selective modulation of GABA Type-A receptor neurotransmission in schizophrenia. *American Journal of Psychiatry* 165: 1585–1593.

Lijffijt, M., Kenemans, J. L., Verbaten, M. N., and van Engeland, H. (2005). A meta-analytic review of stopping performance in attention-deficit/hyperactivity disorder: Deficient inhibitory motor control? *Journal of Abnormal Psychology* 114: 216–222.

McGaughy, J., Dalley, J. W., Morrison, C. H., Everitt, B. J., and Robbins, T. W. (2002). Selective behavioral and neurochemical effects of cholinergic lesions produced by intrabasalis infusions of 192 IgG-saporin on attentional performance in a five-choice serial reaction time task. *Journal of Neuroscience* 22: 1905–1913.

McGaughy, J., Kaiser, T., and Sarter, M. (1996). Behavioral vigilance following infusions of 192 IgG-saporin into the basal forebrain: Selectivity of the behavioral impairment and relation to cortical AChE-positive fiber density. *Behavioral Neuroscience* 110: 247–265.

Marshall, J. F. and Teitelbaum, P. (1977). New considerations in the neuropsychology of motivated behaviors. In *Handbook of Psychopharmacology* (pp. 201–229). Springer US.

Middleton, H. C., Coull, J. T., Sahakian, B. J., and Robbins, T. W. (1994). Clonidine-induced changes in the spectral distribution of heart rate variability correlate with performance on a test of sustained attention. *Journal of Psychopharmacology* 8: 1–7.

Milstein, J. A., Lehmann, O., Theobald, D. E. H., Dalley, J. W., and Robbins, T. W. (2007). Selective depletion of cortical noradrenaline by anti-dopamine beta-hydroxylase-saporin impairs attentional function and enhances the effects of guanfacine in the rat. *Psychopharmacology* 190: 51–63.

Minzenberg, M. J. and Carter, C. S. (2008). Modafinil, a review of neurochemical actions and effects on cognition. *Neuropsychopharmacology* 33: 1477–1502.

Muir, J. L., Dunnett, S. B., Robbins, T. W., and Everitt, B. J. (1992). Attentional functions of the forebrain cholinergic systems: Effects of intraventricular hemicholinium, physostigmine, basal forebrain lesions and intracortical grafts on a multiple-choice serial reaction time task. *Experimental Brain Research* 89: 611–622.

Muir, J. L., Everitt, B. J., and Robbins, T. W. (1994). AMPA-induced excitotoxic lesions of the basal forebrain: A significant role for the cortical cholinergic system in attentional function. *Journal of Neuroscience* 14: 2313–2326.

Muir, J. L., Everitt, B. J., and Robbins, T. W. (1995). Reversal of visual attentional dysfunction following lesions of the cholinergic basal forebrain by physostigmine and nicotine but not by the 5-HT3 receptor antagonist, ondansetron. *Psychopharmacology* 118: 82–92.

Murphy, F. C. and Klein, R. M. (1998). The effects of nicotine on spatial and non-spatial expectancies in a covert orienting task. *Neuropsychologia* 36: 1103–1114.

Nelson, C. L., Sarter, M., and Bruno, J. P. (2005). Prefrontal cortical modulation of acetylcholine release in posterior parietal cortex. *Neuroscience* 132: 347–359.

Newman, L. A., Darling, J., and McGaughy, J. (2008). Atomoxetine reverses attentional deficits produced by noradrenergic deafferentation of medial prefrontal cortex. *Psychopharmacology (Berl)* 200: 39–50.

Nieuwenhuis, S., Gilzenrat, M. S., Holmes, B. D., and Cohen, J. D. (2005). The role of the locus coeruleus in mediating the attentional blink: A neurocomputational theory. *Journal of Experimental Psychology: General* 134: 291–307.

Nieuwenhuis, S., van Nieupoort, I. C., Veltman, D. J., and Drent, M. L. (2007). Effects of the noradrenergic agonist clonidine on temporal and spatial attention. *Psychopharmacology* 193: 261–269.

Noudoost, B. and Moore, T. (2011). The role of neuromodulators in selective attention. *Trends in Cognitive Sciences* 15: 585–591.

Oke, A., Lewis, R., and Adams, R. N. (1980). Hemispheric asymmetry of norepinephrine distribution in rat thalamus. *Brain Research* 188: 269–272.

O'Neill, J., Fitten, L. J., Siembieda, D. W., Ortiz, F., and Halgren, E. (2000). Effects of guanfacine on three forms of distraction in the aging macaque. *Life Sciences* 67: 877–885.

Oranje, B., van Berkel, B. N. M., Kemner, C. et al. (2000). The effects of a sub-anaesthetic dose of ketamine on human selective attention. *Neuropsychopharmacology* 22: 293–302.

Ossandon, T., Jerbi, K., Vidal, J. R. et al. (2011). Transient suppression of broadband gamma power in the default-mode network is correlated with task complexity and subject performance. *Journal of Neuroscience* 31: 14521–14526.

Parasuraman, R. (ed.) (1998). *The Attentive Brain*. Cambridge, Mass.: MIT Press.

Parikh, V., Kozak, R., Martinez, V., and Sarter, M. (2007). Prefrontal acetylcholine release controls cue detection on multiple timescales. *Neuron* 56: 141–154.

Passani, M. B., Bacciottini, L., Mannaioni, P. F., and Blandina, P. (2000). Central histaminergic system and cognition. *Neuroscience and Biobehavioral Reviews* 24: 107–113.

Passetti, F., Dalley, J. W., O'Connell, M. T., Everitt, B. J., and Robbins, T. W. (2000). Increased acetylcholine release in the rat medial frontal cortex during performance of a visual attentional task. *European Journal of Neuroscience* 12: 3051–3058.

Perry, E., Walker, M., Grace, J., and Perry, R. (1999). Acetylcholine in mind: A neurotransmitter correlate of consciousness. *Trends in Neurosciences* 22: 273–280.

Pezze, M. A., Dalley, J. W., and Robbins, T. W. (2007). Differential roles of dopamine D1 and D2 receptors in the nucleus accumbens in attentional performance on the five-choice serial reaction time task. *Neuropsychopharmacology* 32: 273–283.

Posner, M. I. and Petersen, S. E. (1990). The attention system of the human brain. *Annual Review of Neuroscience* 13: 25–42.

Posner, M. I., Walker, J. A., Friedrich, F. J., and Rafal, R. D. (1984). Effects of parietal injury in covert orienting of attention. *Journal of Neuroscience* 4: 1863–1874.

Pozzi, L., Baviera, M., Sacchetti, G. et al. (2011). Attention deficit induced by blockade of N-methyl d-aspartate receptors in the prefrontal cortex is associated with enhanced glutamate release and cAMP response element binding protein phosphorylation: Role of metabotropic glutamate receptors 2/3. *Neuroscience* 176: 336–348.

Puumala, T., Riekkinen, Sr., P., and Sirvio, J. (1997). Modulation of vigilance and behavioral activation by alpha-1 adrenoceptors in the rat. *Pharmacology, Biochemistry, and Behavior* 56: 705–712.

Pycock, C. J., Kerwin, R. W., and Carter, C. J. (1980). Effect of lesion of cortical dopamine terminals on subcortical dopamine receptors in rats. *Nature* 286: 74–77.

Rajkowski, J., Majczynski, H., Clayton, E., and Aston-Jones, G. (2004). Activation of monkey locus coeruleus neurons varies with difficulty and performance in a target detection task. *Journal of Neurophysiology* 92: 361–371.

Rieger, M., Mayer, G., and Gauggel, S. (2003). Attention deficits in patients with narcolepsy. *Sleep-New York Then Westchester* 26(1): 36–43.

Robbins, T. W. (1984). Cortical noradrenaline, attention and arousal. *Psychological Medicine* 14: 13–21.

Robbins, T. W. (2002). The 5-choice serial reaction time task: Behavioural pharmacology and functional neurochemistry. *Psychopharmacology 163*: 362–380.

Robbins, T. W., Everitt, B. J., Marston, H. M., Wilkinson, J., Jones, G. H., and Page, K. J. (1989). Comparative effects of ibotenic acid- and quisqualic acid-induced lesions of the substantia innominata on attentional function in the rat: Further implications for the role of the cholinergic neurons of the nucleus basalis in cognitive processes. *Behavioural Brain Research 35*: 221–240.

Robbins, T. W. and Sahakian, B. J. (1979). 'Paradoxical' effects of psychomotor stimulant drugs in hyperactive children from the standpoint of behavioural pharmacology. *Neuropharmacology 18*: 931–950.

Roberts, A. C., De Salvia, M. A., Wilkinson, L. S. et al. (1994). 6-hydroxydopamine lesions of the prefrontal cortex in monkeys enhance performance on an analog of the Wisconsin Card Sort Test: Possible interactions with subcortical dopamine. *Journal of Neuroscience 14*: 2531–2544.

Robinson, E. S. J. (2012). Blockade of noradrenaline re-uptake sites improves accuracy and impulse control in rats performing a five-choice serial reaction time task. *Psychopharmacology 119*: 303–312.

Robinson, E. S. J., Eagle, D. M., Mar, A. C. et al. (2008). Similar effects of the selective noradrenaline reuptake inhibitor atomoxetine on three distinct forms of impulsivity in the rat. *Neuropsychopharmacology 33*: 1028–1037.

Rokem, A., Landau, A. N., Prinzmetal, W. et al. (2012). Modulation of inhibition of return by the dopamine receptor agonist bromocriptine depends on individual DAt1 genotype. *Cerebral Cortex 22*: 1133–1138.

Rowe, J., Saunders, J. R., Durantou, F., and Robbins, T. W. (1996). Systemic idazoxan impairs performance in a non-reversal shift test: Implications for the role of the central noradrenergic systems in selective attention. *Journal of Psychopharmacology 10*: 188–194.

Sahakian, B. J., Owen, A. M., Morant, N. J. et al. (1993). Further analysis of the cognitive effects of tetrahydroaminoacridine (THA) in Alzheimer's disease: Assessment of attentional and mnemonic function using CANTAB. *Psychopharmacology (Berl) 110*: 395–401.

Sarter, M., Hasselmo, M. E., Bruno, J. P., and Givens, B. (2005). Unraveling the attentional functions of cortical cholinergic inputs: Interactions between signal-driven and cognitive modulation of signal detection. *Brain Research: Brain Research Reviews 48*: 90–111.

Schultz, W. and Dickinson, A. (2000). Neuronal coding of prediction errors. *Annual Review of Neuroscience 23*: 473–500

Seamans, J. K. and Robbins, T. W. (2009). Dopamine modulation of the prefrontal cortex and cognitive function. In K. Neve (ed.), *The Dopamine Receptors*, 2nd edn. (pp. 373–398). New York: Humana Press.

Seamans, J. K. and Yang, C. R. (2004). The principal features and mechanisms of dopamine modulation in the prefrontal cortex. *Progress in Neurobiology 74*: 1–58.

Segal, M. and Bloom, F. E. (1976). The action of norepineprine in the rat hippocampus. IV: The effects of locus coeruleus stimulation on evoked hippocampal activity. *Brain Research 107*: 513–525.

Selden, N. R., Cole, B. J., Everitt, B. J., and Robbins, T. W. (1990a). Damage to ceruleo-cortical noradrenergic projections impairs locally cued but enhances spatially cued water maze acquisition. *Behavioural Brain Research 39*: 29–51.

Selden, N. R., Robbins, T. W., and Everitt, B. J. (1990b). Enhanced behavioral conditioning to context and impaired behavioral and neuroendocrine responses to conditioned stimuli following ceruleocortical noradrenergic lesions: Support for an attentional hypothesis of central noradrenergic function. *Journal of Neuroscience 10*: 531–539.

Sillito, A. M. and Kemp, J. A. (1983). Cholinergic modulation of the functional organization of the cat visual cortex. *Brain Research 289*: 143–155.

Silverstein, D. N. and Lansner, A. (2011). Is attentional blink a byproduct of neocortical attractors? *Frontiers in Computational Neuroscience 5*: 13.

Smith, A. and Nutt, D. (1996). Noradrenaline and attention lapses. *Nature 380*: 291.

Smith, A. P., Wilson, S. J., Glue, P., and Nutt, D. J. (1992). The effects and after effects of the a2-adrenoceptor antagonist idazoxan on mood, memory and attention in normal volunteers. *Psychopharmacology 6*: 376–381.

Swanson, J., Baler, R. D., and Volkow N. D. (2011). Understanding the effects of stimulant medications on cognition in individuals with ADHD: A decade of progress. *Neuropsychopharmacology 36*: 207–226.

Tait, D. S., Brown, V. J., Farovik, A., Theobald, D. E., Dalley, J. W., and Robbins, T. W. (2007). Lesions of the dorsal noradrenergic bundle impair attentional set-shifting in the rat. *European Journal of Neuroscience 25*: 3719–3724.

Tannock, R., Schachar R. J., Carr, R. P., Chajczyk, D., and Logan, G. D. (1989). Effects of methylphenidate on inhibitory control in hyperactive children. *Journal of Abnormal Child Psychology 17*: 473–491.

Turchi, J. and Sarter, M. (1997). Cortical acetylcholine and processing capacity: Effects of cortical cholinergic deafferentation on cross-modal divided attention in rats. *Brain Research: Cognitive Brain Research 6*: 147–158.

Turner, D. C., Robbins, T. W., Clark, L., Aron, A. R., Dowson, J., and Sahakian, B. J. (2003). Cognitive enhancing effects of modafinil in healthy volunteers. *Psychopharmacology 165*: 260–269.

Usher, M., Cohen, J. D., Servan-Schrieber, D., Rajkowski, J., and Aston-Jones, G. (1999). The role of locus coeruleus in the regulation of cognitive performance. *Science 283*: 549–554.

Vossel, S., Thiel, C. M., and Fink, G. R. (2008). Behavioral and neural effects of nicotine on visuospatial attentional reorienting in non-smoking subjects. *Neuropsychopharmacology 33*: 731–738.

Voytko, M. L., Olton, D. S., Richardson, R. T., Gorman, L. K., Tobin, J. R., and Price, D. L. (1994). Basal forebrain lesions in monkeys disrupt attention but not learning and memory. *Journal of Neuroscience 14*: 167–186.

Warburton, D. M. and Brown, K. (1971). Attenuation of stimulus sensitivity induced by scopolamine. *Nature 230*: 126–127.

Warburton, D. M. and Brown, K. (1972). Facilitation of discrimination performance by phsyostigmine sulphate. *Psychopharmacologia (Berl.) 27*: 277–284.

Weiner, I. and Feldon, J. (1987), Facilitation of latent inhibition by haloperidol in rats. *Psychopharmacology 91*: 248–253.

Weiss, B. and Laties, V. G. (1962). Enhancement of human performance by caffeine and the amphetamines. *Pharmacological Reviews 14*: 1–36.

Wesnes, K. and Warburton, D. M. (1984). Effects of scopolamine and nicotine on human rapid information processing performance. *Psychopharmacology 82*: 147–150.

Williamson, P. (2007). Are anti-correlated networks in the brain relevant to schizophrenia? *Schizophrenia Bulletin 33*: 994–1003.

Witte, E. A., Davidson, M. C., and Marrocco, R. T. (1997). Effects of altering brain cholinergic activity on covert orienting of attention: Comparison of monkey and human performance. *Psychopharmacology 132*: 324–334.

Yerkes, R. M. and Dodson, J. D. (1908). The relation of strength of stimulus to rapidity of habit-formation. *Journal of Comparative Neurology and Psychology 18*: 459–448.

Zinke, W., Roberts, M. J., Guo, K., McDonald, J. S., Robertson, R., and Thiele, A. (2006). Cholinergic modulation of response properties and orientation tuning of neurons in primary visual cortex of anaesthetized marmoset monkeys. *European Journal of Neuroscience 24*: 314–328.

CHAPTER 19

DEVELOPING ATTENTION AND SELF-REGULATION IN CHILDHOOD

MICHAEL I. POSNER, MARY K. ROTHBART, AND M. ROSARIO RUEDA

ORGANIZATION OF THE CHAPTER

ATTENTION changes in dramatic ways between infancy and adulthood. Although it is easy to see these changes in the infant and child's behaviour, it is more difficult to apply common tasks at different ages to investigate these changes and explore their basis. In the first section of this chapter, we propose an objective definition of the functions of attention related to those used with adults and non-human animals in other chapters in this volume.

We view attention as an organ system with its own unique anatomy, connectivity, neuromodulators, and functions. We examine the development of three of these functions during infancy and childhood. The three networks carry out the functions of alerting, orienting, and executive attention (Posner and Fan 2008). Alerting refers to achieving and maintaining a state of optimal readiness to process and respond to input. Orienting refers to the selection of information from sensory input. Executive attention includes mechanisms for monitoring and resolving conflict among thoughts, feelings, and responses. In the second section of this chapter we discuss brain imaging studies with human adults and animals that summarize the anatomy of these networks and provide evidence of their operation in the adult.

An important aspect of the study of brain development is the application of resting state fMRI to infants and children during development. The third section reviews how this evidence can contribute to understanding the development of the brain by providing evidence that is not based on having specific tasks that can be performed at different ages. The following section examines the behavioural development studied in specific cognitive tasks and parent questionnaires in relation to changes in brain mechanisms underlying attentional networks. Next we examine later development of attention networks during childhood and adolescence. The role of genetic variation is considered in relation to socialization of the child in the next section. Finally we discuss some future development.

IMAGING ATTENTION NETWORKS

Imaging studies have revealed neural networks related to the three functions of attention. The cortical areas involved are shown in Fig. 19. 1. In this section we briefly discuss each of the networks in turn. A more detailed description is in Petersen and Posner (in press).

Alerting

The brain network involved in achieving and maintaining the alert state is represented by triangles in Fig. 19. 1. Alertness is an important prerequisite for other attentional operations. Adult studies show that the source of the alerting effect appears to be the locus coeruleus (LC). Cells in the LC have two modes of processing. One mode is sustained and is perhaps related to the tonic level of alertness over long time intervals (Aston-Jones and Cohen 2005). This function is known to involve the right cerebral hemisphere more strongly than the left. Alertness is influenced by sensory events and

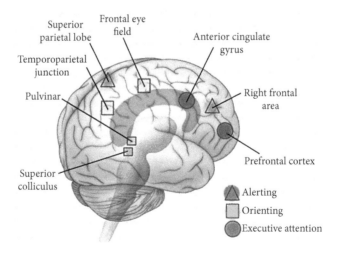

FIGURE 19.1 The alerting, orienting, and executive attention networks. The triangle, circles, and squares indicate nodes of activation of each network.

by the diurnal rhythm. However, its voluntary maintenance during task performance may be orchestrated from the anterior cingulate. More phasic shifts of alerting can result from presenting any environmental signal. However, if the signal is likely to warn about an impending target, this shift results in a characteristic suppression of the intrinsic brain rhythms (e.g. alpha) within a few tens of milliseconds and a strong negative wave (contingent negative variation) recorded from surface electrodes that moves from a frontal generator toward the sensory areas of the hemisphere opposite the expected target (Posner 2008).

Although we often contrast the alert state with sleep it is probably better to consider it in relation to the default state as defined in studies using fMRI with an instruction not to actively process anything (Raichle 2009). The default state is characterized by a slow oscillation between two large-scale networks, one involving medial and one lateral cortical areas. A warning signal moves the brain away from the default state toward a high level of alertness. This change involves widespread variation in autonomic signals such as heart rate (Kahneman 1973) and cortical changes, for example, a negative shift in the scalp recorded EEG called the contingent negative variation (CNV; Walter 1964).

Orienting

Much attention research studies orienting to sensory events. The ease with which the experimenter can control the presentation of visual and auditory stimuli probably accounts for the popularity of studying orienting in different organisms and ages. Precisely controlling the presentation of stimulation also allows studying overt and covert forms of orientation. Overt orienting involves eyes and/or head movements toward the source of stimulation and usually occurs when sufficient time is allowed between the presentation of an orienting cue and the target. Covert orienting involves only orientation of attention and can be studied when not enough time is allowed to move the eyes and/or head or by instructing individuals to attend to the cue without looking at it. The close connection of eye movements to covert shifts of attention has led to studies examining their relation. In general, the same brain areas are active before saccades as are active before covert shifts of attention (Corbetta and Shulman 2002). However, cellular studies in alert monkeys have found that within the frontal eye fields there exist two different but overlapping populations of cells. One is active prior to saccades and the other before attention shifts not leading to saccades (Thompson, Biscoe, and Sato 2005). These findings suggest that eye, head, and covert attention movements become coordinated during early development so that in adults it becomes difficult, but still possible, to separate them.

Every sensory signal provides input both to sensory specific cortical pathways and to brainstem arousal systems related to alerting. The arousal system operates through the brain's norepinephrine system to influence areas of the posterior parietal lobe but does not directly influence the ventral visual pathway (Morrison and Foote 1986). Visual information builds up along the ventral visual pathways allowing recognition of the stimulus. Together these signals may yield changes in a brain network of parietal and frontal areas (see squares in Fig. 19. 1) that orchestrate covert shifts of attention. The orienting network acts so as to boost the strength of input signals in sensory specific pathways in comparison with non-attended signals (Hillyard, Di Russo, and Martinez 2004).

Executive network

The executive attention network is involved in the regulation of feelings (emotions), thoughts (cognition), and actions (see Petersen and Posner in press, for more detail). The anterior cingulate gyrus, one of the main nodes of the executive attention network (see circles in Fig. 19. 1), has been linked to a variety of specific functions related to self-regulation. These include the monitoring of conflict (Botvinick, Braver, Barch, Carter, and Cohen 2001), control of working memory (Duncan et al. 2000), regulation of emotion (Bush, Luu, and Posner 2000), and response to error (Holroyd and Coles 2002). In emotion studies, the cingulate is often seen as part of a network involving orbital frontal cortex and amygdala that regulates our emotional response to input. Activation of the anterior cingulate is observed when people are asked to control their natural reactions to strong positive (Beauregard, Levesque, and Bourgouin 2001) or negative emotions (Ochsner, Bunge, Gross, and Gabrieli 2002). Analysis of functional connectivity between brain areas has shown that when emotionally neutral sensory information is involved there is strong connectivity between the dorsal ACC and the relevant sensory area (Crottaz-Herbette and Mennon 2006). When emotional control is involved there is connectivity between the ventral ACC and the amygdala (Etkin, Egner, Peraza, Kandel, and Hirsch 2006).

Sites and sources of attention

As discussed earlier, all sensory events contribute both to a state of alertness and to orienting of attention. In order to distinguish the brain areas involved in alerting and orienting (*sources*) from the *sites* at which they operate, it is useful to separate the presentation of a cue indicating where a target will occur from the presentation of the target requiring a response (Posner 1978; Corbetta and Shulman 2002). This methodology has been used for behavioural studies with normal individuals (Posner 1978), patients (Posner and Fan 2008), monkeys (Marrocco and Davidson 1998), and in studies using scalp electrical recording and event related neuroimaging (Corbetta and Shulman 2002). Two types of cues are of interest. Some cues provide information only on when the target will occur. These warning signals lead to changes in a network of brain areas related to alerting. Other cues provide information on aspects of the target such as where it will occur and lead to changes in the orienting network.

Studies using event-related fMRI have shown that following the presentation of the cue and before the target is presented, a network of brain areas becomes active

(Corbetta and Shulman 2002). There is widespread agreement about the identity of these areas but there remains work to do in order to understand the function of each area.

When a target is presented in isolation at the cued location it is processed more efficiently than if no cue to its location had been presented (see Posner and Fan 2008, for a review). The brain areas influenced by orienting will be those that would normally be used to process the target. For example, in the visual system, orienting can influence sites of processing in the primary visual cortex, or in a variety of extrastriate visual areas where the computations related to the target are performed (Corbetta, Miezin, Dobmeyer, Shulman, and Petersen 1990). Orienting to target motion influences area MT (V5) while orienting to target colour influences area V4. This principle of activation of brain areas extends to higher-level visual input as well. For example, attention to faces modifies activity in the face-sensitive area of the fusiform gyrus (Wojciulik, Kanwisher, and Driver 1998). The finding that attention can modify activity in the primary visual cortex has been of particular importance because this brain area has been more extensively studied than any other. When multiple targets are presented they tend to suppress the normal level of activity produced when presented in isolation (Desimone and Duncan 1995). One important role of orienting to a particular location is to provide a relative enhancement of the target at that location in comparison with other items presented in the visual field.

Executive attention and self-regulation

The perception of pain, either physical (Rainville, Duncan, Price, Carrier, and Bushnell 1997) or social (Eisenberger, Lieberman, and Williams 2003), processing of reward (Hampton and O'Doherty 2007), monitoring of conflict (Botvinick et al. 2001), error detection (Dehaene, Posner and Tucker 1994), and theory of mind (Kampe, Frith and Frith 2003) in neuroimaging studies activate an area of midfrontal cortex that includes the anterior cingulate gyrus. Many of the same tasks also activate the anterior insula and basal ganglia. Is there also a single function that involves these important input signals? We have argued that the role of this brain area is to regulate the processing of information from other networks, serving as part of an executive attention network involved in the control of both cognition and emotion (Posner and Rothbart 2007a).

In adult studies, the executive attention network is often activated by requiring a person to withhold a dominant response in order to perform a subdominant response (Posner and Rothbart 2007a, 2007b). The ability to control our thoughts, feelings, and behaviour in developmental psychology is called self-regulation. This is a broad function, not easy to test or model. However, the self-regulatory view fits well with the evidence of brain activation, functional and structural connectivity, and individual differences. Moreover, the self-regulatory view helps us understand how brain networks relate to important real life functions and provides a perspective into how the shift takes place between infancy, where regulation is under the control of the caregiver, and later life, where self-control is most important.

Attention network test

In our work we have used the Attention Network Test (ANT) to examine the efficiency of three brain networks underlying attention: alerting, orienting, and executive attention (Fan, McCandliss, Sommer, Raz, and Posner 2002). The task requires the person to press one key if the central arrow points to the left and another if it points to the right. Conflict is introduced by having flankers surrounding the target that point in either the same (congruent) or opposite (incongruent) direction as the target. Cues presented prior to the target provide information on where or when the target will occur. Reaction times for the separate conditions are subtracted, providing three measures that represent efficiency of in alerting, orienting, and executive networks. A child version of this test is very similar but replaces the arrows with fish (Rueda et al. 2004a).

Subsequent work has shown fairly high reliability of the conflict scores, but much lower reliability for the orienting and alerting scores (MacLeod et al. 2010); recent revisions that provide better measure of orienting and alerting might improve these results (Fan et al. 2009). When more complex versions of the ANT have been used, significant interactions have been obtained between networks (Callejas, Lupiáñnez, and Tudela 2004; Fan et al. 2009). It is clear that these networks do communicate and work together in many situations, even though their anatomy is quite different.

BRAIN CHANGES IN HUMAN DEVELOPMENT

Even at rest common brain areas appear to be active together (default state, Raichle 2009). While evidence for connection between brain areas related to attention is found even in infancy (Gao et al. 2009), studies suggest that the connectivity between these areas changes over the course of development. Two sets of attention-related brain networks are connected at rest: a set of fronto-parietal brain areas (related to orienting and to aspects of control) and a cingulo-opercular (related to executive attention) network. The fronto-parietal network (see top left panel of Fig. 19. 2) in adults is involved in short-term control operations common when orienting to sensory signals. The cingulo-parietal network (see top right hand panel of Fig. 19. 2) is involved in longer-term more strategic control that fits well with an executive system (Dosenbach et al. 2007). While there are important differences in detail between these networks (see Dosenbach et al. 2007; Petersen and Posner in press) and the orienting and executive networks found in our studies, it seems likely they play similar roles, particularly during development.

Connections change over the life span. Fig. 19. 2 shows that adults (left panel) have separate networks related to orienting and executive attention. In 7- to 9-year-old children these networks are more integrated (see panel on the right side). Children age 7 to 9 show many shorter connections whereas adults show more segregation of the two networks and longer connections (Dosenbach et al. 2007; Fair et al. 2007, 2008). Since resting connectivity analysis requires no task, it can be studied during infancy (Gao et al. 2009). During the first year of life the anterior cingulate shows little or no connectivity

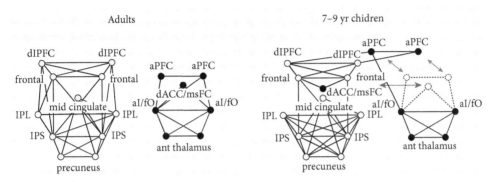

FIGURE 19.2 Functional connectivity between brain areas at rest: (left side) children 9 years of age; (right side) adults. Adapted from Dosenbach, N. U., Fair, D. A., Miezin, F. M., Cohen, A. L., Wenger, K. K., Dosenbach, R. A., Fox, M. D., Snyder, A. Z., Vincent, J. L., Raichle, M. E., Schlaggar, B. L., and Petersen, S. E., Distinct brain networks for adaptive and stable task control in humans, *Proceedings of the National Academy of Sciences of the United States of America*, 104(4), pp. 1073–1978 © 2007, The National Academy of Sciences..

to other areas. After the first year, infants begin the slow process of developing the long-range connectivity that is typical of adults. However, the details of these developmental studies may change since they involve cross-sectional comparisons between varying ages and may reflect other changes besides brain maturation.

Another aspect of attention, especially prominent in the transition between infancy and early childhood is self-regulation. Self-regulation refers to the ability to control one's own emotions, thoughts, or behaviour. It has been possible to show that infants carry out at least one of the important functions related to the anterior cingulate, the recognition of error. In one study, 7-month-old infants were found to look longer at erroneous than correct events (Wynn 1992). Error events also appear to cause a scalp negative electrical potential over a set of electrodes that have been localized in the anterior cingulate (Dehaene et al. 1994) in 7- to 9-month-old infants (Berger, Tzur, and Posner 2006). However, the typical regulation of behaviour found in adults, that is, to slow down following an error, does not seem to emerge until about age 3 years (Jones, Rothbart, and Posner 2003). Together the connectivity and task data fit well with the idea that infants can process information and use executive attention to a limited degree, but are unable to show regulation of their behaviour by this network.

Behavioural Development in Infancy

Attention in infancy is less developed than later in life and the functions of alerting, orienting, and executive control appear to be less independent during infancy. We first examine alerting and orienting and then consider attention in relation to self-regulation.

The measurement of these variables must be different in infancy than later when voluntary responses can be directed by the experimenter. Efforts have been made to design tasks that can be performed by infants that tap into the same networks of brain areas shown in Fig. 19.1.

Alerting and orienting

The early life of the infant is chiefly concerned with changes in state. Sleep dominates at birth and the waking state is relatively rare at first. The newborn spends nearly three-quarters of the time sleeping (Colombo and Horowitz 1987). Many of the changes in the alert state depend upon external input. Arousal of the central nervous system involves input from brainstem systems that modulate activation of the cortex. As in adults, primary among these is the locus coeruleus. It has been demonstrated that the influence of warning signals operates via this brain system, since drugs that block it also prevent the changes in the alert state that lead to improved performance after a warning signal is provided (Marrocco and Davidson 1998). It is likely that the endogenous changes during waking that take place without external input also involve this system.

There is a dramatic change in the percentage of time in the waking state over the first three months of life. By the 12th postnatal week the infant has become able to maintain the alert state during much of the daytime hours. This ability still depends heavily upon external stimulation, much of it provided by the caregiver.

Much of the response to external stimuli also involves orienting toward a stimulus. Newborns show head and eye movements toward novel stimuli. These eye movements are preferentially directed toward moving stimuli and have been shown to involve properties of the stimulus, for example how much they resemble human faces (Johnson and Morton 1991). It has also been demonstrated that newborns can make imitative responses; for example, when shown a face with a protruding tongue they respond with a similar movement (Meltzoff and Moore 1977). However, the reliability and complexity of these responses to sensory input change dramatically over the first few months of life.

The most frequent method of studying orienting in infancy involves tracking of saccadic eye movements. As in adults, there is a close relation, but not identity, between the direction of gaze and the infants' attention. The attention system can be driven by external input from birth (Richards and Hunter 1998); however, the system continues to improve in precision over many years. Infant eye movements often fall short of the target and peripheral targets are often foveated by a series of head and eye movements (Clohessy, Posner, and Rothbart 2001). Although not as easy to track, the covert system likely follows a similar trajectory. Studies examining the covert system by use of brief cues that do not produce an eye movement followed by targets that do, show that the speed of the eye movement to the target is enhanced by the cue and this enhancement improves over the first year of life (Butcher 2000). In more complex situations, for example when there are competing targets, the improvement in orienting ability may continue longer.

Orienting to sensory input is a major mechanism for regulation of distress. Infants often have a hard time disengaging from high spatial frequency targets and may become distressed before they are able to move away from the target (Ruff and Rothbart 1996). Caregivers provide a hint of how attention is used to regulate the state of the infant when they attempt to distract their infants by bringing their attention to other stimuli. As infants orient, they are often quieted, and their distress appears to diminish. In one study (Harman, Rothbart, and Posner 1997), infants were first shown a sound and light display and became distressed, but when oriented to interesting events signs of distress disappeared. However, as soon as the orienting stopped, for example when the object was removed, the infants' distress returned to almost exactly the levels shown prior to presentation of the soothing object. An internal system, which was termed the *distress keeper*, and which we believe involves the amygdala, appears to hold a computation of the initial level of distress, so that it returns if the infant's orientation to the novel event is lost. Interestingly, infants were quieted by distraction for as long as one minute, without changing the eventual level of distress reached once orienting ended (Harman et al. 1997).

For newborns, the control of orienting is initially largely in the hands of caregiver presentations. By four months, however, infants have gained considerable control in disengaging their gaze from one visual location and moving it to another, and greater orienting skill in the laboratory is associated with lower temperamental negative emotion and greater soothability as reported by parents (Johnson, Posner, and Rothbart 1991). Late infancy is the time when self-regulation develops. Infants increasingly are able to gain control of their own emotions and other behaviours. This transition marks the development of the executive attention system.

Executive attention in infancy

It is difficult to assess executive attention in infants because as outlined above the caregivers provide most of the regulation of infant behaviour. Effortful control is a high level factor from parental reports on infant temperament (Rothbart and Rueda 2005). This factor is defined as the ability to withhold a dominant response in order to carry out a non-dominant one. Parents observing their children's specific behaviour in daily life situations (for example, put away toys on command, etc.) can readily rate questions that relate to this factor. This can be done for children about 2 years of age and older. Below this age, temperament questionnaires (Rothbart, Ahadi, and Hershey 1994) are confined to factors like orienting and positive and negative affect (Rothbart 2011), and control of attention is measured as a combination of duration of attention, soothability, etc. (Gartstein and Rothbart 2003; see Rueda in press, for a review). Older children receive scores on effortful control. In addition, children above age 2 can be scored on tasks that involve voluntary responding such as pressing keys to visual input.

As mentioned earlier there is evidence of the executive attention network at about 7 months for the detection of error. Later in the first year of life, there is evidence of further development of executive attention. One example is Adele Diamond's work using the 'A not B' task and the reaching task. These two marker tasks involve inhibition of an action that is strongly elicited by the situation. In the 'A not B' task, the experimenter shifts the location of a hidden object from location A to location B, after the infant's retrieving from location A had been reinforced as correct in the previous trials (Diamond 1991). In the reaching task, visual information about the correct route to a toy is put in conflict with the cues that normally guide reaching. Important changes in the performance of these tasks are observed from 6 to 12 months (Diamond 2006). Another task that reflects the executive system involves anticipatory looking in a visual sequence task (Clohessy et al. 2001; Haith, Hazan, and Goodman 1988). In the visual sequence task, stimuli are placed in front of the infant in a fixed and predictable sequence of locations. The infant's eyes are drawn reflexively to stimuli designed to be attractive and interesting. After a few trials, some infants will begin to anticipate the location of the next target by moving their eyes in anticipation of the target. It has been shown that anticipatory looking occurs with infants as young as 3.5 to 4 months (Clohessy et al. 2001; Haith et al. 1988). When sequences in which a location is followed by one of two or more different locations (e.g. location 1, then location 2, then location 1, then location 3, and so on ... where location 1 can be followed by location 2 or location 3 depending on the previous location), monitoring of context is necessary and attention is required. The ability to respond when this occurs is not present until about 18–24 months of age (Clohessy et al. 2001). At 3 years, the ability to respond correctly when there is conflict in the sequential looking task is related to the ability to resolve conflict in a spatial conflict task (Rothbart, Ellis, Rueda, and Posner 2003). These findings support the slow development of the executive attention network during the first and second year of life.

Summary

Colombo (2001) presented a summary of attentional functions in infancy, which included alertness, orienting to spatial locations and to objects, and endogenous attention. This division is similar to the network approach but divides orienting into space and features and includes the functions of inter-stimulus shifts and sustained attention as part of endogenous attention. He argues that alerting reaches the mature state at about 4 months, orienting by 6–7 months, and endogenous attention by 4–5 years. This schedule is similar to the order of development described above, but as discussed in the next major section all these functions continue developing during childhood. The genetic findings discussed below are new since the Colombo summary and add further substance to the distinctions between functions and their integration in the achievement of self-regulation.

ATTENTIONAL NETWORKS
AND CHILD DEVELOPMENT

Alerting network

Preparation from warning cues (phasic alertness) can be measured by comparing the speed and accuracy of response to stimulation with and without warning signals (Posner 2008). Presentation of warning cues prior to targets allows the individual to get ready to respond by increasing the state of alertness. This commonly results in increased response speed, although it may also cause declines in the accuracy of the response, particularly at short intervals between warning cue and target (Posner 1978).

The difficulty of using reaction time tasks with very young children makes studying developmental differences in preparation from alerting cues more challenging, yet several studies have examined developmental changes in phasic alertness between preschoolers, older children, and adults. Using the Child ANT, Mezzacappa (2004) observed a trend to larger alerting scores (difference between RT in trials with and without warning cues) with age in a sample of 5- to 7-year-old children. Increasing age was associated with larger reductions in RT in response to warning cues. Older children also showed lower rates of omissions overall, indicating greater ability to remain vigilant during the task period. Moreover, young children (5-year-olds) appear to need more time than older children (8-year-olds) and adults to get full benefit from a warning cue, and they also seem to be less able to sustain the optimal level of alertness over time (Morrison 1982). The difficulty of maintaining the alert state without a cue is also observed for older children (10-year-olds) when compared to adults (Rueda et al. 2004a), suggesting that tonic or sustained attention continues developing through late childhood.

The alert state can be elicited by external stimulation, but also varies in a regular rhythm over the course of the day and can be attained in a voluntary endogenously generated way. Infants show a progressive increase in the frequency and duration of alert periods during the first year of life, whereas the ability to voluntarily deploy attention seems to emerge later and shows a steadier developmental course during childhood (Colombo 2001).

Sustained attention is frequently measured by examining variations in performance in a task over a relatively extended period of time, as in the Continuous Performance Tasks (CPT). Variations in the level of alertness can be observed by examining the percentage of correct and/or omitted responses to targets or through indexes of perceptual sensitivity (d) over time. With young children, the percentage of individuals able to complete the task can also indicate maturational differences in the ability to sustain attention. In a study conducted with preschoolers, only 30–50% of the 3- to 4-year-olds were able to complete the task, whereas the percentage rose to 70% for 4- to 4½-year olds and close to 100% from that age up (Levy 1980). However, even though the largest development of vigilance seems to occur during the preschool period, children continue to show larger declines in performance in CPT over time compared to adults through middle and late childhood, especially under more difficult task conditions, reaching the adult level by approximately 13 years of age (Curtindale, Laurie-Rose, Bennett-Murphy, and Hull 2007; Lin, Hsiao, and Chen 1999).

Developmental changes in alertness during childhood and early adolescence appear to relate to continuous maturation of frontal systems during this period. One way to examine brain mechanisms underlying changes in alertness is by registering patterns of brain-generated electrical activation through electrodes placed on the scalp while warning cues are processed. The *Contingent Negative Variation* (CNV) appears to be related to a source of activation in the right ventral and medial frontal (ACC) brain areas (Segalowitz and Davies 2004). The CNV is related to performance in various measures of intelligence and executive functions as well as functional capacity of the frontal cortex (Segalowitz, Unsal, and Dywan 1992). The CNV and other slow waves have been related to changes in activation using fMRI (Raichle 2009). The amplitude of the CNV increases with age, especially during middle childhood. Jonkman (2006) found that the CNV amplitude is significantly smaller for 6-to 7-year-old children compared to adults, but no differences were observed between 9- to 10-year-olds and adults. Moreover, the difference in CNV amplitude between children and adults seems to be restricted to early components of the CNV observed over right fronto-central channels (Jonkman, Lansbergen, and Stauder 2003), suggesting a role of maturation of the frontal alerting network.

Orienting network

Infants are able to orient attention to external stimulation from early in life. Nonetheless, aspects of the attention system that increase precision and voluntary control of orienting continue developing throughout childhood and adolescence. Most infant studies examine overt forms of orienting. By the time children are able to follow instructions and respond to stimulation by pressing keys, both overt and covert orienting can be measured. The cueing task has been widely used to study the development of visual orienting over the life span. Mostly using a cueing paradigm, several studies have examined the development of orienting during childhood. The cueing method allows a separation of benefits from cueing (valid—neutral cue) from the costs of reorienting after a wrong cue (invalid—neutral cue). Despite a progressive increase in orienting speed to valid cues during childhood (Schul, Townsend, and Stiles 2003), data generally show no age differences in the orienting benefit effects between young children (5–6 years of age), older children (8–10), and adults (Enns and Brodeur 1989), regardless of whether the effect is measured in covert or overt orienting conditions (Wainwright and Bryson 2002). However, there seems to be an age-related decrease in the orienting cost (Enns and Brodeur 1989; Schul et al. 2003; Wainwright and Bryson 2002). In addition, the effect of age when disengagement and reorienting to an uncued location are required appears to be larger, particularly with longer intervals between cue and target (Schul et al. 2003; Wainwright and Bryson 2005). This suggests that mostly aspects of orienting related to the control of disengagement and voluntary orientation, which depend on cortical regions of the parietal and temporal lobes, improve with age during childhood. When endogenous orienting was examined for children aged 6 to 14 and adults, all groups but the young children showed larger orienting effects, calculated as the difference in RT to targets appearing at cued and uncued locations, with longer cue–target intervals (Wainwright and Bryson 2005). This indicates that young children seem to have problems endogenously adjusting the scope of their attentional focus. This idea was also suggested by Enns and Girgus (1985), who found that attentional focusing as well as the ability to effectively divide or switch attention between stimuli improves with age between ages 5, 8, and 10 and adults.

Executive attention network

Self-regulation of cognition and action can be measured in the laboratory by registering responses to tasks that involve conflict. Common conflict tasks, like the classic Stroop task, require the participant to avoid paying attention to dominant aspects of the stimulus (for example the word *WHITE*), while responding to non-dominant features (i.e. the colour in which the word is written). From 2 years of age and older, children are able to perform simple conflict tasks in which their reaction time can be measured. The Spatial Conflict Task (SCT; Gerardi-Caulton 2000) induces conflict between the identity and the location of an object. In this task, pictures of houses of two animals (i.e. a duck and a cat) are presented in the bottom left and right sides of the screen, then one of the two animals appears either on the left or right side of the screen in each trial and the child is required to show the animal what its house is by touching it. Location is the dominant aspect of the stimulus though instructions require responding according to its identity. Thus, conflict trials in which the animal appears on the side of the screen opposite to its house usually cause slower responses and larger error rates than non-conflict trials (when the animal appears on the side of its house). Between 2 and 4 years of age, children progress from an almost complete inability to carry out the task to relatively good performance. Although 2-year-old children tend to perseverate on a single response, 3-year-olds perform at high accuracy levels, although, like adults, they respond more slowly and with reduced accuracy to conflict trials (Gerardi-Caulton 2000; Rothbart et al. 2003).

The detection and correction of errors is another form of action monitoring. While performing the SCT, 2½ and 3-year-old children showed longer RTs following erroneous trials than following correct ones, indicating that children were noticing their errors and using them to guide performance in the next trial. However, no evidence of slowing following an error was found at 2 years of age (Rothbart et al. 2003). As mentioned previously, a similar result was found when using a version of the Simple Simon game. In this task, children are asked to execute a response when a command is given by one stuffed animal, while inhibiting responses commanded by a second animal

(Jones et al. 2003). Children of 36–38 months were unable to inhibit their response and showed no slowing following an error, but at 39–41 months, children showed both an ability to inhibit action and a slowing of reaction time following an error. These results suggest that between 30 and 39 months children greatly develop the capacity to correct erroneous responses and that this ability may relate to the development of inhibitory control.

The development of executive attention has also been traced into the primary school period using the child version of the ANT. Overall, child reaction times were much longer than adults', but considerable development in the speed of resolving conflict from age 4 to about 7 years of age was observed (Rueda, Posner, and Rothbart 2005). However, the ability to resolve conflict on the flanker task, as measured by increases in RT and percentage of errors produced by the presence of incompatible compared to compatible flankers, remained about the same from age 7 to adulthood (Rueda et al. 2004a). Nonetheless, studies in which the difficulty of the conflict task is increased by other demands such as switching rules or holding more information in working memory have shown further development of conflict resolution between late childhood and adulthood (Davidson, Amso, Anderson, and Diamond 2006).

To study the brain mechanisms that underlie the development of executive attention some developmental studies have been carried out using event-related potentials (ERP) and conflict tasks. In one of these studies, a flanker task was used to compare conflict resolution in three groups of children aged 5 to 6, 7 to 9, and 10 to 12, and a group of adults (Ridderinkhof and van der Molen 1995). In this study, developmental differences were examined in two ERP components, one related to response preparation (lateralized readiness potential, LRP) and another one related to stimulus evaluation (P3). The authors found differences between children and adults in the latency of the LRP, but not in the latency of the P3 peak, suggesting that developmental differences in the ability to resist interference are mainly related to response competition and inhibition, not to stimulus evaluation.

Brain responses to errors are also informative of the function of the executive attention system. The error-related negativity (ERN) is a potential with a fronto-central scalp distribution that appears some time (usually between 60 and 120 ms) after an error response (Gehring, Gross, Coles, Meyer, and Donchin 1993) and is thought to be generated by the ACC (van Veen and Carter 2002). The amplitude of the ERN seems to reflect detection of an error as well as salience of the error for a particular individual in the context of the task and is subject to individual differences in temperament or motivation. Generally, larger ERN amplitudes are associated with greater engagement in the task and/or greater efficiency of the error-detection system (Santesso, Segalowitz, and Schmidt 2005; Tucker, Hartry-Speiser, McDougal, Luu, and deGrandpre 1999). Developmentally, the amplitude of the ERN shows a progressive increase during childhood into late adolescence (Segalowitz and Davies 2004), with young children (age 7–8 years) being less likely to show the ERN to errors than older children and adults. This is likely to reflect the progressive maturation of the brain system for action-monitoring and regulation.

Another evoked potential, the N2, has been related to situations that require executive control (Koop, Rist, and Mattler 1996) and has been directly associated to activation coming from the anterior cingulate cortex (van Veen and Carter 2002). We have conducted an ERP study in which we used the fish flanker task of the child ANT with 4-year-old children and adults (Rueda, Posner, Rothbart, and Davis-Stober 2004b). Adults showed larger N2 for incongruent trials than congruent trials over the mid frontal leads. Four-year-old children also showed a larger negative deflection for the incongruent condition at the mid frontal electrodes that, compared to adults, had greater amplitude, and was extended over a longer period of time. Whereas the frontal effect was evident for adults at around 300 ms post-target, children did not show any effect until approximately 550 ms after the target. In addition, the effect was sustained over a period of 500 ms before the children's responses, in contrast to only 50 ms in the case of adults. Another important difference between 4-year-old children and adults was the distribution of effects over the scalp. In adults, the frontal effects appear to be focalized on the mid-line, whereas in children the effects were observed mostly at pre-frontal sites and in a broader number of channels, including the mid-line and lateral areas.

The focalization of signals in adults as compared to children is consistent with neuroimaging studies conducted with older children, where children appear to activate the same network of areas as adults when performing similar tasks, but the average volume of activation appears to be remarkably greater in children (Casey, Thomas, Davidson, Kunz, and Franzen 2002; Durston et al. 2002). Altogether, these data suggest that the brain circuitry underlying executive functions becomes more focal as it gains in efficiency. This contrasts with the increase in long-range connectivity discussed in the previous section. However, both longer direction connections and focalization may be compatible with a maturational process that reduces the time these systems need to resolve each of the processes implicated in the task.

Summary

Attention networks show substantial development during childhood. The rates of development appear to differ among the three networks with alerting showing a very slow developmental time course. While the ANT shows most development in the executive network to occur before age 7, the connectivity data (see Fig. 19. 2) indicate increased segregation between orienting and executive networks beyond the age of 9.

GENES AND EXPERIENCE BUILD NETWORKS

The finding that common brain networks of attention show similarities and differences between humans and other organisms (e.g. primates) offers an important approach to evolution. Another approach of equal importance involves an examination of differences in the efficiency of this network between individuals. Such differences could rest in part upon genetic variation known to exist among individuals and in part upon differences in cultural or individual experience between people. The study of temperament examines individual differences in reactivity and self-regulation that are biologically based (Rothbart 2011). As mentioned earlier, effortful control is the construct developed within the temperament literature to study individual differences in self-regulation.

The adult and child versions of the attention network test were discussed previously. A study using fMRI showed that the anatomy of these three networks was for the most part independent (Fan, McCandliss, Fossella, Flombaum, and Posner 2005; see also Fig. 19. 1). In addition, each of the networks has a dominant neuromodulator arising from subcortical brain areas. The alerting network is modulated by norepinephrine arising in the locus coeruleus, the orienting network by acetylcholine from the basal forebrain, and the executive network by dopamine from the ventral tegmental area (Posner and Fan 2008).

Conflict scores obtained with the ANT have been shown to correlate with measures of the temperament factor of effortful control (EC) at several ages during childhood (see Rueda 2012). Gerardi-Caulton (2000) carried out some of the first research linking EC to underlying brain networks of executive attention, using spatial conflict as a laboratory marker task. Similar findings linking parent-reported EC to performance on laboratory attention tasks have been shown for 24-, 30-, and 36-month-olds (Rothbart et al. 2003), 3- and 5-year-olds (Chang and Burns 2005), and 7-year-olds (Gonzalez, Fuentes, Carranza, and Estevez, 2001). Adult studies have also found a correlation between conflict resolution ability and effortful control (Kanske 2008) and some disorders influence both executive (Fernandez-Duque and Black 2006) and effortful control.

Daily life

The correlation between conflict scores in the ANT and parent reports of effortful control form a basis for the association between self-regulation and executive attention. As discussed above, ANT executive attention scores and effortful control have been related to many aspects of child development. Effortful control is related to the empathy children show toward others, their ability to delay an action, and to avoid such behaviours as lying or cheating when given the opportunity (Posner and Rothbart 2007b; Rothbart and Rueda 2005). High levels of effortful control and the ability to resolve conflict are related to fewer antisocial behaviours such as truancy in adolescents (Ellis, Rothbart, and Posner 2004) and better acceptance among peers in the school context (Checa, Rodriguez-Bailon, and Rueda 2008). Additionally, EC has been shown to be an important predictor of school competence. In a study conducted with 12-year-old children, both EC and brain activity during performance of a conflict task predicted academic achievement, particularly in subjects such as mathematics (Checa and Rueda 2011). These findings support the position that self-regulation, a psychological function crucial for child socio-emotional and cognitive development, can also be studied in terms of specific anatomical areas and their connections.

The common nature of brain networks such as those in Fig. 19.1 argue strongly for the role of genes in their construction. This has led cognitive neuroscience to incorporate data from the growing field of human genetics (Green et al. 2008; Posner, Rothbart, and Sheese 2007). One method for doing this involves studying the relation between individual variations in genes (genetic alleles) and aspects of human behaviour. Brain activity can serve as an intermediate level for relating genes to behaviour. As one example, the ANT has been used to examine individual differences in the efficiency of executive attention. Strong heritability of the executive network (Fan et al. 2002) supported the search for genes related to individual differences in network efficiency.

Genetic variation

The association of the executive network with the neuromodulator dopamine provides a way of searching for candidate genes that might be related to the efficiency of the network (Fossella, Posner, Fan, Swanson, and Pfaff 2002; Posner and Fan 2008). For example, several studies employing conflict-related tasks have found that alleles of the catechol-O-methyl transferase (COMT) gene, the dopamine 4 receptor gene (DRD4), as well as the monoamine oxidase A gene (MAOA) and some other dopamine-related genes were associated with the ability to resolve conflict (Blasi et al. 2005; Diamond, Briand, Fossella, and Gehlbach 2004; Posner et al. 2007). It has been possible to show in brain imaging studies that some of these genetic differences are related to the degree to which the anterior cingulate is activated during task performance (Fan et al. 2003). In the future, it may be possible to relate genes to specific nodes within neural networks, allowing a much more detailed understanding of the origins of brain networks.

Longitudinal study

Recently, we conducted a longitudinal study to see if the genes we had shown to influence attention in adults would have specific roles in the development of self-regulation during infancy and childhood. Our study began when the infants were 7 months old. We retested and genotyped the children at age 2 years and also tested them at age 4 when they are able perform the ANT as a measure of executive attention. Because infants are not able to carry out voluntary attention tasks, we used the visual sequence described previously in which a series of attractive stimuli are put on the screen in a repetitive sequence. Infants orient to them by moving their eyes (and head) to the location. On some trials, infants show they anticipate what is coming by orienting prior to the stimulus. It had been shown previously that infants as young as 4 months of age have a significantly better than chance performance in their anticipations (Clohessy et al. 2001), and we thought that anticipations may serve as an early indicant of executive attention.

In agreement with this idea, it was found that infants who make the most anticipatory looks also exhibited a pattern of cautious reaching toward novel objects (Sheese,
Rothbart, Posner, White, and Fraundorf 2008), which in turn predicts effortful control
in older children (Rothbart, Ahadi, Hershey, and Fisher 2000; Rothbart et al. 2003).
In addition, infants with more anticipatory looks showed more spontaneous attempts
at self-regulation when presented with somewhat frightening objects. Along with the
infants' use of the anterior cingulate in detecting errors (Berger et al. 2006; Wynn 1992),
these finding suggested that at 7 months, infants have a rudimentary executive attention
system in place, even though parents are as yet unable to report it and infants do not
carry out instructed behaviours.

Rothbart and Derryberry (1981) proposed a distinction between reactive and
self-regulatory aspects of child temperament. They argued that early in life negative
affect, particularly fear and orienting of attention, served as regulatory mechanisms that
were supplemented by parental regulation. Rothbart and Bates (2006) also argued for
developmental change in which effortful control only arose at about 3–4 years of age
when parents could first report on their children's self-regulatory ability.

Our longitudinal study has confirmed but also revised and extended this analysis. We
found a negative correlation at 7 months between parent reports of infant orienting of
attention and negative affect. Orienting also correlated positively with reports of positive affect. By 2 years, orienting is no longer related to affect, but effortful control showed
modest non-significant negative correlation with both positive and negative affect.
There is substantial evidence that for children, adolescents, and adults, effortful control
is inversely related to negative affect in Western countries, although Ahadi, Rothbart,
and Ye (1993) found that in China effortful control was negatively correlated with positive affect in children. They argued that culture may shape the direction of the interaction of effortful control and emotion.

Results of the longitudinal study suggest that early in life, orienting serves as a regulatory system (Posner, Rothbart, Sheese, and Voelker in press; Rothbart, Sheese, Rueda,
and Posner 2011). It both reduces negative affect and increases positive affect. In this
view, both orienting and executive networks serve parallel regulatory functions during infancy. Later, executive attention appears to dominate in regulating emotions and
thoughts, but orienting still serves as a control system. Parenting may play an important role in the development of the executive attention network, perhaps partly through
the presentation of novel objects that have been shown in adults to activate the executive network (Shulman et al. 2009). This parallel use of the two networks fits with the
findings of Dosenbach et al. (2007) that in adults the fronto-parietal network controls
behaviour at short time intervals while their cingulo-opercular network exercises strategic control over long intervals. The resting state imaging work may also reflect additional fronto-parietal brain areas than have been included in the orienting network
(Petersen and Posner in press).

The association of the executive attention system with dopamine led us to examine
several genes related to dopamine transmission in relation to early development of
attention networks. These are summarized below.

COMT

COMT is a protein-coding gene located at chromosome 22. It plays an important role in dopamine metabolism by modulating extracellular levels of dopamine. Polymorphic variations of the COMT gene have consistently been shown to be related to executive attention in adults and older children (Blasi et al. 2005; Diamond et al. 2004). A finding from our current longitudinal study is that COMT is also related to aspects of attention in toddlers (Voelker et al. 2009). We found that haplotypes of the COMT gene (Diatchenko et al. 2005) influenced both anticipatory looking and nesting cup performance at 18–20 months. At 7 months variations of the COMT gene were also related to positive affect as reported by parents. The finding of a relation of COMT to positive affect together with the influence of this gene on executive attention at 18–20 months could provide a genetic link between reactive emotion and emotional regulation during early development.

DRD4

The DRD4 gene is located at chromosome 11. It is also a protein-coding gene which modulates sensitivity of D4 receptors to extrasynaptic levels of DA in the prefrontal cortex. The 7 repeat allele of the DRD4 gene has been linked to attention deficit hyperactivity disorder (ADHD) and to the temperamental dimension of risk taking. There has been considerable evidence that the environment can have a strong influence in the presence of the 7 repeat allele but not when it is absent (Bakermans-Kranenburg and van Ijzendoorn 2006; van Ijzendoorn and Bakermans-Kranenburg 2006). The same group (Bakermans-Kranenburg, van Ijzendoorn, Pijlman, Mesman, and Juffer 2008) has also performed a parent training intervention. They found that training decreased externalizing behaviour, but only for those children with the 7 repeat allele of the DRD4 gene. This finding is important because assignment to the training group was random, ensuring that the result was not due to something about the parents other than the training.

In our longitudinal study, raters observed caregiver/child interaction and rated the parents on five dimensions of parental quality according to a schedule developed by NICHD (1993): support, autonomy, stimulation, lack of hostility, and confidence in the child. Although all of the parents were likely concerned and caring, they did differ in their scores, and we divided the combined scores at the median into two groups. One of the groups was considered to show a higher quality of parenting, and the other a lower quality. We found a strong interaction between genes and parenting. For children without the 7-repeat polymorphism, variations in parenting within the range we examined were unrelated to the children's scores on impulsivity and risk taking. For children carrying the 7-repeat gene variant, however, variations in parenting quality mattered. Children with this allele and high quality parenting showed normal levels of risk taking, but those with lower quality parenting showed very high values for risk taking (Sheese, Voelker, Rothbart, and Posner 2007).

It seems paradoxical that the 7 repeat allele associated with developmental psychopathology (ADHD) is also under positive selective pressure in recent human evolution

(Ding et al. 2002). Why should an allele related to ADHD be positively selected? One possibility is that positive selection of the 7 repeat allele could well arise from its sensitivity to environmental influences (Belsky and Pluess 2009). Parenting provides training for children in the values favoured by the culture in which they live. In recent years the genetic part of the nature by nurture interaction has been given a lot of emphasis, but if genetic variations are selected according to the sensitivity they give children to cultural influences, this could support a greater balance between genes and environment. Theories of positive selection in the DRD4 gene have stressed the role of sensation seeking in human evolution (Wang, Kodama, Baldi, and Moyzis 2006). Our new findings do not contradict this emphasis, but suggest a form of explanation that could have even wider significance. It remains to be seen whether the other 300 genes estimated to show positive selection would also increase an individual's sensitivity to variations in rearing environments.

How could variation in genetic alleles lead to enhanced influence of cultural factors like parenting? The anterior cingulate receives input on both reward value and pain or punishment, and this information is clearly important in regulating thoughts and feelings. Dopamine is the most important neuromodulator in these reward and punishment pathways. Thus, changes in the availability of dopamine could enhance the influence of signals from parents related to reward and punishment. Another interaction has been reported between the serotonin transporter gene and parent social support on behavioural inhibition or social fear (Fox et al. 2005). To explain this interaction, Fox, Hane, and Pine (2007) argue that those children with a short form of the serotonin transporter gene who also have lower social support from parents show enhanced attention to threat and greater social fear. In our study of the DRD4, however, attention did not appear to be the mechanism by which the genetic variation influenced the child's behaviour. In our study there was no influence of the 7 repeat allele on executive attention; instead, gene and environment interacted to influence the child's behaviour as observed by the caregiver. However, a link between the DRD4 and attention as rated by parents did appear at age 4 and older. We also found that the COMT genotype showed an interaction with parenting quality, and unlike the DRD4 it did operate through attention even at age 2. It is important to consider the multiple mechanisms by which genes may influence behaviour. Clearly, one important mechanism lies in the executive attention network we have been discussing in this chapter, but there must be other pathways that influence behaviour through other non-attentional mechanisms.

CHRNA4

The nicotinic cholinergic receptor also modulates activity of dopamine in the mesolimbic system (Pidoplichko et al. 2004). Polymorphisms in the CHRNA4 gene have been associated with nicotine dependence in humans and with cognitive performance (Rigbi et al. 2008). The *CHRNA4* (C1545T) polymorphism (rs1044396) has been associated with variation in performance of visuospatial attention (Parasuraman, Greenwood, Kumar, and Fossella 2005) and in brain activity when performing a visual oddball task involving the cingulate (Winterer et al. 2007). During infancy the T/T allele of *CHRNA4* is related to greater anticipatory looking, but at 18 months the C/C homozygotes have the highest scores on effortful control (Voelker et al. 2009). In a spatial attention task known to involve the orienting network (Parasuraman et al. 2005) adults with the C/C allele showed higher benefits and lower costs than those with the T/T or T/C alleles. Our genetic findings may provide support for the parallel model of regulation discussed above. Those children with higher levels of control by orienting in infancy could be slower to show the conversion to control by the executive network.

Summary

Particular genes have been associated with individual differences in each of the attentional networks (Green et al. 2008). The expression of these genes may also interact with features of the environment during early development. In some cases, genetic variation appears to be important in how much influence the environment has on behaviour. These findings suggest the importance of genetic variation and genetic/environment interactions in understanding the development of common attention networks and differences in their efficiency among individuals.

FUTURE RESEARCH

In this chapter, we have examined some of the tools for studies of the human brain and mind during development. These tools may allow a deeper understanding of how the developing brain makes possible the changes in attention and self-regulation that occur early in life. Future research should allow us to use these tools to understand how developmental changes in functional activation and connectivity relate to the specific behavioural markers at the same age. For example, how do changes in activation relate to differences found in functional connectivity and in the volume of white and grey matter? Is there a fixed order of these changes or does the speed and order of their occurrence depend on whether they result from development or from practice on a task? Better coordination of human and non-human animal work may also allow us to determine the relationship between changes found with non-invasive imaging and those seen in studies of the microanatomy and circuitry of brain areas in animal research.

It is often difficult to determine how brain changes relate to the behaviour changes found at the same time. Longitudinal studies could allow us to better trace out this relationship. To do so may require the use of methods that remain relatively stable across ages. The use of resting fMRI allows testing of different ages without the need to develop comparable tasks (Fair et al. 2009). The discovery that the EEG signal for error detection involves similar brain areas at 7 months as it does for adults provides another means of examining an event that may be comparable across differences in age. The greater use of analytic behavioural observations (e.g. anticipatory eye movement, the ANT, and parent-reported temperament scales) may foster the mapping of changes in mental operations to brain changes in development.

The growing knowledge of genetic and epigenetic methods has only just begun to influence research in human development. Genetic variation has been related to individual differences in behaviour (Posner et al. 2007). However, it seems likely that the same genes related to individual differences are also involved in building the common networks underlying attention. Thus, studies designed to relate the expression of genes to key aspects of behaviour would help our understanding of how neural networks become organized in development.

While we know that some genetic variants interact with environmental experience we do not yet know the mechanisms involved, since genetic variations are expressed at numerous locations in the brain and rest of the body. As the mechanisms by which genes can be altered by the environment are better understood through study of epigenetics, we may learn more about how training has its influence on development.

REFERENCES

Ahadi, S. A., Rothbart, M. K., and Ye, R. (1993). Children's temperament in the U.S. and China: Similarities and differences. *European Journal of Personality 7*(5): 359–378.

Aston-Jones, G. and Cohen, J. D. (2005). An integrative theory of locus coeruleus-norepinephrine function: Adaptive gain and optimal performance. *Annual Review of Neuroscience 28*: 403–450.

Bakermans-Kranenburg, M. J. and van Ijzendoorn, M. H. (2006). Gene–environment interaction of the dopamine D4 receptor (DRD4) and observed maternal insensitivity predicting externalizing behavior in preschoolers. *Developmental Psychobiology 48*(5): 406–409.

Bakersmans-Kranenburg, M. J., van Ijzendoorn, M. H., Pijlman, F. T. A., Mesman, J., and Juffer, F. (2008). Experimental evidence for differential susceptibility: Dopamine D4 receptor polymorphism (DRD4 VNTR) moderates intervention effects on toddlers' externalizing behavior in a randomized controlled trial. *Developmental Psychology 44*(1): 293–300.

Beauregard, M., Levesque, J., and Bourgouin, P. (2001). Neural correlates of conscious self-regulation of emotion. *Journal of Neuroscience 21*(18): RC 165.

Belsky, J. and Pluess, M. (2009). Beyond diathesis stress: Differential susceptibility to environmental influences. *Psychological Bulletin 135*(6): 624–652.

Berger, A., Tzur, G., and Posner, M. I. (2006). Infant babies detect arithmetic error. *Proceedings of the National Academy of Sciences USA 103*(33): 12649–12553.

Blasi, G., Mattay, G. S., Bertolino, A., Elvevåg, B., Callicott, J. H., Das, S., Kolachana, B. S., Egan, M. F., Goldberg, T. E., and Weinberger, D. R. (2005). Effect of Catechol-O-Methyltransferase val[158] met genotype on attentional control. *Journal of Neuroscience 25*(20): 5038–5045.

Botvinick, M. M., Braver, T. S., Barch, D. M., Carter, C. S., and Cohen, J. D. (2001). Conflict monitoring and cognitive control. *Psychological Review 108*(3): 624–652.

Bush, G., Luu, P., and Posner, M. I. (2000). Cognitive and emotional influences in the anterior cingulate cortex. *Trends in Cognitive Sciences 4*(6): 215–222.

Butcher, P. R. (2000). *Longitudinal Studies of Visual Attention in Infants: The Early Development of Disengagement and Inhibition of Return*. Meppel: Aton.

Callejas, A., Lupiáñnez, J., and Tudela, P. (2005). The three attentional networks: On their independence and interactions. *Brain and Cognition 54*(3): 225–227.

Casey, B., Thomas, K. M., Davidson, M. C., Kunz, K., and Franzen, P. L. (2002). Dissociating striatal and hippocampal function developmentally with a stimulus–response compatibility task. *Journal of Neuroscience* 22(19): 8647–8652.

Chang, F. and Burns, B. M. (2005). Attention in preschoolers: Associations with effortful control and motivation. *Child Development* 76(1): 247–263.

Checa, P., Rodriguez-Bailon, R., and Rueda, M. R. (2008). Neurocognitive and temperamental systems of self-regulation and early adolescents' social and academic outcomes. *Mind, Brain & Education* 2(4): 177–187.

Checa, P. and Rueda, M. R. (2011). Behavioral and brain measures of attention control predict schooling competence in late childhood. *Developmental Neuropsychology* 36(8): 1–15.

Clohessy, A. B., Posner, M. I., and Rothbart, M. K. (2001). Development of the functional visual field. *Acta Psychologica* 106(1–2): 51–68.

Colombo, J. (2001). The development of visual attention in infancy. *Annual Review of Psychology* 52: 337–367.

Colombo, J. and Horowitz, F. D. (1987). Behavioral state as a lead variable in neonatal research. *Merrill-Palmer Quarterly* 33: 423–438.

Corbetta, M., Miezin, F. M., Dobmeyer, S., Shulman, G. L., and Petersen, S. E. (1990). Attentional modulation of neural processing of shape, color, and velocity in humans. *Science* 248: 1556–1559.

Corbetta, M. and Shulman, G. L. (2002). Control of goal-directed and stimulus-driven attention in the brain. *Nature Reviews Neuroscience* 3(3): 201–215.

Crottaz-Herbette, S. and Mennon, V. (2006). Where and when the anterior cingulate cortex modulates attentional response: Combined fMRI and ERP evidence. *Journal of Cognitive Neuroscience* 18(5): 766–780.

Curtindale, L., Laurie-Rose, C., Bennett-Murphy, L., and Hull, S. (2007). Sensory modality, temperament, and the development of sustained attention: A vigilance study in children and adults. *Developmental Psychology* 43(3): 576–589.

Davidson, M. C., Amso, D., Anderson, L. C., and Diamond, A. (2006). Development of cognitive control and executive functions from 4 to 13 years: Evidence from manipulations of memory, inhibition, and task switching. *Neuropsychologia* 44(11): 2037–2078.

Dehaene, S., Posner, M. I., and Tucker, D. M. (1994). Localization of a neural system for error detection and compensation. *Psychological Science* 5(5): 303–305.

Desimone, R. and Duncan, J. (1995). Neural mechanisms of selective visual attention. *Annual Review of Neuroscience* 18: 193–222.

Diamond, A. (1991). Neuropsychological insights into the meaning of object concept development. In S. Carey and R. Gelman (eds.), *The Epigenesis of Mind: Essays on Biology and Cognition* (pp. 67–110). Hillsdale, N.J.: Lawrence Erlbaum Associates.

Diamond, A. (2006). The early development of executive functions. In E. Bialystok and F. I. M. Craik (eds.), *Lifespan Cognition: Mechanisms of Change* (pp. 70–95). New York: Oxford University Press.

Diamond, A., Briand, L., Fossella, J., and Gehlbach, L. (2004). Genetic and neurochemical modulation of prefrontal cognitive functions in children. *American Journal of Psychiatry* 161(1): 125–132.

Diatchenko, L., Slade, G. D., Nackley, A. G. et al. (2005). Genetic basis for individual variations in pain perception and the development of a chronic pain condition. *Human Molecular Genetics* 14(1): 135–143.

Ding, Y. C., Chi, H. C., Grady, D. L., Morishima, A., Kidd, J. R., Kidd, K. K. et al. (2002). Evidence of positive selection acting at the human dopamine receptor D4 gene locus. *Proceedings of the National Academy of Sciences USA* 99(1): 309–314.

Dosenbach, N. U. F., Fair, D. A., Miezin, F. M., Cohen, A. L., Wenger, K. K. R., Dosenbach, A. T., Fox, M. D., Snyder, A. Z., Vincent, J. L., Raichle, M. E., Schlaggar, B. L., and Petersen, S. E. (2007). Distinct brain networks for adaptive and stable task control in humans. *Proceedings of the National Academy of Sciences USA 104*(26): 11073–11078.

Duncan, J., Seitz, R. J., Kolodny, J., Bor, D., Herzog, H., Ahmed, A., Newell, F. N., and Emslie, H. (2000). A neural basis for general intelligence. *Science 289*: 457–460.

Durston, S., Thomas, K. M., Yang, Y., Ulug, A. M., Zimmerman, R. D., and Casey, B. (2002). A neural basis for the development of inhibitory control. *Developmental Science 5*(4): F9–F16.

Eisenberger, N. I., Lieberman, M. D., and Williams, K. D. (2003). Does rejection hurt? An fMRI study of social exclusion. *Science 302*(5643): 290–292.

Ellis, E., Rothbart, M. K., and Posner, M. I. (2004). Individual differences in executive attention predict self-regulation and adolescent psychosocial behaviours. *Annals of the New York Academy of Sciences 1031*: 337–340.

Enns, J. T. and Brodeur, D. A. (1989). A developmental study of covert orienting to peripheral visual cues. *Journal of Experimental Child Psychology 48*(2): 171–189.

Enns, J. T. and Girgus, J. S. (1985). Developmental changes in selective and integrative visual attention. *Journal of Experimental Child Psychology 40*(2): 319–337.

Etkin, A., Egner, T., Peraza, D. M., Kandel, E. R., and Hirsch, J. (2006). Resolving emotional conflict: A role for the rostral anterior cingulate cortex in modulating activity in the amygdala. *Neuron 51*(6): 871–882.

Fair, D., Cohen, A. L., Dosenbach, A. U. F., Church, J. A., Meizin, F. M., Barch, D. M., Raichle, M. E., Petersen, S. E., and Schlagger, B. L. (2008). The maturing architecture of the brain's default network. *Proceedings of the National Academy of Sciences USA 105*(10): 4028–4032.

Fair, D. A., Cohen, A. L., Power, J. D., Dosenbach, N. U., Church, J. A., Miezin, F. M., Schlaggar, B. L., and Petersen, S. E. (2009). Functional brain networks develop from a "local to distributed" organization. *PLoS Computational Biology 5*(5): e1000381.

Fair, D. A., Dosenbach, N. U. F., Church, J. A., Cohen, A. L., Brahmbhatt, S., Miezin, F. M. et al. (2007). Development of distinct control networks through segregation and integration. *Proceedings of the National Academy of Sciences USA 104*(33): 13507–13512.

Fan, J., Fossella, J. A., Summer, T., Wu, Y., and Posner, M. I. (2003). Mapping the genetic variation of executive attention onto brain activity. *Proceedings of the National Academy of Sciences USA 100*(12): 7406–7411.

Fan, J., Gu, X., Guise, K. G., Liu, X., Fossella, J., Wang, H., and Posner, M. I. (2009). Testing the behavior interaction and integration of attentional neworks. *Brain and Cognition 70*(2): 209–220.

Fan, J., McCandliss, B. D., Fossella, J., Flombaum, J. I., and Posner, M. I. (2005). The activation of attentional networks. *NeuroImage 26*(2): 471–479.

Fan, J., McCandliss, B. D., Sommer, T., Raz, M., and Posner, M. I. (2002). Testing the efficiency and independence of attentional networks. *Journal of Cognitive Neuroscience 3*(14): 340–347.

Fernandez-Duque, D. and Black, S. E. (2006). Attentional networks in normal aging and Alzheimer's disease. *Neuropsychology 20*: 133–143.

Fossella, J., Posner, M. I., Fan, J., Swanson, J. M., and Pfaff, D. M. (2002). Attentional phenotypes for the analysis of higher mental function. *The Scientific World Journal 2*: 217–223.

Fox, N. A., Hane, A. A., and Pine, D. S. (2007). Plasticity for affective neurocircuitry: How the environment affects gene expression. *Current Directions in Psychological Science 16*(1): 1–5.

Fox, N. A., Nichols, K. E., Henderson, H. A., Rubin, K. H., Schmidt, L. A., Hamer, D. et al. (2005). Evidence for a gene–environment interaction in predicting behavioral inhibition in middle school children. *Psychological Science 16*(12): 921–926.

Gao, W., Zhu, H., Giovanello, K. S., Smith, J. K., Shen, D., Gilmore, J. H., and Lin, W. (2009). Evidence on the emergence of the brain's default network from 2-week-old to 2-year-old healthy pediatric subjects. *Proceedings of the National Academy of Sciences USA* 106(16): 6790–6795.

Gartstein, M. A. and Rothbart, M. K. (2003). Studying infant temperament via the Revised Infant Behavior Questionnaire. *Infant Behavior and Development* 26(1): 64–86.

Gehring, W. J., Gross, B., Coles, M. G. H., Meyer, D. E., and Donchin, E. (1993). A neural system for error detection and compensation. *Psychological Science* 4: 385–390.

Gerardi-Caulton, G. (2000). Sensitivity to spatial conflict and the development of self-regulation in children 24–36 months of age. *Developmental Science* 3(4): 397–404.

Gonzalez, C., Fuentes, L. J. Carranza, J. A., and Estevez, A. F. (2001). Temperament and attention in the self-regulation of 7-year-old children. *Personality and Individual Differences* 30: 931–946.

Green, A. E., Munafo, M. R., DeYoung, C. G., Fossella, J. A. Fan, J., and Gray, J. R. (2008). Using genetic data in cognitive neuroscience: From growing pains to genuine insights. *Nature Reviews Neuroscience* 9: 710–720.

Haith, M. M., Hazan, C., and Goodman, G. S. (1988). Expectation and anticipation of dynamic visual events by 3.5 month old babies. *Child Development* 59: 467–469.

Hampton, A. N. and O'Doherty, J. P. (2007). Decoding the neural substrates of reward-related decision making with functional MRI. *Proceedings of the National Academy of Sciences* 104(4): 1377–1382.

Harman, C., Rothbart, M. K., and Posner, M. I. (1997). Distress and attention interactions in early infancy. *Motivation and Emotion* 21: 27–43.

Hillyard, S. A., Di Russo, F., and Martinez, A. (2004). The imaging of visual attention. In N. Kanwisher and J. Duncan (eds.), *Functional Neuroimaging of Visual Cognition: Attention and Performance* (vol. 20, pp. 381–390). New York: Oxford University Press.

Holroyd, C. B. and Coles, M. G. H. (2002). The neural basis of human error processing: Reinforcement learning, dopamine and error-related negativity. *Psychological Review* 109: 679–709.

Johnson, M. H. and Morton, J. (1991). *Biology and Cognitive Development: The Case of Face Recognition*. Oxford: Blackwell.

Johnson, M. H., Posner, M. I., and Rothbart, M. K. (1991). Components of visual orienting in early infancy: Contingency learning, anticipatory looking and disengaging. *Journal of Cognitive Neuroscience* 3(4): 335–344.

Jones, L. B., Rothbart, M. K., and Posner, M. I. (2003). Development of executive attention in preschool children. *Developmental Science* 6(5): 498–504.

Jonkman, L. M. (2006). The development of preparation, conflict monitoring and inhibition from early childhood to young adulthood: A go/no-go ERP study. *Brain Research* 1097(1): 181–193.

Jonkman, L. M., Lansbergen, M., and Stauder, J. E. A. (2003). Developmental differences in behavioral and event-related brain responses associated with response preparation and inhibition in a go/no-go task. *Psychophysiology* 40(5): 752–761.

Kahneman, D. (1973). *Attention and Effort*. Englewood Cliffs, N.J.: Prentice Hall.

Kampe, K. K., Frith, C. D., and Frith, U. (2003). 'Hey John': Signals conveying communicative intention toward the self activate brain regions associated with 'mentalizing,' regardless of modality. *The Journal of Neuroscience* 23(12): 5258–5263.

Kanske, P. (2008). *Exploring Executive Attention in Emotion*. Dresden: Sachsisches Digitaldruckzentrum.

Koop, B., Rist, F., and Mattler, U. (1996). N200 in the flanker task as a neurobehavioral tool for investigating executive control. *Psychophysiology* 33: 282–294.

Levy, F. (1980). The development of sustained attention (vigilance) in children: Some normative data. *Journal of Child Psychology and Psychiatry* 21(1): 77–84.

Lin, C. C. H., Hsiao, C. K., and Chen, W. J. (1999). Development of sustained attention assessed using the Continuous Performance Test among children 6–15 years of age. *Journal of Abnormal Child Psychology* 27(5): 403–412.

MacLeod, J. W., Lawrence, M. A., McConnell, M. M., Eskes, G. A., Klein, R. M., and Shore, D. I. (2010). Appraising the ANT: Psychometric and Theoretical Considerations of the Attention Network Test. *Neuropsychology* 24(5): 637–651.

Marrocco, R. T. and Davidson, M. C. (1998). Neurochemistry of attention. In R. Parasuraman (ed.), *The Attentive Brain* (pp. 35–50). Cambridge, Mass.: MIT Press.

Meltzoff, A. N. and Moore, M. K. (1977). Imitation of facial and manual gestures by human neonates. *Science* 198: 74–78.

Mezzacappa, E. (2004). Alerting, orienting, and executive attention: Developmental properties and sociodemographic correlates in an epidemiological sample of young, urban children. *Child Development* 75(5): 1373–1386.

Morrison, F. J. (1982). The development of alertness. *Journal of Experimental Child Psychology* 34(2): 187–199.

Morrison, J. H. and Foote, S. L. (1986). Noradrenergic and serotonergic innervation of cortical, thalamic, and tectal visual structures in old and new world monkeys. *Journal of Comparative Neurology* 243(1): 117–128.

NICHD Early Child Care Research Network (1993). *The NICHD Study of Early Child Care: A Comprehensive Longitudinal Study of Young Children's Lives.* ERIC Document Reproduction Service No. ED3530870.

Ochsner, K. N., Bunge, S. A., Gross, J. J., and Gabrieli, J. D. E. (2002). Rethinking feelings: An fMRI study of the cognitive regulation of emotion. *Journal of Cognitive Neuroscience* 14(8): 1215–1229.

Parasuraman, R., Greenwood, P. M., Kumar, R., and Fossella, J. (2005). Beyond heritability: Neurotransmitter genes differentially modulate visuospatial attention and working memory. *Psychological Science* 16(3): 200–207.

Petersen, S. E. and Posner, M. I. (in press). The attention system of the human brain: Twenty years after. *Annual Review of Neuroscience.*

Pidoplichko, V. I., Noguchi, J., Areola, O. O., Liang, Y., Peterson, J., Zhang, T., and Dani, J. A. (2004). Nicotinic cholinergic synaptic mechanisms in the ventral tegmental area contribute to nicotine addiction. *Learning & Memory* 11(1): 60–69.

Posner, M. I. (1978). *Chronometric Explorations of Mind.* Hillsdale, N.J.: Lawrence Erlbaum Associates.

Posner, M. I. (2008). Measuring alertness. *Annals of the New York Academy of Sciences* 1129 (Molecular and Biophysical Mechanisms of Arousal, Alertness, and Attention): 193–199.

Posner, M. I. (in press). *Attention is a Social World.* New York: Oxford University Press.

Posner, M. I. and Fan, J. (2008). Attention as an organ system. In J. R. Pomerantz (ed.), *Topics in Integrative Neuroscience* (pp. 31–61). New York: Cambridge University Press.

Posner, M. I. and Rothbart, M. K. (2007a). Research on attention networks as a model for the integration of psychological science. *Annual Review of Psychology* 58: 1–23.

Posner, M. I. and Rothbart, M. K. (2007b). *Educating the Human Brain.* Washington, D.C.: APA Books.

Posner, M. I., Rothbart, M. K., and Sheese, B. E. (2007). Attention genes. *Developmental Science* 10(1): 24–29.

Posner, M. I., Rothbart, M. K., Sheese, B. E., and Voelker, P. (in press). Control networks and neuromodulators of early development. *Developmental Psychology*.

Raichle, M. E. (2009). A paradigm shift in functional brain imaging. *Journal of Neuroscience* 29(41): 12729–12734.

Rainville, P., Duncan, G. H., Price, D. D., Carrier, B., and Bushnell, M. C. (1997). Pain affect encoded in human anterior cingulate but not somatosensory cortex. *Science* 277(5328): 968–971.

Richards, J. E. and Hunter, S. K. (1998). Attention and eye movements in young infants: Neural control and development. In J. E. Richards (ed.), *Cognitive Neuroscience of Attention* (pp. 131–162). Mahwah, N.J.: Lawrence Erlbaum Associates.

Ridderinkhof, K. R. and van der Molen, M. W. (1995). A psychophysiological analysis of developmental differences in the ability to resist interference. *Child Development* 66(4): 1040–1056.

Rigbi, A., Kanyas, K., Yakir, A., Greenbaum, L., Pollak, Y., Ben-Asher, E., Lancet, D. et al. (2008). Why do young women smoke? V. Role of direct and interactive effects of nicotinic cholinergic receptor gene variation on neurocognitive function. *Genes, Brain, and Behavior* 7: 164–172.

Rothbart, M. K. (2011). *Becoming Who We Are*. New York: Guilford Press.

Rothbart, M. K., Ahadi, S. A., and Hershey, K. L. (1994). Temperament and social behavior in childhood. *Merrill-Palmer Quarterly* 40: 21–39.

Rothbart, M. K., Ahadi, S. A., and Evans, D. E. (2000). Temperament and personality: origins and outcomes. *Journal of Personality and Social Psychology* 78(1): 122.

Rothbart, M. K., Ahadi, S. A., Hershey, K. L., and Fisher, P. (2001). Investigations of temperament at three to seven years: The Children's Behavior Questionnaire. *Child Development* 72: 1394–1408.

Rothbart, M. K. and Bates, J. E. (2006). Temperament in children's development. In W. Damon, R. Lerner, and N. Eisenberg (eds.), *Handbook of Child Psychology. Vol. 3: Social, Emotional, and Personality Development*, 6th edn. (pp. 99–166). New York: Wiley.

Rothbart, M. K. and Derryberry, D. (1981). Development of individual differences in temperament. In M. E. Lamb and A. L. Brown (eds.), *Advances in Developmental Psychology*. (pp. 37–86). Hillsdale, N.J.: Lawrence Erlbaum Associates.

Rothbart, M. K., Ellis, L. K., Rueda, M. R., and Posner, M. I. (2003). Developing mechanisms of effortful control. *Journal of Personality* 71: 1113–1143.

Rothbart, M. K. and Rueda, M. R. (2005). The development of effortful control. In U. Mayr, E. Awh, and S. W. Keele (eds.), *Developing Individuality in the Human Brain: A Festschrift Honoring Michael I. Posner* (pp. 167–188). Washington, D.C.: American Psychological Association.

Rothbart, M. K., Sheese, B. E., Rueda, M. R., and Posner, M. I. (2011). Developing mechanisms of self-regulation in early life. *Emotion Review* 3: 207–213.

Rueda, M. R. (2012). Effortful control. In M. Zentner and R. Shiner (eds.), *Handbook of Temperament*. New York: Guilford Press.

Rueda, M., Fan, J., McCandliss, B. D., Halparin, J. D., Gruber, D. B., Lercari, L. P. et al. (2004a). Development of attentional networks in childhood. *Neuropsychologia* 42(8): 1029–1040.

Rueda, M. R., Posner, M. I., and Rothbart, M. K. (2005). The development of executive attention: Contributions to the emergence of self-regulation. *Developmental Neuropsychology* 28(2): 573–594.

Rueda, M. R., Posner, M. I., Rothbart, M. K., and Davis-Stober, C. P. (2004b). Development of the time course for processing conflict: An event-related potentials study with 4 year olds and adults. *BMC Neuroscience*. doi: 10.1186/1471-2202-5-39.

Ruff, H. A. and Rothbart, M. K. (1996). *Attention in Early Development*. New York: Oxford University Press.

Santesso, D. L., Segalowitz, S. J., and Schmidt, L. A. (2005). ERP correlates of error monitoring in 10-year-olds are related to socialization. *Biological Psychology 70*: 79–87.

Schul, R., Townsend, J., and Stiles, J. (2003). The development of attentional orienting during the school-age years. *Developmental Science 6*(3): 262–272.

Segalowitz, S. J. and Davies, P. L. (2004). Charting the maturation of the frontal lobe: An electrophysiological strategy. *Brain and Cognition 55*(1): 116–133.

Segalowitz, S. J., Unsal, A., and Dywan, J. (1992). Cleverness and wisdom in 12-year-olds: Electrophysiological evidence for late maturation of the frontal lobe. *Developmental Neuropsychology 8*(2–3): 279–298.

Sheese, B. E., Rothbart, M. K., Posner, M. I., White, L., and Fraundorf, S. (2008). Executive attention in infancy. *Infant Behavior and Development 31*: 501–510.

Sheese, B. E., Voelker, P. M., Rothbart, M. K., and Posner, M. I. (2007). Parenting quality interacts with genetic variation in dopamine receptor DRD4 to influence temperament in early childhood. *Development & Psychopathology 19*: 1039–1046.

Shulman, G. L., Astafiev, S. V., Franke, D., Pope, D. L. W., Snyder, A. Z., McAvoy, M. P., and Corbett, M. (2009). Interaction of stimulus-driven reorienting and expectation in ventral and dorsal frontoparietal and basal ganglia–cortical networks. *Journal of Neuroscience 29*: 4392–4407.

Thompson, K. G., Biscoe, K. L., and Sato, T. R. (2005). Neuronal basis of covert spatial attention in the frontal eye fields. *Journal of Neuroscience 25*: 9479–9487.

Tucker, D. M., Hartry-Speiser, A., McDougal, L., Luu, P., and deGrandpre, D. (1999). Mood and spatial memory: Emotion and right hemisphere contribution to spatial cognition. *Biological Psychology 50*: 103–125.

van Ijzendoorn, M. H. and Bakermans-Kranenburg, M. J. (2006). DRD4 7-repeat polymorphism moderates the association between maternal unresolved loss or trauma and infant disorganization. *Attachment and Human Development 8*: 291–307.

van Veen, V. and Carter, C. S. (2002). The timing of action-monitoring processes in the anterior cingulate cortex. *Journal of Cognitive Neuroscience 14*: 593–602.

Voelker, P., Sheese, B. E., Rothbart, M. K., and Posner, M. I. (2009). Variations in catechol-O-methyltransferase gene interact with parenting to influence attention in early development. *Neuroscience 164*(1): 121–130.

Wainwright, A. and Bryson, S. E. (2002). The development of exogenous orienting: Mechanisms of control. *Journal of Experimental Child Psychology 82*(2): 141–155.

Wainwright, A. and Bryson, S. E. (2005). The development of endogenous orienting: Control over the scope of attention and lateral asymmetries. *Developmental Neuropsychology 27*(2): 237–255.

Walter, G. (1964). The convergence and interaction of visual, auditory and tactile responses in human non-specific cortex. *Annals of the New York Academy of Sciences 112*: 320–361.

Wang, E. T., Kodama, G., Baldi, P., and Moyzis, R. K. (2006). Global landscape of recent inferred Darwinian selection for Homo sapiens. *Proceedings of the National Academy of Sciences USA 103*(1): 135–140.

Winterer, G., Musso, F., Konrad, A., Vucurevuc, G., Stoeter, P., Sander, T., and Gallinat, J. (2007). Association of attentional network function with exon 5 variations of the CHRNA4 gene. *Human Molecular Genetics 16*: 2165–2174.

Wojciulik, E., Kanwisher, N., and Driver, J. (1998). Covert visual attention modulates face-specific activity in the human fusiform gyrus: fMRI study. *Journal of Neurophysiology* 79(3): 1574–1578.

Wynn, K. (1992). Addition and subtraction by human infants. *Nature* 358(6389): 749–750.

PART D

NON-SPATIAL ATTENTION

CHAPTER 20

FEATURE- AND OBJECT-BASED ATTENTIONAL MODULATION IN THE HUMAN VISUAL SYSTEM

MIRANDA SCOLARI, EDWARD F. ESTER, AND JOHN T. SERENCES

INTRODUCTION

THE human visual system has a limited processing capacity. Consequently, mechanisms of selective attention are needed to prioritize behaviourally relevant stimuli. Broadly speaking, the term 'selective attention' refers to a collection of mechanisms that insulate patterns of neural activity evoked by relevant stimuli from the deleterious effects of stochastic synaptic transmission and interference generated by other, irrelevant stimuli (Bisley and Goldberg 2003; Desimone and Duncan 1995; Mitchell, Sundberg, and Reynolds 2009; Moran and Desimone 1985; Pestilli, Carrasco, Heeger, and Gardner 2011; Reynolds and Desimone 1999; Reynolds, Pasternak, and Desimone 2000; Serences and Yantis 2006). Early studies of selective attention focused primarily on spatial attention, or selection that is based solely on a location that is likely to contain relevant information (e.g. Posner 1980). However, we often know the defining feature(s) of a stimulus (e.g. my keychain is red and rectangular) without knowing its specific location (e.g. my keys could be anywhere on the desk). Under these circumstances, relevant information may be selected in one of two ways: (1) on the basis of a single critical feature value (e.g. the colour red) or on the basis of a group of features bound into a holistic representation (e.g. a red rectangle). Here, we review behavioural and neurophysiological studies that examine the consequences and the sources of top-down feature- and object-based attentional control in the human visual system. While we also review a handful of relevant single-unit recording studies in non-human primates, a thorough treatment of this literature can be found in Treue (chapter 21), this volume.

FEATURE-BASED ATTENTION

Behavioural evidence for feature-based attention

When scanning a crowded stadium to locate a friend, a successful search is facilitated by attending to a salient feature, like the colour of her baseball cap. Such anecdotal cases reveal a key property of feature-based attention (FBA): items throughout the visual field that contain the attended feature are prioritized while other features are muted (Egeth, Virzi, and Garbart 1984; Liu and Hou 2011; White and Carrasco 2011). For example, studies examining visual search performance suggest that observers can restrict search to only items that contain a target feature value while ignoring all others (Egeth et al. 1984; Treisman and Gelade 1980; Wolfe 1994; see also Wolfe (chapter 2), this volume). These findings prompted researchers to investigate how an attentional mechanism might act on the visual system in order to prioritize one feature over others. In an early study, Davis and Graham (1981) asked observers to report the presence of a grating in one of two sequential intervals. On 80–95% of all trials, the grating was rendered at a single spatial frequency (primary frequency). On the remaining trials the grating was rendered with a variable spatial frequency (secondary frequencies; randomly chosen from a set of six possibilities). As expected, observers detected the primary frequency with greater accuracy than any of the secondary frequencies. Moreover, detection rates generally declined as the size of the deviation between primary and secondary frequencies increased. Critically, the advantage for the primary frequency was eliminated when all frequencies were presented with equal probability. These findings suggest that observers can selectively monitor the responses of low-level feature-selective neuronal populations at the expense of others when it is behaviourally advantageous; several single-unit recording and human neuroimaging studies have corroborated this finding (Corbetta, Miezin, Dobmeyer, Shulman, and Petersen 1990, 1991; Ho et al. 2012; Liu, Larsson, and Carrasco 2007; Maunsell and Treue 2006; Scolari, Byers, and Serences 2012; Serences and Boynton 2007; Serences, Saproo, Scolari, Ho, and Muftuler 2009; Treue and Maunsell 1996; see 'Neural evidence for feature-based attention' below).

Several researchers have argued that space-based attention (SBA) increases the effective salience of a stimulus akin to a change in local contrast, and this may be true for FBA as well (Carrasco 2011; Carrasco, Ling, and Read 2004). Support for this view has been reported in adaptation studies, where prolonged exposure to a feature or object leads to a potent after-effect. In one example, Lankheet and Verstraten (1995) measured the relative strength of motion after-effects (MAE; the tendency to perceive motion with a trajectory opposite to that of a physical stimulus after prolonged viewing) induced by attended and unattended motion dot fields (kinetograms). During the adaptation phase, subjects were instructed to attend one of two spatially superimposed kinetograms that moved in opposite directions. Following adaptation, subjects performed a discrimination task where they were required to report the direction of a test stimulus that contained some proportion (0–100%) of coherently moving dots. The logic of this approach was as follows: selectively attending to one kinetogram during the adaptation phase of the experiment should enhance its salience relative to the unattended kinetogram and lead to a stronger MAE. Consequently, when presented with a test stimulus moving in the same direction as the attended dot field (and opposite in direction relative to the MAE), observers would require relatively high levels of motion coherence in order to perform the discrimination task with criterion accuracy (compared to trials without prior adaptation). This is precisely what the authors found: despite equivalent sensory stimulation, the strength of adaptation was greater for the attended relative to the unattended kinetogram. This result is consistent with the hypothesis that FBA increases the effective saliency of an attended stimulus.

In a subsequent study, Rossi and Paradiso (1995) asked subjects to discriminate either the orientations or spatial frequencies of two sequentially presented foveal gratings (primary task). On one third of trials, subjects were also prompted to report the presence or absence of a near-threshold peripheral grating (secondary task; see Fig. 20.1a). The spatial frequency and orientation of the peripheral grating sometimes matched (1/5 of target present trials) and sometimes mismatched the features of the foveal stimulus. Note, however, that the features of the peripheral grating were task-irrelevant. Nonetheless, when subjects attended to orientation in the primary task, they detected peripheral gratings at matched orientations (0° for the results depicted in Fig. 20.1b) with higher accuracy than those at mismatched orientations. Conversely, detection performance did not differ across spatial frequencies (i.e. the unattended feature; the matched spatial frequency is 0.5 cycles per degree, or cpd, for the results depicted in Fig. 20.1b). Importantly, these effects disappeared when subjects were not required to attend the central stimulus, suggesting that the advantage for matching peripheral stimuli was not simply a passive sensory effect. These results suggest that feature-based selection facilitates the processing of attended feature values across the entire visual field, and subsequent psychophysical evidence has corroborated this finding (Arman, Ciaramitaro, and Boynton 2006; Liu and Hou 2011; Sàenz, Buračas, and Boynton 2003; White and Carrasco 2011; see also 'Neural evidence for feature-based attention' below).

While FBA can be deployed across all of visual space, many studies have shown that it may also be restricted to only certain features of an object. For example, under certain circumstances attention may select task-relevant features without also selecting irrelevant ones belonging to the same stimulus (Corbetta et al. 1991; Lu and Itti 2005; Rossi and Paradiso 1995). This is illustrated in the Rossi and Paradiso (1995) study described above: the detection results indicated that while subjects attended to only the orientation of the primary grating, they ignored spatial frequency (the behaviourally irrelevant feature). However, one must be careful not to overgeneralize this result,

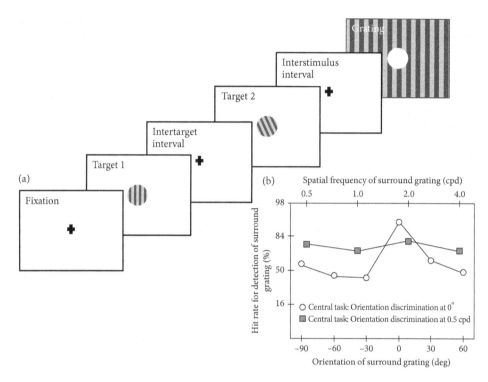

FIGURE 20.1 (a) Schematic representation of the task used in Rossi and Paradiso (1995). Subjects first completed an orientation discrimination task, in which they reported the directional rotation of a second Gabor patch (target 2) relative to the first Gabor patch (target 1). On a random one third of trials, subjects were instructed also to report the presence or absence of a secondary peripheral grating (shown here); it was present on one sixth of all trials and either matched or mismatched the orientation and spatial frequency of target 1. Note that while this illustration is made up of square-wave gratings, the actual experiment utilized sinusoidal waves. (b) Depiction of a single subject's results for the secondary orientation detection task (open circles) and secondary spatial frequency detection task (filled squares) when the subject was attending to orientation in the primary discrimination task.

as other studies have reported enhanced processing of task-irrelevant features paired with a target feature (Arman et al. 2006; Melcher, Papathomas, and Vidnyánszky 2005; Sohn, Chong, Papathomas, and Vidnyánszky 2005), even outside the locus of SBA. In one example (Sohn et al. 2005), subjects were instructed to attend one of two spatially superimposed random dot kinetograms (differentiated by colour) rendered in one visual hemifield ('attended hemifield') in order to detect changes in luminance. Two task-irrelevant spatially superimposed kinetograms were also rendered in the opposite hemifield ('unattended hemifield'), one of which moved in a single direction with 100% coherence. Subjects experienced significantly longer MAE durations when the colour of the high-coherence task-irrelevant kinetogram matched the colour of the attended random dot pattern than when it did not, even though motion was irrelevant to the task. Furthermore, in a similar version of the study adapted for functional magnetic resonance imaging (fMRI), the magnitude of the blood-oxygenation-level-dependent (BOLD) response in MT+ to the task-irrelevant kinetogram was significantly stronger when it shared the target's colour. It should also be noted that some feature-based attentional spreading was similarly evident in the Rossi and Paradiso (1995) study: when subjects attended to the spatial frequency of the central Gabor patch, detection performance for peripheral gratings revealed feature selectivity for both spatial frequency and orientation (though note that this effect was asymmetrical, as similar spreading did not occur while subjects attended orientation).

In a subsequent study, Lu and Itti (2005) measured the relative perceptual benefit afforded to a secondary stimulus when it shared task-relevant and/or task-irrelevant features with a behaviourally prioritized primary stimulus. A shared irrelevant feature across stimuli provided no additional perceptual benefit to the secondary stimulus if the relevant feature was also shared. Conversely, a small benefit was observed when the secondary stimulus shared only a task-irrelevant feature with the primary stimulus, relative to a condition where no features were shared. Based on these results, Lu and Itti argued that paired irrelevant features are only weakly enhanced compared to relevant features. Thus, at present, the boundary conditions determining when attention can be restricted to a subset of features within an object are unclear. We revisit this issue under 'Object-Based Attention', below.

Neural evidence for feature-based attention

Psychophysical demonstrations like those described in the preceding section can point to possible mechanisms of FBA, but they cannot unambiguously reveal how underlying changes in brain activity lead to the observed behavioural effects. Early demonstrations of FBA effects in the visual system primarily came from single-unit recording studies with rhesus monkeys (Haenny and Schiller 1988; Spitzer, Desimone, and Moran 1988). For instance, Haenny and Schiller (1988) documented FBA effects in visual cortex while a monkey attended to a precued orientation. Attentional modulation was observed in V4 and to a lesser extent V1, both of which contain neurons that are selective for orientation. Subsequent single-unit recordings have demonstrated similar modulatory patterns across the visual hierarchy (reviewed by Boynton 2005; Maunsell and Treue 2006; Serences and Yantis 2006). Given the strength of modulation observed in early visual areas, one of the first human neuroimaging studies of FBA targeted regions according to their presumed sensory selectivity (Corbetta et al. 1990, 1991). These positron emission topography (PET) studies revealed that attending to the shape, colour, or velocity of a set of objects during a difficult discrimination task differentially activated corresponding human extrastriate visual areas selective for these features.

In the previous section, we discussed psychophysical evidence to suggest that FBA is deployed across the entire visual field, regardless of target location (Rossi and Paradiso 1995). Evidence from human neuroimaging across visual areas motivates a similar conclusion (Liu, Larsson, and Carrasco 2007; Serences and Boynton 2007). For example, Sàenz, Buraĉas, and Boynton (2002) instructed observers to attend to one of two overlapping dot fields of upward and downward motion respectively, while an ignored dot field on the opposite side of space moved either upward or downward. Consistent with previous findings that support a spatially global recruitment account of FBA (e.g. Rossi and Paradiso 1995; Treue and Martinez-Trujillo 1999), the BOLD responses to the ignored dot field were modulated in accord with the attended dot pattern in the opposite visual field for all tested regions (V1–V3A and MT+). A similar result was observed for colour when subjects attended to either red or green dots. Moreover, subsequent work has demonstrated that cortical areas that were not directly driven by a stimulus also exhibited selectivity for an attended feature (Serences and Boynton 2007; see Fig. 20.2), suggesting that FBA modulates the firing rates of neurons tuned to the relevant feature irrespective of their spatial receptive field (Andersen, Fuchs, and Müller 2009; Liu and Hou 2011; Sàenz et al. 2003; Serences et al. 2009; White and Carrasco 2011).

In a recent study, Schoenfeld et al. (2007) obtained fMRI, electroencephalographic (EEG), and magnetoencephalographic (MEG) measurements while subjects performed a demanding motion or colour discrimination task. This approach allowed the authors

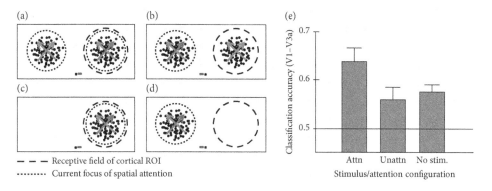

FIGURE 20.2 Adapted from *Neuron*, 55 (2), John T. Serences and Geoffrey M. Boynton, Feature-Based Attentional Modulations in the Absence of Direct Visual Stimulation, pp. 301–12, Copyright (2007), with permission from Elsevier. In this neuroimaging study, subjects attended one of two superimposed kinetograms to detect brief perturbations in speed. A central cue signals the location and direction of motion of the relevant stimulus (as depicted here, the red line at fixation indicates that subjects attend the 45° kinetogram and ignore the 135° one). (a–d.) A depiction of the different possible stimulus configurations, with respect to a cortical region of interest (ROI) under consideration; in these depicted cases, the ROI always receives input from the right visual field (as indicated by the thick dotted line). (a) Spatial attention is directed inside the receptive field (RF) of the ROI, and a second set of kinetograms is presented in the ignored hemifield. (b) Spatial attention is directed away from the RF of the ROI, which is stimulated by a set of ignored kinetograms. (c) Spatial attention is directed inside the RF of the ROI, and the ignored hemifield is empty. (d) Spatial attention is directed away from the RF of the ROI, which is not stimulated. (e) Depiction of classification accuracy for attended motion direction, averaged across V1–V3a, for an attended ROI, an unattended ROI, and an unstimulated ROI.

to (1) verify visual cortical areas whose responses are modulated by FBA (e.g. by iden-tifying regions that show a greater fMRI BOLD response when attention is directed to a single feature), and (2) examine the time course of these attentional effects (by examining changes in the amplitudes of EEG and MEG responses time-locked to the onset of the stimulus array). As in earlier neuroimaging work (e.g. Sàenz et al. 2002), Schoenfeld et al. reported that directing attention to either the motion or colour of a moving dot kine-togram selectively enhanced the amplitude of the fMRI BOLD response in visual cor-tical areas hMT+ and V4, respectively. Concurrent EEG and MEG recordings revealed that the attention-related response enhancement in these specialized cortical areas began as early as 90–120 ms following stimulus onset. This 'between-feature' selection—in which attention is directed to one of two orthogonal feature dimensions—occurred in an earlier epoch than previous observations of feature selection among values within a shared dimension ('within-feature' selection; e.g. Anllo-Vento, Luck, and Hillyard 1998; Liu, Stevens, and Carrasco 2007). This prompted Schoenfeld et al. to conclude that fea-ture selection *between* dimensions is faster than feature selection *within* a dimension. However, Zhang and Luck (2009) demonstrated that at least under some conditions, within-dimension selection can also operate very rapidly following stimulus onset.

Given that FBA can modulate neuronal responses very quickly following stimulus onset, Schneider (2011) hypothesized that it might also manifest at subcortical levels, analogous to spatial attention. Previous studies indicate that retinotopically organized subcortical regions, such as the lateral geniculate nucleus (LGN) and pulvinar, exhibit feature selectivity (Ferster, Chung, and Wheat 1996; Merigan and Maunsell 1993; Petersen, Robinson, and Keys 1985; Wiesel and Hubel 1966). Schneider (2011) there-fore measured FBA effects using high-resolution fMRI at these subcortical levels while subjects detected changes in either the colour (coded by the parvocellular layers of the LGN) or motion (coded by the pulvinar and magnocellular layers of the LGN) of one of two superimposed kinetograms. As expected, the BOLD responses were substantially greater in each region of interest (ROI) when the preferred feature was attended. This suggests that top-down attention operates at multiple levels along the visual hierarchy, including anatomically early regions in the thalamus.

Models of feature-based attention

Single-unit recording studies suggest that FBA enhances the firing rate of neurons that are selectively tuned to a behaviourally relevant feature, regardless of the locus of spa-tial attention (Treue and Martinez-Trujillo 2007; Treue and Martinez-Trujillo 1999). This modulation is thought to amplify responses associated with the attended feature and to attenuate responses associated with the irrelevant feature(s), thus enhancing the separability of the relevant representation from those of competing distractors. These hypotheses are codified in the feature similarity gain model developed by Treue and Martinez-Trujillo (Martinez-Trujillo and Treue 2004; Maunsell and Treue 2006; Treue and Martinez-Trujillo 1999). This account holds that attention modulates all sensory neurons that are tuned along the relevant feature dimension: the level of gain afforded each unit is proportional to its response to the attended feature. This means that maximally driven neurons are enhanced the most (see Fig. 20.3a; Martinez-Trujillo and Treue 2004; Maunsell and Treue 2006; McAdams and Maunsell 1999; Treue and Martinez-Trujillo 1999), while neurons tuned to opposing, irrelevant feature values are suppressed. This mixture of excitation and inhibition effectively 'sharpens' the population response to the attended feature, which presumably then facilitates the detection and discrimination of relevant features.

The feature similarity gain model has had an enormous influence on investigations of FBA (Carrasco 2011). In general, this model provides a good description of data obtained in tasks where subjects are required to make coarse discriminations (e.g. between two orthogonal directions of motion). From a computational perspective, enhancing the gain of the maximally responsive (on-channel) neurons is optimal for discriminating between dissimilar stimuli: the Gaussian-shaped neuronal tuning function peaks at the target orientation while the distractor orientation falls at a local minimum, therefore resulting in the highest signal-to-noise ratio (SNR). However, given the response properties of sensory neurons, two similar orientations (e.g. 90° and 92°; fine discrimination) will elicit similar firing rates from neurons tuned to either orientation (Hol and Treue 2001; Navalpakkam and Itti 2007; Regan and Beverley 1985; Seung and Sompolinsky 1993). This means that applying gain to the neurons tuned to the target feature will not result in much change in the SNR, and will thus likely provide little information in a discrimination task. Recently, models of FBA have incorporated this logic to suggest that attentional gain should be applied to neurons tuned to a flanking (off-channel) orientation during fine discriminations (Navalpakkam and Itti 2007),

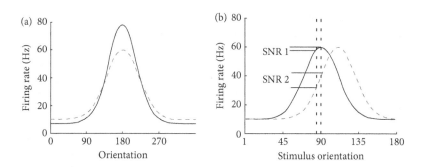

FIGURE 20.3 (a) Illustrations of hypothetical tuning functions for an orientation-selective sensory neuron with a preference for 180° in the absence of attention (dotted line) and when the neuron's preferred orientation is attended (solid line). Here, feature-based attention enhances the response of the maximally responsive neuron as described by the feature similarity gain model. Figure adapted from Boynton (2005). (b) Alternatively, as indicated by optimal gain models, off-channel sensory neurons that flank the behaviourally relevant feature are most informative during a fine discrimination because they yield a relatively high signal-to-noise ratio (SNR) compared to on-channel neurons. Target (90°) and distractor (92°) orientations are marked by vertical dashed lines. Adapted from *Neuron*, 53 (4), Vidhya Navalpakkam and Laurent Itti, Search Goal Tunes Visual Features Optimally, pp. 605–17, Copyright (2007), with permission from Elsevier.

where the firing rate differences between stimuli will be maximized (therefore resulting in a high SNR; see Fig. 20.3b). Scolari and Serences (2009) provided psychophysical evidence suggesting that humans can deploy FBA in this off-channel manner during a difficult fine discrimination, and that such modulation in primary visual cortex aids in decision-making (Scolari et al. 2012; Scolari and Serences 2010). Furthermore, relative off-channel gain predicted behavioural performance, on a between- (Scolari and Serences 2009) and within-subject basis (Scolari et al. 2012; Scolari and Serences 2010). Based on these findings, we suggest that feature-based attentional gain can be deployed in a flexible manner across populations of low-level sensory neurons depending on the nature of the task. Thus, a modification to the feature similarity gain model may be in order that takes into account the current goals of the observer: rather than stipulating that gain is applied to sensory neurons in proportion to the similarity between tuning preference and target, the model may instead stipulate that attentional gain is applied in proportion to the informativeness of sensory neurons.

Efficient selection: Feature-based attention

The goal of FBA, as alluded to throughout this chapter, is to prioritize behaviourally relevant information so that it may be properly utilized in the decision-making process. Indeed, many studies reviewed here have demonstrated that FBA improves performance on a range of perceptual tasks (e.g. Rossi and Paradiso 1995; Sàenz et al. 2003; White and Carrasco 2011). Given the strong evidence that FBA operates at the level of sensory coding, it is also worthwhile to explore how FBA influences decision-making mechanisms. For instance, visual information that is coded in low-level areas must be fed forward to later decision-making regions (e.g. lateral intraparietal area (LIP), dorsal-lateral prefrontal cortex (DLPFC), frontal eye field (FEF), etc.; Gold and Shadlen 2001, 2003, 2007; Hanes and Schall 1996; Horwitz, Batista, and Newsome 2004; Leon and Shadlen 1999; Roitman and Shadlen 2002; Schall 2001; Shadlen and Newsome 2001) and the efficiency of this 'read-out' process will influence the speed and accuracy of perceptual decisions (Das, Giesbrecht, and Eckstein 2010; Palmer, Huk, and Shadlen 2005).

In the preceding section, we discussed how FBA can flexibly modulate the firing rates of the most informative sensory neurons given a specific behavioural task (Navalpakkam and Itti 2007; Scolari et al. 2012; Scolari and Serences 2009). This information could be further amplified by preferentially weighting informative sensory signals during decision-making, which could operate either in lieu of, or concurrently with, sensory gain. For example, during a fine-motion discrimination task, MT neurons tuned to directions of motion that flank the target are found to be the most informative (Jazayeri and Movshon 2006, 2007), and simulations of fine-motion discriminations revealed that these off-channel MT-like neurons (tuned to directions of motion offset from a target direction by ~±40° in this case) may be weighted most strongly by LIP neurons during decision-making (Law and Gold

2008, 2009; Purushothaman and Bradley 2005). Notably, this type of reweighting by later decision mechanisms may account for improved perceptual performance, independent from any changes in sensory gain.

Pestilli et al. (2011) jointly modelled psychophysical and BOLD data to determine how changes in sensory gain, noise reduction, and/or efficient 'read-out' of information could account for changes in contrast detection thresholds. Although the authors observed an additive shift in the BOLD signal measured from visual cortex (V1–hV4) on trials in which a target location was precued (focused attention trials) relative to trials in which all locations were precued (distributed attention trials), this response enhancement could not adequately account for corresponding changes in behavioural performance between conditions; nor could an additional reduction in the variability of the BOLD response. The data instead were best fit by a model that included both additive response changes in early visual areas coupled with a selective read-out rule in which inputs from the most responsive neurons are preferentially weighted by decision mechanisms. Thus, the biased read-out rule effectively amplified the impact of the small additive increase in the evoked BOLD response. While this study focused only on SBA, it is conceivable that similar selective pooling rules may apply to FBA as well. However, future research is required to explore the impact of biased sensory read-out rules, particularly as FBA studies continue to reveal a dynamic, sophisticated system that operates in accordance with behavioural goals.

Control of feature-based attention

While much of the FBA literature has focused extensively on feature-based attentional modulation in visual cortex, recent work has begun to explore where and how top-down control signals might instantiate and mediate these effects. For example, shifts of spatial attention appear to be guided by a distributed frontoparietal network that includes superior parietal lobule (SPL), intraparietal sulcus (IPS), FEF, and supplementary eye field (SEF; Corbetta and Shulman 2002; Kastner and Ungerleider 2000; Szczepanski, Konen, and Kastner 2010; Yantis et al. 2002), and there is some evidence suggesting that shifts of FBA might be mediated by a similar network (Corbetta and Shulman 2002; Greenberg, Esterman, Wilson, Serences, and Yantis 2010; Le, Pardo, and Hu 1998; Liu, Hospadaruk, Zhu, and Gardner 2011; Liu, Slotnick, Serences, and Yantis 2003; Pollmann, Weidner, Müller, and Cramon 2000; Rushworth, Paus, and Sipila 2001). For example, Liu et al. (2003) asked subjects to attend the colour or direction of a dynamic kinetogram that changed colours and directions multiple times during the course of a trial. Certain feature values (e.g. the colour red or upward motion) directed subjects to switch attention from one feature dimension to another ('switch' cues), while others (e.g. green or leftward motion) directed subjects to hold attention on the current feature dimension ('hold' cues). Using fMRI, Liu et al. were able to identify cortical areas that showed stronger responses following 'switch' relative to 'hold' targets, including left precentral gyrus, precuneus, and left IPS. These areas may be involved in attentional control across different mechanisms, as similar patterns of switch-related activity have also been observed when subjects shifted between spatial locations (Yantis et al. 2002), objects (Serences, Schwarzbach, Courtney, Golay, and Yantis 2004), and even modalities (e.g. vision vs audition; Shomstein and Yantis 2004b, 2006).

Greenberg et al. (2010) similarly found a common BOLD signal corresponding to both space-based and feature-based shifts of attention in posterior parietal cortex and prefrontal cortex, including medial SPL, FEF, SEF, and left medial frontal gyrus, while subjects shifted attention either between or within locations and colours. Domain-general attentional control centres in frontal and parietal cortex have also been implicated in other studies (Liu et al. 2011; Liu et al. 2003; Shomstein and Yantis 2004b). In particular, converging evidence from both fMRI and transcranial magnetic stimulation (TMS) studies has added further support to the domain-general role subregions of the parietal lobe play in shifting of attention: Schenkluhn, Ruff, Heinen, and Chambers (2008) reported that stimulating anterior IPS disrupted both spatial and feature-based selection mechanisms (consistent with Wojciulik and Kanwisher 1999), while stimulation to the supramarginal gyrus only disrupted SBA. How the same network controls the selection of multiple features as well as locations within sensory cortex, and how such control may be exerted differently depending on task demands, however, warrants further exploration. One possibility is that subunits within these areas play different roles in mediating each type of control (Greenberg et al. 2010; Liu et al. 2011; Yantis and Serences 2003). For example, Greenberg et al. (2010) demonstrated that patterns of activation within medial SPL could be used to accurately classify attentional shifts between locations and attentional shifts between colours, suggesting that interdigitated populations of cells in SPL may control different forms of selection. Liu and colleagues also found differential patterns of activation in topographically defined IPS (IPS1–4) when subjects attended to either colour or motion, as well as in FEF, suggesting that different features may recruit distinct subpopulations in a frontoparietal network.

OBJECT-BASED ATTENTION

In the previous section, we described how humans can select relevant information on the basis of simple feature values (e.g. a particular colour). However, objects in a visual scene consist of many features, all or part of which may be behaviourally relevant. Although converging evidence from the FBA literature reveals that relevant features within an object are afforded a representational bias, other studies have shown that selective attention can extend to all features in an object. Below, we review behavioural and neural evidence suggesting that attention sometimes operates in an *object-based* manner by simultaneously enhancing the cortical representations of all features within a selected item, even when some of these elements are wholly task-irrelevant. This selection can occur either when all features of a complex object are simultaneously enhanced, or when the boundaries of an object constrain the spread of SBA. We discuss how behavioural goals and task demands might explain why FBA is observed in some cases, while OBA is observed in others.

Behavioural evidence for object-based attention

It is well known that attention can be used to select behaviourally relevant complex objects at the expense of others, even if those objects appear with overlapping distractors (Scholl 2001). In one early demonstration, Neisser and Becklen (1975) instructed subjects to attend to the events depicted in one of two superimposed videos. While subjects focused on one video, unusual events occurring in the unattended video were often missed (see also Simons and Chabris 1999). Given that most objects in the videos occupied the same spatial locations, these findings are most parsimoniously explained by a selection mechanism that operates on object representations rather than spatial positions.

Duncan (1984) later reported more direct evidence for the existence of an object-based selection mechanism. He showed subjects brief displays containing a spatially superimposed box and line and asked them to report either one dimension of a single object (e.g. the size of the box), two dimensions of a single object (e.g. the size of the box and the location of a small gap on its contours), or one dimension from each of the two objects (e.g. the size of the box and the tilt of the line). Subjects were equally good at reporting one or two dimensions of a single object, but task performance declined precipitously when subjects were required to report one attribute from each of the two objects. Subsequent studies have replicated this basic pattern using an impressively diverse array of stimuli and behavioural paradigms (Baylis and Driver 1993; Behrmann, Zemel, and Mozer 1998; He and Nakayama 1995; Kramer and Jacobson 1991; Melcher et al. 2005; Mitchell, Stoner, and Reynolds 2004; Sohn, Papathomas, Blaser, and Vidnyánszky 2004; Valdes-Sosa, Cobo, and Pinilla 2000). Critically, these findings cannot be readily explained by classic models of SBA as all stimuli were spatially superimposed and thus could not be selected purely on the basis of their location. Instead, together they point to the existence of an attentional mechanism that prioritizes whole objects.

Evidence for OBA has also been reported in cueing tasks that are typically used to study spatial selection (Egly, Driver, and Rafal 1994; Moore, Yantis, and Vaughan 1998). In one example, Egly et al. (1994) presented subjects with displays containing two parallel rectangles arranged above and below or to the left and right of fixation (see Fig. 20.4a). On each trial, a target item appeared at one corner of one rectangle, and subjects were asked to report its location as quickly as possible. Shortly before target onset, an exogenous precue was flashed at one corner of one rectangle. On 75% of trials, the cue appeared at the same location as the upcoming target ('valid' trials), and on the remaining 25% of trials, the cue appeared at a non-target location ('invalid' trials). Critically, two types of invalid trials were possible: (1) the cue could appear on

the opposite end of the same rectangle as the upcoming target ('same-object' cues); or
(2) the cue could appear on one end of the other rectangle ('different-object' cues). As
expected from previous SBA studies, subjects' responses were significantly slower on
invalid relative to valid trials. However, this effect was larger for different-object relative
to same-object cues, even though same- and different-object cues appeared at the same
absolute distance from the target (see Fig. 20.4b). This result implies a processing advantage for items that appear within the same structured space as an attended location.

One explanation for the effects reported by Egly et al. is that attention automatically
'spreads' outward from the cued location and ends abruptly at the contours of the cued
object (Abrams and Law 2000; Egly et al. 1994). However, Shomstein and Yantis (2002,
2004a) have argued that sensory enhancement does not necessarily spread to object
boundaries. Based on their interpretation of the Egly et al. findings, the uncued end of
the attended rectangle receives higher priority than the uncued end of the unattended
rectangle, and therefore is searched first on invalid trials (resulting in faster reaction
times). However, if a location within a cued object is reliably irrelevant, it will not be
afforded attentional priority. Consistent with this claim, Shomstein and Yantis (2002)
found that distracting flankers had equally deleterious effects on subjects' ability to
report the identity of a target letter, regardless of whether or not the flankers appeared
on the same object as the target (but see Kramer and Jacobson 1991). In a related study,
Shomstein and Yantis (2004a) presented subjects with displays similar to those used
by Egly et al. while manipulating the amount of time separating the onset of the cue
and target displays (referred to as the stimulus onset asynchrony or SOA). Same-object

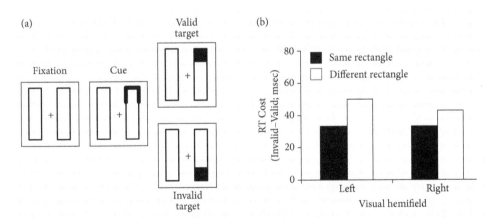

FIGURE 20.4 (a) Schematic representation of the task used in Egly et al. (1994). The thick
black contours in the middle panel represent cues, while the black squares in the final panel
represent targets. During invalidly cued trials, the target could appear on the opposite end
of the cued rectangle ('same-object' trials) or on the same end of the uncued rectangle
('different-object' trials). (b) Depiction of the mean costs of invalid cueing (defined as invalid–valid cue reaction time, or RT) as a function of invalid cue type (same rectangle shown in
black; different rectangle shown in white) and the visual hemifield that contained the target.

advantages similar to those reported by Egly et al. were observed when the cue-to-target SOA was low (200 or 400 ms), but not when it was high (600 ms). This result suggests that attention may initially prioritize whole objects before contracting to encompass only specific cued locations.

Additional evidence for object-based selection has been reported in the multiple-object tracking (MOT) literature. In a typical MOT task, subjects are cued to track a number of independent targets as they move across the display; moving non-targets are also presented, thereby ensuring that subjects cannot select the entire display via a single spatial 'spotlight' (Pylyshyn and Storm 1988). Typically, this task becomes much easier when targets move in a co-linear or otherwise predictable manner, thereby allowing observers to group different targets into a single object (e.g. a single moving square or other polygon; Yantis 1992). It is worth noting that these findings may reflect operations of OBA and/or SBA, as multiple studies have demonstrated that spatial attention may be directed to discrete regions of space without spreading to intervening locations (Awh and Pashler 2000; McMains and Somers 2004). In a related study, Blaser, Pylyshyn, and Holcombe (2000) created a task where subjects tracked stationary objects as they moved through *feature* space in order to remove any SBA contributions. Subjects were shown two spatially superimposed Gabor patches that moved along different trajectories in orientation, colour, and spatial frequency space while remaining fixed in the centre of the screen. To discourage a feature-based tracking strategy, the trajectories of both Gabors were random and independent such that the stimuli frequently 'crossed paths' in feature space. Despite this, subjects were able to track the target Gabor with very high accuracy. In a second experiment using similar displays, subjects detected small discontinuities in one or two stimulus attributes (e.g. a sudden displacement in colour or orientation) on the same or different objects that occurred at unpredictable intervals during the tracking period. The results of this study were nearly identical to those reported by Duncan (1984): specifically, subjects were equally good at detecting either one or two feature displacements within a single object, but were relatively poor at detecting feature displacements on different objects.

Neural evidence for and models of object-based attention

The available evidence suggests that—like FBA—OBA modulates stimulus representations across early stages of the visual processing hierarchy. For example, Wannig, Rodriguez, and Freiwald (2007) recorded from neurons in cortical area MT+ while monkeys performed a surface discrimination task. At the beginning of each trial, a colour cue indicated which one of two superimposed rotating (i.e. clockwise vs counterclockwise) kinetograms to attend. Neurons in MT+ responded more strongly to their preferred direction of motion when it corresponded to the attended relative to the unattended surface. Similar changes in firing rates have also been documented in visual areas V1–V3a and V4 (Ciaramitaro, Mitchell, Stoner, Reynolds, and Boynton 2011; Fallah, Stoner, and Reynolds 2007). Because both surfaces occupied the same spatial location, these findings cannot be explained by a selection mechanism that enhances the cortical representation of all stimuli within a given aperture.

At the cortical level, Duncan (1998) has proposed that OBA results from an integration of competitive interactions across multiple feature-selective modules. According to this integrative competition model, when an observer directs attention to one feature of an object (e.g., colour), mechanisms of selective attention bias ongoing competitive interactions in cortical modules that process this feature as well as the remaining features (e.g. orientation, motion, spatial frequency) of the same object. As a result, the neural representations of all the object's features are enhanced. This perspective is supported by multiple electrophysiological and neuroimaging studies in humans. In one such study, O'Craven, Downing, and Kanwisher (1999) presented subjects with arrays containing superimposed images of faces and houses. On each trial, either the face or house image moved along one of four axes. In separate blocks, subjects were instructed to attend the identity of the face image, the identity of the house image, or the direction of the moving image with the goal of detecting trial-by-trial repetitions of the relevant attribute. The authors examined changes in the amplitude of the BOLD response observed in cortical regions selective for faces (the fusiform face area or FFA), houses (the parahippocampal place area or PPA), and motion (hMT/MST) as a function of what attribute subjects were instructed to attend. The results revealed that attending to one attribute of an object was not only associated with a greater BOLD response in the cortical area selective for this attribute, but also in the cortical area selective for the other, irrelevant attribute of the same stimulus. For example, while subjects detected repetitions in the moving faces array and ignored superimposed houses, both FFA and hMT/MST were activated, while PPA was not. Similarly, Schoenfeld et al. (2003) found evidence for preferential processing of an attended object's behaviourally irrelevant features using EEG and fMRI. Here, subjects were instructed to attend to one of two superimposed white dot kinetograms that were distinguishable by their direction of motion (leftward or rightward) and detect brief changes in speed. On a subset of trials, the dots within the attended or unattended kinetogram changed colour from white to an isoluminant red. Spatiotemporal analyses of event-related potentials and the BOLD signal revealed a rapid increase in neural activity within colour-selective regions of fusiform gyrus when the attended kinetogram changed colour (~50 ms following the initial registration of colour information in the same cortical area) that was not observed for similar colour changes in the unattended kinetogram. These findings suggest that OBA enhances neural responses to both relevant and irrelevant object features in a rapid manner, consistent with the integrated competition model of OBA proposed by Duncan (1998).

The integrated competition model also predicts that the cortical representation of unattended objects should be suppressed (relative to the representation of the attended object), and there is some evidence to support this (Khoe, Mitchell, Reynolds, and Hillyard 2005; Pinilla, Cobo, Torres, and Valdes-Sosa 2001; Valdes-Sosa, Bobes, Rodriguez, and Pinilla 1998). Valdes-Sosa et al. (1998) recorded EEG while human subjects attended to one moving kinetogram (defined by colour) to detect brief perturbations in its rotational direction, while ignoring task-irrelevant perturbations in a

superimposed, unattended kinetogram (defined by a different colour). In one condition, the two fields were made to rotate in opposite directions, resulting in a percept of
two transparent surfaces sliding across one another ('two-surface' condition). In a second condition, both kinetograms rotated in the same direction, yielding a percept of a
single multicoloured object ('one-surface' condition). Attention effects were quantified
by comparing the amplitudes of early, visually evoked potentials (the P_1/N_1 complex)
observed approximately 100 ms following a perturbation of the attended or unattended
fields. In the two-surface condition, P_1/N_1 amplitudes were substantially smaller following a perturbation of the unattended relative to the attended field. Critically, this
effect was eliminated in the one-surface condition: P_1/N_1 amplitudes were statistically equivalent for either field, each reaching the same level of attended fields in the
two-surface condition. Together, these results suggest that processing of superimposed,
irrelevant sensory information can be suppressed in favour of relevant information
when each can be perceived as belonging distinct objects.

Control of object-based attention

In the previous section, we surveyed many studies suggesting that OBA (like FBA)
modulates sensory representations across early stages of the visual processing hierarchy.
Available evidence suggests that these modulations reflect top-down attentional control signals that originate in frontoparietal cortical areas (Friedman-Hill, Robertson,
Desimone, and Ungerleider 2003; Olson 2003; Robertson and Treisman 2006; Serences
et al. 2004; Shomstein and Behrmann 2006; Wojciulik and Kanwisher 1999). In one
study, Serences et al. (2004) showed human subjects displays containing spatially superimposed face and house images (similar to the displays used by O'Craven et al. 1999,
discussed in the last paragraph) that smoothly morphed every one second. Subjects
were instructed to attend to the face or house images in order to detect occasional pre-
specified target images. Two types of targets were presented: 'hold' targets instructed the
subject to maintain attention on the current image category (e.g. faces), while 'switch'
targets indicated the subject to switch attention to the other image category (e.g. from
faces to houses). Event-related fMRI revealed transient increases in activation within
several frontoparietal regions (including IPS, SPL, and superior frontal sulcus or SFS)
immediately following the presentation of 'switch' relative to 'hold' targets, suggesting
that these regions play an important role in mediating object-based shifts of attention.
Interestingly, many of the same regions also showed transient increases in activation following shifts of SBA (e.g. Corbetta and Shulman 2002; Serences and Yantis 2006; Yantis
et al. 2002), suggesting that a common attentional control network might mediate shifts
of both spatial- and object-based attention. In a related study, Shomstein and Behrmann
(2006) presented subjects with arrays similar to those used by Egly et al. (1994; see Fig.
20.4a) and examined transient changes in the BOLD response following instructions
to shift attention to a different location of the same object, or an equidistant location
on a different object. As in earlier work (e.g. Serences et al. 2004), activation within

regions of SPL increased transiently immediately following an instruction to shift attention. Moreover, activation in left SPL was substantially larger following within-object
relative to between-object shifts, suggesting that this region is particularly important
for object-based attentional selection. Similar to attentional control of feature selection, however, object-based attentional control is currently underexplored. Given the
modest evidence that suggests some gross anatomical overlap across SBA, OBA, and
FBA, future studies would benefit from utilizing MVPA methods to determine how subpopulations within the frontoparietal network may differentially control these selection
mechanisms.

Limitations of existing object-based attention demonstrations

Although the findings reviewed in the preceding section are consistent with an
object-based selection mechanism, many of these effects are also consistent with modified feature-based accounts, so caution is warranted before positing two entirely separate mechanisms of selection. For example, consider the findings reported by O'Craven
et al. (1999), where directing attention to one attribute of a stimulus (e.g. the identity of a
moving face image) enhanced the cortical response to other attributes of the same object
(e.g. the motion of the image). Taken at face value, these results suggest that directing
attention to one attribute of an object *automatically* leads to enhanced processing of all
attributes of the object. However, these results can also be explained via the operation
of a feature-based attentional mechanism. For example, in order to track the motion
of the face image, subjects may have chosen to attend the eyes, mouth, or the face as
a whole. Presumably, this strategy would result in an increased response in both face-
and motion-selective cortical regions. On this point, it is worth noting that O'Craven
et al. (1999) observed that neural responses to the task-relevant attribute were always
stronger than those observed to the task-irrelevant attribute of the same object, consistent with the operation of feature selection. Moreover, the high accuracy with which subjects completed the task suggests it was not particularly attention-demanding; therefore,
a second, parsimonious account is that attention was not fully engaged by the face, and
that subjects voluntarily attended to the motion vector as well, which would certainly be
within attentional capacity limits (see discussion of the Xu 2010 study in 'Interactions
Between FBA and OBA' below). Likewise, recall that Wannig et al. (2007) demonstrated that neurons in MT+ responded more strongly to their preferred direction of
motion when it was carried by an attended versus an unattended colour-defined surface. Although these findings are nominally consistent with the operation of a surface or
object-based attentional mechanism, they can also be explained by putative interactions
between spatial- and feature-based attentional mechanisms (see Treue and Katzner
2007). For example, rotating surfaces like those used in the study contain a large number
of locally varying direction signals (e.g. for a counterclockwise-rotating surface, dots on
the right will appear to move upward while those on the left will appear to move downward). When attention is directed to such a surface, neurons with receptive fields (RFs)

that cover only local patches of the surface will be modulated according to the match between the local direction inside the neuron's RF and the neuron's preferred direction of motion (e.g. Martinez-Trujillo and Treue 2004). Across multiple neurons, this will result in a position-dependent pattern of modulation that will selectively enhance processing of the currently attended direction of rotation.

In many studies purporting to document object-based selection, subjects were not explicitly discouraged from attending task-irrelevant features and therefore the extent to which OBA may be automatically deployed cannot be determined. Some studies have reported evidence for OBA even when such selection would offer no benefit to the observer, but neither was this selection necessarily detrimental (e.g. see discussion of O'Craven et al. 1999 above). A small number of studies, however, have shown evidence of OBA even when such selection was disruptive to the observer's goals. Both Kramer and Jacobson (1991) and Scholl, Pylyshyn, and Feldman (2001) found that subjects were less able to ignore distracting features when they belonged to the same object as the target. For example, Kramer and Jacobson (1991) found greater flanking effects when distracting flankers were connected with a central target, while Scholl et al. (2001) found in an MOT task that subjects were more likely to erroneously track a distractor when it belonged to the same object as a target. These data suggest that under some circumstances, OBA may be obligatory. Of note, however, Kramer and Jacobson (1991) found the largest effects when flanking distractors were near the central target (these effects were reduced as distance between stimuli increased); Scholl et al. (2001) found the largest effects when targets and distractors were difficult to differentiate into component parts. Thus, OBA may be automatically deployed when reducing an object into individual features is difficult or effortful.

INTERACTIONS BETWEEN FBA AND OBA

The evidence presented above on object-based selection runs counter to several studies discussed earlier that favour discrete feature selection (see 'Behavioural evidence for feature-based attention'): while OBA studies tend to show preferential selection for both relevant and irrelevant features of an attended object, FBA studies tend to show that only the neuronal representations of relevant features are enhanced (or at least are afforded a greater enhancement). Xu (2010) argues that these disparate results can be accounted for if one considers the capacity limitations of the attentional system. Various studies have converged on a capacity limit of approximately four items (Fisher 1984; Pylyshyn and Storm 1988; Scholl 2001), and there may be some cost associated with encoding multiple features of a given object (Woodman and Vogel 2008). In line with these previous findings, Xu (2010) found that neural responses to an irrelevant feature dimension were modulated only when the number of unique instances along an attended feature dimension did not exceed subjects' capacity. Here, subjects completed a colour visual short-term memory task in which they reported whether a test colour was present or absent in a previously viewed array of six objects. The sample array of to-be-remembered information varied in the number of unique features present, including: one shape rendered in one colour, one shape rendered in six different colours, six shapes rendered in one colour, or six shapes rendered in six different colours (see Fig. 20.5a). As shown in Fig. 20.5b, fMRI responses in the lateral occipital complex (LOC) and the superior IPS were modulated by the number of unique colours present in the sample array. However, responses observed in LOC—a region from which responses have been linked to the relative complexity or 'information load' imposed by an array of to-be-remembered materials (e.g. Xu and Chun 2006)—were also modulated by the number of unique shapes present in the sample array. For example, responses observed when the sample array contained one colour and one shape were substantially lower than those observed when it contained one colour and six unique shapes. This difference was abolished, however, when the sample array contained six unique colours. Assuming that items containing six unique colours or shapes were enough to exhaust mnemonic resources, these data suggest that OBA is not always automatically deployed. Instead, the selection of task-irrelevant information may depend on task demands.

Conclusions

Throughout this chapter, we have generally followed the course of the existing literature by treating FBA and OBA as two distinct selection mechanisms. This separation makes intuitive sense: FBA operates entirely on elementary properties coded by the early visual system, such as colour, shape, orientation, and motion, while OBA can operate on more complex representations such as faces and houses. A second obvious and potentially critical difference between studies of FBA and pure OBA is the spatial extent of modulation. Both psychophysical and neuroimaging studies have reliably established that feature selection globally recruits relevant sensory populations, even those outside the locus of spatial attention (Andersen et al. 2009; Rossi and Paradiso 1995; Serences and Boynton 2007; White and Carrasco 2011), whereas OBA demonstrations are typically restricted to the attended object. However, recent research suggests that at least under some circumstances, OBA may spread to cortical regions with strong foveal biases (e.g. Williams et al. 2008; Williams, Dang, and Kanwisher 2007), although not across the entire field. Thus, even if there is some spatial spread of OBA, it appears to be distinct from the more global spread of FBA, suggesting a mechanistic distinction between these two forms of selection.

Nonetheless, the distinction between FBA and OBA is not entirely clear-cut, and it is not always trivial to classify a single study as evidence in support of one form of selection over another. The main theoretical distinction between feature-based and object-based selection is whether relevant and irrelevant features are afforded a similar attentional benefit when they belong to the same object. However, even this simple distinction breaks down in studies of global feature-based attentional spread, as FBA may sometimes spread from a relevant feature to a paired irrelevant feature, even if they occur

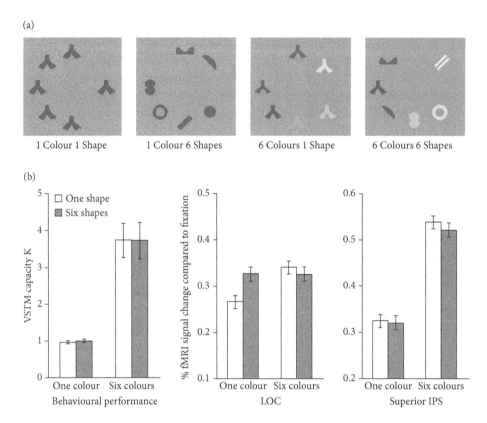

FIGURE 20.5 (a) Schematic of the stimulus arrays used in Xu (2010). Display complexity was manipulated by varying the number of unique colours within the sample array (one or six, respectively). (b) Left panel: Visual short-term memory capacity was modulated by the number of unique colours in the display, but was unaffected by the number of unique shapes. Middle and right panels: fMRI responses in lateral occipital complex (LOC) and superior intraparietal sulcus (IPS) were modulated by the number of unique colours present in the sample array. However, in LOC— where the magnitude of neural responses has been linked to the relative complexity or information load imposed by an array of to-be-remembered information—responses were also modulated by the number of unique shapes in the sample array when only one colour was present. Xu interpreted these findings as evidence for a flexible object-selective encoding mechanism. When processing resources have been exhausted (e.g. when subjects were asked to remember six unique colours) then neural responses to behaviourally irrelevant features (e.g. shape) are attenuated.

together outside the spatial focus of attention (Arman et al. 2006; Melcher et al. 2005; Sohn et al. 2005). In fact, here we have reviewed a myriad of studies that have shown single feature selection (1) entirely at the expense of paired irrelevant features; (2) in conjunction with modest (albeit comparatively reduced) representation of paired irrelevant features; and holistic object selection, in which all features are afforded similar levels of cortical representation.

Given this apparent gradient from single feature to full object selection, we argue against two completely independent attention mechanisms and particularly against the automatic nature of object-based selection. Instead, we propose that relevant information is flexibly selected according to task demands, and that the interplay between observer goals and the nature of the physical display will dictate the nature of selection across the set of features that combine to make an object (see Kravitz and Behrmann 2011). For example, FBA can violate the tenets of OBA when extreme emphasis is placed on accurately characterizing a single feature of a multi-part object. In these cases OBA may *not* be automatic or obligatory, but rather *can* occur when selection demands are not high and no cost is incurred for selecting all the features on an object. Finally, although object-based attention does not appear to be automatic, it may be the rule rather than the exception in many cases where holistic processing is critical for identifying relevant information, such as when searching for a face in a crowd (Richler, Tanaka, Brown, and Gauthier 2008; Tanaka and Farah 1993). In this situation, FBA might still be possible, but relatively useless given processing demands. While each of these questions merits further investigation, the emerging consensus is that feature-based and object-based attentional mechanisms are not distinct systems in any absolute sense. Instead, they operate along a continuum and the extent to which selection is based on a specific feature or an object depends on both the complexity of the stimulus array and on the specific behavioural goals of the observer.

ACKNOWLEDGEMENTS

This work was funded by NIMH RO1–092345 to J.T.S.

REFERENCES

Abrams, R. and Law, M. (2000). Object-based visual attention with endogenous orienting. *Attention, Perception, & Psychophysics* 62(4): 818–833. doi: 10.3758/bf03206925.

Andersen, S. K., Fuchs, S., and Müller, M. M. (2009). Effects of feature-selective and spatial attention at different stages of visual processing. *Journal of Cognitive Neuroscience* 23(1): 238–246. doi: 10.1162/jocn.2009.21328.

Anllo-Vento, L., Luck, S. J., and Hillyard, S. A. (1998). Spatio-temporal dynamics of attention to color: Evidence from human electrophysiology. *Human Brain Mapping* 6(4): 216–238. doi: 10.1002/(sici)1097-0193(1998)6:4>216::aid-hbm3<3.0.co;2-6.

Arman, A. C., Ciaramitaro, V. M., and Boynton, G. M. (2006). Effects of feature-based attention on the motion aftereffect at remote locations. *Vision Research* 46(18): 2968–2976. doi: 10.1016/j.visres.2006.03.003.

Awh, E. and Pashler, H. (2000). Evidence for split attentional foci. *Journal of Experimental Psychology: Human Perception and Performance* 26(2): 834–846. doi: 10.1037/0096-1523.26. 2.834.

Baylis, G. C. and Driver, J. (1993). Visual attention and objects: Evidence for hierarchical coding of location. *Journal of Experimental Psychology: Human Perception and Performance* 19(3): 451–470.

Behrmann, M., Zemel, R. S., and Mozer, M. C. (1998). Object-based attention and occlusion: Evidence from normal participants and a computational model. *Journal of Experimental Psychology: Human Perception and Performance* 24(4): 1011–1036.

Bisley, J. W. and Goldberg, M. E. (2003). Neuronal activity in the lateral intraparietal area and spatial attention. *Science* 299(5603): 81–86. doi: 10.1126/science.1077395.

Blaser, E., Pylyshyn, Z. W., and Holcombe, A. O. (2000). Tracking an object through feature space. *Nature* 408(6809): 196–199. doi: 10.1038/35041567.

Boynton, G. M. (2005). Attention and visual perception. *Current Opinion in Neurobiology* 15(4): 465–469. doi: 10.1016/j.conb.2005.06.009.

Carrasco, M., Ling, S., and Read, S. (2004). Attention alters appearance. *Nature Neuroscience* 7(3): 308–313. doi: 10.1038/nn1194.

Carrasco, M. (2011). Visual attention: The past 25 years. *Vision Research* 51(13): 1484–1525. doi: 10.1016/j.visres.2011.04.012.

Ciaramitaro, V. M., Mitchell, J. F., Stoner, G. R., Reynolds, J. H., and Boynton, G. M. (2011). Object-based attention to one of two superimposed surfaces alters responses in human early visual cortex. *Journal of Neurophysiology* 105(3): 1258–1265. doi: 10.1152/jn.00680.2010.

Corbetta, M., Miezin, F., Dobmeyer, S., Shulman, G., and Petersen, S. (1990). Attentional modulation of neural processing of shape, color, and velocity in humans. *Science* 248(4962): 1556–1559. doi: 10.1126/science.2360050.

Corbetta, M., Miezin, F., Dobmeyer, S., Shulman, G., and Petersen, S. (1991). Selective and divided attention during visual discriminations of shape, color, and speed: Functional anatomy by positron emission tomography. *Journal of Neuroscience* 11(8): 2383–2402.

Corbetta, M. and Shulman, G. L. (2002). Control of goal-directed and stimulus-driven attention in the brain. *Nature Reviews Neuroscience* 3(3): 201–215. doi: 10.1038/nrn755.

Das, K., Giesbrecht, B., and Eckstein, M. P. (2010). Predicting variations of perceptual performance across individuals from neural activity using pattern classifiers. *NeuroImage* 51(4): 1425–1437. doi: 10.1016/j.neuroimage.2010.03.030.

Davis, E.T., and Graham, N. (1981). Spatial frequency uncertainty effects in the detection of sinusoidal gratings. *Vision Research* 21(5): 705–712. doi: 10.1016/0042-6989(81)90079-1.

Desimone, R. and Duncan, J. (1995). Neural mechanisms of selective visual attention [review]. *Annual Review of Neuroscience* 18: 193–222. doi: 10.1146/annurev.neuro.18.1.193.

Duncan, J. (1984). Selective attention and the organization of visual information. *Journal of Experimental Psychology General* 113(4): 501–517.

Duncan, J. (1998). Converging levels of analysis in the cognitive neuroscience of visual attention. *Philosophical Transactions of the Royal Society of London B: Biological Sciences* 353(1373): 1307–1317. doi: 10.1098/rstb.1998.0285.

Egeth, H. E., Virzi, R. A., and Garbart, H. (1984). Searching for conjunctively defined targets. *Journal of Experimental Psychology: Human Perception and Performance* 10(1): 32–39. doi: 10.1037/0096-1523.10.1.32.

Egly, R., Driver, J., and Rafal, R. D. (1994). Shifting visual attention between objects and locations: Evidence from normal and parietal lesion subjects. *Journal of Experimental Psychology General* 123(2): 161–177.

Fallah, M., Stoner, G. R., and Reynolds, J. H. (2007). Stimulus-specific competitive selection in macaque extrastriate visual area V4. *Proceedings of the National Academy of Sciences USA* 104(10): 4165–4169. doi: 10.1073/pnas.0611722104.

Ferster, D., Chung, S., and Wheat, H. (1996). Orientation selectivity of thalamic input to simple cells of cat visual cortex. *Nature* 380(6571): 249–252. doi: 10.1038/380249a0.

Fisher, D. L. (1984). Central capacity limits in consistent mapping, visual search tasks: Four channels or more? *Cognitive Psychology 16*(4): 449–484. doi: 10.1016/0010-0285(84)90017-3.

Friedman-Hill, S. R., Robertson, L. C., Desimone, R., and Ungerleider, L. G. (2003). Posterior parietal cortex and the filtering of distractors. *Proceedings of the National Academy of Sciences USA 100*(7): 4263–4268. doi: 10.1073/pnas.0730772100.

Gold, J. and Shadlen, M. (2001). Neural computations that underlie decisions about sensory stimuli. *Trends in Cognitive Sciences 5*(1): 10–16. doi: citeulike-article-id:86939.

Gold, J. and Shadlen, M. (2003). The influence of behavioral context on the representation of a perceptual decision in developing oculomotor commands. *Journal of Neuroscience 23*(2): 632–651.

Gold, J. and Shadlen, M. (2007). The neural basis of decision making. *Annual Review of Neuroscience 30*: 535–574. doi: 10.1146/annurev.neuro.29.051605.113038.

Greenberg, A. S., Esterman, M., Wilson, D., Serences, J. T., and Yantis, S. (2010). Control of spatial and feature-based attention in frontoparietal cortex. *Journal of Neuroscience 30*(43): 14330–14339. doi: 10.1523/jneurosci.4248-09.2010.

Haenny, P. E. and Schiller, P. H. (1988). State dependent activity in monkey visual cortex. *Experimental Brain Research 69*(2): 225–244. doi: 10.1007/bf00247569.

Hanes, D. P. and Schall, J. D. (1996). Neural control of voluntary movement initiation. *Science 274*(5286): 427–430.

He, Z. J. and Nakayama, K. (1995). Visual attention to surfaces in three-dimensional space. *Proceedings of the National Academy of Sciences USA 92*(24): 11155–11159.

Ho, T., Brown, S., van Maanen, L., Forstmann, B. U., Wagenmakers, E.-J., and Serences, J. T. (2012). The optimality of sensory processing during the speed–accuracy tradeoff. *Journal of Neuroscience 32*(23): 7992–8003. doi: 10.1523/jneurosci.0340-12.2012.

Hol, K. and Treue, S. (2001). Different populations of neurons contribute to the detection and discrimination of visual motion. *Vision Research 41*(6): 685–689. doi: 10.1016/s0042-6989(00)00314-x.

Horwitz, G. D., Batista, A. P., and Newsome, W. T. (2004). Representation of an abstract perceptual decision in macaque superior colliculus. *Journal of Neurophysiology 91*(5): 2281–2296. doi: 10.1152/jn.00872.2003.

Jazayeri, M. and Movshon, J. A. (2006). Optimal representation of sensory information by neural populations. *Nature Neuroscience 9*(5): 690–696. doi: 10.1038/nn1691. Available online at <http://www.nature.com/neuro/journal/v9/n5/suppinfo/nn1691_S1.html>, last accessed 27 June 2013.

Jazayeri, M. and Movshon, J. A. (2007). Integration of sensory evidence in motion discrimination. *Journal of Vision 7*(12): doi: 10.1167/7.12.7.

Kastner, S. and Ungerleider, L. G. (2000). Mechanisms of visual attention in the human cortex. *Annual Review of Neuroscience 23*(1): 315–341. doi:10.1146/annurev.neuro.23.1.315.

Khoe, W., Mitchell, J. F., Reynolds, J. H., and Hillyard, S. A. (2005). Exogenous attentional selection of transparent superimposed surfaces modulates early event-related potentials. *Vision Research 45*(24): 3004–3014. doi: 10.1016/j.visres.2005.04.021.

Kramer, A. F. and Jacobson, A. (1991). Perceptual organization and focused attention: The role of objects and proximity in visual processing. *Perception & Psychophysics 50*(3): 267–284.

Kravitz, D. and Behrmann, M. (2011). Space-, object-, and feature-based attention interact to organize visual scenes. *Attention, Perception, & Psychophysics 73*(8): 2434–2447. doi: 10.3758/s13414-011-0201-z.

Lankheet, M. J. M. and Verstraten, F. A. J. (1995). Attentional modulation of adaptation to two-component transparent motion. *Vision Research 35*(10): 1401–1412. doi: 10.1016/0042-6989(95)98720-t.

Law, C.-T. and Gold, J. I. (2008). Neural correlates of perceptual learning in a sensory-motor, but not a sensory, cortical area. *Nature Neuroscience* 11(4): 505–513. doi: 10.1038/nn2070.

Law, C.-T. and Gold, J. I. (2009). Reinforcement learning can account for associative and perceptual learning on a visual-decision task. *Nature Neuroscience* 12(5): 655–663. doi: 10.1038/nn.2304.

Le, T. H., Pardo, J. V., and Hu, X. (1998). 4 T-fMRI study of nonspatial shifting of selective attention: Cerebellar and parietal contributions. *Journal of Neurophysiology* 79(3): 1535–1548.

Leon, M. I. and Shadlen, M. N. (1999). Effect of expected reward magnitude on the response of neurons in the dorsolateral prefrontal cortex of the macaque. *Neuron* 24(2): 415–425.

Liu, T., Slotnick, S. D., Serences, J. T., and Yantis, S. (2003). Cortical mechanisms of feature-based attentional control. *Cerebral Cortex* 13(12): 1334–1343. doi: 10.1093/cercor/bhg080.

Liu, T., Larsson, J., and Carrasco, M. (2007). Feature-based attention modulates orientation-selective responses in human visual cortex. *Neuron* 55(2): 313–323. doi: 10.1016/j.neuron.2007.06.030.

Liu, T., Stevens, S. T., and Carrasco, M. (2007). Comparing the time course and efficacy of spatial and feature-based attention. *Vision Research* 47(1): 108–113. doi: 10.1016/j.visres.2006.09.017.

Liu, T., Hospadaruk, L., Zhu, D. C., and Gardner, J. L. (2011). Feature-specific attentional priority signals in human cortex. *Journal of Neuroscience* 31(12): 4484–4495. doi: 10.1523/jneurosci.5745-10.2011.

Liu, T. and Hou, Y. (2011). Global feature-based attention to orientation. *Journal of Vision* 11(10): doi: 10.1167/11.10.8.

Lu, J. and Itti, L. (2005). Perceptual consequences of feature-based attention. *Journal of Vision* 5(7): doi: 10.1167/5.7.2.

Martinez-Trujillo, J. C. and Treue, S. (2004). Feature-based attention increases the selectivity of population responses in primate visual cortex. *Current Biology* 14(9): 744–751. doi: 10.1016/j.cub.2004.04.028.

Maunsell, J. H. R. and Treue, S. (2006). Feature-based attention in visual cortex. *Trends in Neurosciences* 29(6): 317–322. doi: 10.1016/j.tins.2006.04.001.

McAdams, C. J. and Maunsell, J. H. R. (1999). Effects of attention on orientation-tuning functions of single neurons in macaque cortical area V4. *Journal of Neuroscience* 19(1): 431–441.

McMains, S. A. and Somers, D. C. (2004). Multiple spotlights of attentional selection in human visual cortex. *Neuron* 42(4): 677–686.

Melcher, D., Papathomas, T. V., and Vidnyánszky, Z. (2005). Implicit attentional selection of bound visual features. *Neuron* 46(5): 723–729. doi: 10.1016/j.neuron.2005.04.023.

Merigan, W. H. and Maunsell, J. H. R. (1993). How parallel are the primate visual pathways? *Annual Review of Neuroscience* 16(1): 369–402. doi: 10.1146/annurev.ne.16.030193.002101.

Mitchell, J. F., Stoner, G. R., and Reynolds, J. H. (2004). Object-based attention determines dominance in binocular rivalry. *Nature* 429(6990): 410–413. doi: 10.1038/nature02584.

Mitchell, J. F., Sundberg, K. A., and Reynolds, J. H. (2009). Spatial attention decorrelates intrinsic activity fluctuations in macaque area V4. *Neuron* 63(6): 879–888. doi: 10.1016/j.neuron.2009.09.013.

Moore, C. M., Yantis, S., and Vaughan, B. (1998). Object-based visual selection: Evidence from perceptual completion. *Psychological Science* 9(2): 104–110. doi: 10.1111/1467-9280.00019.

Moran, J. and Desimone, R. (1985). Selective attention gates visual processing in the extrastriate cortex. *Science* 229(4715): 782–784. doi: 10.1126/science.4023713.

Navalpakkam, V. and Itti, L. (2007). Search goal tunes visual features optimally. *Neuron* 53(4): 605–617. doi: 10.1016/j.neuron.2007.01.018.

Neisser, U. and Becklen, R. (1975). Selective looking: Attending to visually specified events. *Cognitive Psychology* 7(4): 480–494. doi: 10.1016/0010-0285(75)90019-5.

O'Craven, K. M., Downing, P. E., and Kanwisher, N. (1999). fMI evidence for objects as the units of attentional selection. *Nature* 401(6753): 584–587. doi: 10.1038/44134.

Olson, C. R. (2003). Brain representation of object-centered space in monkeys and humans. *Annual Review of Neuroscience* 26(1): 331–354. doi: 10.1146/annurev.neuro.26.041002.131405.

Palmer, J., Huk, A. C., and Shadlen, M. N. (2005). The effect of stimulus strength on the speed and accuracy of a perceptual decision. *Journal of Vision* 5(5): doi: 10.1167/5.5.1.

Pestilli, F., Carrasco, M., Heeger, D. J., and Gardner, J. L. (2011). Attentional enhancement via selection and pooling of early sensory responses in human visual cortex. *Neuron* 72(5): 832–846. doi: 10.1016/j.neuron.2011.09.025.

Petersen, S. E., Robinson, D. L., and Keys, W. (1985). Pulvinar nuclei of the behaving rhesus monkey: Visual responses and their modulation. *Journal of Neurophysiology* 54(4): 867–886.

Pinilla, T., Cobo, A., Torres, K., and Valdes-Sosa, M. (2001). Attentional shifts between surfaces: Effects on detection and early brain potentials. *Vision Research* 41(13): 1619–1630.

Pollmann, S., Weidner, R., Müller, H. J., and Cramon, D. Y. von (2000). A fronto-posterior network involved in visual dimension changes. *Journal of Cognitive Neuroscience* 12(3): 480– 494. doi: 10.1162/089892900562156.

Posner, M.I. (1980). Orienting of attention. *Quarterly Journal of Experimental Psychology* 32(1): 3–25. doi: 10.1080/00335558008248231.

Purushothaman, G. and Bradley, D. C. (2005). Neural population code for fine perceptual decisions in area MT. *Nature Neuroscience* 8(1): 99–106. doi: 10.1038/nn1373. Available online at <http://www.nature.com/neuro/journal/v8/n1/suppinfo/nn1373_S1.html>, last accessed 27 June 2013.

Pylyshyn, Z. W. and Storm, R. W. (1988). Tracking multiple independent targets: Evidence for a parallel tracking mechanism. *Spatial Vision* 3(3): 179–197.

Regan, D. and Beverley, K. I. (1985). Postadaptation orientation discrimination. *Journal of the Optical Society of America A* 2(2): 147–155.

Reynolds, J. H. and Desimone, R. (1999). The role of neural mechanisms of attention in solving the binding problem. *Neuron* 24(1): 19–29. doi: 10.1016/s0896-6273(00)80819-3.

Reynolds, J. H., Pasternak, T., and Desimone, R. (2000). Attention increases sensitivity of V4 neurons. *Neuron* 26(3): 703–714. doi: 10.1016/s0896-6273(00)81206-4.

Richler, J. J., Tanaka, J. W., Brown, D. D., and Gauthier, I. (2008). Why does selective attention to parts fail in face processing? *Journal of Experimental Psychology: Learning, Memory, and Cognition* 34(6): 1356–1368. doi: 10.1037/a0013080.

Robertson, L. C. and Treisman, A. (2006). Attending to space within and between objects: Implications from a patient with Balint's syndrome. *Cognitive Neuropsychology* 23(3): 448–462. doi: 10.1080/02643290500180324.

Roitman, J. D. and Shadlen, M. N. (2002). Response of neurons in the lateral intraparietal area during a combined visual discrimination reaction time task. *Journal of Neuroscience* 22(21): 9475–9489.

Rossi, A. F. and Paradiso, M. A. (1995). Feature-specific effects of selective visual attention. *Vision Research* 35(5): 621–634. doi: 10.1016/0042-6989(94)00156-g.

Rushworth, M. F. S., Paus, T., and Sipila, P. K. (2001). Attention systems and the organization of the human parietal cortex. *Journal of Neuroscience* 21(14): 5262–5271.

Sàenz, M., Buracâs, G. T., and Boynton, G. M. (2002). Global effects of feature-based attention in human visual cortex. *Nature Neuroscience* 5(7): 631–632. doi: 10.1038/nn876. Available online at <http://www.nature.com/neuro/journal/v5/n7/suppinfo/nn876_S1.html>, last accessed 27 June 2013.

Sàenz, M., Buraĉas, G. T., and Boynton, G. M. (2003). Global feature-based attention for motion and color. *Vision Research* 43(6): 629–637. doi: 10.1016/s0042-6989(02)00595-3.

Schall, J. D. (2001). Neural basis of deciding, choosing and acting. *Nature Reviews Neuroscience* 2(1): 33–42. doi: 10.1038/35049054.

Schenkluhn, B., Ruff, C. C., Heinen, K., and Chambers, C. D. (2008). Parietal stimulation decouples spatial and feature-based attention. *Journal of Neuroscience* 28(44): 11106–11110. doi: 10.1523/jneurosci.3591-08.2008.

Schneider, K. A. (2011). Subcortical mechanisms of feature-based attention. *Journal of Neuroscience* 31(23): 8643–8653. doi: 10.1523/jneurosci.6274-10.2011.

Schoenfeld, M. A., Hopf, J. M., Martinez, A., Mai, H. M., Sattler, C., Gasde, A., Heinze, H. J., and Hillyard, S. A. (2007). Spatio-temporal analysis of feature-based attention. *Cerebral Cortex* 17(10): 2468–2477. doi: 10.1093/cercor/bhl154.

Schoenfeld, M. A., Tempelmann, C., Martinez, A., Hopf, J. M., Sattler, C., Heinze, H. J., and Hillyard, S. A. (2003). Dynamics of feature binding during object-selective attention. *Proceedings of the National Academy of Sciences USA* 100(20): 11806–11811. doi: 10.1073/pnas.1932820100.

Scholl, B. J. (2001). Objects and attention: The state of the art. *Cognition 80*: 1–46.

Scholl, B. J., Pylyshyn, Z. W., and Feldman, J. (2001). What is a visual object? Evidence from target merging in multiple object tracking. *Cognition, 80*(1–2), 159–177.

Scolari, M. and Serences, J. T. (2009). Adaptive allocation of attentional gain. *Journal of Neuroscience* 29(38): 11933–11942. doi: 10.1523/jneurosci.5642-08.2009.

Scolari, M. and Serences, J. T. (2010). Basing perceptual decisions on the most informative sensory neurons. *Journal of Neurophysiology* 104(4): 2266–2273. doi: 10.1152/jn.00273.2010.

Scolari, M., Byers, A., and Serences, J. T. (2012). Optimal deployment of attentional gain during fine discriminations. *Journal of Neuroscience* 32(22): 7723–7733. doi: 10.1523/jneurosci.5558-11.2012.

Serences, J. T., Schwarzbach, J., Courtney, S. M., Golay, X., and Yantis, S. (2004). Control of object-based attention in human cortex. *Cerebral Cortex* 14(12): 1346–1357. doi: 10.1093/cercor/bhh095.

Serences, J. T. and Yantis, S. (2006). Selective visual attention and perceptual coherence. *Trends in Cognitive Sciences* 10(1): 38–45. doi: 10.1016/j.tics.2005.11.008.

Serences, J. T. and Boynton, G. M. (2007). Feature-based attentional modulations in the absence of direct visual stimulation. *Neuron* 55(2): 301–312. doi: 10.1016/j.neuron.2007.06.015.

Serences, J. T., Saproo, S., Scolari, M., Ho, T., and Muftuler, L. T. (2009). Estimating the influence of attention on population codes in human visual cortex using voxel-based tuning functions. *NeuroImage* 44(1): 223–231. doi: 10.1016/j.neuroimage.2008.07.043.

Seung, H. S. and Sompolinsky, H. (1993). Simple models for reading neuronal population codes. *Proceedings of the National Academy of Sciences* 90(22): 10749–10753.

Shadlen, M. N. and Newsome, W. T. (2001). Neural basis of a perceptual decision in the parietal cortex (area LIP) of the rhesus monkey. *Journal of Neurophysiology* 86(4): 1916–1936.

Shomstein, S. and Yantis, S. (2002). Object-based attention: Sensory modulation or priority setting? *Attention, Perception, & Psychophysics* 64(1): 41–51. doi: 10.3758/bf03194556.

Shomstein, S. and Yantis, S. (2004a). Configural and contextual prioritization in object-based attention. *Psychonomic Bulletin & Review* 11(2): 247–253. doi: 10.3758/bf03196566.

Shomstein, S. and Yantis, S. (2004b). Control of attention shifts between vision and audition in human cortex. *Journal of Neuroscience* 24(47): 10702–10706. doi: 10.1523/jneurosci.2939-04.2004.

Shomstein, S. and Behrmann, M. (2006). Cortical systems mediating visual attention to both objects and spatial locations. *Proceedings of the National Academy of Sciences USA 103*(30): 11387–11392. doi: 10.1073/pnas.0601813103.

Shomstein, S. and Yantis, S. (2006). Parietal cortex mediates voluntary control of spatial and nonspatial auditory attention. *Journal of Neuroscience 26*(2): 435–439. doi: 10.1523/jneurosci.4408-05.2006.

Simons, D. J. and Chabris, C. F. (1999). Gorillas in our midst: Sustained inattentional blindness for dynamic events. *Perception 28*(9): 1059–1074.

Sohn, W., Papathomas, T. V., Blaser, E., and Vidnyánszky, Z. (2004). Object-based cross-feature attentional modulation from color to motion. *Vision Research 44*(12): 1437–1443. doi: 10.1016/j.visres.2003.12.010.

Sohn, W., Chong, S. C., Papathomas, T. V., and Vidnyánszky, Z. (2005). Cross-feature spread of global attentional modulation in human area MT+. *NeuroReport 16*(12): 1389–1393.

Spitzer, H., Desimone, R., and Moran, J. (1988). Increased attention enhances both behavioral and neuronal performance. *Science 240*(4850): 338–340. doi: 10.1126/science.3353728.

Szczepanski, S. M., Konen, C. S., and Kastner, S. (2010). Mechanisms of spatial attention control in frontal and parietal cortex. *Journal of Neuroscience 30*(1): 148–160. doi: 10.1523/jneurosci.3862-09.2010.

Tanaka, J. W. and Farah, M. J. (1993). Parts and wholes in face recognition. *Quarterly Journal of Experimental Psychology Section A 46*(2): 225–245. doi: 10.1080/14640749308401045.

Treisman, A. M. and Gelade, G. (1980). A feature-integration theory of attention. *Cognitive Psychology 12*(1): 97–136. doi: 10.1016/0010-0285(80)90005-5.

Treue, S. and Maunsell, J. H. R. (1996). Attentional modulation of visual motion processing in cortical areas MT and MST. *Nature 382*(6591): 539–541. doi: 10.1038/382539a0.

Treue, S. and Martinez-Trujillo, J. C. (1999). Feature-based attention influences motion processing gain in macaque visual cortex. *Nature 399*(6736): 575–579. doi: 10.1038/21176.

Treue, S. and Katzner, S. (2007). Visual attention: of features and transparent surfaces. *Trends in Cognitive Sciences 11*(11): 451–453. doi: 10.1016/j.tics.2007.08.012.

Treue, S. and Martinez-Trujillo, J. C. (2007). Attending to features inside and outside the spotlight of attention. *Neuron 55*(2): 174–176. doi: 10.1016/j.neuron.2007.07.005.

Valdes-Sosa, M., Bobes, M. A., Rodriguez, V., and Pinilla, T. (1998). Switching attention without shifting the spotlight object-based attentional modulation of brain potentials. *Journal of Cognitive Neuroscience 10*(1): 137–151.

Valdes-Sosa, M., Cobo, A., and Pinilla, T. (2000). Attention to object files defined by transparent motion. *Journal of Experimental Psychology: Human Perception and Performance 26*(2): 488–505.

Wannig, A., Rodriguez, V., and Freiwald, W. A. (2007). Attention to surfaces modulates motion processing in extrastriate area MT. *Neuron 54*(4): 639–651. doi: 10.1016/j.neuron.2007.05.001.

White, A. L. and Carrasco, M. (2011). Feature-based attention involuntarily and simultaneously improves visual performance across locations. *Journal of Vision 11*(6): 1–10. doi: 10.1167/11.6.15.

Wiesel, T. N. and Hubel, D. H. (1966). Spatial and chromatic interactions in the lateral geniculate body of the rhesus monkey. *Journal of Neurophysiology 29*(6): 1115–1156.

Williams, M. A., Dang, S., and Kanwisher, N. G. (2007). Only some spatial patterns of fMRI response are read out in task performance. *Nature Neuroscience 10*(6): 685–686. doi: 10.1038/nn1900. Available online at <http://www.nature.com/neuro/journal/v10/n6/suppinfo/nn1900_S1.html>, last accessed 27 June 2013.

Williams, M. A., Baker, C. I., Op de Beeck, H. P., Mok Shim, W., Dang, S., Triantafyllou, C., and Kanwisher, N. (2008). Feedback of visual object information to foveal retinotopic cortex. *Nature Neuroscience* 11(12): 1439–1445. doi: 10.1038/nn.2218. Available online at<http://www.nature.com/neuro/journal/v11/n12/suppinfo/nn.2218_S1.html>, last accessed 27 June 2013.

Wojciulik, E. and Kanwisher, N. (1999). The generality of parietal involvement in visual attention. *Neuron* 23(4): 747–764. doi: 10.1016/s0896-6273(01)80033-7.

Wolfe, J. (1994). Guided Search 2.0: A revised model of visual search. *Psychonomic Bulletin & Review* 1(2): 202–238. doi: 10.3758/bf03200774.

Woodman, G. and Vogel, E. (2008). Selective storage and maintenance of an object's features in visual working memory. *Psychonomic Bulletin & Review* 15(1): 223–229. doi: 10.3758/pbr.15.1.223.

Xu, Y. and Chun, M. M. (2006). Dissociable neural mechanisms supporting visual short-term memory for objects. *Nature* 440(7080): 91–95. doi: 10.1038/nature04262. Available online at <http://www.nature.com/nature/journal/v440/n7080/suppinfo/nature04262_S1.html>, last accessed 27 June 2013.

Xu, Y. (2010). The neural fate of task-irrelevant features in object-based processing. *Journal of Neuroscience* 30(42): 14020–14028. doi: 10.1523/jneurosci.3011-10.2010.

Yantis, S. (1992). Multielement visual tracking: Attention and perceptual organization. *Cognitive Psychology* 24(3): 295–340. doi: 10.1016/0010-0285(92)90010-y.

Yantis, S., Schwarzbach, J., Serences, J. T., Carlson, R. L., Steinmetz, M. A., Pekar, J. J., and Courtney, S. M. (2002). Transient neural activity in human parietal cortex during spatial attention shifts. *Nature Neuroscience* 5(10): 995–1002. doi: 10.1038/nn921. Available online at <http://www.nature.com/neuro/journal/v5/n10/suppinfo/nn921_S1.html>, last accessed 27 June 2013.

Yantis, S. and Serences, J. T. (2003). Cortical mechanisms of space-based and object-based attentional control. *Current Opinion in Neurobiology* 13(2): 187–193. doi: 10.1016/s0959-4388(03)00033-3.

Zhang, W. and Luck, S. J. (2009). Feature-based attention modulates feedforward visual processing. *Nature Neuroscience* 12(1): 24–25. doi: 10.1038/nn.2223. Available online at >http://www.nature.com/neuro/journal/v12/n1/suppinfo/nn.2223_S1.html>, last accessed 27 June 2013, last accessed 27 June 2013.

CHAPTER 21

OBJECT- AND FEATURE-BASED ATTENTION: MONKEY PHYSIOLOGY

STEFAN TREUE

VISUAL attention is a powerful mechanism that acts as a central component for sensory information processing and perception. It allows us to select a small subset of the information picked up by our eyes and enhance its processing, thus concentrating scant resources onto those aspects of the incoming deluge of sensory data that we momentarily deem most relevant. This selective processing of bottom-up signals modulates the response of neurons in visual cortex to sensory signals, enhancing the representation of behaviourally significant portions of the input at the expense of those aspects deemed less relevant. This notion of attention as the selective modulation of sensory information processing based on the behavioural relevance of the incoming signals is captured in the popular metaphor of attention as a spotlight, in which those spatial regions falling within the current focus of attention are selected for enhanced processing. Space-based attention has dominated investigations of the neural basis of attention, and is covered extensively in other chapters of this book. However, attention can be allocated not only to locations but also to features, such as a particular colour, an orientation, or a specific direction of motion. Although feature-based attention has received less study than space-based attention, results from electrophysiological studies of the activity of individual neurons in the visual cortex of rhesus monkeys trained to perform attentional tasks ('single-unit studies') suggest that the two types of attention rely on closely related mechanisms. Consequently modern theories of attention try to account for both spatial and feature-based attentional effects.

Feature-based attention, that is, the ability to enhance the representation of those input components throughout the visual field that match a particular feature, should be particularly useful when searching for a stimulus with that feature. This ability to detect such a target—a behaviourally relevant item—amongst distractors is the basis of a very popular paradigm in visual psychophysics: visual search. In visual search experiments targets and distractors differ by at least one feature, such as their colour or orientation, and the target is typically defined in advance of the presentation of the search array. Independent of whether subjects detect a target using a parallel search process or using a serial process that guides a recognition mechanism through a sequence of potential target locations (Wolfe and Horowitz 2004), target detection could be improved by enhancing the representation of image components that match the attended feature (such as the colour red or a vertical orientation) and by suppressing those that do not. One approach to achieve this type of modulation would be to employ feature-based attention to enhance the responses of all neurons that respond preferentially to the attended feature, thereby selectively strengthening the representation of stimuli sharing the attended feature before any stage where objects are recognized.

Many psychophysical studies have demonstrated that feature-based attention improves detection or otherwise enhances behavioural performance across the visual field (see Scolari, Ester, and Serences (chapter 20), this volume). Neural correlates of feature-based attention were identified in some of the earliest brain imaging studies (Corbetta et al. 1990) and continue to be actively investigated in fMRI studies (Beauchamp et al. 1997; Watanabe et al. 1998; Wojciulik et al. 1998; O'Craven et al. 1999; Shulman et al. 1999; Saenz et al. 2002; Serences and Boynton 2007; Liu et al. 2007). We focus here on evidence from single-unit recordings made in the visual cortex of macaque monkeys, which have provided detailed insights into how feature-based attention alters the neuronal representation of the visual scene.

SINGLE-UNIT ELECTROPHYSIOLOGY OF ATTENTIONAL MODULATION IN VISUAL CORTEX

Most single-unit studies of attention have been performed at intermediate levels of the hierarchy of visual cortex, such as area V4 in the ventral pathway and the middle temporal visual area (MT) in the dorsal pathway. These areas are a popular target of such studies not because they are thought to play a special or prominent role in attention, but because they represent a good compromise between earlier stages of visual cortex, where responses to simple stimuli are robust and well understood and where neurons have moderate-sized receptive fields, and later stages of visual cortex, where the effects of attention tend to be more pronounced (Maunsell and Cook 2002) but the sensory properties are less well understood and the receptive fields are very large.

A large number of single-unit studies have examined the effects of spatial-, i.e. location-based attention on responses in visual cortex. An important result from these studies has been that spatial attention changes the strength of neurons' responses, i.e. their gain, without changing their underlying response properties. This multiplicative modulation increases the responses of neurons in V4 without systematically sharpening or broadening their orientation tuning curves: responses to all orientations are scaled proportionally (McAdams and Maunsell 1999). Similarly spatial attention increases the response gain in MT without affecting the tuning width for the direction of motion (Treue and Martinez-Trujillo 1999). Additionally, spatial attention has been shown to enhance synchronization of neuronal activity and this enhancement correlates with enhanced neuronal and behavioural responses to changes in attended stimuli (Fries et al. 2001; Womelsdorf et al. 2006). In contrast to this body of knowledge on spatial attention, relatively few single-unit experiments have focused on feature-based attention.

This chapter will focus on single-unit studies of feature-based attention in areas MT and V4 of primate extrastriate visual cortex. Both of these areas are at an intermediate processing stage along the dorsal and temporal cortical processing pathway respectively. Area MT is of central importance in the perception of visual motion (Newsome and Paré 1988; Britten et al. 1996) and probably the extrastriate area whose sensory encoding properties are best understood. Area V4 is implicated in form recognition and visual search (Schiller and Lee 1991; Schiller 1995). While its sensory encoding properties are slightly less well understood than those in MT, it probably is the area in visual cortex most extensively studied for its modulation by attention.

FEATURE-BASED ATTENTION: THE BEGINNINGS

Initial investigations of neuronal activity in striate and extrastriate visual cortex of awake monkeys, following the ground-breaking work by Hubel and Wiesel in the 1960s, have focused on the sensory encoding of neurons, i.e. the relationship between stimulus properties and the firing rate of individual neurons (captured by the tuning of individual neurons to specific stimulus dimensions). Fortunately, we can now look back at more than two decades in which the research focus has shifted towards studies of attentional modulation, i.e. at how the responses of these neurons to visual stimuli are modulated by the behavioural relevance of the stimulus. A majority of these studies have focused on spatial attention (see the corresponding chapters in this book for reviews). But even some of the earliest studies of influences on V4 responses by factors other than the stimulus properties, so-called extra-retinal effects, documented non-spatial influences of behavioural relevance. An early example are studies where monkeys were shown a series of visual gratings and were trained to respond to gratings that matched the orientation of a cue grating presented at the start of each trial (Haenny et al. 1988; Maunsell et al. 1991). Over half the neurons recorded in V4 had responses that varied depending on which orientation the animal was seeking, even if the cue orientation was only provided to the monkey's tactile system via a grooved plate or bar (Haenny et al. 1988; Maunsell et al. 1991).

Motter (1994a, 1994b) trained monkeys to do a task in which they viewed arrays of mixed stimuli. At an intermediate point in each trial the monkey was provided with some information allowing the animal to focus its attention on the subset of stimuli whose colour or luminance matched a cue stimulus. Most of the responses recorded from V4 neurons were stronger when the stimulus in their receptive field belonged to the selected subset, i.e. matched the feature of the cue. Although this modulation was based on the visual feature that the animal was attending to, this task represents an example of a study where spatial attention may have played a role: It is possible that the change in neuronal activity reflected a spatial selection of those locations that the animal identified as behaviourally relevant based on colour or luminance.

Feature-based attention as a modulation across visual space

The first direct and unambiguous documentation of the systematic modulation of single cell responses in visual cortex by feature-based attention was achieved in area MT, an area that traditionally had been thought to be devoid of extra-retinal influences (Newsome et al. 1988) and where attentional modulations correspondingly had been found much later than in V4 (Treue and Maunsell 1996; Seidemann and Newsome 1999). In a series of studies, Martinez-Trujillo and Treue (Treue and Martinez-Trujillo 1999, 2004) presented a stimulus inside the receptive field moving in the preferred or anti-preferred direction while the rhesus monkey attended to a stimulus in the opposite hemifield that could also move either in the preferred or null direction (Fig. 21.1a). They found that changes in the direction of motion that the animal was attending modulated the response to the behaviourally irrelevant stimulus in the receptive field. Attention to motion in the preferred direction resulted in responses that were on average 13% stronger than those when the animal's attention was on the anti-preferred direction. This modulation was independent of whether the direction inside the receptive field was a match to the attended direction or not. The response in trials where the animal had to attend to the fixation point fell in between the two attentional condition responses.

Feature-based attention within the receptive field

Because in these studies the attended stimulus was far outside the receptive field it was straightforward to change the attended feature as different stimulus directions could be used without them changing a given neuron's sensory response, a prerequisite to be able to interpret changes in neuronal responses as effects of the change in attentional state. For investigating feature-based attention inside the receptive field this is much more difficult to achieve. This is exemplified by the classical spatial attention experiment of Moran and Desimone (1985). They positioned two oriented bars (one with the preferred and one with a less preferred orientation) inside the receptive field of a neuron in area V4 of rhesus monkeys trained in a match-to-sample attentional task and observed that

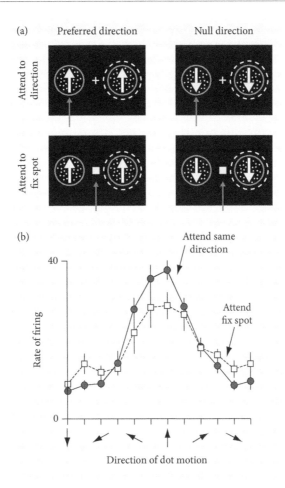

FIGURE 21.1 Feature-based attention in MT. (a) Schematic representation of tasks used to assess the effects of feature-based attention to a direction of motion. Two moving sets of random dot patterns were presented within stationary apertures, one within the receptive field of the neurons being recorded (dashed white line). On a given trial the patches always moved in the same direction, but different directions of motion were presented on different trials. On some trials (lower row) the animal's attention (grey arrows) was directed to the fixation spot to detect a change in luminance. On other trials (upper row), the animal was instructed to pay attention to the motion of the patch outside the receptive field to detect a change in that motion. (b) Responses of a representative MT neuron to different directions of motion during the two states of attention. Attention to the preferred direction of motion increased the neuron's response, but attention to the null direction of motion decreased its response. Thus, attention to a particular direction of motion does not increase responses across all neurons. Rather, it has a push–pull effect that increases responses only for neurons that prefer motion close to the attended direction. Adapted from *Trends in Neurosciences*, 29 (6), John H. R. Maunsell and Stefan Treue, Feature-based attention in visual cortex, pp. 317–22, Copyright (2006), with permission from Elsevier.

when the animals were spatially cued to direct their attention to one of the stimuli, the neurons increased their responses when attention was on the preferred stimulus (i.e. the one producing a strong response) and reduced their response when attention was on the less preferred stimulus (i.e. the one that produced a weaker response) (Moran and Desimone 1985). This effect seemed to indicate a reduced influence of the unattended stimulus on a neuron's response. Moran and Desimone hypothesized that the mechanism underlying this non-sensory response modulation was a change in the neurons' receptive field profile. Essentially, the neurons responded as if the receptive field had shifted towards and shrunk around the attended stimulus, effectively excluding the unattended stimulus from the receptive field. The hypothesized attentional distortions in the spatial profile of receptive fields have indeed been shown (Connor et al. 1997; Womelsdorf et al. 2006, 2008; Anton-Erxleben 2009; Niebergall et al. 2011; see also other chapters on spatial attention). But the discovery of feature-based attention offers an alternative or additional possible explanation for the modulation observed by Moran and Desimone, as their paradigm did not only involve a shift of the spatial spotlight of attention but also a switch between a preferred and a non-preferred stimulus. Thus the attentional response modulation observed could reflect this change in feature similarity without a need to invoke a change in the receptive field profile.

To disentangle these two types of visual attention Patzwahl and Treue (2009) used superimposed random dot patterns moving in opposite directions positioned inside the receptive field of MT neurons and instructed monkeys to attend to one of the random dot patterns and ignore the other. In this design, a shrinking of receptive fields could not account for the attentional modulation of responses since the two moving sets of dots were fully superimposed and both in the fixation disparity plane. Patzwahl and Treue observed an average attentional modulation of responses of about 30% when the animals switched attention from the anti-preferred to the preferred direction, which was about half of that observed when the random dot patterns were spatially separated inside the receptive field of the same neurons. This suggests a combined effect of spatial attention (perhaps equivalent to a shrinking of the receptive field) and feature-based attention.

Core aspects of feature-based attention

The data described above document several core aspects of the neural correlate of feature-based attention that have later been confirmed and extended in other cortical areas (McAdams and Maunsell 2000; Hayden and Gallant 2009), and for which behavioural correlates have been found in human psychophysical studies (see Scolari, Ester, and Serences (chapter 20), this volume chapter): (1) feature-based attention spreads across the visual field as the response modulation was observed in neurons whose receptive field was in the visual hemifield opposite to the attended stimulus; (2) feature-based attention enhances responses of neurons whose feature-preference matches the attended feature while it suppresses responses of those neurons with opposite feature-preference;

(3) feature-based attention does not reflect a match between the attended stimulus feature and the stimulus feature in a given receptive field, even though the consequence of feature-based attention across a population of neurons is the selective enhancement of stimuli whose features match the attended feature; (4) feature-based and spatial attention effects combine quasi-linearly creating the largest response enhancement for attended stimuli that are matching a neuron's feature preference (such as the preferred direction or orientation) and a neuron's spatial preference (i.e. fall in the neuron's receptive field); and (5) the attentional modulation seems to reflect a gain change, creating a multiplicative change in neuronal responses as has been observed for spatial attention.

The feature-similarity gain model of attention

The similarities between feature-based and space-based attention raise the possibility that they are simply different sides of the same coin. This has led to the 'feature-similarity gain model' proposed by Treue and Martinez-Trujillo (1999), in which the attentional change in the gain of a visual neuron depends on the similarity of the features of the current behaviourally relevant target and the response selectivities of the neuron. Similarity might be based on the spatial location or any other feature. Thus, the responses of all those neurons would be enhanced whose sensory selectivity matched the current attentional state (i.e. feature-similarity for the non-spatial feature), and similarly, independent of their stimulus selectivity the responses of all those neurons would be enhanced whose receptive fields overlapped an attended location in the visual field (i.e. feature-similarity for location). These similarities can be combined creating a particularly large gain increase (or decrease) for neurons whose spatial and non-spatial preferences in total provide a large (or small) degree of similarity to the attentional target.

To match the physiological properties listed above, in this scheme stimulus properties determine the basic sensory response of a neuron but not the sign or magnitude of the attentional modulation. That modulation is a gain change that is independent of the stimulus driving the neuron; in fact a stimulus is not even needed, either in the receptive field (as most neurons show some firing even in the absence of any stimulus) or at the attended location (as long as the subject is allocating attention even without a stimulus to focus it on). This could account for the attentional modulations that have been reported in the absence of sensory stimulation (Luck et al. 1997; Reynolds et al. 2000; McMains et al. 2007). The general framework of the feature-similarity gain model can account for a wide range of effects of attention on single-unit responses (Boynton 2005).

It is important to note that while the attentional modulation hypothesized by the feature-similarity gain model (and many other attentional models) is a gain change, in a given attentional condition this gain change will vary across a set of neurons presented with a stimulus as the feature-similarity will be different for every neuron, depending on the relationship between the attended feature and the individual neuron's preference. Therefore the population response to an attended stimulus will be a non-multiplicatively modulated version of the response to the same stimulus when it is unattended (Fig. 21.1).

Feature-based attention during visual search

Visual search is one task where feature-based attention (possibly in conjunction with a moving spatial attentional 'spotlight') should be particularly valuable. Chelazzi and his colleagues (1998, 2001) showed that the activity of individual V4 and inferotemporal neurons is modulated when monkeys search for different targets. For each neuron they recorded, they identified two images. On each trial they cued the animal to respond to one of two stimuli presented within the receptive field of the neuron: one that generated a relatively strong response and one that generated a relatively weak response. Shortly before the animal's response, neural activity was stronger when the searched-for stimulus was the neuron's preferred stimulus. While these findings are consistent with feature-based attention, a more parsimonious explanation accounts for the observed modulation by spatial attention. The enhanced response to preferred stimulus targets shortly before the monkey signalled its choice would then be the animal's 'spotlight of attention', enhancing the effectiveness of the attended stimulus at the expense of the representation of the distractor.

A more recent study (Bichot et al. 2005) was able to avoid this alternative explanation for attentional modulation during a visual search task. Monkeys were trained to search for a target with a particular colour or a particular shape in a crowded display and were allowed to freely move their gaze. Responses were recorded during the brief periods between saccades, when a known stimulus lay in the receptive field of the neuron being recorded. The critical responses were those recorded when the target stimulus fell in the receptive field of the neuron being recorded, but was not detected by the animal, who made an eye movement elsewhere and continued the search. These responses could be compared directly with those recorded on other trials in which the same stimulus was a distractor. Almost all the neurons Bichot et al. examined gave a larger response when the stimulus in their receptive field matched the cued feature, with a median increase of 30%. These investigators also looked at the effects of attention on the local field potential (LFP). Although the firing rate of individual V4 neurons was affected by feature-based attention, there was no effect on the magnitude of the LFP. However, the coherence between the spikes of individual neurons and the LFP increased in the gamma band (30–60 Hz) when animals searched for the stimulus preferred by neurons at the recording site. Thus, feature-based attention matches spatial attention, for which influences on the synchrony of neuronal firing have been documented (Fries et al. 2001).

Normalization models of attention and feature-based attention

The early investigations of attentional modulation in visual cortex led to descriptive models designed to allow qualitative predictions. The most influential of these frameworks is the 'biased competition model' (BCM) proposed by Desimone and Duncan (1995; see also Reynolds et al. 1999). The feature-similarity model (FSM) of attention described above differs from the BCM in that the BCM sees attention as a mechanism to influence the competition between various objects in a visual scene for neural represen-tation while the FSM interprets attention as a mechanism that changes the distribution of response gains of neurons across a whole population of neurons, independently of the stimuli that might be present in the visual field. Despite these conceptual differences both models provide good descriptive accounts of most of the known electrophysiologi-cal effects of attention in visual cortex.

More recently a number of laboratories have proposed more quantitative models of attention (Ghose and Maunsell 2008; Boynton 2009; Ghose 2009; Lee and Maunsell 2009, 2010; Reynolds and Heeger 2009) that are unified by the central role that they attribute to response normalization, the observation that the response of sensory neurons in visual cortex does not increase linearly with increasing stimulus strength, numerosity, or size. While these models differ in where and how the normalization is implemented, they agree in that attentional effects are caused by a systematic manipula-tion of the response normalization process. They also provide quantitative implementa-tions of the BCM and the FSM.

Beyond features: Switching attention between dimensions

Feature-based attention is usually used to denote modulations in neural responses when attention is switched between different features, i.e. between particular properties within a given stimulus dimension (e.g. upwards motion is a feature within the stimulus dimension of motion, and blue is a feature within the stimulus dimension of colour). As it is not uncommon that neurons in visual cortex show tuning for more than one dimen-sion, some experiments have employed dimension switches and found attentional effects that are similar to those observed with feature switches.

An early example is a study of McAdams and Maunsell (2000). They showed effects of shifting attention between the dimensions of colour and orientation. Responses were recorded from V4 neurons with a stimulus of the preferred orientation in the receptive field. In one condition the animal was required to attend to the orientation of another stimulus in a distant location. In a second condition the animal was required to attend to the colour of an unoriented stimulus in the distant location. The responses of most V4 neurons were affected by shifting attention between orientations and colours. Just as has been observed for feature-based attention this result shows an attentional modulation of the neural representations of stimuli in parts of the visual field that have no relevance to the task.

A recent study from the same laboratory (Cohen and Maunsell 2011) used a match-to-sample design where the animals were directed to pay attention to either ori-entation or spatial frequency, rather than one orientation versus another. Nevertheless when looking at comparable indices they found the attentional effects to be similar to those previously reported for feature-based attention. In addition, by recording from a large number of neurons across two hemispheres simultaneously, they were able to show that fluctuations in feature-based attention (but not spatial attention) are coordinated across hemispheres, consistent with distribution of the neuronal preference for a given feature across a cortical area and its contralateral equivalent and the concentration of spatial preference in one location of the retinotopic map within a cortical area. Providing evidence that spatial attention and feature-based attention are behaviourally independent, even though they might each employ the same physiological modulation mechanisms Cohen and Maunsell (2011) also showed that the strength of the two types of attention can fluctuate independently over time. This latter observation is consistent with the observation by Hayden and Gallant (2009) that spatial and feature-based attention do not strongly interact but rather are combined quasi-linearly.

BEYOND FEATURES AND DIMENSIONS: OBJECT-BASED ATTENTION

We are able to attend to a spatial location, a stimulus feature, or a stimulus dimension. It is conceptually straightforward to see how such attentional allocation would systematically modulate sensory neurons in visual cortex. Their preference for location (embodied by their receptive field), for features (embodied by their feature-tuning curves within certain stimulus dimensions), and for dimensions (embodied by giving tuned responses in some dimensions and not in others) ensures that for typical cases of attention to a particular visual object a set of neurons exists which matches the attended object's properties (both in space and in terms of non-spatial properties). As has been outlined above, these are the neurons whose gain is typically increased, while the sensory gain of those neurons with widely differing preferences is typically reduced. Conceptually the neural basis is less clear for another form of visual attention, namely object-based attention. Beginning with the initial investigation by Duncan (1984), psychophysical and brain imaging studies have documented that the perceptual grouping of individual stimulus features into visual objects can influence the allocation of attention (see Scolari, Ester, and Serences (chapter 20), this volume for a full review). In a typical psychophysical demonstration of object-based attention, two or more visual objects are superimposed, such that spatial attention cannot be used to guide the allocation of attention. In such paradigms, features belonging to the same object are generally processed faster and more accurately than features belonging to different objects. Strong evidence for the existence of object-based attentional mechanisms has also been provided by imaging studies comparing activity in functionally defined regions of interest. Here, the visual features of superimposed objects are carefully chosen to differentially activate well-defined cortical regions. Attending to a particular feature can result not only in enhanced activity within the cortical region processing the attended feature, but also in enhanced activity within regions processing other task-irrelevant features of the same object. Therefore, in contrast to feature-based attention, object-based attention is characterized by a transfer of attention from attended to unattended features of the same object, thereby enhancing the processing of even those features that are currently irrelevant (e.g. O'Craven et al. 1999; Blaser et al. 2000). In physiological experiments, it has been difficult to design paradigms that specifically target the neural correlates of object-based attention at the single neuron level. This difficulty is partly because at least up to mid-level, extrastriate cortex neurons do not seem to be tuned to the complex amalgamation of features that make up an object but rather respond to individual features of objects, making it conceptually more difficult to see how object-based attention could be implemented in such visual areas.

Three lines of single-unit studies that have overcome these problems shall be discussed here. The first, and by far the most extensive series of experiments has been conducted by Roelfsema and his colleagues (Roelfsema et al. 1998; Khayat et al. 2006). They recorded responses in primary visual cortex of rhesus monkeys trained to mentally trace one of two curved lines while keeping fixation on one of its endpoints. The animal's motivation for tracing the curve was a search for its endpoint, which the animal had been taught to saccade to. The core finding of these experiments was that the multi-unit activity of V1 recording sites overlapping with different segments of the line was enhanced if the curve crossing the receptive fields was behaviourally relevant as opposed to when it was not. Furthermore the enhancement occurred earlier if the receptive field was close to the beginning of the traced line, suggesting that a spatial process was moving along the line as the animal traced the attended line to find its endpoint for saccade planning. Such findings indicate that responses of neurons in area V1 can depend on whether the stimulus inside their receptive field is part of an attended object.

In a quite different approach, Wannig and colleagues (2007) used moving surfaces as simple visual objects. They trained rhesus monkeys to attend to one of two superimposed moving random dot patterns rotating in opposite directions. This stimulus creates the percept of two surfaces sliding across each other. After rotating for some period, the two dot patterns briefly changed to linear motion, each surface moving in a different randomly selected direction. The monkeys reported the direction of linear motion in the target pattern by making a speeded eye movement in the corresponding direction. Using variants of this paradigm, psychophysical studies of attention in humans have provided strong support for the existence of a surface- or object-based selection mechanism (Valdes-Sosa et al. 2000; and Scolari, Ester, and Serences (chapter 20), this volume).

Wannig et al. (2007) report that the response of MT neurons to the linear motion period was stronger if those dots had been part of the attended rotation direction than when they belonged to the unattended rotating surface. Because of the complete spatial overlap of the two sets of dots this finding provides a physiological demonstration of a non-spatial modulation of responses inside the 'spotlight of attention' in the dorsal pathway, consistent with similar effects reported in the ventral pathway (Fallah et al. 2007) and for overlapping linear motions in MT (Patzwahl and Treue 2009; see above). Contrary to these two studies, Wannig et al.'s (2007) results suggest a high-level binding between the attended dots moving along a circular path and the same dots that suddenly change to a linear motion. Such a binding over time is a requirement for tracking objects over time and through changes in their visual properties.

In a third approach for documenting the neural correlate of object-based attention at the single-neuron level Katzner and colleagues (2009) trained rhesus monkeys to attend either to the colour (responding to colour changes while ignoring irrelevant direction changes) or to the linear motion direction (responding to direction changes while ignoring irrelevant colour changes) of a random dot pattern moving within a stationary aperture. The motion direction was either in the neuron's preferred or anti-preferred direction while the two colours used were isoluminant, i.e. were not differentially preferred by the neuron. In the core experiment of the study the attended pattern was placed outside of a given MT receptive field while the neuron was driven by a second, behaviourally irrelevant moving pattern inside the receptive field. The authors report that the MT neurons showed an enhanced response whenever the attended stimulus was moving in the preferred direction. This is expected whenever the animal's task was to attend to the pattern's motion direction based on the global spread of feature-based attention to motion direction in area MT. On the other hand the observation that attending to the colour of the pattern created a modulation based on the pattern's direction suggests an involuntary transfer of attention from the attended feature (colour) to the unattended feature (direction), one of the hallmarks of object-based attention.

Generating an attentionally modulated topographic representation of the visual environment

Combining the insights gained from single-unit studies of visual attention it is possible to infer the response modulation of a population of neurons with receptive fields at various positions and preferring various values for a particular feature (such as orientation in V4 neurons or direction of motion in MT) caused when attention is directed to a particular stimulus feature at a particular location in a complex visual scene. Let us imagine a scenario where the visual input creates a fairly homogeneous level of activation across the neuronal population. Spatial attention will increase the gain of all neurons whose receptive field overlaps the current attentional focus, creating an enhanced representation at that location. Note that according to the feature-similarity hypothesis this modulation of the retinotopic population would produce a range of modulations because neurons whose receptive fields only partially overlap the focus of attention will experience less of a gain increase than those centred on the focus, a prediction not tested experimentally so far.

In addition to this modulation at the location of the focus of attention in the retinotopic representation of the visual input comes the effect of the attended non-spatial feature. This will cause a differential gain change across the whole retinotopic representation with a particularly strong gain increase for neurons preferring the attended feature and a gain decrease for those of opposite preference. The total effect will be a population response that is no longer homogeneous but has its highest activity in the group of neurons preferring the attended location and feature, intermediate enhancements at retinotopic locations where the visual input matches the attended feature (i.e. potential targets in a visual search situation), and suppressed responses everywhere else.

Combining such modulated population responses across cortical areas could create an integrated saliency map or priority map, that is, a topographic representation of relative stimulus strength and behavioural relevance across visual space (Treue 2003; Maunsell and Treue 2006; Bisley 2011).

The generation of this attentionally enhanced representation of attended objects would be aided by the transfer of attention from relevant to irrelevant stimulus features, within an attended object and across the visual field (Treue and Katzner 2009). By extending the modulation to features that are not directly attended but simply associated with the attended object the system allows for a more sophisticated, multi-dimensional modulation profile across visual space, because the gain change applied to the inputs at a given location in the integrated saliency map would reflect the overlap between *all* features of an attended object and the features present at the given location. As a consequence, the highest attentional gain would apply to those locations in the map that contain objects most like the attended object, without any need to explicitly invoke a sophisticated object-recognition system (Kaping et al. 2007).

Wiring up and guiding attentional modulation to features

Creating complex differential attentional effects across a population of neurons raises the question of how this can be achieved by top-down input from centres responsible for the allocation of attention. For space-based attention, one could imagine a specialized visuotopic map that represents which parts of visual space are currently of greatest behavioural relevance: an attention map. Such a representation of behaviourally relevant locations might be activated by knowledge of the environment, or by interactions between such knowledge and current sensory signals (see Itti and Koch 2001). Excitatory connections between sites in a visuotopic map of attention and neurons in visual cortex with receptive fields in corresponding locations could mediate modulations of sensory responses by space-based attention. Functional imaging studies have identified topographic organization related to spatial attention in parietal and frontal cortex that might serve this purpose (Gitelman et al. 1999; Astafiev et al. 2003). Moore and Armstrong (2003) activated what seems to be part of such a system when they microstimulated the frontal eye field and observed retinotopically matched enhancements in V4 that resembled those observed in attentional studies.

It is more difficult to envision the implementation of feature-based attention. While spatial attention involves the two or possibly three (He and Nakayama 1995; Kasai et al. 2003) dimensions of visual space, a subject might pay attention to any of a potentially enormous number of stimulus features. The brain may be unable to maintain neurons devoted to representing the behavioural relevance of each of these features. For spatial attention, Moore and Armstrong's stimulation of the frontal eye field suggests that a spatial map of attention might be used to enhance the responses of neurons throughout the visual cortex that had receptive fields overlying the attended location (Moore and Armstrong 2003). An analogous arrangement for feature-based attention would require representations for each feature that might be attended (orientation, colour, curvature, patterns, shapes, etc.), such that activation of such a representation (reflecting the allocation of attention to a particular feature value) would modulate the activity of neurons throughout visual cortex that were selective for the particular feature.

Maintaining the analogy to the control of attentional modulation exerted by spatial attention onto sensory areas, two issues appear. First, efficient implementation of top-down control of feature attention might require a topographic organization for the attended feature and a systematic tuning of sensory neurons along the feature. For spatial location these requirements are fulfilled by the retinotopic organization and the well-defined spatial receptive fields in early visual cortex. A topographic organization has been documented for some stimulus features, such as motion direction and stereoscopic disparity (Albright et al. 1984; DeAngelis and Newsome 1999), but it is not known if representations of most features are topographically organized. For neuronal representations of complex features in inferotemporal cortex there is much debate what the tuning dimensions may be (Gross 1969; Gross et al. 1972; Richmond et al. 1983; Desimone et al. 1984; Kobatake and Tanaka 1994).

Second, an important constraint might be the numbers of neurons that would be needed to represent the behavioural relevance of all features. If the attentional resolution needs to be high it seems reasonable to assume that the representation of the behavioural relevance of a feature would require as many neurons as contribute to the sensory representation of that feature. If so, then the behavioural relevance of some features could be represented quite efficiently, but for others we lack the data for such an estimate. For example, the behavioural relevance of features represented in V1 (low-level orientations, colours, etc.) might be accomplished by a hypercolumn-sized piece of cortex. This is because each hypercolumn in V1 contains a complete representation of the encoded features, with the other hypercolumns replicating this representation for other retinal positions. Applying such an estimate to the features only represented in higher areas of extrastriate cortex appears currently impossible given the lack of understanding about feature representations in those areas.

It is possible that representing the behavioural relevance of all the features represented in visual cortex would require more neurons than the brain could afford. Therefore, a critical question is what limits there are on the types of features to which one can direct attention. To our knowledge, no experimental evidence addresses the capacity of feature-based attention. Feature-based attention, and the neuronal representations on which it depends, might be limited to a subset of features that frequently demand attention, such as colours and orientations, and not work for all features that are readily discriminated. Studies that investigate which features are topographically represented might provide important insights. With plasticity, it might be possible to reserve the ability to generate representations that might support attention to any feature, or perhaps combinations of features, after practice. Behavioural improvements in searching for certain patterns with practice (see Wolfe 1998) are consistent with this idea. It will be important to learn more about the limits of feature-based attention as we try to understand how attention is implemented in neuronal representations.

CLOSING COMMENTS

In summary, feature-based and object-based attention are selective modulation processes that, just like spatial attention, affect the responses of sensory neurons throughout the visual cortex of primates. It is an open issue whether the similarity of spatial attention and feature-based attentional effects reflects a unified attentional system that treats the location of a stimulus as one of its features, or whether spatial attention, feature-based attention, and object-based attention, while occurring simultaneously and additively, are separate, increasingly complex processes that jointly constitute physiological mechanisms for changing the gain of cortical neurons. Together, these forms of attention create, without the need to rely on a sophisticated preliminary analysis of the input (such as object segmentation and recognition or long-range stimulus comparisons), an integrated saliency map of the visual input, a representation of the visual environment that enhances aspects that match the current behavioural preference at the expense of the vast portion of the input that is behaviourally irrelevant. Such a representation is an important component for a visual system that needs to concentrate its limited processing resources on the most relevant sensory inputs.

ACKNOWLEDGEMENTS

Preparation of this manuscript was supported by the German Ministry for Education and Science grant BMBF 01GQ1005C to the Bernstein Center for Computational Neuroscience, Göttingen and the DFG Collaborative Research Center 889 'Cellular Mechanisms of Sensory Processing'.

REFERENCES

Albright, T. D., Desimone, R., and Gross, C. G. (1984). Columnar organization of directionally selective cells in visual area MT of the macaque. *Journal of Neurophysiology 51*: 16–31.

Anton-Erxleben, K., Stephan, V. M., and Treue, S. (2009). Attention reshapes center-surround receptive field structure in macaque cortical area MT. *Cerebral Cortex 19*: 2466–2478.

Astafiev, S. V., Shulman, G. L., Stanley, C. M., Snyder, A. Z., Van Essen, D. C., and Corbetta, M. (2003). Functional organization of human intraparietal and frontal cortex for attending, looking, and pointing. *Journal of Neuroscience 23*: 4689–4699.

Beauchamp, M. S., Cox, R. W., and Deyoe, E. A. (1997). Graded effects of spatial and featural attention on human area MT and associated motion processing areas. *Journal of Neurophysiology 78*: 516–520.

Bichot, N. P., Rossi, A. F. and Desimone, R. (2005). Parallel and serial neural mechanisms for visual search in macaque area V4. *Science 308*: 529–534.

Bisley, J. W. (2011). The neural basis of visual attention. *Journal of Physiology* 589: 49–57.

Blaser, E., Pylyshyn, Z. W., and Holcombe, A. O. (2000). Tracking an object through feature space. *Nature 408*: 196–199.

Boynton, G. M. (2005). Attention and visual perception. *Current Opinion in Neurobiology* 15: 465–469.

Boynton, G. M. (2009). A framework for describing the effects of attention on visual responses. *Vision Research 49*: 1129–1143.

Britten, K. H., Newsome, W. T., Shadlen, M. N., Celebrini, S., and Movshon, J. A. (1996). A relationship between behavioral choice and the visual responses of neurons in macaque MT. *Visual Neuroscience 13*: 87–100.

Chelazzi, L., Duncan, J., Miller, E. K., and Desimone, R. (1998). Responses of neurons in inferior temporal cortex during memory-guided visual search. *Journal of Neurophysiology 80*: 2918–2940.

Chelazzi, L., Miller, E. K., Duncan, J., and Desimone, R. (2001). Responses of neurons in macaque area V4 during memory-guided visual search. *Cerebral Cortex 11*: 761–772.

Cohen, M. R. and Maunsell, J. H. (2011). Using neuronal populations to study the mechanisms underlying spatial and feature attention. *Neuron 70*: 1192–1204.

Connor, C. E., Preddie, D. C., Gallant, J. L., and Van Essen, D. C. (1997). Spatial attention effects in macaque area V4. *Journal of Neuroscience 17*: 3201–3214.

Corbetta, M., Miezin, F. M., Dobmeyer, S., Shulman, G. L., and Petersen, S. E. (1990). Attentional modulation of neural processing of shape, color, and velocity in humans. *Science 248*: 1556–1559.

DeAngelis, G. C. and Newsome, W. T. (1999). Organization of disparity-selective neurons in macaque area MT. *Journal of Neuroscience 19*: 1398–1415.

Desimone, R., Albright, T. D., Gross, C. G., and Bruce, C. (1984). Stimulus-selective properties of inferior temporal neurons in the macaque. *Journal of Neuroscience 4*: 2051–2062.

Duncan, J. (1984). Selective attention and the organization of visual information. *Journal of Experimental Psychology: General 113*: 501–517.

Fallah, M., Stoner, G. R., and Reynolds, J. H. (2007). Stimulus-specific competitive selection in macaque extrastriate visual area V4. *Proceedings of the National Academy of Sciences USA 104*: 4165–4169.

Fries, P., Reynolds, J. H., Rorie, A. E., and Desimone, R. (2001). Modulation of oscillatory neuronal synchronization by selective visual attention. *Science 291*: 1560–1563.

Ghose, G. M. (2009). Attentional modulation of visual responses by flexible input gain. *Journal of Neurophysiology 101*: 2089–2106.

Ghose, G. M. and Maunsell, J. H. (2008). Spatial summation can explain the attentional modulation of neuronal responses to multiple stimuli in area V4. *Journal of Neuroscience 28*: 5115–5126.

Gitelman, D. R., Nobre, A. C., Parrish, T. B., Labar, K. S., Kim, Y. H., Meyer, J. R., and Mesulam, M. M. (1999). A large-scale distributed network for covert spatial attention: Further anatomical delineation based on stringent behavioral and cognitive controls. *Brain 122*: 1093–1106.

Gross, C. G., Bender, D. B., and Rocha-Miranda, C. E. (1969). Visual receptive fields of neurons in inferotemporal cortex of the monkey. *Science, 166*: 1303–1306.

Gross, C. G., Rocha-Miranda, C. E., and Bender, D. B. (1972). Visual properties of neurons in inferotemporal cortex of the macaque. *Journal of Neurophysiology 35*: 96–111.

Haenny, P. E., Maunsell, J. H. R., and Schiller, P. H. (1988). State dependent activity in monkey visual cortex II: Retinal and extraretinal factors in V4. *Experimental Brain Research 69*: 245–259.

Hayden, B. Y. and Gallant, J. L. (2009). Combined effects of spatial and feature-based attention on responses of V4 neurons. *Vision Research 49*: 1182–1187.

He, Z. J. and Nakayama, K. (1995). Visual-attention to surfaces in 3-dimensional space. *Proceedings of the National Academy of Sciences USA 92*: 11155–11159.

Itti, L. and Koch, C. (2001). Computational modelling of visual attention. *Nature Reviews Neuroscience 2*: 194–203.

Kaping, D., Tzvetanov, T., and Treue, S. (2007). Adaptation to statistical properties of visual scenes biases rapid categorization. *Visual Cognition 15*: 12–19.

Kasai, T., Morotomi, T., Katayama, J., and Kumada, T. (2003). Attending to a location in three-dimensional space modulates early ERPs. *Cognitive Brain Research 17*: 273–385.

Katzner, S., Busse, L., and Treue, S. (2009) Attention to the color of a moving stimulus modulates motion-signal processing in macaque area MT: Evidence for a unified attentional system. *Frontiers in Systems Neuroscience, 3*: 12.

Khayat, P. S., Spekreijse, H., and Roelfsema, P. R. (2006). Attention lights up new object representations before the old ones fade away. *Journal of Neuroscience 26*: 138–142.

Kobatake, E. and Tanaka, K. (1994). Neuronal selectivities to complex object features in the ventral visual pathway of the macaque cerebral cortex. *Journal of Neurophysiology 71*: 856–867.

Lee, J. and Maunsell, J. H. (2009). A normalization model of attentional modulation of single unit responses. *PLoS One 4*: e4651.

Lee, J. and Maunsell, J. H. (2010). Attentional modulation of MT neurons with single or multiple stimuli in their receptive fields. *Journal of Neuroscience 30*: 3058–3066.

Liu, T., Larsson, J., and Carrasco, M. (2007). Feature-based attention modulates orientation-selective responses in human visual cortex. *Neuron 55*: 313–323.

Luck, S. J., Chelazzi, L., Hillyard, S. A., and Desimone, R. (1997). Neural mechanisms of spatial selective attention in areas V1, V2, and V4 of macaque visual cortex. *Journal of Neurophysiology 77*: 24–42.

McAdams, C. J. and Maunsell, J. H. R. (1999). Effects of attention on orientation-tuning functions of single neurons in Macaque cortical area V4. *Journal of Neuroscience 19*: 431–441.

McAdams, C. J. and Maunsell, J. H. R. (2000). Attention to both space and feature modulates neuronal responses in macaque area V4. *Journal of Neurophysiology 83*: 1751–1755.

McMains, S. A., Fehd, H. M., Emmanouil, T. A., and Kastner, S. (2007). Mechanisms of feature- and space-based attention: Response modulation and baseline increases. *Journal of Neurophysiology 98*: 2110–2121.

Martinez-Trujillo, J. C. and Treue, S. (2004). Feature-based attention increases the selectivity of population responses in primate visual cortex. *Current Biology 14*: 744–751.

Maunsell, J. H. R. and Cook, E. P. (2002). The role of attention in visual processing. *Philosophical Transactions of the Royal Society B: Biological Sciences 357*: 1063–1072.

Maunsell, J. H. R., Sclar, G., Nealey, T. A., and De Priest, D. D. (1991). Extraretinal representations in area V4 in the macaque monkey. *Visual Neuroscience 7*: 561–573.

Maunsell, J. H. R. and Treue, S. (2006). Feature-based attention in visual cortex. *Trends in Neurosciences 29*: 317–322.

Moore, T. and Armstrong, K. M. (2003). Selective gating of visual signals by microstimulation of frontal cortex. *Nature 421*: 370–373.

Motter, B. C. (1994a). Neural correlates of attentive selection for color or luminance in extrastriate area V4. *Journal of Neuroscience 14*: 2178–2189.

Motter, B. C. (1994b). Neural correlates of feature selective memory and pop-out in extrastriate area V4. *Journal of Neuroscience 14*: 2190–2199.

Moran, J. and Desimone, R. (1985). Selective attention gates visual processing in the extrastriate cortex. *Science 229*: 782–784.

Newsome, W. T. and Paré, E. B. (1988). A selective impairment of motion perception following lesions of the middle temporal visual area (MT). *Journal of Neuroscience 8*: 2201–2211.

Niebergall, R., Khayat, P. S., Treue, S., and Martinez-Trujillo, J. C. (2011). Expansion of MT neurons excitatory receptive fields during covert attentive tracking. *Journal of Neuroscience 31*: 15499–15510.

O'Craven, K. M., Downing, P. E., and Kanwisher, N. (1999). fMRI evidence for objects as the units of attentional selection. *Nature 401*: 584–587.

Patzwahl, D. and Treue, S. (2009). Combining spatial and feature-based attention within the receptive field of MT neurons. *Vision Research 49*: 1188–1193.

Reynolds, J. and Heeger, D. J. (2009). The normalization model of attention. *Neuron 61*: 168–185.

Reynolds, J. H., Pasternak, T., and Desimone, R. (2000). Attention increases sensitivity of V4 neurons. *Neuron 26*: 703–714.

Richmond, B. J., Wurtz, R. H., and Sato, T. (1983). Visual responses of inferior temporal neurons in awake rhesus monkey. *Journal of Neurophysiology 50*: 1415–1432.

Roelfsema, P. R., Lamme, V. A. F., and Spekreijse, H. (1998). Object-based attention in the primary visual cortex of the macaque monkey. *Nature 395*: 376–381.

Saenz, M., Buracas, G. T., and Boynton, G. M. (2002). Global effects of feature-based attention in human visual cortex. *Nature Neuroscience 5*: 631–632.

Schiller, P. H. (1995). Effect of lesions in visual cortical area V4 on the recognition of transformed objects. *Nature 376*: 342–344.

Schiller, P. H. and Lee, K. (1991). The role of primate extrastriate area V4 in vision. *Science 251*: 1251–1253.

Seidemann, E. and Newsome, W. T. (1999). Effect of spatial attention on the responses of area MT. *Journal of Neurophysiology 81*: 1783–1794.

Serences, J. T. and Boynton, G. M. (2007). Feature-based attentional modulations in the absence of direct visual stimulation. *Neuron 55*: 301–312.

Shulman, G. L., Ollinger, J. M., Akbudak, E., Conturo, T. E., Snyder, A. Z., Petersen, S. E., and Corbetta, M. (1999). Areas involved in encoding and applying directional expectations to moving objects. *Journal of Neuroscience 19*: 9480–9496.

Treue, S. (2003). Visual attention: The where, what, how and why of saliency. *Current Opinion in Neurobiology 13*: 428–432.

Treue, S. and Katzner, S. (2009). Visual attention. In L. Squire (ed.), *Encyclopedia of Neuroscience* (pp. 243–250). San Diego: Elsevier.

Treue, S. and Martinez-Trujillo, J. C. (1999). Feature-based attention influences motion processing gain in macaque visual cortex. *Nature 399*: 575–579.

Treue, S. and Maunsell, J. H. R. (1996). Attentional modulation of visual motion processing in cortical areas MT and MST. *Nature 382*: 539–541.

Valdes-Sosa, M., Cobo, A., and Pinilla, T. (2000). Attention to object files defined by transparent motion. *Journal of Experimental Psychology: Human Perception and Performance 26*: 488–505.

Wannig, A., Rodriguez, V., and Freiwald, W. A. (2007). Attention to surfaces modulates motion processing in extrastriate area MT. *Neuron 54*: 639–651.

Watanabe, T., Harner, A., Miyauchi, S., Sasaki, Y., Nielsen, M., Palomo, D., and Mukai, I. (1998). Task-dependent influences of attention in the activation of human primary visual cortex. *Proceedings of the National Academy of Sciences USA 95*: 11489–11492.

Wojciulik, E., Kanwisher, N., and Driver, J. (1998). Covert visual attention modulates face-specific activity in the human fusiform gyrus: fMRI study. *Journal of Neurophysiology* 79: 1574–1578.

Wolfe, J. M. 1998. Visual search. In H. Pashler (ed.), *Attention* (pp. 13–74). London: University College London Press.

Wolfe, J. M. and Horowitz, T. S. (2004). What attributes guide the deployment of visual attention and how do they do it? *Nature Reviews Neuroscience* 5: 1–7.

Womelsdorf, T., Anton-Erxleben, K., Pieper, F., and Treue, S. (2006). Dynamic shifts of visual receptive fields in cortical area MT by spatial attention. *Nature Neuroscience* 9: 1156–1160.

Womelsdorf, T., Anton-Erxleben, K., and Treue, S. (2008). Receptive field shift and shrinkage in macaque middle temporal area through attentional gain modulation. *Journal of Neuroscience* 28: 8934–8944.

Womelsdorf, T., Fries, P., Mitra, P. P. and Desimone, R. (2006). Gamma-band synchronization in visual cortex predicts speed of change detection. *Nature* 439: 733–736.

CHAPTER 22

....

THE ROLE OF BRAIN OSCILLATIONS IN THE TEMPORAL LIMITS OF ATTENTION

....

KIMRON SHAPIRO AND SIMON HANSLMAYR

FRAMES OF REFERENCE

....

THE ubiquitous concept of attention has numerous definitions as well as multiple frames of reference. Eriksen (1974) and Posner (1980) were among the first to reveal that attention can have a spatial, i.e. *location*, frame of reference (in chapter 8). For example, Posner showed that either an exogenous (e.g. onset of a spot of light) or endogenous (e.g. arrow pointing in a specific direction) cue can direct attention to a particular location in the visual field. Evidence to support this claim comes from examining reaction time (RT) to detect the occurrence of a cued target in the form of faster RTs (benefit) at the cued, relative to slower RTs (cost) at an uncued location, or relative to when no location is cued (neutral condition). Arriving at the same conclusion but using a different paradigm from what has come to be known as the Posner 'cost–benefit' paradigm just described, Eriksen (1974) found faster RTs to an imperative stimulus when flanked by compatible (i.e. requiring the same response) stimuli than when flanked by incompatible (i.e. requiring a different response) stimuli. That attention can operate within this location frame of reference is important for humans and animals when there is a demand to respond quickly and accurately to the sudden occurrence of a stimulus, e.g. when prey animals must avoid detection.

Location is not the only frame of reference in which attention has been shown to operate. Duncan (1984) revealed that attention can operate in an *object* frame of reference when he found that humans respond more quickly and accurately to two features when both appear as part of one object, relative to when the same two features appear but each on a different object. Coming to the same conclusion, Tipper (1985) used the negative priming paradigm (see below) to show that inhibition, a reciprocal process that facilitates attention, can be attached to an object. By changing the location of the inhibited object but not the object itself, a determination can be made as to which of these frames of reference are controlling behaviour. Although care must be applied when attempting to distinguish between location- and object-based frames of reference, given that an object must occupy a location in space and thus poses a potential confound, the above studies among many others have nevertheless shown the definitive existence of the object frame of reference.

The existence of yet a third, *feature*, frame of reference has been shown by Treisman and her colleagues (cf. Treisman and Gormican 1988). Using the visual search paradigm, Treisman revealed that a specified feature, e.g. a red circle, can be found equally rapidly from among an array of circles uniformly of another colour, e.g. green, regardless of the number of items in the array. Such 'preattentive', or parallel, search performance demonstrates that attention can operate in a feature mode, as differentiated from the location and object modes previously described.

Before turning to examine another frame of reference, it is important to point out that attention can flexibly operate in any of the modes discussed above, even using the same stimuli, but dependent on particular task demands. For example, Tipper (1994) found evidence to suggest that two circular-shaped objects, which revealed a location basis of attention when unconnected, revealed an object basis of attention when connected by a line that suggested the object 'barbell'.

What other frame of reference might there be? In addition and in relation to locations, objects, and features, humans are exquisitely sensitive to the temporal aspects of their environment. By way of example, in another chapter in the present volume, Nobre and Rohenkohl (in chapter 24) presents research suggesting that humans can focus attention based on their *expectation* of when a stimulus will occur. But there is another aspect of time that relates to attention, which examines the temporal *availability* of this construct. This aspect of attention is typically studied by presenting two imperative stimuli for which a response is required to each. By separating the two stimuli in time, the question can be asked, 'What is the availability or effect of attention to detect/identify the second stimulus after attention has been deployed to detect/identify the first?' A variety of paradigms have been developed to address this question and each will be explored here with a focus on one particular approach, the attentional blink (AB), which has been the centre of considerable interest for 20 years. Following a discussion of the AB in the context of the temporal frame of reference, the chapter will take an in-depth look at the role played by neural oscillations in regulating the availability of attention, with particular reference to the AB.

Inhibition of return

The inhibition-of-return paradigm was established by Posner and Cohen (1984) and indexes the spatial location of attention within a short time frame. In the original implementation of this paradigm, attention is centred on a box with two possible equi-distant locations on either side where equally sized boxes are located. The brightening of a randomly chosen box (i.e. the cue) in one of the two locations precedes the bright-ening of a randomly chosen one (i.e. target) of the three boxes with a stimulus onset asynchrony (SOA) of 0, 50, 100, 200, 300, or 500 ms. The centre box had a probability of being chosen as the target on 60% of trials, each peripheral box 10%, and no target (catch trials) occurred on 20% of trials. Participants were required to make an RT response to a single key as soon as they detected the target and to remain fixated on the centre box throughout the duration of the trial.

The results of this experiment revealed that at SOAs less than 300 ms, participants were faster to respond to the location of the cue, suggesting facilitation, but at SOAs greater than 300 ms they were faster to respond to locations opposite to the cue, suggest-ing inhibition. Klein and MacInnes (1999) suggested a foraging metaphor to account for these results; having searched a particular location, there is a reduced likelihood some-thing will be found in the same location once the initial effects of attention to the cued location have subsided (but see Chica, Lupiáñez, and Bartolomeo 2006) for an alterna-tive explanation. For an excellent review of the IOR literature, the reader is directed to Lupiáñez, Klein, and Bartolomeo (2006).

Priming

Priming enables the relationship between two temporally closely spaced stimuli to be investigated. The paradigm of 'priming', both positive and negative, enables investiga-tion into the temporal framework of attention by allowing one to probe the excitatory and inhibitory effects of deploying attention. In the case of priming, these processes are not studied with regard to spatial location, as they are with regard to inhibition of return. In priming, attending to a first stimulus can result in either faster responding (positive priming) or slower (negative priming) responding, for example, to a semantically related second stimulus, in comparison to a control condition where the two stimuli are unre-lated (see examples to follow). Depending on the various factors, the interval between prime and probe can be anywhere from less than 100 ms to as long as 15 minutes, but is typically in the same range as that employed with the inhibition-of-return paradigm just described and the other paradigms whose descriptions follow. Negative priming has been described previously in this chapter in the context of the object frame of refer-ence (cf. Tipper 1985), but has also been shown in the context of the location frame of reference (Tipper, Brehaut, and Driver 1990). Positive priming, on the other hand, is revealed, for example when repetition of a given word results in faster processing of the second relative to a non-repetition (e.g. Scarborough, Cortese, and Scarborough 1977, but see Kanwisher 1987 as described below where the opposite is true). Examples of pos-itive priming may also arise when the presentation of the first word is below conscious awareness, as in masked priming (e.g. Marcel 1983), or even when the two words are semantically related, for example the word 'doctor' priming 'nurse' in a lexical decision task (cf. McKoon and Ratcliff 1979). Accounts of positive and negative priming typically invoke concepts of (pre)activation and inhibition, respectively, although at a cognitive, rather than low level. When negative priming is indexed using the negative priming paradigm, the inhibitory process is argued to arise either at during the first display, i.e. at selection, or during the second display, i.e. at retrieval (cf. Tipper 2001). Once again, as in the case of inhibition of return, we see the effects of attention as viewed from the temporal perspective.

Repetition blindness

As indicated above in the discussion of priming, under some circumstances repetition can lead to a faster response than non-repetition. In stark contrast, Kanwisher (1987) reported a phenomenon she termed 'repetition blindness', where repetition of a letter or word within approximately 1000 ms leads to a failure to report its second occurrence, even if the repetition was in a different case, or if the word was a homophone (e.g. one, won; Bavelier and Potter 1992). Leading accounts of repetition blindness (cf. Kanwisher 1987) favour a type–token account. In this account each occurrence of a repeated letter or word activates a representation or *type* of that word but only the first occurrence activates an episodic (i.e. temporally bound), consciously identifiable *token*, which gives rise to the report of only a single instance having been presented. In keeping with the current discussion, repetition blindness represents another important empirical outcome that underlies the importance of the temporal frame of reference. Repetition blindness has been contrasted to the attentional blink phenomenon (see next section) as the two share certain obvious similarities (cf. Arnell and Shapiro 2011). Although the present discussion is not meant to be all-inclusive, Watson and Humphreys (1997), for example, describe a phenomenon called 'visual marking' that also has a temporal frame of reference.

Psychological refractory period

The psychological refractory period paradigm presents two target tasks in close temporal succession with the participant required to make a speeded response to both. For example, the first task might require a two-alternative forced choice response to whether one of two pre-specified letters was presented with the second task requiring participants to make a similar choice but to the pitch of a tone, i.e. high vs. low. Importantly, and distinguishing it from the attentional blink task (see below), neither target is masked. The interval between the targets is varied over trials, typically within the range of 100–1000 msec. The typical finding (cf. Pashler 1994) is that reaction time to the second target increases as the interval between the two targets (stimulus onset asynchrony, SOA) decreases. Performance to the first target is mostly unaffected by SOA. Various accounts of the psychological refractory period all centre around the notion that processing of the second target to a response must wait on the processing of the first target to be completed (see Tombu and Jolicoeur 2003, for a more complete description of these theories). We now move on to a discussion of the attentional blink.

ATTENTIONAL BLINK

The paradigm

The attentional blink (AB) paradigm (Raymond, Shapiro, and Arnell 1992) requires participants to report the identity, or detect the occurrence, of two targets presented as part of a rapid serial visual presentation (RSVP) sequence of stimuli presented at fixation. Letters and digits have primarily been used as stimuli, with the rate of presentation varying between 6 and 20 items per second. In the canonical dual-task paradigm, participants are presented with a randomly chosen series of letters, from which they have to identify the only white letter in a series of black letters (first target task; T1) and then report whether a black letter 'X' (second target task; T2) occurred in the subsequent letter stream. T2 is presented on 50% of trials, enabling a false alarm rate to be determined, and when presented, occurs with an interval between 100 and 800 ms separating the two targets. Report of both targets, in the correct order, is required after the stimulus stream terminates.

Many specific parameters have been varied across the many published studies but the attentional blink appears robust with only minor variations. For example, the stimulus duration and interstimulus interval of the stream (i.e. non-target) items have been manipulated but generally reveal a similar outcome in terms of the magnitude of the attentional blink. Manipulating the target parameters, however, has been shown to have an effect. McLaughlin, Shore, and Klein (2001) varied in separate experiments the duration of each target and the item (mask) just following the target in a reciprocal relationship holding the total duration of the two constant. Varying the first target in such a manner revealed no effect on the attentional blink, whereas varying the second target revealed an additive effect of difficulty, i.e. longer duration targets yielded less of an attentional blink.

Other manipulations to parameters of the attentional blink paradigm, such as making the two target tasks identical, e.g. identifying letters, or making them different, e.g. one letter, one digit, have yielded different attentional blink functions and given rise to a small cottage industry known as the *Lag-1 sparing* phenomenon (cf. Dux and Marois 2009). Virtually any other parameter one can think of has been manipulated but a full discussion is beyond the scope of the present chapter and the reader is referred to the excellent review by Dux and Marois (2009).

To characterize the magnitude of the attentional blink outcome, performance on T2 (percent correct or d'), conditional on correct T1 performance, is plotted (see Fig. 1) as a function of *lag* (stimulus onset asynchrony, SOA, between T1 and T2). The AB 'signature' is defined as a significant interaction between *lag* and *condition*,

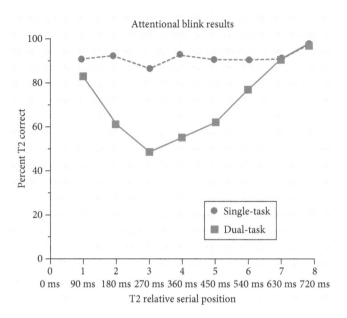

FIGURE 22.1 Results from the attentional blink experiment by Raymond, Shapiro, and Arnell (1992). The Y axis shows percent correct responding to the second target (T2) as a function of the relative serial position and lag of T2 relative to T1. The red circles represent single-task (control) performance where participants were instructed to ignore T1 and respond only to T2. Blue squares represent dual-task (experimental) performance where participants are instructed to respond to both T1 and T2. The attentional blink is evidence by the interaction between Task and Lag. Data from Raymond, J. E., Shapiro, K. L., and Arnell, K. M., 1992, Temporary suppression of visual processing in an RSVP task: An attentional blink? *Journal of Experimental Psychology Human Perception and Performance*, 18(3), pp. 849–860.

where *condition* is comprised of the experimental condition just described and a single-task control condition wherein T1 is ignored and to which no response is made. The typical AB stimulus stream consists of T1 and T2 embedded among filler items before T1, between the two targets, and after T2. A shorter, skeletal version has also been frequently used. It eliminates all the filler items leaving only T1, T2, and the stream items (i.e. masks) immediately following each target (Duncan, Ward, and Shapiro 1994).

There have been many hundreds of studies using near and far variants of the AB method just described. Below we present only a cursory overview of various theoretical accounts of the AB and refer the reader to two relatively recent reviews to gain further insight (cf. Dux and Marois 2009; Olivers and Meeter 2008). The AB has been extensively used to probe the complex processes supporting consciousness (e.g. perception, selective attention, and working memory) and the result of this many-faceted body of empirical data is a significant advance in the development of theory concerning how sensory information becomes represented at the level of consciousness.

Theoretical accounts

Although there are various accounts purporting to explain the AB, most place the mechanism responsible for the failure to identify T2 at a relatively late stage of processing, after sensory but before response processing. These theories fall into three main categories and the reader is once again referred to Dux and Marois (2009) for a full discussion. (1) Filter-based: The AB reflects the workings of a mechanism designed to filter out non-relevant visual information; (2) Consolidation bottleneck: The AB represents a temporal bottleneck in the transfer of highly-processed information into short-term memory that eventually makes information available to consciousness; and (3) Retrieval failures: The AB reflects a temporal bottleneck in retrieval of information from short-term memory into access consciousness.

We begin with filter theories because in the first report of the AB (Raymond et al. 1992) a simple version of this idea was advanced. Raymond and colleagues proposed that the AB resulted when the T1 mask item signalled to a central processor that the potential for representational confusion, e.g. binding errors (Treisman 1996), was too high and that any incoming stimuli should be suppressed. The basic notion of a filtering process evoked as a response to distractors subsequently formed the basis of an account advanced by Olivers and Meeter (2008) and another account proposed by Di Lollo and colleagues (Di Lollo, Kawahara, Shahab Ghorashi, and Enns 2005; Kawahara, Enns, and Di Lollo 2006). As a category, these theories emphasize the role of top-down target selection processes and thus link the AB very closely to selective attention as it might operate prior to durable storage of information in a cache, such a visual working memory, accessible by consciousness.

The second category of filter theories is similar but places greater emphasis on limited capacity mechanisms required to transfer current perceptual representations into a durable short-term memory cache (cf. Chun and Potter 1995). The basic idea is that both a representation and transfer of that representation to working memory is able to occur on the first target due to the availability of attention. The AB arises when a representation of the second target is formed but due to the unavailability of attention is unable to be transferred to working memory. Jolicoeur and his colleagues (Jolicoeur 1998, 1999; Jolicoeur and Dell'Acqua 1998) expanded this account to connect it to the psychological refractory period phenomenon (Pashler 1994), which argues for central capacity limitations in humans' ability to process two temporally adjacent stimuli such as occurs in both psychological-refractory-period and AB tasks. However, key findings distinguish the AB from PRP (but see Jolicoeur 1998 for a counter-argument). First, the attentional blink typically does not occur without masking both targets. Second, using event-related potentials, Luck, Vogel, and Shapiro (1998) showed that the AB occurs postperceptually but before the state of response selection where the PRP effect has been argued to occur.

Formally modelling the Chun and Potter two-stage model, Bowman and Wyble (2007) proposed a 'simultaneous type/serial token model' (see also Wyble, Bowman, and Nieuwenstein 2009) based on the distinction between types and tokens (cf. Kanwisher

1987). At the centre of this account is the notion that the AB arises when two targets are unable to be *episodically* distinguished one from the other.

Recently there have been a series of investigations into neuropharmacological factors that may affect the consolidation process as described above. Nieuwenhuis and his colleagues (Nieuwenhuis, Gilzenrat, Holmes, and Cohen 2005) hypothesized that the AB occurs as a consequence of the refractory nature of the noradrenergic modulatory signal from the locus coeruleus, implicated in supporting attention through phasic alerting and possibly other functions (see chapters in the present volume by Robertson and by Robbins). Although Nieuwenhuis and his colleagues failed to find empirical evidence to support this hypothesis (Nieuwenhuis, van Nieuwpoort, Veltman, and Drent, 2007), Dolan's group (De Martino, Strange, and Dolan 2008) have reported behavioural evidence that the adrenergic system has a modulatory influence on selective attention as revealed with the AB paradigm.

A third category of accounts places the cause of the AB late in processing at the stage where information is retrieved from short-term memory and made available to consciousness. This account was originally expressed by Shapiro, Raymond, and Arnell (1994) on the basis of evidence that T1 difficulty manipulations had no effect on AB magnitude. A subsequent modification to this account (*attentional dwell time*; Duncan et al. 1994; Ward, Duncan, and Shapiro 1996) argued that the AB occurs because the two targets compete for limited attentional resources with the loser giving way to extended processing of the winner. A related idea was put forward by Dehaene and his colleagues (Dehaene, Sergent, and Changeux 2003) who proposed a global workspace account where a stimulus must enter a 'global neuronal' space for it to become consciously accessible.

It is important to point out that many of these theoretical accounts share the notion of a 'bottleneck' (filter theories being a possible exception), though each place the bottleneck at a different locus in the information processing stream. It is as difficult to design experiments to unambiguously distinguish between theories of the attentional blink as it is to design experiments to distinguish between early vs. late attentional selection. Before leaving this topic, it is also important to point out that one must not necessarily confuse empirical findings for the role of a particular brain area, oscillatory frequency, or neurotransmitter in the production of the attentional blink for a theory or even a model of it. Whereas each of these factors may have a vital role to play, the attentional blink outcome is dependent on a significant number of basic processes, e.g. perception, attention, visual short-term memory, such that no one factor is likely to account for such a complex phenomenon.

Neural synchronization and the AB

The attentional blink remains a topic of intense investigation using a variety of methodological approaches, including relatively recent reports involving functional imaging and electrophysiology (EEG, MEG). Although functional magnetic resonance imaging (fMRI) has proven a successful approach to studying the AB, this method is limited due to the difficulty in separating the neural responses to T1 and T2 relying on slow hemodynamic response functions. In contrast, the temporal resolution of M/EEG has afforded important insights into the neural underpinning of the AB, e.g. Luck et al. (1996) revealed that T2 is processed to a level of meaning even when it cannot be reported.

More recently, using MEG and a variant of the standard AB paradigm, Gross et al. (2004) examined long-range synchronization as a means of determining whether such a mechanism could predict when an AB would occur. Synchronization has been proposed as a means of inter-area communication (Varela, Lachaux, Rodriguez, and Martinerie 2001; Fries 2005) and is defined as phase-locked oscillatory activity between two or more cortical areas. Importantly, these cortical areas must be phase-locked to each other, rather than to the external stimulus driving the oscillations. The results (see Fig. 22.2) revealed a varying amount of synchronization to the targets and de-synchronization to the masks at 15 Hz (beta) in a 'network' primarily composed of left frontal and right occipito-parietal areas. Whereas synchronization is thought to reflect an active communication channel, de-synchronization can be interpreted to reflect a lack of communication. The results

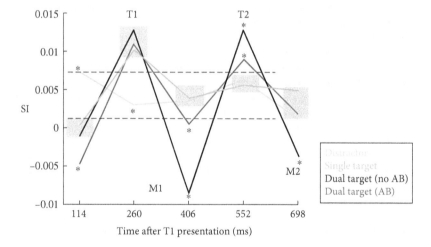

FIGURE 22.2 Mean synchronization (SI) in the target-related network. SI for the components of five successive stimuli. The x-axis specifies time after presentation of the first target. Each point represents the mean SI in a 60-ms window centred at 260 ms after the respective stimulus. Values at 260 ms quantify the network synchronization to the first target, and values at 114 ms represent the network synchronization corresponding to the distractor preceding the first target. Conditions are colour-coded (black, no-AB; red, AB; blue, target; green, distractor). The dashed lines mark the extent of SI in trials containing only distractors. Points marked with an asterisk are significantly different from their neighbours at the same position (P < 0.05, Kruskall–Wallis test), whereas points within the same shaded area are not significantly different. Negative values arise from the filtering of the SI time courses. Reprinted from Gross, J., Schmitz, F., Schnitzler, I., Kessler, K., Shapiro, K., Hommel, B., et al., Modulation of long-range neural synchrony reflects temporal limitations of visual attention in humans, *Proceedings of the National Academy of Sciences of the United States of America*, 101(35), pp. 13050–13055 © 2004, The National Academy of Sciences.

showed an equal amount of synchronization on all trials on which T1 was reported correctly and an equivalent amount on T2 trials when it was reported correctly. Trials, on which T2 was not reported correctly, i.e. an AB occurred or no T2 was presented, revealed a significantly lower degree of synchronization evoked by the second target. The unexpected finding was a significant *de*-synchronization evoked by the T1 and T2 masks on trials when no AB occurred. The significance of this finding requires some explanation. In an important paper early in the history of research on the attentional blink, Seiffert and Di Lollo (1997) found masking both T1 and T2 is critical to the production of the AB. Notionally, masking arises from the subsequent item in the stimulus stream that follows each target, although the mechanism by which the mask exerts its effect on the AB likely differs for T1 and T2. Nevertheless, as masking is known to (negatively) influence target detection via both perceptual and cognitive mechanisms, so it is conceivable that anything which reduces masking should improve target detection. Although speculative, the de-synchronization of the mask on trials on which target detection was accurate is consistent with this view.

Neural oscillations in various frequency bands have been implicated to influence diverse cognitive operations involving perception, attention, and memory (cf. Buzsáki and Draguhn 2004; Hanslmayr, Gross, Klimesch, and Shapiro 2011). One of the principal contributions of the present chapter is to describe how such oscillations work and provide examples of their possible influence on the temporal availability of attention via the phenomenon of the attentional blink. We first give a brief description on the nature of brain oscillations and their importance in determining behaviour, then return to the relationship of one particular frequency band of oscillations, alpha, to the attentional blink phenomenon.

BRAIN OSCILLATIONS: A BRIEF INTRODUCTION

Brain oscillations reflect the coordinated activity of thousands of neurons, and can be recorded in humans non-invasively with EEG/MEG, and invasively with intracranial electrodes in patients with epilepsy, undergoing pre-surgical investigation (Kahana 2006). In general, brain oscillations reflect rhythmic fluctuations between excitatory and inhibitory states of neural assemblies, and are generated by excitatory or inhibitory postsynaptic potentials (IPSPs/EPSPs; Lopes da Silva 1991; Buzsáki, Anastassiou, and Koch 2012). Thereby, brain oscillations open and close the time window for neural firing, and mediate communication between neural assemblies. These rhythmic fluctuations can already be seen with the naked eye in the raw EEG of healthy human subjects, which typically contain a strong signal at around 10 Hz, the so-called alpha frequency (Berger 1929). The EEG signal, however, also contains activity in other frequency ranges, which can be analysed by applying spectral analysis (e.g. Wavelet analysis; Fig. 22.3a). Brain oscillatory activity can unambiguously be described by three different parameters: frequency, amplitude, and phase. In the following, a brief description of these three parameters and their relation to neural mechanisms will be given.

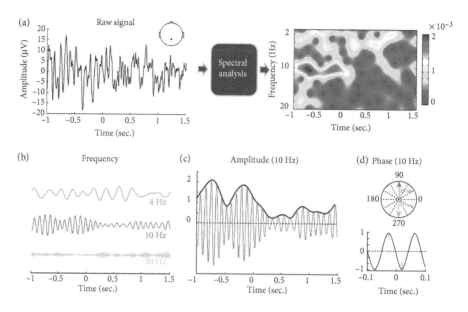

FIGURE 22.3 Brain oscillations and their parameters. (a) An example of a raw signal as recorded with a parietal EEG electrode is shown on the left. A stimulus was presented at time 0. The plot on the right shows the results of a time-frequency analysis in which the amplitude is depicted for each time point (x-axis) and frequency band (y-axis). (b) Theta (4 Hz), alpha (10 Hz), and gamma (40 Hz) oscillations as extracted from the above shown raw signal by means of band-pass filtering. (c) The time-course of alpha (10 Hz) amplitude is shown. Amplitude can be computed from the Hilbert transform of the band-pass filtered signal. (d) Alpha phase at two different time points (25 ms prior, and 25 ms after stimulus presentation) is illustrated. Reprinted from *Brain Research Reviews*, 67(1–2), Simon Hanslmayr, Joachim Gross, Wolfgang Klimesch, and Kimron L. Shapiro, The role of alpha oscillations in temporal attention, pp. 331–43, Copyright (2011), with permission from Elsevier.

Frequency

As mentioned above, the raw EEG signal contains several different brain oscillations characterized by their frequency (Fig. 22.3b). Classically, these frequency bands are divided into delta (1–3 Hz), theta (5–7 Hz), alpha (8–12 Hz), beta (15–35 Hz), and gamma (>40 Hz) oscillations. Earlier studies in EEG/MEG research tried to link the different frequency bands to different cognitive functions, but this approach became more problematic with increasing numbers of studies showing that there is no simple frequency-to-cognition mapping. A more recent, and probably more fruitful, approach is to link the different oscillations to different biophysical and anatomical network properties. Following this account, the frequency of an oscillation is inversely related to the size of the underlying network, with high frequencies reflecting small, and slow frequencies reflecting large networks (Kopell, Ermentrout, Whittington, and Traub 2000; von Stein and Sarnthein 2000; Buzsáki and Draguhn 2004). In a similar way, the frequency of an oscillation can also reflect the action of anatomically different networks, and thereby indicate different processing states. For instance, studies examining the spectral profile of the different layers in the visual cortex showed that the superficial layers tend to oscillate in higher (gamma) frequencies, whereas the deep layers tend to oscillate in lower (beta and alpha) frequencies (Buffalo, Fries, Landman, Buschman, and Desimone 2011). As the superficial layers predominantly receive input from feedforward, and the deep layers receive input from feedback connections, these results suggest that alpha and beta oscillations reflect top-down processing, whereas gamma oscillations reflect bottom-up processing. This notion is in line with prior attention studies (von Stein, Chiang, and König 2000) and is especially relevant for this chapter, which focuses on the role of alpha oscillations for temporal attention.

Amplitude

The amplitude (or power) of an oscillation is directly related to the number of excitatory and inhibitory postsynaptic potentials (EPSPs/IPSPs) that arrive at a given time point at a neural assembly (Varela et al. 2001; Hämäläinen, Hari, Illmoniemi, Knuutila, and Lounasmaa 1993). Thereby, amplitude indicates the number of these postsynaptic potentials, as well as the synchrony between these potentials. Presumably, low amplitudes reflect de-synchronized and high amplitudes reflect synchronized network activity, and measures of stimulus-induced changes in amplitude have therefore been termed event-related synchronization and de-synchronization (ERS/ERD; Pfurtscheller and Aranibar 1977; Hanslmayr, Staudigl, and Fellner 2012). Interestingly, alpha and beta oscillations tend to show stimulus-induced decreases in amplitude, whereas theta and gamma oscillations typically show stimulus-induced increases in amplitude (Fig. 22.3b, c).

Phase

The phase reflects the polarity of an oscillation in the EEG/MEG signal (Fig. 22.3d), and therefore indicates whether the underlying neural assembly is in a relatively excitatory or inhibitory state. This assumption is corroborated by several studies showing that the firing rate of neurons is modulated by the phase of ongoing oscillations (Fries 2005; Lee, Simpson, Logothetis, and Rainer 2005; Jacobs, Kahana, Ekstrom, and Fried 2007; Canolty, Ganguly, Kennerley et al. 2010). The phase of an oscillation therefore imposes rhythmic firing on neural assemblies by providing fine-grained temporal windows of excitation and inhibition. These findings led to the conclusion that neural communication between distant cell assemblies is established via oscillatory phase dynamics (Fries 2005). Phase-coherence (or phase-coupling), which indexes the consistency of phase differences between two recording sites over time/trials, can therefore be taken as a direct measure of neural communication. Besides measuring the phase-consistency between two recording sites, one can also measure the phase-consistency at one recording site across single trials. Although being mathematically closely related, phase-consistency at one recording site across single trials and phase-coherence between two recording sites refer to quite different neural processes. Whereas phase-coherence reflects inter-areal communication, phase-consistency at one recording site across single trials refers to the momentary excitatory or inhibitory state of a neural assembly at a specific time point. As we will point out later, these two measures might reflect the action of different neural circuits.

THE SPECIAL ROLE OF ALPHA OSCILLATIONS

As pointed out above, alpha oscillations (~10 Hz) are the most dominant signal in the human EEG/MEG. They are most pronounced over posterior recording sites, and can be seen with the naked eye. Historically, alpha oscillations have been thought to reflect a passive idling mode of the cortex because they are high during resting periods and decrease in amplitude during sensory stimulation or cognitive effort (Pfurtscheller, Stancák, and Neuper 1996). Recent studies, however, challenged this rather passive view of alpha oscillations, and suggest that alpha plays a very active and important role for cognitive processes. For instance, studies on spatial orienting of attention demonstrated that alpha oscillations decrease at attended visual areas (Worden, Foxe, Wang, and Simpson 2000; Sauseng, Klimesch, Stadler et al. 2005; Thut, Nietzel, Brandt, and Pascual-Leone 2006; Gould, Rushworth, and Nobre 2011; see Müller and Weisz 2012, for similar results in the auditory domain). Interestingly, alpha oscillations show a specific increase in amplitude at recording sites that correspond to distractor stimuli or to-be-ignored spatial locations (Kelly, Lalor, Reilly, and Foxe 2006; Rihs, Michel, and Thut 2007). Together, these findings led to the conclusion that alpha oscillations play an active and important role for cognition by inhibiting task-irrelevant brain regions (Klimesch, Sauseng, and Hanslmayr 2007). Indeed, a recent study in monkeys provided direct evidence for this conclusion, by showing that alpha amplitude is inversely related to neural firing rate (Haegens, Nácher, Luna, Romo, and Jensen 2011).

Prestimulus alpha oscillations predict visual perception

In a typical perception experiment, sensory stimuli are presented repeatedly such that they are hard to detect (e.g. short presentation time, masking stimulus, weak contrast, etc.). Data from such experiments reveal that a given subject perceives identical stimuli on some occasions, and misses them on other occasions even if all presentation parameters are held constant. In classical psychological models this variance is treated as 'noise'. However, recent studies demonstrated that a considerable amount of this variance can be explained by ongoing dynamics in alpha oscillatory activity, suggesting that the current brain state plays a crucial role for perception of external stimuli. In a recent paper, we reviewed these findings and argue that alpha oscillations indicate whether the brain is biased towards processing information of internal representations, or external sensory stimuli (Hanslmayr et al. 2011). In the following section we will give a brief overview of this idea and describe how different parameters of prestimulus oscillatory activity (i.e. amplitude, phase-consistency across single trials, and phase-coherence) are linked to these internally and externally oriented brain states, in turn having a pronounced effect on the temporal availability of attention.

Alpha amplitude and perception

One of the first reports in this field was published by Ergenoglu and colleagues (Ergenoglu, Demiralp, Bayraktaroglu et al. 2004) who observed that the alpha amplitude, prior to the presentation of a briefly flashed stimulus, is negatively correlated with perception performance. In the meantime, this finding has been replicated by others, who showed that this effect was most pronounced over parieto-occipital recording sites (Fig. 22.4a; van Dijk, Schoffelen, Oostenveld, and Jensen 2008; Thut et al. 2006). Consistently, a recent MEG study localized the difference in prestimulus alpha power between detected and non-detected visual stimuli to the precuneus (van Dijk et al. 2008). Others demonstrated that the inverse relationship between alpha power and detection performance not only holds within subjects, on a single trial level, but can also be extended to differences between subjects, with good perception performers showing lower prestimulus alpha power than bad perception performers (Hanslmayr, Klimesch, Sauseng et al. 2005; Hanslmayr, Aslan, Staudigl et al. 2007). In line with the inhibition view of alpha oscillations, these results suggest that a visual stimulus is unlikely to be perceived if posterior, presumably visual processing, regions are in an inhibitory state. Direct evidence for this idea comes from a transcranial magnetic stimulation (TMS) study, showing that phosphenes (i.e. an unstructured sensation of a light flash that is usually perceived when the visual cortex is stimulated) are less likely to occur during periods of high alpha activity (Romei, Brodbeck, Michel et al. 2008). Similar findings have been obtained for the relationship between alpha amplitude over the sensory cortex and the perception of tactile stimuli (Schubert, Haufe, Blankenburg, Villringer, and Curio 2009), suggesting that these mechanisms might generalize to other sensory domains. The question, however, is whether the relationship between alpha amplitude and perception is of a correlational, or a causal nature. Addressing this issue, a recent study showed that driving posterior brain regions in the alpha frequency, but not in other frequencies, prior to stimulus presentation, caused a decrease in perception performance of visual stimuli, which indeed points to a causal influence of alpha oscillations on perception (Romei, Gross, and Thut 2010).

Together these studies indicate that the spontaneous fluctuations of alpha amplitude indicate different levels of excitatory/inhibitory cortical states, which partly determine the fate of a sensory stimulus (Fig. 22.4a). Thereby high levels of alpha amplitudes over sensory processing areas likely indicate inhibition of these areas, which renders these

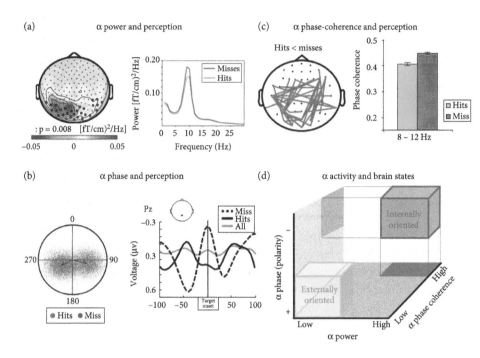

FIGURE 22.4 Prestimulus alpha activity and its relation to visual perception. (a) Enhanced alpha power prior to stimulus presentation is negatively related to visual perception (reproduced with permission from van Dijk, H., Schoffelen, J.-M., Oostenveld, R., & Jensen, O., Prestimulus oscillatory activity in the alpha band predicts visual discrimination ability, *Journal of Neuroscience*, 28 (8), pp. 1816–1823 © 2008, The Society for Neuroscience). (b) Hits show a positive polarity at stimulus onset, whereas misses show a negative polarity at stimulus over a parietal electrode (reproduced with permission from Mathewson, K. E., Gratton, G., Fabiani, M., Beck, D. M., & Ro, T., To see or not to see: prestimulus alpha phase predicts visual awareness. *The Journal of Neuroscience: The Official Journal of the Society for Neuroscience*, 29(9), pp. 2725–2732 © 2009, The Society for Neuroscience). (c) Alpha phase-coherence between frontal and parietal sensors prior to stimulus presentation is negatively related to visual perception. (d) An overview is presented showing how alpha power (x-axis), alpha phase (y-axis), and alpha phase-coherence (z-axis) are linked to externally vs. internally oriented brain states. (a) Reprinted from van Dijk, H., Schoffelen, J.-M., Oostenveld, R., and Jensen, O., Prestimulus oscillatory activity in the alpha band predicts visual discrimination ability, *Journal of Neuroscience*, 28 (8), pp. 1816–1823 © 2008, The Society for Neuroscience. (b) Reprinted from Mathewson, K. E., Gratton, G., Fabiani, M., Beck, D. M., and Ro, T., To see or not to see: prestimulus alpha phase predicts visual awareness. *The Journal of Neuroscience: The Official Journal of the Society for Neuroscience*, 29(9), pp. 2725–2732 © 2009, The Society for Neuroscience.

brain regions less susceptible to external stimulation. Increased alpha amplitudes might thus bias the brain towards processing internal representations, by shutting down external input. In line with this notion, working memory studies showed that alpha amplitude increases linearly as a function of the number of items that have to be internally maintained in working memory (Klimesch, Doppelmayr, Schwaiger, Auinger, and Winkler 1999; Jensen, Gelfand, Kounios, and Lisman 2002).

Alpha phase and perception

As outlined above, the phase of an oscillation imposes rhythmic firing onto a neural assembly by providing fine-grained time windows of excitation and inhibition. As alpha oscillations are so dominant in the human EEG/MEG, the idea that the peaks and troughs of alpha might be related to the perceptual fate of a stimulus can be found in quite early studies (e.g. Varela, Toro, John, and Schwartz 1981; Callaway and Yeager 1960; Dustman and Beck 1965). Together, these studies suggest that visual processing is enhanced when the onset of the stimulus coincides with the positive peak of the alpha oscillation at parietal recording sites. These ideas currently experience a renaissance, due to several recent studies which have further investigated this issue applying more advanced and sophisticated analysis techniques than those that were available in these earlier studies. Corroborating the earlier findings, recent EEG studies demonstrated that the likelihood of a visual stimulus being perceived can be predicted by the phase of the alpha oscillation at stimulus onset (Busch, Dubois, and VanRullen 2009; Busch and VanRullen 2010; Mathewson, Gratton, Fabiani, Beck, and Ro 2009). Specifically, the findings of Mathewson et al. (2009) nicely match the earlier findings in showing that visual stimuli were more likely to be perceived if presented during a positive peak of alpha, as measured over parietal recording sites (Fig. 22.4b). Similar findings were obtained by Busch et al. (2009) and Busch and VanRullen (2010), although the effects in these studies differed slightly with respect to the frequency band (~7 Hz) and topography. Converging evidence comes also from recent simultaneous EEG–fMRI studies showing that the blood oxygenation-level dependent (BOLD) signal and BOLD connectivity in visual and parietal areas varied as a function of the alpha phase at stimulus onset (Scheeringa, Mazaheri, Bojak, Norris, and Kleinschmidt 2011; Hanslmayr, Volberg, Wimber, Dalal, and Greenlee, in press).

Similar to the relationship between alpha amplitude and perception, the crucial question is whether alpha phase at stimulus onset plays a causal role for perception. The experiment by Mathewson et al. (Mathewson, Fabiani, Gratton, Beck, and Lleras 2010) sheds some light on this issue. In their experiment, Mathewson et al. (2010) presented a stream of stimuli at a regular rate within the alpha frequency band (12 Hz), which is known to induce a strong phase alignment at the stimulation frequency (Moratti, Clementz, Gao, Ortiz, and Keil 2007; see Thut, Schyns, and Gross 2011, for a review) known as steady-state-visual evoked potentials (Herrmann 2001; Vialatte, Maurice, Dauwels, and Cichocki 2010). After this prestimulus train of stimuli, a critical stimulus was presented that had to be detected by the participants. This critical stimulus was presented at a delay of 32, 59, 82, 107, or 130 ms after the prestimulus train. The results of Mathewson et al. (2010) reveal that perception performance varied as a sinusoidal function of this delay, exactly matching the period length of 12 Hz. These results are therefore a first hint that the perceptual fate of a stimulus can be modulated by entraining the alpha phase at stimulus onset. Although Mathewson et al. did not measure the EEG and thus cannot show direct evidence for alpha phase entrainment, this study is a first hint for a causal role of alpha phase for perception.

Taken together, the findings reviewed above demonstrate that alpha phase, similar to alpha amplitude, at stimulus onset indicates states that render the brain more or less susceptible to visual stimulation. Similar to alpha amplitude, alpha phase may regulate the excitatory/inhibitory level of visual processing regions, however, at a much faster time scale (Jensen and Mazaheri 2010). Thereby, alpha phase can bias the brain towards processing stimuli from the sensory channels, or towards processing internal representations (Fig. 22.4b). Following this concept, internally and externally oriented brain states are two sides of the same coin, such that the absence of one state automatically implies the other. As we will point out below, the relationship between alpha phase and internally and externally oriented brain states might be crucially important in explaining temporal attention phenomena in RSVP paradigms, such as the attentional blink.

Alpha phase-coherence and perception

In contrast to alpha amplitude and alpha phase, which both indicate the excitatory/inhibitory state of a locally circumscribed neural assembly (e.g. the visual cortex), alpha phase-coherence (or phase-coupling) points towards a more complex measure of brain states. As pointed out above, phase-coherence is a measure of neural communication between distant brain areas. Prestimulus alpha phase-coherence therefore indicates the degree to which distant brain areas exchange information at a given time point. Employing this measure, two prior studies demonstrated that high prestimulus phase-coherence in the alpha frequency range is negatively correlated with the perception of a visual stimulus (Hanslmayr et al. 2007; Kranczioch, Debener, Maye, and Engel 2007). In the study by Hanslmayr et al. (2007) one out of four possible stimuli was briefly presented and followed by a mask. A pronounced correlation between prestimulus alpha phase-coherence and perception was obtained with single trials in which the stimulus was perceived showing significantly less phase-coherence than trials in which the stimulus was not perceived (Fig. 22.4c). This effect was most pronounced between frontal and parietal electrode sites. Sorting the single trials according to the prestimulus phase-coherence, the results demonstrate that alpha phase-coherence could account for a large range of the behavioural variance: ranging from 80% perception performance in the trials with the lowest, and 40% perception performance in the trials with highest phase-coherence. Utilizing the attentional blink phenomenon, Kranczioch and colleagues (2007) obtained similar results, and showed that trials in which an AB was obtained were characterized by increased alpha phase-coherence prior to presentation of the second target stimulus. Parallel results were recently obtained in a multi-sensory study showing that the integration of audio-visual stimuli can be predicted by the prestimulus phase-coherence between auditory and visual processing regions (Keil, Müller, Ihssen, and Weisz 2012).

Although additional studies are needed to explore the role of prestimulus phase-coherence for perception, the studies reviewed so far present compelling evidence that the fluctuations in alpha phase-coherence indicate states that render the brain more or less susceptible to process incoming information. Thereby, high alpha phase-coherence, presumably indicating a high degree of cortico–cortical information transfer, might point towards processing of internal representations, which makes it hard for sensory stimuli to be perceived. In other words, if the brain is talking to itself, it does not listen to the information from the sensory channels. As we will point out in more detail below, this assumption is backed by findings showing that the maintenance or manipulation of internal representations in working memory induces an increase in alpha phase-coherence (Sauseng, Klimesch, Doppelmayr et al. 2005; Palva, Monto, Kulashekhar, and Palva 2010).

Taken together, ongoing measures of alpha amplitude, phase, and phase-coherence jointly reflect the waxing and waning between different brain states. Externally oriented brain states, which promote sensory perception, are characterized by low alpha power, low alpha phase-coherence, and a positive polarity over parietal sensors at stimulus onset. Internally oriented brain states, on the other hand, are characterized by high alpha power, high alpha phase-coherence, and a negative polarity at stimulus onset (Fig. 22.4d).

Alpha amplitude and phase reflect thalamo-cortical information transfer

Historically, alpha oscillations are believed to be generated by thalamo-cortical feedback loops, and several animal studies provide evidence for this assumption (Lopes da Silva, Vos, Mooibroek, and van Rotterdam 1980; Hughes, Lörincz, Cope et al. 2004; Hughes and Crunelli 2007). Particularly interesting for this chapter is the finding that ongoing alpha oscillations in the thalamus gate signal transmission to the cortex (Lorincz, Kékesi, Juhász, Crunelli, and Hughes 2009). In this study, Lorincz et al. demonstrated that the firing of thalamo-cortical neurons is modulated by the phase of the ongoing alpha oscillation. It might thus well be that the effect of alpha phase on perception as described above reflects exactly this thalamo-cortical gating mechanism. If this is true, the alpha phase in the thalamus at stimulus onset should predict whether or not a visual stimulus will be perceived. Recording the EEG directly from the thalamus, in an epileptic patient undergoing surgery for deep brain stimulation, recent data indeed support such a relationship (Staudigl, Hanslmayr, Voges et al. 2013). As shown in Fig. 20.5, a pronounced difference between perceived and not-perceived stimuli in the thalamic alpha phase around stimulus onset was obtained.

However, not only variations in alpha phase but also variations in alpha amplitude might reflect different states of thalamo-cortical loops. This assumption would be in line with ideas suggesting that the thalamus serves as a pacemaker for the posterior alpha rhythm (Hughes and Crunelli 2007). Indeed several recent studies, employing simultaneous EEG–fMRI demonstrated a positive correlation between fluctuations in alpha amplitude and the BOLD signal in the thalamus (Sadaghiani, Scheeringa, Lehongre et al. 2010; Moosmann, Ritter, Krastel et al. 2003; Goldman, Stern, Engel, and Cohen 2002). Additional evidence comes from intracranial recordings in patients, showing that the pathological slowing of the alpha rhythm is due to abnormal thalamo-cortical network activity (Sarnthein and Jeanmonod 2007; Sarnthein, Stern, Aufenberg, Rousson, and Jeanmonod 2006).

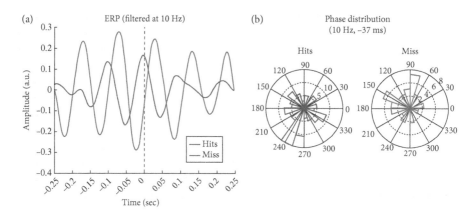

FIGURE 22.5   Data from EEG recordings in the thalamus (medio-dorsal nucleus, left) are shown for one patient during a visual perception task (Staudigl et al. unpublished data). (a) Hits are characterized by a positive polarity at stimulus onset, whereas misses show a negative polarity. (b) The phase distributions at 10 Hz, shortly before stimulus presentation (−35 ms), are shown plotted across single trials.

Together, the studies presented above suggest that the alpha phase and amplitude at stimulus onset indicate different states of thalamo-cortical feedback loops. These dynamics render the thalamo-cortical loops more or less permeable for external sensory stimuli, and thereby gate signal transmission from the sensory channels to higher cortical processing regions. This idea would suggest that alpha amplitude and phase both reflect the same underlying neural circuit and should thus jointly be linked to perception performance. Indeed, the data of Mathewson et al. (2009) are in line with this notion in showing that the effect of alpha phase on stimulus perception varied as a function of alpha amplitude. Specifically, the impact of alpha phase on perception performance increased with increasing alpha amplitude.

Alpha phase-coherence reflects cortico–cortical information exchange

Any higher order cognitive function requires the communication between the cortical regions involved, assumed to be mediated by phase-coherence (Fries 2005; Varela et al. 2001). Phase-coherence in the alpha frequency range in particular has been linked to top-down attentional control as well as working memory processes. For instance, in their seminal paper von Stein et al. (2000) demonstrate that alpha phase-coherence specifically reflects the flow of information from higher to lower visual processing regions during attentional selection. A number of human EEG/MEG studies reported increased alpha phase-coherence during working memory tasks, requiring maintenance or manipulation of internal representations (Sauseng et al. 2005; Palva et al. 2010).

Interestingly, Palva et al. demonstrated that alpha phase-coherence between frontal and parietal regions increased parametrically as a function of working memory load and was positively correlated with individual working memory capacity. Together with the results by Hanslmayr et al. (2007), showing that increased fronto-parietal alpha phase-coherence predicts poor perception performance, these results suggest that increased alpha phase-coherence indicates the processing of internal representations, thus preventing the perception of sensory stimuli. This notion is in line with behavioural and fMRI work showing that increased working memory load can induce inattentional blindness (i.e. the failure to perceive salient sensory stimuli; Todd, Fougnie, and Marois 2005).

Linking Alpha Oscillations and Temporal Attention

As pointed out before, the attentional blink paradigm utilizes the rapid serial visual presentation of stimuli at a regular rate in a frequency range between 7 and 13 Hz, which exactly matches the classical alpha band. As we argue below, this paradigm may influence all three parameters of alpha oscillatory activity (amplitude, phase, and phase-coherence) such that they are maximally in their least favourable state at the time the second target occurs.

First, perception of the first target likely triggers complex cognitive processes such as top-down attentional selection mechanisms and encoding of the stimulus into working memory. Studies in visual masking demonstrate that the successful perceptual identification of a stimulus requires the match between a template held in working memory and the sensory representation in the visual cortex (Enns and Di Lollo 2000). Such processes likely require the communication between frontal and parietal cortical regions, which is mediated by alpha phase-coherence. It is therefore conceivable that the processing of the first target induces an increase in alpha phase-coherence, reflecting an internally oriented processing state where T1 is being transferred into working memory (cf. Chun and Potter 1995). If true, the dynamics of increased alpha phase-coherence induced by the perception of the first target should match the time course of the attentional blink. Indeed an EEG study showed that the perception of a visual stimulus (followed by a mask) triggers an increase in alpha phase-coherence which peaks at 250 ms, perfectly matching the time point where the maximal AB usually is obtained (Mima, Oluwatimilehin, Hiraoka, and Hallett 2001).

Second, in the AB paradigm a steady state visual evoked potential in the alpha frequency range is induced at visual processing regions. Although it is still a matter of debate whether it is indeed the genuine alpha oscillation that is entrained by such stimulation, or whether it is just a series of additive visual evoked components (Capilla, Pazo-Alvarez, Darriba, Campo, and Gross 2011; Thut et al. 2011), such stimulation

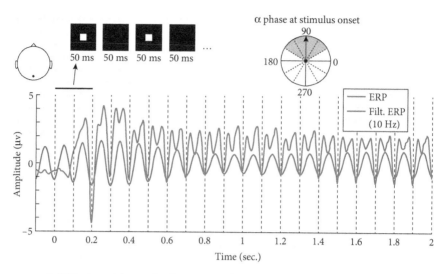

FIGURE 22.6 ERP data (electrode Oz; averaged over 17 participants) are shown during a steady state visual potential experiment. A stimulus (square) flickering at 10 Hz was presented. The blue line shows the unfiltered ERP, and the red line shows the bandpass-filtered ERP (8–12 Hz). Data from Wimber, M., Maaß, A., Staudigl, T., Richardson-Klavehn, A., Hanslmayr, S. (2012) Rapid memory reactivation revealed by oscillatory entrainment. *Current Biology*, 22, 1482–1486.

induces a strong phase alignment in alpha and also might increase alpha amplitude in general. Fig. 22.6 shows an example of a steady state visual evoked potential during an experiment in which subjects (N = 17) viewed a 10 Hz flickering stimulus (Wimber, Maaß, Staudigl, Richardson-Klavehn, and Hanslmayr 2012). These data demonstrate that the flicker stimulation entrains alpha activity such that the onset of each stimulus exactly matches the negative peak of the alpha phase. As discussed earlier, and as shown in Fig. 22.5, this resembles an internally oriented brain state during which thalamo-cortical information transfer is diminished. Thus, the entrainment of alpha phase and amplitude by the regular stream of stimuli might be one critical ingredient in generating the attentional blink. Indeed, recent results support this conclusion in showing that the attentional blink is virtually abolished by presenting the stimuli at an irregular rate, thus not entraining alpha oscillations (Fig. 7; Martin, Enns, and Shapiro 2011).

Taken together, alpha amplitude, phase, and phase-coherence reflect internally and externally oriented brain states, which determine the perceptual fate of a sensory stimulus. These parameters of alpha oscillations might be jointly driven by external stimulation and internal cognitive processes, and in turn exert a significant influence on the availability of attention for external stimuli over time. This relationship becomes most apparent in the attentional blink paradigm, where all these parameters are driven by the experimental procedure such that they resemble a worst-case condition (i.e. internally oriented brain state) for the perception of a sensory stimulus (T2; Fig. 22.4d).

Alpha and the AB

Recent investigations into the effects of alpha on the AB have confirmed a number of the predictions that arise from the preceding discussion. For instance, MacLean, Arnell, and Cote (2012) demonstrated that the magnitude of the AB blink was positively correlated with resting state alpha power. Interestingly, they also found that beta was negatively correlated with AB magnitude.

Martin et al. (2011) further investigated the role of the alpha in the AB by varying the temporal regularity of the non-target stimulus stream comprising the AB task. The logic is that disrupting the brain from going into a state of high alpha following identification of T1 should attenuate the AB and reveal a higher percentage of correct report of T2 relative to a control condition where alpha is not disrupted. Toward this goal, Martin et al. manipulated the temporal characteristics of every non-target element in the RSVP stream, leaving intact the timing of *critical* items, i.e. T1, T2, and their respective masks, as in the canonical AB paradigm. The SOA between all other items in the stream varied around a mean of 100 ms (ranging between 34 and 221 ms), creating an arrhythmic percept. The participants' task was to identify the only two coloured (target) letters in a (non-target) stream of black letters.

As shown in Fig. 22.7 (square symbols), AB magnitude was dramatically reduced by the arrhythmic stream, relative to the canonical (regular) condition (circle symbols). Martin and colleagues wished to rule out an alternative account for the attenuation of the AB, i.e. perhaps the arousal caused by the unpredictability of the RSVP stream required more attentional resources to be devoted to the task, thus enhancing performance. If this were true, then unpredictability on a different aspect of the stimulus stream should lead to the same outcome. To test this hypothesis, in a subsequent experiment Martin et al. returned the AB to its canonical regular temporal rhythm (100 ms SOA between all stimuli), but created unpredictability by varying the *size* (font) of the non-target RSVP stream. The critical (target) items were presented in the same size (18 point) as used in the previous experiment, but all other stream items varied randomly between 14 and 22 point, in a spatial manipulation that mirrored the temporal manipulation of the previous condition. Instead of attenuating the AB, as was seen with the temporally arrhythmic non-target stream, a dramatic and significant *increase* in AB magnitude relative to the canonical AB task was found (Fig. 7, triangle symbols). Clearly, arousal was inadequate to explain this pattern of results because there was no reason to predict more arousal in the temporally unpredictable condition than in the spatially unpredictable condition. Accordingly, Martin et al. concluded that preventing alpha entrainment was the key factor in attenuating the AB outcome.

Although the results of the study just described suggest a role for alpha in the AB, it does not exclude a similar role for a different frequency band. To address this issue, Shapiro et al. (submitted) created RSVP streams of non-targets to entrain frequencies in four different bands: theta (6.25 Hz); alpha (10.3 Hz); beta (16.0 Hz); and gamma (36.0 Hz). At the end of every trial, observers reported which of six possible alternative red letters (T1: B, G, S; T2: X, K, Y) were presented. Importantly, target duration was equated

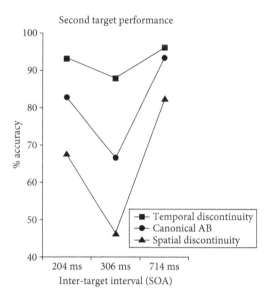

FIGURE 22.7 Percent accuracy on T2 as a function of SOA between T1 and T2 in the experiment by Martin, Enns, and Shapiro (2011). Square symbols represent performance in the arrhythmic (temporal discontinuity) stream; circle symbols indicate performance in the regular (canonical) AB condition; and triangles show performance in the condition (spatial discontinuity) where stimulus size was varied. Data from Martin, E. W., Enns, J. T., and Shapiro, K. L. (2011), Turning the Attentional Blink On and Off: Opposing Effects of Spatial and Temporal Discontinuity. Psychonomic, *Bulletin, & Review,* 18(2), pp. 295–301. Reproduced from Shapiro, K. L., Kerlin, J., Martin, E., Hanslmayr, S., Enns, J., and Lleras, A. (submitted). Alpha, beta: The rhythm of the attentional blink.

and the T1–T2 SOA was approximately matched (SOA; ~100, 300, or 700 msec) across all frequencies. In a second control experiment, we presented a set of identical stimulus conditions but instructed the participants to ignore T1 and respond only to T2. AB magnitude was calculated as the difference between correct T2 responses at SOA 700–SOA 300 msec. Results revealed a striking outcome (Fig. 8). Only when the stimulus stream was presented in the alpha and beta frequency band, was a significant AB obtained (both p's < 0.001), suggesting that these frequency bands play an important role in perception. Remarkably, although T1 'visibility' became increasingly difficult as the stimulation frequency increased, T1 bore no systematic relationship to T2 (i.e. AB) performance (see Fig. 8; dotted line). These results suggest that access to conscious awareness is gated by one of the brain's dominant frequencies (alpha) and by only one other frequency (beta), which often reveals outcomes paralleling those of alpha (Hanslmayr et al. 2012).

As previously argued, maintaining a moderate level of power and/or coherence sustains a brain state conducive to external perception, with evidence previously discussed suggesting synchronization occurring between the thalamus and cortex. On the other hand, when alpha (and beta) oscillatory power and/or coherence is high, as occurs when a target has been detected and whose identity is in the process of being consolidated into working memory, perception is significantly attenuated.

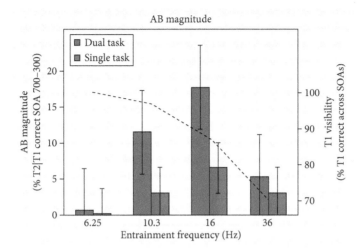

FIGURE 22.8 Bar plot of AB magnitude (SOA 700–300) for each frequency condition and task plotted with T1 visibility (dotted line) revealing T1 visibility inversely related to frequency and unrelated to AB magnitude. Error bars represent 95% confidence intervals. Reproduced from Shapiro, K. L. , Kerlin, J., Martin, E., Hanslmayr, S., Enns, J., and Lleras, A. (submitted). Alpha, beta: The rhythm of the attentional blink.

SUMMARY AND CONCLUSIONS

The goal of the present chapter was to provide a framework, based on neural oscillations in the alpha frequency band, for understanding the role played by such oscillations in determining the waxing and waning of perception. Various behavioural phenomena that exhibit such fluctuations in perception, such as priming—both positive and negative—inhibition of return, repetition blindness, and the attentional blink, were described. Whereas it is beyond the scope of this chapter to describe in detail how oscillations may underlie each of these cognitive phenomena, the role of alpha oscillations in the AB phenomenon was described in detail to provide a platform from which to present empirical findings in support of this basic contention. It is important to note that alpha is by no means the only frequency that has been related to cognitively based behaviours or the paradigms used to generate them. The reader is referred to an excellent recent review by Siegel, Donner, and Engel (2012) that describes the role of other frequencies in the context of reviewing the literature on the role of oscillations as they relate to cognitive function. It is also important to point out that alpha (and sometimes beta) oscillations bear a potentially causal and inverse relationship to both higher and lower frequency oscillations (cf. Siegel, Donner, Oostenveld, Fries, and Engel 2008).

Although the results of these studies lend support to the theoretical framework described herein, we hasten to point out that many important questions remain. At the top of the list would be the fundamental question of why the AB is revealed on only approximately half of all trials. This outcome suggests that the AB is not a mechanistic outcome based on imperturbable hard-wired neural properties. Future experiments able to study the role of oscillations on a trial-by-trial basis will be necessary to answer this question and will no doubt illuminate the stochastic nature of the brain's ability to segregate signal from noise (in Summerfield and Egner, chapter 29, this volume).

Investigation into the role of neural oscillations in perception, attention, and visual short-term memory is just beginning to hit its stride if the number of reports appearing in cognitive neuroscience journals and at recent major conferences is any indication. Importantly, although alpha oscillations play a very significant role, for which hopefully we have made the case in the present chapter, oscillations in other frequency bands play an equally important role and ultimately should be studied alongside that played by alpha. Although structural and functional imaging approaches to studying cognitive neuroscience have illuminated many important findings concerning the anatomical and functional locus of brain–behaviour relationships, EEG/ERP and MEG are the approaches of choice to study the role of oscillations and thus will come into even further prominence in the near future.

References

Arnell, K. M. and Shapiro, K. L. (2011). Attentional blink and repetition blindness. *Wiley Interdisciplinary Reviews: Cognitive Science* 2: 336–344.

Bavelier, D. and Potter, M. C. (1992). Visual and phonological codes in repetition blindness. *Journal of Experimental Psychology: Human Perception and Performance* 18(1): 134–147.

Berger, H. (1929). Über das Electroenkephalogramm des Menschen. 1st report. *Archiv für Psychiatrie und Nervenkrankheiten* 97: 6–26.

Bowman, H. and Wyble, B. (2007). The simultaneous type, serial token model of temporal attention and working memory. *Psychological Review* 114(1): 38–70.

Buffalo, E. A., Fries, P., Landman, R., Buschman, T. J., and Desimone, R. (2011). Laminar differences in gamma and alpha coherence in the ventral stream. *Proceedings of the National Academy of Sciences USA* 108(27): 11262–11267.

Busch, N. A., Dubois, J., and VanRullen, R. (2009). The phase of ongoing EEG oscillations predicts visual perception. *Journal of Neuroscience: The Official Journal of the Society for Neuroscience* 29(24): 7869–7876.

Busch, N. A. and VanRullen, R. (2010). Spontaneous EEG oscillations reveal periodic sampling of visual attention. *Proceedings of the National Academy of Sciences USA* 107(37): 16048–16053.

Buzsáki, G., Anastassiou, C. A., and Koch, C. (2012). The origin of extracellular fields and currents: EEG, ECoG, LFP and spikes. *Nature Reviews Neuroscience* 13: 407–420.

Buzsáki, G. and Draguhn, A. (2004). Neuronal oscillations in cortical networks. *Science* 304: 1926–1929.

Callaway, E. and Yeager, C. L. (1960). Relationship between reaction time and electroencephalographic alpha phase. *Science* 132: 1765–1766.

Canolty, R. T., Ganguly, K., Kennerley, S. W., Cadieu, C. F., Koepsell, K., Wallis, J. D., et al. (2010). Oscillatory phase coupling coordinates anatomically dispersed functional cell assemblies. *Proceedings of the National Academy of Sciences USA* 107(40): 17356–17361.

Capilla, A., Pazo-Alvarez, P., Darriba, A., Campo, P., and Gross, J. (2011). Steady-state visual evoked potentials can be explained by temporal superposition of transient event-related responses. *PloS One* 6(1): e14543.

Chica, A. B., Lupiáñez, J., and Bartolomeo, P. (2006). Dissociating IOR from endogenous orienting of spatial attention: Evidence from detection and discrimination tasks. *Cognitive Neuropsychology* 23: 1015–1034.

Chu, T., Hanslmayr, S., and Shapiro, K. L. (2012). Stimulation at alpha frequency affects visual search. Manuscript in preparation.

Chun, M. M. and Potter, M. C. (1995). A two-stage model for multiple target detection in rapid serial visual presentation. *Journal of Experimental Psychology: Human Perception and Performance* 21(1): 109–127.

De Martino, B., Strange, B. A., and Dolan, R. J. (2008). Noradrenergic neuromodulation of human attention for emotional and neutral stimuli. *Psychopharmacology (Berlin)* 197(1): 127–136.

Dehaene, S., Sergent, C., and Changeux, J. P. (2003). A neuronal network model linking subjective reports and objective physiological data during conscious perception. *Proceedings of the National Academy of Sciences USA* 100(14): 8520–8525.

Di Lollo, V., Kawahara, J., Shahab Ghorashi, S. M., and Enns, J. T. (2005). The attentional blink: Resource depletion or temporary loss of control? *Psychological Research* 69(3): 191–200.

Duncan, J. (1984). Selective attention and the organization of visual information. *Journal of Experimental Psychology* 13: 501–517.

Duncan, J., Ward, R., and Shapiro, K. L. (1994). Direct measurement of attentional dwell time in human vision. *Nature* 369(6478): 313–315.

Dustman, R. E. and Beck, E. C. (1965). Phase of alpha brain waves, reaction time and visually evoked potentials. *Electroencephalography and Clinical Neurophysiology* 18: 433–440.

Dux, P. E. and Marois, R. (2009). The attentional blink: A review of data and theory. *Attention, Perception, & Psychophysics* 71(8): 1683–1700.

Enns, J. T. and Di Lollo V (2000). What's New in Visual Masking? *Trends in Cognitive Sciences* 4(9): 345–352.

Ergenoglu, T., Demiralp, T., Bayraktaroglu, Z., Ergen, M., Beydagi, H., and Uresin, Y. (2004). Alpha rhythm of the EEG modulates visual detection performance in humans. *Brain Research: Cognitive Brain Research* 20(3): 376–383.

Fries, P. (2005). A mechanism for cognitive dynamics: Neuronal communication through neuronal coherence. *Trends in Cognitive Sciences* 9(10): 474–480.

Goldman, R. I., Stern, J. M., Engel, J., and Cohen, M. S. (2002). Simultaneous EEG and fMRI of the alpha rhythm. *NeuroReport* 13(18): 2487–2492.

Gould, I. C., Rushworth, M. F., and Nobre, A. C. (2011). Indexing the graded allocation of visuospatial attention using anticipatory alpha oscillations. *Journal of Neurophysiology* 105(3): 1318–1326.

Gross, J., Schmitz, F., Schnitzler, I., Kessler, K., Shapiro, K., Hommel, B., et al. (2004). Modulation of long-range neural synchrony reflects temporal limitations of visual attention in humans. *Proceedings of the National Academy of Sciences USA* 101(35): 13050–13055.

Haegens, S., Nácher, V., Luna, R., Romo, R., and Jensen, O. (2011). α-oscillations in the monkey sensorimotor network influence discrimination performance by rhythmical inhibition of neuronal spiking. *Proceedings of the National Academy of Sciences USA* 108(48): 19377–19382.

Hämäläinen, M., Hari, R., Ilmoniemi, R. J., Knuutila, J., and Lounasmaa, O. V. (1993). Magnetoencephalography—theory, instrumentation, and applications to noninvasive studies of the working human brain. *Reviews of Modern Physics*, 65(2), 413–497.

Hanslmayr, S., Aslan, A., Staudigl, T., Klimesch, W., Herrmann, C. S., and Bäuml, K.-H. (2007). Prestimulus oscillations predict visual perception performance between and within subjects. *NeuroImage* 37(4): 1465–1473.

Hanslmayr, S., Gross, J., Klimesch, W., and Shapiro, K. L. (2011). The role of alpha oscillations in temporal attention. *Brain Research Reviews* 67(1–2): 331–343.

Hanslmayr, S., Klimesch, W., Sauseng, P., Gruber, W., Doppelmayr, M., Freunberger, R., et al. (2005). Visual discrimination performance is related to decreased alpha amplitude but increased phase locking. *Neuroscience Letters* 375(1): 64–68.

Hanslmayr, S., Staudigl., T., and Fellner, M. C. (2012). Oscillatory power decreases and long-term memory: The information via desynchronization hypothesis. *Frontiers in Human Neuroscience* 6: 74.

Hanslmayr, S., Volberg, G., Wimber, M., Dalal, S. S., and Greenlee, M. W. (in press). Prestimulus oscillatory phase at 7 Hz gates cortical information flow and perception. *Current Biology*.

Herrmann, C. S. (2001). Human EEG responses to 1–100 Hz flicker: Resonance phenomena in visual cortex and their potential correlation to cognitive phenomena. *Experimental Brain Research/Experimentelle Hirnforschung/Expérimentation cérébrale* 137(3–4): 346–353.

Hughes, S. W. and Crunelli, V. (2007). Just a phase they're going through: The complex interaction of intrinsic high-threshold bursting and gap junctions in the generation of thalamic alpha and theta rhythms. *International Journal of Psychophysiology: Official Journal of the International Organization of Psychophysiology* 64(1): 3–17.

Hughes, S. W., Lörincz, M., Cope, D. W., Blethyn, K. L., Kékesi, K. A., Parri, H. R., et al. (2004). Synchronized oscillations at alpha and theta frequencies in the lateral geniculate nucleus. *Neuron* 42(2): 253–268.

Jacobs, J., Kahana, M. J., Ekstrom, A. D., and Fried, I. (2007). Brain oscillations control timing of single-neuron activity in humans. *Journal of Neuroscience: The Official Journal of the Society for Neuroscience* 27(14): 3839–3844.

Jensen, O., Gelfand, J., Kounios, J., and Lisman, J. E. (2002). Oscillations in the alpha band (9–12 Hz) increase with memory load during retention in a short-term memory task. *Cerebral Cortex* 12(8): 877–882.

Jensen, O. and Mazaheri, A. (2010). Shaping functional architecture by oscillatory alpha activity: Gating by inhibition. *Frontiers in Human Neuroscience* 4: 186.

Jolicoeur, P. (1998). Modulation of the attentional blink by on-line response selection: Evidence from speeded and unspeeded Task-sub-1 decisions. *Memory & Cognition* 26(5): 1014–1032.

Jolicoeur, P. (1999). Concurrent response-selection demands modulate the attentional blink. *Journal of Experimental Psychology: Human Perception and Performance* 25(4): 1097–1113.

Jolicoeur, P. and Dell'Acqua, R. (1998). The demonstration of short-term consolidation. *Cognitive Psychology* 36(2): 138–202.

Kahana, M. J. (2006). The cognitive correlates of human brain oscillations. *Journal of Neuroscience: The Official Journal of the Society for Neuroscience* 26(6): 1669–1672.

Kanwisher, N. G. (1987). Repetition blindness: Type recognition without token individuation. *Cognition* 27: 117–143.

Kawahara, J., Enns, J. T., and Di Lollo, V. (2006). The attentional blink is not a unitary phenomenon. *Psychological Research* 70(6): 405–413.

Keil, J., Müller, N., Ihssen, N., and Weisz, N. (2012). On the variability of the McGurk effect: Audiovisual integration depends on prestimulus brain states. *Cerebral Cortex* 22(1): 221–231.

Kelly, S. P., Lalor, E. C., Reilly, R. B., and Foxe, J. J. (2006). Increases in alpha oscillatory power reflect an active retinotopic mechanism for distractor suppression during sustained visuospatial attention. *Journal of Neurophysiology* 95(6): 3844–3851.

Klein, R. M. and MacInnes, W. J. (1999). Inhibition of return is a foraging facilitator in visual search. *Psychological Science* 10: 346–352.

Klimesch, W., Doppelmayr, M., Schwaiger, J., Auinger, P., and Winkler, T. (1999). 'Paradoxical' alpha synchronization in a memory task. *Brain Research: Cognitive Brain Research* 7(4): 493–501.

Klimesch, W., Sauseng, P., and Hanslmayr, S. (2007). EEG alpha oscillations: The inhibition-timing hypothesis. *Brain Research Reviews* 53(1): 63–88.

Kopell, N., Ermentrout, G. B., Whittington, M. A., and Traub, R. D. (2000). Gamma rhythms and beta rhythms have different synchronization properties. *Proceedings of the National Academy of Sciences USA* 97(4): 1867–1872.

Kranczioch, C., Debener, S., Maye, A., and Engel, A. K. (2007). Temporal dynamics of access to consciousness in the attentional blink. *NeuroImage* 37(3): 947–955.

Lee, H., Simpson, G. V., Logothetis, N. K., and Rainer, G. (2005). Phase locking of single neuron activity to theta oscillations during working memory in monkey extrastriate visual cortex. *Neuron* 45(1): 147–156.

Lopes da Silva, F. (1991). Neural mechanisms underlying brain waves: From neural membranes to networks. *Electroencephalography and Clinical Neurophysiology* 79(2): 81–93.

Lopes da Silva, F. H., Vos, J. E., Mooibroek, J., and van Rotterdam, A. (1980). Relative contributions of intracortical and thalamo-cortical processes in the generation of alpha rhythms, revealed by partial coherence analysis. *Electroencephalography and Clinical Neurophysiology* 50(5–6): 449–456.

Lorincz, M. L., Kékesi, K. A., Juhász, G., Crunelli, V., and Hughes, S. W. (2009). Temporal framing of thalamic relay-mode firing by phasic inhibition during the alpha rhythm. *Neuron* 63(5): 683–696.

Luck, S. J., Vogel, E. K., and Shapiro, K. L. (1996). Word meanings can be accessed but not reported during the attentional blink. *Nature* 383(6601): 616–618.

Lupiáñez, J., Klein, R. M., and Bartolomeo, P. (2006). Inhibition of return: Twenty years after. *Cognitive Neuropsychology* 23(7), 1003–1014.

McKoon, G. and Ratcliff, R. (1979). Priming in episodic and semantic memory. *Journal of Verbal Learning and Verbal Behavior* 18: 463–480.

McLaughlin, E. N., Shore, D., and Klein, R. M. (2001). The attentional blink is immune to masking-induced data limits. *Quarterly Journal of Experimental Psychology* 54(1): 169–196.

MacLean, M. H., Arnell, K. M., and Cote, K. A. (2012). Resting EEG in alpha and beta bands predicts individual differences in attentional blink magnitude. *Brain and Cognition* 78(3): 218–229.

Marcel, A. (1983). Conscious and unconscious perception: An approach to the relations between phenomenal experience and perceptual processes. *Cognitive Psychology* 15: 238–300.

Martin, E. W., Enns, J. T., and Shapiro, K. L. (2011). Turning the attentional blink on and off: Opposing effects of spatial and temporal discontinuity. *Psychonomic Bulletin & Review* 18(2): 295–301.

Mathewson, K. E., Fabiani, M., Gratton, G., Beck, D. M., and Lleras, A. (2010). Rescuing stimuli from invisibility: Inducing a momentary release from visual masking with pre-target entrainment. *Cognition* 115(1): 186–191.

Mathewson, K. E., Gratton, G., Fabiani, M., Beck, D. M., and Ro, T. (2009). To see or not to see: Prestimulus alpha phase predicts visual awareness. *Journal of Neuroscience: The Official Journal of the Society for Neuroscience* 29(9): 2725–2732.

Mima, T., Oluwatimilehin, T., Hiraoka, T., and Hallett, M. (2001). Transient interhemispheric neuronal synchrony correlates with object recognition. *Journal of Neuroscience: The Official Journal of the Society for Neuroscience* 21(11): 3942–3948.

Moosmann, M., Ritter, P., Krastel, I., Brink, A., Thees, S., Blankenburg, F., et al. (2003). Correlates of alpha rhythm in functional magnetic resonance imaging and near infrared spectroscopy. *NeuroImage* 20(1): 145–158.

Moratti, S., Clementz, B. A., Gao, Y., Ortiz, T., and Keil, A. (2007). Neural mechanisms of evoked oscillations: Stability and interaction with transient events. *Human Brain Mapping* 28(12): 1318–1333.

Müller, N. and Weisz, N. (2012). Lateralized auditory cortical alpha band activity and interregional connectivity pattern reflect anticipation of target sounds. *Cerebral Cortex* 22(7): 1604–1613.

Nieuwenhuis, S., Gilzenrat, M. S., Holmes, B. D., and Cohen, J. D. (2005). The role of the locus coeruleus in mediating the attentional blink: A neurocomputational theory. *Journal of Experimental Psychology: General* 134(3): 291–307.

Nieuwenhuis, S., van Nieuwpoort, I. C., Veltman, D. J., and Drent, M. L. (2007). Effects of the noradrenergic agonist clonidine on temporal and spatial attention. *Psychopharmacology* 193(2): 261–269.

Olivers, C. N. and Meeter, M. (2008). A boost and bounce theory of temporal attention. *Psychological Review* 115(4): 836–863.

Padoa-Schioppa, C. and Assad, J. A. (2006). Neurons in orbitofrontal cortex encode economic value. *Nature* 441: 223–226.

Palva, J. M., Monto, S., Kulashekhar, S., and Palva, S. (2010). Neuronal synchrony reveals working memory networks and predicts individual memory capacity. *Proceedings of the National Academy of Sciences USA* 107(16): 7580–7585.

Pashler, H. (1994). Dual-task interference in simple tasks: Data and theory. *Psychological Bulletin* 116(2): 220–244.

Pfurtscheller, G. and Aranibar, A. (1977). Event-related cortical desynchronization detected by power measurements of scalp EEG. *Electroencephalography and Clinical Neurophysiology* 42(6): 817–826.

Pfurtscheller, G., Stancák, A., and Neuper, C. (1996). Event-related synchronization (ERS) in the alpha band: An electrophysiological correlate of cortical idling—a review. *International Journal of Psychophysiology: Official Journal of the International Organization of Psychophysiology* 24(1–2): 39–46.

Posner, M. I. (1980). Orienting of attention. *Quarterly Journal of Experimental Psychology* 32: 3–25.

Posner, M. I. and Cohen, Y. (1984). Components of visual orienting. In H. Bouma and D. G. Bouwhuis (eds.), *Attention and Performance X* (pp. 531–536). Hillsdale, N.J.: Lawrence Erlbaum Associates.

Raymond, J. E., Shapiro, K. L., and Arnell, K. M. (1992). Temporary suppression of visual processing in an RSVP task: An attentional blink? *Journal of Experimental Psychology: Human Perception and Performance* 18(3): 849–860.

Rihs, T. A., Michel, C. M., and Thut, G. (2007). Mechanisms of selective inhibition in visual spatial attention are indexed by alpha-band EEG synchronization. *European Journal of Neuroscience* 25(2): 603–610.

Romei, V., Brodbeck, V., Michel, C., Amedi, A., Pascual-Leone, A., and Thut, G. (2008). Spontaneous fluctuations in posterior alpha-band EEG activity reflect variability in excitability of human visual areas. *Cerebral Cortex* 18(9): 2010–2018.

Romei, V., Gross, J., and Thut, G. (2010). On the role of prestimulus alpha rhythms over occipito-parietal areas in visual input regulation: Correlation or causation? *Journal of Neuroscience: The Official Journal of the Society for Neuroscience* 30(25): 8692–8697.

Sadaghiani, S., Scheeringa, R., Lehongre, K., Morillon, B., Giraud, A.-L., and Kleinschmidt, A. (2010). Intrinsic connectivity networks, alpha oscillations, and tonic alertness: A simultaneous electroencephalography/functional magnetic resonance imaging study. *Journal of Neuroscience: The Official Journal of the Society for Neuroscience* 30(30): 10243–10250.

Sarnthein, J. and Jeanmonod, D. (2007). High thalamocortical theta coherence in patients with Parkinson's disease. *Journal of Neuroscience: The Official Journal of the Society for Neuroscience* 27(1): 124–131.

Sarnthein, J., Stern, J., Aufenberg, C., Rousson, V., and Jeanmonod, D. (2006). Increased EEG power and slowed dominant frequency in patients with neurogenic pain. *Brain: A Journal of Neurology* 129(Pt 1): 55–64.

Sauseng, P., Klimesch, W., Stadler, W., Schabus, M., Doppelmayr, M., Hanslmayr, S., et al. (2005). A shift of visual spatial attention is selectively associated with human EEG alpha activity. *European Journal of Neuroscience* 22(11): 2917–2926.

Sauseng, P., Klimesch, W., Doppelmayr, M., Pecherstorfer, T., Freunberger, R., and Hanslmayr, S. (2005). EEG alpha synchronization and functional coupling during top-down processing in a working memory task. *Human Brain Mapping* 26(2): 148–155.

Scarborough, D. L., Cortese, C., and Scarborough, H. S. (1997). Frequency and repetition effects in lexical memory. *Journal of Experimental Psychology: Human Perception and Performance* 3(1): 1–17.

Scheeringa, R., Mazaheri, A., Bojak, I., Norris, D. G., and Kleinschmidt, A. (2011). Modulation of visually evoked cortical fMRI responses by phase of ongoing occipital alpha oscillations. *Journal of Neuroscience: The Official Journal of the Society for Neuroscience* 31(10): 3813–3820.

Schubert, R., Haufe, S., Blankenburg, F., Villringer, A., and Curio, G. (2009). Now you'll feel it, now you won't: EEG rhythms predict the effectiveness of perceptual masking. *Journal of Cognitive Neuroscience* 21(12): 2407–2419.

Seiffert, A. E. and Di Lollo, V. (1997). Low-level masking in the attentional blink. *Journal of Experimental Psychology: Human Perception and Performance* 23(4): 1061–1073.

Shapiro, K. L., Kerlin, J., Martin, E., Hanslmayr, S., Enns, J., and Lleras, A. (submitted). Alpha, beta: The rhythm of the attentional blink.

Shapiro, K. L., Raymond, J. E., and Arnell, K. M. (1994). Attention to visual pattern information produces the attentional blink in rapid serial visual presentation. *Journal of Experimental Psychology: Human Perception and Performance* 20(2): 357–371.

Siegel, M., Donner, T. H., and Engel, A. K. (2012). Spectral fingerprints of large-scale neuronal interactions. *Nature Reviews Neuroscience* 13: 121–134.

Siegel, M., Donner, T. H., Oostenveld, R., Fries, P., and Engel, A. K. (2008). Neuronal synchronization along the dorsal visual pathway reflects the focus of spatial attention. *Neuron* 60: 709–719.

Staudigl, T., Hanslmayr, S., Voges, J., Hinrichs, H., Schmitt, F. C., Heinze, H. J., Richardson-Klavehn, A., and Zaehle, T. (2013). Thalamo-cortical alpha synchrony during human visual perception. Manuscript in preparation.

Telford, C. (1931). The refractory phase of voluntary and associative response. *Journal of Experimental Psychology* 14: 1–35.

Thut, G., Nietzel, A., Brandt, S. A., and Pascual-Leone, A. (2006). Alpha-band electroencepha-lographic activity over occipital cortex indexes visuospatial attention bias and predicts visual target detection. *Journal of Neuroscience: The Official Journal of the Society for Neuroscience* 26(37): 9494–9502.

Thut, G., Schyns, P. G., and Gross, J. (2011). Entrainment of perceptually relevant brain oscil-lations by non-invasive rhythmic stimulation of the human brain. *Frontiers in Psychology* 2: 170.

Tipper, S. P. (1985). The negative priming effect: Inhibitory priming by ignored objects. *Quarterly Journal of Experimental Psychology: Human Experimental Psychology* 37(4): 571–590.

Tipper, S. P. (2001). Does negative priming reflect inhibitory mechanisms? A review and inte-gration of conflicting views. *Quarterly Journal of Experimental Psychology* 54(2): 321–343.

Tipper, S. P., Brehaut, J. C., and Driver, J. (1990). Selection of moving and static objects for the control of spatially directed action. *Journal of Experimental Psychology: Human Perception and Performance* 16: 492–504.

Tipper, S. P., Weaver, B., Jerreat, L., and Burak, A. (1994). Object-based and environment-based inhibition of return of visual attention. *Journal of Experimental Psychology: Human Perception and Performance* 20: 478–499.

Todd, J. J., Fougnie, D., and Marois, R. (2005). Visual short-term memory load suppresses temporo-parietal junction activity and induces inattentional blindness. *Psychological Science* 16(12): 965–972.

Tombu, M. and Jolicoeur, P. (2003). A central capacity sharing model of dual-task performance. *Journal of Experimental Psychology: Human Perception and Performance* 29: 3–18.

Treisman, A. (1996). The binding problem. *Current Opinion in Neurobiology* 6: 171–178.

Treisman, A. and Gormican, S. (1988). Feature analysis in early vision: Evidence from search asymmetries. *Psychological Review* 95(1): 15–48.

van Dijk, H., Schoffelen, J.-M., Oostenveld, R., and Jensen, O. (2008). Prestimulus oscillatory activity in the alpha band predicts visual discrimination ability. *Journal of Neuroscience: The Official Journal of the Society for Neuroscience* 28(8): 1816–1823.

Varela, F., Lachaux, J. P., Rodriguez, E., and Martinerie, J. (2001). The brainweb: Phase synchro-nization and large-scale integration. *Nature Reviews Neuroscience* 2(4): 229–239.

Varela, F. J., Toro, A., John, E. R., and Schwartz, E. L. (1981). Perceptual framing and cortical alpha rhythm. *Neuropsychologia* 19(5): 675–686.

Vialatte, F.-B., Maurice, M., Dauwels, J., and Cichocki, A. (2010). Steady-state visually evoked potentials: Focus on essential paradigms and future perspectives. *Progress in Neurobiology* 90(4): 418–438.

Vogel, E. K., Luck, S. J., and Shapiro, K. L. (1998). Electrophysiological evidence for a post-perceptual locus of suppression during the attentional blink. *Journal of Experimental Psychology: Human Perception and Performance* 24: 1656–1674.

von Stein, A., Chiang, C., and König, P. (2000). Top-down processing mediated by interareal synchronization. *Proceedings of the National Academy of Sciences USA* 97(26): 14748–14753.

von Stein, A. and Sarnthein, J. (2000). Different frequencies for different scales of cortical inte-gration: From local gamma to long range alpha/theta synchronization. *International Journal of Psychophysiology: Official Journal of the International Organization of Psychophysiology* 38(3): 301–313.

Ward, R., Duncan, J., and Shapiro, K. (1996). The slow time-course of visual attention. *Cognitive Psychology* 30(1): 79–109.

Watson, D. G. and Humphreys, G. W. (1997). Visual marking: Prioritizing selection for new objects by top-down attentional inhibition. *Psychological Review 104*: 90–122.

Wimber, M., Maaß, A., Staudigl, T., Richardson-Klavehn, A., and Hanslmayr, S. (2012). Rapid memory reactivation revealed by oscillatory entrainment. *Current Biology 22*(16): 1482–1486.

Worden, M. S., Foxe, J. J., Wang, N., and Simpson, G. V. (2000). Anticipatory biasing of visuospatial attention indexed by retinotopically specific alpha-band electroencephalography increases over occipital cortex. *Journal of Neuroscience: The Official Journal of the Society for Neuroscience 20*(6): RC63.

Wyble, B., Bowman, H., and Nieuwenstein (2009). The attentional blink provides episodic distinctiveness: Sparing at a cost. *Journal of Experimental Psychology: Human Perception and Performance 35*(3): 787–807.

....

CHAPTER 23

DYNAMIC ATTENTION

....

PATRICK CAVANAGH, LORELLA BATTELLI, AND ALEX O. HOLCOMBE

INTRODUCTION: TRACKING EVENTS AS THEY UNFOLD IN TIME

....

IN order to process the events around us we must select and keep track of the objects of current interest, ignoring others around them. This indexing or individuation of targets is a central function of attention and here we will examine how it operates during dynamic events, some as simple as a moving dot, others as complex as moving human forms. This indexing of targets maintains the continuity of their identity as they change and move. This requirement of continuity was defined by Ternus (1926, 1938) as 'the problem of phenomenal identity' and since then there have been several proposals to fill this role: object files (Kahneman, Treisman, and Gibbs 1992), Fingers of Instantiation or FINSTs (Pylyshyn 1989, 2000, 2001), deictic codes (Ballard, Hayhoe, Pook, and Rao 1997), and attention pointers (Cavanagh, Hunt, Afraz, and Rolfs 2010). These concepts are closely related, all providing temporary representations of the objects of interest— representations that index or point to the properties of the object, such as its features, history, location, and identity. This is of critical importance if the target is moving, as we can no longer interrogate its properties by accessing the same location in space. We must know where it has gone. In this chapter, we trace the evidence that these temporary representations are the functional core of attention: they control the selection of input and they have limited capacity. We will review six key properties of dynamic attention: (1) its 'identity' operation that individuates moving, changing targets; (2) the role of the motion trajectory; (3) spatiotemporal limits; (4) anatomical locus; (5) temporal structure; and (6) temporal salience maps. Two differences emerge that distinguish dynamic attention from standard spatial attention: first, temporal limits on selection become spatiotemporal limits, extending over space and time; and second, the controlling anatomical structures show bilateral rather than contralateral properties.

TRACKING TARGETS: IS IT ATTENTION OR IS IT LOW-LEVEL MOTION?

Dynamic attention keeps the location of selection focused on the target of interest as it moves. In doing so, it fills the fundamental role of keeping track of the target, maintaining the continuity of the target's identity as it moves. This tracking operation has been most widely studied in the multiple-object tracking task (Pylyshyn and Storm 1988; see review, Cavanagh and Alvarez 2005). In these experiments, several items are moving independently, a few of which are the targets. These targets are distinguished from the distractors only by their history—they began life in the display highlighted with a different colour or with flicker. Once this marking is extinguished, however, they are identical to the non-targets in the display, and differentiated only in the subject's mind. The task is of course a spatial as well as temporal one and if the items are too close together, the tracking fails for reasons of crowding—the identity of the targets and distractors cannot be kept independent if the targets cannot be individuated. But it is in the pure sense spatiotemporal. When the speed of items increases, the ability to keep track is reduced (Alvarez and Franconeri 2007; Holcombe and Chen 2012) even though the spacing is not changed.

Tracking multiple objects with attention certainly feels effortful. However, on its own, that is not actual evidence that the tracking is an attentional process. Nevertheless, recent results (e.g. Drew, McCollough, Horowitz, and Vogel, 2010) now strongly favour the direct role of attention in tracking. These results overturned the earlier findings that surprisingly did not show any evidence of the role of attention for tracking the targets. In particular, Pylyshyn and Annan (2006) presented test probes either on the tracked targets, on the distractors, or in empty space to see if there was a performance advantage for probe detection on the tracked targets. These results showed a deficit for probes on the distractors but no advantages and no differences for probes in empty space or on the tracked targets. However, Drew et al. (2010) argued that the dual task nature of this experiment disrupted normal allocation of attention. Specifically, having to detect probes on the distractors and in empty space forced subjects to unnaturally allocate attention away from the targets. To address this, they used event-related potential (ERP) measures of response to brief probes that the subjects were told to ignore. In this case, attentional enhancement of the ERP response was seen strongly on the tracked targets, weakly on the distractors, and most weakly in empty space (and on static distractors). These results provided direct evidence for what seems obvious to anyone who tries the multiple object-tracking task: spatial attention is strongly allocated to each target.

Brain imaging as well as transcranial magnetic stimulation (TMS) experiments also show the involvement of attentional areas during the multiple object-tracking task (Culham, Brandt, Cavanagh et al. 1998; Culham, Cavanagh, and Kanwisher 2001; Howe, Horowitz, Morocz et al. 2009; Jovicich, Peters, Koch et al. 2001; Shim, Alvarez, Vickery, and Jiang 2010; Battelli, Alvarez, Carlson, and Pascual-Leone 2009). More specifically, certain areas in frontal and parietal cortex modulate their activity as a function of the number of items being tracked. Roelfsema, Lamme, and Spekreijse (1998) have shown in a related curve-tracing task that enhanced neural activity can be detected moving along the path over which attention would be expected to move during the task. Overall, the behavioural, electrophysiological, and neurophysiological evidence all support the hypothesis that tracking is accomplished by maintaining a focus of attention over each target as it moves (attention pointers, Cavanagh et al. 2010). These results argue against Pylyshyn's original claims (1989) that the targets are indexed by non-attentional processes.

While attention is clearly involved in tracking, there is something special about the motion of the targets that helps keep attention locked on to its position. For example, Horowitz, Holcombe, Wolfe et al. (2004) asked subjects to move their attention across a set of targets arranged in a circle around fixation. They found that the subjects could shift attention much more rapidly if the targets appeared to be jumping than if they were static and attention had to switch from one to the next. Hogendoorn, Carlson, and Verstraten (2007) made essentially the same point in a similar experiment. This suggests that the motion of the targets is critical in engaging a much more nimble, mobile attention, one that stays with a single target as it moves, rather than slowly disengaging from one and re-engaging with the next as it steps through a series of separate targets.

If motion is the key, however, it comes in two varieties: low-level and high-level (Anstis 1980; Braddick 1974; Julesz 1971; Cavanagh 1992; Lu and Sperling 1995). The low-level motion signals are provided by directionally tuned neurons in early visual areas. These units are activated when there is motion in their preferred direction within their small area of surveillance, their 'receptive field'. Low-level units respond to energy in the input without having to identify or categorize anything. They also respond whether or not attention is directed to the moving stimulus, although attention can produce improvements in response (e.g. 20% in area MT; Treue and Maunsell, 1996). The second variety is called high-level motion but some have argued that is really just another name for attentive tracking (Verstraten, Cavanagh, and Labianca 2000; Wertheimer 1912). It makes little sense to ask whether high-level motion (attentive tracking) is critical for attentive tracking but we can ask whether this high-level motion system just collates low-level signals and attributes them to the target object; or whether it solves the tracking problem on its own.

Continuously moving targets will certainly activate low-level motion mechanisms. Do these responses help to keep attention focused (Cavanagh et al. 2010) on the target? In fact, it is easy to show that low-level mechanisms are of little or no use in tracking objects. The first evidence that the tracking process is independent of low-level mechanisms is that subjects can track stimuli that do not drive low-level motion responses (St. Clair, Huff, and Seiffert 2010). However, there is a second and more fundamental argument against the contribution of low-level signals. Specifically, low-level motion is a local measurement based in retinal coordinates, not an object property. In order to use low-level motion signals, the object in question has to be segmented from the background in order to pick up only the object's signals independently of background

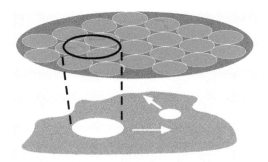

FIGURE 23.1 Low-level motion problematic for tracking targets. The visual system has to know where an object is to read out its low-level motion signals and avoid mixing them with other motions. This segmentation requires knowing where the object is at each moment. But if the object location is known on a moment-by-moment basis, there is no need to read out low-level motion. The object tracking problem is already solved.

motion. The segmentation therefore requires moment-to-moment knowledge of the object's location, in effect, requiring that the successful tracking of the object occur before the appropriate low-level signals can be encoded (see Fig. 23.1). Clearly, low-level motion cannot be of much help with tracking if tracking is a prerequisite for the help.

Fine, but could the low-level signal, once analysed from within the object's current boundaries, still help to determine the likely next location to find the target? Possibly, but clearly it is not essential (St. Clair et al. 2010), and often it is not possible because the recovery of global direction from low-level signals is frequently intractable (Rubin and Hochstein 1993). So it is not clear what the low-level signals could add, except perhaps, an after-the-fact sensation of the direction of the object's motion, in those cases where global motion extraction is possible. Here again, there is no need to extract motion from low-level signals, as the object's motion can be recovered from the attentive tracking signals. This is a process much like the one that recovers a target's motion when we track it with our eyes (smooth pursuit). In this case, when the pursuit is accurate, the target has little or no motion on the retina, and so little or no low-level motion signal. We nevertheless see it move. The signals that keep the eye on the target (efference copy) must provide the perception of motion for the target (e.g. Freeman and Banks 1998). Similarly, the signals that keep attention on a moving target, 'covert efference copy' (Cavanagh 1992), can provide a perception of motion for the target when the eyes are not moving. This is especially useful when the target does not activate low-level mechanisms (St. Clair et al. 2010). In this case, the objects are seen to slow or stop if they are not tracked, but when tracked they are perceived to move at close to their actual speed (Cavanagh 1992). In the study by St. Clair et al. (2010), the targets were patches of texture that had their own internal motion that could be consistent with the motion of the target itself or inconsistent. The internal motion was low-level, carried by local displacements of the luminance-defined texture, whereas the target's motion was high-level (not luminance defined). When the internal motion was inconsistent with the target's direction, tracking was impaired. This could suggest either that the low-level motion signals were contributing to the tracking, perhaps helping to predict the next location for the target, or that the target's perceived locations were distorted by the low-level signals (Ramachandran and Antis 1990) making it more difficult to keep track of target locations. The role of inconsistent low-level motion remains to be decided here, but the important point is that the absence of low-level motion does not impair tracking.

To summarize, stimuli that do not drive low-level motion mechanisms are nevertheless seen to move and can be tracked with attention. Moreover, the extraction of a target's motion (from displacement of an attention pointer that tracks it) is simpler than the extraction of global motion from low-level signals. In particular, the solution of target direction based on low-level motion requires an object segmentation that renders the low-level solution redundant, even if it were available.

Therefore, it would be more accurate to say that attentive tracking, high-level motion, is an independent system. This suggests that when contributions of low-level motion can be ruled out, research on high-level motion can be used to characterize the properties of dynamic attention, how it works, and how fast, and how far objects can be tracked as they move in continuous motion (multiple object-tracking tasks), or discrete jumps (apparent motion). We do not yet know how this tracking is accomplished but one outcome of the process is likely the updating of the target's activation, or attention pointer, on saccade maps (Cavanagh et al. 2010) to keep it locked on the target.

Spatial Attention Operates on Objects; Dynamic Attention Operates on 'Sprites'

Motion can tell us more than where an object is going; it can also tell us what the object is. The characteristic motions of familiar objects like a pencil bouncing on a table, a butterfly in flight, or a closing door can support the recognition of these objects. In return, once the object and its stereotypical motion are recognized, knowledge of that motion can support the continuing percept. Like the first notes of a familiar tune, our knowledge can guide our hearing of the remainder of the melody, filling in missing notes. Selfridge (1959) had argued that shape recognition was supported by legions of 'daemons' each of which detected whether a particular feature was present. We proposed dynamic versions of these agents, 'sprites' that would underlie the detection and representation of objects undergoing characteristic, stereotyped motions (Cavanagh, Labianca, and Thornton 2001). The suggestion is that dynamic attention does not operate on inert objects but on dynamic models that carry information not only about their identity and features but also about their expected motions. Point-light walkers make this point compellingly. A human form is easily recognized from the motions of a set of lights attached to a person filmed while walking in the dark (Johansson 1973; Neri, Morrone, and Burr 1998). Most importantly, Johansson (1973) proposed that the analysis relied specifically on an automatic and spontaneous extraction of mathematically lawful spatiotemporal relations. However, this does not hold up. Search for point-light walkers is very inefficient, suggesting only one can be analysed at a time (Cavanagh et al. 2001). Perception of this compelling, characteristic motion requires attention and that is a key argument for bringing these processes under the umbrella of attention.

The central point of the sprite proposal is that dynamic attention must actively model the motions of targets rather than simply passively follow them. One hundred years ago, Max Wertheimer (1912) reported a percept of motion that could not be explained in terms of low-level motion. Using a tachistoscope, he presented a configuration of two intersecting lines and alternated this stimulus (a cross) with one that was rotated 45 degrees. In space-time, the lines of the cross have correlations of equal strength in both the clockwise and the counterclockwise direction. This results in an ambiguous percept where back and forth motion between the lines is often the initial impression. However, Wertheimer (1912) also noticed that this was not always true. In the case where 'the lines stand normal to one another, and the distances are objectively equally favored, then it is *set and posture of attention* [. ..] that proved decisive in determining whether the rotation was seen towards the right or towards the left' (our italics, translated in Shipley 1961: 1070).

This observation points out the importance of attentional mechanisms in perceiving motion under ambiguous stimulus conditions. Despite its early discovery, this phenomenon was not studied again until recently (e.g. Ramachandran and Anstis 1983; Cavanagh 1992; Verstraten et al. 2000).

These phenomena suggest that dynamic attention uses models of familiar or characteristic motions to track moving objects, whether the motion of a wheel or the stride of a person walking. We claim that the animations are played out by attentive processes in the same way that we can animate a mental image. With the object present in the visual field, the input image data act like set points in the progress of the animation, a technique often used in computer graphics. The advantage of the motion models is the same advantage that is offered by any recognition of a familiar pattern. Once enough of the pattern is acquired to recognize it, the rest can be filled in from memory. Sparse inputs can support rich percepts and in the case of a moving object, filling in implies a prediction of likely motions and tracking them with fewer data than would otherwise be necessary. These advantages have formed the basis of many theories of perception from schemata and schema theory (Bartlett 1932; Neisser 1967) to frames and scripts (Minsky 1975; Schank and Abelson 1977).

These results suggest that the visual system acquires and uses stored motion patterns, sprites, which are characteristic of familiar events or objects. We use these stored patterns to recognize and then animate our perception of familiar events. Our experience of these animation routines might suggest that they are effortless; however, our studies showed that they are not (Cavanagh et al. 2001; Battelli, Cavanagh, and Thornton 2003b).

The internal modelling of trajectories and speed can underlie the perception of simple motions as well as complex ones. A tracked object in smooth (Verstraten et al. 2000) or random motion (Pylyshyn and Storm 1988) may be supported by the internal representation of its current and expected trajectory. We have proposed that high-level motion (cf. Anstis 1980; Braddick 1980) is realized by this type of model-based attention tracking. In other words, it relies on sets of attention routines that acquire and track targets (Cavanagh 1992) and it is bounded by the capacity limits and temporal resolution of attention (Verstraten et al. 2000).

WHAT ARE THE SPATIOTEMPORAL LIMITS OF DYNAMIC ATTENTION AND HOW DO THEY DIFFER FROM THOSE OF STATIC ATTENTION?

The importance of mobile attention for perceiving a dynamic scene is revealed when viewing a display created by Holcombe, Linares, and Vaziri-Pashkam (2011). Two circular arrays of coloured patches, centred on fixation, revolved continuously at the same rate. In the example shown in Fig. 23.2, the green patch in the inner ring is always aligned with the red patch in the outer ring. At slow rotation rates, that spatial relation (green aligned with red) is easy to perceive, as are the relative positions of all the other objects. However, above about 1.5 revolutions per second, one can no longer see which colours are adjacent. Yet the colours present are still easily recognized, and the motion direction easily perceived. The speed limit for attentionally tracking a single disc is approximately equivalent to that for judging their spatial relations. This is unlikely to be a coincidence, and this limit and other evidence (Holcombe et al. 2011; Franconeri, Scimeca, Roth et al. 2011) indicate that attentional tracking is required to perceive spatial relationships. Attentional tracking allows one to select an individual object with attention, which is required to apprehend its spatial relationships with other objects, possibly by shifting attention among them (Holcombe et al. 2011; Franconeri et al. 2011). The temporal limits on selection that constrain this process are reviewed below.

The temporal limits for attention are quite severe (Holcombe 2009; Shapiro this volume) and they are already in evidence for a stimulus that changes in place without moving. The shortest duration that can be isolated with attention within a stream of events has been called the dwell time of attention (Duncan, Ward, and Shapiro 1994; Moore, Egeth, Berglan, and Luck 1996). If two events fall within that time, they are irretrievably combined—they cannot be individuated. This duration is reported variously as 150 to 250 ms (Duncan et al. 1994; Moore et al. 1996). This same temporal limit constrains attention when a target moves. For example, if a dot turns off at one location and a second one turns on at a different location, observers report the apparent motion of a single target. If the two dots continue to alternate at the two locations, the impression of a dot moving back and forth is compelling as long as the rate of alternation remains under 5 to 8 Hz (equivalent to dwell times of 125 to 200 ms). Above that rate, the on and off phases

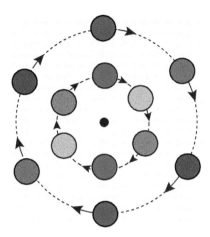

FIGURE 23.2 Spatial judgements between moving targets require attentive tracking. The coloured discs revolve about fixation, all at the same rate. Thus, two colours that are adjacent remain adjacent throughout the display. Above the speed limit for attentional tracking, however, observers are unable to judge which colours are adjacent.

for each dot are no longer resolved and so cannot be compared from the first dot to the second, making it impossible to check whether the offset of the first is coincident with the onset of the second, an essential requirement for seeing motion. Without this timing information the 'correspondence problem' cannot be solved, the offset of one dot cannot be linked to the onset of the other. The two locations now appear as two separate, flickering dots rather than one dot in motion (e.g. Anstis, Giaschi, and Cogan 1984: their Fig. 23.4b).

In temporal terms, the limits for selection of a static and a moving target are similar—attention has the same 'dwell time' in both cases. However, where they differ is in how the dwell time is spread over space. Specifically, in the static case, attention remains at a fixed location and requires about 200 ms to individuate single events at that location. However, in the moving case, as we will describe below, attention at any one location along the path can access events as brief as 50 ms (Cavanagh, Holcombe, and Chou 2008). The dwell time is spread out along the spatiotemporal path and moving attention can select brief stimuli along the path that could not otherwise be individuated.

Unlike recognition of certain elementary features that can be perceived at very fast rates of over 20 per second (Holcombe 2009), the maximum rate at which a single item can be recognized in a rapid sequence is around 10–12 items per second, or 5–6 Hz (White and Harter 1969; Potter 1993; Vagharchakian, Dehaene-Lambertz, Pallier, and Dehaene 2012). This limit is the same if the information is presented alternately to each eye, suggesting that the limitation is not due to peripheral constraints, but the temporal resolution of attention (White, Cheatham, and Armington 1953; Andrews, White, Binder, and Purves 1996). As well as limiting performance in rapid-serial-visual-presentation (RSVP) tasks that involve rapid presentation of individual objects, this maximum rate can also constrain discriminations of the relations between simultaneously presented simple features. Temporal rates for phase discrimi-nation of flickering lights show this low temporal limit (He, Intriligator, Verstraten, and Cavanagh 1998; He and MacLeod 1996; Rogers-Ramachandran and Ramachandran 1998). These and other data have led several authors to propose both a slow and a fast mechanism for detecting phase differences (Rogers-Ramachandran and Ramachandran 1998; Forte, Hogben, and Ross 1999; Victor and Conte 2002) where the fast mechanism can only work over short distances whereas the slow mechanism can operate over very large distances. The temporal limit of the slow mechanism has been linked to the tem-poral resolution of attention where the individuation of the light and dark phases of the flicker is likely to be mediated by visual attention (Battelli, Cavanagh, Martini, and Barton 2003a; Verstraten et al. 2000; Aghdaee and Cavanagh 2007). Note that this tem-poral limit is much lower than the temporal resolution of vision, which is around 30–50 Hz (Andrews et al. 1996; Rovamo and Raninen 1984; see review Holcombe 2009). Thus, just as the spatial resolution of attention is much worse than the spatial resolution of vision (Intriligator and Cavanagh 2001), the temporal resolution of visual attention is also much coarser than the temporal resolution of vision.

Similar limits are found for high-level motion tasks. Whereas simple luminance-defined motion can be perceived at fast rates of over 30 Hz (Burr and Ross 1982), for tracking a target in ambiguous motion (Verstraten et al. 2000; Battelli, Cavanagh, Intriligator et al. 2001), or in apparent motion (Verstraten et al. 2000), or a bar in a continuously drifting, sinusoidal grating, the upper rate for tracking is about 4–8 Hz (Verstraten et al. 2000). In their test with continuously moving targets, there was also an indication of a maximum speed for tracking of about 2 rotations per second (about the fovea). The limiting rate of 4–8 Hz is quite close to the well-documented limits on apparent motion (more specifically, at this rate and spacing, phi motion, Neuhaus 1930; Caelli and Finlay 1979, 1981; Tyler 1973), on phase discrimination of flickering lights (He and MacLeod 1996; He et al. 1998; Rogers-Ramachandran and Ramachandran 1998), on motion of drifting stereo-defined and motion-defined gratings (Patterson, Ricker, McGary, and Rose 1992; Lu and Sperling 1995), and on smooth pursuit for sam-pled motion (Morgan and Turnbull 1978). These phenomena may all be limited by a common factor: the temporal resolution of attention.

Battelli, Pascual-Leone, and Cavanagh (2007) proposed that the limiting factor is the access to the individual events in a rapid stream of events. In the case of ambiguous or apparent motion, each disc in the display is turning on and off and the task is to pair the offset of one disc with the onset of the next, adjacent disc. If each disc is turning on and off very rapidly, it is possible that the relative timing of the offsets and onsets of dif-ferent discs is no longer available, making it impossible to judge if one disc turns on at about the same time as the other turns off, a requirement for combining the two discs in the perception of a single disc in motion. At low rates of flicker, say, 1 or 2 Hz, an indi-vidual disc appears to turn on and turn off at discrete moments. Tracking at these rates is relatively easy. At higher rates of flicker, the same disc may appear to be continuously present but flickering—there is no access to the separate on and off intervals, and no way to link the offset of one disc to the onset of the neighbouring disc. Tracking fails at these rates, 4–8 Hz and higher.

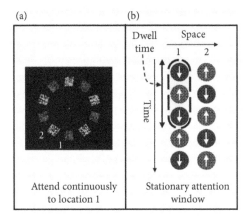

FIGURE 23.3 Attention sampling from a fixed location. (a) Each coloured, moving texture patch switches between red inward motion and green outward motion. (b) When attention is focused on location 1, sampling information from that patch, it has a minimum duration or dwell time before it can stop sampling, typically no less than 200 msec (Theeuwes, Godijn, and Pratt 2004; Duncan, Ward, and Shapiro 1994). During that time, the patch alternates between the two values and the resulting mixture degrades the ability to pair the colours with their motions. Adapted from *Journal of Vision*, 8(12), article 1, Cavanagh, P., Holcombe, A. O., & Chou, W., Mobile computation : spatiotemporal integration of the properties of objects in motion, pp. 1–23, figure 13 (2008), The Association for Research in Vision and Ophthalmology.

In one tracking experiment (Verstraten et al. 2000: experiment 3), the stimuli were in continuous motion, so low-level motion signals were available. The direction of the rotation of the grating could be reported at much faster rates than the 4–8 Hz where tracking failed. Just as some mechanism exists that responds to flicker even when separate on and off intervals are no longer experienced, some mechanism exists, undoubtedly low-level direction-selective units, that responds to motion at rates beyond those that support tracking individual targets.

We return now to the dwell time of attention. This refers to the minimum temporal interval that can be attended independently of preceding and following stimulation (Duncan et al. 1994). The dwell time for selecting and combining the colours and motions is fairly long, 300 ms or more (Moradi and Shimojo 2004; Arnold 2005), as it is for other attention-dependent tasks (e.g. Duncan et al. 1994; Holcombe and Cavanagh 2001). In an experiment by Cavanagh, Holcombe, and Chou (2008), colours and motion were alternated rapidly at each location in an array. At higher rates of alternation, 4 Hz or more, both of the alternating colours and both of the alternating motions are present within the dwell time (Fig. 23.3) so that processing of the colour–motion combination cannot be completed before the next pair arrives. Performance was severely degraded for rates above 3 Hz as would be expected from the standard view of attentional dwell time.

However, quite different results were seen when attention was moving. Figure 23.4 shows the alternating displays and the sampling window for attention as it moves across locations when the display is constructed so that each successive patch acquired

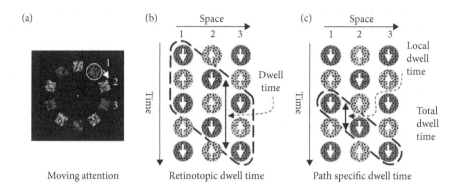

FIGURE 23.4 Attention sampling from a moving location. (a) On the simple dwell time account, when attention is moving over the alternating patches, it opens an attention window at each location that stays open for the dwell time before closing again. (b) With this simple dwell time theory, alternating stimuli at each location would be integrated to the same extent whether attention is moving or stationary. (c) The results instead showed that moving attention can offer substantial performance advantages, suggesting that once attention starts sampling at a given location, it does not continue to sample there for the whole dwell time, but rather it samples along the trajectory of motion. It may access a given location only very briefly (local dwell time as little as 50 ms), allowing attention to sample brief instants from a rapidly changing stream whose elements would otherwise be inaccessible to attention. Reproduced from *Journal of Vision*, 8(12), article 1, Cavanagh, P., Holcombe, A. O., & Chou, W., Mobile computation : spatiotemporal integration of the properties of objects in motion, pp. 1–23, figure 14 (2008), The Association for Research in Vision and Ophthalmology.

by moving attention is the same. Performance improved dramatically, indicating that attention no longer dwelled at a single location for an extended period, but rather its ≈300 ms dwell time is spread over different locations at different times so that it continually samples a single colour–motion pairing. It seems that when attention is moving, the dwell time is spread over space, covering 8° to 12° of visual angle at an eccentricity of 6.5° for the speeds used in that experiment. At even higher speeds, access by attention to any one location (local dwell time) may last as little as the 50 msec. The implication is that once attention arrives at a location and opens a channel to sample information from that position, that sampling channel is not local but moves on as attention moves on. It does not remain open for the full 300 ms at that location once attention has moved on.

WHAT ARE THE ANATOMICAL
UNDERPINNINGS OF DYNAMIC ATTENTION?

Two distinctive properties characterize spatial attention and distinguish it from dynamic, spatiotemporal attention. First, a wide variety of imaging, patient, and normal behavioural studies have shown that the networks controlling visual spatial attention, in

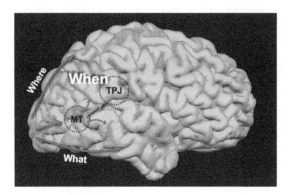

FIGURE 23.5 The 'When' pathway. Studies on neglect patients and TMS on normals suggest that there is a right parietal centre for interpreting the temporal order of events on the sub-second scale. This right hemisphere centre analyses temporal events in both hemifields.

the dorsal frontal and parietal areas (Battelli et al. 2001; Corbetta and Shulman 2002; see Corbetta and Shulman 2011 for a review), are generally contralaterally organized. That is, areas in the right hemisphere oversee spatial attention in the left visual field and vice versa. Second, the acuity of spatial attention scales with eccentricity. We can pay attention to, and select in isolation very small targets among closely spaced distractors when they are near the fovea but as targets move into the periphery, the spacing required for individual selection gets very large very quickly (Intriligator and Cavanagh 2001).

In contrast, the right hemisphere has a special role in the control of temporal aspects of dynamic attention for discrete stimuli and it appears to be bilaterally organized (Fig. 23.6, Battelli et al. 2001, 2003a, 2007, 2008). The temporal aspect that we focus on is the sorting and ordering of transients into the meaningful structure of an event stream. Objects appear, move, and disappear and all of these changes produce transients that on their own are not very informative. They need to be grouped together so an onset at one location and an offset at another are seen as the motion path of a single object. Each object on its own also needs to be individuated from preceding and following objects. The ability to individuate single events in a rapidly changing stream can be seen as a temporal equivalent to spatial acuity, as discussed in the previous section. But the temporal limit for the individuation of events as separate rather than an unintelligible flicker is much lower. This ability to detect the order of events, whether two events are seen as simultaneous or successive, sets the stage for the moment-to-moment interpretation of the visual world. Evidence from parietal patients, functional magnetic resonance imaging (fMRI), and TMS of the parietal lobe suggests that the right parietal lobe underlies this analysis of event timing for events in both left *and* right visual fields. Judgement of temporal order, simultaneity, and high-level motion (Fig. 23.6) are all impaired after right parietal lesions, but not left (Rorden et al 1997; Battelli et al. 2003a; Reddy, Rémy, Vayssière, and VanRullen 2011) and degraded after TMS over the right inferior parietal lobe (VanRullen, Pascual-Leone, and Battelli 2008). The experimental evidence suggests that the right inferior parietal lobe serves as part of a *when* pathway that mediates the timing component of many sensory capabilities from visual to auditory object discrimination across time (Rauschecker 2011).

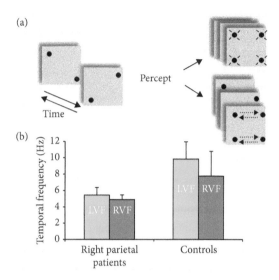

FIGURE 23.6 Bilateral impairment in apparent motion. (a) A quartet apparent motion stimulus. Two frames with two dots each are alternated at a variable frequency (left, arrows indicate
alternation in time). When the interval between the frames is very short (at high frequency,
more than 10 Hz), subjects can perceive only flickering dots and no motion is reported (top
right). At appropriate time intervals (around a frequency of alternation of 7 or 8 Hz), subjects
report motion (bottom right). (b) Patients who have right parietal lesions (average data from
three patients) show a severe deficit in perceiving apparent motion both in the left visual field
(LVF) and in the right visual field (RVF). Their threshold is about half that of normal controls
(average of six age-matched controls are reported). The patients cannot distinguish between
four flashing and two moving dots unless the alternation rate is as low as 4 or 5 Hz, which corresponds to an average of 200 ms interval between frames. Reprinted from *Trends in Cognitive
Sciences*, 11(5), Lorella Battelli, Alvaro Pascual-Leone, and Patrick Cavanagh, The 'when' pathway of the right parietal lobe, pp. 204–10, Copyright (2007), with permission from Elsevier.

In addition, the temporal resolution of attention does not appear to change much
with eccentricity (Aghdaee and Cavanagh 2007), decreasing only moderately in the
periphery. The *spatial* resolution of attention varies dramatically across the visual field;
a variation may arise from the properties of the cortices where attention operates. The
underlying assumption is that an 'attentive field' has a constant size on the visual cortex
on which it operates, so that the scaling of the attentional field with eccentricity reflects
the cortical magnification factor of that particular cortex. Parietal areas are often implicated in the control of spatial attention (Culham et al. 1998; Posner, Walker, Friedrich,
and Rafal 1984, 1987). There is no corresponding temporal cortical magnification factor
yet identified. The flicker fusion rate does not vary much across the visual field either as
a function of eccentricity or as a function of visual field (upper vs. lower) (Rovamo and
Raninen 1984), although the spatial integration area that sets it does (Granit and Harper
1930). This suggests that the temporal resolution of low-level (visual) mechanisms is
relatively homogeneous across the visual field. Aghdaee and Cavanagh (2007) showed

that high-level (attentional) resolution was relatively unchanged with eccentricity as well. They measured the temporal resolution of attention using long-range phase judgements, based on the assumption that attention is required to individuate the phases of spatially widely separated flickering stimuli. They concluded that the variation of the temporal limits of visual attention across the visual field differs markedly from that of the spatial resolution of attention.

Battelli et al. (2007) demonstrated another loss in temporal processing for detecting an odd item, a white square among black squares where all the squares alternate together in contrast, white to black and black to white. We might imagine that the odd square should be easy to notice as a single white square 'pops out' among black squares and vice versa. However, just as the 'effortless' processing of biological motion turned out to require attention (Cavanagh et al, 2001), so too does the discrimination of the 'odd' contrast item in an alternating display. In particular, a patient with a right parietal lesion is severely impaired at this task unless the alternation rate is below 3 Hz, while normal subjects fail on the task at alternation rates above 7/8 Hz (Fig. 23.7).

Patients appear to be able to discriminate temporal changes of objects with a much lower resolution relative to healthy subjects and studies with normal subjects and cerebrally lesioned patients show that brain regions in the parietal lobe are involved in the analysis of time as well as space, for both visual (Husain, Shapiro, Martin, and Kennard 1997; Battelli et al. 2001; Hillstrom, Husain, Shapiro, and Rorden 2004) and auditory (Rao, Mayer, and Harrington 2001; Harrington, Haaland, and Knight 1998) stimuli (see Husain and Rorden 2003, for a review). Studies with non-human primates are consistent with this view (Janssen and Shadlen, 2005; Herrington and Assad 2009, 2010) and they demonstrate the role of the monkey lateral intraparietal sulcus (LIP) in orienting of attention to sudden change of events in time. The human homologue of monkey LIP is presumably part of the posterior portion of the inferior parietal lobe (Orban, Claeys, Nelissen et al. 2006) and this brain area plays a major role in detecting visual events at unexpected locations (Kincade, Abrams, Astafiev et al. 2005). In particular, studies on patients with lesions in the right inferior parietal lobe suggest a specific role for this area of the brain in perceptual abilities that require the analysis of time (Husain et al. 1997; Magnani, Oliveri, Mancuso et al. 2011).

A fMRI (Claeys, Lindsey, De Schutter, and Orban 2003) study has demonstrated that the right inferior parietal lobe is significantly more active while perceiving a stimulus moving in apparent motion compared to the same dots flashing at identical frequency. The authors used the same stimulus we used with parietal patients and their results were in very good agreement with our data (Fig. 23.5, from Battelli et al. 2001). Furthermore another fMRI study has shown more significant activity in the right inferior parietal lobe while subjects were asked to covertly orient visual attention toward sudden visual stimuli (Yantis, Schwarzbach, Serences et al. 2002) and a similar result was also obtained in an MEG study (Martinez-Trujillo, Cheyne, Gaetz et al. 2007) where subjects were asked to report a transient change in speed in a moving random dot pattern in the left or in the right visual field. An EEG study (VanRullen, Reddy, and Koch 2006) showed a correlation between EEG signal in the right parietal lobe and the illusory perception of a rotating wheel that required discrete motion processing. TMS studies have also shown

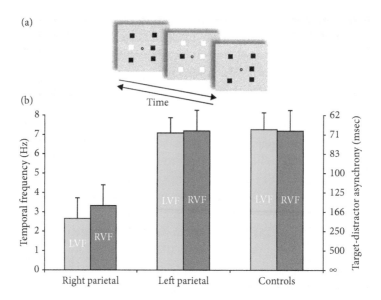

FIGURE 23.7 Phase discrimination task: bilateral deficit of identification of a visual event. (a) Subjects were asked to identify the odd target among six squares that alternated black and white at the same frequency as the target (middle item in the column left of fixation, top panel; arrows indicate alternation in time). The phase of the target square was shifted in time relative to the other five squares (when the target was black, the distractors were white). The target is easily seen at low alternation rates, but the task becomes more difficult at high alternation rates (for demonstrations of the task and patients' performance, see <http://visionlab. harvard.edu/Members/Lorella/movies/movies.htm>). (b) Normal controls and patients who had left parietal lesions could perform the task up to a speed of 7 or 8 Hz, whereas patients who had right parietal lesions had a threshold speed of 3 Hz for both the left visual field (LVF) and the right visual field (RVF). Asynchrony (ms) between the target and the distractors is reported on the right axis. Reprinted from *Trends in Cognitive Sciences*, 11(5), Lorella Battelli, Alvaro Pascual-Leone, and Patrick Cavanagh, The 'when' pathway of the right parietal lobe, pp. 204–10, Copyright (2007), with permission from Elsevier.

that the right parietal lobe must be specialized in performing tasks requiring the discrimination of discrete events in visual and auditory timing (Beck, Muggleton, Walsh, and Lavie 2006; Alexander, Cowey, and Walsh, 2005). Finally, a recent fMRI study (Reddy et al. 2011) showed activity in the right parietal lobe during the illusory perception of a rotating wheel that required discrete motion processing. The activity was independent of the side of stimulus presentation. Moreover, a TMS study using the same stimuli (VanRullen, Pascual-Leone, and Battelli, 2008) confirmed the role of the right inferior parietal lobe in perceiving the spatiotemporal structure of events, in this case discriminating forward from reverse motion. Altogether these data show evidence of a special role of the right inferior parietal lobe in visual event timing using both non-spatially lateralized dynamic and stationary stimuli.

From these studies, Battelli et al. (2007) concluded that the deficit involves the accuracy in parsing offsets and onsets as belonging to or not belonging to the same event. If the structure of offsets and onsets could not be paired together at higher rates, it would not be possible to link the offset of one dot with the onset of the other as a single item in motion. Note that the patients perceive smooth motion normally and show deficits only in the contralesional visual field in other attention-related motion tasks (Battelli et al. 2001).

Does Dynamic Attention Have a Temporal Structure?

Increasing evidence suggests that attention can concurrently select multiple locations (e.g. Pylyshyn and Storm 1988), yet it is not clear whether this ability relies on continuous allocation of attention to the different targets (a 'parallel' strategy) or whether attention switches rapidly between the targets (a periodic 'sampling' strategy). With respect to visual search tasks, in which a single target must be detected among a variable number of elements, this debate has divided the community for quite some time, with no accepted conclusion. A similarly unresolved argument has been made regarding multiple-object tracking paradigms (Tripathy, Ogmen, and Narasimhan 2011).

A recent article by VanRullen, Carlson, and Cavanagh (2007) addressed this question in a task where a 'probe' event of variable duration was detected by the observer. When only a single location was cued, the observer could allocate their attentional resources entirely to this location ('full attention' condition). In other trials, there were two or more cued locations ('divided attention'). Finally, on catch trials, the probe occurred on an uncued, unexpected location ('minimal attention' condition). Within a 'parallel' model, attention is shared across the targets so performance for a given probe duration should lie somewhere between the performance levels obtained with full and with minimal attention at this same duration. As the number of cued locations increases, the performance should move uniformly closer to the function found for minimal attention. For a 'sampling' strategy, however, performance with any given target could be at the full or minimal attention level depending on the location of attention. This latter case is what was found.

These results showed that attention might resolve a difficult, attentionally demanding task by periodically sampling information from the different target locations, at a rate of approximately seven elements per second. A related study by Landau and Fries (2012) has provided further support. The results also indicated that attention operated with periodic sampling even when it was focused on a single target location. If attention, when focused on a single location, samples information periodically like a blinking spotlight, then why did hundreds of previous studies of attentional mechanisms not reveal this property? The fact that most experimental paradigms (even those involving electrophysiology) rely on averaging signals across several trials is probably one reason. If the onset of each periodic attentional sample (an internal process) bears no relation to stimulus onset (an external event), such averaging would conceal the effects of periodic attentional sampling from the experimenter.

It is nevertheless puzzling that attention should sample cyclically when only one location is attended. Periodic sampling is often seen in sensory systems: saccades in vision, sniffs in olfaction, whisker movements in rat somatosensation, and even echolocation in bats or electrolocation in electric fish are all examples of explicit cycling of perceptual uptake (Uchida, Kepecs, and Mainen, 2006). Attentional sampling might have evolved from these periodic processes. There may also be multiple stages in sampling that require periodic breaks in uptake from an attended stimulus. Perhaps sampling must alternate with transmission or other control processes. Whatever the reason, the long debate over serial versus parallel processing will continue for the question of attention itself.

Is There a Salience Map of Local Time that Is Sometimes Distorted by Strong Attentional Focus?

A number of studies report that the subjective experience of time is slowed at traumatic or attention-grabbing events (see review, Eagleman 2008). One interpretation of this phenomenon is that perceived duration is a function of the amount of information processed per unit of objective time. Attention may boost the amount of information processed above baseline level so that it generates more information per unit of objective time (Fig. 23.8). Consequently, the attended event may seem to last longer than a less attended event of the same objective duration. Tse, Intriligator, Rivest, and Cavanagh (2004) used an oddball paradigm to explore this phenomenon. A stream of repeating stimuli were presented, one per second for example, each lasting 500 ms (these durations were varied). Occasionally a novel item was presented and subjects had to adjust its duration until it appeared to last as long as the repeating stimulus. Overall, the novel item appeared to last 50% longer. More extreme versions of this experiment were conducted by Stetson and his colleagues (Stetson, Fiesta, and Eagleman 2007) where subjects were released from a tall tower for 50 metres (3 seconds) of freefall (into a net). They again judged the interval as longer than a control (non-terrifying) interval that was matched in objective time. Stetson et al. tried to test whether this expansion of time was accompanied by a greater amount of information processed per unit of time, using a test related to measurement of flicker fusion rate. However, the lack of eye movement controls for the rapidly falling observers compared to the calmly sitting observers leaves the question regarding flicker fusion unresolved. Additional tests should also be done on the rate of processing at rates beyond the flicker fusion limit.

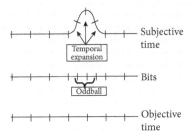

FIGURE 23.8 Attention-induced, time dilation. When an attention-grabbing event occurs, more information is processed over the stimulus per unit of objective time. If subjective time is gauged in terms of the amount of perceptual information processed, subjective time will seem to expand relative to objective time, as shown at the top region indicated 'temporal expansion'. Reproduced from *Perception & Psychophysics*, 6(7), 2004 pp 1171–1189, Attention and the subjective expansion of time, Tse, P., Intriligator, J., Rivest, J., and Cavanagh, P., © Springer Science and Business Media. With kind permission from Springer Science and Business Media.

CONCLUSIONS

We reviewed the role of attention in tracking and processing dynamic events. We showed that attention has a mobile point of operation or 'pointer' that follows moving targets, picking up pieces of evidence along the way to determine not just what a target is, but what it is doing. Familiar trajectories help identify a target and guide encoding of continuing input from its path. Attention has coarse temporal resolution but when the focus of selection is on the move, a given location on a moving target's path can be selected for as little as 50 ms, compared to the typical 'dwell time' or minimum duration of attention selection at a fixed location of 200 ms or more. This indicates that the temporal capacity limits of attention are imposed in a target-specific frame of reference, not a retinal coordinate frame. When individuating targets in a rapidly changing scene, a critical limit is the necessity to assess each transient as a target offset or an onset. This is not as simple as encoding and cataloguing luminance transients because the onset of an object that is darker than its surround will produce a decrement in luminance whereas the onset of an object that is lighter than its surround will produce an increment. Instead, objects must be segmented, identified, and tracked, a process that is slower than simple detection of transients by a factor of about 10. This step of temporal selection is fundamental in our rich visual environment where suddenly appearing (and disappearing) salient objects must be continually and rapidly discriminated from the background. This process has been localized to the right parietal region, a cortical structure that was then seen as a central part of a 'when' pathway. Patient studies show that this temporal selection is a qualitatively different system from spatial attention, where right parietal patients affected by neglect show a strong spatial impairment in the contralateral hemifield *only*. In contrast, this temporal selection and tracking of object identity is completely based in the right inferior parietal lobe for events in both hemifields.

Finally, attention may have a cyclical nature, sampling its input, whether static or dynamic, in a series of snapshots at a preferred sampling rate of around 8 Hz, and may be able to allocate more resources to upcoming moments of expected salience, with one consequence being a dilation in the subjective experience of time during those moments.

ACKNOWLEDGEMENTS

The preparation of this review was supported in part by NIH grants EY09258 (PC) and EY15960 (LB), ANR Chaire d'Excellence (PC), and an ARC Future Fellowship (AOH).

REFERENCES

Aghdaee, S. M. and Cavanagh, P. (2007). Temporal limits of long-range phase discrimination across the visual field. *Vision Research 47*: 2156–2163.

Alexander, I., Cowey, A., and Walsh, V. (2005). The right parietal cortex and time perception: Back to Critchley and the Zeitraffer phenomenon. *Cognitive Neuropsychology 22*: 306–315.

Alvarez, G. A. and Franconeri, S. L. (2007). How many objects can you track? Evidence for a resource-limited attentive tracking mechanism. *Journal of Vision 7*(13): 14.1–10.

Andrews, T. J., White, L. E., Binder, D., and Purves, D. (1996). Temporal events in cyclopean vision. *Proceedings of the National Academy of Sciences USA 93*(8): 3689–3692.

Anstis, S. M. (1980). The perception of apparent movement. *Philosophical Transactions of the Royal Society B: Biological Sciences 290*: 153–168.

Anstis, S., Giaschi, D., and Cogan, A. I. (1984). Adaptation to apparent motion. *Vision Research 25*: 1051–1062.

Arnold, D. H. (2005). Perceptual pairing of colour and motion. *Vision Research 45*: 3015–3026.

Ballard, D. H., Hayhoe, M. M., Pook, P. K., and Rao, R. P. (1997). Deictic codes for the embodiment of cognition. *Behavioral and Brain Sciences 20*: 723–742; discussion 743–767.

Bartlett, S. F. (1932). *Remembering: A Study in Experimental and Social Psychology.* Cambridge: Cambridge University Press.

Battelli L., Alvarez G., Carlson T., and Pascual-Leone A. (2009). The role of the parietal lobe in visual extinction studied with transcranial magnetic stimulation. *Journal of Cognitive Neuroscience 21*(10): 1946–1955.

Battelli, L., Cavanagh, P., Intriligator, J., Tramo, M. J., Hénaff, M.-A., Michèl, F., and Barton, J. J. S. (2001). Unilateral right parietal damage leads to bilateral deficit for high-level motion. *Neuron 32*: 985–995.

Battelli, L., Cavanagh, P., Martini, P., and Barton, J. S. S. (2003a). Bilateral deficits of transient visual attention in right parietal patients. *Brain 126*: 2164–2174.

Battelli, L., Cavanagh, P., and Thornton, I. M. (2003b). Perception of biological motion in parietal patients. *Neuropsychologia 41*(13): 1808–1816.

Battelli, L., Pascual-Leone, A., and Cavanagh, P. (2007). The 'when' pathway of the right parietal lobe. *Trends in Cognitive Science 11*: 204–210.

Battelli, L., Walsh, V., Pascual-Leone, A., and Cavanagh, P. (2008). The 'when' parietal pathway explored by lesion studies. *Current Opinion in Neurobiology 18*: 120–126.

Beck, D. M., Muggleton, N., Walsh, V., and Lavie, N. (2006). Right parietal cortex plays a critical role in change blindness. *Cerebral Cortex 16*(5): 712–717.

Braddick, O. (1974). A short-range process in apparent motion. *Vision Research 14*: 519–527.

Braddick, O. J. (1980). Low-level and high-level processes in apparent motion. *Philosophical Transactions of the Royal Society Biological Sciences*, 290: 137–151.

Burr, D. C. and Ross, J. (1982). Contrast sensitivity at high velocities. *Vision Research 22*: 479–484.

Caelli, T. and Finlay, D. (1979). Frequency, phase, and colour coding in apparent motion. *Perception 8*: 59–68.

Caelli, T. and Finlay, D. (1981). Intensity, spatial frequency, and temporal frequency determinants of apparent motion. *Perception 10*: 183–189.

Cavanagh, P. (1992). Attention-based motion perception. *Science 257*: 1563–1565.

Cavanagh, P. and Alvarez, G. (2005). Tracking multiple targets with multifocal attention. *Trends in Cognitive Sciences 9*: 349–354.

Cavanagh, P., Holcombe, A. O., and Chou, W. (2008). Mobile computation: Spatiotemporal integration of the properties of objects in motion. *Journal of Vision 8*(12): 1.1–23.

Cavanagh, P., Hunt, A., Afraz, A., and Rolfs, M. (2010). Visual stability based on remapping of attention pointers. *Trends in Cognitive Sciences 14*: 147–153.

Cavanagh, P., Labianca, A. T., and Thornton, I. M. (2001). Attention-based visual routines: Sprites. *Cognition 80*: 47–60.

Claeys, K. G., Lindsey, D. T., De Schutter, E., and Orban, G. A. (2003). A higher order motion region in human inferior parietal lobule: Evidence from fMRI. *Neuron 40*(3): 631–642.

Corbetta, M. and Shulman, G. L. (2002). Control of goal-directed and stimulus-driven attention in the brain. *Nature Reviews Neuroscience 3*(3): 201–215.

Corbetta, M. and Shulman, G. L. (2011). Spatial neglect and attention networks. *Annual Review of Neuroscience 2011*(34): 569–599.

Culham, J. C., Brandt, S. A., Cavanagh, P., Kanwisher, N. G., Dale, A. M., and Tootell, R. B. H. (1998). Cortical fMRI activation produced by attentive tracking of moving targets. *Journal of Neurophysiology 80*: 2657–2670.

Culham, J. C., Cavanagh, P., and Kanwisher, N. G. (2001). Attention response functions: Characterizing brain areas with fMRI activation during parametric variations of attentional load. *Neuron 32*: 737–745.

Drew, T., McCollough, A. W., Horowitz, T. S., and Vogel, E. K. (2010). Attentional enhancement during multiple-object tracking. *Psychonomic Bulletin & Review 16*(2): 411–417

Duncan, J., Ward, R., and Shapiro, K. (1994). Direct measurement of attentional dwell time in human vision. *Nature 369*: 313–315.

Eagleman, D. M. (2008). Human time perception and its illusions. *Current Opinions in Neurobiology*, 18(2):131–136. doi: 10.1016/j.conb.2008.06.002.

Forte, J., Hogben, J. H., and Ross, J. (1999). Spatial limitations of temporal segmentation. *Vision Research 39*(24): 4052–4061.

Franconeri, S. L., Scimeca, J. M., Roth, J. C., Helseth, S. A., and Kahn, L. E. (2011). Flexible visual processing of spatial relationships. *Cognition 122*(2): 210–227.

Freeman, T. C. and Banks, M. S. (1998). Perceived head-centric speed is affected by both extra-retinal and retinal errors. *Vision Research 38*: 941–945.

Granit, R. and Harper, P. (1930). Comparative studies on the peripheral and central retina. II: Synaptic reactions in the eye. *American Journal of Physiology 95*: 211–228.

Harrington, D. L., Haaland, K. Y., and Knight, R. T. (1998). Cortical networks underlying mechanisms of time perception. *Journal of Neuroscience* 18(3): 1085–1095.

He, S. and MacLeod, D. I. (1996). Local luminance nonlinearity and receptor aliasing in the detection of high-frequency gratings. *Journal of the Optical Society of America A: Optics, Image Science, and Vision* 13(6): 1139–1151.

He, S., Intriligator, J., Verstraten, F. A. J., and Cavanagh, P. (1998). Slow mechanism for phase discrimination of both luminance and color flicker. *Investigative Ophthalmology and Visual Science* 39: 1110 (suppl).

Herrington, T. M. and Assad, J. A. (2009). Neural activity in the middle temporal area and lateral intraparietal area during endogenously cued shifts of attention. *Journal of Neuroscience* 29(45): 14160–14176.

Herrington, T. M. and Assad, J. A. (2010). Temporal sequence of attentional modulation in the lateral intraparietal area and middle temporal area during rapid covert shifts of attention. *Journal of Neuroscience* 30(9): 3287–3296.

Hillstrom, A. P., Husain, M., Shapiro, K. L., and Rorden, C. (2004). Spatiotemporal dynamics of attention in visual neglect: A case study. *Cortex* 40(3): 433–440.

Hogendoorn, H., Carlson, T. A., and Verstraten, F. A. (2007). The time course of attentive tracking. *Journal of Vision* 7: 2.1–10.

Holcombe, A. O. (2009). Seeing slow and seeing fast: Two limits on perception. *Trends in Cognitive Sciences* 13(5): 216–221.

Holcombe, A. O., and Cavanagh, P. (2001). Early binding of feature pairs for visual perception. *Nature Neuroscience*, 4: 127–128.

Holcombe, A. O. and Chen, W. Y. (2012). Exhausting attentional tracking resources with a single fast-moving object. *Cognition* 123(2): 218–228.

Holcombe, A. O., Linares, D., and Vaziri-Pashkam, M. (2011). Perceiving spatial relations via attentional tracking and shifting. *Current Biology* 21(13): 1135–1139. doi: 10.1016/j.cub.2011.05.031.

Horowitz, T. S., Holcombe, A. O., Wolfe, J. M., Arsenio, H. C., and DiMase, J. S. (2004). Attentional pursuit is faster than attentional saccade. *Journal of Vision* 4(7): 585–603.

Howe, P. D., Horowitz, T. S., Morocz, I. A., Wolfe, J., and Livingstone, M. S. (2009). Using fMRI to distinguish components of the multiple object tracking task. *Journal of Vision* 9(4): 10.1–11.

Husain, M. and Rorden, C. (2003). Non-spatially lateralized mechanisms in hemispatial neglect. *Nature Reviews Neuroscience* 4(1): 26–36.

Husain, M., Shapiro, K. Martin. J., and Kennard, C. (1997). Abnormal temporal dynamics of visual attention in spatial neglect patients. *Nature* 385(6612): 154–156.

Intriligator, J. and Cavanagh, P. (2001). The spatial resolution of visual attention. *Cognitive Psychology* 43: 171–216.

Janssen P. and Shadlen, M. N. (2005). A representation of the hazard rate of elapsed time in macaque area LIP. *Nature Neuroscience* 8(2): 234–241.

Johansson, G. (1973). Visual perception of biological motion and a model for its analysis. *Perception & Psychophysics* 14: 201–211.

Jovicich, J., Peters, R. J., Koch, C., Braun, J., Chang, L., and Ernst, T. (2001). Brain areas specific for attentional load in a motion-tracking task. *Journal of Cognitive Neuroscience* 13: 1048–1058.

Julesz, B. (1971). *Foundations of Cyclopean Perception*. Chicago: University of Chicago Press.

Kahneman, D., Treisman, A., and Gibbs, B. J. (1992). The reviewing of object files: Object specific integration of information. *Cognitive Psychology* 24: 175–219.

Kincade, J. M., Abrams, R. A., Astafiev, A. V., Shulman, G. L., and Corbetta, M. (2005). An event-related functional magnetic resonance imaging study of voluntary and stimulus-driven orienting of attention. *Journal of Neuroscience* 25(18): 4593–4604.

Landau, A. N. and Fries, P. (2012). Attention samples stimuli rhythmically. *Current Biology* 22(11): 1000–1004. doi: 10.1016/j.cub.2012.03.054.

Lu, Z.-L. and Sperling, G. (1995). Attention-generated apparent motion. *Nature* 377: 237–239.

Lu, Z.-L. and Sperling, G. (1996). Three systems for visual motion perception. *Current Directions in Psychological Science* 5: 44–53.

Magnani, B., Oliveri, M., Mancuso, G., Galante, E., and Frassinetti, F. (2011). Time and spatial attention: Effects of prism adaptation on temporal deficits in brain damaged patients. *Neuropsychologia* 49(5): 1016–1023.

Martinez-Trujillo, J. C., Cheyne, D., Gaetz, W., Simine, E., and Tsotsos, J. K. (2007). Activation of area MT/V5 and the right inferior parietal cortex during the discrimination of transient direction changes in translational motion. *Cerebral Cortex* 17(7): 1733–1739.

Minsky, M. (1975). A framework for representing knowledge. In P. H. Winston (ed.), *The Psychology of Computer Vision* (pp. 211–280). New York: McGraw-Hill.

Moore, C. M., Egeth, H., Berglan, L., and Luck, S. J. (1996). Are attentional dwell times inconsistent with serial visual search? *Psychonomic Bulletin & Review* 3: 360–365.

Moradi, F. and Shimojo, S. (2004). Perceptual-binding and persistent surface segregation. *Vision Research* 44: 2885–2899.

Morgan, M. J. and Turnbull, D. F. (1978). Smooth eye tracking and the perception of motion in the absence of real movement. *Vision Research* 18: 1053–1059.

Neisser, U. (1967). *Cognitive Psychology*. New York: Prentice Hall.

Neri, P., Morrone M. C., and Burr, D. C. (1998). Seeing biological motion. *Nature* 395: 894–896.

Neuhaus, W. (1930). Experimentelle Studien über das Schein von Bewegung. *Pflügers Archiv für die Gesamte Psychologie des Menschen und der Tiere* 75: 315–458.

Orban, G. A., Claeys, K., Nelissen, K., Smans, R., Sunaert, S., Todd, J. T., Wardak, C., Durand, J. B., and Vanduffel, W. (2006). Mapping the parietal cortex of human and non-human primates. *Neuropsychologia* 44(13): 2647–2667.

Patterson, R., Ricker, C., McGary, J., and Rose D. (1992). Properties of cyclopean motion perception. *Vision Research* 32: 149–156.

Posner, M. I., Walker, J. A., Friedrich, F. J., and Rafal, R. D. (1984). Effects of parietal injury on covert orienting of attention. *Journal of Neuroscience* 4: 1863–1874.

Posner, M. I., Walker, J. A., Friedrich, F. A., and Rafal, R. D. (1987). How do the parietal lobes direct covert attention? *Neuropsychologia* 25: 135–145.

Potter, M. C. (1993). Very short-term conceptual memory. *Memory & Cognition* 21: 156–161.

Pylyshyn, Z. W. (1989). The role of location indexes in spatial perception: A sketch of the FINST spatial indexing model. *Cognition* 32: 65–97.

Pylyshyn, Z. W. (2000). Situating vision in the world. *Trends in Cognitive Sciences* 4: 197–207.

Pylyshyn, Z. W. (2001). Visual indexes, preconceptual objects, and situated vision. *Cognition* 80(1/2): 127–158.

Pylyshyn, Z. W. and Annan, Jr, V. (2006). Dynamics of target selection in multiple object tracking (MOT). *Spatial Vision* 19(6): 485–504.

Pylyshyn, Z. W. and Storm, R. W. (1988). Tracking multiple independent targets: Evidence for a parallel tracking mechanism. *Spatial Vision* 3: 151–224.

Ramachandran, V. S. and Anstis, S. M. (1983). Perceptual organization in moving patterns. *Nature* 304(5926): 529–531.

Ramachandran, V. S. and Anstis, S. M. (1990). Illusory displacement of equiluminous kinetic edges. *Perception* 19(5): 611–616.

Rao, S. M., Mayer, A. R., and Harrington, D. L. (2001). The evolution of brain activation during temporal processing. *Nature Neuroscience* 4(3): 317–323.

Rauschecker, J. P. (2011). An expanded role for the dorsal auditory pathway in sensorimotor control and integration. *Hearing Research* 271(1–2): 16–25.

Reddy, L., Rémy, F., Vayssière, N., and VanRullen, R. (2011). Neural correlates of the continuous Wagon Wheel Illusion: A functional MRI study. *Human Brain Mapping* 32(2): 163–170.

Roelfsema, P. R., Lamme, V. A., and Spekreijse, H. (1998). Object-based attention in the primary visual cortex of the macaque monkey. *Nature* 395: 376–381.

Rogers-Ramachandran, D. C. and Ramachandran, V. S. (1998). Psychophysical evidence for boundary and surface systems in human vision. *Vision Research* 38: 71–77.

Rorden, C., Mattingley, J. B., Karnath, H. O., and Driver, J. (1997). Visual extinction and prior entry: Impaired perception of temporal order with intact motion perception after unilateral parietal damage. *Neuropsychologia* 35(4): 421–433.

Rovamo, J. and Raninen, A. (1984). Critical flicker frequency and M-scaling of stimulus size and retinal illuminance. *Vision Research* 24(10): 1127–1131.

Rubin, N. and Hochstein, S. (1993). Isolating the effect of one-dimensional motion signals on the perceived direction of moving two-dimensional objects. *Vision Research* 3(10): 1385–1396.

Schank, R. and Abelson R. (1977). *Scripts, Plans, Goals and Understanding*. Hillsdale, N.J.: Lawrence Erlbaum Associates.

Selfridge, O. G. (1959). Pandemonium: A paradigm for learning. In D. V. Blake and A. M. Uttley (eds.), *Proceedings of the Symposium on the Mechanisation of Thought Processes* (pp. 511–529). London: Her Majesty's Stationery Office.

Shim, W. M., Alvarez, G. A., Vickery, T. J., and Jiang, Y. V. (2010). The number of attentional foci and their precision are dissociated in the posterior parietal cortex. *Cerebral Cortex* 20(6): 1341–1349.

Shipley, T. (ed.) (1961). *Classics in Psychology*. New York: Philosophical Library.

St. Clair, R., Huff, M., and Seiffert, A. E. (2010). Conflicting motion information impairs multiple object tracking. *Journal of Vision* 10(4): 18.1–13.

Stetson, C., Fiesta, M. P., and Eagleman, D. M. (2007). Does time really slow down during a frightening event? *PLoS One* 2(12): e1295.

Ternus, J. (1926). Experimentelle Untersuchungen über phänomenale Identität. *Psychologische Forschung* 7: 81–136. [Abridged English translation: Ternus, J. (1938). The problem of phenomenal identity. In W. D. Ellis (ed.), *A Source Book of Gestalt Psychology* (pp. 149–160). London: Routledge & Kegan Paul.]

Theeuwes, J., Godijn, R., and Pratt, J. (2004). A new estimation of the duration of attentional dwell time. *Psychonomic Bulletin & Review* 11: 60–64.

Treue, S. and Maunsell, J. H. (1996). Attentional modulation of visual motion processing in cortical areas MT and MST. *Nature* 382: 539–541.

Tripathy, S. P., Ogmen, H., and Narasimhan, S. (2011). Multiple-object tracking: A serial attentional process? In C. Mole, D. Smithies, and W. Wu (eds.), *Attention: Philosophical and Psychological Essays* (pp. 117–144). Oxford: Oxford University Press.

Tse, P., Intriligator, J., Rivest, J., and Cavanagh, P. (2004). Attention and the subjective expansion of time. *Perception & Psychophysics* 66: 1171–1189.

Tyler, C. W. (1973). Temporal characteristics in apparent movement: Omega movement vs. phi movement. *Quarterly Journal of Experimental Psychology* 25: 182–192.

Uchida, N., Kepecs, A., and Mainen, Z. F. (2006). Seeing at a glance, smelling in a whiff: Rapid forms of perceptual decision making. *Nature Reviews Neuroscience*, 7(6): 485–491.

Vagharchakian, L., Dehaene-lambertz, G., Pallier, C., Dehaene, S., and France, D. (2012). A temporal bottleneck in the language comprehension network. *Journal of Neuroscience* 32(26): 9089–9102. doi: 10.1523/JNEUROSCI.5685-11.2012.

VanRullen, R., Carlson, T., and Cavanagh, P. (2007). The blinking spotlight of attention. *Proceedings of the National Academy of Sciences USA* 104: 19204–19209.

VanRullen, R., Pascual-Leone, A., and Battelli, L. (2008). The Continuous Wagon Wheel Illusion and the 'When' pathway of the right parietal lobe: A repetitive transcranial magnetic stimulation study. *Plos One* 3(8): e2911.

VanRullen, R., Reddy, L., and Koch, C. (2006). The Continuous Wagon Wheel Illusion is associated with changes in electroencephalogram power at approximately 13 Hz. *Journal of Neuroscience* 26(2): 502–507.

Verstraten, F. A. J., Cavanagh, P., and Labianca, A. T. (2000). Limits of attentive tracking reveal temporal properties of attention. *Vision Research* 40: 3651–3664.

Victor, J. D. and Conte, M. M. (2002). Temporal phase discrimination depends critically on separation. *Vision Research* 42(17): 2063–2071.

Wertheimer, M. (1912). Experimentelle Studien über das Sehen von Bewegung. *Zeitschrift für Psychologie* 61: 161–265. Partial English translation in T. Shipley (ed.), *Classics in Psychology* (pp. 1032–1089). New York: Philosophical Library, 1961.

White, C. T., Cheatham, P. G., and Armington, J. C. (1953). Temporal numerosity. II: Evidence for central factors influencing perceived number. *Journal of Experimental Psychology* 46: 283–287.

White, C. T. and Harter, M. R. (1969). Intermittency in reaction time and perception, and evoked response correlates of image quality. *Acta Psychologica* 30: 368–377.

Yantis, S., Schwarzbach J., Serences, J. T., Carlson, R. L., Steinmetz, M. A., Pekar, J. J., and Courtney, S. M. (2002). Transient neural activity in human parietal cortex during spatial attention shifts. *Nature Neuroscience* 5(10): 995–1002.

CHAPTER 24

TIME FOR THE FOURTH DIMENSION IN ATTENTION

ANNA C. NOBRE AND GUSTAVO ROHENKOHL

SELECTIVE attention, understood as the processes that focus neural processing in service of current goals and requirements, is inherently and necessarily dynamic. As we navigate along, our receptor surfaces move, events in the environment unfold, and the relationships between our receptors and events change. Ironically perhaps, our core theoretical and computational models of attention are primarily static. They consider mechanisms for selecting relevant or conspicuous target events and inhibiting irrelevant or interfering distraction within freeze-frame instants of experience. As the many chapters in this Handbook attest, tremendous progress has been made in revealing these snapshot mechanisms of attention control and modulation at various levels of organization. However, still largely missing is the consideration of whether and how predictive information in the temporal structure of events can contribute to optimizing perception.

Considering how predictive temporal information can influence perceptual analysis necessitates contemplating new types of modulatory mechanisms. To date, most snapshot mechanisms revealed to enhance perceptual analysis involve regulating and coordinating neuronal excitability according to receptive field properties in anticipation of relevant events. However, we still understand little about whether and how receptive field properties are specifically tuned to temporal intervals within sensory areas. Furthermore, it is unclear how pre-activation of neurons with temporal specificity would preserve temporal estimates. How then can the anticipated timings of relevant events be used to regulate neuronal excitability during perceptual analysis? This chapter reviews the early steps of a burgeoning literature addressing this intriguing and fundamental question.

EARLY STUDIES

The role played by the temporal structure of events in guiding perception was not always ignored. The temporal interval between events, known as the foreperiod, has long been acknowledged to be one of the main determinants of response speeds in a variety of tasks (see Teichner 1954; Niemi and Näätänen 1981). According to our reading, Wilhelm Wundt (1874/1904) may have been the first to show that response times are faster in the presence of a warning signal that predicts the occurrence of a target after a constant and predictable interval. He gave participants the task of releasing a key upon hearing the sound of a steel ball hitting a metal plate. They were significantly faster when they had the opportunity to view the release mechanism that dropped the ball. (The foreperiod was manipulated by adjusting the height of the release mechanism.) Extending Wundt's investigation, Woodrow (1914) manipulated the regularity of the interval between a warning signal and a target on a trial-by-trial basis. Response times were faster when intervals were constant and predictable, than when they were variable and unpredictable (Fig. 24.1a). Subsequent investigations showed that though benefits are larger when the nature of the stimulus and response are predetermined, they also occur in choice reaction-time tasks when the identity of the stimulus and the response remain uncertain (Bertelson and Boons 1960).

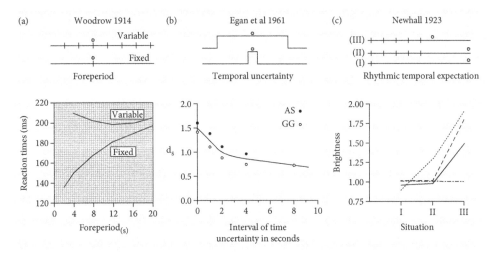

FIGURE 24.1 Pioneer investigations on the effect of time in perception and action. (a) Effect of regular and irregular foreperiods on reaction times found by Woodrow (1914: 43). Foreperiod intervals are presented on the X-axis, and reaction times on the Y-axis. The upper curve represents the results with irregular foreperiods, showing consistently high reaction times. The lower line shows faster reaction times with regular foreperiods, which also increase as foreperiods are lengthened (attributed to increasing difficulty to estimate longer intervals accurately). Adapted from Woodrow H., *The Measurement of Attention*, p. 43 © 1914, Whitefish. (b) Results reported by Egan et al. (1961: 774) showing decrements in discriminability (ds) performance as a function of increasing temporal uncertainty. Markers indicate mean values for each observer (AS and GG). Adapted from *Archives of Psychology* 61, Newhall, S. N., Effects of attention on the intensity of cutaneous pressure and on visual brightness pp. 5–75, 1923. (c) Subjective brightness report for each participant in the three experimental conditions ('Situations') presented in Newhall (1923: 60). 'Situations' represent different levels of temporal expectation, from high (III) to low (I). Adapted from, *The Journal of Acoustical Society of America* 33(6), Egan, J. P., Greenberg, G. Z., Schulman, A. I., Interval of Time Uncertainty in Auditory Detection, pp. 771–778 © 1961, Acoustical Society of America.

Benefits carried by temporal prediction in these early tasks were usually interpreted as resulting from increases in the level of readiness of a general type of attention. The degree of preparation was proposed to increase as certainty of the foreperiods increased and as the length of the foreperiod on a particular trial increased (Woodrow 1914; Karlin 1959). An alternative account proposed an additional specific process of temporal 'anticipation', in which the prospective intervals of events are estimated from the time of warning cue (Nickerson 1965; Snodgrass 1969).

Egan et al. (1961) developed a simple and elegant design to explore further the role of temporal un/certainty in perception. They varied temporal expectation parametrically across experimental blocks by presenting an auditory stimulus sometime during the persistence of a light signal of varying duration (e.g. 1 / 2 / 4 / 8 secs in Experiment 1). Detectability deteriorated progressively with the increasing temporal uncertainty associated with increasing interval durations (Fig. 24.1b). Findings were later confirmed and extended in similar experiments in the visual domain by Lowe (1967), Lasley and Cohn (1981), and Westheimer and Ley (1996). Together, these studies suggested that temporal prediction could improve perceptual judgements about target events, and have effects beyond merely speeding response times.

Newhall (1923) introduced the use of rhythms to manipulate temporal expectations. He showed that the brightness perception of a visual stimulus was increased if the stimulus occurred at the next temporal interval of a regular, isochronous rhythm induced by a series of auditory clicks. The three experimental conditions of the experiment involved the visual target occurring 1 sec after a series of five auditory clicks separated by 1-sec intervals (i.e. on the sixth beat of the rhythm), occurring 4 secs after the train of five auditory clicks, or occurring after a 9-sec interval with no leading rhythm (Fig. 24.1c). As the reader may have noted, not all relevant experimental variables were well controlled in this early experiment. Furthermore, behavioural performance was measured subjectively and compared without statistical methods. Nevertheless, the intent was to manipulate temporal expectations—to 'create three different pre-stimulus situations which differed among other things in that they made the observer aware of the time at which the stimulus would occur' (Newhall 1923: 55).

As is plain to see, these pioneering studies started tapping into some fundamental issues about how temporal predictability and structure of events influence performance. For example, they indicate different ways of manipulating temporal expectations and suggest that there may be multiple points of influence along sensory-motor processing. Inexplicably, somehow, there was insufficient momentum, and investigations into the selective attention based on the timing of events lagged behind those of spatial and object-based attention, leaving the temporal dimension largely out of the established contemporary models. The landscape is changing again. Scholars interested in the selective biasing of information processing have rediscovered, sometimes *de novo*, the importance of temporal expectations in shaping perception. Present-day methods enable a detailed characterization of behavioural consequences of temporal expectations, and are beginning to provide a glimpse into the neural modulatory and control mechanisms.

RHYTHMS

Rhythms provide arguably the most natural and common source of temporal predictions of events. These come from the structure of events in the environment (e.g. cadence of speech, the tempo of music, the breaking of waves) as well as from our means to sample and interact with the environment (e.g. saccadic eye movements, walking, breathing) (see Schroeder et al. 2010).

Jones and her colleagues are modern-day pioneers in investigating how rhythms modulate perceptual excitability over time (Jones 1976; Jones and Boltz 1989; Jones et al. 2002, 2006). Using a similar approach to that initially introduced by Newhall (1923), Jones's tasks typically manipulate the timing of auditory target events relative to a regular isochronic rhythm. The results have consistently shown optimal perceptual discrimination for auditory targets coinciding with the predicted beat of the rhythm, with performance degrading exponentially with increasing leading or lagging intervals between the target and the predicted moment (Jones et al. 2002) (Fig. 24.2a). Rhythmically induced expectations have been found to confer behavioural advantages even when they are not predictive of the timing of the target, suggesting that temporal anticipation triggered by isochronous rhythms may operate through an automatic, exogenous process (for a review see Jones 2010). Using pre-exposure to a rhythm to induce temporal expectations, Sanabria and colleagues have also reported improvements in response times to auditory targets occurring at the beat of the leading isochronous rhythm, even when the rhythm did not reliably predict the timing of the target stimulus (Sanabria et al. 2011). The automatic nature of the benefits conferred by rhythms was supported by a further study by the same group showing that simultaneously performing a demanding working-memory task did not interfere with the effects of rhythmic temporal expectations (de la Rosa et al. 2012).

Perceptual Modulation

Similar patterns of facilitation for events coinciding with regular isochronous rhythms have also been reported in the visual modality. Mathewson and colleagues (2010) used a series of zero, two, four, or eight visual cues presented at a regular pace (12.1 Hz) to entrain rhythmic visual attention. Next came the target event, containing a visual stimulus or a blank followed by metacontrast masking. The target occurred either at the beat, or at increasing leading or lagging intervals (25 or 50 ms). Target detectability, measured by d′, was maximal when the target coincided with the preceding rhythm (Fig. 24.2b). Perceptual facilitation for targets occurring after eight entrainers was substantial compared to a control condition that equated the foreperiod duration for target onset and forward masking effects (i.e. 55% increase in d′). Praamstra and colleagues (2006) recorded EEG during a related task in which a train of regularly presented 11–21 imperative stimuli (at 1.5 or 2.0s stimulus-onset asynchrony (SOA)) was followed by a temporally deviant target (at 1.75s SOA). Response times to deviant targets were slowed relative

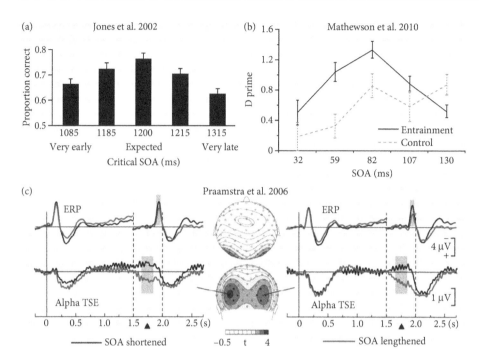

FIGURE 24.2 Using rhythms to orient attention in time. (a) Findings from Jones et al. (2002) showing mean proportion correct to discriminate auditory targets as a function of its interval relative to a preceding rhythm. Maximum performance occurs on the expected rhythmic beat interval and falls off systematically as the target occurs increasingly early or late. Adapted from Mari Riess Jones, Heather Moynihan, Noah MacKenzie, and Jennifer Puente, *Psychological Science*, 13(4), pp. 313–319, copyright © 2002 by SAGE Publications. Reprinted by permission of SAGE Publications. (b) Findings reported in Mathewson et al. (2010). Solid line shows the tuning of detection rate for visual targets preceded by predictive rhythms. Performance is maximal for events at the predicted interval and falls off systematically for progressively early or late events. Dashed line shows performance at equivalent intervals in a control condition with no preceding rhythm. Reprinted from Praamstra, P., Kourtis, D., Kwok, H. F., Oostenveld, R., Neurophysiology of implicit timing in serial choice reaction-time performance, *The Journal of Neuroscience: The Official Journal of the Society for Neuroscience*, 26(20), pp. 5448–5455 © 2006, The Society for Neuroscience. (c) Event-related potentials (ERP) and time course of alpha-band activity (Alpha TSE (temporal spectral evolution)) over occipital electrodes in Praamstra et al. (2006). Alpha-band activity decreases sharply at the time of the expected stimulus (1500 ms) in the short SOA condition, as highlighted by shading in the Alpha TSE plots. This desynchronization in the alpha band was accompanied by an increase in visual evoked activity, as highlighted by shading in the ERP plots. Reprinted from *Cognition*, 115(1), Kyle E. Mathewson, Monica Fabiani, Gabriele Gratton, Diane M. Beck, and Alejandro Lleras, Rescuing stimuli from invisibility: Inducing a momentary release from visual masking with pre-target entrainment, pp. 186–91, Copyright (2010), with permission from Elsevier.

to the regular stimuli, and electrophysiological recordings showed evidence of anticipatory activity related to the rhythm of the initial stimuli (Fig. 24.2c). Alpha-band desynchronization, linked to anticipation of visual targets (Foxe et al. 1998; Kelly et al. 2006,

2009; Worden et al. 2000; Snyder and Foxe 2010; Bollimunta et al. 2008, 2011; Wyart and Tallon-Baudry 2008; Yamagishi et al. 2008; Mathewson et al. 2009; O'Connell et al. 2009; Gould et al. 2011), was accentuated from the time the target was predicted by the rhythm. Slow preparatory brain activity related to motor preparation in the contingent negative variation (Walter et al. 1964) also developed more steeply toward the end of the interval in the context of faster compared to slower rhythms. Visual event-related potentials (ERPs) evoked by the targets also showed modulation by preceding temporal rhythm, with larger N1 potentials occurring for targets occurring later versus earlier than predicted by the preceding short versus long rhythm respectively.

In our laboratory we have used a complementary approach to investigate the effects of temporal expectation on perceptual processing—manipulating the regularity of the temporal context of target events. Our findings show that temporal expectations combine with spatial expectations to enhance perceptual processing, and implicate ongoing oscillatory brain activity in mediating the effects of temporal expectations.

In one series of studies (see Fig. 24.3), we manipulated the regularity of the timing with which a target (a small disc) moved in discrete jumps across a display containing an occluding band. When the disc moved at a regular, isochronous pace, it was possible to predict exactly when the target would re-emerge after disappearing behind the occluding band. The basic task involved making a fine visual discrimination within the target disc when it re-emerged and executing a speeded detection (go/no-go) or forced-choice response accordingly. In the first study, temporal and spatial predictability of the target were manipulated orthogonally in a factorial design. The disc moved with regular or irregular pace along a linear or erratic trajectory across the display. Temporal and spatial expectations conferred similar benefit to response times. Recordings of event-related potentials showed that the similar behavioural effects of isolated temporal or spatial expectations came about through distinct patterns of neural modulation. Of specific relevance to perceptual modulation, isolated spatial expectations (i.e. under temporal uncertainty) increased the magnitude of visual P1 potentials contralateral to spatially expected targets, in line with spatial orienting effects in spatial cueing tasks (Mangun and Hillyard 1987; Eimer 1994). In contrast, isolated temporal expectations had no effect on the first visual potential (see also Correa and Nobre 2008). Strikingly, however, temporal expectation greatly potentiated the P1 gain modulation by spatial attention (Fig. 24.3b). Furthermore, amplitude of the contralateral P1 potential correlated significantly with the average response time in go trials across participants. Modulation of later stages of processing (N1, N2, and P3 potentials) by temporal versus spatial expectations occurred in dissociable ways. The findings from this study suggested that temporal expectations combine synergistically with predictive information about other stimulus attributes (in this case location) that can be mapped onto receptive field properties to time the biasing of excitability in a top-down fashion. We are currently exploring the reliability and generalizability of this hypothesis.

Using a streamlined and optimized design (Fig. 24.3a), we subsequently replicated the perceptual facilitation conferred by temporal expectations to spatially predicted targets and were able to examine effects of combined spatiotemporal expectations on anticipatory brain activity during the occlusion period (Rohenkohl and Nobre 2011). Analysis of induced oscillatory activity during the period when the target remained

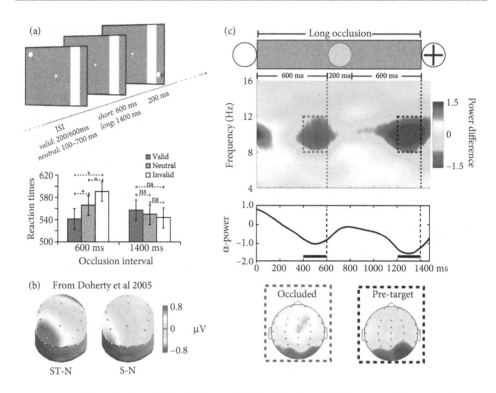

FIGURE 24.3   Results from Rohenkohl and Nobre (2011) and Doherty et al. (2005) showing the synergistic effect between temporal and spatial expectations. (a) Schematic of the task used in Rohenkohl and Nobre (2011) based on the original task by Doherty et al. (2005). Bar plot showing reaction times for valid, neutral, and invalid temporal expectation. Note how valid rhythmic temporal expectation shortens reaction times for targets appearing after the short occlusion. Temporal expectations are equated at the long-occlusion interval, and there are no reaction-time differences then. Reprinted from Doherty, J. R., Rao, A., Mesulam, M. M., Nobre, A. C., Synergistic effect of combined temporal and spatial expectations on visual attention, *The Journal of Neuroscience: The Official Journal of the Society for Neuroscience*, 25(36), pp. 8259–8266 © 2005, The Society for Neuroscience. (b) Topographies presented in Doherty et al. (2005) showing enhanced attentional modulation of early visual P1 potential (between 100 and 130 ms) by combined spatial and temporal expectations (ST-N) relative to spatial expectation alone (S-N). Reprinted from Rohenkohl, G., Nobre, A. C., Alpha oscillations related to anticipatory attention follow temporal expectations, *The Journal of Neuroscience: The Official Journal of the Society for Neuroscience*, 31(40), pp. 14076–14084 © 2011, The Society for Neuroscience. (c) Time course and topographies of alpha-band activity found in Rohenkohl and Nobre (2011) in regular vs. irregular conditions during the long-occlusion period. The schematic above shows the timings of events: the moment when the disc disappears under the occluding band (0 ms), the moment of the invisible step under the occluding band (600 ms), and the moment when the disc reappears (1400 ms). Temporal expectations developed from a regular rhythmic pattern of stimulation led to time-modulation of alpha-band activity over visual electrodes in anticipation of the target onset.

occluded showed that alpha-band activity over occipital electrodes became temporally structured in the regular, rhythmic condition. Alpha-band desynchronization followed the time course of temporal expectation induced by the preceding rhythmic pace, being maximal at the predicted times of disc occurrence under the occluding band and of its reappearance after occlusion (Fig. 24.3c). Our findings support the ability of oscillatory activity to mediate changes in neural excitability according to temporal expectations induced by the regular timing of events.

In a related behavioural experiment, we demonstrated that the facilitatory effect of temporal expectations on response times induced by rhythmic apparent motion occurred relatively automatically, and independently of strategic factors (Rohenkohl et al. 2011). The temporal manipulation induced by the regularity of motion (valid, rhythmic versus neutral, arrhythmic conditions) was crossed with a manipulation whereby the colour of the disc acted as a symbolic cue that predicted the timing for target reappearance (valid, 100% predictive versus neutral, non-predictive). In addition to the manipulations of rhythmic and symbolic cueing, we also introduced instructions to attend to the speed (rhythm) or the colour of the disc. The results showed that both rhythmic and symbolic temporal cues speeded response times, but in dissociable ways. Rhythmic cues facilitated performance regardless of the instructions, but symbolic cues were only effective when participants attended to the symbolic, colour information. These findings indicate that there may be multiple, qualitatively distinct sources of temporal expectations operating upon information processing.

In a second series of studies, we used a psychophysical approach combined with computational modelling to investigate the consequences of rhythmic temporal expectations on visual perceptual discrimination (Cravo et al. 2013; Rohenkohl et al. 2012a). Participants had to discriminate the orientation of a Gabor grating, presented at one of seven contrast levels and embedded within a patch of Gaussian noise. Targets appeared within foveal streams of Gaussian-noise patches presented in a 'regular', isochronous rhythm (50 ms duration, 400 ms SOA) or in an 'irregular', jittered fashion (50 ms duration, 200/300/400/500/600 ms SOA) (Fig. 24.4a). Importantly, the timing around the target stimulus was equated between the two conditions, with 400 ms SOA between the target and the preceding and subsequent adjacent noise patches. Contrast levels for targets were calibrated to individuals' thresholds, anchored at 75% accuracy and varying 1–3 units above and below in steps of 0.1 on a logarithmic scale. The occurrence of targets was signalled by a coloured annulus around the stimulus patch to prompt a forced-choice response. In our first behavioural investigation (Rohenkohl et al. 2012a), response times were faster in the regular, rhythmic condition. In addition, psychometric functions for the proportion of correct responses estimated for individual participants showed that rhythmic temporal expectation significantly increased the contrast sensitivity for target detection (lowering threshold values). A simple diffusion model (Palmer et al. 2005) indicated that temporal expectation improved the quality of sensory information by enhancing the signal-to-noise contrast of the sensory evidence upon which decisions were made. Our subsequent study combining the same design

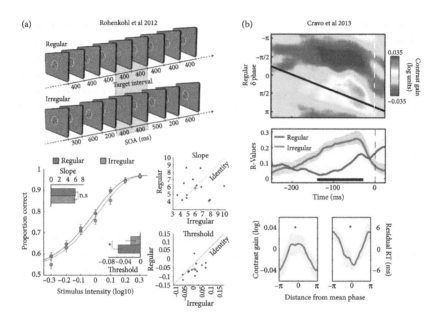

FIGURE 24.4 Rhythmic temporal expectation enhances perceptual processing of visual events. (a) Schematic of the task used in Rohenkohl et al. (2012). Stimuli appeared exactly every 400 ms in the regular condition, and appeared between 200 and 600 ms in the irregular condition. Occasional target stimuli were indicated by a pink circumference, and participants discriminated the orientation of a Gabor grating embedded within a Gaussian noise patch. Psychometric functions described performance in regular and irregular temporal expectation conditions as a function of target contrast. Stimulus contrasts were set for each participant using a staircase procedure in an irregular stream of events; Stimulus intensity = 0 corresponds to the contrast value yielding 75% performance threshold. A shift in threshold, but not slope, of the psychometric function indicates that temporal expectation increases the contrast sensitivity for target events. Differences in slope (non-significant) and threshold (significant) are also plotted for regular and irregular temporal conditions in the bar graphs. Scatterplots show the effect of temporal expectation on slope and threshold values for each participant (bluedots indicate the group average). Reprinted from Rohenkohl, G., Cravo, A. M., Wyart, V., and Nobre, A. C., Temporal expectation improves the quality of sensory information, 32(24), pp. 8424–8428 © 2012, The Society for Neuroscience. (b) Results from in Cravo et al. (2013) showing how the entrainment of delta oscillations over visual areas was closely related to a concurrent enhancement of perceptual discrimination to relevant events. Colour map shows the relationship between delta phase and contrast gain in the regular, rhythmic condition. Black line superimposed onto colour map indicates the mean delta phase across participants. R-values line plots show the time course of the correlation between delta phase and contrast gain. Black line along the X-axis (time) indicates when correlation between delta phase and contrast gain was significantly higher in the regular than in the irregular condition (cluster p < 0.05). Lower line plots show contrast gain and residual response times as a function of the distance from mean phase in the pre-target period (–140 to –30 ms) in the regular condition. This figure shows clearly a decrease in contrast gain and increase in reaction times as distance from mean phase increases. Reprinted from Cravo, A. M., Rohenkohl, G., Wyart, V., Nobre, A. C., Temporal expectation enhances contrast sensitivity by phase entrainment of low-frequency oscillations in visual cortex, 33(9), pp. 4002–4010 © 2013, The Society for Neuroscience.

with EEG recordings replicated these psychophysical and modelling effects, and provided evidence that entrainment of low-frequency oscillatory brain activity to regular stimulus timings may mediate the perceptual benefits (Cravo et al. 2013). Oscillatory activity in the frequency range of the stimulus trains (delta-band activity, 1–4 Hz) became more synchronized in the regular, rhythmic condition over occipital electrodes. Furthermore, delta phase was tightly related to target discriminability, and the optimal delta phase became aligned to target presentation in the regular, rhythmic condition (Fig. 24.4b). Entrainment of delta phase was closely related to increases in contrast gain and the modelling parameter for the sensory accumulation rate. Subsequent visual potentials evoked by target stimuli also became more sensitive to target contrast in the regular, rhythmic condition.

Mathewson and colleagues (2012) conducted a similar experiment using EEG to test whether and how oscillatory brain activity mediated effects of rhythmic temporal expectation. The task was based on their previous study (Mathewson et al. 2010), using rapidly presented streams of stimuli followed by metacontrast masks. In the regular, rhythmic condition, the target followed eight entrainer stimuli appearing at a regular rate (~12 Hz, every 82.3 ms). In the irregular condition, stimulus-onset asynchronies between entrainers varied, but the overall time until target appearance was equated to that of the regular condition. Targets appeared at the time predicted by the regular rhythm or in progressively leading or lagging offsets. As in their previous study, visibility was maximal for targets at the predicted time for the rhythmic condition and fell off with increasing offsets. The effect varied with the degree of regularity in variable entraining rhythms, and was absent in a no-rhythm control condition. Power and phase-locking of oscillatory activity within the frequency of stimulus presentation (~12 Hz, in the alpha band) was significantly higher in the regular rhythmic condition over posterior occipital and parietal electrodes, and phase-locked fluctuations co-varied with fluctuations in visual awareness.

Entrainment of oscillatory activity has also been reported in the auditory domain. Henry and Obleser (2012) found that ability of listeners to detect short gaps within a 3 Hz frequency modulated stimulus clustered around specific preferred phases of the frequency modulation, and was best predicted by the phase of delta-band activity entrained to the temporal structure of the stimulus (see also Will and Berg 2007). Using magnetoencephalogram in rhythmic auditory tasks, Large and colleagues have also proposed that activity in the gamma (Snyder and Large 2005; Fujioka et al. 2009) and beta (Fujioka et al. 2012) band is induced in anticipation of temporally regular events.

Neuronal Mechanisms

By combining laminar recordings of local field potentials (LFPs) and multi-unit recordings in macaques, Lakatos, Schroeder, and colleagues provided some of the first evidence suggesting that entrainment of neuronal activity to external events is an important attentional mechanism—regulating neuronal excitability according to temporal expectation (see also Schroeder, Herrero and Haegens (in chapter 17), this volume). In a set of pioneering studies, Lakatos and colleagues (2008, 2009) recorded neural responses in primary visual (V1) and primary auditory (A1) cortices during performance of an inter-modal attention task in which near-rhythmic streams of visual and auditory stimuli were interdigitated. On average, the interval between successive stimuli in each modal-ity was 650 ms (500–800 ms range, 1.5 Hz, in the delta frequency), and the two stimu-lus streams remained 180° out of phase over trials. As expected, current-source density and multi-unit responses in V1 were significantly enhanced when the visual stream was task-relevant compared with when the auditory stream was relevant. In addition, they also discovered that low-frequency oscillations became entrained to the carrier rhythm of the task-relevant, attended stimuli and that higher frequency gamma-band activity became coupled to these delta oscillations. Single-trial analysis of the influence of delta-phase on event-related responses showed visual responses to be systematically related to the pre-stimulus delta phase. Based on their findings and previous literature, the authors proposed a mechanism by which task-relevant events are capable of reset-ting ongoing oscillatory activity. In contexts containing rhythmic events, entrainment of low frequency oscillatory activity plays an active part in regulating neuronal excitability through hierarchical cross-frequency coupling that leads to increases in response gains and amplification of neuronal responses to task-relevant stimuli (Lakatos et al. 2008, 2009; Schroeder and Lakatos 2009b; see also Lakatos et al. 2005; Canolty et al. 2006). In the absence of a rhythmic context, when attention needs to be sustained tonically over time, low-frequency oscillations may be suppressed (e.g. see Fries et al. 2001).

A recent study by Lakatos and colleagues (2013) further suggests how temporal entrain-ment of low-frequency activity aids differentiation between competing stimuli occurring at similar times. Macaques were cued to attend to one of two competing auditory streams of different frequency content that differed in their rate of presentation (1.6 vs. 1.8 Hz). As in the intermodal studies, low-frequency oscillation became entrained to the attended auditory stream. However, the phase of entrainment depended on the tone frequency, with counter phase entrainment to attended versus unattended tones. The result was amplifica-tion and sharpening of neuronal responses to relevant tones at attended time points.

Working Hypotheses and Open Questions

Together, findings in humans and in macaques support recent proposals that entrain-ment of neural excitability to environmental rhythms is a fundamental aspect of suc-cessful perceptual selection. Entrainment of brain activity to sensory input may be a pervasive mechanism across animal species. For example, it has been observed in the optic tectum in the larvae of zebra fish (Sumbre et al. 2008), in retinal ganglion cells of sal-amanders (Schwartz and Berry 2008), as well as in sensory areas in humans (Herrmann 2001; Williams et al. 2004; Mathewson et al. 2012; Cravo et al. 2013; Nozaradan et al. 2011).

However, a major open question is whether specific frequency bands play privi-leged roles in regulating neural excitability according to the rhythmic temporal struc-ture of events. So far, the results suggest entrainment of neural activity to the pace of external events, but there may be constraints according to intrinsic brain rhythms and entrainment within different frequency ranges may have different modulatory conse-quences. Schroeder and Lakatos (2009a, 2009b; Schroeder et al. 2010) suggest a primary role for endogenous low-frequency delta and theta rhythms in guiding active sensing of environmental stimuli. Active sensing mechanisms may, in turn, be shaped by or aligned to motor sampling mechanisms, such as the rates of saccades (Bosman et al. 2009) or speech prosody (Ghazanfar et al. 2013). Separately, entrainment of alpha-band activity, which has been particularly implicated in mediating visual excitability, has been pro-posed as a mechanism for selective temporal attention based on rhythms (Mathewson et al. 2009; Jensen et al. 2012; Hanslmayr et al. 2011). Future studies varying entrainment rhythms systematically will be needed in order to explore this basic and important issue.

The sources and extent of neural modulation by rhythmic context also remain to be characterized. The endeavour may prove challenging, as the temporal correlations inherent in tasks manipulating stimulus rhythms complicate the use of hemodynamic imaging methods with low temporal resolution, such as functional magnetic-resonance imaging (fMRI), which provide good spatial sampling across the brain. Furthermore, hemodynamic measures may not be sensitive to mechanisms relying on changes in tim-ing or synchronization of brain activity. Besle and colleagues (2011) were able to observe large-scale entrainment of brain areas by using intracranial electrocortical recordings in human epilepsy patients. They used an adaptation of the intermodal attention task used by Lakatos (2008, 2009). Modulation of low-frequency activity entrained to the stimulation was not confined to primary visual areas, but instead occurred over a large number of brain areas, including higher order cortices implicated in control functions. The authors noted considerable overlap in the network of modulated areas with those implicated in cued temporal orienting tasks (Coull and Nobre 1998; see below). This large-scale rhythmic entrainment of brain areas may occur locally and become coordi-nated across brain areas through bootstrapping. Alternatively, there may be a central-ized mechanism, which in turn coordinates oscillatory entrainment. A combination of both local and central mechanisms is also possible.

Studies are also beginning to explore the role temporal expectations play in organ-izing and facilitating higher order cognitive functions involving rhythmic patterns of stimulation, such as music (e.g. Gordon et al. 2011; Nozaradan et al. 2011; Large and Snyder 2009; Tillmann 2012), language (e.g. Ghazanfar et al. 2013; Hoch et al. 2013; Astheimer and Sanders 2009, 2011, 2012; Schmidt-Kassow and Kotz 2009; Power et al. 2012; Kotz et al. 2009), and sensory-motor coordination (Fujioka et al. 2012). As inves-tigations progress, it will be interesting to investigate temporal expectations that occur in the context of complex, non-isochronous rhythms (Chapin et al. 2010; Large et al. 2002). Initial studies have started to reveal interesting effects of temporal sequences involving non-isochronous repeating patterns of intervals on implicit learning (Olson and Chun 2001; O'Reilly et al. 2008a). Interestingly, a striking interaction was also noted between implicit learning of a repeating sequence of temporal intervals and a sequence of stimulus locations in facilitating response times in a serial reaction-time task (O'Reilly et al. 2008a)—echoing the synergistic effects noted between tempo-ral and spatial expectations in the visual task by Doherty and colleagues (2005), and between temporal expectations and task-relevant tone frequencies in the auditory task by Lakatos and colleagues (2013). Whereas no implicit learning of temporal sequences was observed when the stimulus location was uncertain, temporal sequences amplified the implicit learning of spatial sequences enormously.

Hazards

Predictable temporal structure of events is not confined to rhythmic contexts. Any reoc-curring episode may contain temporal predictions about the sequence and timing of its events. The conditional probability of an event occurring at a specified time given that it has not yet occurred is known as the 'hazard function' (Luce 1986).

Most psychophysical or cognitive tasks have temporal predictions embedded within their task structure (see Griffin and Nobre 2005). In warning-signal tasks, conditional probabilities of target events increase with the passage of time, and can become sharply tuned to specific moments when the foreperiod before the target is fixed. The impor-tance of foreperiod duration and regularity has been acknowledged since the classic warning-period studies (Woodrow 1914; reviewed in Niemi and Näätänen 1981). In tasks with variable foreperiods, the sequence of intervals across trials may also influence response times (Woodrow 1914), and the resulting response time is dictated by a combi-nation of foreperiod sequence effects and hazard rates (e.g. Los and Agter 2005). In the earlier literature, foreperiod effects were often treated as reflecting general mechanisms for non-specific preparation for the target (e.g. Bertelson 1967; Niemi and Näätänen 1981), and sometimes linked to effects of general alertness (Posner and Boies 1971). More recently, active and selective mechanisms of temporal anticipation are increas-ingly acknowledged to contribute to foreperiod effects (see Nobre et al. 2007).

Perceptual Modulation

Hazard rates have been shown to influence many types of behaviour. Proactive anticipation of target timings is clearly evident in smooth-pursuit tasks, in which eye position often leads a temporally anticipated change in target trajectory (e.g. de Hemptinne et al. 2007, 2010; Barnes and Asselman 1991). Anticipatory saccades (Kingstone and Klein 1993) and man-ual responses (Nickerson 1965) are also common in simple detection tasks using constant, predictable intervals. Regular, predictable timings for target appearance can also affect per-ceptual judgements: improving thresholds for luminance, orientation, and stereoscopic dis-criminations (Lasley and Cohn 1981; Westheimer and Ley 1996); increasing accuracy for discriminating targets under high perceptual demands Rolke and Hofmann 2007; reviewed in Rolke and Ulrich 2010); and attenuating attentional blink (Shen and Alain 2012).

Sophisticated psychophysical experiments combined with computational model-ling are beginning to be carried out to characterize the effects of hazard rates on different stages of information processing. At this stage, it is worth bearing in mind that multiple levels of influence may occur and differentially influence performance depending on the perceptual, mnemonic, and motoric demands in the task. Using an unspeeded task and modelling of processing parameters according to the 'theory of visual attention' (TVA) (Bundesen 1990; Bundesen et al. 2011) (see also Bundesen and Habekost (in chapter 37), this volume), Vangkilde and colleagues (2012) found that hazard-rate manipulations primarily affected the speed of encoding items into visual short-term memory, rather than the temporal threshold for perception (but see also Seifried et al. 2010; Bausenhart et al. 2008, 2010). Using a fixed-foreperiod manipulation as well as a temporal cueing paradigm (see below) combined with a type of drift-diffusion model (Ratcliff and Rouder 1998), Jepma and colleagues (2012) concluded that temporal expectation affected the duration of non-decision processes, such as target encoding or response preparation, but had little effect on the rate of evidence accumulation or on setting the response threshold (see also Seibold et al. 2011). These results are qualitatively different from our results using rhythms to manipulate temporal expectations (Cravo et al. 2013; Rohenkohl et al. 2012a, 2012b). These interesting discrepancies call for additional rigorous and systematic studies using computational models to compare the effects of temporal expectations induced by different procedures (e.g. rhythmic contexts vs. hazard rates) and under differing perceptual, mnemonic, and motor demands. For now, it is safe to conclude that manipulations of hazard rates, like rhythmic contexts, exert strong and reliable influences over information processing in tasks emphasizing perceptual discrimination or speeded responses.

Neuronal Mechanisms

Hazard rates have been shown to influence activity across multiple brain areas. Single-unit and local field potential studies in animal models have revealed modulations in striate and extrastriate visual cortices (Ghose and Bearl 2010; Ghose and Maunsell 2002; Shuler and Bear 2006); parietal area LIP (Janssen and Shadlen 2005; Premereur et al. 2012), motor and premotor cortices (Riehle et al. 1997; Lucchetti and Bon 2001; Heinen and Liu 1997; Renoult et al. 2006); striatal and prefrontal cortices (Jin et al. 2009; Tsujimoto and Sawaguchi 2005; Roesch and Olson 2005); and subcortical reward-related areas (Hollerman and Schultz 1998; Fiorillo et al. 2003; Bermudez et al. 2012). Non-invasive studies in humans have also indicated modulation across large networks of brain areas, including sensory and motor areas, depending on task parameters (e.g. Bueti et al. 2010; Schubotz and von Cramon 2001; Cui et al. 2009; Coull and Nobre 2008; Cravo et al. 2011b; Schoffelen et al. 2005). Findings using single-unit recordings in sensory cortices and in sensorimotor areas implicated in the control of attention are of particular interest to understanding how temporal expectations can contribute to attentional modulation of perception.

Sensory areas

Ghose and Maunsell (2002) were the first to note modulation of neuronal activity in a visual area by temporal expectation. They observed that the top-down anticipatory effects of spatial attention on the firing rates of neurones in visual area V4 followed the hazard rate predicting the timing of the change in a target stimulus that the monkey had

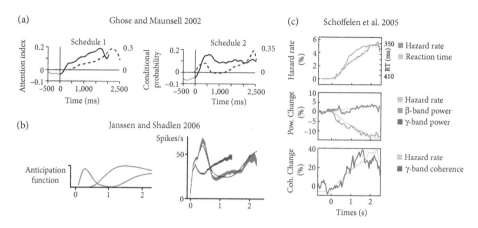

FIGURE 24.5 Effect of hazard rates on neural activity related to perception and action. (a) Findings from Ghose and Maunsell (2002) showing that activity in V4 (solid line) follows the conditional probability distribution (dashed line) of target occurrence in a spatial attention task. Reprinted by permission from Macmillan Publishers Ltd: *Nature*, 419 (6907), Geoffrey M. Ghose and John H. R. Maunsell, Attentional modulation in visual cortex depends on task timing, pp. 616–620, copyright 2002, Macmillan Publishers Ltd. (b) Findings from Janssen and Shadlen (2006). Two distinct 'anticipation functions' for target appearance, and LIP responses corresponding to the anticipation functions in a delayed-saccade task. Reprinted by permission from Macmillan Publishers Ltd: *Nature Neuroscience*, 8(2), Peter Janssen and Michael N Shadlen, A representation of the hazard rate of elapsed time in macaque area LIP, pp. 234–241, copyright 2005, Macmillan Publishers Ltd. (c) Results reported by Schoffelen et al. (2005). Top panel shows hazard rate (grey line) with the resulting reaction times (pink line). Note the inverted reaction-time axis at the right. Middle panel shows the time course of power change in gamma (red) and beta (blue) band. Grey lines represent scaled copies of the hazard rate. Bottom panel shows that the time course of corticospinal coherence in the gamma-band (40 to 70 Hz) also follows the hazard rate. From *Science*, 308 (5718), Wendy Winckler, Simon R. Myers, Daniel J. Richter, Robert C. Onofrio, Gavin J. McDonald, Ronald E. Bontrop, Gilean A. T. McVean, Stacey B. Gabriel, David Reich, Peter Donnelly, and David Altshuler, Comparison of Fine-Scale Recombination Rates in Humans and Chimpanzees, pp. 111–113 (c) 2005, The American Association for the Advancement of Science. Reprinted with permission from AAAS.

to report (Fig. 24.5a). They demonstrated convincingly the modulation of the spatial attention effect by temporal expectations by introducing bimodal hazard rates, which yielded a bimodal amplification pattern of the spatial attention effects. These results, like those in the human ERP study by Doherty and colleagues (2005) manipulating temporal and spatial expectations, point to the ability of temporal expectations to tune modulation of neuronal activity based on other receptive-field properties.

More recently, Ghose and Bearl (2010) measured neuronal activity in visual area MT in a task requiring detection of a very brief motion pulse in one of two locations. The probability of the pulse occurring at each location (with 0.95 to 0.98 certainty) alternated in a square-wave function of a constant period (0.5 Hz or 1.33 Hz in different conditions). In addition, the direction and duration of the motion pulse were kept constant, so that it was also possible to predict the nature of the anticipated stimulus. Behavioural performance was strongly correlated to the spatial and temporal probability of pulse appearance, with animals displaying near optimal spatiotemporal integration when pulses were likely (see also Ghose 2006). Reverse-correlation analysis showed dynamic modulation of receptive field properties in MT over a sub-second timescale according to changing spatiotemporal expectations. Again, these findings indicate strong interactions between temporal and spatial expectations.

A recent study by Lima and colleagues (2011) demonstrates that temporal expectation can modulate sensory processing as early as in primary visual cortex (V1). A simple detection task was used, requiring monkeys to release a lever upon a change in the colour of the fixation point. Task-irrelevant visual stimuli were presented to drive and measure changes in visual excitability according to temporal expectations. Temporal expectations were manipulated in different ways over three experimental protocols. One experiment in particular introduced a clear hazard-rate manipulation (Experiment 2, block protocol), in which the probability for the imperative stimulus appearing at one of two intervals (1600 or 3600 ms) was changed between experimental blocks (Fig. 24.6a). Targets occurred at the probable interval on 85% of trials. Power and coherence of gamma-band activity increased during the foreperiod and was modulated by the hazard rates (see also Liang et al. 2005). Increases in gamma-band activity were paralleled by decreases in alpha-band activity. Gamma and alpha modulation developed significantly earlier in blocks in which targets were expected early (Fig. 24.6a). Changes of oscillatory activity were not confined to the spatially attended location. Instead, comparable effects on gamma-band activity occurred for stimuli at attended, foveal, as well as for unattended, peripheral locations.

Jaramillo and Zador (2011) studied the neuronal mechanisms of temporal expectations in primary auditory cortex (A1) of rats. Auditory targets occurred embedded in tone sequences at one of two interval periods (300–450 or 1350–1500 ms). Temporal expectation was manipulated in a blocked manner, so that targets appeared early or late on 85% of trials in 'expect-early' or 'expect-late' blocks respectively. Behavioural results revealed temporal expectation improved both reaction times and accuracy. Temporal expectations also modulated local field potentials and firing rates in primary auditory cortex, and these effects correlated with the behavioural performance on a trial-by-trial basis (Fig. 24.6b). Reversible lesions of the auditory cortex diminished the behavioural effect, confirming its causal involvement in using temporal predictions to enhance performance. Together, these results indicate that modulation of early sensory areas can mediate behavioural advantages conferred by temporal expectations.

Sensorimotor and motor areas

Parietal area LIP has been strongly implicated in regulating control of spatial attention (see Bisley and Goldberg 2010; Gottlieb 2007; see also Gottlieb (in chapter 12), this volume). This area may provide a nexus for integrating signals from different perceptual modalities, reward prediction, motor intention, and task set. These qualities, combined

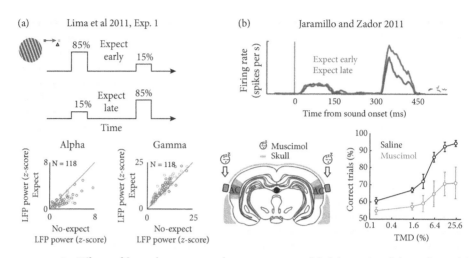

FIGURE 24.6   Effects of hazard rates on early sensory areas. (a) Schematic of the task used in Lima et al. (2011). In a block design, monkeys were required to respond to a small change in the fixation point. During expect-early blocks, the fixation point change occurred for most of the cases (85%) early in the trial, at 1600 ms. Only rarely (15% of the cases, catch trials) did the change occur late in the trial, at 3600 ms. In expect-late blocks, the probabilities of fixation point change were reversed. Scatterplots comparing LFP power in the alpha and gamma band on expected versus unexpected stimuli in V1 (Lima et al. 2011). Note how there is a decrease in alpha and an increase in gamma power for high compared with low temporal expectation. Reprinted by permission from Macmillan Publishers Ltd: *Nature Neuroscience*, 14(2), Santiago Jaramillo and Anthony M. Zador, The auditory cortex mediates the perceptual effects of acoustic temporal expectation, pp. 246–251, copyright 2011, Macmillan Publishers Ltd. (b) Findings from Jaramillo and Zador (2011). Similarly to the protocol used in Lima et al. (2011), here rats were rewarded for discriminating target sounds presented at 350 or 450 ms in expect-early blocks and 1350 or 1500 ms during late blocks. Responses of a single neuron in A1 show increased spiking rate in anticipation of the target under early (blue) compared to late (red) temporal expectations when the stimulus parameters were equated. Note how the greatest difference in evoked activity is seen for the tone that immediately preceded the early target (450 ms). Bottom panel shows the results of the inactivation experiments presented by Jaramillo and Zador (2011), showing that bilateral inactivation of A1 reliably impaired the performance in the task. Reprinted from Lima, B., Singer, W., Neuenschwander, S., Gamma responses correlate with temporal expectation in monkey primary visual cortex, 31(44), pp. 15919–15931 © 2011, The Society for Neuroscience.

with its involvement in sensorimotor integration for oculomotor control, place LIP in a strong position to influence ongoing perceptual analysis. Janssen and Shadlen (2005) showed that firing rates in LIP neurons vary systematically with hazard-rate functions in anticipation of 'go' stimuli prompting saccade in a delayed saccade task (Fig. 24.5b). More recently, Janssen and colleagues have started investigating the effects of temporal expectation on local field potentials and induced oscillations during visually guided and memory-guided saccade tasks and during passive visual fixation (Premereur et al. 2012). They found that gamma-band activity encoded the location of the saccade, but decreased during the foreperiod before the saccade. In contrast, alpha- and beta-band activity were less sensitive to saccade location but increased with temporal probability during the foreperiod. Interestingly, significant time-locked local field potentials and multi-unit responses also occurred at the anticipated time of the go stimulus, even when this stimulus was omitted.

Schoffelen and colleagues (2005) showed strong effects of hazard rates at the end of the information-processing pathway. They examined the effects of hazard-rate manipulations on motor excitability in a simple reaction-time task, measuring the temporal evolution of coherence between motor cortex and spinal cord neurons. Both reaction times and the strength of cortico–spinal coherence in the gamma-band followed the hazard-rate function (Fig. 24.5c). A study of ours in humans using a simple reaction-time task and EEG recordings also showed co-variation of response times and motor excitability with the hazard rates (Cravo et al. 2011b).

Working Hypotheses and Open Questions

How modulations by temporal expectations in sensorimotor areas, like LIP, relate to those in sensory areas, like V4, MT, V1, or A1, is unknown. Principles of organization in modulatory mechanisms of temporal expectation still remain to be revealed. At this point it is unclear whether coordination of modulatory mechanisms across large networks of regions is required to bring about behavioural benefits; whether central sources of temporal expectation are required to drive these effects; or whether localized mechanisms occurring at stages of processing that are most relevant for task performance are sufficient. In order to tease apart the degree and direction of influence among different brain areas across different frequency bands and firing rates, it will be important to use similar measures of spiking and oscillatory neuronal activity across different sites and under varying task parameters. Studies using simultaneous recordings across sites (Buschman and Miller 2009; Bosman et al. 2012; Zhou and Desimone 2011) will be particularly useful. For example, one interesting puzzle to solve is the observation that alpha-band activity in LIP increases in anticipation of the imperative signal (Premereur et al. 2012), whereas alpha becomes desynchronized in V1 (Lima et al. 2011; see also Rohenkohl and Nobre 2011).

It will also be important to understand whether influences of temporal expectations driven by rhythms and hazard rates are supported by co-extensive mechanisms. Some of the mechanisms proposed to support increases in sensory excitability in rhythmic context do not translate onto hazard-rate contexts in a trivial way. Activity in lower-frequency, delta and theta, bands is often suppressed in perceptual tasks that may be subject to hazard-rate effects. Furthermore, it is difficult to conceive how up-regulation of a specific frequency band, and cross-frequency coupling to that carrier frequency, can account for facilitatory effects of complex manipulations of hazard rates, such as bimodal (Ghose and Maunsell 2002; Janssen and Shadlen 2005) or alternating (Ghose and Bearl 2010) distributions of stimulus intervals. It is possible that common underlying mechanisms for regulation of neuronal excitability account for effects in predictable rhythmic and hazard-rated contexts. For example, these could rely on dynamic combinations of oscillatory activity across different frequencies. However, it is also prudent to entertain the possibility of multiple, dissociable sources of influences related to the temporal expectations.

Cues

The early foreperiod studies, as well as the more recent work on rhythms and hazard rates, left open the question about whether temporal expectations are under flexible, voluntary control. One possible interpretation was that increases in preparatory processes with the passage and predictability of time occur automatically and outside voluntary control. Another, more interesting possibility was that foreknowledge about predicted or relevant time intervals could be used to orient attention voluntarily and flexibly to a point in time in order to optimize behaviour.

Coull and Nobre (1998) adapted the spatial orienting task developed by Posner (1978, 1980) in order to investigate whether it was possible to orient attention voluntarily to temporal instants, analogously to our ability to orient attention to spatial locations, objects, or features (Fig. 24.7a). Symbolic cues were introduced to predict the time interval after which a target stimulus would appear. In this first experiment, predictive temporal cues (80% validity) were crossed factorially with predictive spatial cues (80% validity). Targets could appear at one of two intervals (300 or 1500 ms) and at one of two locations (left or right peripheral locations), and required a simple detection response. Relative to a neutral-cue condition, both temporal and spatial valid cues conferred significant behavioural advantages. In fact, behavioural benefits for temporal cues were larger than those for spatial cues. Because of changes in the hazard rates over time, targets are always 100% certain to occur at the long interval if they have not already occurred earlier. Accordingly, temporal cues led to equivalent performance at the long-interval condition, independently of whether the cue was valid (long-interval cued) or invalid (short-interval cued). This study opened up the investigation of voluntary orienting of attention based on the predicted timing of events.

Several behavioural studies have replicated and extended the effects of temporal orienting. In our laboratory, effects were shown with peripheral and foveal targets; in simple detection and in discrimination tasks; using predictive and instructive cues; using cues of different shapes; and over different interval ranges (see Griffin et al. 2001, 2002; Miniussi et al. 1999). In a related experiment, Correa and colleagues (2004) demonstrated that the benefits of temporal cues were not dependent on effects of foreperiod duration or sequence. All of our early experiments emphasized response speed and used tasks with relatively low perceptual demands. Using event-related potentials in these types of task, we found that the substantial benefits of temporal orienting were supported by a set of mechanisms that was qualitatively different from the modulatory mechanisms described for spatial orienting. In the absence of spatial certainty or spatial cueing, the early visual P1 potential was unaffected by temporal orienting. The most reliable modulatory effects were the attenuation of a frontally distributed N2 potential followed by an earlier rise and peak of the late positive centro-parietal 'P3' potential, as well as an increase in its amplitude (Griffin et al. 2002; Miniussi et al. 1999). This pattern of effects is similar to that which we observed in experiments using rhythmic apparent motion to manipulate

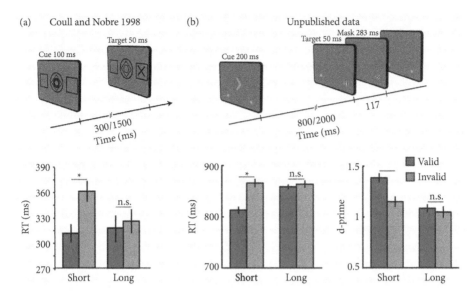

FIGURE 24.7   Behavioural effects of temporal cueing. (a) Schematic of the temporal orienting task, and interaction between temporal cues (valid × invalid) and cue-target interval
(short × long) obtained in Coull and Nobre (1998). Temporal orienting cues significantly
diminished response times to targets appearing at the short interval. (b) Results of an ongoing study using symbolic temporal orienting cues in a perceptually demanding task requiring
participants to discriminate a peripheral target (low contrast) followed by a backward pattern mask. The cues in this task were 100% spatially predictive, according to the direction
of the arrow, and 80% temporally predictive, according to its colour. The results indicate
that under these conditions, temporal orienting not only speeds response times, but also
improves perceptual discrimination. In line with the manipulations of conditional temporal
probability, effects of temporal orienting in (a) and (b) are confined for targets occurring at
the short interval. Reprinted from Coull, J. T., Nobre, A. C., Where and when to pay attention: the neural systems for directing attention to spatial locations and to time intervals as
revealed by both PET and fMRI, 18(18), pp. 7426–7435 © 1998, The Society for Neuroscience.

temporal expectation in the absence of spatial certainty (Doherty et al. 2005; Correa and
Nobre 2008; see above). Using a series of foveal temporal cueing tasks of this type, Zanto
and colleagues (2011) replicated the behavioural and neural effects of temporal orienting
under detection, discrimination, and go/no-go conditions. Interestingly, they found that
these effects were highly sensitive to ageing; proactive voluntary use of temporal cues was
not observed in groups of elderly (62–82-year-old) participants.

Perceptual Modulation

Studies using visual tasks with higher perceptual demands suggest that it may be possible for cued temporal orienting to influence early stages of visual perceptual processing. For example, Correa and colleagues (2005) found that valid temporal cues

enhanced perceptual sensitivity (d′) measures for detecting a target letter embedded within a stream of letters under rapid serial visual presentation (RSVP) conditions. Using a shape discrimination task, this group also reported modulation of the early visual P1 potential (Correa et al. 2006). However, some caution is required in interpreting these findings, since cues predicting short versus long intervals were also blocked, making this experiment a combination of a cueing and a blocked hazard-function manipulation.

Jepma and colleagues (2012) used computational modelling to reveal the information processing parameters influenced by predictive temporal cueing (400 or 1400 ms, 75% validity) to foveal visual targets requiring a simple, speeded detection response. Responses were significantly speeded to validly cued targets; the effects were pronounced at the short foreperiod and for dimmer targets. Model fitting indicated that temporal orienting affected the duration of processes such as stimulus encoding and/or motor preparation, which are unrelated to the critical decision-related variables: rate of evidence accumulation or setting of the decision threshold. These results argue against early perceptual modulation by temporal cueing in simple visual tasks, and are consistent with the authors' findings using a fixed-foreperiod manipulation of the hazard rate during a lexical-decision task (Jepma et al. 2012; Experiment 1, see above). They are, however, qualitatively different from our results using a rhythmic manipulation of temporal expectation in a perceptually demanding psychophysical task sensitive to changes in contrast sensitivity (see above Cravo et al. 2013: Rohenkohl et al. 2012a). We have pointed out (Rohenkohl et al. 2012b) that there may be multiple reasons for the difference in results; for example, rhythmic temporal expectations may be more potent at influencing early visual excitability and/or effects of temporal expectations may differentially reflect bottlenecks in perceptual analysis or response parameters depending on the demands of the task.

Studies of temporal cueing in the auditory modality, combined with ERP recordings, have consistently suggested modulation of early perceptual analysis. Valid temporal cues have been reported to enhance the auditory N1 potential, linked to perceptual analysis in auditory cortex (Lange et al. 2006; Lange and Röder 2006; Lampar and Lange 2011; Sanders and Astheimer 2008; reviewed in Lange and Röder 2010). Similar auditory modulation has also been observed in an audio-tactile cross-modal study of temporal cueing (Lange and Röder 2006). However, again, strong conclusions must remain curbed. Most auditory cueing tasks also contain conflated blocked manipulations of hazard rate, in which cues predicting short or long intervals occur with higher probability in separate blocks (Lange et al. 2003, 2006; Sanders and Astheimer 2008). No enhancement of the auditory N1 was observed in a predictive temporal cueing experiment using equiprobable short and long foreperiods within blocks and a target-discrimination task (Lampar and Lange 2011, Experiment 1), though significant N1 modulation was observed when cues were instructive (rather than predictive) and signalled which target interval was relevant for task performance (Experiment 2). Furthermore, to strengthen conclusions about the role of temporal cueing in modulating early auditory analysis, it will be necessary to measure effects even earlier, during the first stages of sensory processing in primary auditory cortex, which has been shown to be modulated by spatial attention (mid-latency potentials; see Woldorff et al. 1987).

The ability of predictive temporal cues to enhance perceptual analysis is also suggested by their strong influence on visibility of second targets in attentional blink tasks. Identification of a second target (T2) presented in a stream presented under RSVP conditions is usually significantly compromised when it follows a previous target (T1) within a brief temporal window (Raymond et al. 1992). However, cues predicting short intervals between the successive targets greatly diminish this effect in both vision (Martens and Johnson 2005) and audition (Shen and Alain 2011). Influences of temporal cueing have also been noted in tasks tapping into higher levels of stimulus analysis, such as unconscious categorical or semantic priming in RSVP tasks (Naccache et al. 2002; Kiefer and Brendel 2006; Fabre et al. 2007) or spatial Stroop tasks (Correa et al. 2010).

We are yet to characterize the gamut of mechanisms by which cued temporal expectations may influence different stages of stimulus analysis. Whether early, perceptual or later, motor-preparation stages are affected may heavily depend on whether, at one extreme, perceptual limits dictate variability in performance or whether, on the other extreme, perceptual requirements are trivial but instead motor preparation and selection limit performance. In addition, predictions about other properties of the anticipated stimulus, such as its location or constituent features, may also interact with temporal orienting effects (see Nobre et al. 2012). We are currently investigating some of these issues in the laboratory. In an ongoing study (unpublished observations), we observe strong effects of trial-by-trial temporal cueing when combined with spatial cues on perceptual sensitivity to discriminate the orientation of masked peripheral visual targets (Fig. 24.7b).

To complete the picture, it will also be important to compare and contrast effects under similar tasks between different modalities. It is highly probable, for example, that temporal orienting impacts visual and auditory processing differently (Nobre 2010). Vision and audition have complementary levels of spatial and temporal acuity, and it is reasonable to propose that these modalities have evolved to sense the organization and changes of events along these dimensions differentially. Audition is characterized by high temporal sensitivity and acuity, and temporal parameters of stimuli are coded from the earliest, subcortical processing stages (Viemeister and Plack 1993; Poeppel 2003; Theunissen 2003; Theunissen et al. 2000; King and Nelken 2009). This sense may therefore contain earlier substrates for and greater sensitivity to temporal expectations.

Neuronal Mechanisms

To the best of our knowledge, only two studies have used intracranial recordings to investigate how neuronal activity is modulated by temporal cues used to orient attention flexibly, in a trial-by-trial manner. The first study was by Anderson and Sheinberg (2008), recording from the inferior temporal visual area IT. Two visual pictures appeared in succession, separated by an interval of one or two seconds (Fig. 24.8a). The first picture acted as a predictive temporal cue (80% validity) and the second picture, which could be presented at different levels of contrast, prompted the execution of a previously associated left or right button-press response. Similar to speeded discrimination studies in humans, macaques showed evidence of using temporally predictive cues in a flexible manner. They were significantly faster in validly cued trials, especially at the short foreperiod and for dimmer stimuli. Spiking rates in IT neurons were also significantly enhanced for validly cued target pictures appearing at the short foreperiod compared to invalidly cued targets appearing at the same time. Increases in anticipatory beta-band power also occurred during heightened temporal expectation, and there was greater coherence between neuronal firing elicited by the target and both low (~4 Hz) and higher (beta and gamma band, 32–40 Hz) frequencies of the underlying field potential.

Lima and colleagues (2011, see above) also included a temporal cueing condition in their investigation of temporal expectations in primary visual cortex (Experiment 3, cue protocol). Cues appeared early (1000 ms) or late (3000 ms) into the trial, and indicated the appearance of the target 800 ms later on the majority of trials. However, on 10% of trials, cues appeared early (1000 ms) but were only followed by targets 2800 ms later. Modulations of gamma-band and alpha-band activity were similar to those observed in the blocked modulation of hazard rates (Experiment 1, sequence protocol), except that no gamma-band enhancement was observed in anticipation of the target when no stimulus was present within the receptive field of the recorded neuron. Gamma-band modulation was dependent on there being a stimulus present to drive the gamma response (Fig. 24.8b), suggesting that a covert change in the excitability state in visual cortex only becomes manifest once the cortical circuit is activated by the stimulus. In contrast, anticipatory desynchronization of alpha-band activity occurred in the presence or absence of a stimulus in the receptive field.

Of course, there are striking differences between these two studies, which make it difficult to extract overall patterns of neuronal modulation by cued temporal expectations. Recordings are made from different visual areas, using different cueing manipulations. Whereas stimuli driving neuronal responses being investigated are task-relevant and associated with responses and rewards in the study by Anderson and Sheinberg (2008), the stimuli are unrelated to the task in the study by Lima and colleagues (2011).

More studies will be required, therefore, for defining the set of cellular modulatory mechanisms of temporal cueing. It would be straightforward to introduce predictive temporal cues into future single-unit and field-potential studies of perception and attention in macaques. Such manipulation would likely yield hugely informative data that would shed light not only on the putative mechanisms of cued temporal expectations, but also on the characteristics of the other perceptual and attentional mechanisms under study, with which temporal expectations may interact.

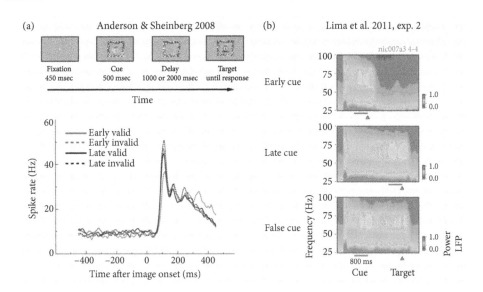

FIGURE 24.8   Perceptual effects of temporal cueing. (a) Schematic of the task used in Anderson and Sheinberg (2008). In this study, a first image of an object cued a temporal delay before a second target image appeared (1000 or 2000 ms later). Cue validity was 80%. As in human behavioural studies, effects of temporal orienting were confined to the early foreperiod condition. Spiking rates were significantly elevated for predicted, attended targets (Early Valid, solid red line) compared to unexpected, invalidly cued targets at the same time (Early Invalid, dashed red line). Reprinted from Neuropsychologia, 46(4), Britt Anderson and David L. Sheinberg, Effects of temporal context and temporal expectancy on neural activity in inferior temporal cortex, pp. 947–57, Copyright (2008), with permission from Elsevier. (b) Results in the second experiment reported by Lima et al. (2011) using symbolic cues. Here, a slight increase of fixation point luminance predicted that a change in fixation colour (target) would occur 800 ms later. In the Early and Late Cue conditions, the onset of the cue occurred either early or late in the trial, at 1000 ms or at 3000 ms respectively, and the target occurred at the predicted time, 800 ms later (at 1800 or 3800 ms). In the remaining 10% of the cases (false-cue condition), the cue appeared early in the trial (at 1000 ms), but the fixation point colour change was delayed until the end of the trial (3800 ms). Gamma power was highest preceding target presentation. Interestingly, note how under the false-cue condition, gamma oscillations transiently ceased when the target was not presented at the interval indicated by the cue, then gradually increased again toward the end of the trial. Reprinted from Lima, B., Singer, W., and Neuenschwander, S., Gamma responses correlate with temporal expectation in monkey primary visual cortex, 31(44), pp. 15919–31 © 2011, The Society for Neuroscience.

Control networks

Brain-imaging studies using hemodynamic methods (positron emission tomography (PET) and fMRI) have implicated the left posterior parietal cortex along the intraparietal sulcus (IPS) and in the anterior inferior parietal lobule, as well as the inferior premotor cortex, in the control of temporal orienting (Cotti et al. 2011; Davranche et al.

2011; Coull et al. 2000, 2001, 2013; Coull and Nobre 1998). This frontoparietal network appears to reflect a qualitatively distinct sensorimotor circuit compared to that involved in oculomotor control, which has been strongly implicated in the control of spatial orienting. Its left-hemispheric dominance and more inferior location suggest that it may comprise inferior parietal and frontal areas related with preparation and control of manual responses for reaching and grasping (see Krams et al. 1998; Rushworth et al. 1997). Timing is of particular importance to manual dexterity, and frontoparietal circuits for manual control may therefore contain fine-scale temporal computations that can support temporal orienting of attention. Accordingly, it has been suggested that temporal orienting may rely on manual control circuits in an analogous way to how spatial orienting relies on the oculomotor circuitry (see O'Reilly et al. 2008b).

The reliability of the involvement of this network in temporal orienting, and especially of the left parietal cortex, is increasingly clear. The pattern of parietal activations across temporal cueing, and related, tasks is plotted in a meta-analysis we produced for this chapter (Fig. 24.9). The analysis includes eight studies, and plots activations induced by the main or simple effect of temporal orienting. The resulting pattern confirms the reliability of activations in left IPS, anterior inferior parietal lobule, and premotor cortex. In addition, reliable activations are also observed in the cerebellum (see also O'Reilly et al. 2008b), although unfortunately cerebellar activations have not been systematically reported or discussed across studies.

Left parietal cortex is arguably the most reliable site of activation, and tends to be preferentially involved in temporal orienting compared to other types of orienting. Its activation strength is higher when conditions of temporal cueing are contrasted to spatial cueing (Coull and Nobre 1998) and when conditions of temporal cueing are contrasted to cueing of the motor effector for responding (Cotti et al. 2011). In the latter experiment, partial overlap was observed between parietal areas involved in temporal orienting and in preparing to use manual (vs. saccadic) responses, supporting a possible functional overlap between temporal orienting and manual preparation (Cotti et al. 2011; O'Reilly et al. 2008b). Left intraparietal activation is observed in tasks requiring unspeeded difficult perceptual discriminations as well as in tasks requiring speeded motor responses (Davranche et al. 2011). Furthermore, by comparing functional connectivity between tasks, Davranche and colleagues found that parietal cortex was more strongly correlated with extrastriate visual cortex in the perceptually demanding task and with premotor cortex in the speeded motor task. Consistent parietal activations have also been noted in tasks in which temporal expectations about event timings are induced by predictions based on stimulus motion (Assmus et al. 2003, 2005; Coull et al. 2008b; O'Reilly et al. 2008b).

In contrast, patterns of brain activation in temporal cueing tasks differ from those in tasks that require participants explicitly to estimate and produce temporal intervals in order to make judgements about the timing of stimuli or execute timed responses (Coull et al. 2004, 2013). Explicit timing tasks of this sort have been reported to engage right frontostriatal networks, as well as auditory cortex (see Coull and Nobre 2008; Nobre and O'Reilly 2004).

Coull and colleagues have interpreted the pattern of results across studies, sensibly and parsimoniously, as implicating the left parietal cortex as an important source of

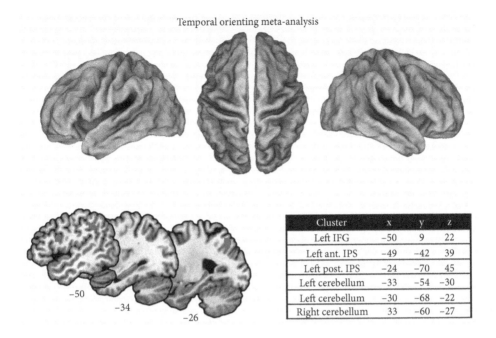

Temporal orienting meta-analysis

Cluster	x	y	z
Left IFG	−50	9	22
Left ant. IPS	−49	−42	39
Left post. IPS	−24	−70	45
Left cerebellum	−33	−54	−30
Left cerebellum	−30	−68	−22
Right cerebellum	33	−60	−27

FIGURE 24.9 Activation likelihood estimation (ALE—GingerALE 2.0 software) maps for temporal orienting studies. Eight studies were included in the meta-analysis (Coull and Nobre 1998—Exp. 1 and 2; Coull et al. 2000, 2001, 2012a, 2012b; Cotti et al. 2011; Davranche et al. 2012). Values are significant at FDR q < 0.05, minimum cluster size > 200 mm³.

temporal expectations in cueing tasks (Coull et al. 2008a, 2011; Coull and Nobre 2008). However, it is still worth bearing in mind possible alternatives. fMRI studies so far have not isolated neural activations specifically triggered by cues, nor shown direct influence of cue-related parietal activations on activations along the information processing stream and behaviour. The closest we get to this is the recent study by Davranche and colleagues (2011). A competing possible explanation is that parietal involvement in temporal cueing tasks reflects modulation of target-related processes. Multiple candidate functions remain in play, since similar posterior parietal areas have been implicated in accumulation of sensory evidence (Gold and Shadlen 2007; Yang and Shadlen 2007; Gould et al. 2012), limitations in perceptual detection or working-memory capacity (Marois and Ivanoff 2005; Tosoni et al. 2004; Heekenren et al. 2004), and motor preparation (Krams et al. 1998; Rushworth et al. 1997).

The limitations of the fMRI methodology pose particular problems when trying to pinpoint the specific functional contributions of parietal and other putative areas to top-down control of temporal orienting. Hemodynamic measures are slow and therefore susceptible to effects of differential temporal correlations among task events. Temporal cueing, by its very nature, requires systematic manipulations of temporal correlations. The rapid pace, and differential correlations among events in temporal cueing tasks greatly complicate the dissecting out of activations specifically related to top-down control versus target-related analysis. Complementary problems in spatial resolution plague studies using electroencephalography or event-related potentials. We are currently using magnetoencephalography with the goal of investigating the time course of involvement of parietal and other brain areas during temporal orienting based on trial-by-trial cues.

Temporal cueing studies using event-related potentials have consistently shown modulation of the contingent negative variation (CNV) (Walter et al. 1964) during selective temporal anticipation of target events (e.g. Zanto et al. 2011; Miniussi et al. 1999; Los and Heslenfeld 2005; Capizzi et al. 2013). The time course of the CNV follows that of cued temporal expectation. The potential develops more sharply in anticipation of target events at shorter intervals, building up to a common maximum level at the anticipated time of the target event. Similar CNV modulation is observed in explicit timing tasks, for example, in which participants have to judge the duration of a target stimulus relative to a standard (Macar et al. 2004; Pfeuty et al. 2005). It is difficult to conclude whether the CNV modulation in cued temporal orienting tasks and in explicit timing tasks taps into a common timing mechanism used both for orienting and for timing, or whether temporal orienting is used to optimize perceptual and decision-making processes in explicit timing tasks. This common pattern of CNV build-up mirrors the gradual and systematic increases in neuronal firing rates in parietal (Janssen and Shadlen 2005; Leon and Shadlen 2003), motor (Renoult et al. 2006; Riehle et al. 1997), premotor (Akkal et al. 2004; Lucchetti and Bon 2001), and prefrontal (Niki and Watanabe 1979) regions in motor and timing tasks. Most likely, CNV modulation in temporal cueing tasks reflects proactive preparation and/or synchronization processes linked to sensorimotor integration and motor preparation; which can occur independently of perceptual modulation (Nobre and Coull 2010; Nobre and O'Reilly 2004; Nobre 2001).

Not many human temporal cueing studies have reported anticipatory effects related to optimization of perceptual analysis. However, this may simply reflect the use of tasks with low perceptual demands and the lack of analysis of induced oscillatory activity in earlier studies (e.g. Miniussi et al. 1999). More recently, Zanto and colleagues (2011) found enhanced alpha-band desynchronization when young adults anticipated targets at shorter versus longer intervals (see also Babiloni et al. 2004). These findings are similar to what is observed with rhythmic modulation of temporal expectations for visual stimuli (Praamstra et al. 2006; Rohenkohl and Nobre 2011), and in intracranial recordings during temporal cueing or blocked foreperiod manipulations in the macaque (Lima et al. 2011). More reports of anticipatory modulatory mechanisms are expected as more studies get under way.

Working Hypotheses and Open Questions

The growing literature on temporal cueing has already made some significant contributions to our understanding of attentional biasing. Going beyond the literatures on foreperiod, rhythms, and hazard rates, cueing studies show that temporal anticipation of events is under flexible and voluntary control. The effects are robust and occur across a variety of task settings and in different modalities.

Investigations of neural modulatory mechanisms are still relatively few. We lack a full picture, and it is likely that more temporal modulatory mechanisms will be discovered. But we have already learned that similar benefits of spatial and temporal orienting observed at the behavioural level can result from markedly different underlying neural mechanisms (Griffin et al. 2002). Cueing studies will be particularly useful in determining whether there are dedicated networks for top-down control of temporal expectations, and for separating these from mechanisms at the sites of modulation. It is a real possibility that the flexible deployment of temporal expectations relies on flexible temporal organization of activity within networks of brain areas participating in the task. Assuming there are dedicated networks for top-down control, these may be difficult to isolate because of methodological difficulties. Convergence across tasks and across methods, including imaging (magnetoencephalography) and interference (transcranial magnetic stimulation) methods with high temporal resolution, will be essential.

So far, studies in different modalities suggest that we are not heading toward an equivalence of modulatory mechanisms. Instead, temporal biases may influence different stages of information processing, and in different ways across the senses. Temporal biases may also interact differently with other biases about other stimulus attributes or action intentions. The initial findings remind us that our senses are not redundant, but most likely evolved to provide complementary sources of information about the external environment.

Conclusions and Open Questions

Types of temporal biases

We have discussed three types of temporal biases, but now we have to admit that this subdivision is somewhat arbitrary, possibly acting as a placeholder for subsequent, better-informed categorizations. We have focused on temporal biases concerned with short temporal intervals that frame the timing of cognitive functions (sub-second to seconds). These operate within slower fluctuations that may alter the cognitive and emotional state in our system, such as those related to circadian rhythms. There may also be much faster temporal regulatory mechanisms that fine-tune perceptual or motor processing beyond the scope of our awareness.

Within the 'interval timing' stretch we discussed, behavioural modulations—'foreperiod effects'—can arise from the length, regularity, sequence, contextual conditional probability, cued probability, and cued relevance of an event. At the moment it is unclear how many underlying types of temporal biases may carry these effects. Behavioural performance may also be affected by temporally non-specific transient changes in alertness (Posner and Boies 1971; Petersen and Posner 2012; Posner and Petersen 1990), which may interact with selective temporal biases (as well as other types of biases) to modulate their effects (see Nobre et al. 2012). We have proposed three major classes of selective temporal biases, guided by the subdivisions and distinctions in the literature, combined with our synthesis and analyses of the various findings. Refining our understanding of the number and nature of the essential temporal biasing mechanisms that adapt our perception on a moment-to-moment basis should remain a priority area for research.

Looking back at the effects of temporal expectations produced by rhythms, hazards, and cues, we can note many similarities. All types of manipulations lead to modulations of anticipatory CNV potentials, at least in tasks that require speeded responses (Praamstra et al. 2006; Cravo et al. 2011b; Miniussi et al. 1999; Hackley et al. 2007; Los and Heslenfeld 2005; Muller-Gethmann et al. 2003). Temporal expectations also tune desynchronization of alpha-band activity in anticipation of targets in a variety of tasks manipulating rhythms, hazards, and cueing (Rohenkohl and Nobre 2011; Praamstra et al. 2006; Lima et al. 2011). This effect, however, is not apparent in all rhythmic tasks (e.g. Cravo et al. 2013; Lakatos et al. 2008), and has not been well investigated in human studies using temporal cues. Modulations of event-related potentials triggered by targets are also similar in rhythmic and cued attention tasks (e.g. Correa and Nobre 2008; Doherty et al. 2005; Griffin et al. 2002; Miniussi et al. 1999).

But there are also some differences. For example, in audition, regular rhythms were found to attenuate the N1 potential elicited by targets falling on the predicted beat (Lange 2009, 2010), while temporally predictive cues (presented in a blocked fashion) lead to enhancement of the auditory N1 potential (Lange and Röder 2006; Lange et al. 2003, 2006). By directly comparing cued versus rhythmic temporal expectations in a visual task, we showed that benefits were functionally dissociable. In a rhythmic motion task, additive performance benefits were provided by temporal predictions based on the colour (cueing) or the pace (rhythm) of the moving disc (Rohenkohl et al. 2011). Furthermore, effects of rhythmic expectations were independent of strategic factors, whereas effects of cueing were dependent upon instructions to attend to the colour cues. We concluded that rhythmic cues triggered an automatic, exogenous type of temporal orienting, while symbolic cues relied on an endogenous mechanism; and proposed an analogy to the distinction made between exogenous vs. endogenous orienting of spatial attention (Posner 1980; Posner and Boies 1971). De la Rosa and colleagues (2012) also found effects of rhythmic temporal orienting to be independent of cognitive control. A concurrent working-memory task interferes with performance benefits conferred by temporal cueing but not with benefits from temporal rhythms. Similarly, sequential effects are unaffected by concurrent working memory tasks that disrupt temporal cueing (Capizzi et al. 2012, 2013). Deficits in patients with lesions in the left vs. right frontal lobes also suggest functional dissociations among temporal effects related to rhythms, hazards, and cues (Trivino et al. 2010). Right frontal lesions were found to disrupt temporal cueing selectively, and left frontal lesions to disrupt benefits from rhythms and constant foreperiods. Sequential effects remained unaffected by either type of lesion.

Different sources and mechanisms contributing to temporal expectations may contribute to discrepancies noted in performance benefits in different studies. For example, stronger and more automatic effects of temporal rhythm may make it easier to modulate early levels of stimulus analysis, such as those related to contrast sensitivity and accumulation of perceptual evidence for subsequent decision-making (Cravo et al. 2013; Rohenkohl et al. 2012a, 2012b). However, in order to understand the contributions of temporal expectations generated by different task manipulations, it will be necessary to compare these using stimulus parameters and task demands that are otherwise controlled.

Interactions between temporal and other biases

When manipulated separately, effects of temporal expectations often appear to be independent from those of spatial expectations (Griffin et al. 2002; MacKay and Juola 2007; Bruchmann et al. 2011; Lange et al. 2006). Cueing temporal intervals also yielded additive effects to cueing the motor effector for responding to a target in a task eliminating specific spatial expectations about the stimulus or the action to be performed (Cotti et al. 2011). In contrast, strong interactions are observed when expectations about timing of events are combined with other selective expectations. In our first rhythmic manipulation of temporal and spatial expectations, we noted a striking interaction between these two sources of biases on early stages of analysis (Doherty et al. 2005). In the absence of spatial certainty, rhythmic temporal expectations had no effect on the visual P1 potential. In contrast, temporal expectations greatly magnified the effect of spatial attention on P1 amplitude. The synergy between temporal and spatial expectations was not observed at the behavioural level, in which additive effects were obtained; but this may be because the bottleneck for performance in that particular task may not have been early perceptual analysis. We are currently investigating whether synergistic effects of temporal and spatial expectations become manifest in tasks requiring fine perceptual discriminations under perceptually challenging conditions (see also Milliken et al. 2003, discrimination task). Strong interactions have also been observed between learning temporal and spatial/motor sequences, even when the sequences in the different dimensions are completely orthogonal (O'Reilly et al. 2008a).

These kinds of observations suggest an intuitive way by which temporal expectations may help guide selective perception. It is difficult to imagine how isolated temporal expectations can modulate sensory processing in a proactive and anticipatory manner. Overall changes in sensory excitability by temporal expectations may be possible, in the form of a transient alerting-like mechanism. However, on its own this kind of mechanism would not only be metabolically costly, it would also be highly non-selective, magnifying processing of any and all events, targets and distractors alike, at predicted relevant moments. However, by interacting with other receptive-field properties, temporal expectations can adjust proactive anticipatory biases over time in order to optimize the state of excitability of relevant items at the right time. Temporal modulation of spatial-attention biases has been noted in single-unit studies in the macaque (Ghose and Bearl 2010; Ghose and Maunsell 2002) and in human EEG studies (Rohenkohl and Nobre 2011; van Ede et al. 2011). Effects of temporal expectation in non-spatial attention tasks are also suggestive of interactions between temporal and feature-based expectations (Lakatos et al. 2013; White et al. 2010). Enhanced preparation of specific movements and associated neural activity has long been noted in motor tasks (e.g. Riehle et al. 1997; Lucchetti and Bon 2001; Heinen and Liu 1997; Schoffelen et al. 2005; Cravo et al. 2011a).

Stepping back, the idea that temporal expectations combine with foreknowledge about other attributes makes obvious sense. We struggle to conceive or understand the nature of time in isolation—indeed some scholars negate its very existence (e.g. Rovelli 2007). In cognition, encoding and sensing of timing may be intrinsically bound to events and their constituent properties. Expectations are about events and not about timings or spatial locations in isolation. Events in turn are situated in time and space, and contain spatiotemporal structure. It will be interesting to continue to explore the synergies between temporal expectations and expectations about other attributes of task relevant events, such as their locations or features, as well as expectations about decisions and actions to be taken in response to these events. Looking at interactions among different types of biasing signals will enrich the study of attention in general, and not only the study of temporal expectations.

Proposed mechanisms

There is still a difficult puzzle to solve: how are temporal expectations coded in the brain in the first place so that they can interact with other biases, or change neuronal excitability in their own right? It is early days to attempt any definitive answer, but it is probably worth airing briefly different types of mechanisms that have been envisaged so far.

One common starting point is to consider whether temporal expectations rely on the same or similar mechanisms that might be in place for explicit timing functions in the brain—whatever those turn out to be (for discussion see Coull and Nobre 2008). If we had a clear understanding of the neural systems and mechanisms responsible for explicit timing functions, it would be possible to design experiments to measure or manipulate activity in these areas during tasks manipulating temporal expectations. However, in its current state, the timing literature provides little guidance. There is still no accepted view on the networks and mechanisms that support perception of temporal intervals. Traditional proposals for the existence of an internal clock (Gibbon et al. 1984; Treisman 1963), for keeping time and enabling retrieval and comparison of stored time intervals, still frame much of contemporary research. Dedicated timing networks have been proposed to involve frontostriatal circuits (Buhusi and Meck 2005; Coull et al. 2004, 2011). The cerebellum has also been suggested to participate specifically in the timing of events (Ivry and Spencer 2004). In contrast, other researchers propose that timing functions occur in a much more widely distributed fashion, as a common property of many or all neural systems (Mauk and Buonomano 2004; Nobre and O'Reilly 2004). Distortions in temporal perception that are highly specific to events occurring within specific sensory modalities and in specific locations (e.g. Morrone et al. 2005; Johnston et al. 2006) suggest the involvement of highly localized mechanisms for time perception. These could support timing functions in isolation, or interact with centralized timing mechanisms to bring about highly specific effects (Coull et al. 2011).

Within timing systems, be they centralized or distributed, temporal intervals have been proposed to rely on periodic or oscillatory neural activity (e.g. Buhusi and Meck 2005; Miall 1989; Treisman 1963). Others have noted that temporal intervals and regularities within a given context may also be encoded through time-dependent neuronal properties and short-term plasticity mechanisms embedded within neuronal assemblies (Buonomano and Maass 2009; Karmarkar and Buonomano 2007; Crowe et al. 2010). If such state-dependent dynamics and plasticity exist, timing signals could be intrinsic to information processing systems, and these could contribute to optimizing neural processing at anticipated relevant events.

Our current review of the emerging literature on temporal expectations clearly suggests that oscillatory brain activity may provide an important medium for the coding and integration of temporal expectations in the brain. The most developed theoretical proposal so far is that of 'active sensing' based on rhythmic sensory sampling of the environment (see above Lakatos et al. 2008, 2009, 2013; Zion Golumbic et al. 2013; Schroeder et al. 2010; Schroeder and Lakatos 2009b). This proposal combines classic ideas about the importance of motor control and intention in guiding perception (Liberman and Mattingly 1985; Rizzolatti et al. 1987, 1994: Schubotz 2007) with the appreciation that many of our effector systems display rhythmic activity within frequencies similar to our intrinsic low-frequency oscillations (Schroeder et al. 2010; Bosman et al. 2009). It suggests that low-frequency oscillations become entrained to the timing of rhythmic sensory input, occurring naturally within the environment or as a result of rhythmic sampling. This entrainment regulates neuronal excitability so that it is maximal at the predicted times of relevant events, and may also serve to coordinate rhythmic changes of neuronal excitability across different brain areas involved in a given task (see Buzsáki 2006). Because of the ebbing and flowing of neuronal excitability, higher frequency oscillations related to stimulus processing or anticipation become nested within the periods of higher excitability. This process can be repeated, regulating neuronal excitability at multiple temporal scales. Mounting evidence from human and animal studies supports the viability of such a mechanism in the context of regular, rhythmic stimulation (e.g. Cravo et al. 2013; Rohenkohl et al. 2012a; Lakatos et al. 2008, 2009, 2013; Mathewson et al. 2010; Henry and Obleser 2012; de Graaf et al. 2013). Recent work further points to the ability of such mechanisms to enhance selectively signals related to task-relevant events, sharpening the contrast between target and distractor processing (Lakatos et al. 2013).

However, it remains unclear whether and how this kind of rhythmic nesting mechanism can be generalized to conditions in which more complicated hazard functions predict event onsets (e.g. Ghose and Maunsell 2002; Janssen and Shadlen 2005), or during predicted sequences of events (e.g. Olson and Chun 2001; O'Reilly et al. 2008a).

In principle, it is possible that elemental rhythmic entrainment mechanisms can become combined to generate more complex temporal predictions, in a Fourier-like fashion. The biological plausibility of such a mechanism would have to be ascertained. Conversely, or additionally, short-term plasticity mechanisms working upon temporal dynamics of neuronal assemblies could reinforce temporal states of relevant events within given contexts (Buonomano and Maass 2009). To test whether summation of oscillatory activity at different frequencies and/or reinforcement of dynamical states contribute to complex temporal expectation functions, it may be worth investigating modulation of oscillatory activity within temporal prediction contexts that vary systematically from isochronous rhythms to complex predictable temporal sequences of events.

Alpha-band activity has also been consistently linked to anticipatory states in perceptual tasks in visual (Worden et al. 2000; Thut et al. 2006; van Dijk et al. 2008; Ergenoglu et al. 2004; Hanslmayr et al. 2007; Romei et al. 2010; Gould et al. 2011) and also other modalities (van Ede et al. 2011; Haegens et al. 2011, 2012). Different theoretical accounts have been suggested for how alpha-band regulates the excitability for sensory events. For example, Jensen and colleagues have suggested that alpha-band activity reflects activity in an inhibitory circuit, such that cortical uptake of sensory processing is mainly limited to the periodic windows of alpha-band desynchronization (Jensen et al. 2012; see also Ray and Cole 1985; Klimesch et al. 2007; Pfurtscheller and Lopes da Silva 1999; Pfurtscheller et al. 1994, 1996). Others have suggested that alpha desynchronization may also contribute to the organization and support of awareness and maintenance of sensory representations in short-term memory (Jensen et al. 2012; Palva and Palva 2007). As we have reviewed, the timing of alpha-band activity in anticipation of sensory stimuli is often modulated by temporal expectations, with effects noted in rhythmic (Rohenkohl and Nobre 2011; Praamstra et al. 2006; Mathewson et al. 2012), hazard-rate (van Ede et al. 2011; Lima et al. 2011), and temporal cueing (Lima et al. 2011; Zanto et al. 2011) tasks. Modulation in the anticipatory alpha-band activity, however, does not always co-occur with modulation of lower frequency bands suggestive of entrainment to the timing of task-relevant events (Cravo et al. 2013; Besle et al. 2011; Lakatos et al. 2008). It will be important, therefore, to test the extent to which modulations of oscillations in alpha and in lower-frequency (delta and theta) bands express common versus dissociable mechanisms for adjusting and coordinating neural excitability according to temporal expectations.

Fries and colleagues have recently proposed that alignment of phase coherence among distinct populations of neurons involved in a task is of central importance for the selection and integration of relevant events during perception (Bosman et al. 2012; Fries 2009). Modulation of neural activity according to the predicted timings of events, either through rhythmic entrainment or through other mechanisms, is likely to play a significant role in modulating the efficacy of neuronal communication through their coherence. It will be of great interest to introduce manipulations of temporal expectation into large-scale multi-site recording studies of selective attention (e.g. Bosman et al. 2012).

References

Akkal, D., Escola, L., Bioulac, B., and Burbaud, P. (2004). Time predictability modulates pre-supplementary motor area neuronal activity. *NeuroReport* 15: 1283–12836.

Anderson, B. and Sheinberg, D. L. (2008). Effects of temporal context and temporal expectancy on neural activity in inferior temporal cortex. *Neuropsychologia* 46: 947–957.

Assmus, A., Marshall, J. C., Noth, J., Zilles, K., and Fink, G. R. (2005). Difficulty of perceptual spatiotemporal integration modulates the neural activity of left inferior parietal cortex. *Neuroscience* 132: 923–927.

Assmus, A., Marshall, J. C., Ritzl, A., Noth, J., Zilles, K., and Fink, G. R. (2003). Left inferior parietal cortex integrates time and space during collision judgments. *NeuroImage* 20 Suppl. 1: S82–S88.

Astheimer, L. B. and Sanders, L. D. (2009). Listeners modulate temporally selective attention during natural speech processing. *Biological Psychology* 80: 23–34.

Astheimer, L. B. and Sanders, L. D. (2011). Predictability affects early perceptual processing of word onsets in continuous speech. *Neuropsychologia* 49: 3512–3516.

Astheimer, L. B. and Sanders, L. D. (2012). Temporally selective attention supports speech processing in 3- to 5-year-old children. *Developmental Cognitive Neuroscience* 2: 120–128.

Babiloni, C., Miniussi, C., Babiloni, F., Carducci, F., Cincotti, F., Del Percio, C., Sirello, G., Fracassi, C., Nobre, A. C., and Rossini, P. M. (2004). Sub-second 'temporal attention' modulates alpha rhythms: A high-resolution EEG study. *Brain Research: Cognitive Brain Research* 19: 259–268.

Barnes, G. R. and Asselman, P. T. (1991). The mechanism of prediction in human smooth pursuit eye movements. *Journal of Physiology* 439: 439–461.

Bausenhart, K. M., Rolke, B., Seibold, V. C., and Ulrich, R. (2010). Temporal preparation influences the dynamics of information processing: Evidence for early onset of information accumulation. *Vision Research* 50: 1025–1034.

Bausenhart, K. M., Rolke, B., and Ulrich, R. (2008). Temporal preparation improves temporal resolution: Evidence from constant foreperiods. *Perception & Psychophysics* 70: 1504–1514.

Bermudez, M. A., Gobel, C., and Schultz, W. (2012). Sensitivity to temporal reward structure in amygdala neurons. *Current Biology* 22: 1839–1844.

Bertelson, P. (1967). The time course of preparation. *Quarterly Journal of Experimental Psychology* 19: 272–279.

Bertelson, P. and Boons, J. P. (1960). Time uncertainty and choice reaction time. *Nature* 187: 531–532.

Besle, J., Schevon, C. A., Mehta, A. D., Lakatos, P., Goodman, R. R., McKhann, G. M., Emerson, R. G., and Schroeder, C. E. (2011). Tuning of the human neocortex to the temporal dynamics of attended events. *Journal of Neuroscience* 31: 3176–3185.

Bisley, J. W. and Goldberg, M. E. (2010). Attention, intention, and priority in the parietal lobe. *Annual Review of Neuroscience* 33: 1–21.

Bollimunta, A., Chen, Y., Schroeder, C. E., and Ding, M. (2008). Neuronal mechanisms of cortical alpha oscillations in awake-behaving macaques. *Journal of Neuroscience* 28: 9976–9988.

Bollimunta, A., Mo, J., Schroeder, C. E., and Ding, M. (2011). Neuronal mechanisms and attentional modulation of corticothalamic alpha oscillations. *Journal of Neuroscience* 31: 4935–4943.

Bosman, C. A., Schoffelen, J. M., Brunet, N., Oostenveld, R., Bastos, A. M., Womelsdorf, T., Rubehn, B., Stieglitz, T., De Weerd, P., and Fries, P. (2012). Attentional stimulus selection through selective synchronization between monkey visual areas. *Neuron* 75: 875–888.

Bosman, C. A., Womelsdorf, T., Desimone, R., and Fries, P. (2009). A microsaccadic rhythm modulates gamma-band synchronization and behavior. *Journal of Neuroscience: The Official Journal of the Society for Neuroscience* 29: 9471–9480.

Bruchmann, M., Hintze, P., and Mota, S. (2011). The effects of spatial and temporal cueing on metacontrast masking. *Advances in Cognitive Psychology/University of Finance and Management in Warsaw* 7: 132–141.

Bueti, D., Bahrami, B., Walsh, V., and Rees, G. (2010). Encoding of temporal probabilities in the human brain. *Journal of Neuroscience* 30: 4343–4352.

Buhusi, C. and Meck, W. (2005). What makes us tick? Functional and neural mechanisms of interval timing. *Nature Reviews Neuroscience* 6: 755–765.

Bundesen, C. (1990). A theory of visual attention. *Psychological Review* 97: 523–547.

Bundesen, C., Habekost, T., and Kyllingsbaek, S. (2011). A neural theory of visual attention and short-term memory (NTVA). *Neuropsychologia* 49: 1446–1457.

Buonomano, D. and Maass, W. (2009). State-dependent computations: Spatiotemporal processing in cortical networks. *Nature Reviews Neuroscience* 10: 113–125.

Buschman, T. J. and Miller, E. K. (2009). Serial, covert shifts of attention during visual search are reflected by the frontal eye fields and correlated with population oscillations. *Neuron* 63: 386–396.

Buzsáki, G. (2006). *Rhythms of the Brain*. Oxford: Oxford University Press.

Canolty, R. T., Edwards, E., Dalal, S. S., Soltani, M., Nagarajan, S. S., Kirsch, H. E., Berger, M. S., Barbaro, N. M., and Knight, R. T. (2006). High gamma power is phase-locked to theta oscillations in human neocortex. *Science* 313: 1626–1628.

Capizzi, M., Correa, A., and Sanabria, D. (2013). Temporal orienting of attention is interfered by concurrent working memory updating. *Neuropsychologia* 51: 326–339.

Capizzi, M., Sanabria, D., and Correa, A. (2012). Dissociating controlled from automatic processing in temporal preparation. *Cognition* 123: 293–302.

Chapin, H. L., Zanto, T., Jantzen, K. J., Kelso, S. J., Steinberg, F., and Large, E. W. (2010). Neural responses to complex auditory rhythms: The role of attending. *Frontiers in Psychology* 1: 224.

Correa, A., Cappucci, P., Nobre, A. C., and Lupiáñez, J. (2010). The two sides of temporal orienting: Facilitating perceptual selection, disrupting response selection. *Experimental Psychology* 57: 142–148.

Correa, A., Lupiáñez, J., Madrid, E., and Tudela, P. (2006). Temporal attention enhances early visual processing: A review and new evidence from event-related potentials. *Brain Research* 1076: 116–128.

Correa, A., Lupiáñez, J., Milliken, B., and Tudela, P. (2004). Endogenous temporal orienting of attention in detection and discrimination tasks. *Perception & Psychophysics* 66: 264–278.

Correa, A., Lupiáñez, J., and Tudela, P. (2005). Attentional preparation based on temporal expectancy modulates processing at the perceptual level. *Psychonomic Bulletin & Review* 12: 328–334.

Correa, A. and Nobre, A. (2008). Neural modulation by regularity and passage of time. *Journal of Neurophysiology* 100: 1649–1655.

Cotti, J., Rohenkohl, G., Stokes, M., Nobre, A. C., and Coull, J. T. (2011). Functionally dissociating temporal and motor components of response preparation in left intraparietal sulcus. *NeuroImage* 54: 1221–1230.

Coull, J. T., Cheng, R. K., and Meck, W. H. (2011). Neuroanatomical and neurochemical substrates of timing. *Neuropsychopharmacology: Official Publication of the American College of Neuropsychopharmacology* 36: 3–25.

Coull, J. T., Davranche, K., Nazarian, B., and Vidal, F. (2013). Functional anatomy of timing differs for production versus prediction of time intervals. *Neuropsychologia 51*: 309–319.

Coull, J. T., Frith, C. D., Büchel, C., and Nobre, A. C. (2000). Orienting attention in time: Behavioural and neuroanatomical distinction between exogenous and endogenous shifts. *Neuropsychologia 38*: 808–819.

Coull, J. T., Nazarian, B., and Vidal, F. (2008a). Timing, storage, and comparison of stimulus duration engage discrete anatomical components of a perceptual timing network. *Journal of Cognitive Neuroscience 20*: 2185–2197.

Coull, J. T. and Nobre, A. C. (1998). Where and when to pay attention: The neural systems for directing attention to spatial locations and to time intervals as revealed by both PET and fMRI. *Journal of Neuroscience 18*: 7426–7435.

Coull, J. T. and Nobre, A. C. (2008). Dissociating explicit timing from temporal expectation with fMRI. *Current Opinion in Neurobiology 18*: 137–144.

Coull, J. T., Nobre, A. C., and Frith, C. D. (2001). The noradrenergic alpha2 agonist clonidine modulates behavioural and neuroanatomical correlates of human attentional orienting and alerting. *Cerebral Cortex 11*: 73–84.

Coull, J. T., Vidal, F., Goulon, C., Nazarian, B., and Craig, C. (2008b). Using time-to-contact information to assess potential collision modulates both visual and temporal prediction networks. *Frontiers in Human Neuroscience 2*: 10.

Coull, J. T., Vidal, F., Nazarian, B., and Macar, F. (2004). Functional anatomy of the attentional modulation of time estimation. *Science 303*: 1506–1508.

Cravo, A. M., Claessens, P. M., and Baldo, M. V. (2011a). The relation between action, predictability and temporal contiguity in temporal binding. *Acta Psychologica 136*: 157–166.

Cravo, A. M., Rohenkohl, G., Wyart, V., and Nobre, A. C. (2011b). Endogenous modulation of low frequency oscillations by temporal expectations. *Journal of Neurophysiology 106*: 2964–2972.

Cravo, A. M., Rohenkohl, G., Wyart, V., and Nobre, A. C. (2013). Temporal expectation enhances contrast sensitivity by phase entrainment of low-frequency oscillations in visual cortex. *Journal of Neuroscience: The Official Journal of the Society for Neuroscience 33*: 4002–4010.

Crowe, D. A., Averbeck, B. B., and Chafee, M. V. (2010). Rapid sequences of population activity patterns dynamically encode task-critical spatial information in parietal cortex. *Journal of Neuroscience: The Official Journal of the Society for Neuroscience 30*: 11640–11653.

Cui, X., Stetson, C., Montague, P. R., and Eagleman, D. M. (2009). Ready … go: Amplitude of the fMRI signal encodes expectation of cue arrival time. *PLoS Biology 7*: e1000167.

Davranche, K., Nazarian, B., Vidal, F., and Coull, J. (2011). Orienting attention in time activates left intraparietal sulcus for both perceptual and motor task goals. *Journal of Cognitive Neuroscience 23*: 3318–3330.

De Graaf, T. A., Gross, J., Paterson, G., Rusch, T., Sack, A. T., and Thut, G. (2013). Alpha-band rhythms in visual task performance: Phase-locking by rhythmic sensory stimulation. *PLoS One 8*: e60035.

De Hemptinne, C., Barnes, G. R., and Missal, M. (2010). Influence of previous target motion on anticipatory pursuit deceleration. *Experimental Brain Research/Experimentelle Hirnforschung/Experimentation cérébrale 207*: 173–184.

De Hemptinne, C., Nozaradan, S., Duvivier, Q., Lefevre, P., and Missal, M. (2007). How do primates anticipate uncertain future events? *Journal of Neuroscience: The Official Journal of the Society for Neuroscience 27*: 4334–4341.

De La Rosa, M. D., Sanabria, D., Capizzi, M., and Correa, A. (2012). Temporal preparation driven by rhythms is resistant to working memory interference. *Frontiers in Psychology 3*: 308.

Doherty, J. R., Rao, A., Mesulam, M. M., and Nobre, A. C. (2005). Synergistic effect of combined temporal and spatial expectations on visual attention. *Journal of Neuroscience* 25: 8259–8266.

Egan, J. P., Greenberg, G. Z., and Schulman, A. I. (1961). Interval of time uncertainty in auditory detection. *Journal of Acoustical Society of America* 33: 771–778.

Eimer, M. (1994). 'Sensory gating' as a mechanism for visuospatial orienting: Electrophysiological evidence from trial-by-trial cuing experiments. *Perception & Psychophysics* 55: 667–675.

Ergenoglu, T., Demiralp, T., Bayraktaroglu, Z., Ergen, M., Beydagi, H., and Uresin, Y. (2004). Alpha rhythm of the EEG modulates visual detection performance in humans. *Brain Research: Cognitive Brain Research* 20: 376–383.

Fabre, L., Lemaire, P., and Grainger, J. (2007). Attentional modulation of masked repetition and categorical priming in young and older adults. *Cognition* 105: 513–532.

Fiorillo, C. D., Tobler, P. N., and Schultz, W. (2003). Discrete coding of reward probability and uncertainty by dopamine neurons. *Science* 299: 1898–1902.

Foxe, J. J., Simpson, G. V., and Ahlfors, S. P. (1998). Parieto-occipital approximately 10 Hz activity reflects anticipatory state of visual attention mechanisms. *NeuroReport* 9: 3929–3933.

Fries, P. (2009). Neuronal gamma-band synchronization as a fundamental process in cortical computation. *Annual Review of Neuroscience* 32: 209–224.

Fries, P., Reynolds, J. H., Rorie, A. E., and Desimone, R. (2001). Modulation of oscillatory neuronal synchronization by selective visual attention. *Science* 291: 1560–1563.

Fujioka, T., Trainor, L. J., Large, E. W., and Ross, B. (2009). Beta and gamma rhythms in human auditory cortex during musical beat processing. *Annals of the New York Academy of Sciences* 1169: 89–92.

Fujioka, T., Trainor, L. J., Large, E. W., and Ross, B. (2012). Internalized timing of isochronous sounds is represented in neuromagnetic beta oscillations. *Journal of Neuroscience: The Official Journal of the Society for Neuroscience* 32: 1791–1802.

Ghazanfar, A. A., Morrill, R. J., and Kayser, C. (2013). Monkeys are perceptually tuned to facial expressions that exhibit a theta-like speech rhythm. *Proceedings of the National Academy of Sciences USA* 110: 1959–1963.

Ghose, G. M. (2006). Strategies optimize the detection of motion transients. *Journal of Vision* 6: 429–440.

Ghose, G. M. and Bearl, D. W. (2010). Attention directed by expectations enhances receptive fields in cortical area MT. *Vision Research* 50: 441–451.

Ghose, G. M. and Maunsell, J. H. (2002). Attentional modulation in visual cortex depends on task timing. *Nature* 419: 616–620.

Gibbon, J., Church, R. M., and Meck, W. H. (1984). Scalar timing in memory. *Annals of the New York Academy of Sciences* 423: 52–77.

Gold, J. I. and Shadlen, M. N. (2007). The neural basis of decision making. *Annual Review of Neuroscience* 30: 535–574.

Gordon, R. L., Magne, C. L., and Large, E. W. (2011). EEG correlates of song prosody: A new look at the relationship between linguistic and musical rhythm. *Frontiers in Psychology* 2: 352.

Gottlieb, J. (2007). From thought to action: The parietal cortex as a bridge between perception, action, and cognition. *Neuron* 53: 9–16.

Gould, I. C., Nobre, A. C., Wyart, V., and Rushworth, M. F. (2012). Effects of decision variables and intraparietal stimulation on sensorimotor oscillatory activity in the human brain. *Journal of Neuroscience: The Official Journal of the Society for Neuroscience* 32: 13805–13818.

Gould, I. C., Rushworth, M. F., and Nobre, A. C. (2011). Indexing the graded allocation of visuospatial attention using anticipatory alpha oscillations. *Journal of Neurophysiology* 105: 1318–1326.

Griffin, I. C., Miniussi, C., and Nobre, A. C. (2001). Orienting attention in time. *Frontiers in Bioscience 6*: D660–D671.

Griffin, I. C., Miniussi, C., and Nobre, A. C. (2002). Multiple mechanisms of selective attention: Differential modulation of stimulus processing by attention to space or time. *Neuropsychologia 40*: 2325–2340.

Griffin, I. C. and Nobre, A. C. (2005). Temporal orienting of attention. In L. Itti, G. Rees, and J. K. Tsotsos (eds.), *Neurobiology of Attention* (pp. 257–263). San Diego: Elsevier Academic Press.

Hackley, S. A., Schankin, A., Wohlschlaeger, A., and Wascher, E. (2007). Localization of temporal preparation effects via trisected reaction time. *Psychophysiology 44*: 334–338.

Haegens, S., Handel, B. F., and Jensen, O. (2011). Top-down controlled alpha band activity in somatosensory areas determines behavioral performance in a discrimination task. *Journal of Neuroscience: The Official Journal of the Society for Neuroscience 31*: 5197–5204.

Haegens, S., Luther, L., and Jensen, O. (2012). Somatosensory anticipatory alpha activity increases to suppress distracting input. *Journal of Cognitive Neuroscience 24*: 677–685.

Hanslmayr, S., Aslan, A., Staudigl, T., Klimesch, W., Herrmann, C. S., and Bauml, K. H. (2007). Prestimulus oscillations predict visual perception performance between and within subjects. *NeuroImage 37*: 1465–1473.

Hanslmayr, S., Gross, J., Klimesch, W., and Shapiro, K. L. (2011). The role of alpha oscillations in temporal attention. *Brain Research Reviews 67*: 331–343.

Heinen, S. J. and Liu, M. (1997). Single-neuron activity in the dorsomedial frontal cortex during smooth-pursuit eye movements to predictable target motion. *Visual Neuroscience 14*: 853–865.

Henry, M. J. and Obleser, J. (2012). Frequency modulation entrains slow neural oscillations and optimizes human listening behavior. *Proceedings of the National Academy of Sciences USA 109*: 20095–20100.

Herrmann, C. S. (2001). Human EEG responses to 1–100 Hz flicker: Resonance phenomena in visual cortex and their potential correlation to cognitive phenomena. *Experimental Brain Research 137*: 346–353.

Hoch, L., Tyler, M. D., and Tillmann, B. (2013). Regularity of unit length boosts statistical learning in verbal and nonverbal artificial languages. *Psychonomic Bulletin & Review 20*: 142–147.

Hollerman, J. R. and Schultz, W. (1998). Dopamine neurons report an error in the temporal prediction of reward during learning. *Nature Neuroscience 1*: 304–309.

Ivry, R. B. and Spencer, R. M. (2004). The neural representation of time. *Current Opinion in Neurobiology 14*: 225–32.

Janssen, P. and Shadlen, M. (2005). A representation of the hazard rate of elapsed time in macaque area LIP. *Nature Neuroscience 8*: 234–241.

Jaramillo, S. and Zador, A. M. (2011). The auditory cortex mediates the perceptual effects of acoustic temporal expectation. *Nature Neuroscience 14*: 246–251.

Jensen, O., Bonnefond, M., and Vanrullen, R. (2012). An oscillatory mechanism for prioritizing salient unattended stimuli. *Trends in Cognitive Sciences 16*: 200–206.

Jepma, M., Wagenmakers, E. J., and Nieuwenhuis, S. (2012). Temporal expectation and information processing: A model-based analysis. *Cognition 122*: 426–441.

Jin, D. Z., Fujii, N., and Graybiel, A. M. (2009). Neural representation of time in cortico-basal ganglia circuits. *Proceedings of the National Academy of Sciences USA 106*: 19156–19161.

Johnston, A., Arnold, D. H., and Nishida, S. (2006). Spatially localized distortions of event time. *Current Biology 16*: 472–479.

Jones, M. R. (1976). Time, our lost dimension: Toward a new theory of perception, attention, and memory. *Psychological Review 83*: 323–355.

Jones, M. R. (2010). Attending to sound patterns and the role of entrainment. In A. C. Nobre and J. T. Coull (eds.), *Attention and Time* (pp. 317–330). Oxford: Oxford University Press.

Jones, M. R. and Boltz, M. (1989). Dynamic attending and responses to time. *Psychological Review* 96: 459–491.

Jones, M. R., Johnston, H. M., and Puente, J. (2006). Effects of auditory pattern structure on anticipatory and reactive attending. *Cognitive Psychology* 53: 59–96.

Jones, M. R., Moynihan, H., Mackenzie, N., and Puente, J. (2002). Temporal aspects of stimulus-driven attending in dynamic arrays. *Psychological Science* 13: 313–319.

Karlin, L. (1959). Reaction time as a function of foreperiod duration and variability. *Journal of Experimental Psychology* 58: 185–191.

Karmarkar, U. R. and Buonomano, D. (2007). Timing in the absence of clocks: Encoding time in neural network states. *Neuron* 53: 427–438.

Kelly, S. P., Gomez-Ramirez, M., and Foxe, J. J. (2009). The strength of anticipatory spatial biasing predicts target discrimination at attended locations: A high-density EEG study. *European Journal of Neuroscience* 30: 2224–2234.

Kelly, S. P., Lalor, E. C., Reilly, R. B., and Foxe, J. J. (2006). Increases in alpha oscillatory power reflect an active retinotopic mechanism for distractor suppression during sustained visuospatial attention. *Journal of Neurophysiology* 95: 3844–3851.

Kiefer, M. and Brendel, D. (2006). Attentional modulation of unconscious 'automatic' processes: Evidence from event-related potentials in a masked priming paradigm. *Journal of Cognitive Neuroscience* 18: 184–198.

King, A. J. and Nelken, I. (2009). Unraveling the principles of auditory cortical processing: Can we learn from the visual system? *Nature Neuroscience* 12: 698–701.

Kingstone, A. and Klein, R. M. (1993). What are human express saccades? *Perception & Psychophysics* 54: 260–273.

Klimesch, W., Sauseng, P., and Hanslmayr, S. (2007). EEG alpha oscillations: The inhibition-timing hypothesis. *Brain Research Reviews* 53: 63–88.

Kotz, S. A., Schwartze, M., and Schmidt-Kassow, M. (2009). Non-motor basal ganglia functions: A review and proposal for a model of sensory predictability in auditory language perception. *Cortex* 45: 982–990.

Krams, M., Rushworth, M. F., Deiber, M. P., Frackowiak, R. S., and Passingham, R. E. (1998). The preparation, execution and suppression of copied movements in the human brain. *Experimental Brain Research* 120: 386–398.

Lakatos, P., Karmos, G., Mehta, A., Ulbert, I., and Schroeder, C. (2008). Entrainment of neuronal oscillations as a mechanism of attentional selection. *Science* 320: 110–113.

Lakatos, P., Musacchia, G., O'Connell, M. N., Falchier, A. Y., Javitt, D. C., and Schroeder, C. E. (2013). The spectrotemporal filter mechanism of auditory selective attention. *Neuron* 77: 750–761.

Lakatos, P., O'Connell, M. N., Barczak, A., Mills, A., Javitt, D. C., and Schroeder, C. E. (2009). The leading sense: Supramodal control of neurophysiological context by attention. *Neuron* 64: 419–430.

Lakatos, P., Shah, A. S., Knuth, K. H., Ulbert, I., Karmos, G., and Schroeder, C. E. (2005). An oscillatory hierarchy controlling neuronal excitability and stimulus processing in the auditory cortex. *Journal of Neurophysiology* 94: 1904–1911.

Lampar, A. and Lange, K. (2011). Effects of temporal trial-by-trial cuing on early and late stages of auditory processing: Evidence from event-related potentials. *Attention, Perception, & Psychophysics* 73: 1916–1933.

Lange, K. (2009). Brain correlates of early auditory processing are attenuated by expectations for time and pitch. *Brain and Cognition 69*: 127–137.

Lange, K. (2010). Can a regular context induce temporal orienting to a target sound? *International Journal of Psychophysiology: Official Journal of the International Organization of Psychophysiology 78*: 231–238.

Lange, K., Kramer, U. M., and Röder, B. (2006). Attending points in time and space. *Experimental Brain Research 173*: 130–140.

Lange, K. and Röder, B. (2006). Orienting attention to points in time improves stimulus processing both within and across modalities. *Journal of Cognitive Neuroscience 18*: 715–729.

Lange, K. and Röder, B. (2010). Temporal orienting in audition, touch, and across modalities. In A. C. Nobre and J. Coull (eds.), *Attention and Time* (pp. 393–406). Oxford: Oxford University Press.

Lange, K., Rosler, F., and Röder, B. (2003). Early processing stages are modulated when auditory stimuli are presented at an attended moment in time: An event-related potential study. *Psychophysiology 40*: 806–817.

Large, E. W., Fink, P., and Kelso, J. A. (2002). Tracking simple and complex sequences. *Psychological Research 66*: 3–17.

Large, E. W., and Snyder, J. S. (2009). Pulse and meter as neural resonance. *Annals of the New York Academy of Sciences 1169*: 46–57.

Lasley, D. J. and Cohn, T. (1981). Detection of a luminance increment: Effect of temporal uncertainty. *Journal of the Optical Society of America 71*: 845–850.

Leon, M. I. and Shadlen, M. (2003). Representation of time by neurons in the posterior parietal cortex of the macaque. *Neuron 38*: 317–327.

Liang, H., Bressler, S. L., Buffalo, E. A., Desimone, R., and Fries, P. (2005). Empirical mode decomposition of field potentials from macaque V4 in visual spatial attention. *Biological Cybernetics 92*: 380–392.

Liberman, A. M. and Mattingly, I. G. (1985). The motor theory of speech perception revised. *Cognition 21*: 1–36.

Lima, B., Singer, W., and Neuenschwander, S. (2011). Gamma responses correlate with temporal expectation in monkey primary visual cortex. *Journal of Neuroscience 31*: 15919–15931.

Los, S. A. and Agter, F. (2005). Reweighting sequential effects across different distributions of foreperiods: Segregating elementary contributions to nonspecific preparation. *Perception & Psychophysics 67*: 1161–1170.

Los, S. A. and Heslenfeld, D. J. (2005). Intentional and unintentional contributions to nonspecific preparation: Electrophysiological evidence. *Journal of Experimental Psychology: General 134*: 52–72.

Lowe, G. 1967. Interval of time uncertainty in visual detection. *Perception & Psychophysics 2*: 278–280.

Lucchetti, C. and Bon, L. (2001). Time-modulated neuronal activity in the premotor cortex of macaque monkeys. *Experimental Brain Research 141*: 254–260.

Luce, R. (1986). *Response Times: Their Role in Inferring Elementary Mental Organization.* New York: Oxford University Press.

Macar, F., Anton, J. L., Bonnet, M., and Vidal, F. (2004). Timing functions of the supplementary motor area: An event-related fMRI study. *Brain Research: Cognitive Brain Research 21*: 206–215.

Mackay, A. and Juola, J. F. (2007). Are spatial and temporal attention independent? *Perception & Psychophysics 69*: 972–979.

Mangun, G. R. and Hillyard, S. (1987). The spatial allocation of visual attention as indexed by event-related brain potentials. *Human Factors: Cognitive Psychophysiology* 29: 195–211.

Marois, R. and Ivanoff, J. (2005). Capacity limits of information processing in the brain. *Trends in Cognitive Sciences* 9: 296–305.

Martens, S. and Johnson, A. (2005). Timing attention: Cuing target onset interval attenuates the attentional blink. *Memory & Cognition* 33: 234–240.

Mathewson, K. E., Fabiani, M., Gratton, G., Beck, D. M., and Lleras, A. (2010). Rescuing stimuli from invisibility: Inducing a momentary release from visual masking with pre-target entrainment. *Cognition* 115: 186–191.

Mathewson, K. E., Gratton, G., Fabiani, M., Beck, D. M., and Ro, T. (2009). To see or not to see: Prestimulus alpha phase predicts visual awareness. *Journal of Neuroscience: The Official Journal of the Society for Neuroscience* 29: 2725–2732.

Mathewson, K. E., Prudhomme, C., Fabiani, M., Beck, D. M., Lleras, A., and Gratton, G. (2012). Making waves in the stream of consciousness: Entraining oscillations in EEG alpha and fluctuations in visual awareness with rhythmic visual stimulation. *Journal of Cognitive Neuroscience* 24: 2321–2333.

Mauk, M. and Buonomano, D. (2004). The neural basis of temporal processing. *Annual Review of Neuroscience* 27: 307–340.

Miall, C. (1989). The storage of time intervals using oscillating neurons. *Neural Computation* 1: 359–371.

Milliken, B., Lupiáñez, J., Roberts, M., and Stevanovski, B. (2003). Orienting in space and time: Joint contributions to exogenous spatial cuing effects. *Psychonomic Bulletin & Review* 10: 877–883.

Miniussi, C., Wilding, E. L., Coull, J. T., and Nobre, A. C. (1999). Orienting attention in time: Modulation of brain potentials. *Brain* 122: 1507–1518.

Morrone, M., Ross, J., and Burr, D. (2005). Saccadic eye movements cause compression of time as well as space. *Nature Neuroscience* 8: 950–954.

Müller-Gethmann, H., Ulrich, R., and Rinkenauer, G. (2003). Locus of the effect of temporal preparation: Evidence from the lateralized readiness potential. *Psychophysiology* 40: 597–611.

Naccache, L., Blandin, E., and Dehaene, S. (2002). Unconscious masked priming depends on temporal attention. *Psychological Science* 13: 416–424.

Newhall, S. N. (1923). Effects of attention on the intensity of cutaneous pressure and on visual brightness. *Archives of Psychology* 61: 5–75.

Nickerson, R. S. (1965). Response time to the second of two successive signals as a function of absolute and relative duration of intersignal interval. *Perceptual & Motor Skills* 21: 3–10.

Niemi, P. and Näätänen, R. (1981). Foreperiods and simple reaction time. *Psychological Bulletin* 89: 133–162.

Niki, H. and Watanabe, M. (1979). Prefrontal and cingulate unit activity during timing behavior in the monkey. *Brain Research* 171: 213–224.

Nobre, A. C. (2001). Orienting attention to instants in time. *Neuropsychologia* 39: 1317–1328.

Nobre, A. C. (2010). How can temporal expectations bias perception and action? In A. C. Nobre and J. Coull (eds.), *Attention and Time* (pp. 371–392). Oxford: Oxford University Press.

Nobre, A., Correa, A., and Coull, J. (2007). The hazards of time. *Current Opinion in Neurobiology* 17: 465–470.

Nobre, A. C. and Coull, J. T. (eds.) (2010). *Attention and Time*. Oxford: Oxford University Press.

Nobre, A. C. and O'Reilly, J. (2004). Time is of the essence. *Trends in Cognitive Sciences* 8: 387–389.

Nobre, A. C., Rohenkohl, G., and Stokes, M. (2012). Nervous anticipation: Top-down biasing across space and time. In M. I. Posner (ed.), *Cognitive Neuroscience of Attention*, 2nd edn. (pp. 159–186). New York: Guilford Press.

Nozaradan, S., Peretz, I., Missal, M., and Mouraux, A. (2011). Tagging the neuronal entrainment to beat and meter. *Journal of Neuroscience: The Official Journal of the Society for Neuroscience* 31: 10234–10240.

O'Connell, R. G., Dockree, P. M., Robertson, I. H., Bellgrove, M. A., Foxe, J. J., and Kelly, S. P. (2009). Uncovering the neural signature of lapsing attention: Electrophysiological signals predict errors up to 20 s before they occur. *Journal of Neuroscience: The Official Journal of the Society for Neuroscience* 29: 8604–8611.

O'Reilly, J. X., McCarthy, K. J., Capizzi, M., and Nobre, A. C. (2008a). Acquisition of the temporal and ordinal structure of movement sequences in incidental learning. *Journal of Neurophysiology* 99: 2731–2735.

O'Reilly, J. X., Mesulam, M., and Nobre, A. (2008b). The cerebellum predicts the timing of perceptual events. *Journal of Neuroscience* 28: 2252–2260.

Olson, I. and Chun, M. (2001). Temporal contextual cuing of visual attention. *Journal of Experimental Psychology: Learning, Memory, and Cognition* 27: 1299–1313.

Palmer, J., Huk, A. C., and Shadlen, M. N. (2005). The effect of stimulus strength on the speed and accuracy of a perceptual decision. *Journal of Vision* 5: 376–404.

Palva, S. and Palva, J. M. (2007). New vistas for alpha-frequency band oscillations. *Trends in Neurosciences* 30: 150–158.

Petersen, S. E. and Posner, M. I. (2012). The attention system of the human brain: 20 years after. *Annual Review of Neuroscience* 35: 73–89.

Pfeuty, M., Ragot, R., and Pouthas, V. (2005). Relationship between CNV and timing of an upcoming event. *Neuroscience Letters* 382: 106–111.

Pfurtscheller, G. and Lopes Da Silva, F. H. (1999). Event-related EEG/MEG synchronization and desynchronization: Basic principles. *Clinical Neurophysiology* 110: 1842–1857.

Pfurtscheller, G., Neuper, C., and Mohl, W. (1994). Event-related desynchronization (ERD) during visual processing. *International Journal of Psychophysiology: Official Journal of the International Organization of Psychophysiology* 16: 147–153.

Pfurtscheller, G., Stancak, A., Jr, and Neuper, C. (1996). Event-related synchronization (ERS) in the alpha band: An electrophysiological correlate of cortical idling—a review. *International Journal of Psychophysiology: Official Journal of the International Organization of Psychophysiology* 24: 39–46.

Poeppel, D. (2003). The analysis of speech in different temporal integration windows: Cerebral lateralization as 'asymmetric sampling in time'. *Speech Communication* 41: 245–255.

Posner, M. I. (1978). *Chronometric Explorations of Mind.* Hillsdale, N.J.: Lawrence Erlbaum Associates.

Posner, M. I. (1980). Orienting of attention. *Quarterly Journal of Experimental Psychology* 32: 3–25.

Posner, M. I. and Boies, S. J. (1971). Components of attention. *Psychological Review* 78: 391–408.

Posner, M. I. and Petersen, S. E. (1990). The attention system of the human brain. *Annual Review of Neuroscience* 13: 25–42.

Posner, M. I., Snyder, C. R., and Davidson, B. J. (1980). Attention and the detection of signals. *Journal of Experimental Psychology* 109: 160–174.

Power, A. J., Mead, N., Barnes, L., and Goswami, U. (2012). Neural entrainment to rhythmically presented auditory, visual, and audio-visual speech in children. *Frontiers in Psychology* 3: 216.

Praamstra, P., Kourtis, D., Kwok, H. F., and Oostenveld, R. (2006). Neurophysiology of implicit timing in serial choice reaction-time performance. *Journal of Neuroscience: The Official Journal of the Society for Neuroscience* 26: 5448–5455.

Premereur, E., Vanduffel, W., and Janssen, P. (2012). Local field potential activity associated with temporal expectations in the macaque lateral intraparietal area. *Journal of Cognitive Neuroscience* 24: 1314–1330.

Ratcliff, R. and Rouder, J. N. (1998). Modeling response times for two-choice decisions. *Psychological Science* 9: 347–356.

Ray, W. J. and Cole, H. W. (1985). EEG alpha activity reflects attentional demands, and beta activity reflects emotional and cognitive processes. *Science* 228: 750–752.

Raymond, J. E., Shapiro, K. L., and Arnell, K. M. (1992). Temporary suppression of visual processing in an RSVP task: An attentional blink? *Journal of Experimental Psychology: Human Perception and Performance* 18: 849–860.

Renoult, L., Roux, S., and Riehle, A. (2006). Time is a rubberband: Neuronal activity in monkey motor cortex in relation to time estimation. *European Journal of Neuroscience* 23: 3098–3108.

Riehle, A., Grun, S., Diesmann, M., and Aertsen, A. (1997). Spike synchronization and rate modulation differentially involved in motor cortical function. *Science* 278: 1950–1953.

Rizzolatti, G., Riggio, L., Dascola, I., and Umiltà, C. (1987). Reorienting attention across the horizontal and vertical meridians: Evidence in favor of a premotor theory of attention. *Neuropsychologia* 25: 31–40.

Rizzolatti, G., Riggio, L., and Sheliga, B. M. (1994). Space and selective attention. In C. Umiltà and M. Moscovitch (eds.), *Attention and Performance XV* (pp. 421–452). Cambridge, Mass.: MIT Press.

Roesch, M. R. and Olson, C. R. (2005). Neuronal activity dependent on anticipated and elapsed delay in macaque prefrontal cortex, frontal and supplementary eye fields, and premotor cortex. *Journal of Neurophysiology* 94: 1469–1497.

Rohenkohl, G., Coull, J. T., and Nobre, A. C. (2011). Behavioural dissociation between exogenous and endogenous temporal orienting of attention. *PLoS One* 6: e14620.

Rohenkohl, G., Cravo, A. M., Wyart, V., and Nobre, A. C. (2012a). Temporal expectation improves the quality of sensory information. *Journal of Neuroscience: The Official Journal of the Society for Neuroscience* 32: 8424–8428.

Rohenkohl, G., Cravo, A. M., Wyart, V., and Nobre, A. C. (2012b). Re: Temporal expectation may affect the onset, not the rate, of evidence accumulation. Reply to Nieuwenhuis, S., Jepma, M., and Wagenmakers, E.-J. Temporal expectation may affect the onset, not the rate, of evidence accumulation. *Journal of Neuroscience* 32: 8424–8428.

Rohenkohl, G. and Nobre, A. C. (2011). Alpha oscillations related to anticipatory attention follow temporal expectations. *Journal of Neuroscience* 31: 14076–14084.

Rolke, B. and Hofmann, P. (2007). Temporal uncertainty degrades perceptual processing. *Psychonomic Bulletin & Review* 14: 522–526.

Rolke, B. and Ulrich, R. (2010). On the locus of temporal preparation: Enhancement of premotor processes? In A. C. Nobre and J. T. Coull (eds.), *Attention and Time* (pp. 227–242). Oxford: Oxford University Press.

Romei, V., Gross, J., and Thut, G. (2010). On the role of prestimulus alpha rhythms over occipito-parietal areas in visual input regulation: Correlation or causation? *Journal of Neuroscience: The Official Journal of the Society for Neuroscience* 30: 8692–8697.

Rovelli, C. (2007). *Quantum Gravity*. Cambridge: Cambridge University Press.

Rushworth, M. F., Nixon, P. D., Renowden, S., Wade, D. T., and Passingham, R. E. (1997). The left parietal cortex and motor attention. *Neuropsychologia* 35: 1261–1273.

Sanabria, D., Capizzi, M., and Correa, A. (2011). Rhythms that speed you up. *Journal of Experimental Psychology: Human Perception and Performance* 37: 236–244.

Sanders, L. and Astheimer, L. (2008). Temporally selective attention modulates early perceptual processing: Event-related potential evidence. *Perception & Psychophysics* 70: 732–742.

Schmidt-Kassow, M. and Kotz, S. A. (2009). Event-related brain potentials suggest a late interaction of meter and syntax in the P600. *Journal of Cognitive Neuroscience* 21: 1693–1708.

Schoffelen, J. M., Oostenveld, R., and Fries, P. (2005). Neuronal coherence as a mechanism of effective corticospinal interaction. *Science* 308: 111–113.

Schroeder, C. E. and Lakatos, P. (2009a). The gamma oscillation: Master or slave? *Brain Topography* 22: 24–26.

Schroeder, C. E. and Lakatos, P. (2009b). Low-frequency neuronal oscillations as instruments of sensory selection. *Trends in Neurosciences* 32: 9–18.

Schroeder, C. E., Wilson, D. A., Radman, T., Scharfman, H., and Lakatos, P. (2010). Dynamics of active sensing and perceptual selection. *Current Opinion in Neurobiology* 20: 172–176.

Schubotz, R. I. (2007). Prediction of external events with our motor system: Towards a new framework. *Trends in Cognitive Sciences* 11: 211–218.

Schubotz, R. I. and Von Cramon, D. Y. (2001). Functional organization of the lateral premotor cortex: fMRI reveals different regions activated by anticipation of object properties, location and speed. *Brain Research: Cognitive Brain Research* 11: 97–112.

Schwartz, G. and Berry, M. J., 2nd (2008). Sophisticated temporal pattern recognition in retinal ganglion cells. *Journal of Neurophysiology* 99: 1787–1798.

Seibold, V. C., Bausenhart, K. M., Rolke, B., and Ulrich, R. (2011). Does temporal preparation increase the rate of sensory information accumulation? *Acta Psychologica* 137: 56–64.

Seifried, T., Ulrich, R., Bausenhart, K. M., Rolke, B., and Osman, A. (2010). Temporal preparation decreases perceptual latency: Evidence from a clock paradigm. *Quarterly Journal of Experimental Psychology* 63: 2432–2451.

Shen, D. and Alain, C. (2011). Temporal attention facilitates short-term consolidation during a rapid serial auditory presentation task. *Experimental Brain Research/Experimentelle Hirnforschung/Experimentation cérébrale* 215: 285–292.

Shen, D. and Alain, C. (2012). Implicit temporal expectation attenuates auditory attentional blink. *PLoS One* 7: e36031.

Shuler, M. G. and Bear, M. F. (2006). Reward timing in the primary visual cortex. *Science* 311: 1606–1609.

Snodgrass, J. G. (1969). Foreperiod effects in simple reaction time: Anticipation or expectancy? *Journal of Experimental Psychology* 79: 1–19.

Snyder, A. C. and Foxe, J. J. (2010). Anticipatory attentional suppression of visual features indexed by oscillatory alpha-band power increases: A high-density electrical mapping study. *Journal of Neuroscience: The Official Journal of the Society for Neuroscience* 30: 4024–4032.

Snyder, J. S. and Large, E. W. (2005). Gamma-band activity reflects the metric structure of rhythmic tone sequences. *Brain Research: Cognitive Brain Research* 24: 117–126.

Sumbre, G., Muto, A., Baier, H., and Poo, M. (2008). Entrained rhythmic activities of neuronal ensembles as perceptual memory of time interval. *Nature* 456: 102–106.

Teichner, W. H. (1954). Recent studies of simple reaction time. *Psychological Bulletin* 51: 128–149.

Theunissen, F. E. (2003). From synchrony to sparseness. *Trends in Neurosciences* 26: 61–64.

Theunissen, F. E., Sen, K., and Doupe, A. J. (2000). Spectral-temporal receptive fields of nonlinear auditory neurons obtained using natural sounds. *Journal of Neuroscience: The Official Journal of the Society for Neuroscience* 20: 2315–2331.

Thut, G., Nietzel, A., Brandt, S. A., and Pascual-Leone, A. (2006). Alpha-band electroencepha-lographic activity over occipital cortex indexes visuospatial attention bias and predicts visual target detection. *Journal of Neuroscience 26*: 9494–9502.

Tillmann, B. (2012). Music and language perception: Expectations, structural integration, and cognitive sequencing. *Topics in Cognitive Science 4*: 568–584.

Treisman, M. (1963). Temporal discrimination and the indifference interval: Implications for a model of the 'internal clock'. *Psychological Monographs 77*: 1–31.

Trivino, M., Correa, A., Arnedo, M., and Lupiáñez, J. (2010). Temporal orienting deficit after prefrontal damage. *Brain 133*: 1173–1185.

Tsujimoto, S. and Sawaguchi, T. (2005). Neuronal activity representing temporal prediction of reward in the primate prefrontal cortex. *Journal of Neurophysiology 93*: 3687–3692.

Van Dijk, H., Schoffelen, J. M., Oostenveld, R., and Jensen, O. (2008). Prestimulus oscillatory activity in the alpha band predicts visual discrimination ability. *Journal of Neuroscience: The Official Journal of the Society for Neuroscience 28*: 1816–1823.

Van Ede, F., De Lange, F., Jensen, O., and Maris, E. (2011). Orienting attention to an upcoming tactile event involves a spatially and temporally specific modulation of sensorimotor alpha-and beta-band oscillations. *Journal of Neuroscience 31*: 2016–2024.

Vangkilde, S., Coull, J. T., and Bundesen, C. (2012). Great expectations: Temporal expectation modulates perceptual processing speed. *Journal of Experimental Psychology: Human Perception and Performance 38*: 1183–1191.

Viemeister, N. F. and Plack, C. J. (1993). Time analysis. In W. Yost, A. Popper, and R. Fay (eds.), *Human Psychophysics* (pp. 116–154). New York: Springer-Verlag.

Walter, W. G., Cooper, R., Aldridge, V. J., McCallum, W. C., and Winter, A. L. (1964). Contingent negative variation: An electric sign of sensorimotor association and expectancy in the human brain. *Nature 203*: 380–384.

Westheimer, G. and Ley, E. (1996). Temporal uncertainty effects on orientation discrimination and stereoscopic thresholds. *Journal of the Optical Society of America 13*: 884–886.

White, R. C., Aimola Davies, A. M., Halleen, T. J., and Davies, M. (2010). Tactile expecta-tions and the perception of self-touch: An investigation using the rubber hand paradigm. *Consciousness and Cognition 19*: 505–519.

Will, U. and Berg, E. (2007). Brain wave synchronization and entrainment to periodic acoustic stimuli. *Neuroscience Letters 424*: 55–60.

Williams, P. E., Mechler, F., Gordon, J., Shapley, R., and Hawken, M. J. (2004). Entrainment to video displays in primary visual cortex of macaque and humans. *Journal of Neuroscience 24*: 8278–8288.

Woldorff, M., Hansen, J. C., and Hillyard, S. A. (1987). Evidence for effects of selective attention in the mid-latency range of the human auditory event-related potential. *Electroencephalography and Clinical Neurophysiology Supplement 40*: 146–154.

Woodrow, H. (1914). *The Measurement of Attention*. Whitefish, Mont.: Kessinger.

Worden, M. S., Foxe, J. J., Wang, N., and Simpson, G. V. (2000). Anticipatory biasing of visu-ospatial attention indexed by retinotopically specific alpha-band electroencephalography increases over occipital cortex. *Journal of Neuroscience 20*: RC63.

Wundt, W. (1874/1904). *Principles of Physiological Psychology*. London: Swan Sonnenschein.

Wyart, V. and Tallon-Baudry, C. (2008). Neural dissociation between visual awareness and spatial attention. *Journal of Neuroscience 28*: 2667–2679.

Yamagishi, N., Callan, D. E., Anderson, S. J., and Kawato, M. (2008). Attentional changes in pre-stimulus oscillatory activity within early visual cortex are predictive of human visual performance. *Brain Research 1197*: 115–122.

Yang, T. and Shadlen, M. N. (2007). Probabilistic reasoning by neurons. *Nature 447*: 1075–1080.

Zanto, T. P., Pan, P., Liu, H., Bollinger, J., Nobre, A. C., and Gazzaley, A. (2011). Age-related changes in orienting attention in time. *Journal of Neuroscience: The Official Journal of the Society for Neuroscience 31*: 12461–12470.

Zhou, H. and Desimone, R. (2011). Feature-based attention in the frontal eye field and area V4 during visual search. *Neuron 70*: 1205–1217.

Zion Golumbic, E. M., Ding, N., Bickel, S., Lakatos, P., Schevon, C. A., McKhann, G. M., Goodman, R. R., Emerson, R., Mehta, A. D., Simon, J. Z., Poeppel, D., and Schroeder, C. E. (2013). Mechanisms underlying selective neuronal tracking of attended speech at a 'cocktail party'. *Neuron 77*: 980–991.

PART E

INTERACTIONS BETWEEN ATTENTION & OTHER PSYCHOLOGICAL DOMAINS

CHAPTER 25

ATTENTION, MOTIVATION, AND EMOTION

LUIZ PESSOA

DURING the past decade, we have witnessed a veritable explosion of the research on the effects of emotion and motivation on both perception and cognition. In the first part of this chapter, I will review studies that have investigated the relationship between attention and motivation. In particular, the review will focus on recent findings that have studied how potential reward (and at times punishment) influences visual performance during attentional tasks. Traditional psychological models have described motivation as involving a global *energization* factor that is a rather blunt instrument. Under this view, motivation influences the vigour and frequency of behavioural output, but typically would not have more *selective* effects. As will be reviewed, in the case of attention, this is far from being the case. In fact, motivation has been shown to display specific effects that clearly go beyond changes in response criterion or general speeding up of reaction time.

The processing of emotional stimuli is fast and takes place under conditions of inattention and decreased visibility. In the second part of the chapter, I will review evidence both for and against the idea that their processing is independent of attention. Although the research on emotion and attention is quite broad, the question of 'automaticity' has been a central one that has attracted immense interest. This is likely the case because potentially automatic processing is not only of great interest from a basic research perspective, but is also of considerable clinical relevance. This is because, for instance, defects in this 'automatic processing system' are suggested to underlie phobias, mood disorders, and post-traumatic stress syndrome.

ATTENTION AND MOTIVATION

In the past two decades there has been considerable interest in the neural basis of reward and motivation. This line of research has highlighted the importance of the dopamine system and its cortical projection sites in behavioural control (Schultz et al. 1992), led to the formulation of computational models of valuation (Montague, Hyman, and Cohen 2004), and contributed to the development of the field of neuroeconomics (e.g. Platt and Glimcher 1999; Berns et al. 2001). The vigorous progress in our understanding of mechanisms of reward and motivation has also translated into research attempting to unravel how motivation interacts with cognitive systems broadly conceived. The reasoning is that if valuation processes shape behaviour, they would be expected to influence perceptual and cognitive processes that are central to the production of behaviour.

Behavioural effects

In an initial study from my lab, we investigated the effects of motivation on task performance by probing the impact of parametric changes in incentive value on behaviour during a difficult spatial localization task (Engelmann and Pessoa 2007). Participants were asked to indicate the location of a target stimulus (a red dot) as quickly and accurately as possible. Exogenous attention was manipulated by using a peripheral cue that predicted target location with 70% validity (such that 30% of the time the cue indicated the incorrect target location)—in such cases, performance during validly cued trials is known to exceed that during invalidly cued ones. Motivation was parametrically manipulated in a blocked fashion by linking pay-off to behavioural performance. Both reward and punishment were employed; in the latter, participants could avoid losing money when performance was both fast and accurate. The findings revealed improved detection performance as a function of absolute incentive value (Fig. 25.1a). Notably, because behaviour was characterized via the detection sensitivity measure *dprime*, the results revealed a *specific* effect of motivation on behavioural performance, instead of unspecific influences such as general *activation*[1] (e.g. purely faster response times) or response bias (e.g. more conservative responses). The same basic pattern of behavioural results was observed in distinct versions of the task that varied in difficulty level, type of target and distractor stimuli, and cue type (exogenous vs. endogenous; the latter was investigated in Engelmann et al. 2009, as will be discussed).

Based on these results, the argument was made that motivation improved visual attention. In general, however, the reasons for enhanced performance are difficult to ascertain, because improved performance can result from diverse mechanisms. As pointed out by Hubner and Schlosser (2010), incentives can speed up stimulus coding and/or motoric responding, and the saved time can then be spent to extend the response selection phase, which, in turn, could improve sensitivity. To investigate this question further, Huebner and Schlosser probed a version of the flanker task (Eriksen and Eriksen 1974) under reward and control conditions. The flanker task is a response interference task in which participants are asked to determine the direction of a central arrow embedded in identical symbols (for instance, '>>>>>') or in arrows pointing to the opposite direction (for instance, '<<><>'). Participants who received a performance-contingent monetary reward had significantly higher accuracy than did participants who earned a fixed amount of money. By varying response deadlines (i.e. the time by when a response

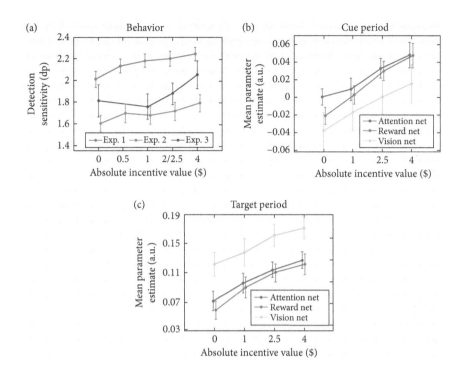

FIGURE 25.1 Behavioural and brain effects of incentive motivation. (a) In all experiments, the detection sensitivity measure dprime (dp) increased as a function of absolute incentive magnitude. Red line: Experiment 1 of Engelmann and Pessoa (2007); light orange line: Experiment 2 of Engelmann and Pessoa (2007); dark red line: parallel increases in evoked brain responses observed in the study by Engelmann et al. (2009) during the cue (b) and target (c) task phases in three types of regions, namely attentional, visual, and valuation-related (see Fig. 25.2 for some of the sites). Results were obtained by pooling the responses from regions within these three region types. Net: network. Reproduced from Pessoa and Engelmann (2010) with permission. Figure as originally published in Weiss, S.A. and Faber, D.S. (2010) Field effects in the CNS play functional roles Front. Neural Circuits 4:15. doi: 10.3389/fncir.2010.00015

had to be provided), the authors were able to evaluate speed–accuracy trade-offs, which suggested that participants had better information for decisions during the rewarded condition—consistent with an enhancement in the *quality* of sensory coding. However, they did not observe a reduction in the flanker effect with reward, which indicated that reward did not tighten the spatial focus of attention. Taken together, their findings suggested a specific effect of motivation on sensory processing that likely did not alter the size of the attentional focus (for further discussion, see Hubner and Schlosser 2010).

These two studies illustrate the strategy of manipulating motivation in a performance-contingent manner: participants are informed up front that they will receive extra monetary compensation if they perform at certain levels. The impact of motivation on behavioural performance has also been investigated when incentive levels are *dissociated* from task performance. In one investigation (Della Libera and Chelazzi 2009; see also Della Libera and Chelazzi 2006), participants performed three training sessions on consecutive days, followed by a test session. Visual items whose correct selection as targets had typically been followed by high reward during training became more dif-ficult to reject when serving as distractors, and easier to select when serving as targets. In contrast, items whose correct selection as targets had typically been followed by low reward during training, became easier to reject when serving as distractors and more difficult to select when serving as targets. The study results suggest that visual process-ing is adjusted according to the reward history of the visual items in question. Therefore, the long-term learning to select and to ignore specific objects in the environment is shaped by the *reward history* tied to past encounters with those objects. In a related study, Doallo, Patai, and Nobre (2013) showed that past rewards potentiate the effects of spatial memories upon the discrimination of target objects embedded within complex scenes starting from early perceptual stages.

In a related *value-learning* study, Anderson and colleagues reported that non-salient, task-irrelevant stimuli previously associated with reward slowed visual search even dur-ing a later phase of the experiment in which rewards did not occur (B. A. Anderson, Laurent, and Yantis 2011). Notably, the magnitude of slowing was spatially specific, such that when a target appeared in a location occupied by a high-value distractor on the previous trial, slowing was especially prolonged. Furthermore, value-driven attentional capture operated on a basic (and task-irrelevant) stimulus feature, namely colour.

Value learning was also employed in the context of the *attentional blink* paradigm (Raymond and O'Brien 2009). During an initial learning phase, participants viewed faces that were paired with low or high probability of monetary reward or punishment. Whereas faces associated with losses or zero gain/loss exhibited the standard attentional blink, those associated with reward did not. Therefore, association with prior reward counteracted the attentional blink, such that performance for those stimuli was equiva-lent at short vs. long lags between the first and second targets.

A final example of the interaction between motivation and attention involved the so-called *priming of pop-out* paradigm (Kristjansson, Sigurjonsdottir, and Driver 2010). Participants performed a visual search for a colour-singleton target (e.g. a red item among green distractors), whose shape was then discriminated (was the small notch on the target at its top or bottom?). Priming of pop-out refers to the fact that when a target colour is repeated, participants perform better—even though pop-out is an extremely basic task (discussed later). The observers were told that they would be rewarded for fast and accurate performance, but without the relative values of spe-cific target colours being explained. For half the participants, a correct response for a red target trial yielded 10 points on 75% of such trials, 1 point for the other 25%, and vice versa for green targets. For the other participants, this was reversed. Incorrect responses gave 0 points. The findings revealed that the benefit of successive target rep-etitions (i.e. the priming of pop-out effect) was larger for the more highly rewarded target colour. Thus, priming of pop-out can be significantly enhanced for targets asso-ciated with higher reward. Moreover, in a second experiment, the extent of priming of pop-out dynamically tracked reversals in reward levels when these were changed unpredictably, leading to significant changes within a few trials of the reversal. These results are important (see also Shen and Chun 2011) because priming of pop-out is considered largely immune to voluntary control or task priorities and to involve a low-level passive memory mechanism. The findings of the second experiment are particularly noteworthy as they suggest that implicit mechanisms were at play—upon debriefing, nearly all participants reported that they thought the reward schedules were random.

To summarize, in this section, I briefly reviewed behavioural paradigms that have explored the manner by which motivation affects performance during attentional tasks. Early studies in signal detection manipulated reward pay-offs, but focused on under-standing changes in response criterion (e.g. Green and Swets 1966). It was proposed that participants shift to a more conservative criterion during rewarded conditions. Recent research has attempted to elucidate several aspects by which motivation impacts performance in visual tasks: Does motivation enhance attention or does it have only other, less specific effects, such as speeding up reaction time? Are the effects of motiva-tion on attention related to changes in sensory processing, or are they related to more decision-related processes? The answer to the first question is that *selective* effects are indeed found. Examples include the increase in visual sensitivity (dprime) in both endogenous and exogenous attention tasks, enhanced stimulus coding, and target/dis-tractor effects. The impact of motivation on visual performance has been found both in studies in which reward was administered in a performance-contingent manner and in studies in which reward was not contingent on behaviour. The latter includes stud-ies that employed value learning, which shows that the effects of reward are not only manifested when participants are encouraged to perform better, but also via associative learning mechanisms. Stimuli associated with reward in this manner behave as if they had increased *salience* (discussed later). The second question is harder to answer with behavioural studies (see discussion by Hubner and Schlosser 2010), and possibly better addressed by cognitive neuroscience studies, as reviewed later.[2] Nevertheless, Hubner and Schlosser (2010) have argued that the pattern of results of their speed-accuracy trade-offs is indicative of 'better information' being available for a decision, that is, the mobilization of attentional resources by reward improved the *quality* of sensory coding. Furthermore, findings that a basic feature, like stimulus colour, can affect visual perfor-mance when linked to reward even when task-irrelevant, suggest that motivation alters sensory processing.

Attention: Brain-recording findings

Further advances in our understanding of motivation–attention interactions come from event-related potential (ERP) studies, which provide millisecond-level temporal resolution. These studies have capitalized on the previous characterization of several response components, often response peaks or troughs that have been linked to specific psychological processes.

Kiss et al. (2009) investigated the impact of reward on a basic detection task in which participants performed a visual search for a colour-singleton target (e.g. a red item among grey distractors), whose shape was then discriminated (is the small notch on the target at its top or bottom?)—as in the pop-out task reviewed earlier. Participants were told that a larger reward could be earned for correct fast response to a target in the high-reward colour (e.g. red), and a smaller reward could be earned for a target in the low-reward colour (e.g. green). The authors investigated the so-called N2pc component, which has been tied to visual target selection and is observed approximately 200 ms after display onset. The N2pc was earlier and larger for high- than for low-reward targets. Notably, the N2pc amplitude correlated positively with the impact of reward level on performance efficiency (an index that takes into account both speed and accuracy). Later post-selection processing was also affected by reward level, specifically, a component around 350–400 ms believed to be involved in additional processing of target stimuli, including their maintenance in visual short-term memory. These results demonstrate that visual selection of task-relevant items is rapidly modulated by reward-related priorities, even when the possibility of a reward is not announced in advance by a cue signalling potential reward.

In another ERP study, Hickey, Chelazzi, and Theeuwes (2010) sought to investigate interactions between reward and attention in a manner that allowed a clearer dissociation between 'strategic' and 'incidental' effects of reward. In many experimental paradigms, as seen in several of the previous examples, participants are explicitly informed that they may earn additional reward depending on their performance during certain task conditions. Although influences of reward have been documented in such circumstances, it is difficult to separate the neural effects of reward from those of attention. As pointed out by Maunsell (2004), 'in most cases, attention-related modulation could equally well be described in terms of expectation about rewards because the two are inextricably confounded'. Because participants are more highly engaged and motivated to perform better when rewards are involved, the concomitant effects may reflect the up-regulation of attention. Therefore, to separate the effects of attention from those of reward more clearly, it is necessary to devise tasks in which reward may have an effect that is not simply due to 'extra' engagement during the reward condition.

To do so, Hickey, Chelazzi, and Theeuwes (2010) probed how reward in one trial affected visual processing in the next one. Participants were asked to detect a target visual stimulus among an array of distractors, and the target was always defined in terms of a uniquely shaped object among same-shape distractors. The impact of reward was investigated by determining performance and ERPs during trials that *followed* low or high reward. Following a high-reward trial, the P1 component was enhanced contralateral to targets of the same colour rewarded on the *previous trial*. The P1 component, which occurs approximately 100 ms post-stimulus onset, is believed to reflect an amplification of early visual processing stages in extrastriate visual cortex (for review, see Hillyard and Anllo-Vento 1998), thus indicating facilitated perceptual responses for reward-associated stimuli. Results of the N2pc component, which as already stated is believed to index the deployment of attention to a spatial location, corroborated the idea that objects characterized by reward-associated features are more likely to be attended. Critically, P1 and N2pc effects were observed regardless of whether the stimulus (on trials following high reward) was the search target: when a salient *distractor* was shown in the reward-associated colour, additional visual resources were allocated to this task-irrelevant object. Taken together, the results reinforce the notion that reward has an impact on vision that is independent of its role in the top-down establishment of endogenous attention (because it was observed for distractors). Furthermore, the early effects observed in the P1 response component are also consistent with the idea that reward enhances visual *salience*.

Peck and colleagues also attempted to disentangle the contributions of attention and reward to neural signals (Peck et al. 2009). Monkeys performed a task in which a peripheral visual cue predicted the reward value of the trial, but to be rewarded, they had to make a saccade to a separate target whose location was independent of the cue. In this manner, a cue predicting reward was spatially separate from, and could interfere with, a required action (Fig. 25.2a). Cues predicting reward attracted attention to their location and evoked sustained excitation in posterior parietal cortex (Fig. 25.2b), whereas cues predicting no reward repulsed attention and evoked sustained inhibition. Thus, although the cues indicating the possibility of reward had no operant significance (i.e. they did not specify saccade location), they biased attention in a value-specific manner. Critically, these biases were maladaptive, as they interfered with the required saccade to the target. It has been argued that posterior parietal cortex contains a *salience map*, such that the area of the visual field associated with the greatest activity corresponds to the locus of visual attention (Goldberg et al. 2002; Serences and Yantis 2006). In this context, the results by Peck and colleagues suggest that, in the monkey, the posterior parietal cortex contains a visuospatial map that takes into account reward expectations for the purpose of guiding attention. Furthermore, reward associations conferred on the reward cues an intrinsic salience that was akin to the *bottom-up salience* of a conspicuous object—because reward cues were spatially separate from, and interfered with, the required action.

Functional MRI has also contributed to our understanding of attention–motivation interactions. In one study, participants performed a visual orientation discrimination task during low- and high-reward blocks (Weil et al. 2010). Behaviourally, task performance was better during high- vs. low-reward trials but only for easier visual discriminations, not hard ones. Trial-by-trial analysis revealed that receiving reward on a given trial was associated with improved accuracy on the subsequent trial (for both difficulty levels). In terms of brain responses, visual cortex beyond retinotopic regions showed differential signals only during reward feedback, a trial phase that involved an auditory stimulus. In other words, no effect of reward was detected during visual stimulation itself. Notably, however, early retinotopic visual cortex (areas V1, V2, and V3) showed instead enhanced signals in response to the visual grating on the *next* trial, after receipt of rewarding feedback on the previous one. Thus, early retinotopic and later non-retinotopic visual areas showed distinct patterns of reward influence, which manifested themselves at different task phases (next trial and same trial, respectively).

(a)

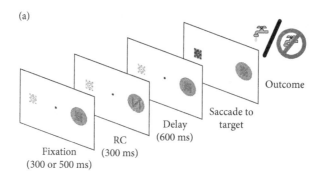

Fixation
(300 or 500 ms)

RC
(300 ms)

Delay
(600 ms)

Saccade to
target

Outcome

(b)

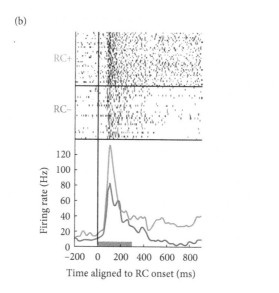

FIGURE 25.2 Behavioural task and cell responses in the lateral intraparietal area. (a) Two patterns, one to the right and one to the left of fixation, were shown throughout the trial. After a fixation period, a cue appears (inverted N in red, followed by a delay period. At the end of the delay, one of the patterns was brightened (see arrow), indicating the saccade target location. On correct reward trials, the reward was then administered. The grey circle indicates the area of the receptive field of the cell being recorded. (b) Response of a representative neuron. Trial onset is aligned with the presentation of the cue stimulus. Average firing rate during reward (blue) and no-reward (red) conditions are shown. The black horizontal bar denotes the cue duration. Reprinted from Peck, C. J., Jangraw, D. C., Suzuki, M., Efem, R., and Gottlieb, Reward modulates attention independently of action value in posterior parietal cortex, *Journal of Neuroscience*, 29(36), pp. 11182–11191 © 2009, The Society for Neuroscience.

Furthermore, brain responses to reward feedback were clearly distinct from well-known effects of spatial attention observed during visual discrimination. For instance, the contrast of reward vs. no-reward trials during the feedback phase revealed differential activation in orbitofrontal cortex and ventral striatum, regions that are centrally involved in valuation processes (this is discussed later).

In another functional MRI study, fast target detection could lead to monetary wins or avoidance of monetary losses and, in the control condition, did not involve monetary outcomes (Small et al. 2005; for a related study, see Mohanty et al. 2008). Better performance during the disengagement of attention was associated with enhanced activity in the inferior parietal lobe in the vicinity of the temporo-parietal junction, a region that has been implicated in the reorienting of attention (Corbetta, Patel, and Shulman 2008; Corbetta and Shulman 2002). Importantly, this effect was enhanced during trials in which participants could win or avoid losing money, and were accompanied by activations in valuation-related regions, including the orbitofrontal cortex. Of particular interest, responses in the posterior cingulate cortex were correlated with visual spatial expectancy (defined as the degree to which the cue improved performance), an effect that was enhanced by incentive motivation. Given the connectivity of this region with areas of the brain involved in attention and motivational processing, it was proposed that the posterior cingulate cortex serves as a 'neural interface' between motivation and the top-down control of attention (see also Engelmann et al. 2009; Pessoa and Engelmann 2010).

A final functional MRI study reviewed here investigated the interaction between endogenous attention and motivation during functional MRI (Engelmann et al. 2009)—using an endogenous attention variant of the study reviewed earlier (Engelmann and Pessoa 2007). Attention was manipulated by using a central arrow cue that predicted target location with 70% validity, and motivation was parametrically varied. The study design allowed the separate estimation of responses to cue and target task phases. In a manner parallel to the behavioural findings, parametric influences of incentive value on brain responses were observed during both the cue (Fig. 25.1b) and target (Fig. 25.1c) periods. Interestingly, these neuroimaging results revealed effects of incentive value across many brain regions, including occipito-temporal visual areas, parietal and frontal sites that are important for the control of attention, and several areas that are important for stimulus valuation, including the caudate and midbrain.

In summary, in the past decade, there has been great progress in advancing our understanding of the neural bases of attention–motivation interactions. ERP studies have demonstrated that the impact of reward on attention can be extremely fast, involving early response components, such as the P1 and the N2pc. Whereas the contributions of reward and attention to neural signals are often difficult to disentangle, recent paradigms have made important inroads into this question. For instance, in the monkey physiology study by Peck et al. (2009), the spatially specific influence of reward was separated from the behavioural requirements for successful task completion. Furthermore, the findings from both monkey physiology and human ERP studies demonstrate that, in several paradigms, reward acts in a manner that is similar to what would be expected for a physical change in stimulus salience. Broadly speaking, functional MRI studies have identified three types of brain region engaged during motivation–attention tasks (Fig. 25.3): (i) occipito-temporal visual cortical sites that are involved in sensory processing (including V1); (ii) fronto-parietal sites that are important for the control of attention (e.g. frontal eye field); (iii) nodes of the reward/valuation system (e.g. orbitofrontal cortex, caudate, and midbrain).

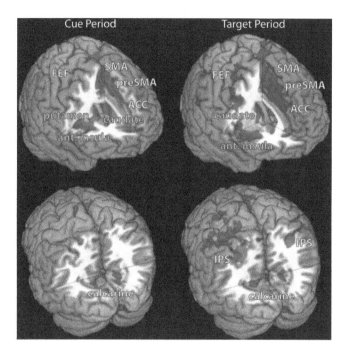

FIGURE 25.3 Brain regions exhibiting correlations with absolute incentive magnitude during cue and target task periods. Some of the attentional (blue font), visual (light green font), and valuation (orange font) regions from the study by Engelmann et al. (2009) are shown. ACC, anterior cingulate cortex; FEF, frontal eye field; IPS, intraparietal sulcus; pre-SMA, pre-supplementary motor area; and preSMA, pre-supplementary motor area. Reproduced from Engelmann et al. (2009) with permission. Figure as originally published in Weiss, S. A. and Faber, D. S. (2010) Field effects in the CNS play functional roles Front. Neural Circuits 4:15. doi: 10.3389/fncir.2010.00015

Conflict processing

In this section, I will briefly discuss interactions between motivation and attention from a slightly broader perspective, namely by considering conflict-processing tasks.

Does motivation influence the selection of information pertinent to the task at hand? To probe this question, we investigated the effects of reward during a response-conflict task (Padmala and Pessoa 2011). Participants were asked to indicate if the stimulus contained a picture of a house or building while ignoring the superimposed words (Fig. 25.4). The strings 'house', 'bldng', and 'xxxxx' were used to produce congruent, incongruent, and control trials. Based on previous studies, it was anticipated that motivation would enhance processing in attentional regions in fronto-parietal cortex and, consequently, that these regions would be better positioned to exert top-down control favouring the processing of task-relevant information in visual cortex. This would be accomplished by amplifying task-relevant information (Egner and Hirsch 2005) and/or by improving filtering of task-irrelevant information (Polk et al. 2008). Behaviourally, participants exhibited a motivation by cognition interaction. In other words, response

Trial structure

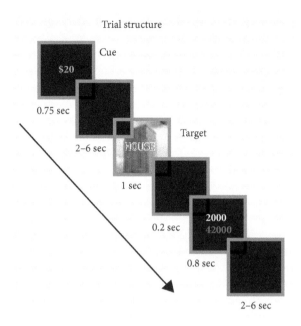

Cue

$20

0.75 sec

2–6 sec   HOUSE

Target

1 sec

0.2 sec   2000
            42000

0.8 sec

2–6 sec

FIGURE 25.4 Response-conflict paradigm. Subjects performed a response conflict task under two motivational contexts. During the reward condition (shown here), a cue stimulus ('$20') signalled that participants would be rewarded for fast and correct performance; during the control condition (not shown here), a cue stimulus ('$00') signalled that no reward was involved. During the target phase, a stimulus containing a picture of a house or building was shown together with a task-irrelevant word (an incongruent condition is illustrated here). After the target stimulus, subjects were informed about the reward and about the total number of points accrued. Reprinted from Padmala, S., and Pessoa, L., Affective learning enhances visual detection and responses in primary visual cortex, *Journal of Neuroscience*, 28(4), pp. 3419–3432 © 2011, The Society for Neuroscience.

interference (i.e. the slowing during incongruent relative to control trials) was reduced during reward trials (relative to no-reward). Given that reward also decreased facilitation (i.e. the speeding during congruent relative to control trials), the results were consistent with the notion that motivation enhanced attentional filtering, thereby reducing the influence of the task-irrelevant word item.[3]

The brain imaging findings revealed that, during the cue phase, responses in fronto-parietal regions were stronger with reward. During the target phase, similar to the behavioural data, a motivation-by-cognition interaction was observed in medial PFC, such that interference-related responses (as revealed by contrasting incongruent and neutral trials) decreased during reward trials. Notably, cue and target responses were correlated, such that larger *cue*-related responses were associated with larger decreases in interference-related responses in medial PFC during the *target* phase. The pattern of cue and target responses was thus consistent with the idea that the up-regulation of control during the cue phase led to decreased interference during the target phase. In fact, the relationship between cue and target responses was consistent with a *mediation* role for target-phase responses in visual cortex sensitive to word-related processing (in the left

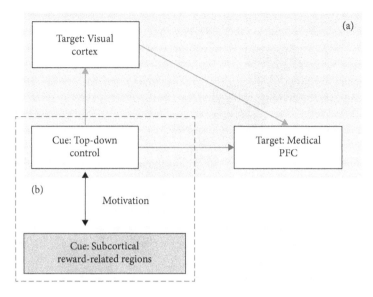

FIGURE 25.5 Region interactions. (a) The relationship between attentional control implemented in fronto-parietal cortex during the cue phase and conflict-related activity in MPFC
during the subsequent target phase was mediated via the amount of target/distractor processing in visual cortex. (b) We also hypothesized that the functional coupling between
fronto-parietal cortex and subcortical regions involved in reward processing would be
affected by motivational context. Reprinted from Padmala, S., and Pessoa, L., Affective learning enhances visual detection and responses in primary visual cortex, *Journal of Neuroscience*,
28(4), pp. 3419–3432 © 2011, The Society for Neuroscience.

parahippocampal gyrus, a region that is sensitive to word stimuli). Taken together, the
findings suggest that participants were able to employ motivationally salient cues to upreg-
ulate top-down control processes that bias the selection of visual information in a way that
reduces both behavioural conflict and conflict-related brain responses (Fig. 25.5a).

Cue-related responses were also observed in several subcortical sites that are frequently engaged during reward processing, including caudate and putamen in the dorsal
striatum, nucleus accumbens in the ventral striatum, as well as midbrain. We reasoned
that, if motivationally salient cues engage fronto-parietal regions more robustly during
the cue phase, they would exhibit increased *functional coupling* with some of the above
regions, which are sensitive to the motivational significance of the cues (Fig. 25.5b).
Indeed, increased *functional connectivity* (a measure of correlated signals) evaluated on
a trial-by-trial basis between the intraparietal sulcus in parietal cortex and putamen,
caudate (at a slightly more relaxed statistical threshold), and nucleus accumbens was
observed during the reward relative to no-reward condition. Notably, the strength of the
coupling between cortical and subcortical areas was linearly related to individual differences in reward sensitivity, indicating that the interaction between these regions was
stronger for participants who scored higher in reward sensitivity trait.

In a subsequent paper, we investigated the same dataset with graph-theoretic methods (Kinnison et al. 2012). Our goal was to understand network properties of a focused
set of regions engaged by the reward cue. Community detection (Newman 2010)

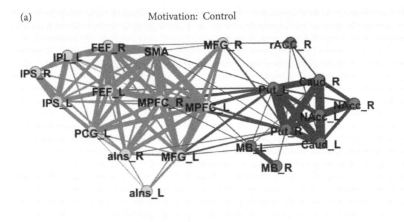

(a)   Motivation: Control

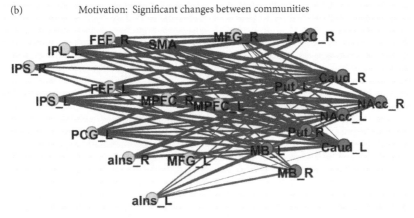

(b)   Motivation: Significant changes between communities

FIGURE 25.6   Network analysis. (a) Force layout depiction of the group-level network during the control condition. Nodes are coloured to show community organization (red for
subcortical community, teal for cortical community). Edges are also coloured according
to communities with between-community edges coloured purple. (b) Between-community
edges with significant reward versus control connectivity changes are shown (FDR corrected). Node positions and colours as in part (a). For abbreviations, see Table 2 of original
paper. Reprinted from Kinnison, J., Padmala, S., Choi, J. M., and Pessoa, L., Network analysis reveals increased integration during emotional and motivational processing, *Journal of
Neuroscience*, 32(24), pp. 8361–8372 © 2012, The Society for Neuroscience.

applied to regions that responded more strongly to reward versus control cues identified
two partitions (or clusters), one comprising cortical regions and another comprising
subcortical regions in addition to the right rostral ACC (Fig. 25.6a). Global efficiency
(a measure of integration) increased and graph-modularity (a measure of how easily a
network can be divided in terms of smaller subnetworks or 'communities') decreased
with reward. Furthermore, average between-community functional connections
increased with reward (Fig. 25.6b). The involvement of the nucleus accumbens and the
caudate in reward-related processing is well documented (Haber and Knutson 2010). In
our paradigm, these regions consistently increased their functional connectivity with
cortical regions.

In a pair of related behavioural and imaging studies, Krebs et al. (2011) and Krebs, Boehler, and Woldorff (2010) investigated the influence of reward associations on conflict processing during the classic Stroop task, which asks participants to determine the ink colour of a word. The words are displayed in different ink colour and these two stimulus dimensions at times conflict with each other (the word 'red' in blue ink). A subset of ink colours was associated with the potential of reward (e.g. green and blue), while other ink colours were not (e.g. red and yellow) (word meaning was not linked to reward). Reward linked to the ink colour of the word led to performance facilitation, as reflected by overall faster responses and lower error rates. Importantly, the typical conflict-induced slowing of responses was *reduced* during trials involving reward-associated ink colours. In contrast, reward associations related to the *irrelevant* word-meaning dimension inflicted costs on performance if they were incongruent with ink colour. Expressed in a different way, incongruent words semantically related to reward-associated colours (e.g. the words 'green' and 'blue') interfered more strongly with performance than words semantically unrelated to reward (e.g. 'red' and 'yellow'). This was observed despite the word meaning always being entirely task-irrelevant. In terms of brain responses, irrelevant reward associations increased activity in a medial PFC, likely reflecting increased demands to select the response when encountering irrelevant reward-related words.

The studies briefly reviewed in this section demonstrate that reward shapes the selection of information in a manner that impacts conflict processing, illustrating that an important area of research will involve characterizing how motivation interacts with executive functions more broadly (e.g. Jimura, Locke, and Braver 2010; Savine and Braver 2010; Aarts et al. 2010).

ATTENTION AND EMOTION

In this second half of the chapter, the role of attention during the processing of emotion-laden stimuli will be reviewed. Although emotion and motivation are often treated fairly independently of one another, they are clearly related. Both depend on the relationship between the organism and its environment. In the case of emotion, the emphasis might be on the evaluative aspect of the organism–environment relationship, whereas in the case of motivation it might be on how the organism acts in a given situation. Yet both task manipulations of valence (e.g. neutral and fearful faces) and the use of incentives (e.g. pairing with reward) imbue stimuli with 'motivational value' and influence attentional processing (Pessoa 2009).

Emotion helps shape information gathering, such that behaviourally relevant items receive heightened attention (Lang and Davis 2006). But how does emotion depend on attention? Here, to focus the review, this problem is considered mostly from a cognitive/affective neuroscience perspective as informed by experimental paradigms that have investigated this question by manipulating attention during the processing of (mostly) emotion-laden visual items. (For related reviews, please consult Adolphs 2008; Palermo and Rhodes 2007; Vuilleumier 2005; for the roles of attention and awareness, please see Pessoa 2005.)

The processing of emotion-laden visual stimuli is often proposed to take place in an 'automatic' fashion. More generally, although 'automaticity' is a concept that is operationalized in quite different ways across studies in cognitive and social psychology, it can be characterized as involving processing occurring independently of the availability of processing resources, not affected by intentions and strategies, and not necessarily tied to conscious processing (Jonides 1981; Posner and Snyder 1975). From a more clinical perspective, cognitive models of anxiety also assume the existence of a prioritized and largely automatic threat-processing system, and propose that anxiety is characterized by attentional biases that favour the processing of threat cues. These biases are proposed to be associated with individual differences in anxiety susceptibility (e.g. Mogg and Bradley 1998; Williams et al. 1997).

A host of experimental paradigms have documented the many ways in which the processing of emotion-laden visual stimuli is prioritized. These include detection, search, interference, masking, and the attentional blink, to name but a few. For instance, during the attentional blink paradigm, subjects are asked to report both a first (T1) and a second (T2) visual target within a stream of distractor items. Detecting a second target in close temporal proximity (300–500 ms) is believed to be hampered by the initial T1 processing (due to limited processing resources). Interestingly, an emotional T2 item is better detected than a corresponding neutral one, demonstrating that the affective dimension of the item *counteracts* the 'blink' (A. K. Anderson 2005; A. K. Anderson and Phelps 2001). Emotional stimuli elicit stronger 'attentional blinks' themselves, suggesting that their processing is prioritized (and that the processing leaves fewer resources for other stimuli). For instance, negative arousing pictures capture and hold attention, impairing participants' ability to perform a simple task on a subsequent target stimulus in a rapid stream of visual items (Most et al. 2005).

The mechanisms underlying affective prioritization continue to be the target of much research, but are generally believed to involve increased sensory processing to affective stimuli. Indeed, relative to neutral stimuli, emotional stimuli evoke increased fMRI responses across all of ventral occipito-temporal cortex, including early retinotopic and late non-retinotopic visual areas. For instance, Bradley and colleagues reported more extensive visual cortex activity when participants viewed emotional, compared to neutral, pictures (Bradley et al. 2003). More recently, Padmala and I showed a close link between improvements in behavioural performance and trial-by-trial responses in early visual cortex (including primary visual cortex) during the processing of affective visual items (Padmala and Pessoa 2008). Increased cortical responses in visual cortex to affective stimuli may be due to modulatory signals from the amygdala, consistent with the existence of efferent projections from this structure that reach many levels of the visual cortex (Amaral, Behniea, and Kelly 2003; Freese and Amaral 2005). Other sources of modulation may involve, for instance, the orbitofrontal cortex and the basal forebrain, as well as indirect circuits that involve the hypothalamus and pulvinar (Pessoa 2010a 2010b).

In the following sections, evidence for and against the need for attention during the processing of emotion-laden stimuli is presented. The goal is not to provide a comprehensive review of this growing literature, but to provide examples that illustrate the central issues.

Attention is not required for emotional perception

Emotional stimuli effectively divert processing resources and interfere with performance even when they are task-irrelevant (Pessoa and Ungerleider 2004; Vuilleumier 2005). For instance, reaction times when subjects performed auditory tasks (e.g. word discrimination) were slower when they viewed distractor pictures that were unpleasant relative to neutral ones (Bradley, Cuthbert, and Lang 1996; Buodo, Sarlo, and Palomba 2002). Strikingly, interference has been observed even when the primary task is very basic, such as the detection of a simple visual stimulus (Pereira et al. 2006). Interference effects are not only evident in terms of behavioural performance, but are also manifested physiologically. For example, specific ERP components due to picture viewing were modulated by emotional content even when the main task involved simply detecting a chequerboard stimulus that was interspersed with picture presentation (Schupp et al. 2003a). Together, these studies are often interpreted as supporting the notion that the processing of emotional stimuli is *obligatory* and that increased resources are allocated towards their processing although they are irrelevant to the task at hand.

A stronger argument can be advanced that emotional processing is obligatory based on studies in which the spatial focus of attention is explicitly manipulated—note that in the experiments of the previous paragraph, although task-irrelevant, emotional stimuli were fully attended. In a well-known study (Vuilleumier et al. 2001), the attentional focus was manipulated by having subjects maintain central fixation while they were asked to compare either two faces or two houses presented eccentrically. On each trial, subjects either compared the faces to each other or the houses to each other. Thus, the focus of attention was varied by having subjects attend to the left and the right of fixation (while ignoring top/bottom stimuli) or above and below fixation (while ignoring left/right stimuli). In each case, they indicated whether the attended stimuli were the same or different. When conditions involving fearful faces were contrasted to those involving neutral ones, differential responses in the amygdala—which are often considered as a 'signature' of emotional processing—were not modulated by the focus of attention, consistent with the view that the processing of emotional items does not require attention. Related findings were observed when manipulating object-based attention while maintaining the spatial locus of attention constant (A. K. Anderson et al. 2003). Amygdala responses evoked by fearful faces were equivalent whether or not the faces were attended. Interestingly, however, during unattended conditions, responses evoked by fear and disgust faces were comparable to each other, consistent with the idea that attention is needed to discriminate emotional content (both expressions evoked greater responses than neutral faces). We now turn to reviewing evidence that suggests that emotional perception requires attention.

Attention is required for emotional perception

Based on the findings summarized in the previous section, it has been surmised that emotional stimuli comprise a privileged stimulus category that is not only prioritized but their processing also takes place in an obligatory fashion that is independent of attention. However, it is also known that, in general, visual processing capacity is limited. Because of this finite capacity, competition among visual items is proposed to 'select' the most important information at any given time (Desimone and Duncan 1995; Grossberg 1980). When resources are not fully consumed, it has been suggested that spare processing capacity is utilized for the processing of unattended items (Lavie 1995). This line of reasoning, which has been successfully applied to regular, non-emotional stimuli, suggests that the automaticity of affective processing can be tested by attentional manipulations that more fully consume processing resources. More generally, multiple factors determine how information competes in visual cortex and beyond, including task difficulty, set size, spatial arrangement, cueing, and so on. Indeed, the general practice of associating set size with overall 'load' is also potentially problematic (Tsal and Benoni 2010; Wilson, Muroi, and MacLeod 2011). Given that the contributing factors are diverse, in the studies I will be discussing I refer to situations of *low/high competition*, or *low/high demand*.

Several fMRI studies have attempted to follow the strategy outlined earlier. For example, the responses evoked by centrally presented emotional faces were evaluated when a very demanding peripheral task was performed. Under these conditions, differential responses to fearful vs. neutral faces were eliminated in both the amygdala and visual cortex (Pessoa et al. 2002). Consistent with the notion that task demand was important in determining the extent of processing of the face stimuli, when the difficulty of the peripheral task was parametrically manipulated, a valence effect (i.e. fearful > neutral) was observed during low task-demand conditions, but not during medium- or high-demand conditions (Pessoa, Padmala, and Morland 2005). The dependence of emotional perception on attention was also observed in studies that employed centrally presented, overlapping competing stimuli (i.e. paradigms that manipulate object-based attention) (Mitchell et al. 2007), including emotional stimuli of higher affective significance that were paired with shock (Lim, Padmala, and Pessoa 2008; see also Yates, Ashwin, and Fox 2010)—or by using highly aversive, mutilation pictures (Erthal et al. 2005). Posner-type manipulations of attention also indicate that amygdala activation depends on the focus of attention (Brassen et al. 2010). Furthermore, attentional modulation of emotional perception has also been observed for peripherally presented faces (Silvert et al. 2007).

ERP studies, which unlike fMRI studies offer temporal information on the order of milliseconds, have also investigated how emotional perception depends on attentional factors. In one study (Schupp et al. 2007), the processing of emotional pictures from the International Affective Picture System (IAPS) was strongly attenuated (as measured by an early ERP component labelled the 'EPN') when participants performed demanding attention tasks. On the contrary, passively viewing the same emotional images generated increased responses relative to those evoked by neutral stimuli. Likewise, differential ERP responses to peripheral, emotional IAPS pictures also relied on the availability of processing resources (De Cesarei, Codispoti, and Schupp 2009). Emotional pictures in the near periphery modulated brain activity only when they were attended (though passively viewed), but not when participants were engaged in a distractor task (determining whether a rectangular outline contained a gap or not).

Attention is not required for emotional perception, again

The results suggesting that emotional perception is automatic or that it depends on attention can be reconciled by making use of the concept of competition. When task demand is low, 'spillover' capacity is available to the processing of task-irrelevant emotional stimuli. As task demand is increased, however, fewer resources will be available and, in the limit, emotional perception will be eliminated. Whereas this framework can be used to explain a broad set of results, some findings appear to resist this explanation. In one study, subjects performed a difficult target-detection task while task-irrelevant, though emotionally arousing, pictures were shown in the background (Muller, Andersen, and Keil 2008). Despite the difficulty of the task, emotional pictures interfered behaviourally with the main task. Parallel findings were registered in steady-state visual evoked potentials, which were reduced during the presentation of emotional relative to neutral background images (such reduction was suggested to reflect the withdrawal of processing resources from the main task by the emotional distractors).

Another recent MEG study provided evidence for mandatory processing of fearful faces (Fenker et al. 2010). Both low- and high-demand conditions were investigated in separate experiments. During the high-demand condition, the target was defined by a conjunction of features, such as a red-green (vs. blue-yellow) vertical bar. In the low-demand condition, subjects determined the orientation of an oriented bar (vertical vs. horizontal) presented in a given colour (indicated at the beginning of the block). During the low-demand condition, task-irrelevant fearful faces slowed down reaction time when they were presented in the same visual field as the bar target (relative to when faces were presented in the opposite visual field). To investigate the neural impact of the task-irrelevant faces, the authors probed the so-called N2pc component, which is believed to reflect attentional selection in visual search. They observed that lateralized fearful faces elicited an N2pc approximately 240–400 ms in contralateral visual cortex. Importantly, the N2pc was observed during conditions of high demand, although no behavioural effects were detected.

Finally, it has been suggested that, whereas competition does dampen the impact of emotion-laden items in typical individuals, they are not easily reduced in specific populations. Indeed, behavioural and ERP results in spider-fearful individuals were not altered by standard set size manipulations (Norberg, Peira, and Wiens 2010). In addition, an fMRI study with spider phobics reported unchanged amygdala responses as a function of attention (Alpers et al. 2009), although the attentional manipulation was not strong.

Temporal paradigms and mechanisms of prioritization

A particularly rich paradigm to study capacity limitations is the attentional blink, a paradigm that is especially interesting given its temporal dimension—as opposed to the spatial nature of several of the manipulations discussed in earlier sections. As noted, the strength of the attentional blink is influenced by the emotional content of the stimuli involved, such that participants are better at detecting the second target when it is emotionally laden. However, until recently, the neural mechanisms by which emotional content influences perceptual processing remained unclear.

In a recent study (Lim, Padmala, and Pessoa 2009), we investigated how affective significance shapes visual perception during an attentional blink paradigm combined with aversive conditioning. The experimental session begun with an initial phase during which houses (CS+) or buildings (CS−; counterbalanced) were paired with mild shock. Behaviourally, following aversive learning, affectively significant T2 scenes (CS+) were better detected than neutral (CS−) ones (72% vs. 62%, respectively) during the blink period. In terms of mean brain responses, both amygdala and visual cortical responses were stronger during CS+ relative to CS− trials. Increased responses in these regions were associated with improved behavioural performance across participants. Specifically, although amygdala responses were predictive of behavioural performance, once responses in visual cortex were taken into account (via statistical mediation analysis), the initial relationship was no longer statistically significant, consistent with the idea that the influence of the amygdala was mediated via visual cortex.

We hypothesized that if fluctuations in evoked responses in the brain determine the accuracy of the detection of the second target, *trial-by-trial* variability in response amplitude should predict behavioural reports. In addition, because T2 performance was better during the CS+ relative to the CS− condition, this relationship should be stronger for the former. To evaluate these predictions, we performed logistic regression analysis and modelled the probability of a hit trial (i.e. correctly reporting 'house' or 'building') as a function of single-trial amplitude. In visual cortex, the mean logistic regression slopes, which represented the strength of the predictive effect, were significant for both CS+ and CS− trials, indicating that trial-by-trial fluctuations in fMRI signals reliably predicted perceptual T2 decisions. Importantly, a direct comparison of the CS+ and CS− conditions revealed that the predictive power of the logistic regression fit was stronger during CS+ relative to CS− scenes. An analogous trial-by-trial analysis was performed for the amygdala. The mean logistic regression slope was significant for CS+ trials, but not for CS− trials, indicating that variability in fMRI signals in the amygdala contributed to perceptual T2 decisions more robustly when these stimuli were affectively significant (a direct paired comparison was also significant).

Taken together with other findings, our results suggest that affective significance potentially determines the fate of a visual item during competitive interactions by enhancing sensory processing. By helping establish affective significance, the amygdala helps separate the significant from the mundane. One way to interpret these results is in terms of an attentional function of the amygdale (Pessoa 2010b). For example, in studies of attention and visual cortical function, fluctuation of responses in visual cortex is often conceptualized as dependent on 'source' regions in parietal and frontal cortices (Corbetta and Shulman 2002; Kastner and Ungerleider 2000), and these mechanisms are typically viewed as linked to how the processing of attended objects is prioritized. In our study of the attentional blink, something quite similar was observed insofar as fluctuations in the amygdala were predictive of the strength of the link between visual cortex and behaviour. In this case, the amygdala was found to behave much like an 'attentional device' would be expected to—namely, as a device that helps prioritize the processing of certain stimuli over others (Pessoa 2010b).

An especially pertinent finding of the study was that the contrast between emotional and neutral Miss trials did not reveal significant differential responses in the amygdala. In contrast, the comparison between emotional and neutral Hit trials exhibited differential responses. In other words, differential responses were not produced unless a T2 scene was detected. More generally, this finding suggests that affective perception is indeed under the control of attentional mechanisms during temporal 'bottleneck' conditions, in addition to during spatial competition conditions. These findings are of particular interest because they involve stimuli that were particularly potent (given the history of pairing with shock).

A recent attentional blink study introduced a clever manipulation in an attempt to influence the load associated with processing the first target (Stein et al. 2010). Specifically, perceptual load of the blink-inducing target was manipulated by varying flanker interference. During the low-demand T1 condition, the centre face was flanked by identical copies of that face. During the high-demand T1 condition, the centre face was flanked by randomly sampled faces. For the first (T1) task, observers were instructed to report the sex of the central face. For the second (T2) task, observers were asked to detect (present vs. absent) faces presented during the attentional blink period that could depict either a fearful or a happy expression. For the low-demand condition, fearful faces were detected more often than happy faces, replicating previous reports. Importantly, this advantage for fearful faces disappeared for the high-demand condition, during which fearful and happy faces were detected equally often. These results suggest that the privileged access of fearful faces to awareness does not occur mandatorily, but instead depends on attentional resources. It is important to note, furthermore, that in all conditions, a blink was observed—a property that appears to be shared by all affective emotional blink experiments. It was just the advantage for fearful faces that was eliminated during the high-demand T1 condition. In other words, capacity limitations for the processing of emotional faces were obtained for both conditions. At the relatively low-demand condition, even though fearful faces blinked, they counteracted the blink to a greater extent than happy faces. At the more stringent high-demand condition, this advantage disappeared.

Anderson and Phelps reported that patients with amygdala lesion do not exhibit the typical enhancement for T2 detection during attentional blink tasks (A. K. Anderson and Phelps 2001). Since then, it has been assumed that the amygdala is *necessary* for the competitive advantage of emotion-laden stimuli during the attentional blink. However, the 'necessary' status of the amygdala has been called into question by recent studies. For instance, one study revealed that two individuals with selective bilateral amygdala lesions exhibited normal pattern of enhanced detection of aversive words during the attentional blink (Bach et al. 2011). More broadly, the latter study is part of a growing number of studies demonstrating typical effects of emotional stimuli in patients with amygdala lesions (Bach et al. 2011; Piech et al. 2011; Piech et al. 2010; Tsuchiya et al. 2009). Elsewhere, it has been argued that other brain structures, including the pulvinar nucleus of the thalamus, contribute to the fast and efficient processing of emotion-laden stimuli (Pessoa and Adolphs 2010).

In summary, the results from attentional blink experiments suggest that emotion-laden stimuli are also subject to the blink, counter to the notion of strong automaticity. However, as in the case of spatial paradigms, some have interpreted results of the emotional attentional blink in terms of automaticity (A. K. Anderson 2005).

Attention and emotion: Summary

Taken together, results from behavioural and neuroimaging methods suggest that while emotional processing is prioritized, in many contexts it depends on processing resources. In general, the discrepancy between studies suggesting that emotional perception is automatic and those illustrating the dependence on attention is accounted by the concepts of capacity limitation and competition. Thus, to reveal that emotional perception is not immune to the effects of attention, processing resources need to be largely consumed—otherwise, performance will *appear* to be relatively automatic.

As outlined previously, this account may not explain all cases, and there may be circumstances in which more automaticity is observed. At present, the reasons for this discrepancy are unclear, suggesting that it would be profitable for future studies to tackle this issue more directly. One possibility is that individual differences are important predictors of amygdala sensitivity to emotional stimuli and help explain the impact of emotional stimuli. For instance, studies from the literature on anxiety have revealed that anxious participants exhibit greater interference from threat-related stimuli (MacLeod, Mathews, and Tata 1986). More recent studies have investigated the extent to which amygdala responses to threat-related distractors depend upon individual anxiety levels (Bishop et al. 2004). Whereas low-anxious individuals only showed increased amygdala responses to attended fearful faces, high-anxious individuals showed increased amygdala responses to both attended and unattended threat-related stimuli. These findings suggest that the threat value of a stimulus varies as a function of a participant's anxiety level, although attention appears to be important even for high-anxious individuals (Bishop, Jenkins, and Lawrence 2007; Fox, Russo, and Georgiou 2005).

An additional issue is that a better understanding of competition is greatly needed. As emphasized by several recent studies, a simple notion of 'load' is insufficient (Benoni and Tsal 2010; Tsal and Benoni 2010; Wilson, Muroi, and MacLeod 2011) as a vast array of factors contributes to the unfolding of competitive interactions. In the context of investigations of the role of attention during emotional perception, this type of knowledge is particularly relevant given the substantial number of studies that have varied task difficulty simply by varying set sizes of distractor arrays. Given that 'reverse load' effects have been reported with neutral stimuli, this type of manipulation needs to be revisited in the context of attention–emotion studies.

Conclusions

The goal of this chapter was to review how motivation and emotion interact with attention. The review was limited in scope because, given the growing corpus of findings, only some of the results could be described.

The more recent literature on motivation and attention has reported findings that one could say are somewhat surprising. Earlier studies had focused on changes in response criterion and whether participants employed an optimal decision criterion (for further discussion, see Navalpakkam, Koch and Perona 2009). These more decisional effects are qualitatively different from recent studies reporting, for example, increased visual sensitivity (dprime) in both endogenous and exogenous attention tasks, enhanced stimulus coding, and target/distractor effects. The recent findings are also surprising insofar as traditional psychological models described motivation as involving a global energization factor that typically varies independently of control demands and behaviour direction (Duffy 1962; Hull 1943). As reviewed in the first part of this chapter, recent studies have revealed results that are far from global. Instead they reflect specific mechanisms that are manifested both behaviourally and in terms of brain responses.

In the second part of this chapter, we focused mainly on the interaction between emotion and attention from the standpoint of the literature evaluating the ostensible automaticity of emotional perception. A review of how emotion-laden visual stimuli enhance visual processing and capture attention is available elsewhere (Pourtois, Schettino, and Vuilleumier 2012). It was concluded that, when one considers the bulk of the evidence, emotional processing is revealed to be capacity-limited. That having been said, it is still important to understand why attention did not appear to be required in some experimental paradigms in which stronger demand manipulations were employed. This is particularly important given recent studies that have challenged the idea that task 'load' adequately captures when distractor interference will occur (Tsal and Benoni 2010; Wilson, Muroi, and MacLeod 2011).

Finally, an important question for future research concerns the relationship between the impact of motivation, on the one hand, and emotion, on the other, on visual processing. For instance, both reward-associated (Raymond and O'Brien 2009) and aversively conditioned (Lim Padmala, and Pessoa 2009) stimuli counter the attentional blink. Increases in visual detection sensitivity have been reported under both motivated conditions (Engelmann and Pessoa 2007) and in the context of aversive conditioning (Padmala and Pessoa 2008). Furthermore, early effects on evoked responses, including the P1 ERP component, have been reported in the context of motivation (Hickey, Chelazzi, and Theeuwes 2010) and emotion (Schupp et al. 2003b) studies. These parallels illustrate that an important area for future research will involve understanding both the similarities and differences of the mechanisms of interaction between attention and motivation and emotion.

Notes

1. *Activation* is here employed in the sense of an 'energizing' function, one that is linked to, for instance, the vigour and frequency of behavioural output. Activation is a better term than *arousal* given that the latter has several connotations that are associated with reticular systems involved in sleep-wake cycles.
2. The sensory vs. decisional distinction is, at any rate, artificial as these processes are closely related (Churchland, Ramachandran, and Sejnowski 1994).
3. In contrast, the study by Hubner and Schlosser (2010) reviewed earlier did not observe a reduction of response interference (during a flanker task) when reward was provided.

Bibliography

Aarts, E., Roelofs, A., Franke, B., Rijpkema, M., Fernandez, G., Helmich, R. C., and Cools, R. (2010). Striatal dopamine mediates the interface between motivational and cognitive control in humans: evidence from genetic imaging. *Neuropsychopharmacology* 35(9): 1943–1951. doi: 10.1038/npp.2010.68.

Adolphs, R. (2008). Fear, faces, and the human amygdala. *Current Opinion in Neurobiology* 18(2): 166–172.

Alpers, G. W., Gerdes, A. B., Lagarie, B., Tabbert, K., Vaitl, D., and Stark, R. (2009). Attention and amygdala activity: an fMRI study with spider pictures in spider phobia. *Journal of Neural Transmission* 116(6): 747–757. doi: 10.1007/s00702-008-0106-8.

Amaral, D. G., Behniea, H., and Kelly, J. L. (2003). Topographic organization of projections from the amygdala to the visual cortex in the macaque monkey. *Neuroscience* 118(4): 1099–1120.

Anderson, A. K. (2005). Affective influences on the attentional dynamics supporting awareness. *Journal of Experimental Psychology: General* 134(2): 258–281.

Anderson, A. K., Christoff, K., Panitz, D., De Rosa, E., and Gabrieli, J. D. (2003). Neural correlates of the automatic processing of threat facial signals. *Journal of Neuroscience* 23(13): 5627–5633.

Anderson, A. K. and Phelps, E. A. (2001). Lesions of the human amygdala impair enhanced perception of emotionally salient events. *Nature* 411(6835): 305–309.

Anderson, B. A., Laurent, P. A., and Yantis, S. (2011). Value-driven attentional capture. *Proceedings of the National Academy of Sciences USA* 108(25): 10367–10371. doi: 10.1073/pnas.1104047108.

Bach, D. R., Talmi, D., Hurlemann, R., Patin, A., and Dolan, R. J. (2011). Automatic relevance detection in the absence of a functional amygdala. *Neuropsychologia* 49(5): 1302–1305. doi: 10.1016/j.neuropsychologia.2011.02.032.

Benoni, H. and Tsal, Y. (2010). Where have we gone wrong? Perceptual load does not affect selective attention. *Vision Research* 50(13): 1292–1298. doi: 10.1016/j.visres.2010.04.018.

Berns, G. S., McClure, S. M., Pagnoni, G., and Montague, P. R. (2001). Predictability modulates human brain response to reward. *Journal of Neuroscience* 21(8): 2793–2798.

Bishop, S., Duncan, J., Brett, M., and Lawrence, A. D. (2004). Prefrontal cortical function and anxiety: controlling attention to threat-related stimuli. *Nature Neuroscience* 7(2): 184–188.

Bishop, S., Jenkins, R., and Lawrence, A. D. (2007). Neural processing of fearful faces: effects of anxiety are gated by perceptual capacity limitations. *Cerebral Cortex* 17(7): 1595–1603.

Bradley, M. M., Cuthbert, B. N., and Lang, P. J. (1996). Picture media and emotion: effects of a sustained affective context. *Psychophysiology* 33(6): 662–670.

Bradley, M. M., Sabatinelli, D., Lang, P. J., Fitzsimmons, J. R., King, W., and Desai, P. (2003). Activation of the visual cortex in motivated attention. *Behavioral Neuroscience* 117(2): 369–380.

Brassen, S., Gamer, M., Rose, M., and Buchel, C. (2010). The influence of directed covert attention on emotional face processing. *NeuroImage* 50(2): 545–551.

Buodo, G., Sarlo, M., and Palomba, D. (2002). Attentional resources measured by reaction times highlight differences within pleasant and unpleasant, high arousing stimuli. *Motivation and Emotion* 26: 123–138.

Churchland, P. S., Ramachandran, V. S., and Sejnowski, T. J. (1994). A critique of pure vision. In C. Koch and J. L. Davis (eds.), *Large-scale neuronal theories of the brain* (pp. 23–60). Cambridge, Mass.: MIT Press.

Corbetta, M., Patel, G., and Shulman, G. L. (2008). The reorienting system of the human brain: from environment to theory of mind. *Neuron* 58(3): 306–324.

Corbetta, M., and Shulman, G. L. (2002). Control of goal-directed and stimulus-driven attention in the brain. *Nature Reviews Neuroscience* 3(3): 201–215.

De Cesarei, A., Codispoti, M., and Schupp, H. T. (2009). Peripheral vision and preferential emotion processing. *NeuroReport* 20(16): 1439–1443.

Della Libera, C. and Chelazzi, L. (2006). Visual selective attention and the effects of monetary rewards. *Psychological Science* 17(3): 222–227.

Della Libera, C. and Chelazzi, L. (2009). Learning to attend and to ignore is a matter of gains and losses. *Psychological Science* 20(6): 778–784. doi: 10.1111/j.1467-9280.2009.02360.x.

Desimone, R. and Duncan, J. (1995). Neural mechanisms of selective attention. *Annual Review of Neuroscience*, 18, 193–222.

Doallo, S., Patai, Z., and Nobre, A. C. (2013). Reward associations magnify memory-based biases on perception. *Journal of Cognitive Neuroscience* 25(2): 245–257. doi: 10.1162/jocn_a_00314.

Duffy, E. (1962). *Activation and behavior*. New York: Wiley.

Egner, T. and Hirsch, J. (2005). Cognitive control mechanisms resolve conflict through cortical amplification of task-relevant information. *Nature Neuroscience* 8(12): 1784–1790.

Engelmann, J. B., Damaraju, E. C., Padmala, S., and Pessoa, L. (2009). Combined effects of attention and motivation on visual task performance: Transient and sustained motivational effects. *Frontiers in Human Neuroscience* 3(4): doi: 10.3389/neuro.3309.3004.2009.

Engelmann, J. B., and Pessoa, L. (2007). *Behavioral and neural interactions between reward and attention.* Paper presented at the Society for Neuroscience, San Diego.

Eriksen, B. A., and Eriksen, C. W. (1974). Effects of noise letters upon the identification of a target letter in a nonsearch task. *Attention, Perception, & Psychophysics* 16(1): 143–149. doi: 10.3758/BF03203267.

Erthal, F. S., de Oliveira, L., Mocaiber, I., Pereira, M. G., Machado-Pinheiro, W., Volchan, E., and Pessoa, L. (2005). Load-dependent modulation of affective picture processing. *Cognitive, Affective, & Behavioral Neuroscience* 5(4): 388–395.

Fenker, D. B., Heipertz, D., Boehler, C. N., Schoenfeld, M. A., Noesselt, T., Heinze, H. J., and Hopf, J. M. (2010). Mandatory processing of irrelevant fearful face features in visual search. *Journal of Cognitive Neuroscience* 22(12): 2926–2938. doi: 10.1162/jocn.2009.21340.

Fox, E., Russo, R., and Georgiou, G. A. (2005). Anxiety modulates the degree of attentive resources required to process emotional faces. *Cognitive, Affective, & Behavioral Neuroscience* 5(4): 396–404.

Freese, J. L., and Amaral, D. G. (2005). The organization of projections from the amygdala to visual cortical areas TE and V1 in the macaque monkey. *Journal of Comparative Neurology* 486(4): 295–317.

Green, D. M. and Swets, J. A. (1966). *Signal detection theory and psychophysics.* New York: Wiley.

Grossberg, S. (1980). How does a brain build a cognitive code? *Psychological Review* 87(1): 1–51.

Haber, S. N. and Knutson, B. (2010). The reward circuit: linking primate anatomy and human imaging. *Neuropsychopharmacology* 35(1): 4–26. doi: 10.1038/npp.2009.129.

Hickey, C., Chelazzi, L., and Theeuwes, J. (2010). Reward changes salience in human vision via the anterior cingulate. *Journal of Neuroscience* 30(33): 11096–11103. doi: 10.1523/jneurosci.1026-10.2010.

Hillyard, S. A. and Anllo-Vento, L. (1998). Event-related brain potentials in the study of visual selective attention. *Proceedings of the National Academy of Sciences USA* 95(3): 781–787.

Hubner, R. and Schlosser, J. (2010). Monetary reward increases attentional effort in the flanker task. *Psychonomic Bulletin & Review* 17(6): 821–826. doi: 10.3758/PBR.17.6.821.

Hull, C. L. (1943). *Principles of Behavior: An Introduction to Behavior Theory.* New York: Appleton-Century-Crofts.

Jimura, K., Locke, H. S., and Braver, T. S. (2010). Prefrontal cortex mediation of cognitive enhancement in rewarding motivational contexts. *Proceedings of the National Academy of Sciences of the United States of America* 107(19): 8871–8876. doi: 10.1073/pnas.1002007107.

Jonides, J. (1981). In M. I. Posner and O. Marin (eds.), *Attention and Performance XI* (pp. 187–205). Hillsdale, N.J.: Erlbaum.

Kastner, S. and Ungerleider, L. G. (2000). Mechanisms of visual attention in the human cortex. *Annual Review of Neuroscience* 23: 315–341.

Kinnison, J., Padmala, S., Choi, J. M., and Pessoa, L. (2012). Network analysis reveals increased integration during emotional and motivational processing. *Journal of Neuroscience* 32(24): 8361–8372. doi: 10.1523/jneurosci.0821-12.2012.

Kiss, M., Driver, J., and Eimer, M. (2009). Reward priority of visual target singletons modulates event-related potential signatures of attentional selection. *Psychological Science* 20(2): 245–251. doi: 10.1111/j.1467-9280.2009.02281.x.

Krebs, R. M., Boehler, C. N., Egner, T., and Woldorff, M. G. (2011). The neural underpinnings of how reward associations can both guide and misguide attention. *Journal of Neuroscience* 31(26): 9752–9759. doi: 10.1523/JNEUROSCI.0732-11.2011.

Krebs, R. M., Boehler, C. N., and Woldorff, M. G. (2010). The influence of reward associations on conflict processing in the Stroop task. *Cognition* 117(3): 341–347. doi: 10.1016/j.cognition.2010.08.018.

Kristjansson, A., Sigurjonsdottir, O., and Driver, J. (2010). Fortune and reversals of fortune in visual search: Reward contingencies for pop-out targets affect search efficiency and target repetition effects. *Attention, Perception, & Psychophysics* 72(5): 1229–1236. doi: 10.3758/APP.72.5.1229.

Lang, P. J. and Davis, M. (2006). Emotion, motivation, and the brain: reflex foundations in animal and human research. *Progress in Brain Research* 156: 3–29.

Lavie, N. (1995). Perceptual load as a necessary condition for selective attention. *Journal of Experimental Psychology: Human Perception and Performance* 21(3): 451–468.

Lim, S. L., Padmala, S., and Pessoa, L. (2008). Affective learning modulates spatial competition during low-load attentional conditions. *Neuropsychologia* 46(5): 1267–1278.

Lim, S. L., Padmala, S., and Pessoa, L. (2009). Segregating the significant from the mundane on a moment-to-moment basis via direct and indirect amygdala contributions. *Proceedings of the National Academy of Sciences USA* 106(39): 16841–16846.

MacLeod, C., Mathews, A., and Tata, P. (1986). Attentional bias in emotional disorders. *Journal of Abnormal Psychology* 95(1): 15–20.

Maunsell, J. H. (2004). Neuronal representations of cognitive state: reward or attention? *Trends in Cognitive Sciences* 8(6): 261–265.

Mitchell, D. G., Nakic, M., Fridberg, D., Kamel, N., Pine, D. S., and Blair, R. J. (2007). The impact of processing load on emotion. *NeuroImage* 34(3): 1299–1309.

Mogg, K. and Bradley, B. P. (1998). A cognitive-motivational analysis of anxiety. *Behaviour Research and Therapy* 36(9): 809–848.

Mohanty, A., Gitelman, D. R., Small, D. M., and Mesulam, M. M. (2008). The spatial attention network interacts with limbic and monoaminergic systems to modulate motivation-induced attention shifts. *Cerebral Cortex* 18(11): 2604–2613.

Montague, P. R., Hyman, S. E., and Cohen, J. D. (2004). Computational roles for dopamine in behavioural control. *Nature* 431(7010): 760–767. doi: 10.1038/nature03015.

Most, S. B., Chun, M. M., Widders, D. M., and Zald, D. H. (2005). Attentional rubbernecking: cognitive control and personality in emotion-induced blindness. *Psychonomic Bulletin & Review* 12(4): 654–661.

Muller, M. M., Andersen, S. K., and Keil, A. (2008). Time course of competition for visual processing resources between emotional pictures and foreground task. *Cerebral Cortex* 18(8): 1892–1899.

Navalpakkam, V., Koch, C., and Perona, P. (2009). Homo economicus in visual search. *Journal of Vision* 9(1): 31. 1–16. doi: 10.1167/9.1.31.

Newman, M. E. J. (2010). *Networks: An introduction*. New York City: Oxford University Press.

Norberg, J., Peira, N., and Wiens, S. (2010). Never mind the spider: late positive potentials to phobic threat at fixation are unaffected by perceptual load. *Psychophysiology* 47(6): 1151–1158. doi: 10.1111/j.1469-8986.2010.01019.x.

Padmala, S. and Pessoa, L. (2008). Affective learning enhances visual detection and responses in primary visual cortex. *Journal of Neuroscience* 28(24): 6202–6210.

Padmala, S. and Pessoa, L. (2011). Reward Reduces Conflict by Enhancing Attentional Control and Biasing Visual Cortical Processing. *Journal of Cognitive Neuroscience* 23(11): 3419–3432. doi: 10.1162/jocn_a_00011.

Palermo, R. and Rhodes, G. (2007). Are you always on my mind? A review of how face perception and attention interact. *Neuropsychologia* 45(1): 75–92.

Peck, C. J., Jangraw, D. C., Suzuki, M., Efem, R., and Gottlieb, J. (2009). Reward modulates attention independently of action value in posterior parietal cortex. *Journal of Neuroscience* 29(36): 11182–11191. doi: 10.1523/jneurosci.1929-09.2009.

Pereira, M. G., Volchan, E., de Souza, G. G., Oliveira, L., Campagnoli, R. R., Pinheiro, W. M., and Pessoa, L. (2006). Sustained and transient modulation of performance induced by emotional picture viewing. *Emotion* 6(4): 622–634.

Pessoa, L. (2005). To what extent are emotional visual stimuli processed without attention and awareness? *Current Opinion in Neurobiology* 15(2): 188–196.

Pessoa, L. (2010a). Emergent processes in cognitive-emotional interactions. *Dialogues in Clinical Neuroscience* 12(4): 433–448.

Pessoa, L. (2010b). Emotion and cognition and the amygdala: from 'what is it?' to 'what's to be done?'. *Neuropsychologia* 48(12): 3416–3429. doi: 10.1016/j.neuropsychologia.2010.06.038.

Pessoa, L. and Adolphs, R. (2010). Emotion processing and the amygdala: from a 'low road' to 'many roads' of evaluating biological significance. *Nature Reviews Neuroscience* 11(11): 773–783. doi: 10.1038/nrn2920.

Pessoa, L. and Engelmann, J. B. (2010). Embedding reward signals into perception and cognition. *Frontiers in Neuroscience* 4.

Pessoa, L., McKenna, M., Gutierrez, E., and Ungerleider, L. G. (2002). Neural processing of emotional faces requires attention. *Proceedings of the National Academy of Sciences USA* 99(17): 11458–11463.

Pessoa, L., Padmala, S., and Morland, T. (2005). Fate of unattended fearful faces in the amygdala is determined by both attentional resources and cognitive modulation. *NeuroImage* 28(1): 249–255.

Pessoa, L. and Ungerleider, L. G. (2004). Neuroimaging studies of attention and the processing of emotion-laden stimuli. *Progress in Brain Research* 144: 171–182.

Piech, R. M., McHugo, M., Smith, S. D., Dukic, M. S., Van Der Meer, J., Abou-Khalil, B., and Zald, D. H. (2011). Attentional capture by emotional stimuli is preserved in patients with amygdala lesions. *Neuropsychologia*. doi: 10.1016/j.neuropsychologia.2011.08.004.

Piech, R. M., McHugo, M., Smith, S. D., Dukic, M. S., Van Der Meer, J., Abou-Khalil, B., and Zald, D. H. (2010). Fear-enhanced visual search persists after amygdala lesions. *Neuropsychologia* 48(12): 3430–3435. doi: 10.1016/j.neuropsychologia.2010.07.009.

Platt, M. L. and Glimcher, P. W. (1999). Neural correlates of decision variables in parietal cortex. *Nature* 400(6741): 233–238.

Polk, T. A., Drake, R. M., Jonides, J. J., Smith, M. R., and Smith, E. E. (2008). Attention enhances the neural processing of relevant features and suppresses the processing of irrelevant features in humans: a functional magnetic resonance imaging study of the stroop task. *Journal of Neuroscience* 28(51): 13786–13792.

Posner, M. I., and Snyder, C. R. R. (1975). Attention and cognitive control. In R. L. Solso (ed.), *Information processing and cognition: The Loyola symposium* (pp. 55–85). Hillsdale, N.J.: Erlbaum.

Pourtois, G., Schettino, A., and Vuilleumier, P. (2012). Brain mechanisms for emotional influences on perception and attention: What is magic and what is not. *Biological Psychology*. doi: 10.1016/j.biopsycho.2012.02.007.

Raymond, J. E., and O'Brien, J. L. (2009). Selective visual attention and motivation: the consequences of value learning in an attentional blink task. *Psychological Science* 20(8): 981–988. doi: 10.1111/j.1467-9280.2009.02391.x.

Savine, A. C., and Braver, T. S. (2010). Motivated cognitive control: reward incentives modulate preparatory neural activity during task-switching. *Journal of Neuroscience* 30(31): 10294–10305. doi: 10.1523/JNEUROSCI.2052-10.2010.

Schultz, W., Apicella, P., Scarnati, E., and Ljungberg, T. (1992). Neuronal activity in monkey ventral striatum related to the expectation of reward. *Journal of Neuroscience* 12(12): 4595–4610.

Schupp, H. T., Junghofer, M., Weike, A. I., and Hamm, A. O. (2003a). Attention and emotion: an ERP analysis of facilitated emotional stimulus processing. *NeuroReport* 14(8): 1107–1110.

Schupp, H. T., Junghofer, M., Weike, A. I., and Hamm, A. O. (2003b). Emotional facilitation of sensory processing in the visual cortex. *Psychological Science* 14(1): 7–13.

Schupp, H. T., Stockburger, J., Bublatzky, F., Junghofer, M., Weike, A. I., and Hamm, A. O. (2007). Explicit attention interferes with selective emotion processing in human extrastriate cortex. *BMC Neuroscience* 8: 16.

Shen, Y. J., and Chun, M. M. (2011). Increases in rewards promote flexible behavior. *Attention, Perception, & Psychophysics* 73(3): 938–952. doi: 10.3758/s13414-010-0065-7.

Silvert, L., Lepsien, J., Fragopanagos, N., Goolsby, B., Kiss, M., Taylor, J. G., and Nobre, A. C. (2007). Influence of attentional demands on the processing of emotional facial expressions in the amygdala. *NeuroImage* 38(2): 357–366.

Small, D. M., Gitelman, D., Simmons, K., Bloise, S. M., Parrish, T., and Mesulam, M. M. (2005). Monetary incentives enhance processing in brain regions mediating top-down control of attention. *Cerebral Cortex* 15(12): 1855–1865.

Stein, T., Peelen, M. V., Funk, J., and Seidl, K. N. (2010). The fearful-face advantage is modulated by task demands: evidence from the attentional blink. *Emotion* 10(1): 136–140.

Tsal, Y., and Benoni, H. (2010). Diluting the burden of load: perceptual load effects are simply dilution effects. *Journal of Experimental Psychology: Human Perception and Performance* 36(6): 1645–1656. doi: 10.1037/a0018172.

Tsuchiya, N., Moradi, F., Felsen, C., Yamazaki, M., and Adolphs, R. (2009). Intact rapid detection of fearful faces in the absence of the amygdala. *Nature Neuroscience* 12(10): 1224–1225.

Vuilleumier, P. (2005). How brains beware: neural mechanisms of emotional attention. *Trends in Cognitive Sciences* 9(12): 585–594.

Vuilleumier, P., Armony, J. L., Driver, J., and Dolan, R. J. (2001). Effects of attention and emotion on face processing in the human brain: An event-related fMRI study. *Neuron* 30(3): 829–841.

Weil, R. S., Furl, N., Ruff, C. C., Symmonds, M., Flandin, G., Dolan, R. J., and Rees, G. (2010). Rewarding feedback after correct visual discriminations has both general and specific influences on visual cortex. *Journal of Neurophysiology* 104(3): 1746–1757. doi: 10.1152/jn.00870.2009.

Williams, J. M. G., Watts, F. N., MacLeod, C., and Mathews, A. (1997). *Cognitive Psychology and Emotional Disorders*. Chichester: Wiley.

Wilson, D. E., Muroi, M., and MacLeod, C. M. (2011). Dilution, not load, affects distractor processing. *Journal of Experimental Psychology: Human Perception and Performance* 37(2): 319–335. doi: 10.1037/a0021433.

CHAPTER 26

WORKING MEMORY BIASES IN HUMAN VISION

DAVID SOTO AND GLYN W. HUMPHREYS

INTRODUCTION

WORKING memory (WM) is a key concept for understanding human cognition. Originally conceived as a storage system for temporary retention of information while other tasks are being performed (Baddeley 1986), current theories suggest that this form of temporary storage system is critical for imaging information when we recall it from long-term memory (see Chun and Kuhl, this volume) and that it also plays a more general role in the control of goal-directed behaviour, for example by keeping task-priorities and relevant feature information 'online'. This chapter is concerned with the role of WM in behavioural control, and we focus on the somewhat counterintuitive possibility that, although WM is usually helpful for guiding ongoing behaviour, it can also be disruptive in particular circumstances. Those circumstances are informative about the interplay between WM and task control.

To illustrate a case where WM may be disruptive rather than helpful for performance, consider the following armchair example. Imagine driving to the market and thinking of the list of items you need to buy; you may rehearse the items to be used in cooking dinner, and this could involve, for example, holding a representation of a hamburger in WM. This representation of a hamburger could be disruptive, however, if you happen to be passing a Burger King advertisement at the time, as your attention might stray to this rather than the task at hand (driving). Having items active in memory may inadvertently affect the stimuli you select for action. Under such conditions, the contents of WM may control action but the action is not integrated with the greater context of ongoing behaviour. This would suggest that WM can operate 'locally' to control attention, and in some conditions it can be divorced from broader aspects of task control. Here we will review the evidence for this contention, and consider the broader implications for understanding the relations between WM, attention, and task control.

An important initial conceptualization of WM was developed by Baddeley (see Baddeley and Hitch 1974; Baddeley 2000). Baddeley has proposed the operation of different 'maintenance' components (phonological, visuospatial, and episodic buffers), plus an 'executive' component which acts to control the operation of the maintenance mechanisms. The executive component of WM is similar to the idea of an attentional supervisory system (Norman and Shallice 1986), which acts to modulate processing in routine cognitive processes (driven bottom-up from the environment) to bias activity to favour the goals of the current task. However, although central to the conceptualization of WM, the executive component of WM remains poorly understood. The work we will discuss, on how WM interacts with visual attention, speaks to this issue by showing how components of this 'WM executive' can be fractionated, according to which aspects of WM affect stimulus selection. In particular, and in line with our everyday example, the evidence indicates that WM representations can affect stimulus selection even when they are irrelevant, or even misleading, for the primary task at hand. The results, as we shall review below, call for a re-evaluation of the relations between executive functions, attentional control, and WM.

MODELS OF VISUAL SELECTION

Our knowledge of how we select from vision objects for action has made enormous strides over the past 30 years, drawing on converging evidence from behavioural studies, functional brain imaging, studies of attentional disorders, and electrophysiological studies of attention in animal models. These empirical developments have been matched by the generation of explicit models of selection. Models such as the 'guided search' account (Wolfe et al. 1989), the 'biased competition' framework (Desimone and Duncan 1995), the 'selective attention for identification model' (Heinke and Humphreys 2003), and the 'theory of visual attention' (TVA) (Bundesen 1990) postulate the notion of 'attentional templates', which act to guide the selection of visual stimuli. These templates hold an internal representation set-up for behaviourally relevant targets and, though not always described in these terms, they can be thought akin to representations held in WM. In neural accounts, it is often assumed that cognitive control operates through cell assemblies, coded in the prefrontal cortex, which maintain and manipulate goal-related information (Miller and Cohen 2001). In the context of a visual selection task, the prefrontal activity may reflect the 'template', which regulates responses in visual processing pathways, selectively enhancing neural pathways associated, for example, with the most relevant location in the visual field (Kastner et al. 1999). Classic neurophysiological evidence comes from single-unit recording studies within the inferior temporal (IT) cortex of monkeys performing a memory-guided search task. In Chelazzi et al. (1998), a memory cue instructed the monkeys about the target for a forthcoming eye movement. This target had to be kept 'online' during a delay period of several seconds until a search display containing the saccade target and a distractor appeared. During the delay interval the sustained firing rate of IT neurons reflected maintenance and/or an expectancy of target-related information. Critically, after the onset of the search array, the response of the pre-activated neuron came to reflect only information related to the relevant target object in its receptive field and the neural responses to irrelevant distractors in the search display were suppressed. These data suggest that WM-based feedback helped IT neurons respond selectively to the target which 'won' the competition for representation with the distractor. Similar patterns of results for spatially defined targets have been documented in extrastriate cortex (V4) (Luck et al. 1997) and in prefrontal neurons (Rao et al. 1997; Rainer et al. 1998). Such results support the general contention that attentional templates, established as a WM representation in prefrontal cortex, bias selection towards expected targets.

Now, in these single-unit studies, the contents of WM overlap with the target of attention, making it difficult to judge if WM is necessarily linked to task-based guidance of behaviour. In an attempt to pull WM and attentional task factors apart, a recent body of research has used new paradigms where the contents of WM and selective attention for a given target are varied in an orthogonal fashion—creating conditions where the information in WM is irrelevant or even directly disruptive of performance in another ongoing (primary) task. Does WM still determine selection? If it does, what are the conditions generating such effects? By asking such questions, we can learn about the relations between WM, task control, and attentional selection. Here we review this research, highlighting the psychological and the neural mechanisms that support WM biases in visual selective attention and the extent to which they are subjected to cognitive control. We subsequently consider the consequences for theories of visual selection.

COMMONALITIES BETWEEN WM AND ATTENTION

Machizawa and Driver (2011) examined individual differences in the efficiency with which participants showed effects of (i) an alerting signal, (ii) cues to orient attention to the spatial location of a target, and (iii) response competition between a target and distractors (Fan et al. 2002). The same participants also performed a battery of tests measuring visual WM capacity, precision, and vulnerability to interference (from irrelevant items). Using principal component analysis to pull out common factors underlying performance in the attention and WM tests, Machizawa and Driver showed that these aspects of attention (alerting, orienting, and response conflict) mapped onto a common component that also reflected WM capacity, precision, and vulnerability to interference (Vogel et al. 2005; Bays and Husain 2008; Zhang and Luck 2008). These results point to a functional overlap between WM and attention.

There is also ample evidence of functional interactions between WM and attention. For example, our ability to ignore distractors during visual selection tasks depends on the availability of WM capacity; loading that capacity by giving participants a secondary task leads to a reduced ability to withstand distractor competition (de Fockert et al. 2001). The study by de Fockert and colleagues presented observers with a visual selection task (attend to a target whilst ignoring distractors) that had to be performed under a concurrent WM task of either high or low processing load. The visual target of the attention task could be surrounded by distractors, which could be either congruent or incongruent with the response associated with the target. When the capacity of WM was highly taxed, performance in attentional selection decreased (i.e. response interference by incongruent distractors increased). This finding indicates that stressing the capacity of WM can lead to impairments in control processes that help to filter out distractors and to focus attention on a task-relevant target. This provides converging evidence to the results using principal component analysis (Machizawa and Driver 2011), in this case by showing that a variable that affects WM (increasing load) also disrupts attentional selection.

However, not all ways of stressing the capacity of WM are equal, as indicated by evidence of crossover effects based upon the type of mental representation in WM and the representations on which selection is carried out. There are instances where high processing loads in WM can either disrupt or boost selection, depending on whether the load in WM extenuates target or distractor information processing. For example, when the representations filling WM capacity match with distractors rather than targets in a task, then distractor processing is reduced and hence target processing is facilitated (Kim et al. 2005; Park et al. 2007). Such evidence indicates WM can de-couple from (and override) task control. We now discuss the conditions under which this happens.

Coupling WM and Attention and De-coupling Task Control

The paradigm depicted in Fig. 26.1a illustrates a scenario used to assess whether the biasing effects of WM on visual selection are under task control. In this paradigm, search is defined as the primary task which must be undertaken whilst participants hold an irrelevant item in WM. This irrelevant item can reappear in the search task, aligned either with the search target or a distractor. The primary goal of visual selection (prioritize the target in the search task) can be orthogonally varied with the contents of WM, so that WM can be set against the task goals (e.g. when the item in WM reappears in the search display alongside a search distractor). What happens under these conditions?

In this paradigm search performance can be indexed by indirect measures of attentional selection such as the response latencies to find the target or via direct measures of overt attentional orienting such as the direction of the first eye movement made in the search display. The typical finding is that, when the WM item reappears in the search display alongside a distractor, search is slower and less accurate when compared with a neutral baseline, where the search display contains the same items but they no longer

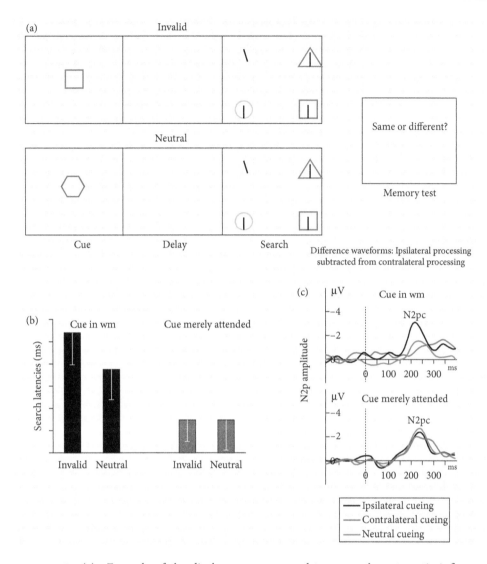

FIGURE 26.1 (a) Example of the display sequences used to assess the automatic influence of the contents of WM on visual selection. Observers are presented with a cue and subsequently the task is to search for a tilted line target. In the invalid condition, the pre-cued object again reappears but this time it contains a distractor. In the neutral condition the memory item does not reappear in the search display. (b) Search is slowed on invalid relative to neutral trials when the irrelevant cue is kept in WM, and this effect is stronger under WM conditions relative to when the cue is merely attended but not held in WM for later report. (c) The WM bias modulates the N2pc. Waveforms were obtained by subtracting activity in electrodes ipsilateral to the target from those contralateral to the target. Reproduced from Sanjay Kumar, David Soto, Glyn W. Humphreys, Electrophysiological evidence for attentional guidance by the contents of working memory, European Journal of Neuroscience, 30(2) pp. 307–317, Copyright © 2003, The Authors (2009). Journal Compilation © Federation of European Neuroscience Societies and Blackwell Publishing Ltd.

match the memory cue (Fig. 26.1b) (Downing 2000; Soto et al. 2005, 2006; Olivers et al. 2006; Pan and Soto 2010). In these studies the working memory item is at best irrelevant to the search task and at worst it can be consistently detrimental (e.g. in experiments where the memory item only ever reappears at a distractor location rather than at the location of the target; Soto et al. 2005, 2007); nevertheless the re-presented WM stimulus still affects selection of the search target.

These effects of holding an item in memory can be contrasted with performance in another baseline condition (the 'mere repetition' condition), when the same visual events precede the search display but participants do not have to hold the cue in memory (the cue can be 'merely repeated' in the search display). This baseline condition controls for the effect of the mere presentation of an initial cue, in the WM condition. Despite this, biases from the cue are attenuated under mere repetition conditions (Soto et al. 2005; Olivers et al. 2006). These data indicate that the biases on selection reflect the presence of the cue in WM and not mere bottom-up priming from the initial presentation of the cue itself. Furthermore, the biasing effects from WM cannot be easily modulated by task-based attention to search targets; in such cases the strong association between WM and attention trumps task-based control. The data suggest that WM can operate in a relatively modular way and is not necessarily part of the structures that generate task control. We now go on to discuss the parameters of these effects.

WM Biasing: Early or Late?

The capture of attention by irrelevant items in WM happens rapidly. This is indicated by several pieces of data. One finding is based on the measurement of visual evoked electrophysiological responses based on electrical activity measures on the scalp. Spatial selection of a target within one visual field has an electrophysiological marker known as the N2pc, which reflects a greater negative going waveform over the hemisphere opposite to the selected location in the visual field and arises about 250 ms after the onset of a display (Hopf et al. 2000; Luck and Hillyard 1994). It has been shown that the amplitude of the N2pc is modulated if a search display contains an item matching another irrelevant stimulus being held in WM, and this effect is much stronger than that found when a stimulus is repeated but not initially held in WM (Kumar et al. 2009; Mazza et al. 2011). Fig. 26.1c illustrates the N2pc profiles for the search bias driven by WM and by (mere) repetition priming. As can be seen, the amplitude of the N2pc is larger when the irrelevant WM item falls on the same side of space as the search target (i.e. ipsilateral cueing) relative to when the cue does not reappear in the search display (on neutral cueing trials) or when the irrelevant WM cue appears on the opposite side of space (and presumably competes for selection with) the search target. These results are consistent with the WM item affecting early selection of items in the search display.

Matching these electrophysiological data are results of studies measuring eye movements. Here it has been found that the first eye movement made in search is affected if the search display repeats an item currently held in WM (Soto et al. 2005). A recent study by Mannan and colleagues (Mannan, Kennard, Potter, Pan, and Soto 2010) investigated saccadic performance in a variation of the combined WM–Attention paradigm of Fig. 26.1. In this study, a search distractor appeared abruptly in the search display. There is much research indicating that the abrupt onset of a stimulus can capture attention (e.g. Yantis and Jonides 1984). In addition to the abrupt onset distractor being a potent bottom-up cue to attention, Mannan found that initial saccades were still modulated by whether the new onset distractor matched the contents of WM (the effect of the onset distractor was greater when the same stimulus was held in WM; Fig. 26.2a and b). Interestingly, the timing of this effect matched the time course of the N2pc, affecting eye movements initiated around 200–250 ms after the appearance of the search display. Mannan et al. also measured the trajectory of the saccade to the search target. They found that saccades directed to the target curved away from the location of the irrelevant onset distractor (Fig. 26.2c), and this effect was strongest when the irrelevant distractor matched the item in WM. This result indicates that even salient distractors (distractor onsets), otherwise thought to capture attention, can be affected by matching an irrelevant item held in WM. Interestingly, the curving of saccades away from distractors has been taken as evidence for the distractors being inhibited (Van der Stigchel et al. 2006), suggesting that, at least on trials where targets are selected rather than the item repeated from WM, there is rapid inhibition of the repeated distractor. On such occasions, there is evidence of attentional control affecting performance but in a manner that is independent of WM, which still biases selection to matching items. We will return to this point.

A third piece of evidence for WM exerting an early effect on visual selection comes from studies demonstrating that stimuli in WM can modulate perceptual sensitivity to visual targets (Soto et al. 2010 in the same manner as spatial selective attention) (Downing 1988; Carrasco et al. 2000; Blanco and Soto 2002) (but see Theeuwes and Van der Burg 2007; Cosman and Vecera 2011). Perceptual sensitivity can be measured when the search display is briefly presented and masked, when report accuracy can be used to derive the d' index. d' has been shown to be enhanced when an item in WM is re-presented at the location of the search target, compared with the re-presented WM item falling at the location of a search distractor (Soto et al. 2010). Note that, in these studies, participants do not know the location where the repeated WM item will fall, so attentional guidance is based on a match between the features of stimuli in the search display and the WM item. This suggests that stimuli held in WM may produce neural 'baseline' shifts in the activation of perceptual channels for corresponding features, so that the subsequent processing of stimuli along those channels is automatically enhanced. Search targets falling at such locations also benefit.

These results from items being held in WM are mirrored by other results in visual search where the match between a stimulus and a 'template' can direct attention even when it is detrimental to the task. For example, Moores, Laiti, and Chelazzi (2003) found that telling people to search for a particular target (e.g. for a motor bike) led to them sometimes selecting an associated distractor (e.g. a crash helmet), even though

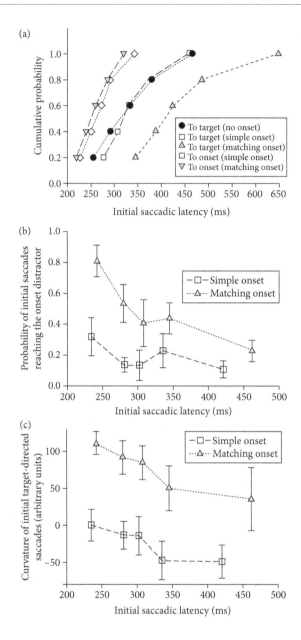

FIGURE 26.2 The WM bias modulates early eye movement performance in the presence of salient stimulus-onset signals. (a) Cumulative distribution of initial latencies of eye movements directed to the target and an onset distractor. (b) Probability of the initial saccade being directed to the onset as a function of saccade latency. (c) Curvature of initial target-directed saccades as function of saccade latency. Reprinted from *Vision Research*, 50(16), Sabira K. Mannan, Christopher Kennard, Daniela Potter, Yi Pan, and David Soto, Early oculomotor capture by new onsets driven by the contents of working memory, pp. 1590–1597, Copyright (2010), with permission from Elsevier.

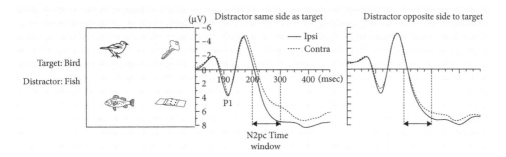

Target: Bird

Distractor: Fish

(μV) Distractor same side as target   Distractor opposite side to target

—— Ipsi

····· Contra

P1

N2pc Time
window

FIGURE 26.3 Example displays used to assess semantic interference in visual search. N2pc waveforms at electrodes contralateral and ipsilateral to the target as a function of the position of the distractor in the search display. Reproduced from Anna L. Telling, Sanjay Kumar, Antje S. Meyer and Glyn W. Humphreys, 'Electrophysiological Evidence of Semantic Interference in Visual Search', *Journal of Cognitive Neuroscience*, 22:10 (October, 2010), pp. 2212–2225. © 2010 by the Massachusetts Institute of Technology.

such a distractor could never be the target. One account of this result is that the attentional template does not only specify a proposed target but also associates of that target. The associated information, held in the template, can direct search to the distractor outside of task control. Telling et al. (2010) further showed that interference from associated distractors modulated the amplitude of the N2pc amplitude (see Fig. 26.3) in the same manner as found by Kumar et al. (2009) using an irrelevant WM cue. The N2pc was higher when the distractor and the search target fell in the same hemifield relative to when they appeared in different hemifields (Telling et al. 2010). Taken together, these findings indicate that information held in memory can modulate visual selection even when it is irrelevant to the primary task (visual search).

Not all results support this contention, however. Carlisle and Woodman (2011a) used a similar WM–Attention paradigm but found no modulation of the N2pc when they re-presented as distractors items that matched the contents of WM. Caution should be exerted, however, as WM biases on attention were found in search latencies (i.e. search was slower on invalid-WM trials relative to the neutral condition, when the WM cue did not reappear).

FEATURES IN WM THAT BIAS ATTENTION

The studies of Moores et al. (2003) and Telling et al. (2010), noted above, indicate that attention may be biased by distractors that are semantically associated with target information coded in an attentional template (Moores and Maxwell 2008; Telling et al. 2010). Several studies have additionally shown that abstract cues in WM (e.g. words or even labelled stimulus dimensions) can be sufficient to bias subsequent visual selection (Pan et al. 2009; Balani et al. 2011). For example, having participants hold the words 'red square' in WM is sufficient for attention subsequently to go to a red square when it is presented as a distractor in a search display (Soto and Humphreys 2007). Thus WM biases can be driven not only by visual but also by more abstract information held in WM. These effects suggest that WM can bias selection through multiple levels of representation, which may include automatic linkages between semantic and visual codes. Some studies have even reported similar magnitudes of bias from visual and verbal information held in WM (Soto and Humphreys 2007; Soto et al. 2010). Interestingly, visual WM biases have been documented to occur with both short and long time intervals between the memory cue and the search task (Olivers et al. 2006; Soto and Humphreys 2008), as long as the WM cue is actively maintained. However, the effects of verbal WM cues may be less sustained than the visual counterpart (Dombrowe et al. 2010). This last result could arise if the verbal information is initially held in an executive representation in WM but is subsequently coded into a phonological 'slave' system (cf. Baddeley 1986). Once in the 'slave' representation, the verbal cue is less effective at directing attention. Here we begin to de-couple attention from some forms of WM, complementing our earlier distinction between WM and task control.

WM Biasing: Intentional Memory Resampling or True Capture?

Though the evidence we have reviewed fits with the idea that items held in WM automatically bias attention to matching stimuli, counter-arguments can be made. As these alternatives would change any interpretation of the relation between WM, task goals, and attention, they need to be considered. One proposal is that the critical data reflect strategic rather than automatic linkages between WM and attention. For example, possibly participants try to refresh their memory trace when the WM reappears in a search display and so they deliberately attend to re-presented WM cues (Woodman and Luck 2007) (see Fig. 26.1). The evidence, however, indicates that this is not the case. First, WM biases of selection are greatly attenuated or even abolished as the capacity of WM is taxed by larger memory loads (Soto and Humphreys 2008; Soto et al. 2012a; Zhang et al. 2011). This finding goes against any 'strategic' memory-refreshing account because memory resampling would be most beneficial to sustain the memory representation when the capacity of WM is taxed, yet this is clearly not the case. Second, Bahrami-Balani, Soto, and Humphreys (2010) had participants hold a specific object exemplar in WM and re-presented in the search display a different exemplar of that search item (e.g. a labrador dog might be held in WM and a setter might appear in the search display). In the subsequent memory test, participants had to discriminate the exemplar they had originally seen in WM and to reject distractors that were different exemplars. Balani et al. found that search was affected when a different exemplar of the WM item appeared, even though it would have been detrimental to memory performance to strategically attend to this different exemplar. Finally, Kiyonaga et al. (2012)

used surprise memory tests which replaced the search display, abolishing any potential strategy to use the reappearance of the WM item in search to boost the memory trace for a subsequent test. Re-presentation of the WM item still affected visual selection. We conclude that a strategic resampling account is not viable; rather, information held in at least some components of WM (not the phonological slave system) can bias attention outside of the bounds of task control.

THE BOUNDS OF TASK CONTROL

Do items in the appropriate WM state always escape task control? Above we discussed evidence that the effects of items held in WM weaken as the WM load increases (Soto and Humphreys 2008). This is interesting, because it is typically harder to implement task control as the load on working memory increases (de Fockert et al. 2001). Yet, here, an increasing WM load is associated with greater task control in the sense that there are weaker distraction effects from WM. One way to explain this is to suggest that, when there are multiple items held in WM, the representation of each item is weakened. The weakened WM representation has a less potent effect on directing attention.

Other evidence points to additional conditions where WM effects weaken and task-based control over selection is increased. One factor is whether the search target remains the same or changes across trials. Several studies have shown that strong biases from WM are apparent when the search target remains the same from trial to trial and the WM stimuli are updated on a trial-by-trial basis. In contrast, when the search target also changes on a trial-by-trial-basis, biasing effects from WM decrease (Downing and Dodds 2004; Houtkamp and Roelfsema 2006). This is again counterintuitive. Varying the search target on a trial-by-trial basis makes search harder; hence you might expect task control to then be reduced (de Fockert et al. 2001). However, what seems critical here is how the WM cue and the (primary) search target are represented in WM. The result tells us about the nature of WM in relation to attention and task control.

Olivers and colleagues (2011) have argued that the interplay between WM and visual selection is determined by distinct states in WM. Although it has typically been argued that, for example, visual WM may hold three or four items (Bundesen 1990), Olivers proposed that only a single item is represented in at the 'forefront' of WM at any one time (Oberauer 2002). It is this item that is intimately linked to attention. Hence, attention is directed to the WM cue if this cue is in the forefront of WM; however, if the search target is at the forefront, search will be directed to that and be less affected by the (irrelevant) WM cue. How does this fit with the data on keeping the search target constant or changing it on a trial-by-trial basis? The proposal is that changing the target on a trial-by-trial basis highlights the search target in WM rather than the irrelevant WM item, and this reduces the effectiveness of the WM cue for the subsequent guidance of attention (Olivers et al. 2011). This is supported by other data. Peters and colleagues (2009) asked observers to keep two items in WM, each of which changed on a trial-by-trial basis; one item had to be detected in a visual stream at central fixation, the other item had to be held for a subsequent memory test after the search response. The WM item could sometimes appear in the central stream, when they should have been treated as distractors. The authors measured the P3 event-related potential, and they interpreted this ERP component with matching stimuli to memory contents (Duncan-Johnson and Donchin 1977). There was a change in the P3 response when the search target occurred, while there was no change in the P3 response when WM stimuli appeared, when compared with the responses to non-matching distractors (Peters et al. 2009). These data indicate that, when the search item was constantly updated, it was immediately available to modulate the P3 response. There is a final caveat, however, which is how general these effects are. In a recent study using a similar paradigm to Peters et al., Zhang and colleagues (2011) had participants hold a colour rather than a letter shape in WM and found that the colour in WM did affect responses to a matching colour in the central stream of items. Apparently, some properties of items in WM may still permeate attentional guidance even if the representation in WM is held in a 'background' rather than a 'foreground' state. Nevertheless, at least for complex shape stimuli, it appears that WM can be compartmentalized into foreground and background components, and that the coupling of the WM state to attention is most effective for the foreground representation. This foreground representation can be dissociated from task-based control, though, given the evidence so far presented in this chapter that the foreground stimulus in WM directs attention to matching distractors.

There is evidence that frontal lobe structures are important for this compartmentalization of WM into foreground and background components. Soto et al. (2006) tested patients with frontal lobe lesions on the WM–Attention paradigm. They expected that frontal lobe patients might show weaker effects of WM-based guidance of attention, given that the frontal lobes may be critical for representing stimuli in WM (Miller, this volume). This is not what was found. Instead Soto and colleagues reported *exaggerated* WM biases. To account for this, Soto et al. proposed that the frontal lobe patients had problems in 'compartmentalizing' the WM cue and the search target in WM. We suggest that normal participants do compartmentalize the representations of these items to some degree, even if the WM item is held in the foreground of WM under appropriate conditions. Having the items compartmentalized enables participants to switch attention rapidly from an irrelevant WM item to the search target. However, if the search item is not separated from the WM cue, then WM biases may be exacerbated.

Aside from cases where WM stimuli are held in the 'background' of WM, are there other conditions in which behaviour can be controlled by the primary search task, and not by items in WM? The evidence here is that task control can be exerted under the appropriate circumstances. For example, Han and Kim (2009) examined conditions in which the WM cue was always invalid (falling at the location of a distractor) when it reappeared in a search display and they varied the time between when the WM cue was given and when the same item reappeared in the search display. They found that the cost from the invalid WM cue changed to a facilitation effect as the interval between the cue and the search display increased. The change from the standard cost from re-presenting the WM item to a facilitation effect (faster RTs on trials when the WM cue appeared and was invalid relative to when it did not reappear, on neutral trials) is striking. The result suggests that participants were able to inhibit the cue in WM over time, so that search was more likely to be directed away from this item and towards the search target (see also Woodman and Luck 2007). Apparently, even if an item is initially placed in the forefront of WM, it can be suppressed over time when participants know that it is always going to be irrelevant for the primary task (here visual search).

Further evidence demonstrates that cognitive control over WM biases can operate through modulation of the memory trace itself (Kiyonaga et al. 2012). Kiyonaga and colleagues orthogonally varied the probability of whether WM cues were valid or invalid. In some blocks of the task participants could reliably anticipate that the WM item would be irrelevant. The WM bias was weaker in this condition relative to when the WM cue could sometimes be valid in the search task (see also Carlisle and Woodman 2011b). Interestingly, Kiyonaga's study showed that, when WM items were expected to be invalid, responses were slowed to the items on a surprise memory test. This result is consistent with the memory representation itself being weaker, perhaps due to memory suppression taking place. WM biases can be also 'controlled' by the demands imposed by the attentional task, for example by training observers in visual search tasks under conditions of high perceptual demand (e.g. by using brief exposures of the search items), which arguably enhances the prioritization of search goals over memory goals (Dalvit and Eimer 2011). Also, by spatially pre-cueing the location of the upcoming search target, the influence of an irrelevant WM-matching item in the search display can be eliminated (Pan and Soto 2010; Soto et al. 2011b).

Taken together, the above findings indicate that WM biases of attention can be subject to task-based control; specifically, WM biases can be partly enhanced or inhibited based on expectations about either the distractor (its likely validity), the spatial location of the target, and the time available for control processes to be recruited.

Role of Conscious Awareness in WM Biases

As well as being linked to attentional guidance, information in WM has also been linked to awareness (Baddeley 1986). However, just as the link between WM and attention can be questioned under some conditions (when task-based control is maximized and when items are held in the background of WM; see above), so the link between WM and awareness can also be challenged. Several questions are relevant to this issue. One is whether WM biases in visual search are dependent on conscious awareness of the search display items. Consider work on patients with 'visual extinction' following a brain lesion. Patients with extinction are typically unaware of an item presented in the contralesional field if a competing stimulus is shown simultaneously on the ipsilesional side. Despite this problem in awareness, the patients can have improved report of contralesional targets if those targets match the contents of WM (Soto and Humphreys 2006). This evidence indicates that WM biases may boost access of non-conscious information into awareness. Research on the phenomenon of 'inattentional blindness' also supports this notion. Inattentional blindness is the failure to be aware of the presence of stimuli that are not attended. Studies have demonstrated that inattentional blindness may be reduced when participants are directed to look for a particular stimulus and the unattended stimulus is either visually or semantically related to the behaviourally relevant stimulus being held in memory (Most et al. 2005; Koivisto and Revonsuo 2007). Here we have a result reminiscent of the findings for semantic guidance of attention in visual search (selecting the distractor 'crash helmet' when searching for a motorbike; Moores et al. 2003; Telling et al. 2010), but even more striking since participants appear not to be aware of the stimulus unless this match is made to the representation in memory. Memory-driven biases appear therefore capable of increasing the signal strength of items that would otherwise remain non-conscious, thus determining which information gains access into conscious awareness.

We can also ask whether awareness of the memory cues themselves is necessary to observe a WM bias. Intuitively you would think this would be the case but recent work suggests otherwise. Soto et al. (2012c) presented participants with an oriented Gabor patch acting as a cue, which was followed by a further oriented Gabor as a test stimulus. The task was to report whether the test Gabor was tilted clockwise or anti-clockwise relative to the cued Gabor. The first cue was masked so that participants were not aware of its orientation. Despite this, participants could perform the delayed discrimination task well above chance in the absence of awareness of the initial Gabor cue and even in the presence of intervening distractor Gabors across a 4 second cue–target delay. This effect contrasts with what are often reported to be short-lived effects from merely repeating non-conscious items (typically found with prime-target intervals of around 0.2–0.3 seconds (Kouider and Dehaene 2007; though see Kunst-Wilson and Zajonc 1980; Bar and Biederman 1998) which have also been shown to capture the deployment of spatial attention (Astle et al. 2009). This finding indicates that unseen items may be maintained in WM in a non-conscious state and still affect the subsequent deployment of attention and awareness (see Pan, Lin, Zhao and Soto, in press). This will be an interesting avenue for future research.

The Neural Basis of WM-based Guidance of Attention

Our understanding of the relations between WM, attention, and task control has also been enhanced by studies of the neural basis of WM-based attentional guidance. Soto and colleagues (2007) used functional MRI in conjunction with the WM–Attention paradigm (see Fig. 26.1). They compared activity when the WM item reappeared in the search display compared with a neutral condition, when the WM stimulus did not reappear. Relative to this neutral condition, the reappearance of the WM item in the search display led to increased activity in frontal, temporal, and visual cortical regions. In contrast, when cues were attended but not held in WM (in a 'mere repetition' condition), the same regions responded in the opposite manner—in this case there was a reduction in the neural response to the reappearance of the initial cue in the search display. This pattern of results is illustrated in Fig. 26.4a. This last effect is reminiscent of 'neural adaptation' effects, reflective of a reduced neural response to repeated stimulation, which may in turn be associated with facilitated perceptual processing ('priming') of previously experienced items (Wiggs and Martin 1998; Grill-Spector et al. 2006). In contrast, the *enhanced* neural response to the reappearance of the WM cue in search appears to reflect the WM bias, namely, the capture of attention by the WM stimulus (again note that this is not due just to carrying an item in WM, as this arises in the neutral baseline condition too). This dissociation in neural repetition effects by the memory context has now been replicated in several studies (Soto et al. 2011b, 2012a; Greene and Soto 2012). The data confirm that holding an item in WM engages distinct neural processes to effects of mere repetition.

Brain interference methods, for example using transcranial magnetic stimulation (TMS), have provided added evidence that holding an item in WM and merely repeating the same item reflect distinct functional states in the cortex. Soto and colleagues (Soto et al. 2012c) used a similar paradigm to the one depicted in Fig. 26.1 and included trials where the WM item was valid (and cued the target) as well as when it was invalid. TMS was applied to early visual cortex at the onset of the search display. This modulated the impact of the memory cue on search. When a feature cue was held in WM and re-presented in the search task, then TMS to visual cortex enhanced search performance on valid relative to invalid cueing trials (and relative to a TMS control condition). When the cue was merely repeated without being held in WM, however, TMS to visual cortex produced the opposite pattern of results. Now occipital TMS impaired search performance on valid relative to invalid trials. This dissociation of the occipital TMS influence on selection may be accounted for by short-term changes in the neural state of the visual cortex under WM and mere repetition conditions. TMS may enhance the capture of attention by items in WM because the WM stimuli contents are represented in a heightened state in visual cortex; TMS may increase the strength of these visual representations (Silvanto and Cattaneo 2010). In the mere-repetition condition, however, TMS may interfere with the process of neural adaptation, observed in fMRI studies (Soto et al. 2007), lessening and even reversing the cue-validity effect. Fig. 26.4b illustrates this finding.

Several studies have also shown that WM biases modulate activity in the thalamus and prefrontal cortex (Grecucci et al. 2010; Soto et al. 2007, 2012a, 2012b). However, in these studies the thalamus and prefrontal cortex did not merely respond to the reappearance of the WM cue in search display but rather activity reflected the congruity of the WM cue in relation to the search goal—that is, the regions were differentially active according to whether the WM item was valid or invalid (see Fig. 26.4a). Taken together the data suggest that a fronto-thalamic pathway may be important to integrate the contents of WM and perceptual input based on the goals imposed by the selection task.

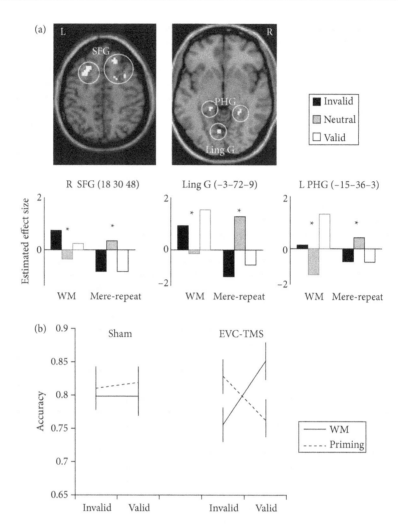

FIGURE 26.4 (a) Example of the brain network linked with WM biases. Superior frontal, parahippocampal regions, and the lingual gyrus were modulated by the reappearance in the search display of a previously experience feature cue. When the cue was kept in WM, reappearance of the WM item in the search display enhanced activity in these areas. In contrast, when the initial cue had to be attended but not held in WM, the same regions showed decreased responses to the reappearance of the cue in the search display (relative to the neutral condition, when the cue did not reappear in the search display). Reproduced from Soto, D., Humphreys, G. W., and Rotshtein, P., Dissociating the neural mechanisms of memory-based guidance of visual selection, Proceedings of the National Academy of Sciences USA, 104, pp. 17186–17191 .Copyright, (c) 2007 National Academy of Sciences, USA <http://www.nasonline.org>. (b) Target discrimination following TMS to the occipital cortex (right) or sham TMS, showing opposite effects of stimulation under WM and mere identification conditions. Reproduced from Soto, D., Llewelyn, D., and Silvanto, J., Distinct causal mechanisms of attentional guidance by working memory and repetition priming in early visual cortex, Journal of Neuroscience, 32, pp. 3447–3452 © 2012, The Society for Neuroscience. <http://www.jneurosci.org>.

Are the neural regions the same for different types of information in WM? Soto et al. (2012d) assessed the neural regions involved in biasing visual selection by verbal and visual items in WM. In the verbal condition, the visual cue and the memory probe tests in Fig. 26.1 were replaced by coloured words (i.e. 'Red', 'Green'). Soto et al. found that biases of visual attention linked to visual cues in WM were associated with increased activity in the left superior frontal gyrus (SFG), while biases of visual attention driven by verbal information in WM modulated responses in the lateral occipital cortex (LOC) (Soto et al. 2012d). This finding suggests two things. One is that biases may come from distinct sources, determined by whether visual or verbal information is represented in WM. The second is that WM biases may operate through neuroanatomical substrates that provide top-down support of earlier visual processing regions; the SFG is a good potential source for biasing visual coding from WM biasing signals because it contains regions (e.g. around the frontal eye fields) which are densely connected to visual cortex (Schall et al. 1995; Moore and Armstrong 2003). The LOC is a visual processing area associated with object recognition (Grill-Spector et al. 1998; Kourtzi and Kanwisher 2000) and visual WM (Xu and Chun 2006) plus also cross-modal sensory processing (Amedi et al. 2007) and semantic processing (Mechelli et al. 2007). Verbal WM may bias visual selection by modulating neural regions associated with semantic analysis of perceptual input.

fMRI studies are also informative for understanding why WM biases are reduced at high memory loads. Soto et al. (2012d) varied the load in WM before participants undertook visual search. Confirming previous results, Soto et al. (2012d) found a robust attentional bias when a single item was held in WM and then repeated in the search display (as in Fig. 26.1). This WM bias then virtually disappeared when WM capacity was taxed with three items. We have argued above that this reduction in WM bias was unlikely to be due to cognitive control structures becoming more engaged under high load conditions. Consistent with this, Soto et al. (2012a) found no increase in activity in prefrontal regions associated with cognitive control as the memory load increased. It could also not simply be the case that representations of the memory cues are lost due to inter-item competition at high WM loads because the presence of WM biases was examined only when participants correctly remembered the information retained on every trial. In addition, even though the WM biases of behaviour were eliminated, there was increased activation in visual cortical regions when WM cues were re-presented in search at high memory loads. This did not reflect the greater load in WM as the increase in visual activation was greater when the WM item was re-presented than when it did not reappear (in a neutral condition). However, the functional coupling between pre-frontal regions (around the ventral anterior inferior prefrontal cortex) and the visual cortex reduced as the load increased. These data suggest that WM biases on attention are brought about through functional cross-talk between frontal and visual brain regions. Items held in the foreground of WM generate stronger coupling even when irrelevant to the task, while increases in memory load decrease this coupling.

In contrast to the neural regions implicated in WM-based guidance of attention, the operation of task-based control of behaviour is typically thought to operate through a network of areas within parietal and frontal brain regions (Corbetta and Shulman 2002). Task-based control of visual attention, for example, may reflect the modulation of visual cortical regions through this fronto-parietal network. For example, this network shows enhanced activity prior to the onset of expected stimuli reflecting task-based prioritiza- tion of upcoming stimuli (Corbetta and Shulman 2002). Intriguingly, involvement of the posterior parietal cortex (PPC) has not been associated with the presence of WM biases on visual selection (Soto et al. 2007, 2011b). For instance, PPC activity has not been found to be sensitive either to the reappearance of the WM cue in search, or to the validity of the cue in imaging studies of WM biases on attention. Also, visual extinction is strongly associated with damage to the PPC (e.g. Chechlacz et al. 2013) yet, as we have noted, visual 'extinction' patients can nevertheless display WM biases in visual selec- tion tasks (Soto and Humphreys 2006; Soto et al. 2011a). These last data indicate that the PPC is not necessary for WM to guide attention. However, as we have noted, there are conditions where there is task control over WM. A cautious interpretation would be that, in these imaging studies, the conditions did not strongly promote strategic cog- nitive control over WM—for example, the validity of the WM stimulus for search has typically varied randomly on a trial-by-trial basis and therefore cue validity could not be actively anticipated by observers (Soto et al. 2007, 2011b; Grecucci et al. 2010).

The behavioural work indicates that task-based control processes are recruited more strongly when the relation between the WM cue and the subsequent task can be predicted (e.g. when the cue is always invalid; Kiyonaga et al., 2012; Han and Kim 2009). Studies need to assess whether the PPC is recruited to modulate the interaction between WM and attention under such conditions before we conclude that the PPC plays no role. Some evi- dence that is consistent with this possibility has been recently reported (Soto et al. 2012b). Specifically, Soto and colleagues (2012b) delineated a novel parieto-medial temporal pathway, involving the posterior parietal cortex, the hippocampus proper, and also the posterior cingulate cortex, which may be critical for the wilful regulation of WM biases on visual selection. In particular, the PPC showed anticipatory activity based on foreknowl- edge of the validity of WM for search, with activity in the PPC enhanced when the WM items were highly predictive of the target or the search distractor. In a similar manner, the hippocampus along with the posterior cingulate were associated with the individu- al's ability to either enhance or inhibit the influence of WM on the search task based on foreknowledge of whether the WM cue was predictive (see Fig. 26.5 for more details). The data provide some indication that parietal areas concerned with task-based control are recruited in conjunction with memory regions to modulate WM biases on attention, which may otherwise be established through fronto-thalamic links with visual cortex.

CONCLUSION

Our review has highlighted the relations between WM, attention, and task-based con- trol of behaviour. Traditionally, WM has been assigned a key role in cognition in which it is thought to modulate task-based biases on attentional selection. We have argued that

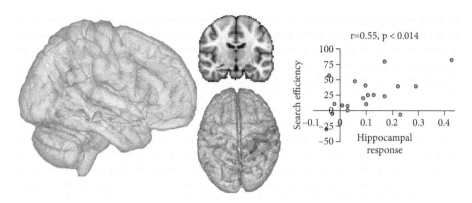

FIGURE 26.5 Regions involved in strategic cognitive control over WM biases of selection based on foreknowledge of WM validity for search. Middle temporal regions, including the hippocampus proper and also the posterior cingulate cortex, showed increased activation when the WM cues reliably coincided on a trial-by-trial basis with targets or distractors than when cue–target relations could not be anticipated. We also depict the correlation between the hippocampal response and the benefits in search efficiency gained from suppressing expected WM distractors or by enhancing WM items that are known to surround the forthcoming target. Interestingly, posterior parietal cortices were modulated by the cue period only, showing anticipatory signals when observers have foreknowledge that the WM cue is a valid predictor of the search target (in green) or when it reliably predicted an invalid search distractor (in red), relative to when there was no such foreknowledge. Reproduced from Soto et al. (2012b) <http://www.jneurosci.org> Reproduced from Soto, D., Greene, C. M., Kiyonaga, A., Rosenthal, C. R., and Egner, T., A parieto-medial temporal pathway for the strategic control over working memory biases in human visual attention, *Journal of Neuroscience*, 32, pp. 17563–17571 © 2012, The Society for Neuroscience.

the situation is more complex than this. We have suggested that WM can operate in a relatively modular manner, divorced from the effects of task-based control—though task-based control can be brought to bear under suitable conditions and, under everyday conditions, WM is often recruited to help implement task-based control. We also propose that WM itself can be fractionated not only into modality-specific components (visual and verbal components) but also into foreground and background representations. Items held in the foreground of WM modulate attentional selection in a relatively automatic way that can be distinct from effects of task control. This compartmentalization of WM into foreground and background components may have additional benefits; notably this compartmentalization can facilitate the switching of attention between task-specific and task-irrelevant stimuli by separating task-specific representations from the representations of other stimuli. In addition, there are intriguing suggestions that non-conscious items may nevertheless permeate into WM systems and be maintained and used to control subsequent behaviour. Further stimuli can be brought into consciousness by contact with WM representations. The results indicate how, by studying how WM interacts with attention and task-based control processes, we can learn about the structure and operation of WM itself.

ACKNOWLEDGEMENTS

This work was supported by grants from the MRC (89631), the Stroke Association, NIHR, and the European Research Council (Project PePE 323883).

REFERENCES

Amedi, A., Stern, W. M., Camprodon, J. A., Bermpohl, F., Merabet, L., Rotman, S., Hemond, C., Meijer, P., and Pascual-Leone, A. (2007). Shape conveyed by visual-to-auditory sensory substitution activates the lateral occipital complex. *Nature Neuroscience 10*: 687–689.

Astle, D. E., Nobre, A. C., and Scerif, G. (2009). Subliminally presented and stored objects capture spatial attention. *Journal of Neuroscience 30*: 3567–3571.

Baddeley, A. D. (1986). *Working Memory*. Oxford: Oxford University Press.

Baddeley, A. D. (2000). The episodic buffer: A new component of working memory? *Trends in Cognitive Sciences 4*(11): 417–423.

Baddeley, A. D., and Hitch, G. J. (1974). Working memory. In G. A. Bower (ed.), *The Psychology of Learning and Motivation: Advances in Research and Theory 8*(pp. 47–89). New York: Academic Press.

Bahrami-Balani, A., Soto, D., and Humphreys, G. W. (2010). Working memory and target-related distractor effects on visual search. *Memory & Cognition, 38*(8): 1058–1076.

Balani, A. B., Soto, D., and Humphreys, G. W. (2011). Working memory and target-related distractor effects on visual search. *Memory and Cognition 38*: 1058–1076.

Bar, M. and Biederman, I. (1998). Subliminal visual priming. *Psychological Science 9*: 464–469.

Bays, P. M. and Husain, M. (2008). Dynamic shifts of limited working memory resources in human vision. *Science 321*: 851–854.

Blanco, M. J. and Soto, D. (2002). Effects of spatial attention on detection and identification of oriented lines. *Acta Psychologica (Amsterdam) 109*: 195–212.

Bundesen, C. (1990). A theory of visual attention. *Psychological Review 97*(4): 523–547.

Carlisle, N. B. and Woodman, G. F. (2011a). When memory is not enough: Electrophysiological evidence for goal-dependent use of working memory representations in guiding visual attention. *Journal of Cognitive Neuroscience 23*: 2650–2664.

Carlisle, N. B. and Woodman, G. F. (2011b). Automatic and strategic effects in the guidance of attention by working memory representations. *Acta Psychologica (Amsterdam) 137*: 217–225.

Carrasco, M., Penpeci-Talgar, C., and Eckstein, M. (2000). Spatial covert attention increases contrast sensitivity across the CSF: Support for signal enhancement. *Vision Research 40*: 1203–1215.

Chechlacz, M., Terry, A., Demeyere, N., Douis, H., Bickerton, W. L., Rotshtein, P., and Humphreys, G. W. (2013). Common and distinct neural mechanisms of visual and tactile extinction: A large scale VBM study in sub-acute stroke. *NeuroImage: Clinical 2*: 291–302.

Chelazzi, L., Duncan, J., Miller, E. K., and Desimone, R. (1998). Responses of neurons in inferior temporal cortex during memory-guided visual search. *Journal of Neurophysiology 80*: 2918–2940.

Corbetta, M. and Shulman, G. L. (2002). Control of goal-directed and stimulus-driven attention in the brain. *Nature Reviews Neuroscience* 3(3): 201–215.

Cosman, J. D. and Vecera, S. P. (2011). The contents of visual working memory reduce uncertainty during visual search. *Attention, Perception, & Psychophysics* 73: 996–1002.

Dalvit, S. and Eimer, M. (2011). Mechanisms of percept–percept and image–percept integration in vision: Behavioral and electrophysiological evidence. *Journal of Experimental Psychology: Human Perception and Performance* 37(1): 1–11.

de Fockert, J. W., Rees, G., Frith, C. D., and Lavie, N. (2001). The role of working memory in visual selective attention. *Science* 291: 1803–1806.

Desimone, R., and Duncan, J. (1995). Neural mechanisms of selective visual attention. *Annual Review of Neuroscience* 18(1): 193–222.

Dombrowe, I., Olivers, C. N. L., and Donk, M. (2010). The time course of working memory effects on visual attention differs depending on memory type. *Visual Cognition* 18: 1089–1112.

Downing, C. J. (1988). Expectancy and visual-spatial attention: Effects on perceptual quality. *Journal of Experimental Psychology: Human Perception and Performance* 14: 188–202.

Downing, P. E. (2000). Interactions between visual working memory and selective attention. *Psychological Science* 11: 467–473.

Downing, P. E. and Dodds, C. M. (2004). Competition in visual working memory for control of search. *Visual Cognition* 11: 689–703.

Duncan-Johnson, C. C. and Donchin, E. (1977). On quantifying surprise: The variation of event-related potentials with subjective probability. *Psychophysiology* 14: 456–467.

Fan, J., McCandliss, B. D., Sommer, T., Raz, A., and Posner, M. I. (2002). Testing the efficiency and independence of attentional networks. *Journal of Cognitive Neuroscience* 14: 340–347.

Grecucci, A., Soto, D., Rumiati, R. I., Humphreys, G. W., and Rotshtein, P. (2010). The interrelations between verbal working memory and visual selection of emotional faces. *Journal of Cognitive Neuroscience* 22: 1189–1200.

Greene, C. M. and Soto, D. (2012). Neural repetition effects in the medial temporal lobe complex are modulated by previous encoding experience. *PLoS One* 7: e40870.

Grill-Spector, K., Henson, R., and Martin, A. (2006). Repetition and the brain: Neural models of stimulus-specific effects. *Trends in Cognitive Sciences* 10: 14–23.

Grill-Spector, K., Kushnir, T., Edelman, S., Itzchak, Y., and Malach, R. (1998). Cue-invariant activation in object-related areas of the human occipital lobe. *Neuron* 21: 191–202.

Han, S. W. and Kim, M. S. (2009). Do the contents of working memory capture attention? Yes, but cognitive control matters. *Journal of Experimental Psychology: Human Perception and Performance* 35(5): 1292–1302.

Hopf, J. M., Luck, S. J., Girelli, M., Hagner, T., Mangun, G. R., Scheich, H., and Heinze, H. J. (2000). Neural sources of focused attention in visual search. *Cerebral Cortex* 10(12): 1233–1241.

Houtkamp, R. and Roelfsema, P. R. (2006). The effect of items in working memory on the deployment of attention and the eyes during visual search. *Journal of Experimental Psychology: Human Perception and Performance* 32: 423–442.

Kastner, S., Pinsk, M. A., De Weerd, P., Desimone, R., and Ungerleider, L. G. (1999). Increased activity in human visual cortex during directed attention in the absence of visual stimulation. *Neuron* 22: 751–761.

Kim, S. Y., Kim, M. S., and Chun, M. M. (2005). Concurrent working memory load can reduce distraction. *Proceedings of the National Academy of Sciences USA* 102: 16524–16529.

Kiyonaga, A., Egner, T., and Soto, D. (2012). Cognitive control over working memory biases of selection. *Psychonomic Bulletin & Review* 19: 639–646.

Koivisto, M. and Revonsuo, A. (2007). How meaning shapes seeing. *Psychological Science* 18: 845–849.

Kouider, S. and Dehaene, S. (2007). Levels of processing during non-conscious perception: A critical review of visual masking. *Philosophical Transactions of the Royal Society of London B: Biological Sciences* 362: 857–875.

Kourtzi, Z. and Kanwisher, N. (2000). Cortical regions involved in perceiving object shape. *Journal of Neuroscience* 20: 3310–3318.

Kumar, S., Soto, D., and Humphreys, G. W. (2009). Electrophysiological evidence for attentional guidance by the contents of working memory. *European Journal of Neuroscience* 30: 307–317.

Kunst-Wilson, W. R. and Zajonc, R. B. (1980). Affective discrimination of stimuli that cannot be recognized. *Science* 207: 557–558.

Luck, S. J. and Hillyard, S. A. (1994). Spatial filtering during visual search: Evidence from human electrophysiology. *Journal of Experimental Psychology: Human Perception and Performance* 20(5): 1000.

Luck, S. J., Chelazzi, L., Hillyard, S. A., and Desimone, R. (1997). Neural mechanisms of spatial selective attention in areas V1, V2, and V4 of macaque visual cortex. *Journal of Neurophysiology* 77: 24–42.

Machizawa, M. G. and Driver, J. (2011). Principal component analysis of behavioural individual differences suggests that particular aspects of visual working memory may relate to specific aspects of attention. *Neuropsychologia* 49(6): 1518–1526.

Mannan, S. K., Kennard, C., Potter, D., Pan, Y., and Soto, D. (2010). Early oculomotor capture by new onsets driven by the contents of working memory. *Vision Research* 50(16): 1590–1597.

Mazza, V., Dallabona, M., Chelazzi, L., and Turatto, M. (2011). Cooperative and opposing effects of strategic and involuntary attention. *Journal of Cognitive Neuroscience* 23: 2838–2851.

Mechelli, A., Josephs, O., Lambon Ralph, M. A., McClelland, J. L., and Price, C. J. (2007). Dissociating stimulus-driven semantic and phonological effect during reading and naming. *Human Brain Mapping* 28: 205–217.

Miller, E. K. and Cohen, J. D. (2001). An integrative theory of prefrontal cortex function. *Annual Review of Neuroscience* 24: 167–202.

Moore, T. and Armstrong, K. M. (2003). Selective gating of visual signals by microstimulation of frontal cortex. *Nature* 421: 370–373.

Moores, E. and Maxwell, J. P. (2008). The role of prior exposure on the capture of attention by items in working memory. *Visual Cognition* 16: 675–695.

Moores, E., Laiti, L., and Chelazzi, L. (2003). Associative knowledge controls deployment of visual selective attention. *Nature Neuroscience* 6(2): 182–189.

Most, S. B., Scholl, B. J., Clifford, E. R., and Simons, D. J. (2005). What you see is what you set: Sustained inattentional blindness and the capture of awareness. *Psychological Review* 112: 217–242.

Norman, D. A. and Shallice, T. (1986). Attention to action: Willed and automatic control of behaviour. In R. J. Davidson, G. E. Schwartz, and D. Shapiro (eds.), *Consciousness and Self Regulation* (pp. 1–18). New York: Plenum Press.

Oberauer, K. (2002). Access to information in working memory: Exploring the focus of attention. *Journal of Experimental Psychology: Learning, Memory, and Cognition* 28: 411–421.

Olivers, C. N., Meijer, F., and Theeuwes, J. (2006). Feature-based memory-driven attentional capture: Visual working memory content affects visual attention. *Journal of Experimental Psychology: Human Perception and Performance* 32: 1243–1265.

Olivers, C. N., Peters, J., Houtkamp, R., and Roelfsema, P. R. (2011). Different states in visual working memory: When it guides attention and when it does not. *Trends in Cognitive Sciences* 15: 327–334.

Pan, Y., Lin, B., Zhao, Y., and Soto, D. (in press). Working memory biasing of visual perception without awareness. *Attention, Perception, & Psychophysics*.

Pan, Y. and Soto, D. (2010). The modulation of perceptual selection by working memory is dependent on the focus of spatial attention. *Vision Research* 50: 1437–1444.

Pan, Y., Xu, B., and Soto, D. (2009). Dimension-based working memory-driven capture of visual selection. *Quarterly Journal of Experimental Psychology (Hove)* 62: 1123–1131.

Park, S., Kim, M. S., and Chun, M. M. (2007). Concurrent working memory load can facilitate selective attention: Evidence for specialized load. *Journal of Experimental Psychology: Human Perception and Performance* 33: 1062–1075.

Peters, J. C., Goebel, R., and Roelfsema, P. R. (2009). Remembered but unused: The accessory items in working memory that do not guide attention. *Journal of Cognitive Neuroscience* 21: 1081–1091.

Rainer, G., Asaad, W. F., and Miller, E. K. (1998). Selective representation of relevant information by neurons in the primate prefrontal cortex. *Nature* 393: 577–579.

Rao, S. C., Rainer, G., and Miller, E. K. (1997). Integration of what and where in the primate prefrontal cortex. *Science* 276: 821–824.

Schall, J. D., Morel, A., King, D. J., and Bullier, J. (1995). Topography of visual cortex connections with frontal eye field in macaque: Convergence and segregation of processing streams. *Journal of Neuroscience* 15: 4464–4487.

Silvanto, J. and Cattaneo, Z. (2010). Transcranial magnetic stimulation reveals the content of visual short-term memory in the visual cortex. *NeuroImage* 50: 1683–1689.

Soto, D. and Humphreys, G. W. (2006). Seeing the content of the mind: Enhanced awareness through working memory in patients with visual extinction. *Proceedings of the National Academy of Sciences USA* 103: 4789–4792.

Soto, D. and Humphreys, G. W. (2007). Automatic guidance of visual attention from verbal working memory. *Journal of Experimental Psychology: Human Perception and Performance* 33: 730–737.

Soto, D. and Humphreys, G. W. (2008). Stressing the mind: The effect of cognitive load and articulatory suppression on attentional guidance from working memory. *Perception & Psychophysics* 70: 924–934.

Soto, D., Heinke, D., Humphreys, G. W., and Blanco, M. J. (2005). Early, involuntary top-down guidance of attention from working memory. *Journal of Experimental Psychology: Human Perception and Performance* 31: 248–261.

Soto, D., Humphreys, G. W., and Heinke, D. (2006). Working memory can guide pop-out search. *Vision Research* 46: 1010–1018.

Soto, D., Humphreys, G. W., and Rotshtein, P. (2007). Dissociating the neural mechanisms of memory-based guidance of visual selection. *Proceedings of the National Academy of Sciences USA* 104: 17186–17191.

Soto, D., Mannan, S. K., Malhotra, P., Rzeskiewicz, A., and Humphreys, G. W. (2011a). Distinguishing non-spatial from spatial biases in visual selection: neuropsychological evidence. *Acta Psychologica (Amsterdam)* 137: 226–234.

Soto, D., Mok, A. Y., McRobbie, D., Quest, R., Waldman, A., and Rotshtein, P. (2011b). Biasing visual selection: Functional neuroimaging of the interplay between spatial cueing and feature memory guidance. *Neuropsychologia* 49: 1537–1543.

Soto, D., Wriglesworth, A., Bahrami-Balani, A., and Humphreys, G. W. (2010). Working memory enhances visual perception: Evidence from signal detection analysis. *Journal of Experimental Psychology: Learning, Memory, and Cognition* 36: 441–456.

Soto, D., Greene, C. M., Chaudhary, A., and Rotshtein, P. (2012a). Competition in working memory reduces frontal guidance of visual selection. *Cerebral Cortex* 22: 1159–1169.

Soto, D., Greene, C. M., Kiyonaga, A., Rosenthal, C. R., and Egner, T. (2012b). A parieto-medial temporal pathway for the strategic control over working memory biases in human visual attention. *Journal of Neuroscience* 32: 17563–17571.

Soto, D., Llewelyn, D., and Silvanto, J. (2012c). Distinct causal mechanisms of attentional guidance by working memory and repetition priming in early visual cortex. *Journal of Neuroscience* 32: 3447–3452.

Soto, D., Rotshtein, P., Hodsoll, J., Mevorach, C., and Humphreys, G. W. (2012d). Common and distinct neural regions for the guidance of selection by visuoverbal information held in memory: Converging evidence from fMRI and rTMS. *Human Brain Mapping* 33: 105–120.

Telling, A. L., Kumar, S., Meyer, A. S., and Humphreys, G. W. (2010). Electrophysiological evidence of semantic interference in visual search. *Journal of Cognitive Neuroscience* 22: 2212–2225.

Theeuwes, J. and Van der Burg, E. (2007). The role of spatial and nonspatial information in visual selection. *Journal of Experimental Psychology: Human Perception and Performance* 33: 1335–1351.

Van der Stigchel, S., Meeter, M., and Theeuwes, J. (2006). Eye movement trajectories and what they tell us. *Neuroscience & Biobehavioural Reviews* 30: 666–679.

Vogel, E. K., McCollough, A. W., and Machizawa, M. G. (2005). Neural measures reveal individual differences in controlling access to working memory. *Nature* 438: 500–503.

Wiggs, C. L. and Martin, A. (1998). Properties and mechanisms of perceptual priming. *Current Opinion in Neurobiology* 8: 227–233.

Wolfe, J. M., Cave, K. R., and Franzel, S. L. (1989). Guided search: An alternative to the feature integration model for visual search. *Journal of Experimental Psychology: Human Perception and Performance* 15: 419–433.

Woodman, G. F. and Luck, S. J. (2007). Do the contents of visual working memory automatically influence attentional selection during visual search? *Journal of Experimental Psychology: Human Perception and Performance* 33: 363–377.

Xu, Y. and Chun, M. M. (2006). Dissociable neural mechanisms supporting visual short-term memory for objects. *Nature* 440: 91–95.

Yantis, S. and Jonides, J. (1984). Abrupt visual onsets and selective attention: Evidence from visual search. *Journal of Experimental Psychology: Human Perception & Performance* 10: 601–621.

Zhang, B., Zhang, J. X., Huang, S., Kong, L., and Wang, S. (2011). Effects of load on the guidance of visual attention from working memory. *Vision Research* 51: 2356–2361.

Zhang, W. and Luck, S. J. (2008). Discrete fixed-resolution representations in visual working memory. *Nature* 453: 233–235.

CHAPTER 27

NEURAL MECHANISMS FOR THE EXECUTIVE CONTROL OF ATTENTION

EARL K. MILLER AND TIMOTHY J. BUSCHMAN

INTRODUCTION

TOP-down, or 'executive' control is the ability to use previously acquired internal information to select a (typically unseen) goal, plan corresponding actions, and then keep thought and action 'on task' while achieving it. This is the core of intelligent, rational, behaviour—a brain that doesn't just react to the world, but acquires information and uses it to act on the world in order to obtain future objectives.

To do so, the brain needs to deal with its limited capacity: The mental sketchpad where all this planning and organization occurs (known as 'working memory') is severely limited in its capacity. While we can store apparently unlimited amounts of items in a latent form (i.e. in long-term memory and as habits), many studies have shown that the neural mechanisms employed when we consciously 'think' can only hold a few (three to four) items simultaneously. The central challenge of executive control, then, is how finite cognitive resources are brought to bear on the information (sensory inputs, stored memories, action plans, strategies, etc.) that is currently important for the goal at hand and how potential distractions are excluded. When this is applied to the external world, we call it attention.

The distractions are often inherently salient stimuli (such as a police siren or a looming object). Our brains reflexively orient to such strong, 'bottom-up' sensory inputs because they often signal events that need an immediate response (like ducking). By contrast, the type of attention that is synonymous with executive control is called 'top-down' because it is based on acquired knowledge. We choose to pay attention to something (like a lecture or a clock on the wall) because we have learned it is important for achieving a goal.

This is the subject of this chapter. We review evidence that top-down attention signals originate from a brain region thought to be central to executive control, the prefrontal cortex. We will discuss candidate neural mechanisms that may mediate focusing of attention. Then, we will broaden the discussion to the neural mechanisms that allow the brain to learn what is important and worth attending to. But first, we begin with a discussion of why attention is needed in the first place: the limitation in cognitive capacity.

SELECTIVE ATTENTION COMPENSATES FOR LIMITED COGNITIVE CAPACITY

The finite resources of cognition have been well known since the classic George Miller paper describing the capacity of working memory as the 'magic number' of seven plus or minus two (Miller 1956). More recent work, using stimuli that cannot be easily combined or 'chunked', has lowered the magic number to three to four for the average adult human (Cowan 2001; similar to the average monkey, as we will see below). In a typical task, subjects are asked to hold a varying number of visual stimuli 'in mind' for a brief period and then report the contents (Luck and Vogel 1997). When the number of stimuli increase to the point that subjects make errors (they begin to lose one or more of the stimuli), their capacity has been exceeded. The exact capacity of a person varies from individual to individual; some can remember only 1–2 items and others can remember up to 7 (Vogel and Machizawa 2004; Vogel et al. 2005). An individual's capacity is highly correlated with measures of fluid intelligence, reflecting the fact that these capacity limits are a fundamental restriction in high-level cognition (Engle et al. 1999; Fukuda et al. 2010). This makes sense: the more thoughts that can be simultaneously held 'in mind' and manipulated, the more associations, connections, and relationships can be made, and the more sophisticated thought can be.

Not only is attention the 'gate-keeper' to these finite resources, it may itself be the bottleneck. This was nicely illustrated by Edward Vogel and colleagues. They showed that much of the variability in cognitive capacity among individuals reflects differences in how well they can filter out distracting information (Vogel et al. 2005). Human subjects briefly saw two arrays, up to eight coloured squares, separated by a memory delay (Fig. 27.1a). On half of the trials one of the squares changed colour from the first array to the second. The subjects' task was to report whether a change occurred. In order to test the impact of attention on the variance in capacity, the authors directed subjects to attend to one half of the display, indicating the colour change was more likely to occur in that half. Using electrophysiological and behavioural measures, Vogel and colleagues were able to determine the amount of information subjects were able to retain (Fig. 27.1b). They found that subjects with low capacities were ineffective in excluding irrelevant

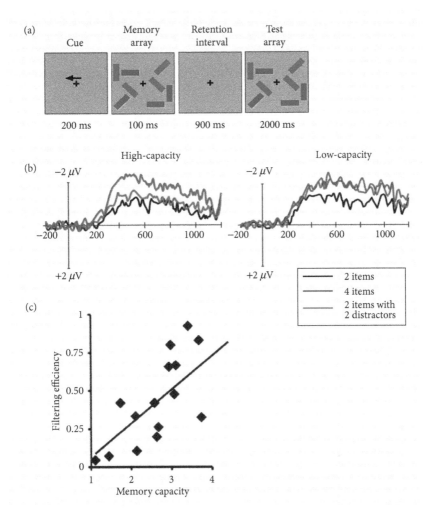

FIGURE 27.1 Human test and correlates of cognitive capacity limitations. (a) The subject needs to detect if one of the coloured bars changes from one display to the next. An arrow indicates the likely side of the change. (b) The magnitude of human evoked potential recordings from the scalp showed dependence on the number of items that need to be processed and retained. Note that the evoked potential for high-capacity subjects (left) showed the same level for two items as for two items with two irrelevant distractors. By contrast, in low-capacity subjects, the evoked potential for two items with two distractors is the same as when four items needed to be retained. This indicates that the low-capacity subjects could not filter out the two irrelevant distractors. (c) The relation between filtering and capacity. Subjects that are better at filtering out items that were not cued show greater capacity limits. Reprinted by permission from Macmillan Publishers Ltd: *Nature*, 438 (7067), Edward K. Vogel, Andrew W. McCollough and Maro G. Machizawa, Neural measures reveal individual differences in controlling access to working memory, pp. 500–503, copyright (2005), Nature Publishing Group.

information that they were directed to ignore. In contrast, high-capacity individuals were not capable of storing more total information; they were just more effective in filtering out distracting information (Fig. 27.1c). In other words, it is not the capacity of individuals that varies but their ability to use attention to control the contents of working memory.

The close relationship between cognitive capacity and attentional capacity has been underscored by other studies as well. For example, adult humans can typically attend to, and track, about four moving objects at a time, a task that has no explicit working memory requirement but rather requires dividing attention (Pylyshyn and Storm 1988; Cavanagh and Alvarez 2005; Drew and Vogel 2008). This capacity is also correlated with their fluid intelligence (Oksama and Hyana 2004). In fact, even when items are absent (and therefore in working memory) there is an intimate relationship between attention and the ability to maintain those memories (Awh and Jonides 2001; Postle et al. 2004). For example, engaging spatial working memory improves visual recognition at remembered locations, similar to directing attention to items when they are actually present. When attention is shifted to a second, parallel, task, spatial memory in the primary task is compromised (Awh et al. 1998). The reverse is also true: holding items in working memory compromises attention. For example, Woodman and Luck asked humans to perform a visual search task (requiring directing attention) while concurrently performing a visual-spatial working memory task and found that increasing a person's working memory load slowed their attentional search speed (Woodman and Luck 2004). Such interactions between working memory and attention suggest a singular capacity is tapped by both behaviours.

An attention bottleneck is also suggested by neurophysiological studies in monkeys that show that when capacity is exceeded, the information loss is in initial encoding of stimuli, not their subsequent retention. Buschman et al. (2011) trained monkeys on a task similar to that used by Vogel and colleagues (see above). Two arrays of two to five coloured squares were separated by a brief memory delay. In this case, one of the squares always changed colour and monkeys had to indicate which one by making an eye movement to it. When capacity was exceeded (as with humans, this occurred around four items) the loss of neural information about the squares was apparent right from the beginning of neural activation to the stimuli. That is, information was lost as the stimuli were being attended and encoded, well before the memory delay. Buschman et al. also found that the monkeys' apparent overall capacity of four items was actually composed of two separate capacities of two and two in the right and left halves of visual space that were independent of each other. In other words, the ability to encode and retain an item on the right half of space, for example, was unaffected by items in the left half of space, regardless of how many items there were on the left (and vice versa). But adding even one more item on the same (right) side impaired performance. This suggests that the right and left cerebral hemispheres can independently process the two halves of visual space and have independent finite resources. The apparent split between the two hemispheres recalls some of the initial observations of humans who had their cerebral hemispheres split to control epilepsy. Without careful testing these subjects usually appear normal. Thus, there may be something of a split even in the intact brain.

Hemifield independence further underscores the close relationship between attentional capacity and general cognitive capacity. Neurophysiological studies, for example, have demonstrated that in visual cortex, attentional filtering is strongest (indeed, often only apparent) when the attended object or location is on the same half of visual space as the to-be-filtered item (Desimone and Duncan 1995). Only at the level of prefrontal cortex do attentional effects seem to bridge the vertical visual meridian (Everling et al. 2002) but, even then, there is a strong bias toward contralateral representation (Rainer et al. 1998a). Finally, the strongest evidence for human hemifield independence comes from divided-attention tasks like multiple object tracking, where attention can be split between the visual hemifields (Alvarez and Cavanagh 2005; Cavanagh and Alvarez 2005).

What all this suggests is that cognitive capacity limitations are not due to limitations in working memory per se. Rather, it reflects a fundamental limitation in the number of separate items that can be represented simultaneously in neural activity, particularly in an active state that is accessible to high-level cognition. But why exactly is this format of neural coding so limited in capacity? One hint comes from the mounting evidence that information encoding during cognitively demanding tasks may depend on the temporal dynamics *between* neurons, a format that has a natural limitation in bandwidth. It has long been known that the electrical potentials that reflect the summed activity of many neurons show a wide range of rhythmic synchronized oscillations (from 1 to 100 Hz), often called 'brain waves'. A number of brain areas in monkeys, humans, and rodents show increases in oscillations during cognitively demanding tasks (Tallon-Baudry et al. 1998; Lee et al. 2005; Jensen et al. 2007; Pesaran et al. 2008). Information may be encoded by alignment of spikes from individual neurons to specific phases of neuronal population oscillations (O'Keefe 1993; Hopfield and Herz 1995; Konig et al. 1995; Laurent 2002; Mehta et al. 2002; Brody et al. 2003; Lee et al. 2005; Fries et al. 2007; Montemurro et al. 2008; Kayser et al. 2009). For example, in the rat hippocampus, spatial information may be encoded at specific phases of ongoing population theta-oscillations (O'Keefe 1993; Mehta et al. 2002; Dragoi and Buzsaki 2006). This has led to the hypothesis that multiple items are simultaneously held 'in mind' by multiplexing them at different phases of population oscillations (Lisman and Idiart 1995; Jensen and Lisman 2005). In other words, the mechanisms for conscious thought 'juggle' separate items by oscillating them out of phase of one another. This has an inherent capacity limitation because, presumably, only so much information can fit within an oscillatory cycle (that is, only a few 'balls' can be juggled at once). Evidence for this multiplexing was recently reported by Siegel et al. (2009): when monkeys held multiple objects in working memory, prefrontal neurons encoded information about each object at different phases of an ongoing, ~32 Hz, oscillation. More work is needed, but all this suggests that making thoughts conscious may depend on generation of oscillatory rhythms and the precise temporal relationships between them and the spiking of neurons representing the conscious thoughts. In short, attention may gate access to brain waves.

The central problem of attention, then, is the same as that of executive control in general: How does the brain's executive mechanism figure out what information is important enough to be in this active state? We will consider that later in this review. But first we have to find out where the executive may be.

Finding the 'Top' in the Top-Down Control of Attention

The term 'executive' implies a hierarchy with a certain brain area or areas providing top-down control to other less-executive brain areas. A good place to look for this is the frontal-parietal network, which is thought to play a central role in attention (Corbetta et al. 1993, 1995, 1998; Coull and Nobre 1998; Donner et al. 2000, 2002; Nobre et al. 2002). In humans, there are regions in the parietal cortex (specifically within the intraparietal sulcus) and prefrontal cortex (including the human analogue of the monkey frontal eye fields in the precentral sulcus) that show increased blood flow when attention is shifted or focused (Corbetta et al. 1993; Coull and Nobre 1998; Corbetta and Shulman 2002; Liu et al. 2003). Damage to these brain regions can cause deficits in attention (Eglin et al. 1991; Knight et al. 1995; Knight 1997).

In monkeys, both top-down and bottom-up shifts of attention modulate neural activity in the parietal (particularly in the lateral intraparietal area, or LIP) and frontal cortex (both the lateral prefrontal cortex, LPFC and the frontal eye fields, FEF; Bichot and Schall 1999; Hasegawa et al. 2000; Bisley and Goldberg 2003; Buschman and Miller 2007; Johnston and Everling 2009; Moore et al. 2009). Neurons in these areas respond more vigorously to visual stimuli that are task relevant (and therefore must be attended) and show little or no activity to irrelevant stimuli (that must be ignored; Rainer et al. 1998b; Everling et al. 2006). A highly influential theory, Desimone and Duncan's Biased Competition Model, suggests that this occurs because neural representations of different stimuli compete for activation by inhibiting one another (Desimone and Duncan 1995). Top-down or bottom-up signals add extra neural energy to the to-be-attended stimuli. This tips the balance of the competition and results in the attended representations winning the competition.

But which is on top, the prefrontal or parietal cortex? Evidence suggests that the parietal cortex is more involved in the bottom-up capture of attention whereas the prefrontal cortex is more central to top-down executive control of attention. LIP seems to have a saliency map—a topographic map of the visual field where each position is weighted by the saliency, or noticeability, of a stimulus at that location. Neurons in LIP reflect the attentional priority of stimuli in their receptive field (Bisley and Goldberg 2003) and are known to respond transiently to flashed stimuli, which can automatically draw attention (Bisley and Goldberg 2006). Further, LIP neurons reflect the target location of a pop-out stimulus very quickly, at about 80 ms after the onset of the stimulus array (Ipata et al. 2006). By contrast, PFC neurons carry more information about a task-relevant stimulus than a salient, but irrelevant, visual stimulus (Hasegawa et al. 2000). Inactivating the lateral PFC with muscimol disrupts top-down visual search tasks, but not simple detection tasks (Iba and Sawaguchi 2003).

Many of the neurophysiological studies of PFC and LIP have employed single electrodes to study single neurons in each area alone. This approach is valuable for learning the properties of each but it makes it difficult to determine the relative roles of different areas. Thus, while both top-down and bottom-up attention shifts are reflected in both frontal and parietal cortex, it is possible that the neural effects seen in one or the other may have been computed in one and simply inherited by the other. To help sort this out, Buschman and Miller recorded from multiple electrodes simultaneously in PFC, FEF, and LIP of monkeys (Buschman and Miller 2007) while they performed a visual search task. This allowed for precise comparison of the timing of neural effects in each area. The logic is straightforward: An area with a shorter latency to show an effect (e.g. reflect a top-down shift of attention) is more likely to be the source of that signal than one with a longer latency.

In visual search, subjects search a visual field for a particular target stimulus (see Fig. 27.2; Treisman and Gelade 1980; Duncan and Humphreys 1989; Wolfe et al. 1989). When distractors (non-target stimuli) all differ from the target in a single dimension (Fig. 27.2a, top row) the target will stand out, or 'pop-out', from distracting stimuli, capturing attention in an automatic bottom-up manner. By contrast, when the distractors differ from the target in more than one dimension, and do so independently from one another (Fig. 27.2a, bottom row), the target no longer automatically grabs the subject's attention based on its inherent qualities. Instead, it must be selected by the subject's knowledge of which stimulus is the target (by top-down mechanisms). This results in an overall slower search speed and, generally, the time to find the target is a function of the number of total items in the search array (Treisman and Gelade 1980). We trained monkeys to alternate between the easy 'pop-out' condition and the difficult 'search' condition (Fig. 27.2). As has been found in humans, we found search time to be longer and more variable in search than pop-out (see also Iba and Sawaguchi 2003). Simultaneous neural recordings revealed that when attention was automatically captured by a salient stimulus in the bottom-up, pop-out, condition, the shift of attention appeared with a shorter latency in LIP than in the LPFC and FEF (Fig. 27.2b). This suggests the bottom-up attention signals flowed anteriorly in the brain from the parietal to the frontal cortex. By contrast, we found the opposite pattern of latencies for the top-down condition, when monkeys had to find the target based on their knowledge, rather than its salience. In that case, neural signals reflecting the shift of attention to the target appeared with a shorter latency in the frontal cortex (both LPFC and FEF) than LIP (Buschman and Miller 2007; Fig. 27.2b). Taken together, these results suggest that when attention is captured by external stimuli, selection of the target is 'bottom-up': fed forward from LIP (possibly as part of a saliency map) to frontal cortex. In contrast, during the internal direction of attention, the signals flow in the opposite direction: 'top-down' from the frontal lobe and fed back to the parietal cortex. Similar results have recently been found in humans (Li et al. 2010).

Other evidence for a frontal source of top-down signals comes from the work of Tirin Moore and colleagues (see Clark, Noudoost, Schafer, and Moore (chapter 13),

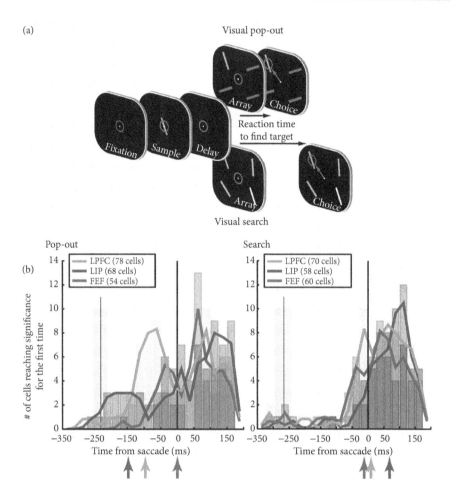

FIGURE 27.2 Pop-out vs. search tasks and neural correlates of the shift of attention to a visual target. (a) Monkeys were trained to find a target that matched a previously seen sample under search and pop-out conditions. The red circle indicates the monkey's eye position. See text for more details. (b) Distribution of times at which neurons first began to carry significant information about the target location (i.e. reflect the shift of attention to the target), relative to the saccade. Vertical black line indicates saccade, grey shaded regions indicate mean and +/− one standard deviation of distribution of visual array onset. The coloured arrows indicate when the shift of attention was first reflected in each cortical area. LPFC: lateral prefrontal cortex, LIP: lateral intraparietal area, FEF: frontal eye fields. As detailed in the text, parietal cortex reflects external capture of attention (pop-out) first, while prefrontal cortex (LPFC and FEF) direct internally guided shifts in attention (search).

this volume). Their work focuses on FEF, a portion of the posterior PFC that seems to be responsible for voluntary eye movements. They found that stimulating FEF neurons at sub-threshold levels (i.e. levels that would not elicit an eye movement) induces attention-like effects in V4 neurons: responses were increased for V4 neurons with receptive fields that overlap with the stimulated FEF neurons (Moore and Armstrong

2003). It was as if the stimulation elicited a top-down attention that acted on visual cortex. Further, microstimulation in FEF will also boost the animal's behavioural discriminability at the target location, suggesting the allocation of attentional resources to that location (Moore and Fallah 2001, 2004). These results suggest that FEF, a PFC sub-area known to play a role in generating volitional eye movements, plays a direct role in top-down attention.

Neural Synchrony and Attention

We previously discussed a possible role for oscillatory activity in holding multiple items in mind and how this may explain why cognition is capacity-limited. Oscillations seem to be involved in attention as well. Above, we mentioned how attentional selection occurs when to-be-attended stimuli gain a competitive edge over other representations (Desimone and Duncan 1995). This could occur by simply raising the level of overall activity of neurons. But there is mounting evidence that another way to boost neural representations is by synchronizing neural activity. Oscillations are a good way to do that.

Synchrony has been proposed to boost neural representations because spikes arriving simultaneously at downstream neurons have a greater impact than unsynchronized spikes (Aertsen et al. 1989b; Usrey and Reid 1999; Salinas and Sejnowski 2001; Fries 2005). Coincidence of spikes from multiple neurons converging on a post-synaptic neuron has a super-additive effect (Aertsen et al. 1989a; Usrey and Reid 1999; Engel et al. 2001; Salinas and Sejnowski 2001; Fries 2005). Therefore, if sensory neurons tuned to the same stimulus synchronize their firing, that stimulus will be more strongly represented in downstream areas (as its impact on those neurons is enhanced). In this fashion, local synchrony may help the brain to improve its signal-to-noise ratio while, at the same time, reducing the number of spikes needed to represent a stimulus (Aertsen et al. 1989a; Tiesinga et al. 2002; Siegel and Konig 2003). This mechanism seems ideal for focal attention which involves enhancing some stimulus representations at the expense of others.

Support for this idea comes from observations that attention correlates with increased spiking synchrony in visual cortex (Fries et al. 2001; Womelsdorf et al. 2006) and somatosensory cortex (Steinmetz et al. 2000; Bauer et al. 2006). For example, when a monkey's attention was directed to a particular visual stimulus, neurons in area V4 with receptive fields encompassing the attended stimulus showed increased synchrony in the gamma band (30–90 Hz) and a reduction in low frequency (<17 Hz) synchronization (Fries et al. 2001). Synchrony can also enhance neural processing by putting the brain and the external world in lockstep. Lakatos et al. (2008) presented monkeys with a stream of sequential visual and auditory stimuli and found that when monkeys attended to the visual or auditory stream, LFPs and spikes in visual cortex synchronized to the rhythm of the attended stream and not to the rhythm of an unattended stream.

Synchrony between regions may also regulate and sculpt communication between brain areas, helping top-down signals find their intended neural representations. If two brain areas oscillate in phase they are more likely to influence one another. If they are out of phase, they are less likely to influence each other. This has led to the suggestion that inter-areal synchrony could be used to flexibly change the effective connection between regions (Bressler 1996; Engel et al. 2001; Salinas and Sejnowski 2001; Fries 2005). Support for this notion comes from observations that inter-areal oscillatory coherence between 'cognitive' regions (such as LIP or FEF) and sensory areas (such as MT or VT) has been found to increase with attention (Saalmann et al. 2007; Siegel et al. 2008; Gregoriou et al. 2009).

Another role of oscillations in top-down attention comes from Buschman and Miller (Buschman and Miller 2007, 2009), who found evidence for a role in controlling when top-down attention is shifted. During top-down visual search, there was a greater increase in ~25 Hz oscillations in the frontal-parietal network relative to bottom-up pop-out. These oscillations corresponded well with behavioural and neural observations that the locus of attention shifted about every 40 ms (40 ms = 25 Hz) during the search. This suggests a relationship between the oscillations and shifts in attention. One hypothesis is that each period of the oscillation encapsulates a shift in attention. To test this, a decoding approach was used to determine how well the locus of attention could be determined in the spiking activity of neurons in the FEF. Decoding was best when the analysis window was centred on and synchronized to each 25 Hz oscillatory cycle on each trial (relative to using time windows fixed to an external event, like the behavioural response). This supports our hypothesis: shifts of attention during search were synchronized to the 25 Hz LFP oscillations (Buschman and Miller 2009). These oscillations could have been extrinsically or intrinsically generated: either reflecting a mechanism specifically generated to regulate the timing of attentional shifts, or, alternatively, it could have been generated by the process of serially attending to different locations in a rhythmic manner. Either way, these oscillations were synchronized across frontal and parietal cortex (Buschman and Miller 2007), and would be ideal for providing a 'timing' or 'clocking' signal that helps coordinate shifts of attention across different brain areas (Buschman and Miller 2010). This is analogous to the bus clock on a computer that coordinates the timing of operations in the computer's many different circuits.

DECIDING WHAT TO ATTEND: NEURAL MECHANISMS FOR EXECUTIVE CONTROL

Now we take up the central question we raised earlier: How does the brain determine what is important and needs attending? For bottom-up attention, selection is more straightforward: our brain has evolved to provide more neural energy to salient stimuli that are loud, looming, sudden, etc. However, navigating complex situations to achieve long-term goals cannot rely on uncoordinated reactions to the environment. Rather, this must be orchestrated 'top-down' from within oneself. And to put it simply, you can't play this game without learning the rules.

Rules are central to our ability to coordinate thought and action and direct them toward a goal. Virtually all long-term, goal-directed behaviours are learned, and thus depend on a cognitive system that can acquire and represent elaborate representations that reflect all the information needed to achieve a goal: what outcomes are possible, what actions have been successful at achieving them or similar goals in the past, information stored in long-term memory, and, of course, what things in the environment require our attention. Consider the set of rules invoked when we dine in a restaurant, such as 'wait to be seated', 'order', and 'pay the bill'. These rules give us an idea about what to expect and what is expected of us when we try a new restaurant (for example, paying attention to the waiter to hear the specials). Thus, rules are needed to orchestrate processing in diverse brain regions along a common, internal theme. The challenge is a model that can explain this neurobiologically, without resorting to a homunculus. Over the rest of this review, we will try to offer one.

Rules and the prefrontal cortex

The PFC seems anatomically well situated to play a role in rule learning. It receives and sends projections to most of the cerebral cortex (with the exception of primary sensory and motor cortices) as well as the hippocampus, amygdala, cerebellum, and, most importantly for our model, the basal ganglia (abbreviated as BG; Porrino et al. 1981; Amaral and Price 1984; Amaral 1986; Selemon and Goldman-Rakic 1988; Barbas and De Olmos 1990; Eblen and Graybiel 1995; Croxson et al. 2005). Thus, the PFC seems to be a hub of cortical processing, able to synthesize a wide range of external and internal information and also exert control over much of the cortex. Although different PFC subdivisions have distinct patterns of interconnections with other brain systems (e.g. lateral—sensory and motor cortex; orbital—limbic), there are prodigious connections both within and between PFC subdivisions, ensuring a high degree of integration of information (Pandya and Barnes 1987; Barbas and Pandya 1989; Pandya and Yeterian 1990; Barbas and Pandya 1991; Petrides and Pandya 1999). Such a dense network of connections could allow PFC to act as a large associative network for detecting and storing associations between diverse events, experiences, and internal states (Fig. 27.3).

There is a large amount of evidence supporting the role of the frontal cortex in rule learning and use (for reviews see Wise et al. 1996; Miller and Cohen 2001). Neurophysiological studies in animals and imaging studies in humans have shown that the PFC has many of the needed attributes. First, the neurons sustain their activity across short, multisecond memory delays (Pribram et al. 1952; Fuster and Alexander 1971; Fuster 1973; Funahashi et al. 1989; Miller et al. 1996). This 'working memory' property is crucial for goal-directed behaviour, which, unlike 'ballistic' reflexes, typically extends over time and allows associations to be formed between items that are not

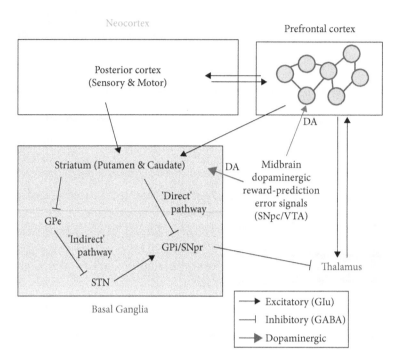

FIGURE 27.3 Schematic diagram of cortical–basal ganglia loops that allow for iterative learning between the slow, associative networks in prefrontal cortex (upper right) and the fast, reward-based networks of the basal ganglia (lower left, see text for details).

simultaneously present. Second, the PFC is highly plastic. After training, a large proportion of neurons in the monkey PFC acquire selectivity for the task contingencies (typically one third to one half of the population; White and Wise 1999; Asaad et al. 2000; Wallis et al. 2001; Mansouri et al. 2006). A computational model by Rigotti et al. (Rigotti et al. 2011) argued that the PFC needs large proportions of neurons with mixed selectivity. Random connections result in arbitrary mixes of external and internal information. These broad representations endow the PFC with a large, perhaps unlimited, capacity to learn new rules. It may also endow cognitive flexibility by allowing the PFC brain to re-utilize the same pool of neurons for different tasks. This has been supported by observations that large proportions of PFC neurons can 'multitask' and play a role in representing disparate, independent categorical rules (Cromer et al. 2010; Roy et al. 2010).

How the PFC may acquire rule information is considered next.

Rule learning and dopamine

Rule learning requires feedback about which behaviours have been successful. The brain must strengthen co-activations that are successful at achieving a goal (rewarded) while breaking associations that are ineffective. This needs to be guided by feedback so that relevant events and predictive relationships can be distinguished from spurious coincidences. This guidance appears to come in the form of a 'reinforcement signal', thought to be provided by DA neurons in the midbrain.

Dopaminergic neurons are located in both the ventral tegmental area and the substantia nigra, pars compacta (Schultz et al. 1992; Schultz et al. 1997; Schultz 1998), and show activity that directly corresponds to the reward prediction error signals suggested by models of animal learning. Midbrain DA neurons send heavy projections into both the frontal cortex and the striatum, the main input of the BG. The projections into the frontal cortex show a gradient connectivity with heavier inputs anteriorly that drop off posteriorly, suggesting a preferential input of reward information into the PFC relative to posterior cortex (Thierry et al. 1973; Goldman-Rakic et al. 1989). Evidence suggests that neither strengthening nor weakening of synapses in the striatum by long-term potentiation or depression can occur without DA input (Calabresi et al. 1992, 1997; Otani et al. 1998; Kerr and Wickens 2001). After training, DA neurons in the midbrain will learn to increase activity to an unexpected stimulus that directly predicts a reward: the event 'stands in' for the reward (Schultz et al. 1993). DA neurons will now respond to the predictive event when it is unexpected, but will no longer respond to the actual, now expected, reward event.

In short, the activity of dopaminergic neurons corresponds to a teaching signal that says, 'Something good happened and you did not predict it, so remember what just happened so you can predict it in the future.' Alternatively, if a reward is expected, but not received, the signal provides feedback that whatever behaviour was just taken is not effective in getting rewarded. This teaching signal is thought to guide the learning of the associations that are the building blocks of rules. If these reward signals affect connections that were recently active, and therefore likely involved in recent behaviour, then the result may be to help strengthen reward-predicting associations within the network, while reducing associations that do not increase benefits. In this way, the brain can learn what rules are effective in producing desirable outcomes.

Top-down control depends on a balance between different styles of learning

Normal learning has to balance different demands. One might expect that the greatest evolutionary benefit would be gained from learning as quickly as possible—adapting at a faster rate than competing organisms lends a definite edge, whereas missed opportunities can be costly (even deadly). However, there are also disadvantages to learning too quickly: one loses the ability to integrate across multiple experiences to form a generalized, less error-prone prediction. Take the classic example of one-trial learning: conditioned taste aversion. Many of us have had the experience of eating a particular food and then becoming ill for an unrelated reason. However, in many cases, the person develops an aversion to that food, even though the attribution is erroneous.

Extending learning across multiple episodes allows organisms to detect the regularities of predictive relationships and leave behind spurious associations and coincidences. Further, networks that learn at a slower rate also tend to be more stable. Artificial neural networks with small changes in synaptic weights at each learning episode converge very slowly. Networks with large synaptic weight changes can quickly capture some patterns; however, the resulting networks tend to be more volatile and exhibit erratic behaviour. This is due to the fact that a high learning rate can overshoot minima in the error function, even oscillating between values on either side of the minima, but never reaching the minima (for more information on artificial neural networks, see Hertz et al. 1991; Dayan and Abbott 2001).

In addition to avoiding errors, slower, more deliberate learning also provides the opportunity to integrate associations across many different experiences to detect common structures across them. It is these commonalities that form abstractions, general principles, concepts, and symbolisms that are the medium of the sophisticated, 'big-picture' thought needed for truly long-term goals. Indeed, this is fundamental to proactive thought and action. Generalizing among many past experiences gives us the ability to generalize to the future, to imagine possibilities that we have not yet experienced—but would like to—and given the generalized rules, we can predict the actions and behaviours needed to achieve our goal. In addition, abstraction may aid in cognitive flexibility, because generalized representations are concise (by definition), lacking the details of more specific representations. These compressed representations should make it easier to maintain multiple generalized representations within a given network and ease switching between them, particularly in contrast to when representations are elaborate and detailed.

Given the advantages and disadvantages associated with both forms of learning, the brain must balance the obvious pressure to learn as quickly as possible with the advantages of slower learning. One possible solution to this conundrum comes from O'Reilly and colleagues, who suggested that fast learning and slow learning systems interact with one another (McClelland et al. 1995; O'Reilly and Munakata 2000). Studying the consolidation of long-term memories, McClelland et al. (McClelland et al. 1995) specifically suggested that fast plasticity mechanisms within the hippocampus are able to quickly capture new memories while 'training' the slower-learning cortical networks. In this way, the brain is able to balance the need to initially grasp new memories with the advantages of a generalized, distributed representation of long-term memories. The idea is that the hippocampus is specialized for the rapid acquisition of new information; each learning trial produces large weight changes. The output of the hippocampus will then repeatedly activate cortical networks that have smaller weight changes per episode. Continued hippocampal-mediated reactivation of cortical representations allows the cortex to gradually connect these representations with other experiences. That way, the shared structure across experiences can be detected and stored, and the memory can be interleaved with others so that it can be readily accessed.

In fact, this architecture (fast learning in more primitive, non-cortical structures training the slower, more advanced, cortex) may be a general brain strategy; in addition to being suggested for the relationship between the hippocampus and cortex, it has also been proposed for the cerebellum and cortex (Houk and Wise 1995). This makes sense: the first evolutionary pressure on our cortex-less ancestors was presumably toward faster learning, whereas only later did we add on a slower, more judicious and flexible cortex. We propose that rule learning occurs through similar interactions between the PFC and the basal ganglia, a set of subcortical structures that is anatomically and functionally related to the PFC, as discussed next.

Interactions between different styles of plasticity in the PFC and basal ganglia

The BG is a collection of subcortical nuclei that, similar to the PFC, have a high degree of cortical convergence. Cortical inputs arrive largely via the striatum (which includes both the caudate and the putamen); are processed through the globus pallidus, the subthalamic nucleus (STN), and the substantia nigra; and are then directed back into the cortex via the thalamus (see Fig. 27.3). The segregated nature of BG inputs is maintained throughout the different nuclei such that the output from the BG (via the thalamus) is largely to the same cortical areas that gave rise to the initial inputs into the BG (Selemon and Goldman-Rakic 1985). Crucially, the frontal cortex receives the largest portion of BG outputs, suggesting a close collaboration between these structures (Middleton and Strick 1994, 2000, 2002). Lesions of the striatum produce impairments in learning new operant behaviours (or concrete rules) and show that damage to different parts of the striatum generally causes deficits similar to those caused by lesions of the area of the cortex that loop with the affected region of the striatum (Divac et al. 1967; Goldman and Rosvold 1972). For example, lesions of the regions of the caudate associated with the frontal cortex result in cognitive impairments. This all suggests that reciprocal connections between the BG and PFC play a significant role in PFC (and therefore cognitive) function.

Interestingly, the input of midbrain DA into the striatum is much heavier than that of the PFC, by as much as an order of magnitude (Lynd-Balta and Haber 1994). Further, DA neurons make connections close to the synapse that striatal neurons form with cortical neurons. By contrast, DA inputs to the cortex synapse out on the dendrites. Thus, DA may play a strong role in gating plasticity in the striatum whereas DA may have a more subtle influence in cortex, in shading, not gating, plasticity. This may reflect the trade-off (discussed above) between the demands of fast plasticity (in the striatum) versus slow plasticity (in the PFC). The result of these different learning styles was suggested by a computational model by Daw et al. (2006).

Daw et al. contrasted learning in the striatum with that in the PFC. They suggested that the rules represented in the PFC are the entire logical structure of a task in a tree-like model from initial state to goal achievement. Behaviours begin in an initial state with two or more possible response alternatives. Choosing one response leads to another state with new response alternatives, with this process continuing through-out the task, ultimately leading to a reward. The PFC is able to capture this entire tree structure, essentially providing the animal with an internal model of the entire task. This endows the characteristics of sophisticated goal-directed behaviour. It allows prediction of long-term outcomes by chaining together short-term predictions (direct associa-tions) into multistep long-range predictions. It also allows mental flexibility. Chaining together predictions on the fly allows the system to flexibly react to changing circum-stances. Further, a change in the value of a goal propagates back through the tree-model, changing which choices might be made.

In contrast to the PFC, the BG is thought to represent acquired information with a cache, not a tree-like model system. That is, the striatum learns not the entire structure of a task; rather it learns the most valuable alternative at each decision point in isolation. It is as if the BG learns each fork in the road whereas the PFC learns the whole route. The BG cache system is computationally simple (and therefore fast) but it is inflexible because the learning is divorced from any change in the outcome. This may explain why the BG is associated with inflexible habit learning.

We suggest that these two representational styles result from differences in plastic-ity in the striatum vs. PFC: namely, fast, DA-gated plasticity in the striatum vs. slower plasticity in the PFC that is DA-shaded. Support for different speeds of plasticity in each comes from an experiment by Pasupathy and Miller (2005). Monkeys were trained to associate a visual cue with a directional eye movement (Fig. 27.4a). Learning occurred over a period of approximately 60 trials (Fig. 27.4b), after which the associations were reversed and the animals had to re-learn the new associations. This allowed Pasupathy and Miller to study how single neurons in the prefrontal cortex and striatum learned (and re-learned) these associations during the trial (Fig. 27.4c/d). Neural activity in the striatum showed rapid, almost bi-stable, learning-related changes in the timing of selec-tivity (Fig. 27.4e). This is in contrast to the PFC where changes were much slower, with selective responses slowly advancing across trials (Fig. 27.4e). These results support the hypothesis that rewarded associations are first identified by the striatum, the output of which 'trains' slower learning mechanisms in the PFC.

Thus, the relationship between the BG and PFC may be similar to the relationship between the hippocampus and cortex as suggested by O'Reilly (discussed above). As the animal learns specific stimulus–response associations they are quickly acquired by the basal ganglia which, in turn, slowly train the prefrontal cortex. In this case, the fast (strong weight changes) plasticity in the striatum is better suited for the rapid formation of associations between a specific cue and response. However, as noted above, fast learn-ing tends to be error prone, and indeed, striatal neurons began predicting the forth-coming behavioural response early in learning when that response was often wrong. By contrast, the smaller weight changes in the PFC may have allowed it to accumulate more evidence and arrive more slowly and judiciously at the correct answer. As has been pro-posed for the hippocampus and cortex, the fast striatal plasticity may be more suited for a quick stamping-in of immediate, direct associations (a cache system). By contrast, the slow PFC plasticity may be suitable for building elaborate rule representations that

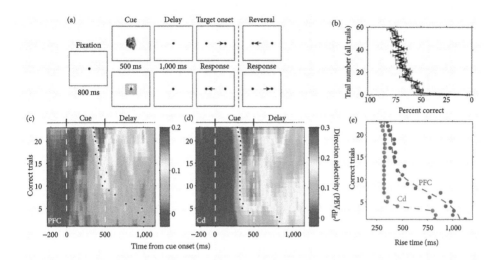

FIGURE 27.4 Fast versus slow learning in prefrontal cortex and basal ganglia. (a) Sample–response association task. Animals were presented with a cue and then made the associated saccade (left or right) to receive a reward. After being learned, the associations would reverse directions. (b) The saccade associated with each cue was learned over time. Performance (x-axis) increased and saturated over the first 60 trials (y-axis). (c and d) Neural selectivity for associated saccade direction (colour axis) evolved during the trial (x-axis) in both (c) prefrontal cortex and (d) caudate nucleus. Selectivity in both regions increased as the animal learned over correct trials (y-axis). However, learning occurred quicker in the caudate: selectivity was seen early in the trial after just a few correct trials. (e) Faster learning in caudate is captured by plotting the evolution of rise time (x-axis) over trials (y-axis). The caudate nucleus (red) not only learns faster than prefrontal (blue), but learning is almost bi-stable. While learning is slower in prefrontal cortex, this more closely matches behaviour (see b).

gradually link in more information (i.e. tree-like representations). The slower PFC plasticity may also be critical for finding the commonalities and regularities among the simpler representations acquired by the striatum that are the basis for abstractions and general principles (see above).

Support for the specific vs. generalized trade-off between the striatum and the PFC during learning comes from Antzoulatos and Miller (2011), who recorded from multiple electrodes in the lateral prefrontal cortex and dorsal striatum while animals learned two categories of stimuli. Each day, monkeys learned to associate novel, abstract dot-based categories with a right vs. left saccade (Fig. 27.5a and b). Early on, when they could acquire specific stimulus–response associations, striatum activity was an earlier predictor of the corresponding saccade (Fig. 27.5c). However, as the number of exemplars was increasing, and monkeys had to form abstractions to classify them, PFC began predicting the saccade associated with each category before the striatum (Fig. 27.5d). Thus, it seems that the striatum was leading the acquisition early on when behaviour could be supported by simple stimulus–response learning. However, when the abstraction requirements exceeded that of the simple striatum cache representations, the PFC

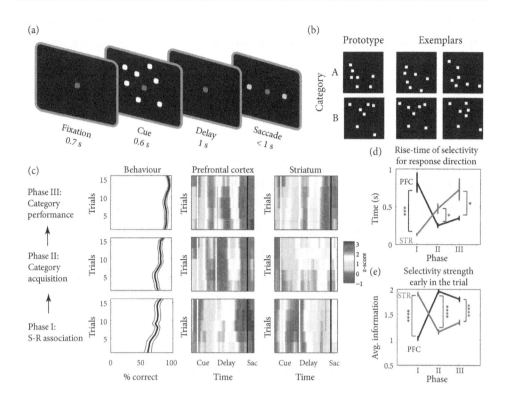

FIGURE 27.5 Specific versus generalized learning in prefrontal cortex and basal ganglia. (a) Category–response association task. Animals were presented with a cue stimulus (an array of dots) that were exemplar stimuli created by morphing stimuli from one of two category prototypes (b). The animals learned to associate each category with either a leftward or rightward saccade (c, left column). After learning the associations for a given set of exemplars, new exemplars were added to the set, requiring the animal to generalize the learned association to these new stimuli. Therefore, earlier in training the animals were able to associate individual stimuli with a response (c, bottom row) but then, as the number of exemplars increased, they were forced to acquire the category (c, middle row), eventually generalizing to new stimuli (c, top row). Selectivity for the associated response was found in both prefrontal cortex (c, middle column) and striatum (c, right column). Early in training, during the stimulus–response phase, selectivity was seen (d) earlier and (e) stronger in striatum. However, prefrontal cortex took a lead role after generalized categories were learned (phases II and III).

took over. In this case the slower-learning, associative activity of PFC is ideal for the integration of stimulus properties over many exemplars, allowing for a generalized 'concept' of categories to be learned. This dual-learner strategy allows the animal to perform optimally throughout the task—early on striatum can learn associations quickly while later in the task, when learning associations is no longer viable, prefrontal cortex guides behaviour.

The interactions of the PFC and the BG might explain several aspects of goal-directed learning and habit formation. The initial learning of a complex operant task invariably begins with the establishment of a simple response immediately proximal to reward (i.e. a single state). Then, as the task becomes increasingly complex with more and more antecedents and qualifications (states and alternatives) the PFC shows greater involvement. It facilitates this learning via its slower plasticity, allowing it to stitch together the relationships between the different states. This is useful because uncertainty of the correct action at any given state adds across the many states within a complex task. Thus, in complex tasks the ability of reinforcement to control behaviour is lessened with the addition of more states. However, model-building in the PFC may provide the overarching infrastructure—the thread weaving between states—that facilitates learning of the entire course of action. Many tasks will remain dependent on the PFC and the models it builds, especially those requiring flexibility (e.g. when the goal often changes or there are multiple goals to choose among) or when a strongly established behaviour in one of the states (e.g. a habit) is incompatible with the course of action needed to obtain a specific goal. However, if a behaviour, even a complex one, is unchanging, then the actions at each state are constant and, once these are learned, control can revert to a piecemeal caching system in the BG. That is, the behaviour becomes a 'habit' and it frees up the more executive PFC model-building system for behaviours requiring the flexibility it provides.

Primates, especially humans, can engage in elaborate goal-directed behaviours. Plus, we can be creative and unique in finding new goals and strategies to pursue them. This means that the mechanisms that build the PFC rule representations must have a corresponding ability for open-ended growth. We propose that the anatomical loops through the PFC and BG support this via recursive, bootstrapping interactions, as we will discuss next.

Recursive processing and bootstrapping in corticoganglia loops

'Bootstrapping' is the process of building increasingly complex representations from simpler ones. The recursive nature of the loops between the BG and PFC may lend itself to this process. As described earlier, anatomical connections between the PFC and BG seem to suggest a closed loop—channels within the BG return outputs, via the thalamus, into the same cortical areas that gave rise to their initial cortical input (Fig. 27.3). This anatomy seems well suited for recursive processing. That is, the neural representations that are results from PFC–BG interactions are fed back into the loop as fodder for further learning. In this manner, new experiences can be added onto previous ones, linking in more information to build more elaborate rule representations. It can allow the discovery of commonalities among more experiences and thus more high-level concepts and principles. Indeed, a hallmark of human intelligence is the propensity for us to ground new concepts in familiar ones because it seems to ease our understanding of novel ideas—we learn to multiply by serial addition, exponentiation by serial multiplication, etc.

The frontal cortex–BG loops suggest an auto-associative type network, similar to that seen in the CA3 of the hippocampus. The looping back of outputs on the inputs allows the network to learn to complete (i.e. recall) previously learned patterns given a degraded version or a subset of the original inputs (Hopfield 1982). In the hippocampus, this network has been suggested to play a role in the formation of memories. The PFC–BG loops are heavily influenced by dopaminergic inputs, and therefore may be more goal-oriented than hippocampal learning and memory. Indeed, the cortical–BG loops may also explain the DA reward prediction signals. As previously described, midbrain DA neurons respond to earlier and earlier events in a predictive chain leading to a reward. Both the frontal cortex and the striatum send projections into the midbrain DA neurons, possibly underlying their ability to bootstrap to early predictors of reward (however, although this is suggestive, it is still unknown whether these descending projections are critical for this behaviour).

The loops may also explain another important aspect of goal-directed behaviour: the stringing together of sequences of thought and action. A key feature of auto-associative networks is their ability to learn temporal sequences of patterns and thus make predictions. This feature relies on the activity pattern being fed back into the network with a temporal delay, allowing the next pattern in the sequence to arrive as the previous pattern is fed back, building an association (Kleinfeld 1986; Sompolinsky and Kanter 1986). Inhibitory synapses in the pathways through the BG may add the temporal delay needed as they have a slower time constant than excitatory synapses (Couve et al. 2000). A second way to add lag is through a memory buffer. The PFC is well known for this type of property; its neurons can sustain their activity to act as a bridge for learning contingencies across several seconds, even minutes. The introduction of lag into the recursive loop through either (or both) mechanism(s) may be enough to tune the network for sequencing and prediction. This would seem to be key to the development of tree-like rule representations that describe an entire sequence of goal-directed actions.

SUMMARY: THE PFC AS A GENERAL EXECUTIVE CONTROLLER

We have reviewed why we need attention (our very finite cognitive resources) and shown that the PFC is a major source of the top-down attention signals that select the sensory (and other) information important for our current goal. This may occur by the top-down signals boosting the representations of the to-be-attended stimuli by raising their activity and/or by synchronizing the activity of those neurons so that they have a greater impact on downstream neurons. In addition, oscillatory coherence in and between brain areas may help route traffic throughout cortex, control or signal when attention is shifted, and, by playing a role in juggling multiple active neural representations, could explain why we have a cognitive capacity limitation in the first place. Finally, we discussed the neural mechanisms that allow the PFC, along with the BG, to learn the rules of the game that determine what is potentially important and in need of selection. To complete the circle, we need to address one more issue: How (and why) do rule representations in the PFC result in top-down selection?

Miller and Cohen (Miller and Cohen 2001) argued that rule representations in the PFC are not arbitrary, esoteric descriptions of a task's logical structure. Rather, the PFC represents rules in a particular format: as a map of the cortical pathways needed to perform the task ('rulemaps') (Fig. 27.6). In other words, the tree-like set of a task's rules in the PFC is also a tree-like map of the neural pathways in and between other brain regions that need to be activated to engage in the current task. In a given situation, cues about context and other current external and internal information activate and complete the corresponding PFC rulemap. Activation of the rulemap (which can be sustained, if needed) sets up bias signals that feed back to other brain areas, affecting sensory systems as well as the systems responsible for response execution, memory retrieval, and emotional evaluation. The aggregate effect is the selection of neural circuits that guide the flow of neural activity along pathways that establish the proper mappings between inputs, internal states, and outputs to reach the goal. It is as if the PFC is a conductor in a railroad yard and learns a map that it uses to guide trains (neural activity) along the right tracks (neural pathways). And when these signals act on sensory systems, we call it top-down attention.

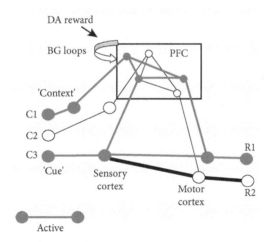

FIGURE 27.6 Miller and Cohen's model of executive control. Shown are processing units representing cues such as sensory inputs, current motivational state, memories, etc. (C1, C2, and C3), and those representing two voluntary actions (e.g. 'responses', R1 and R2). Excitatory signals from the PFC feed back to other brain systems to enable task-relevant neural pathways. Thick lines indicate well-established pathways mediating a prepotent behaviour that can be overcome by top-down PFC signals that activate an alternative pathway. Red indicates active units or pathways. See Miller and Cohen (2001) for details. Data from Miller, E. K. and Cohen, J. D., An integrative theory of prefrontal function, *Annual Review of Neuroscience*, 24, pp.167–202, © 2001, Annual Review of Neuroscience.

ACKNOWLEDGEMENTS

Supported by the Intelligence Advanced Research Projects Activity (IARPA) via Department of the Interior (DOI) contract number D10PC20023. The US Government is authorized to reproduce and distribute reprint for governmental purposes notwithstanding any copyright annotation thereon. The views and conclusions contained herein are those of the authors and should not be interpreted as necessarily representing the official policies or endorsements, either expressed or implied, of IARPA, DOI, or the US Government.

REFERENCES

Aertsen, A. M., Gerstein, G. L., Habib, M. K., and Palm, G. (1989a). Dynamics of neuronal firing correlation: Modulation of 'effective connectivity'. *Journal of Neurophysiology* 61: 900–917.

Aertsen A. M. H. J., Gerstein, G. L., Habib, M. K., Palm, G., and Gochin, P. M. (1989b). Dynamics of neuronal firing correlation: Modulation of 'effective connectivity'. *Journal of Neurophysiology* 61: 900–917.

Alvarez, G. A. and Cavanagh, P. (2005). Independent resources for attentional tracking in the left and right visual hemifields. *Psychological Science* 16: 637–643.

Amaral D. G. (1986). Amygdalohippocampal and amygdalocortical projections in the primate brain. *Advances in Experimental Medicine and Biology* 203: 3–17.

Amaral D. G. and Price, J. L. (1984). Amygdalo-cortical projections in the monkey (Macaca fascicularis). *Journal of Comparative Neurology* 230: 465–496.

Antzoulatos, E. G. and Miller, E. K. (2011). Differences between neural activity in prefrontal cortex and striatum during learning of novel abstract categories. *Neuron* 71: 243–249.

Asaad, W. F., Rainer, G., and Miller, E. K. (2000). Task-specific activity in the primate prefrontal cortex. *Journal of Neurophysiology* 84: 451–459.

Awh, E. and Jonides, J. (2001). Overlapping mechanisms of attention and spatial working memory. *Trends in Cognitive Sciences* 5: 119–126.

Awh, E., Jonides, J., and Reuter-Lorenz, P. A. (1998). Rehearsal in spatial working memory. *Journal of Experimental Psychology: Human Perception and Performance* 24: 780–790.

Barbas, H. and De Olmos, J. (1990). Projections from the amygdala to basoventral and mediodorsal prefrontal regions in the rhesus monkey. *Journal of Comparative Neurology* 300: 549–571.

Barbas, H. and Pandya, D. N. (1989). Architecture and intrinsic connections of the prefrontal cortex in the rhesus monkey. *Journal of Comparative Neurology* 286: 353–375.

Barbas, H. and Pandya, D. N. (1991). Patterns of connections of the prefrontal cortex in the rhesus monkey associated with cortical architecture. In H. S. Levin, H. M. Eisenberg, and A. L. Benton (eds.), *Frontal Lobe Function and Dysfunction* (pp. 35–58). New York: Oxford University Press.

Bauer, M., Oostenveld, R., Peeters, M., and Fries, P. (2006). Tactile spatial attention enhances gamma-band activity in somatosensory cortex and reduces low-frequency activity in parieto-occipital areas. *Journal of Neuroscience* 26: 490–501.

Bichot, N. P. and Schall, J. D. (1999). Effects of similarity and history on neural mechanisms of visual selection. *Nature Neuroscience* 2: 549–554.

Bisley, J. W. and Goldberg, M. E. (2003). Neuronal activity in the lateral intraparietal area and spatial attention. *Science* 299: 81–86.

Bisley, J. W. and Goldberg, M. E. (2006). Neural correlates of attention and distractibility in the lateral intraparietal area. *Journal of Neurophysiology* 95: 1696–1717.

Bressler, S. L. (1996). Interareal synchronization in the visual cortex. *Behavioural Brain Research* 76: 37–49.

Brody, C. D., Hernandez, A., Zainos, A., and Romo, R. (2003). Timing and neural encoding of somatosensory parametric working memory in macaque prefrontal cortex. *Cerebral Cortex* 13: 1196–1207.

Buschman, T. J. and Miller, E. K. (2007). Top-down versus bottom-up control of attention in the prefrontal and posterior parietal cortices. *Science* 315: 1860–1862.

Buschman, T. J. and Miller, E. K. (2009). Serial, covert shifts of attention during visual search are reflected by the frontal eye fields and correlated with population oscillations. *Neuron* 63: 386–396.

Buschman, T. J. and Miller, E. K. (2010). Shifting the spotlight of attention: Evidence for discrete computations in cognition. *Frontiers in Human Neuroscience* 4: Article 194.

Buschman, T. J., Siegel, M., Roy, J. E., and Miller, E. K. (2011). Neural substrates of cognitive capacity limitations. *Proceedings of the National Academy of Sciences USA* 108: 11252–11255.

Calabresi, P., Maj, R., Pisani, A., Mercuri, N. B., and Bernardi, G. (1992). Long-term synaptic depression in the striatum: Physiological and pharmacological characterization. *Journal of Neuroscience* 12: 4224–4233.

Calabresi, P., Saiardi, A., Pisani, A., Baik, J. H., Centonze, D., Mercuri, N. B., Bernardi, G., Borrelli, E., and Maj, R. (1997). Abnormal synaptic plasticity in the striatum of mice lacking dopamine D2 receptors. *Journal of Neuroscience* 17: 4536–4544.

Cavanagh, P. and Alvarez, G. A. (2005). Tracking multiple targets with multifocal attention. *Trends in Cognitive Sciences* 9: 349–354.

Corbetta, M., Akbudak, E., Conturo, T. E., Snyder, A. Z., Ollinger, J. M., Drury, H. A., Linenweber, M. R., Petersen, S. E., Raichle, M. E., Van Essen, D. C., and Shulman, G. L. (1998). A common network of functional areas for attention and eye movements. *Neuron* 21: 761–773.

Corbetta, M., Miezin, F. M., Shulman, G. L., and Petersen, S. E. (1993). A PET study of visuospatial attention. *Journal of Neuroscience* 13: 1202–1226.

Corbetta, M. and Shulman, G. L. (2002). Control of goal-directed and stimulus-driven attention in the brain. *Nature Reviews Neuroscience* 3: 201–215.

Corbetta, M., Shulman, G. L., Miezin, F. M., and Petersen, S. E. (1995). Superior parietal cortex activation during spatial attention shifts and visual feature conjunction. *Science* 270: 802–805.

Coull, J. T. and Nobre, A. C. (1998). Where and when to pay attention: The neural systems for directing attention to spatial locations and to time intervals as revealed by both PET and fMRI. *Journal of Neuroscience* 18: 7426–7435.

Couve, A., Moss, S. J., and Pangalos, M. N. (2000). GABAB receptors: A new paradigm in G protein signaling. *Molecular and Cellular Neuroscience* 16: 296–312.

Cowan, N. (2001). The magical number 4 in short-term memory: A reconsideration of mental storage capacity. *Behavioral and Brain Sciences* 24: 87–114; discussion 114–185.

Cromer, J. A., Roy, J. E., and Miller, E. K. (2010). Representation of multiple, independent categories in the primate prefrontal cortex. *Neuron* 66: 796–807.

Croxson, P. L., Johansen-Berg, H., Behrens, T. E. J., Robson, M. D., Pinsk, M. A., Gross, C. G., Richter, W., Richter, M. C., Kastner, S., and Rushworth, M. F. S. (2005). Quantitative investigation of connections of the prefrontal cortex in the human and macaque using probabilistic diffusion tractography. *Journal of Neuroscience* 25: 8854–8866.

Daw, N. D., O'Doherty, J. P., Dayan, P., Seymour, B., and Dolan, R. J. (2006). Cortical substrates for exploratory decisions in humans. *Nature* 441: 876–879.

Dayan, P. and Abbott, L. F. (2001). *Theoretical Neuroscience: Computational and Mathematical Modeling of Neural Systems (Computational Neuroscience)*. Cambridge, Mass.: MIT Press.

Desimone, R. and Duncan, J. (1995). Neural mechanisms of selective visual attention. *Annual Review of Neuroscience* 18: 193–222.

Divac, I., Rosvold, H. E., and Szwarcbart, M. K. (1967). Behavioral effects of selective ablation of the caudate nucleus. *Journal of Comparative and Physiological Psychology* 63: 184–190.

Donner, T., Kettermann, A., Diesch, E., Ostendorf, F., Villringer, A., and Brandt, S. A. (2000). Involvement of the human frontal eye field and multiple parietal areas in covert visual selection during conjunction search. *European Journal of Neuroscience* 12: 3407–3414.

Donner, T., Kettermann, A., Diesch, E., Ostendorf, F., Villringer, A., and Brandt, S. A. (2002). Visual feature and conjunction searches of equal difficulty engage only partially overlapping frontoparietal networks. *NeuroImage* 15: 16–25.

Dragoi, G. and Buzsaki, G. (2006). Temporal encoding of place sequences by hippocampal cell assemblies. *Neuron* 50: 145–157.

Drew, T. and Vogel, E. K. (2008). Neural measures of individual differences in selecting and tracking multiple moving objects. *Journal of Neuroscience* 28: 4183–4191.

Duncan, J. and Humphreys, G. W. (1989). Visual search and stimulus similarity. *Psychological Review* 96: 433–458.

Eblen, F. and Graybiel, A. (1995). Highly restricted origin of prefrontal cortical inputs to striosomes in the macaque monkey. *Journal of Neuroscience* 15: 5999–6013.

Eglin, M., Robertson, L. C., and Knight, R. T. (1991). Cortical substrates supporting visual search in humans. *Cerebral Cortex* 1: 262–272.

Engel, A. K., Fries, P., and Singer, W. (2001). Dynamic predictions: Oscillations and synchrony in top-down processing. *Nature Reviews Neuroscience* 2: 704–716.

Engle, R. W., Tuholski, S. W., Laughlin, J. E., and Conway, A. R. (1999). Working memory, short-term memory, and general fluid intelligence: A latent-variable approach. *Journal of Experimental Psychology: General* 128: 309–331.

Everling, S., Tinsley, C. J., Gaffan, D., and Duncan, J. (2002). Filtering of neural signals by focused attention in the monkey prefrontal cortex. *Nature Neuroscience* 5: 671–676.

Everling, S., Tinsley, C. J., Gaffan, D., and Duncan, J. (2006). Selective representation of task-relevant objects and locations in the monkey prefrontal cortex. *European Journal of Neuroscience* 23: 2197–2214.

Fries, P. (2005). A mechanism for cognitive dynamics: Neuronal communication through neuronal coherence. *Trends in Cognitive Sciences* 9: 474–480.

Fries, P., Nikolic, D., and Singer, W. (2007). The gamma cycle. *Trends in Neurosciences* 30: 309–316.

Fries, P., Reynolds, J. H., Rorie, A. E., and Desimone, R. (2001). Modulation of oscillatory neuronal synchronization by selective visual attention. *Science* 291: 1560–1563.

Fukuda, K., Vogel, E., Mayr, U., and Awh, E. (2010). Quantity, not quality: The relationship between fluid intelligence and working memory capacity. *Psychonomic Bulletin & Review* 17: 673–679.

Funahashi, S., Bruce, C. J., and Goldman-Rakic, P. S. (1989). Mnemonic coding of visual space in the monkey's dorsolateral prefrontal cortex. *Journal of Neurophysiology* 61: 331–349.

Fuster, J. M. (1973). Unit activity in prefrontal cortex during delayed-response performance: Neuronal correlates of transient memory. *Journal of Neurophysiology* 36: 61–78.

Fuster, J. M. and Alexander, G. E. (1971). Neuron activity related to short-term memory. *Science* 173: 652–654.

Goldman, P. S. and Rosvold, H. E. (1972). The effects of selective caudate lesions in infant and juvenile Rhesus monkeys. *Brain Research* 43: 53–66.

Goldman-Rakic, P. S., Leranth, C., Williams, S. M., Mons, N., and Geffard, M. (1989). Dopamine synaptic complex with pyramidal neurons in primate cerebral cortex. *Proceedings of the National Academy of Sciences USA* 86: 9015–9019.

Gregoriou, G. G., Gotts, S. J., Zhou, H., and Desimone, R. (2009). High-frequency, long-range coupling between prefrontal and visual cortex during attention. *Science* 324: 1207–1210.

Hasegawa, R. P., Matsumoto, M., and Mikami, A (2000). Search target selection in monkey prefrontal cortex. *Journal of Neurophysiology* 84: 1692–1696.

Hertz, J. A., Krogh, A. S., and Palmer, R. G. (1991). *Introduction to Neural Computation Theory.* Santa Fe, N.Mex.: Westview Press.

Hopfield, J. J. (1982). Neural networks and physical systems with emergent collective computational abilities. *Proceedings of the National Academy of Sciences USA* 79: 2554–2558.

Hopfield, J. J. and Herz, A. V. (1995). Rapid local synchronization of action potentials: Toward computation with coupled integrate-and-fire neurons. *Proceedings of the National Academy of Sciences USA* 92: 6655–6662.

Houk, J. C. and Wise, S. P. (1995). Distributed modular architectures linking basal ganglia, cerebellum, and cerebral cortex: Their role in planning and controlling action. *Cerebral Cortex* 5: 95–110.

Iba, M. and Sawaguchi, T. (2003). Involvement of the dorsolateral prefrontal cortex of monkeys in visuospatial target selection. *Journal of Neurophysiology* 89: 587–599.

Ipata, A. E., Gee, A. L., Gottlieb, J., Bisley, J. W., and Goldberg, M. E. (2006). LIP responses to a popout stimulus are reduced if it is overtly ignored. *Nature Neuroscience* 9: 1071–1076.

Jensen, O., Kaiser, J., and Lachaux, J. P. (2007). Human gamma-frequency oscillations associated with attention and memory. *Trends in Neurosciences* 30: 317–324.

Jensen, O. and Lisman, J. E. (2005). Hippocampal sequence-encoding driven by a cortical multi-item working memory buffer. *Trends in Neurosciences* 28: 67–72.

Johnston, K. and Everling, S. (2009). Task-relevant output signals are sent from monkey dorsolateral prefrontal cortex to the superior colliculus during a visuospatial working memory task. *Journal of Cognitive Neuroscience* 21: 1023–1038.

Kayser, C., Montemurro, M. A., Logothetis, N. K., and Panzeri, S. (2009). Spike-phase coding boosts and stabilizes information carried by spatial and temporal spike patterns. *Neuron* 61: 597–608.

Kerr, J. N. D. and Wickens, J. R. (2001). Dopamine D-1/D-5 receptor activation is required for long-term potentiation in the rat neostriatum in vitro. *Journal of Neurophysiology* 85: 117–124.

Kleinfeld, D. (1986). Sequential state generation by model neural networks. *Proceedings of the National Academy of Sciences USA* 83: 9469–9473.

Knight, R. T. (1997). Distributed cortical network for visual attention. *Journal of Cognitive Neuroscience* 9: 75–91.

Knight, R. T., Grabowecky, M. F., and Scabini, D. (1995). Role of human prefrontal cortex in attention control. *Advances in Neurology* 66: 21–34; discussion 34–26.

Konig, P., Engel, A. K., and Singer, W. (1995). Relation between oscillatory activity and long-range synchronization in cat visual cortex. *Proceedings of the National Academy of Sciences USA* 92: 290–294.

Lakatos, P., Karmos, G., Mehta, A. D., Ulbert, I., and Schroeder, C. E. (2008). Entrainment of neuronal oscillations as a mechanism of attentional selection. *Science* 320: 110–113.

Laurent, G. (2002). Olfactory network dynamics and the coding of multidimensional signals. *Nature Reviews Neuroscience* 3: 884–895.

Lee, H., Simpson, G. V., Logothetis, N. K., and Rainer, G. (2005). Phase locking of single neuron activity to theta oscillations during working memory in monkey extrastriate visual cortex. *Neuron* 45: 147–156.

Li, L., Gratton, C., Yao, D., and Knight, R. T. (2010). Role of frontal and parietal cortices in the control of bottom-up and top-down attention in humans. *Brain Research* 1344: 173–184.

Lisman, J. E. and Idiart, M. A. (1995). Storage of 7 short-term memories in oscillatory subcycles. *Science* 267: 1512–1515.

Liu, T., Slotnick, S. D., Serences, J. T., and Yantis, S. (2003). Cortical mechanisms of feature-based attentional control. *Cerebral Cortex* 13: 1334–1343.

Luck, S. J. and Vogel, E. K. (1997). The capacity of visual working memory for features and conjunctions. *Nature* 390: 279–281.

Lynd-Balta, E. and Haber, S. N. (1994). The organization of midbrain projections to the ventral striatum in the primate. *Neuroscience* 59: 609–623.

McClelland, J., McNaughton, B., and O'Reilly, R. (1995). Why there are complementary learning systems in the hippocampus and neocortex: Insights from the successes and failures of connectionist models of learning and memory. *Psychological Review* 102: 419–457.

Mansouri, F. A., Matsumoto, K., and Tanaka, K. (2006). Prefrontal cell activities related to monkeys' success and failure in adapting to rule changes in a Wisconsin card sorting test analog. *Journal of Neuroscience* 26: 2745–2756.

Mehta, M. R., Lee, A. K., and Wilson, M. A. (2002). Role of experience and oscillations in transforming a rate code into a temporal code. *Nature* 417: 741–746.

Middleton, F. A. and Strick, P. L. (1994). Anatomical evidence for cerebellar and basal ganglia involvement in higher cognitive function. *Science* 266: 458–461.

Middleton, F. A. and Strick, P. L. (2000). Basal ganglia and cerebellar loops: Motor and cognitive circuits. *Brain Research Reviews* 31: 236–250.

Middleton, F. A. and Strick, P. L. (2002). Basal-ganglia 'projections' to the prefrontal cortex of the primate. *Cerebral Cortex* 12: 926–935.

Miller, E. K. and Cohen, J. D. (2001). An integrative theory of prefrontal function. *Annual Review of Neuroscience* 24: 167–202.

Miller, E. K., Erickson, C. A., and Desimone, R. (1996). Neural mechanisms of visual working memory in prefrontal cortex of the macaque. *Journal of Neuroscience* 16: 5154–5167.

Miller, G. A. (1956). The magical number seven plus or minus two: Some limits on our capacity for processing information. *Psychological Review* 63: 81–97.

Montemurro, M. A., Rasch, M. J., Murayama, Y., Logothetis, N. K., and Panzeri, S. (2008). Phase-of-firing coding of natural visual stimuli in primary visual cortex. *Current Biology* 18: 375–380.

Moore, T. and Armstrong, K. M. (2003). Selective gating of visual signals by microstimulation of frontal cortex. *Nature* 421: 370–373.

Moore, T. and Fallah, M. (2001). Control of eye movements and spatial attention. *Proceedings of the National Academy of Sciences USA* 98: 1273–1276.

Moore, T. and Fallah, M. (2004). Microstimulation of the frontal eye field and its effects on covert spatial attention. *Journal of Neurophysiology* 91: 152–162.

Moore, T. L., Schettler, S. P., Killiany, R. J., Rosene, D. L., and Moss, M. B. (2009). Effects on executive function following damage to the prefrontal cortex in the rhesus monkey (Macaca mulatta). *Behavioral Neuroscience* 123: 231–241.

Nobre, A. C., Sebestyen, G. N., Gitelman, D. R., Frith, C. D., and Mesulam, M. M. (2002). Filtering of distractors during visual search studied by positron emission tomography. *NeuroImage* 16: 968–976.

Noudoost, B. and Moore, T. (2011). Control of visual cortical signals by prefrontal dopamine. *Nature* 474: 372–375.

O'Keefe, J. (1993). Hippocampus, theta, and spatial memory. *Current Opinion in Neurobiology* 3: 917–924.

Oksama, L. and Hyönä, J. (2004). Is multiple object tracking carried out automatically by an early vision mechanism independent of higher-order cognition? An individual difference approach. *Visual Cognition* 11: 631–671.

O'Reilly, R. C. and Munakata, Y. (2000). *Computational Explorations in Cognitive Neuroscience: Understanding the Mind*. Cambridge, Mass.: MIT Press.

Otani, S., Blond, O., Desce, J. M., and Crépel F. (1998). Dopamine facilitates long-term depression of glutamatergic transmission in rat prefrontal cortex. *Neuroscience* 85: 669–676.

Pandya, D. N. and Barnes, C. L. (1987). Architecture and connections of the frontal lobe. In E. Perecman (ed.), *The Frontal Lobes Revisited* (pp. 41–72). New York: The IRBN Press.

Pandya, D.N. and Yeterian, E. H. (1990). Prefrontal cortex in relation to other cortical areas in Rhesus monkey: Architecture and connections. *Progress in Brain Research* 85: 63–94.

Pasupathy, A. and Miller, E. K. (2005). Different time courses of learning-related activity in the prefrontal cortex and striatum. *Nature* 433: 873–876.

Pesaran, B., Nelson, M. J., and Andersen, R. A. (2008). Free choice activates a decision circuit between frontal and parietal cortex. *Nature* 453: 406–409.

Petrides, M. and Pandya, D. N. (1999). Dorsolateral prefrontal cortex: Comparative cytoarchitectonic analysis in the human and the macaque brain and corticocortical connection patterns. *European Journal of Neuroscience* 11: 1011–1036.

Porrino, L. J., Crane, A. M., and Goldman-Rakic, P. S. (1981). Direct and indirect pathways from the amygdala to the frontal lobe in rhesus monkeys. *Journal of Comparative Neurology* 198: 121–136.

Postle, B. R., Awh, E., Jonides, J., Smith, E. E., and D'Esposito, M. (2004). The where and how of attention-based rehearsal in spatial working memory. *Brain Research: Cognitive Brain Research* 20: 194–205.

Pribram, K. H., Mishkin, M., Rosvold, H. E., and Kaplan, S. J. (1952). Effects on delayed-response performance of lesions of dorsolateral and ventromedial frontal cortex of baboons. *Journal of Comparative and Physiological Psychology* 45: 565–575.

Pylyshyn, Z.W. and Storm, R. W. (1988). Tracking multiple independent targets: Evidence for a parallel tracking mechanism. *Spatial Vision* 3: 179–197.

Rainer, G., Asaad, W. F., and Miller, E. K. (1998a). Memory fields of neurons in the primate prefrontal cortex. *Proceedings of the National Academy of Sciences USA* 95: 15008–15013.

Rainer, G., Asaad, W. F., and Miller, E. K. (1998b). Selective representation of relevant information by neurons in the primate prefrontal cortex. *Nature* 393: 577–579.

Rigotti, M., Rubin, D. B., Wang, X. J., and Fusi, S. (2011). Internal representation of task rules by recurrent dynamics: The importance of the diversity of neural responses. *Frontiers in Computational Neuroscience* 4: 24.

Roy, J. E., Riesenhuber, M., Poggio, T., and Miller, E. K. (2010). Prefrontal cortex activity during flexible categorization. *Journal of Neuroscience 30*: 8519–8528.

Saalmann, Y. B., Pigarev, I. N., and Vidyasagar, T. R. (2007). Neural mechanisms of visual attention: How top-down feedback highlights relevant locations. *Science 316*: 1612–1615.

Salinas, E. and Sejnowski, T. J. (2001). Correlated neuronal activity and the flow of neural information. *Nature Reviews Neuroscience 2*: 539–550.

Schultz, W. (1998). Predictive reward signal of dopamine neurons. *Journal of Neurophysiology 80*: 1–27.

Schultz, W., Apicella, P., and Ljungberg, T. (1993). Responses of monkey dopamine neurons to reward and conditioned stimuli during successive steps of learning a delayed response task. *Journal of Neuroscience 13*: 900–913.

Schultz, W., Apicella, P., Scarnati, E. and Ljungberg, T. (1992). Neuronal activity in monkey ventral striatum related to the expectation of reward. *Journal of Neuroscience 12*: 4595–4610.

Schultz, W., Dayan, P., and Montague, P. R. (1997). A neural substrate of prediction and reward. *Science 275*: 1593–1599.

Selemon, L. D. and Goldman-Rakic, P. S. (1985). Longitudinal topography and interdigitation of corticostriatal projections in the rhesus monkey. *Journal of Neuroscience 5*: 776–794.

Selemon, L. D. and Goldman-Rakic, P. S. (1988). Common cortical and subcortical targets of the dorsolateral prefrontal and posterior parietal cortices in the rhesus monkey: Evidence for a distributed neural network subserving spatially guided behavior. *Journal of Neuroscience 8*: 4049–4068.

Siegel, M., Donner, T. H., Oostenveld, R., Fries, P., and Engel, A. K. (2008). Neuronal synchronization along the dorsal visual pathway reflects the focus of spatial attention. *Neuron 60*: 709–719.

Siegel, M. and Konig, P. (2003). A functional gamma-band defined by stimulus-dependent synchronization in area 18 of awake behaving cats. *Journal of Neuroscience 23*: 4251–4260.

Siegel, M., Warden, M. R., and Miller, E. K. (2009). Phase-dependent neuronal coding of objects in short-term memory. *Proceedings of the National Academy of Sciences USA 106*: 21341–21346.

Sompolinsky, H. and Kanter, I. (1986). Temporal association in asymmetric neural networks. *Physical Review Letters 57*: 2861–2864.

Steinmetz, P. N., Roy, A., Fitzgerald, P. J., Hsiao, S. S., Johnson, K. O., and Niebur, E. (2000). Attention modulates synchronized neuronal firing in primate somatosensory cortex. *Nature 404*: 187–190.

Tallon-Baudry, C., Bertrand, O., Peronnet, F., and Pernier, J. (1998). Induced gamma-band activity during the delay of a visual short-term memory task in humans. *Journal of Neuroscience 18*: 4244–4254.

Thierry, A. M., Blanc, G., Sobel, A., Stinus, L., and Glowinski, J. (1973). Dopaminergic terminals in the rat cortex. *Science 182*: 499–501.

Tiesinga, P. H., Fellous, J. M., Jose, J. V., and Sejnowski, T. J. (2002). Information transfer in entrained cortical neurons. *Network 13*: 41–66.

Treisman, A. M. and Gelade, G. (1980). A feature-integration theory of attention. *Cognitive Psychology 12*: 97–136.

Usrey, W. M. and Reid, R. C. (1999). Synchronous activity in the visual system. *Annual Review of Physiology 61*: 435–456.

Vogel, E. K. and Machizawa, M. G. (2004). Neural activity predicts individual differences in visual working memory capacity. *Nature 428*: 748–751.

Vogel, E. K., McCollough, A. W., and Machizawa, M. G. (2005). Neural measures reveal individual differences in controlling access to working memory. *Nature 438*: 500–503.

Wallis, J. D., Anderson, K. C., and Miller, E. K. (2001). Single neurons in the prefrontal cortex encode abstract rules. *Nature 411*: 953–956.

White, I. M. and Wise, S. P. (1999). Rule-dependent neuronal activity in the prefrontal cortex. *Experimental Brain Research 126*: 315–335.

Wise, S. P., Murray, E. A., and Gerfen, C. R. (1996). The frontal-basal ganglia system in primates. *Critical Reviews in Neurobiology 10*: 317–356.

Wolfe, J. M., Cave, K. R., and Franzel, S. L. (1989). Guided search: An alternative to the feature integration model for visual search. *Journal of Experimental Psychology: Human Perception and Performance 15*: 419–433.

Womelsdorf, T., Fries, P., Mitra, P. P., and Desimone, R. (2006). Gamma-band synchronization in visual cortex predicts speed of change detection. *Nature 439*: 733–736.

Woodman, G. F. and Luck, S. J. (2004). Visual search is slowed when visuospatial working memory is occupied. *Psychonomic Bulletin & Review 11*: 269–274.

....

CHAPTER 28

MEMORY AND ATTENTION

....

BRICE A. KUHL AND MARVIN M. CHUN

INTRODUCTION

A primary theme in attention research is that there is too much information in our environment for everything to be processed and, as a consequence, information processing is selective (Chun et al. 2011). While memory is traditionally thought of as distinct from attention, memory is also subject to processing constraints and necessarily requires selection. That is, we cannot encode into long-term memory all elements of our environment, nor is it possible—or desirable—during acts of retrieval to simultaneously bring to mind all of the information we have encoded. Rather, at every stage of memory, processing constraints are present and selection is required.

In this chapter, we review various properties of memory from the perspective of selective attention. Rather than considering memory and attention as two independent systems that cooperate with one another, we argue that the ways in which we form, retrieve, and work with our memories largely represent *acts of attention* (Chun and Johnson 2011). For example, our ability to selectively bring to mind specific details of a past event is not a phenomenon that simply *co-opts* attention; instead, the act of directing thought to specific mental representations of past events is, itself, a form of internally oriented attention. One obvious advantage of framing mnemonic processes as attentional phenomena is that it underscores the processing limits that are central to memory and the necessity of selection. Another advantage is that this framework can aid our understanding of the neural mechanisms that guide memory and their relation to neural mechanisms of perceptual attention.

The basic conceptualization of the relationship between memory and attention described here draws from two recent theoretical frameworks. The first framework (Chun et al. 2011) argues for multiple forms of attention, distinguishing between attention that is externally oriented (i.e. directed to perceptual stimuli in our environment) vs. internally oriented (i.e. focused on our thoughts or memories). According to a second, complementary framework (Chun and Johnson 2011), memory encoding generally represents the consequence of externally oriented *perceptual attention*, while our ability to bring past experiences to mind represents a form of internally oriented *reflective attention*.

Although the distinction between reflective and perceptual attention is a central theme here, we organize the present review according to different forms and stages of memory. We begin by considering the relationship between attention and long-term episodic memory—that is, explicit memory for past events or episodes. We divide this topic into two distinct stages of episodic memory: encoding and retrieval. We next consider how attention relates to working memory, or the online storage and manipulation of information. Finally, we review how past experience influences the way we allocate attention in current environments.

ATTENTION AND ENCODING

We need only consult our intuition to recognize the importance of attention to memory encoding. When lost in thought for a few minutes, we may find that we have near amnesia for the external events that occurred just moments before. Similarly, two people that experienced the same event may have very different memories for that event according to the specific information that each person attended. Simply, attention at encoding profoundly influences what we remember. Hence, studying the relationship between attention and encoding provides important insight into the requirements for successful remembering.

We first consider a powerful neuroimaging paradigm that has yielded considerable insight into the encoding factors that promote successful remembering. We then focus on two specific themes addressing the relationship between attention and encoding. One theme has focused on how performing a secondary (distracting) task impacts encoding success. These 'divided attention' studies are based on the logic that when a secondary task impairs encoding, this indicates that a common form of attention is required by the two tasks. A second theme has focused on how attention is selectively oriented to individual elements of our perceptual environment. That is, how is memory encoding biased via top-down control (e.g. strategic encoding goals) or bottom-up factors (e.g. the salience of perceptual elements)?

Predictors of successful remembering

What are the neural mechanisms that determine whether an event will later be remembered versus forgotten? This fundamental question has been addressed by well over a hundred studies using the *subsequent memory paradigm*. In this paradigm, fMRI or electroencephalography (EEG) data are recorded as subjects encode various events—for example as subjects encode words or pictures. These neural measures during encoding are then separated and contrasted according to whether the events are later remembered or later forgotten (Brewer et al. 1998; Wagner et al. 1998). This allows for specification of neural regions that support memory formation (i.e. regions that display greater, or lower, responses for subsequently remembered events).

Positive subsequent memory effects have consistently been observed in medial temporal lobe regions, lateral prefrontal cortex, and posterior cortical areas (Kim 2011; Paller and Wagner 2002; Spaniol et al. 2009) (Fig. 28.1a). Critically, the specific regions that display subsequent memory effects are partially dependent on *how* subjects orient attention to encoded information—for example, whether subjects focus attention on the phonological or semantic representation of a word (Paller and Wagner 2002). Thus, relationships between neural encoding responses and subsequent remembering are likely to reflect contributions of attentional mechanisms. Indeed, variance in neural activity just *before* an event is experienced predicts later memory (Guderian et al. 2009; Otten et al. 2006; Turk-Browne et al. 2006). For example, in scene-selective cortical regions, activity prior to the encoding of a scene is greater if the scene is subsequently remembered as compared to forgotten (Turk-Browne et al. 2006). Thus, subsequent memory paradigms have the potential to identify attentional states that facilitate successful encoding.

While the majority of subsequent memory analyses have, to date, focused on univariate contrasts of response amplitude as measured by fMRI or electroencephalography, several exciting new variants of the subsequent memory paradigm have recently

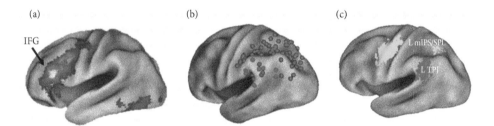

(a)   (b)   (c)

IFG

L mIPS/SPL

L TPJ

FIGURE 28.1 Neural regions that predict later memory. (a) A meta-analysis by Kim (2011) found a robust positive relationship between encoding responses within left inferior frontal gyrus (IFG) and subsequent memory. (b) Distribution of positive (red) and negative (blue) subsequent memory effects in lateral parietal cortex. Positive subsequent memory effects are regularly observed in dorsal parietal cortex, including the superior parietal lobule (SPL) and intraparietal sulcus (IPS); negative subsequent memory effects have been restricted to the inferior parietal lobule (IPL). From Uncapher and Wagner (2009). (c) Conjunction of subsequent memory analyses and effects of attention. A region of left medial IPS (mIPS)/SPL was associated with top-down orienting of spatial attention (in response to spatial cues) and was positively associated with later memory for objects that appeared at cued locations. A region of left temporo-parietal junction (TPJ) in ventral parietal cortex was associated with bottom-up capture of attention (when objects appeared at uncued locations) and was negatively related to subsequent memory for objects. Adapted from Uncapher, M. R., Hutchinson, J. B., and Wagner, A. D., Dissociable effects of top-down and bottom-up attention during episodic encoding, *Journal of Neuroscience*, 31, pp. 12613–12628 © 2011, The Society for Neuroscience. Note: for all panels, only the left hemisphere is shown; effects in the right hemisphere are qualitatively similar.

appeared. For example, intracranial recordings from human subjects have revealed that greater oscillatory power in theta and gamma bands during event encoding is associated with a higher probability of subsequent remembering (Sederberg et al. 2003). Because increases in oscillatory power reflect greater synchronization of neuronal firing, these patterns may reflect increased attentional processing that enhances memory (Jensen et al. 2007).

Another recent trend has been to characterize patterns of neural activity during successful event encoding using multivariate analyses. For example, fMRI has been used to measure distributed patterns of neural activity across repeated viewings of visual stimuli in order to test whether pattern similarity across repeated viewings is associated with better memory outcomes (Xue et al. 2010). Indeed, greater similarity across viewings of a stimulus was associated with better subsequent memory. In a related study, Kuhl et al. used pattern classification analyses to measure the strength of visual category information in prefrontal and temporal lobe structures during the encoding of images of faces and scenes (Kuhl et al. 2012). They found that subtle differences in the strength of visual category information, as reflected in patterns of activity in prefrontal and temporal lobe regions, were predictive of later memory. Thus, these studies suggest methods for probing how the fidelity of information representation during encoding—and, therefore how attention is allocated—relates to later memory.

Together, the above findings highlight the utility of the subsequent memory paradigm for identifying neural mechanisms that contribute to encoding success. As we discuss in more detail below, variants of this paradigm have been used to characterize how encoding mechanisms—and the corresponding likelihood of remembering encoded information—are influenced by manipulations of attention during encoding.

Competition across tasks

To understand the relationship between attention and memory encoding, an obvious starting point is to ask how limiting attentional resources impacts encoding. One of the classic findings in memory research is that performing a secondary task during encoding reliably and often robustly impairs encoding success—a 'dual task' cost that is usually much weaker or absent during retrieval (Baddeley et al. 1984; Craik et al. 1996). These observations show that encoding is particularly resource demanding whereas retrieval may be relatively automatic (a topic we consider in more detail below). The notion that encoding is resource demanding is consistent with the well-known finding that episodic memory benefits from more elaborated encoding (Craik and Tulving 1975). That is, simply registering that an item appears will yield relatively poor memory, but actively incorporating that item into ongoing mental activities through strategic allocation of attention will increase the probability that it is later remembered.

Several neuroimaging studies have sought to specify which neural encoding mechanisms are disrupted in dual task situations by comparing encoding activity when a secondary task is easy or absent, relative to when it is more difficult and challenging. A consistent finding across these studies is that encoding activity in left lateral prefrontal cortex is reduced when a challenging secondary task is concurrently performed (Anderson et al. 2000; Fletcher et al. 1995; Kensinger et al. 2003; Shallice et al. 1994). These findings suggest that encoding mechanisms supported by left lateral prefrontal cortex rely on general attentional mechanisms, which become taxed during a challenging secondary task. These observations support more general evidence that lateral prefrontal cortex contributes to memory encoding by enabling control processes (Simons and Spiers 2003).

Although divided attention paradigms often present subjects with a seemingly unnatural situation—for example, trying to learn pairs of words while rehearsing an arbitrary string of numbers—in 'real world' contexts we are frequently distracted from to-be-learned information by other tasks we try to perform simultaneously. For example, failures to remember details of a conversation may be attributable to attention being simultaneously allocated to driving or to thoughts that drift to other topics. Indeed, even in experimental situations where an overt secondary task is not present, subjects may nonetheless 'divide' their attention between the experimental task and other thoughts or perceptual information. This idea has been offered as a potential explanation for 'negative subsequent memory effects' that have often been reported. That is, in contrast to neural regions whose encoding activity *positively* predicts later memory, activity in some regions *negatively* predicts later memory (Blumenfeld and Ranganath 2007; Turk-Browne et al. 2006; Uncapher and Wagner 2009; Wagner and Davachi 2001). For example, negative subsequent memory effects have been consistently observed in ventral posterior parietal cortex (PPC) (Uncapher and Wagner 2009) (Fig. 28.1b), a region that is frequently associated with the bottom-up capture of attention (Corbetta and Shulman 2002). Thus, encoding events associated with increased activity in ventral PPC may reflect situations where attention has been captured by task-irrelevant information, therefore accounting for the negative relation with later memory.

Building on the basic finding that episodic encoding is impaired when attention is divided, subsequent work has tried to better characterize the forms of long-term memory which are most impacted by distraction. One finding is that divided attention disproportionately affects binding of different elements of an event. For example, divided attention produces greater deficits in memory for associations between items than in memory for items themselves (Castel and Craik 2003; Troyer et al. 1999; cf. Naveh-Benjamin et al. 2003). These findings suggest that encoding associations between items places greater demands on general attentional mechanisms and parallels evidence that perceptual attention is necessary for perceptual feature integration (Treisman and Gelade 1980). A second finding is that whereas divided attention has robust costs for *explicit* memory (e.g. item recognition, cued recall, free recall), costs to *implicit* memory (e.g. measures of priming) may be reduced or, in some cases, absent (Mulligan 1997, 1998; Wolters and Prinsen 1997). These observations illustrate the attentional demands associated with various types of encoding.

Competition between perceptual events

We cannot attend to every source of information in the environment, and, correspondingly, we will not remember everything. Thus, we should consider how attention is allocated among competing perceptual elements and how these acts of selective attention relate to later remembering. The questions here largely parallel questions asked in the domain of perceptual decision-making. For example, whereas in perceptual decision-making competition among stimuli has been considered in terms of neural activity in representational structures, here we consider how the modulations of representational structures during encoding relate to what is later remembered. Similarly, what are the neural mechanisms that guide attention in a top-down manner to promote the formation of long-term memories that are consistent with our goals? How does the bottom-up capture of attention by salient perceptual information influence later memory? And how much, or how little, do we learn about unattended elements in our environment?

Modulation of representational structures during encoding. A basic principle of selective attention is that when multiple elements in our perceptual environment compete for attention, the elements that are ultimately attended are afforded stronger neural representation (Kanwisher and Wojciulik 2000). For example, when face and scene stimuli are simultaneously presented, neural responses within face- and scene-sensitive regions of ventral temporal cortex track which of the stimuli is being attended (Gazzaley et al. 2005; O'Craven et al. 1999; Yi and Chun 2005). To the extent that these modulations are a marker of attentional allocation, and because episodic encoding depends on successful attention, it should follow that successful encoding is related to these modulations. Indeed, in studies that have measured modulation in representational structures as well as subsequent memory, attended stimuli have been associated with both stronger neural representation and better subsequent memory, relative to unattended competing stimuli (Dudukovic et al. 2011; Johnson and Zatorre 2005; Yi and Chun 2005). Notably, selective attention is also associated with greater neural adaptation for attended stimuli (Yi and Chun 2005) (Fig. 28.2)—that is, reduced fMRI responses when attended stimuli are repeated—suggesting that attention-related modulations of neural activity may capture both implicit and explicit forms of memory (Turk-Browne et al. 2006).

Other studies have more directly assessed whether trial-by-trial variance in the strength of attention-related modulation is predictive of subsequent memory. In a task where either object location or object colour was task relevant on a given trial, the strength of modulation in relevant cortical areas was associated with later memory success (Uncapher and Rugg 2009). For example, selective attention to colour was associated with increased activity in visual areas that represent colour (V4) and the greater this modulation, the higher the probability of later remembering colour information. This complements more general evidence that encoding activity within category-sensitive visual cortical regions is predictive of subsequent memory when a stimulus from a preferred category is encoded (Prince et al. 2009). Thus, the success with which cortical

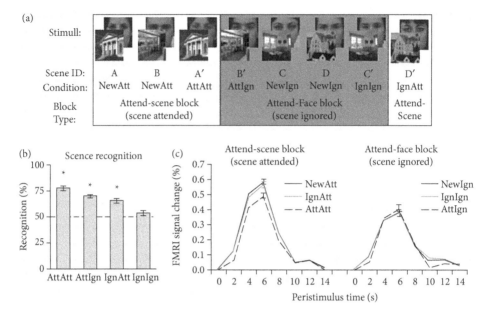

FIGURE 28.2 Attention is required for both memory encoding and expression; from Yi and Chun (2005). In the experiment, subjects performed a task that required attention to either scenes or faces. (a) Illustration of the experimental design that manipulated whether scenes were attended or ignored during first presentation (initial encoding) and/or during second presentation (re-exposure). Each scene–face pair stands for a trial in which two identical composite stimuli were presented in rapid sequence; here, the scene and face images are spatially segregated for illustration purposes. Scenes were repeated across two separate trials, each paired with a different face. During the initial presentation, novel scenes were either attended (i.e. appeared in an 'attend-scene block', NewAtt; e.g. A and B) or ignored (i.e. appeared in an 'attend-face block', NewIgn; e.g. C and D). Likewise, when these scenes were repeated in subsequent trials, they were either attended (A' and D') or ignored (B' and C'), providing four old conditions with different attention histories (AttAtt, attended and attended; AttIgn, attended and ignored; IgnAtt, ignored and attended; IgnIgn, ignored and ignored). (b) Scene-recognition performance outside the scanner revealed best memory for scenes attended during both appearances, poorer memory for scenes attended only once, and chance performance for scenes that were never attended. The dashed line indicates the 50% chance level. Asterisks indicate above-chance recognition. (c) Activations in a parahippocampal place area ROI revealed significant repetition attenuation/adaptation (index of implicit memory) only when scenes were attended during initial encoding and during the second presentation (when adaptation is measured). The error bars indicate SEM. Reproduced from Yi, D. J., and Chun, M. M., Attentional modulation of learning-related repetition attenuation effects in human parahippocampal cortex, *Journal of Neuroscience*, 25, pp. 3593–3600 © 2005, The Society for Neuroscience.

representational areas are modulated by attention may serve as a marker of the success with which selective encoding has occurred.

The relationship between the modulation of representational areas and subsequent memory is strongly consistent with the idea that episodic memory is a direct consequence of—or represents a trace of—prior acts of externally oriented attention (Chun and Johnson 2011). Notably, by this view, the relationship between attention and later memory does not depend on a deliberate intention to encode for the sake of later remembering; rather, memory will be a by-product of how attention was previously oriented, whether or not these prior acts of attention were related to an explicit motivation to form long-term memories.

Top-down control during encoding. If memory is a result of attention, what are the mechanisms that drive these acts of attention in a top-down manner? As reviewed above, mechanisms that support top-down allocation of attention should positively contribute to encoding success.

A recent study directly tested for a relationship between top-down shifts of spatial attention and memory encoding by using a spatial cueing paradigm in which pictures of objects appeared at cued or uncued locations (Uncapher et al. 2011). Top-down orientation of attention to a cued location was associated with activity in the intraparietal sulcus (IPS) and superior parietal lobule (SPL), consistent with prior findings (Corbetta and Shulman 2002). Critically, these top-down shifts of attention in dorsal parietal cortex were positively associated with subsequent memory, but only when objects appeared at validly cued locations (i.e. cued location = object location); in contrast, when objects appeared at invalidly cued locations (i.e. cued location ≠ object location), the magnitude of dorsal parietal cueing activity was *negatively* associated with subsequent memory (Fig. 28.1c). In other words, successfully orienting attention to a cued location benefited memory for objects that appeared at the cued locations, but these shifts of attention actually resulted in costs when objects did not appear at the cued locations.

While top-down allocation of attention benefits long-term memory, a flipside is that failures of selective attention during encoding may be associated with *increased* learning of goal-irrelevant information. Indeed, relative to younger adults, older adults display impaired filtering of goal-irrelevant visual stimuli—as reflected in weaker modulation of representational areas in ventral temporal cortex—and when responses in ventral temporal cortex indicate that modulation is particular deficient, older adults are *more likely* to encode and later remember goal-irrelevant stimuli (Gazzaley et al. 2005 (in chapter 32)). Thus, top-down acts of attention are essential for encoding relevant information about our environment as well as preventing the encoding of irrelevant information. Successfully achieving these acts of selective encoding relies on functional interactions between fronto-parietal cortical mechanisms and posterior representational areas (Gazzaley et al. 2007; Uncapher et al. 2011; Zanto et al. 2011).

Bottom-up influences during encoding. In contrast to top-down goals that determine what features of an event we attend to and remember, some elements of our perceptual experience result in a bottom-up capture of attention and corresponding biases in memory. One particularly striking illustration of this is that when people view pictures of scenes that either contain or do not contain a weapon (e.g. a restaurant with a man holding a handgun vs. a man holding a cheque), attention is strongly drawn to the weapon—i.e. 'weapon focus'—resulting in poorer memory for the scene (Loftus et al. 1987). Similarly, when a scene contains a central element that is of strong negative valence (e.g. a car crash), that element will be well remembered while memory for background information about the scene is impaired, relative to when the central element is emotionally neutral (Kensinger et al. 2007). These observations complement evidence that dual task costs during encoding are reduced if to-be-encoded information is negatively arousing (Kern et al. 2005). Thus, highly salient elements in our environment can robustly bias how attention is oriented and what we ultimately remember.

Unexpected stimuli also capture attention in a bottom-up manner that influences memory. Ventral PPC regions, including the temporal parietal junction (TPJ) show increased activity when stimuli appear at unexpected locations (Corbetta and Shulman 2002). A number of studies have shown that ventral PPC activity during encoding negatively correlates with subsequent remembering, leading to suggestions that activity in ventral PPC reflects capture of attention by task irrelevant representations (Uncapher and Wagner 2009; Turk-Browne et al. submitted). But how do ventral PPC responses relate to later memory when *task-relevant* stimuli appear at unexpected locations?

Interestingly, a recent study found that TPJ activity was particularly robust when an object appeared at an unexpected location *and* was later forgotten (Uncapher et al. 2011) (Fig. 28.1c). While this observation is consistent with prior evidence that TPJ activity during encoding is negatively associated with subsequent memory, it raises the following question: if stimuli that elicit bottom-up capture of attention are often well remembered (as in weapon focus), and if TPJ activity reflects bottom-up capture of attention, why would TPJ responses to stimuli at unexpected locations be *negatively* correlated with later memory? One possibility is that when objects appear at an unexpected location, TPJ activity indexes bottom-up attention to *spatial information*, which may come at the expense of attending to non-spatial features of the stimulus. Thus, an area of future interest will be to identify whether there are situations in which TPJ responses to unexpected stimuli are positively associated with subsequent memory.

Memory for unattended information. What do we learn about the elements of our environment that we do not attend? How much, or how little, do we remember about selected-against (ignored) information?

Behavioural measures of memory have typically indicated that unattended information is poorly learned. For example, when memory for unattended information is measured by explicit tests (e.g. recognition memory), there is often *little to no evidence* of learning (Eich 1984; Merikle and Reingold 1991; Rock and Gutman 1981; Yi and Chun 2005). Similarly, neuroimaging evidence indicates that neural adaptation is absent when stimuli are repeated but not attended (Eger et al. 2004; Yi and Chun 2005), indicating that even low-level forms of perceptual learning may not occur for ignored stimuli. Interestingly, however, recent evidence indicates that even when unattended stimuli are explicitly classified as unfamiliar, confidence in these judgements is lower, relative to stimuli that were not presented at all (Hoffman et al. 2011), suggesting a very subtle form of learning for unattended stimuli. Similarly, in situations where unattended information may not be explicitly recognized, there is evidence that at least some forms of implicit learning (e.g. forms of priming) may occur for unattended information (Eich 1984; Jiang and Leung 2005; Merikle and Reingold 1991).

Together the literature concerning learning of unattended information indicates that while unattended stimuli are poorly remembered when considering typical measures of recognition memory, some forms of learning may nonetheless occur and can be revealed when memory is probed in subtle ways. An interesting question worth future investigation is whether the absence of explicit memory for ignored information can be fully explained in terms of 'lack or attention' at encoding or whether unattended information is actively inhibited as a means of suppressing distraction (Gazzaley et al. 2005). Furthermore, one should always consider that inattention is a relative, not an absolute, state, and that the availability of attention in divided attention situations is affected by concurrent task type and task difficulty (Chun and Turk-Browne 2007; Chun et al. 2011; Lavie 2005).

Attention and Retrieval

Arguably, the most remarkable feature of human memory is our ability to selectively retrieve and bring to mind individual memories of past events from the vast stores of information we retain. Because we hold so much information about the past, interference between memories is often the main obstacle to successful retrieval (Anderson 2003; Kuhl and Wagner 2009). Thus, successful retrieval critically depends on *selective* retrieval—that is, favouring goal-relevant memories over competing or interfering alternatives. This leads to the proposal that memory retrieval is, in fact, an act of selective attention (Anderson and Spellman 1995; Chun and Turk-Browne 2007; Chun and Johnson 2011). In contrast to the form of attention required at encoding—externally oriented or *perceptual attention*—memory retrieval requires internally oriented or *reflective attention*. Here we consider the relationship between attention and retrieval by first considering how retrieval is impacted when attention is divided across tasks and then considering how attention is allocated among individual, competing memories.

Competition across tasks

Retrieval of episodic memories has traditionally been viewed as less reliant on general attentional mechanisms than encoding because of the relatively small costs to retrieval that are observed when a secondary task is performed (Baddeley et al. 1984; Craik et al. 1996). However, while sometimes subtle, dual task costs are often present during retrieval, and it is informative to consider the forms of retrieval that are most impaired by a secondary task.

As with encoding, explicit recognition or retrieval is more disrupted by a secondary task than implicit memory (Clarke and Butler 2008; Jacoby et al. 1989). In a classic demonstration of this dissociation, Jacoby and colleagues (1989) presented subjects with names of famous and non-famous individuals during an encoding task; at retrieval subjects were presented with a list of names and asked to judge whether the names corresponded to famous or non-famous individuals. Critically, when retrieval was performed with a secondary task, subjects were more likely to mistakenly claim that previously encoded non-famous names were actually names of famous individuals (relative to retrieval without a secondary task). It was argued that the secondary task selectively impaired subjects' ability to consciously recollect the source of familiarity (i.e. is this a name I encountered earlier in the experiment, or a name I have seen in the news?); thus, when names appeared familiar but recollection of the source of this familiarity was impaired, these names had an increased probability of being misclassified as famous.

Although memory retrieval may often succeed in dual task situations, one interesting question is whether successful retrieval under full versus divided attention has a similar influence on *later* memory. In particular, because the act of retrieval functions as a powerful (re-)encoding event that typically benefits later memory (Karpicke and Roediger 2008), and because encoding is strongly impacted by divided attention, dividing attention during retrieval may reduce the benefit to later memory that retrieval usually affords. Indeed, successful recognition of an item in a dual task situation reduces the probability of recognizing that item again at a future point in time, relative to successful recognition with full attention (Dudukovic et al. 2009). Thus, even if retrieval succeeds when attention is divided, there are costs for future remembering.

Another factor that is relevant to dual task costs during retrieval is the type of secondary task that is performed. In particular, when the secondary task directly competes with the retrieval task for common representational information, costs to retrieval are more apparent (Fernandes and Moscovitch 2000, 2003). For example, retrieval of verbal information is more impaired when a secondary task involves word monitoring than digit monitoring (Fernandes and Moscovitch 2000). Indeed, representational competition can impair retrieval even when the 'dual task' is not a task at all: for example, detailed retrieval of visual memories is impaired when retrieval cues are accompanied by the presentation of completely irrelevant background visual images (i.e. background images that have no relevance to subjects' behavioural responses) (Wais et al. 2010). This behavioural impairment is associated with reduced functional interactivity of lateral prefrontal and visual cortical regions, suggesting disrupted access to visual memories. Indeed, transcranial magnetic stimulation of the inferior frontal gyrus selectively increases the impairment caused by visual distraction, indicating a direct role for the inferior frontal gyrus in overcoming interfering information (Fig. 28.3) (Wais et al. 2012).

Thus, relative to encoding, dual task costs at retrieval are, on the whole, less pronounced but are not absent. To summarize: dual task costs will be higher when the retrieval task involves more attention-demanding processes (e.g. retrieval of source information), when retrieval is viewed as an encoding event, or when the secondary task—or even background perceptual information—competes with the retrieval task for representational information.

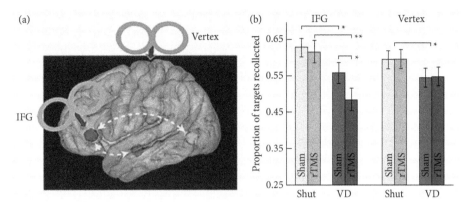

FIGURE 28.3 Visual distraction during retrieval is exacerbated by repetitive transcranial magnetic stimulation (rTMS) perturbation of inferior frontal gyrus (IFG); from Wais et al. (2012). In the experiment, subjects first studied displays of objects (e.g. four pumpkins or one piece of pie). Following study, rTMS or sham (pulses oriented away from brain site) was applied either to the inferior frontal gyrus (IFG) or a control site (vertex). Immediately afterward, subjects were presented with auditory cues (e.g. pumpkin) and asked to report the number of corresponding objects they had previously studied (e.g. how many pumpkins were in the display?). Retrieval was either performed with eyes shut or while subjects viewed background scenes that were completely irrelevant to subjects' task. (a) Illustration of rTMS sites (IFG, vertex) along with regions previously identified as functionally connected with IFG: left hippocampus (magenta) and lateral occipital cortex (green), as reported by Wais et al. (2010). (b) Object memory shown as a function of sham/rTMS and brain site (IFG/vertex). Visual distraction (VD) was associated with overall lower recollection, but rTMS applied to IFG was associated with a selective exaggeration of this interference cost. Reproduced from Wais, P. E., Kim, O. Y., and Gazzaley, A., Distractibility during Episodic Retrieval Is Exacerbated by Perturbation of Left Ventrolateral Prefrontal Cortex, *Cerebral Cortex*, 22(3), pp. 717–724, figure 3 © 2012, Oxford University Press.

Competition between mnemonic representations

While episodic memory is powerful because it is highly associative, its associative nature also creates the potential for interference (McClelland et al. 1995). Moreover, it is precisely in these situations of interference that the parallel between selective perceptual attention and selective reflective attention is most compelling. In this section, we consider the mechanisms that guide retrieval to relevant (target) memories amidst interference. We begin by describing some of the paradigms commonly used to study interference during retrieval—that is, situations in which retrieval most strongly involves selective attention.

The most extensively studied paradigm in the memory interference literature is the classic A–B, A–C learning paradigm. In this paradigm, an initial association between two items is first acquired (A–B pair; e.g. the word pair 'DOG–HAT'). Following A–B learning, subjects may study a new unrelated pair (D–E pair; e.g. 'CAR–TABLE'), a new related pair (A–C pair; e.g. 'DOG-SHOE'), or no new association. When memory for the A–B association is tested (A–?), retrieval success is typically lowest in the A–C condition, reflecting interference between the B and C terms that share a common cue (i.e. the A term). This form of interference is known as *retroactive interference*. Conversely, when memory for an A–C association is tested, having previously learned an A–B pair also creates interference—termed *proactive interference*. The retrieval difficulty—and accompanying forgetting—in these tasks can be explained in terms of competition between the relevant and irrelevant associations that arises during the time of retrieval (Mensink and Raaijmakers 1988).

Retrieval interference has also been studied in a related paradigm in which subjects encode various propositions with overlapping elements (e.g. 'the fireman is in the park', 'the lawyer is in the park'); the reaction time to recognize a proposition increases as a function of the number of elements associated with that proposition (e.g. as a function of how many people were in the park). This finding, termed the 'fan effect', has been described in computational models in terms of a finite amount of activation that must be shared among all associated elements of a proposition (Anderson 1974). Thus, paralleling situations of selective perceptual attention, memory retrieval in these associative interference paradigms represents a situation of selecting among competing representations.

Below, we consider several specific questions regarding competition between memories. As in the section describing competition during encoding, we begin by asking whether selective retrieval—or, selective attention to individual memories—is reflected in activity within representational structures. Second, we describe fronto-parietal mechanisms that guide retrieval in the face of competition. Finally, we consider the fate of memories that are *selected against* (ignored) during acts of retrieval.

Modulation of representational structures during retrieval. As described above, when perceptual stimuli compete during encoding, neural activity tracks representations that are attended (e.g. O'Craven et al. 1999; Yi and Chun 2005) and may serve as a marker of lapses in filtering (Gazzaley et al. 2005). Because memory retrieval involves reactivating neural regions that were engaged during the encoding or perception of an event (for review see Danker and Anderson 2010), one can ask how or whether activity in these representational regions is modulated according to competition during retrieval. Does modulation of neural activity serve as a marker of how reflective attention is allocated?

As described above, the fan effect is thought to occur because competing associations become active during a retrieval event—and, in particular because limited processing resources are shared among these representations. This interpretation predicts that activity in representational regions will reflect the activation of competing associations. Indeed, in a fan paradigm where associations consist of faces or locations, retrieval activity in neural regions that represent faces or locations increases when the number of faces or locations, respectively, that are associated with a given retrieval cue increases (i.e. the size of the fan) (Khader et al. 2005a, 2005b). Similarly, when older memories share a semantic category with newer memories, retrieval of newer (target) memories—a situation that is subject to proactive interference—elicits a particularly strong neural representation of the shared semantic category (Öztekin and Badre 2011). Moreover, the magnitude of this increase in category representation correlates with retrieval failures in behaviour. Thus, when memories that share representational information compete during retrieval, stronger activity in representational regions may serve as a marker of non-selective retrieval of—or attention to—the target memory.

An alternative approach to studying neural measures of competition is to consider cases where competing associations correspond to *distinct* categories—and, therefore, distinct neural representations. In a pair of studies, Kuhl and colleagues employed an A–B, A–C learning paradigm in which the B and C terms corresponded to distinct visual categories—faces and scenes in one study; faces, scenes, or objects in another study (Kuhl et al. 2011, 2012). Multivoxel pattern analysis was applied to fMRI data collected during retrieval in order to assess whether visual category representation during retrieval of the most recent association (i.e. the A–C pair) was influenced by the prior (A–B) association. Indeed, when a prior association competed with a newer (target)

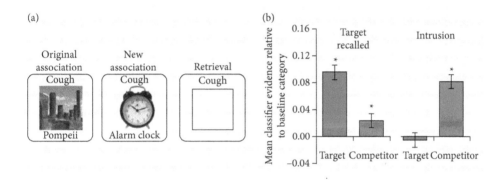

FIGURE 28.4 Neural reactivation reveals competition during memory retrieval, from Kuhl, Bainbridge, and Chun (2012). (a) In the experiment, subjects first encoded initial word-image pairings (original associations). Images were drawn from one of three categories: faces, objects, scenes. Subjects then encoded some of the same words paired with new images (new associations). At retrieval, subjects were presented with words and attempted to retrieve the most recent (target) image paired with each word. Older associations, which were no longer relevant, functioned as competing memories. Of critical interest were cases where subjects were successful at retrieving the target image and cases where older, competing images were erroneously reported (intrusions). (b) A pattern classifier was applied to retrieval trials to measure the degree to which patterns of encoding activity reflecting visual category information were reactivated at retrieval. During successful memory retrieval (left panel), target reactivation (as indexed by classifier evidence) was strongest, but competing memories also showed significant reactivation. Indeed, the strength of competitor reactivation was positively correlated with reaction time (stronger competitor reactivation = slower reaction time). On intrusion trials (right panel), reactivation of the competitor was robust, with no evidence for target reactivation. Thus, these error trials were associated with strong reactivation of the competing memory and a failure to reactivate the target memory. Reproduced from Kuhl, B. A., Bainbridge, W. A., and Chun, M. M., Neural reactivation reveals mechanisms for updating memory, *Journal of Neuroscience*, 32, pp. 3453–3461 © 2012, The Society for Neuroscience.

association, patterns of activity within ventral temporal cortex indicated that older (competing) associations were simultaneously reinstated—or *reactivated*—in ventral temporal cortex (Fig. 28.4). Notably, stronger reactivation of competing memories was associated with more retrieval errors and slower reaction time (Kuhl et al. 2012), and a higher probability that the competing memory would later be remembered (Kuhl et al. 2011). Thus, complementing observations that ventral temporal cortical activity is modulated according to how *perceptual* attention is oriented to competing *external visual stimuli* (O'Craven et al. 1999; Yi and Chun 2005), these findings indicate that ventral temporal cortex is modulated according to how *reflective* attention is oriented to competing *internal representations of past events*.

Top-down control during retrieval. Given the vast number of memories we retain, the need for selection during retrieval is obvious; but how is selection achieved? Bearing on this question, humans with damage to prefrontal cortex exhibit memory retrieval deficits that are most pronounced in situations that can be characterized as competitive (for review see Baldo and Shimamura 2002). For example, relative to control subjects, frontal lobe patients are particularly sensitive to interference that arises in A–B, A–C learning paradigms (Shimamura et al. 1995). That is, whereas initial associations (A–B) may be learned with normal success, memory impairments become apparent once a second list (A–C) is acquired and retrieval involves selecting among competing alternatives (B vs. C).

Building on the neuropsychological literature, neuroimaging studies have investigated specific subregions of prefrontal cortex that contribute to competitive retrieval. In particular, inferior frontal gyrus (IFG) activity—most typically left IFG—increases as a function of retrieval competition (Badre and Wagner 2007). For example, in studies of the fan effect, left IFG activity at retrieval increases with fan size (i.e. the number of associates of a retrieval cue) (Danker et al. 2011; Sohn et al. 2003, 2005). Similarly, left IFG retrieval activity is modulated by interference in A–B, A–C learning paradigms (Henson et al. 2002). Moreover, when competition exists among associates of a retrieval cue, repeated retrieval of target memories—which corresponds to behavioural evidence of reductions in competition—is associated with reductions in left IFG engagement (Kuhl et al. 2007, 2008). These findings are complemented by observations that left IFG activity is also modulated by competition during semantic retrieval (Badre et al. 2005; Thompson-Schill et al. 1999).

The above findings suggest an important role for left IFG in contributing to competitive retrieval; but how, in mechanistic terms, does left IFG support retrieval? Left IFG has been hypothesized to support two distinct mechanisms: (1) a mechanism that operates *pre-retrieval* to specify or elaborate retrieval cues to bias the information that gets retrieved or reactivated, and (2) a mechanism that operates *post-retrieval* to select among competing active representations (Badre and Wagner 2007). The former mechanism is thought to be supported by the most anterior aspect of left IFG (Brodmann's area (BA) 47) whereas the latter mechanism is thought to be supported by a more dorsal and caudal aspect of left IFG (BA 45). While this framework suggests that these two mechanisms would be engaged at different points in time during retrieval (with BA 47 activity preceding BA 45), this hypothesis awaits empirical support.

At a conceptual level, the top-down mechanisms supported by left IFG during memory retrieval may parallel selective attention in the perceptual domain. That is, pre-retrieval biasing in memory (Thompson-Schill and Botvinick 2006) may parallel allocation of perceptual attention that can occur before stimuli appear (Kastner et al. 1999). Similarly, selecting among active mnemonic representations (i.e. post-retrieval selection) may parallel selecting among perceptual elements in our environment (Anderson and Spellman 1995; Chun and Turk-Browne 2007; Chun and Johnson 2011). An important area for future research is to specify the specific prefrontal and posterior regions that interact during memory retrieval and the nature of these top-down biases. While direct evidence for these interactions in humans is, at present, limited, there is compelling evidence from studies of monkeys that prefrontal cortex directly modulates temporal lobe structures during retrieval (Tomita et al. 1999), and, as reviewed above, recent human neuroimaging studies have suggested powerful techniques for probing which memories become active in temporal lobe structures during retrieval (Kuhl et al. 2011, 2012; Öztekin and Badre 2011).

Beyond the role of prefrontal cortex during memory retrieval, there is considerable interest in potential similarities in parietal lobe mechanisms that contribute to memory and attention. This interest stems from consistent neuroimaging evidence that activity in lateral parietal cortex increases during successful mnemonic retrieval (for a review see Wagner et al. 2005). In particular, ventral PPC is frequently activated when specific details of an event are recollected, whereas dorsal PPC is active when a stimulus is recognized as having been encountered but without recollection of specific event details (Cabeza et al. 2008; Hutchinson et al. 2009; Wagner et al. 2005). One influential account of these findings is that they reflect the two forms of attention described by Corbetta and Shulman (2002). That is, ventral PPC activity may signal bottom-up capture of attention by retrieval of event details whereas dorsal PPC activity may signal effortful search to recover goal-relevant information (Cabeza 2008; Cabeza et al. 2008). This framework has been termed the 'attention to memory' model.

While the attention to memory model has the advantage of parsimony, in that it explains parietal contributions to both memory retrieval and standard tasks of attention in terms of the same neural mechanisms, focused investigations have challenged this model. For example, Hutchinson et al. (2009) tested for overlap between neural regions that support memory retrieval and attention by conducting a meta-analysis of neuro-imaging studies. They compared activation foci during two forms of remembering (recollection of event details versus item memory without recollection) and two types of attention (top-down visual attention versus bottom-up visual attention). Importantly, they found that memory retrieval and attention foci were more segregated than overlapping (Fig. 28.5a). Within ventral PPC, bottom-up attention effects were clearly more prevalent in anterior regions, including the temporo-parietal junction and supramarginal gyrus, whereas recollection effects were situated in more posterior aspects, including the angular gyrus. Similarly, in dorsal PPC, top-down attention effects tended to be more medial than item recognition effects. Within-subject comparisons of top-down perceptual attention versus top-down memory search provide further support for this

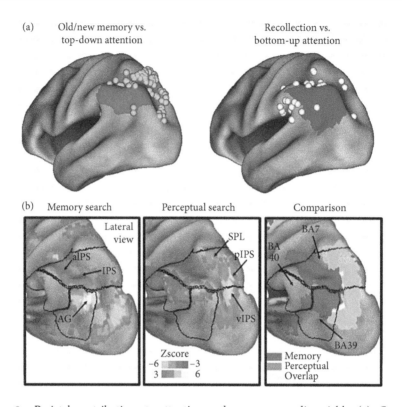

FIGURE 28.5 Parietal contributions to attention and memory are dissociable. (a). Comparison of memory and attention effects in parietal cortex, adapted from Hutchinson, Uncapher, and Wagner, 2009. Left panel: red blob indicates region of parietal cortex associated with old vs. new discriminations at retrieval (item recognition); pink dots indicate foci from studies of top-down visual object/feature attention. Foci from attention studies are largely superior and medial to the region associated with old/new memory effects. Right panel: blue blob indicates region of parietal cortex associated with recollection-based retrieval (i.e., retrieval of item details or context); light blue dots indicate foci from studies of bottom-up visual object/feature attention. Foci from attention studies are largely anterior or superior to the region associated with recollection-based retrieval. Reproduced from Hutchinson, J. B., Uncapher, M. R., and Wagner, A. D., Posterior parietal cortex and episodic retrieval: convergent and divergent effects of attention and memory, *Learning & Memory*, 16 (6), pp. 343–356, Fig. 28.4 © 2009, Cold Spring Harbor Laboratory Press. (b). Within-study comparison of top-down control of memory and perceptual attention reveals more segregation than overlap, from Sestieri et al. (2010). In the experiment, subjects engaged in two tasks: memory search and perceptual search. Memory search involved verifying the accuracy of statements describing previously viewed video clips; perceptual search involved searching for the presence/absence of a specified target in an upcoming video clip. Memory search (left panel) was associated with activation in anterior IPS (aIPS) and angular gyrus (AG); perceptual search (middle panel) was associated with activation in SPL, posterior IPS (pIPS) and ventral IPS (vIPS). Direct comparison of memory and perceptual search (right panel) revealed much stronger segregation than overlap in the regions activated by each task. Reproduced from Sestieri, C., Shulman, G. L., and Corbetta, M., Attention to memory and the environment: Functional specialization and dynamic competition in human posterior parietal cortex, Journal of Neuroscience, 30 (10), pp. 8445–8456 © 2010, The Society for Neuroscience.

segregation within dorsal PPC (Sestieri et al. 2010, Fig. 28.5b). At an even finer level of analysis, comparison of subject-specific spatial attention maps to recollection and item recognition responses has revealed strikingly little overlap in PPC (Hutchinson et al. forthcoming). Notably, however, PPC regions identified from spatial attention maps did exhibit a modulation of activity that corresponded to retrieval demands—perhaps reflecting recruitment of top-down attention to retrieval. Together, these findings indicate that there is clearly segregation among the lateral parietal mechanisms that track recollection and item recognition and those that support attention. Nevertheless, top-down perceptual attention is likely to be recruited when mnemonic decisions require careful scrutiny of perceptual information (Guerin et al. 2012).

If the parietal lobe mechanisms that contribute to memory retrieval are not isomorphic with mechanisms of perceptual attention, how does parietal cortex contribute to memory retrieval? One hypothesis is that parietal responses—particularly those in ventral PPC—reflect the binding of retrieved event details (Shimamura 2011). By this account, ventral PPC functions as a convergence zone that allows discrete elements of an experience to be linked. Two additional hypotheses are that PPC acts as (1) an output buffer, representing retrieved information so that this information can be utilized by decision-making responses, or (2) a mnemonic accumulator, with PPC activity reflecting the strength of memory evidence (Wagner et al. 2005). An additional challenge to understanding parietal lobe contributions to memory retrieval is the fact that damage to PPC often yields very subtle or no obvious deficits in retrieval (for reviews see Cabeza et al. 2008; Shimamura 2011; Wagner et al. 2005). Thus, further work is necessary to establish the precise nature of parietal lobe contributions to memory retrieval.

Fate of selected-against memories. One of the ways in which perceptual selection may be facilitated is through the inhibition of irrelevant representations. For example, when selecting among competing objects, selected-against objects are often associated with a brief period of time during which future processing of that object is impaired (Tipper 1985). This phenomenon of 'negative priming' is thought to reflect transient inhibition of the selected-against object, putatively facilitating processing of the selected object. Similarly, when attention is shifted *away from* a spatial location, it is more difficult to shift attention *back* to that location, relative to another location—a phenomenon termed 'inhibition of return' (Posner et al. 1985). An interesting question is whether similar inhibitory mechanisms may operate during memory retrieval. That is: when a memory is selected against, is it more difficult to subsequently return to or retrieve that memory?

The idea that selected-against memories may be inhibited during acts of retrieval has been studied in the retrieval practice paradigm (M.C. Anderson et al. 1994). In this paradigm, various retrieval cues are each paired with several associates, similar to the fan effect described earlier (J. R. Anderson 1974). Critically, for some of the retrieval cues, *some* of the associates are repeatedly retrieved (target memories); for these cues, the non-retrieved associates function as competing memories. For cues where none of the associates are retrieved, these associates function as baseline memories. After targets are repeatedly retrieved, memory for all items is then assessed. The standard finding is that retrieval of targets promotes forgetting of competing memories, relative to baseline memories—a phenomenon termed *retrieval-induced forgetting*. That is, selective retrieval of one memory can promote forgetting of closely associated, non-retrieved memories.

Critically, retrieval-induced forgetting is thought to reflect an active inhibitory mechanism that is a direct reaction to competition. If, for example, target memories are repeatedly studied (encoded) instead of repeatedly retrieved, 'competing' memories do not actually compete and no forgetting is observed (M. C. Anderson et al. 2000). Additionally, when competing memories are particularly strong associates, retrieval-induced forgetting is, surprisingly, greater (M. C. Anderson et al. 1994; Levy and Anderson 2002). These phenomena have recently been described in a neurobiologically plausible computational model in which individual retrieval attempts both strengthen and weaken synaptic connections such that relevant associations grow stronger and irrelevant associations grow weaker (Norman et al. 2007). In this model, weight changes occur within the hippocampus, and prefrontal cortex serves to bias competition such that relevant memories 'win' the retrieval competition (Miller and Cohen 2001). Thus, when compared to evidence of inhibition during object selection, retrieval-induced forgetting provides an interesting parallel between acts of perceptual and reflective attention (Anderson and Spellman 1995).

ATTENTION FROM MEMORY

Thus far we have considered how long-term memory encoding and retrieval are influenced by—or represent forms of—attention. Here we consider how the allocation of perceptual attention may, in turn, be influenced by memory. Such situations of *attention from memory* have been observed when regularities in perceptual information are gradually learned and this learning then biases how attention is allocated.

A well-documented example of attention from memory is contextual cueing, which refers to facilitated visual search of a target when its location or identity is predictable from its surrounding context (Chun and Jiang 1998; Chun 2000). As an example, when visual search displays are repeated, observers learn both the spatial layout of the items and the location of an embedded target, facilitating attention to the target. Notably, learning of spatial information in this paradigm occurs implicitly; if subjects are explicitly asked to identify familiar versus novel arrays, performance is at chance. Interestingly, and in contrast to most forms of implicit learning, contextual cueing is disrupted by hippocampal amnesia (Chun and Phelps 1999, Fig. 28.6c). Thus, the hippocampal system is functionally important for learning of configural information, or binding, independent of whether the learned information reaches awareness. Neuroimaging evidence has further implicated the hippocampus as being involved in contextual cueing despite the lack of conscious learning (Greene et al. 2007). Similarly, prior exposure to naturalistic scenes improves search for embedded target objects, and such attention from memory is predicted by fMRI responses within the hippocampus (Summerfield et al. 2006, Fig. 28.6a–b). EEG measures indicate that this memory-based facilitation produces

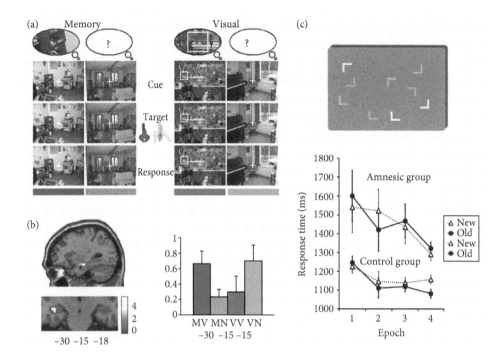

FIGURE 28.6 Attention from memory. (a, b). Orienting from attention vs. memory. Reprinted from *Neuron*, 49 (6), Jennifer J. Summerfield, Jöran Lepsien, Darren R. Gitelman, M. Marsel Mesulam, and Anna C. Nobre, Orienting Attention Based on Long-Term Memory Experience, pp. 905–16, Copyright (2006), with permission from Elsevier. (a) In the experiment, subjects attempted to locate a target stimulus (gold key = target; banana = catch). Left panel: orienting from memory task. When a target-location pairing had previously been learned (left column), subjects could use these 'valid' memory cues to facilitate search (memory valid condition: MV); when the scene was novel (right column), a memory cue was, by definition, absent (memory neutral condition: MN). Right panel: orienting from attention. When a scene was accompanied by a valid spatial cue (left column; cue = white box), subjects could use this visual cue to facilitate search (visual valid, VV); when a spatial cue was not present (right column), there was no information to predict target location (visual neutral, VN). Overall, subjects were successful in using cues to facilitate (i.e., speed up) target detection. (b) Valid memory cues (MV)—relative to valid visual cues (VV)—were associated with greater activity in the left hippocampus, indicating that the hippocampus supported memory for target locations, thereby facilitating search. (c) Contextual cueing in hippocampal amnesics. Top panel: learning about the location of a target stimulus (a rotated T) embedded in a visual display typically improves across repetitions of the display, reflecting a form of implicit learning (contextual cueing). Bottom panel: control subjects become faster to identify targets in repeated (Old) vs. novel (New) displays. However, patients with hippocampal amnesia (Amnesic Group) fail to show this contextual cueing effect. Thus, while contextual cueing is not a conscious form of learning, it depends on a hippocampus-mediated ability to learn contextual information about the environment. Reproduced from Nature Neuroscience, 2 (9), Chun, M. M. and Phelps, E. A., Memory deficits for implicit contextual information in amnesic subjects with hippocampal damage, pp. 844–847, © 1999, Nature Publishing Group.

a spatial bias in alpha-band oscillatory activity in anticipation of target appearance, enhancing the earliest component of the event-related potential when the target appears (Summerfield et al. 2011).

Attention-from-memory effects described above rely on predictive associations between visual elements; however, predictive non-visual factors such as monetary reward can also facilitate visual attention (Awh et al. 2012). Interestingly, reward effects may be double-edged: while target detection is facilitated if targets were previously associated with reward, if current distractors were previously associated with reward, performance is instead *impaired* (Della Libera and Chelazzi 2009). Thus, memory for past experiences can either facilitate or impair attentional orienting in the present according to whether learned information is consistent or inconsistent with current goals.

Previously we considered whether unattended information is encoded and subsequently remembered. Similarly, several studies have considered how/whether memory for unattended information in perceptual attention tasks influences future perception and attention. For example, in contextual cueing when one colour (e.g. red) is task relevant and another colour is not (e.g. green), repeated spatial configurations in the relevant colour yield a contextual cueing effect, but when spatial relationships in the irrelevant colour predict target location, no contextual cueing is observed (Jiang and Chun 2001). While this result suggests that implicit learning of spatial information (and corresponding benefits to target detection) does not occur for ignored information, if a previously irrelevant colour now becomes relevant, a benefit occurs for previously unattended configurations that are repeated and are now relevant/attended (Jiang and Leung 2005). Thus, unattended information may be latently learned and may only influence current acts of attention if and when the learned information is actually attended or relevant to current behaviour.

An intriguing qualification to the idea that repeated unattended information may influence future perceptual attention is that this effect may depend, in a counter-intuitive way, on the strength of the unattended information. Namely, perceptual learning may actually be *greater* when unattended information is weak (e.g. weakly coherent motion of visual stimuli) relative to when it is strong (Tsushima et al. 2008). Putatively, when unattended information is strong, attentional mechanisms detect and successfully suppress this distraction; but when it is weak, suppression is not elicited and learning occurs. Consistent with this view, lateral prefrontal cortex is preferentially recruited when unattended information is strong, relative to when it is weak (Tsushima et al. 2006). Thus, there are situations in which previously unattended information will and will not influence future perceptual attention, and an important area for future research is to continue to specify the parameters that influence such relationships.

ATTENTION AND WORKING MEMORY

Above we have reviewed the many ways that attention and memory are interrelated, with an important distinction drawn between perceptual attention and reflective attention according to whether the targets of attentional processing are currently available in the sensory input or not. At the interface of this distinction between perception and reflection lies working memory, which enables the maintenance and manipulation of information during the moments immediately after sensory information has passed (Chun et al. 2011; D'Esposito et al. 1995; Smith and Jonides 1999).

Key features of working memory include its limited capacity and separate stores for different types of information, mainly distinguished into phonological and visuospatial stores (Baddeley 2003). Each storage and maintenance mechanism not only maintains different kinds of information, but they have different capacities. Verbal working memory mediated by the phonological loop has a capacity of about seven chunks of information (Miller 1956), and it is affected by factors such as phonological similarity and syllabic length. Visuospatial working memory, also described as visual short-term memory, generally has a capacity of about four objects (Luck and Vogel 1997), and its efficiency depends on the similarity and visual complexity of these objects (Alvarez and Cavanagh 2004; Awh et al. 2007; Todd and Marois 2004; Xu and Chun 2006).

Because of the limited capacity of working memory, information competes for selection and maintenance. In fact, working memory may be understood as the active maintenance of attention to information important for behaviour (Chun 2011; Chun et al. 2011). This thesis is based on seminal work that tightly linked spatial attention with spatial working memory (Awh and Jonides 2001). Actively maintaining spatial locations in mind causes spatial attention to be directed to those locations, and filling spatial working memory to capacity impairs perceptual attention operations that require spatial attention (Oh and Kim 2004; Woodman and Luck 2004). Moreover, neural mechanisms for spatial working memory and spatial attention overlap (Awh and Jonides 2001; LaBar et al. 1999).

Thus, we view working memory as sustained attention that serves to extend no-longer-present perceptual information in the mind and brain—a gateway to internal attentional processes. For example, when specific visual features of an object such as orientation or colour are maintained in working memory, these features can be decoded in early visual areas throughout working memory maintenance, indicating sustained processing of perceptual information (Harrison and Tong 2009; Serences et al. 2009). Similarly, 'refreshing' or re-visualizing a stimulus you just saw (Johnson et al. 2007)—which involves working memory operations—increases responses in neural regions that were active when viewing that stimulus (Johnson and Johnson 2009). Likewise, refreshing a just-seen stimulus elicits neural adaptation (a form of perceptual memory) similar to what would be observed if the stimulus had been visually re-presented (Yi et al. 2008).

Importantly, attentional priorities may be established either *before/while* perceptual information is available or *after* the perceptual information has disappeared. In the former case, selective attention robustly modulates what information is encoded into working memory (Gazzaley and Nobre 2012); but in the latter case, attention must be oriented to information that is no longer perceptually available—that is, information only maintained in memory. Comparison of *pre-cueing* and *retro-cueing* indicates that selective attention can be effectively deployed either in advance of perceptual information (pre-cueing) or after perceptual information has disappeared (retro-cueing), with both acts of attention resulting in similar behavioural consequences and involving similar modulations of neural activity (Griffin and Nobre 2003; Lepsien et al. 2005; Lepsien and Nobre 2006, 2007). Thus, attention is intimately related to what is maintained in working memory, whether attentional priorities are established in advance of perception or after perception is complete.

To the extent that working memory contents are a product of attentional allocation, working memory may provide a window into how effectively selective attention is being employed. Indeed, working memory performance across individuals and age groups positively correlates with the ability to suppress perceptual distraction (Gazzaley et al. 2005; Vogel et al. 2005). On the flipside, the information that is maintained in working memory can also powerfully bias how attention is allocated (e.g. Soto et al. 2008), similar to biases in attention driven by long-term memory (as discussed above). From a biased competition perspective (Desimone and Duncan 1995), information that is active in working memory may represent a template that influences which perceptual stimuli are likely to 'win' the competition. Thus, a bi-directional relationship exists between external perceptual attention and internal working memory representations.

Conclusions

There is increasing appreciation for the interrelationship between memory and attention. Indeed, as we argue, memory can be viewed as a form of attention in which acts of selective *perceptual attention* result in enduring traces that can be accessed at later points in time via acts of selective *reflective attention* (Chun and Johnson 2011). Importantly, both perceptual and reflective attention are characterized by a limited capacity and therefore involve selecting among competing alternatives (Chun and Turk-Browne 2007; Chun et al. 2011). In concluding this chapter, we review the degree to which these parallel forms of attention involve common neural substrates.

Accumulating evidence indicates that retrieving an event from memory involves reactivating some of the same neural regions engaged during encoding (for a review see Danker and Anderson 2010). As we describe above, there is evidence that selective retrieval—that is retrieval in the face of competition—modulates activity in what are typically viewed as perceptual regions in a manner similar to selective perceptual attention (Kuhl et al. 2011, 2012; Öztekin and Badre 2011). Indeed, across perceptual and reflective attention common fronto-parietal mechanisms may translate evidence from representational structures into behavioural responses (Kuhl et al. 2011). Similarly, working memory—which is at the intersection of reflective and perceptual attention—involves modulation of the same sensory areas that are modulated by attention (Awh and Jonides 2001; Harrison and Tong 2009; Serences et al. 2009), suggesting an interrelationship in these processes. Thus, reflective and perceptual attention are associated with modulation of common representational regions.

A second point of comparison across perceptual and reflective attention is whether they are guided by similar mechanisms of prefrontal cortex. During memory retrieval, prefrontal cortex implements control by selecting target memories and filtering or inhibiting competing memories (Badre and Wagner 2007; Kuhl and Wagner 2009; Levy and Anderson 2002; Shimamura 2000), which parallels prefrontal contributions to top-down perceptual attention (Corbetta and Shulman 2002; Desimone and Duncan 1995; Miller and Cohen 2001). However, whereas considerable evidence suggests that the inferior frontal gyrus is particularly important for selective memory retrieval (Badre and Wagner 2007), top-down perceptual attention has more typically been associated with dorsal prefrontal cortex (Corbetta and Shulman 2002). Thus, while there is a common role for prefrontal cortex in selection/filtering across acts of top-down reflective and perceptual attention, it is not clear that there is overlap in the specific prefrontal mechanisms that implement control across these domains. More targeted investigations will be useful for establishing the degree to which there is commonality versus segregation in these mechanisms.

Finally, neuroimaging studies consistently demonstrate parietal cortex activity during tasks demanding perceptual attention (Corbetta and Shulman 2002) or during memory retrieval (Wagner et al. 2005). However, the mechanistic contributions of parietal cortex to memory remain ambiguous (Cabeza et al. 2008; Shimamura 2011). Namely, whereas both memory retrieval and top-down acts of attention engage the intraparietal sulcus and superior parietal lobule, direct comparisons suggest dissociations in the specific localization of these mechanisms (Hutchinson et al. 2009; Sestieri et al. 2010). Additionally, it remains to be determined why damage to parietal cortex is associated with minimal or inconsistent impairments to memory retrieval (for discussions of this point see Cabeza et al. 2008; Shimamura 2011; Wagner et al. 2005). Thus, an important area for future research concerns the role of parietal cortex in memory retrieval and the degree to which there are parallel or even common parietal mechanisms that guide memory retrieval and top-down attention.

REFERENCES

Alvarez, G. A. and Cavanagh, P. (2004). The capacity of visual short-term memory is set both by visual information load and by number of objects. *Psychological Science* 15: 106–111.

Anderson, J. R. (1974). Retrieval of propositional information from long-term memory. *Cognitive Psychology* 6: 451–474.

Anderson, M. C. (2003). Rethinking interference theory: Executive control and the mechanisms of forgetting. *Journal of Memory and Language* 49: 415–445.

Anderson, M. C., Bjork, E. L., and Bjork, R. A. (2000). Retrieval-induced forgetting: Evidence for a recall-specific mechanism. *Psychonomic Bulletin & Review* 7: 522–530.

Anderson, M. C., Bjork, R. A., and Bjork, E. L. (1994). Remembering can cause forgetting: Retrieval dynamics in long-term memory. *Journal of Experimental Psychology: Learning, Memory, and Cognition* 20: 1063–1087.

Anderson, M. C. and Spellman, B. A. (1995). On the status of inhibitory mechanisms in cognition: Memory retrieval as a model case. *Psychological Review* 102: 68–100.

Anderson, N. D., Iidaka, T., Cabeza, R., Kapur, S., McIntosh, A. R., and Craik, F. I. M. (2000). The effects of divided attention on encoding- and retrieval-related brain activity: A PET study of younger and older adults. *Journal of Cognitive Neuroscience* 12: 775–792.

Awh, E., Barton, B., and Vogel, E. K. (2007). Visual working memory represents a fixed number of items regardless of complexity. *Psychological Science* 18: 622–628.

Awh, E., Belopolsky, A. V., and Theeuwes, J. (2012). Top-down versus bottom-up attentional control: A failed theoretical dichotomy. *Trends in Cognitive Sciences* 16: 437–443.

Awh, E. and Jonides, J. (2001). Overlapping mechanisms of attention and spatial working memory. *Trends in Cognitive Sciences* 5: 119–126.

Baddeley, A. (2003). Working memory: Looking back and looking forward. *Nature Reviews Neuroscience* 4: 829–839.

Baddeley, A., Lewis, V., Eldridge, M., and Thomson, N. (1984). Attention and retrieval from long-term memory. *Journal of Experimental Psychology: General* 113: 518–540.

Badre, D., Poldrack, R. A., Paré-Blagoev, E. J., Insler, R. Z., and Wagner, A. D. (2005). Dissociable controlled retrieval and generalized selection mechanisms in ventrolateral prefrontal cortex. *Neuron* 47: 907–918.

Badre, D. and Wagner, A. D. (2007). Left ventrolateral prefrontal cortex and the cognitive control of memory. *Neuropsychologia* 45: 2883–2901.

Baldo, J. V. and Shimamura, A. P. (2002). Frontal lobes and memory. In A. D. Baddeley, M. D. Kopelman, and B. A. Wilson (eds.), *The Handbook of Memory Disorders* (pp. 363–379). New York: John Wiley.

Blumenfeld, R. S. and Ranganath, C. (2007). Prefrontal cortex and long-term memory encoding: An integrative review of findings from neuropsychology and neuroimaging. *Neuroscientist* 13: 280–291.

Brewer, J. B., Zhao, Z., Desmond, J. E., Glover, G. H., and Gabrieli, J. D. E. (1998). Making memories: Brain activity that predicts how well visual experience will be remembered. *Science* 281: 1185–1187.

Cabeza, R. (2008). Role of parietal regions in episodic memory retrieval: The dual attentional processes hypothesis. *Neuropsychologia* 46: 1813–1827.

Cabeza, R., Ciaramelli, E., Olson, I. R., and Moscovitch, M. (2008). The parietal cortex and episodic memory: An attentional account. *Nature Reviews Neuroscience* 9: 613–625.

Castel, A. D. and Craik, F. I. (2003). The effects of aging and divided attention on memory for item and associative information. *Psychology and Aging* 18: 873–885.

Chun, M. M. (2000). Contextual cueing of visual attention. *Trends in Cognitive Sciences* 4: 170–178.

Chun, M. M. (2011). Visual working memory as visual attention sustained internally over time. *Neuropsychologia* 49: 1407–1409.

Chun, M. M., Golomb, J. D., and Turk-Browne, N. B. (2011). A taxonomy of external and internal attention. *Annual Review of Psychology* 62: 73–101.

Chun, M. M. and Jiang, Y. (1998). Contextual cueing: Implicit learning and memory of visual context guides spatial attention. *Cognitive Psychology* 36: 28–71.

Chun, M. M. and Johnson, M. K. (2011). Memory: Enduring traces of perceptual and reflective attention. *Neuron* 72: 520–535.

Chun, M. M. and Phelps, E. A. (1999). Memory deficits for implicit contextual information in amnesic subjects with hippocampal damage. *Nature Neuroscience* 2: 844–847.

Chun, M. M. and Turk-Browne, N. B. (2007). Interactions between attention and memory. *Current Opinion in Neurobiology* 17: 177–184.

Clarke, A. J. and Butler, L. T. (2008). Dissociating word stem completion and cued recall as a function of divided attention at retrieval. *Memory* 16: 763–772.

Corbetta, M. and Shulman, G. L. (2002). Control of goal-directed and stimulus-driven attention in the brain. *Nature Reviews Neuroscience* 3: 201–215.

Craik, F. I. M., Govoni, R., Naveh-Benjamin, M., and Anderson, N. D. (1996). The effects of divided attention on encoding and retrieval processes in human memory. *Journal of Experimental Psychology: General* 125: 159–180.

Craik, F. I. M. and Tulving, E. (1975). Depth of processing and the retention of words in episodic memory. *Journal of Experimental Psychology: General* 104: 268–294.

Danker, J. F. and Anderson, J. R. (2010). The ghosts of brain states past: Remembering reactivates the brain regions engaged during encoding. *Psychological Bulletin* 136: 87–102.

Danker, J. F., Fincham, J. M., and Anderson, J. R. (2011). The neural correlates of competition during memory retrieval are modulated by attention to the cues. *Neuropsychologia* 49: 2427–2438.

Della Libera, C. and Chelazzi, L. (2009). Learning to attend and to ignore is a matter of gains and losses. *Psychological Science* 20: 778–784.

Desimone, R. and Duncan, J. (1995). Neural mechanisms of selective visual attention. *Annual Review of Neuroscience* 18: 193–222.

D'Esposito, M., Detre, J. A., Alsop, D. C., Shin, R. K., Atlas, S., and Grossman, M. (1995). The neural basis of the central executive system of working memory. *Nature* 378: 279–281.

Dudukovic, N. M., Dubrow, S., and Wagner, A. D. (2009). Attention during memory retrieval enhances future remembering. *Memory & Cognition* 37: 953–961.

Dudukovic, N. M., Preston, A. R., Archie, J. J., Glover, G. H., and Wagner, A. D. (2011). High-resolution fMRI reveals match enhancement and attentional modulation in the human medial temporal lobe. *Journal of Cognitive Neuroscience* 23: 670–682.

Eger, E., Henson, R. N., Driver, J., and Dolan, R. J. (2004). BOLD repetition decreases in object-responsive ventral visual areas depend on spatial attention. *Journal of Neurophysiology* 92: 1241–1247.

Eich, E. (1984). Memory for unattended events: Remembering with and without awareness. *Memory & Cognition* 12: 105–111.

Fernandes, M. A. and Moscovitch, M. (2000). Divided attention and memory: Evidence of substantial interference effects at retrieval and encoding. *Journal of Experimental Psychology: General* 129: 155–176.

Fernandes, M. A. and Moscovitch, M. (2003). Interference effects from divided attention during retrieval in younger and older adults. *Psychology and Aging* 18: 219–230.

Fletcher, P. C., Frith, C. D., Grasby, P. M., Shallice, T., Frackowiak, R. S. J., and Dolan, R. J. (1995). Brain systems for encoding and retrieval of auditory—verbal memory: An in vivo study in humans. *Brain* 118: 401–416.

Gazzaley, A., Cooney, J. W., Rissman, J., and D'Esposito, M. (2005). Top-down suppression deficit underlies working memory impairment in normal aging. *Nature Neuroscience* 8: 1298–1300.

Gazzaley, A. and Nobre, A. C. (2012). Top-down modulation: Bridging selective attention and working memory. *Trends in Cognitive Sciences* 16: 129–135.

Gazzaley, A., Rissman, J., Cooney, J., Rutman, A., Seibert, T., Clapp, W., and D'Esposito, M. (2007). Functional interactions between prefrontal and visual association cortex contribute to top-down modulation of visual processing. *Cerebral Cortex* 17: i125–i135.

Greene, A. J., Gross, W. L., Elsinger, C. L., and Rao, S. M. (2007). Hippocampal differentiation without recognition: an fMRI analysis of the contextual cueing task. *Learning & Memory* 14: 548–553.

Griffin, I. C. and Nobre, A. C. (2003). Orienting attention to locations in internal representations. *Journal of Cognitive Neuroscience 15*: 1176–1194.

Guderian, S., Schott, B. H., Richardson-Klavehn, A., and Düzel, E. (2009). Medial temporal theta state before an event predicts episodic encoding success in humans. *Proceedings of the National Academy of Sciences USA 106*: 5365–370.

Guerin, S. A., Robbins, C. A., Gilmore, A. W., and Schacter, D. L. (2012). Interactions between visual attention and episodic retrieval: Dissociable contributions of parietal regions during gist-based false recognition. *Neuron 75*: 1122–1134.

Harrison, S. A. and Tong, F. (2009). Decoding reveals the contents of visual working memory in early visual areas. *Nature 458*: 632–635.

Henson, R. N., Shallice, T., Josephs, O., and Dolan, R. J. (2002). Functional magnetic resonance imaging of proactive interference during spoken cued recall. *NeuroImage 17*: 543–558.

Hoffman, Y., Bein, O., and Maril, A. (2011). Explicit memory for unattended words: The importance of being in the 'no'. *Psychological Science 22*: 1490–1493.

Hutchinson, J. B., Uncapher, M. R., and Wagner, A. D. (2009). Posterior parietal cortex and episodic retrieval: Convergent and divergent effects of attention and memory. *Learning & Memory 16*: 343–356.

Hutchinson, J. B., Uncapher, M. R., Weiner, K. S., Bressler, D. W., Silver, M. A., Preston, A. R., and Wagner, A. D. (forthcoming). Functional heterogeneity in posterior parietal cortex across attention and episodic memory retrieval. *Cerebral Cortex.*

Jacoby, L. L., Woloshyn, V., and Kelley, C. (1989). Becoming famous without being recognized: Unconscious influences of memory produced by dividing attention. *Journal of Experimental Psychology: General 118*: 115–125.

Jensen, O., Kaiser, J., and Lachaux, J. P. (2007). Human gamma-frequency oscillations associated with attention and memory. *Trends in Neurosciences 30*: 317–324.

Jiang, Y. and Chun, M. M. (2001). Selective attention modulates implicit learning. *Quarterly Journal of Experimental Psychology 54*: 1105–1124.

Jiang, Y. and Leung, A. W. (2005). Implicit learning of ignored visual context. *Psychonomic Bulletin & Review 12*: 100–106.

Johnson, J. A. and Zatorre, R. J. (2005). Attention to simultaneous unrelated auditory and visual events: Behavioral and neural correlates. *Cerebral Cortex 15*: 1609–1620.

Johnson, M. R. and Johnson, M. K. (2009). Top-down enhancement and suppression of activity in category-selective extrastriate cortex from an act of reflective attention. *Journal of Cognitive Neuroscience 21*: 2320–2327.

Johnson, M. R., Mitchell, K. J., Raye, C. L., D'Esposito, M., and Johnson, M. K. (2007). A brief thought can modulate activity in extrastriate visual areas: Top-down effects of refreshing just-seen visual stimuli. *NeuroImage 37*: 290–299.

Kanwisher, N. and Wojciulik, E. (2000). Visual attention: Insights from brain imaging. *Nature Reviews Neuroscience 1*: 91–100.

Karpicke, J. D. and Roediger, H. L. (2008). The critical importance of retrieval for learning. *Science 319*: 966–968.

Kastner, S., Pinsk, M. A., De Weerd, P., Desimone, R., and Ungerleider, L. G. (1999). Increased activity in human visual cortex during directed attention in the absence of visual stimulation. *Neuron 22*: 751–761.

Kensinger, E. A., Clarke, R. J., and Corkin, S. (2003). What neural correlates underlie successful encoding and retrieval? A functional magnetic resonance imaging study using a divided attention paradigm. *Journal of Neuroscience 23*: 2407–2415.

Kensinger, E. A., Garoff-Eaton, R. J., and Schacter, D. L. (2007). Effects of emotion on memory specificity: Memory trade-offs elicited by negative visually arousing stimuli. *Journal of Memory and Language* 56: 575–591.

Kern, R. P., Libkuman, T. M., Otani, H., and Holmes, K. (2005). Emotional stimuli, divided attention, and memory. *Emotion* 5: 408–417.

Khader, P., Burke, M., Bien, S., Ranganath, C., and Rösler, F. (2005). Content-specific activation during associative long-term memory retrieval. *NeuroImage* 27: 805–816.

Khader, P., Heil, M., and Rösler, F. (2005). Material-specific long-term memory representations of faces and spatial positions: Evidence from slow event-related brain potentials. *Neuropsychologia* 43: 2109–2124.

Kim, H. (2011). Neural activity that predicts subsequent memory and forgetting: A meta-analysis of 74 fMRI studies. *NeuroImage* 54: 2446–2461.

Kuhl, B. A., Bainbridge, W. A., and Chun, M. M. (2012). Neural reactivation reveals mechanisms for updating memory. *Journal of Neuroscience* 32: 3453–3461.

Kuhl, B. A., Dudukovic, N. M., Kahn, I., and Wagner, A. D. (2007). Decreased demands on cognitive control reveal the neural processing benefits of forgetting. *Nature Neuroscience* 10: 908–914.

Kuhl, B. A., Kahn, I., Dudukovic, N. M., and Wagner, A. D. (2008). Overcoming suppression in order to remember: Contributions from anterior cingulate and ventrolateral prefrontal cortex. *Cognitive, Affective, & Behavioral Neuroscience* 8: 211–221.

Kuhl, B. A., Rissman, J., Chun, M. M., and Wagner, A. D. (2011). Fidelity of neural reactivation reveals competition between memories. *Proceedings of the National Academy of Sciences USA* 108: 5903–5908.

Kuhl, B. A., Rissman, J., and Wagner, A. D. (2012). Multi-voxel patterns of visual category representation during encoding are predictive of subsequent memory. *Neuropsychologia* 50: 458–469.

Kuhl, B. A. and Wagner, A. D. (2009). Forgetting and retrieval. In G. G. Bentson and J. T. Cacioppo (eds.), *Handbook of Neurosciences for the Behavioral Sciences* (pp. 586–605). Hoboken, N.J.: John Wiley.

LaBar, K. S., Gitelman, D. R., Parrish, T. B., and Mesulam, M. (1999). Neuroanatomic overlap of working memory and spatial attention networks: A functional MRI comparison within subjects. *NeuroImage* 10: 695–704.

Lavie, N. (2005). Distracted and confused? Selective attention under load. *Trends in Cognitive Sciences* 9: 75–82.

Lepsien, J., Griffin, I. C., Devlin, J. T., and Nobre, A. C. (2005). Directing attention in mental representations: Interactions between attentional orienting and working-memory load. *NeuroImage* 26: 733–743.

Lepsien, J. and Nobre, A. C. (2006). Cognitive control of attention in the human brain: Insights from orienting attention to mental representations. *Brain Research* 1105: 20–31.

Lepsien, J. and Nobre, A. C. (2007). Attentional modulation of object representations in working memory. *Cerebral Cortex* 17: 2072–2083.

Levy, B. J. and Anderson, M. C. (2002). Inhibitory processes and the control of memory retrieval. *Trends in Cognitive Sciences* 6: 299–305.

Loftus, E. F., Loftus, G. R., and Messo, J. (1987). Some facts about 'weapon focus'. *Law and Human Behavior* 11: 55–62.

Luck, S. J. and Vogel, E. K. (1997). The capacity of visual working memory for features and conjunctions. *Nature* 390: 279–281.

McClelland, J. L., McNaughton, B. L., and O'Reilly, R. C. (1995). Why there are complementary learning systems in the hippocampus and neocortex: Insights from the successes and failures of connectionist models of learning and memory. *Psychological Review* 102: 419–457.

Mensink, G. J. and Raaijmakers, J. G. (1988). A model for interference and forgetting. *Psychological Review* 95: 434–455.

Merikle, P. M. and Reingold, E. M. (1991). Comparing direct (explicit) and indirect (implicit) measures to study unconscious memory. *Journal of Experimental Psychology: Learning, Memory, and Cognition* 17: 224–233.

Miller, E. K. and Cohen, J. D. (2001). An integrative theory of prefrontal cortex function. *Annual Review of Neuroscience* 24: 167–202.

Miller, G. A. (1956). The magical number seven, plus or minus two: Some limits on our capacity for processing information. *Psychological Review* 63: 81–97.

Mulligan, N. W. (1997). Attention and implicit memory tests: The effects of varying attentional load on conceptual priming. *Memory & Cognition* 25: 11–17.

Mulligan, N. W. (1998). The role of attention during encoding in implicit and explicit memory. *Journal of Experimental Psychology: Learning, Memory, and Cognition* 24: 27–47.

Naveh-Benjamin, M., Guez, J., and Marom, M. (2003). The effects of divided attention at encoding on item and associative memory. *Memory & Cognition* 31: 1021–1035.

Norman, K. A., Newman, E. L., and Detre, G. (2007). A neural network model of retrieval-induced forgetting. *Psychological Review* 114: 887–953.

O'Craven, K. M., Downing, P. E., and Kanwisher, N. (1999). fMRI evidence for objects as the units of attentional selection. *Nature* 401: 584–587.

Oh, S. H. and Kim, M. S. (2004). The role of spatial working memory in visual search efficiency. *Psychonomic Bulletin & Review* 11: 275–281.

Otten, L. J., Quayle, A. H., Akram, S., Ditewig, T. A., and Rugg, M. D. (2006). Brain activity before an event predicts later recollection. *Nature Neuroscience* 9: 489–491.

Öztekin, I. and Badre, D. (2011). Distributed patterns of brain activity that lead to forgetting. *Frontiers in Human Neuroscience* 5: 86.

Paller, K. A. and Wagner, A. D. (2002). Observing the transformation of experience into memory. *Trends in Cognitive Sciences* 6: 93–102.

Posner, M. I., Rafal, R. D., Choate, L. S., and Vaughan, J. (1985). Inhibition of return: Neural basis and function. *Cognitive Neuropsychology* 2: 211–228.

Prince, S. E., Dennis, N. A., and Cabeza, R. (2009). Encoding and retrieving faces and places: Distinguishing process- and stimulus-specific differences in brain activity. *Neuropsychologia* 47: 2282–2289.

Rock, I. and Gutman, D. (1981). The effect of inattention on form perception. *Journal of Experimental Psychology: Human Perception and Performance* 7: 275–285.

Sederberg, P. B., Kahana, M. J., Howard, M. W., Donner, E. J., and Madsen, J. R. (2003). Theta and gamma oscillations during encoding predict subsequent recall. *Journal of Neuroscience* 23: 10809–10814.

Serences, J. T., Ester, E. F., Vogel, E. K., and Awh, E. (2009). Stimulus-specific delay activity in human primary visual cortex. *Psychological Science* 20: 207–214.

Sestieri, C., Shulman, G. L., and Corbetta, M. (2010). Attention to memory and the environment: Functional specialization and dynamic competition in human posterior parietal cortex. *Journal of Neuroscience* 30: 8445–8456.

Shallice, T., Fletcher, P., Frith, C. D., Grasby, P., Frackowiak, R. S. J., and Dolan, R. J. (1994). Brain regions associated with acquisition and retrieval of verbal episodic memory. *Nature* 368: 633–635.

Shimamura, A. P. (2000). The role of the prefrontal cortex in dynamic filtering. *Psychobiology* 28: 207–218.

Shimamura, A. P. (2011). Episodic retrieval and the cortical binding of relational activity. *Cognitive, Affective, & Behavioral Neuroscience* 11: 277–291.

Shimamura, A. P., Jurica, P. J., Mangels, J. A., Gershberg, F. B., and Knight, R. T. (1995). Susceptibility to memory interference effects following frontal lobe damage: Findings from tests of paired-associate learning. *Journal of Cognitive Neuroscience* 7: 144–152.

Simons, J. S. and Spiers, H. J. (2003). Prefrontal and medial temporal lobe interactions in long-term memory. *Nature Reviews Neuroscience* 4: 637–648.

Smith, E. E. and Jonides, J. (1999). Storage and executive processes in the frontal lobes. *Science* 283: 1657–1661.

Sohn, M. H., Goode, A., Stenger, V. A., Carter, C. S., and Anderson, J. R. (2003). Competition and representation during memory retrieval: Roles of the prefrontal cortex and the posterior parietal cortex. *Proceedings of the National Academy of Sciences USA* 100: 7412–7417.

Sohn, M. H., Goode, A., Stenger, V. A., Jung, K. J., Carter, C. S., and Anderson, J. R. (2005). An information-processing model of three cortical regions: Evidence in episodic memory retrieval. *NeuroImage* 25: 21–33.

Soto, D., Hodsoll, J., Rothstein, P., and Humphreys, G. W. (2008). Automatic guidance of attention from working memory. *Trends in Cognitive Sciences* 12: 342–348.

Spaniol, J., Davidson, P. S., Kim, A. S., Han, H., Moscovitch, M., and Grady, C. L. (2009). Event-related fMRI studies of episodic encoding and retrieval: Meta-analyses using activation likelihood estimation. *Neuropsychologia* 47: 1765–1779.

Summerfield, J. J., Lepsien, J., Gitelman, D. R., Mesulam, M. M., and Nobre, A. C. (2006). Orienting attention based on long-term memory experience. *Neuron* 49: 905–916.

Summerfield, J. J., Rao, A., Garside, N., and Nobre, A. C. (2011). Biasing perception by spatial long-term memory. *Journal of Neuroscience* 31: 14952–14960.

Thompson-Schill, S. L. and Botvinick, M. M. (2006). Resolving conflict: A response to Martin and Cheng (2006). *Psychonomic Bulletin & Review* 13: 402–408.

Thompson-Schill, S. L., D'Esposito, M., and Kan, I. P. (1999). Effects of repetition and competition on activity in left prefrontal cortex during word generation. *Neuron* 23: 513–522.

Tipper, S. P. (1985). The negative priming effect: Inhibitory priming by ignored objects. *Quarterly Journal of Experimental Psychology* 37: 571–590.

Todd, J. J. and Marois, R. (2004). Capacity limit of visual short-term memory in human posterior parietal cortex. *Nature* 428: 751–754.

Tomita, H., Ohbayashi, M., Nakahara, K., Hasegawa, I., and Miyashita, Y. (1999). Top-down signal from prefrontal cortex in executive control of memory retrieval. *Nature* 401: 699–703.

Treisman, A. M. and Gelade, G. (1980). A feature-integration theory of attention. *Cognitive Psychology* 12: 97–136.

Troyer, A. K., Winocur, G., Craik, F. I., and Moscovitch, M. (1999). Source memory and divided attention: Reciprocal costs to primary and secondary tasks. *Neuropsychology* 13: 467–474.

Tsushima, Y., Sasaki, Y., and Watanabe, T. (2006). Greater disruption due to failure of inhibitory control on an ambiguous distractor. *Science* 314: 1786–1788.

Tsushima, Y., Seitz, A. R., and Watanabe, T. (2008). Task-irrelevant learning occurs only when the irrelevant feature is weak. *Current Biology* 18: R516–R517.

Turk-Browne, N. B., Golomb, J., and Chun, M. M. (2013). Complementary attentional components of successful memory encoding. *NeuroImage* 66: 553–562.

Turk-Browne, N. B., Yi, D. J., and Chun, M. M. (2006). Linking implicit and explicit memory: Common encoding factors and shared representations. *Neuron* 49: 917–927.

Uncapher, M. R., Hutchinson, J. B., and Wagner, A. D. (2011). Dissociable effects of top-down and bottom-up attention during episodic encoding. *Journal of Neuroscience* 31: 12613–12628.

Uncapher, M. R. and Rugg, M. D. (2009). Selecting for memory? The influence of selective attention on the mnemonic binding of contextual information. *Journal of Neuroscience* 29: 8270–8279.

Uncapher, M. R. and Wagner, A. D. (2009). Posterior parietal cortex and episodic encoding: Insights from fMRI subsequent memory effects and dual-attention theory. *Neurobiology of Learning and Memory* 91: 139–154.

Vogel, E. K., McCollough, A. W., and Machizawa, M. G. (2005). Neural measures reveal individual differences in controlling access to working memory. *Nature* 438: 500–503.

Wagner, A. D. and Davachi, L. (2001). Cognitive neuroscience: Forgetting of things past. *Current Biology* 11: R964–R967.

Wagner, A. D., Schacter, D. L., Rotte, M., Koutstaal, W., Maril, A., Dale, A. M., Rosen, B. R., and Buckner, R. L. (1998). Building memories: Remembering and forgetting of verbal experiences as predicted by brain activity. *Science* 281: 1188–1191.

Wagner, A. D., Shannon, B. J., Kahn, I., and Buckner, R. L. (2005). Parietal lobe contributions to episodic memory retrieval. *Trends in Cognitive Sciences* 9: 445–453.

Wais, P. E., Kim, O. Y., and Gazzaley, A. (2012). Distractibility during episodic retrieval is exacerbated by perturbation of left ventrolateral prefrontal cortex. *Cerebral Cortex* 22: 717–724.

Wais, P. E., Rubens, M. T., Boccanfuso, J., and Gazzaley, A. (2010). Neural mechanisms underlying the impact of visual distraction on retrieval of long-term memory. *Journal of Neuroscience* 30: 8541–8550.

Wolters, G. and Prinsen, A. (1997). Full versus divided attention and implicit memory performance. *Memory & Cognition* 25: 764–771.

Woodman, G. F. and Luck, S. J. (2004). Visual search is slowed when visuospatial working memory is occupied. *Psychonomic Bulletin & Review* 11: 269–274.

Xu, Y. and Chun, M. M. (2006). Dissociable neural mechanisms supporting visual short-term memory for objects. *Nature* 440: 91–95.

Xue, G., Dong, Q., Chen, C., Lu, Z., Mumford, J. A., and Poldrack, R. A. (2010). Greater neural pattern similarity across repetitions is associated with better memory. *Science* 330: 97–101.

Yi, D. J. and Chun, M. M. (2005). Attentional modulation of learning-related repetition attenuation effects in human parahippocampal cortex. *Journal of Neuroscience* 25: 3593–3600.

Yi, D. J., Turk-Browne, N. B., Chun, M. M., and Johnson, M. K. (2008). When a thought equals a look: Refreshing enhances perceptual memory. *Journal of Cognitive Neuroscience* 20: 1371–1380.

Zanto, T. P., Rubens, M. T., Thangavel, A., and Gazzaley, A. (2011). Causal role of the prefrontal cortex in top-down modulation of visual processing and working memory. *Nature Neuroscience* 14: 656–661.

CHAPTER 29

....

ATTENTION AND
DECISION-MAKING

....

CHRISTOPHER SUMMERFIELD AND TOBIAS EGNER

Introduction

....

Decisions are commitments to mental states that prescribe a course of future action, and *decision-making* is the name given to the neural, cognitive, and computational mechanisms by which such commitments are made. When asked to consider real-world decisions, we might think of the specific choices faced by a consumer purchasing a product, a voter electing a politician, a juror judging a defendant, or a doctor making a medical diagnosis. However, decisions are a ubiquitous feature of ongoing cognition and behaviour in all species from invertebrates to humans and other primates. Firstly, almost all laboratory-based tasks and paradigms commonly employed in experimental psychology, from those tapping low-level sensation to those measuring executive function, require commitments to cognitive or perceptual states that can reasonably be described as choices. For example, in the field of sensory psychophysics, participants are asked to make detection or discrimination judgements about simple stimuli such as visual gratings or auditory tones, typically by indicating their choice with a button press or eye movement. Indeed, a prominent tradition in psychology argues that perception is the process by which we decide which hypothesis best explains currently incoming sensory information (Helmholtz 1909). For example, perceptual reversals experienced when viewing multi-stable stimuli such as the Necker cube may indicate alternating commitment to competing interpretations of the sensory information (Gregory 1980). Thus, one important current in the decision-making literature has been the attempt to define the mechanisms by which we categorize sensory information into discrete classes ('perceptual decision-making') (Green and Swets 1966; Gold and Shadlen 2007).

Secondly, in the real world our behaviour is driven by the imperatives of obtaining resources and avoiding potential threats. Similarly, in most laboratory tasks, participants work to maximize positive feedback, or explicit rewards of both a primary (e.g.

juice) or secondary (e.g. money) nature. The field of decision-making in psychology and economics has tried to provide an account of motivated behaviour, for example by investigating the mechanisms by which agents evaluate and compare the possible positive or negative outcomes associated with different stimuli or courses of action ('economic decision-making') (Kahneman and Tversky 1979; Glimcher et al. 2005). Decision-making is thus a central constituent of our mental life, and understanding how it is interconnected with other psychological phenomena, such as perception, memory, and attention, is a key goal of behavioural and neural scientists.

Principles of decision-making

Mechanistic (cognitive- or computational-level) accounts of choice behaviour attempt to describe the various steps by which a decision unfolds, and the quantities that are computed en route to a choice (we term this a *decision-theoretic* approach). While the precise mechanisms by which decisions are made continue to provoke considerable debate, nevertheless researchers have been able to agree on some fundamental principles. Among these is the notion that decisions depend on *evidence*, which takes the form of absolute or relative information that is relevant to the identification or valuation of a sensory stimulus, and that is often called the 'decision variable' or DV. Many models assume that the DV is normalized in some way, transformed nonlinearly, or (in 'sequential sampling' models) that it is integrated over time. Subsequently, the DV is subjected to a *comparison* process, in which it is judged relative to a criterion or standard (a decision *threshold* or *bound*). If the evidence exceeds the decision bound, then a decision is made, that is, an interpretation of a stimulus is being committed to and/or a course of action is initiated. Finally, researchers assume that decisions respect a *value function*, which specifies the probable outcomes associated with particular stimuli, actions, or goals which the agent is likely to encounter, and that agents employ a *decision policy* that attempts to maximize positive reinforcement and minimize both loss and risk. The family of decision-theoretic approaches to category judgements, their formal equivalences, and relationship to optimality are summarized comprehensively elsewhere (Bogacz et al. 2006; Deco et al. 2013).

The normative framework

One key advantage of the decision-theoretic approach is that it allows us to characterize how an agent *should* behave, given the available (and typically, noisy or volatile) evidence from perception and memory, and the value function. *Normative* models of choice assume that the agent makes optimal inferences about the external world, given the available information; in other words, that he or she computes the probability of a certain hypothesis (e.g. 'If I accept this gamble, I will win £10'; 'the rightmost stimulus was a vertical grating'), given the data $p(H \mid d)$. Bayes' rule, which dictates how such conditional probabilities should be calculated, is thus a ubiquitous tool in the modelling of choice behaviour (see below). The normative framework offers a mathematically elegant approach to understanding the higher-level computational principles guiding perception and cognition. Even where experimental subjects are demonstrably suboptimal, as appears to be the case for many high-level judgement tasks (Kahneman et al. 1982), normative approaches may be useful, in that they allow observed behavioural phenomena to be characterized as deviations from optimality. However, normative accounts are often less informative about the precise mechanisms by which such processes might be implemented than *heuristic* accounts which eschew optimality, and instead simply seek to provide the best fit to subjects' behaviour (Gigerenzer and Gaissmaier 2011).

Scope of this review

Here, we will consider how the deployment of *attention* to a sensory stimulus influences decisions made about it. Attention has been defined in a variety of overlapping ways, typically in terms of a mechanism that preferentially allocates processing resources to percepts, memories, or tasks on the basis of a current goal (Broadbent 1958; Treisman and Gelade 1980; Bundesen 1990; Posner and Petersen 1990; Desimone and Duncan 1995; Carrasco 2011). A related definition of attention—explored below—is that it constitutes a mechanism by which sensory information is weighted according to its motivational relevance. For simplicity, in this review we focus on paradigms in which observers are asked to make simple detection, discrimination, or categorization judgements about visual stimuli that are rendered relevant or salient by an advance cue of some sort. Nevertheless, many of the models described here have been applied to more complex situations, for example where information has to be maintained in a short-term store, or where a target has to be found in a field of distractors (Rensink 2002; Cavanagh and Alvarez 2005; Wolfe 2010). To further constrain the scope of our review, we focus on the visual modality, because it is the most intensively studied and provides the richest body of empirical work on which to base our summary.

We will begin with a brief overview of models that have been proposed to account for decision-making in humans and other primates. We emphasize the classic accounts provided by signal detection theory (Green and Swets 1966), serial sampling models (Wald and Wolfowitz 1949; Ratcliff and McKoon 2008), ideal observer approaches (Shaw 1980; Pelli 1985; Sperling and Dosher 1986; Eckstein et al. 2009), and perceptual 'template' models (Lu and Dosher 2008). Our goal is to then use these models as a framework for contemplating how attention might influence perceptual, cognitive, and motor processes occurring during decision-making. In particular, we will focus on the question of how prior knowledge about the stimulus or task influences perceptual choices. To this end, we will revisit a long-standing debate concerning whether enhanced processing of information that is cued in advance reflects a reduction in uncertainty about where the decision-relevant information will arrive, or a prioritization of processing in a sensory system with limited capacity. In the latter part of the chapter, we go on to describe new theories and empirical data that suggest that it is fruitful to distinguish between two decision-relevant quantities, the *statistical probability* of a sensory event ('expectation') and its *motivational relevance* ('attention'), which may have dissociable influences on choices about sensory stimuli (Summerfield and Egner 2009; Feldman and Friston 2010). We discuss this view in the light of another model of decision-making, which emphasizes reciprocal interactions between top-down and bottom-up information during perceptual inference ('predictive coding') (Mumford 1992; Friston 2005; Clark 2013). Finally, we conclude by highlighting open questions and potentially fruitful avenues for future research.

SIGNAL DETECTION THEORY

Decision-making has long been studied from a multi-disciplinary perspective, and many of the tools that are used to model the psychological processes underlying decision-making were first developed in the fields of statistics, economics, or engineering. This is true of the earliest and perhaps most successful models of perceptual choice, which proposed that binary judgements are made according to a statistically optimal process that determines which of two alternative hypotheses (H_1 or H_2) is most likely, given the sensory evidence d. The decision variable (DV) reflects the log of the likelihood ratio of these two hypotheses:

$$DV = \ln\left[\frac{P(d\,|\,H_1)}{P(d\,|\,H_2)}\right]$$

For example, signal detection theory (hereafter, SDT) maintains that decisions about whether a stimulus occurred or not ('yes–no' or detection judgements) depend on the relative likelihood that the observed decision-relevant evidence d was drawn from a distribution of evidence observed on signal-present trials, or the distribution of evidence observed on signal-absent trials (Green and Swets 1966) (Fig. 1a). When an observer makes repeated binary choices about a stimulus, SDT affords the opportunity to characterize his or her decisions with two key statistics. The first of these, known as d′, indexes the *sensitivity* of the observer, and is a direct measure of the overlap between the distributions of evidence associated with the two perceptual alternatives; the smaller the overlap, the higher the sensitivity. The second, known as β, indexes the log-likelihood value at which an observer discriminates between the two choices. The decision policy in SDT is thus to favour H_1 if $DV > \beta$, and to choose H_2 if $DV < \beta$.

Assuming that both choices are equally likely and symmetrically rewarded, an ideal observer will show a β of zero, i.e. will decide in favour of H_1 when H_1 is more likely, and vice versa for H_2. However, observed values of β may vary, and can thus be seen as an index of observer *bias*. For instance, in a situation where H_1 was much more frequently true than H_2, or was associated with a larger reward, a participant might develop a bias

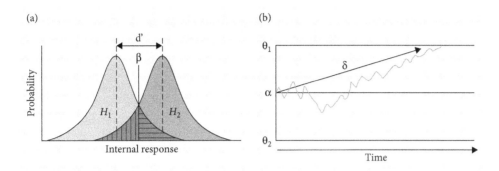

(a)

(b)

FIGURE 29.1 Signal detection theory and sequential sampling models. (a) In signal detection theory, a binary perceptual choice (e.g. is a signal present or not?) is guided by whether an observation ('internal response') was more likely drawn from one out of two distributions (here, H_1 and H_2—where H_1 could map onto a 'noise only' distribution and H_2 onto a 'noise + signal' distribution). The decision taken depends on the setting of criterion β: the observer considers H_1 to be true (signal absent) for any observations falling to the left of the criterion and H_2 to be true (signal present) for observations falling to its right. Due to overlap between the distributions, the observer will commit errors—in the vertically shaded region (left of β) these would correspond to misses, and in the horizontally shaded region (right of β) to false alarms. The observer's sensitivity (d') in discriminating between H_1 and H_2 is a function of the overlap between the distributions (i.e. the difference between the means of the distributions divided by their standard deviation). (b) Serial sampling models temporally unpack the process of evidence accumulation (illustrated as the 'random walk' of the grey line) in favour of either one of two alternatives in the perceptual decision-making process. Key parameters in these models include the starting point of evidence accumulation (α) and the bounds or response thresholds (θ_1, θ_2) whose crossing corresponds to a decision in favour of the respective hypothesis. Most crucially, the drift rate (δ) of evidence accumulation (corresponding to signal strength) determines the speed at which a decision is reached.

for choosing H_1, such that a greater amount of sensory evidence would be required to sway his or her choice in favour of H_2 than H_1.

Attention and signal detection theory

Among the first demonstrations of the influence of covert attention on detection and recognition was provided by Helmholtz, who noted that when viewing briefly illuminated objects in a box through two small apertures, his subjective impression of the objects was richer at the aperture which he attended, even in the absence of any eye movement (Helmholtz 1896). More formal laboratory-based investigation of covert attention, however, was only initiated in the 1970s and 1980s, with the development of the attentional cueing paradigm, in which advance cues provide information about the location at which the task-relevant stimulus is to appear, thereby allowing the comparison of detection performance at cued and uncued spatial locations. Using this paradigm, Posner classically demonstrated that advance cues priming or predicting the spatial location of a to-be-categorized stimulus speeded detection and discrimination judgements relative to unprimed or unpredicted locations (Posner et al. 1980), inspiring the view that attention has a facilitatory effect on perceptual decisions, for example by boosting sensory signals at the attended location (sensory facilitation). This research contributed to a wider programme in nascent cognitive science that viewed attention as a filter that gated the passage of information into a limited-capacity processing system (Broadbent 1958; Neisser 1967).

However, although faster response latencies in the Posner task could have occurred because the cues rendered participants more sensitive to stimulation, they could equally be due to a reduction in the level of information required to make a decision, i.e. a shift in the criterion, β (Sperling and Dosher 1986). Decision-theoretic approaches, such as that offered by SDT, provide a means of disentangling these two accounts, and studies in the 1980s were among the first to demonstrate that detection sensitivity (measured by d′) was enhanced at the cued relative to the uncued location, or was enhanced when the cues were informative (i.e. validly signalled where the target would appear with p > 0.5) relative to when they were uninformative or 'neutral' (p = 0.5) (Bashinski and Bacharach 1980; Downing 1988; Hawkins et al. 1990). This occurred irrespective of whether cues were endogenous (i.e. centrally presented, but probabilistically associated with a given location) or exogenous (i.e. presented transiently at the stimulus location). Although initial reports suggested that this effect might be confined to the discrimination of relatively high-level stimuli, such as letters, over subsequent years it has become clear that d′ is enhanced at the cued location even for relatively low-level stimuli, such luminance increments (Muller and Humphreys 1991). This finding called into question the traditional view that detection is a pre-attentive process that neither requires nor benefits from attention (Broadbent 1958).

IDEAL OBSERVER MODELS OF ATTENTION

However, normative models of attention offer another alternative explanation for the apparent increase in sensitivity at a cued relative to an uncued location that need not invoke the notion of sensory facilitation (Shaw 1980; Pelli 1985; Tsotsos 1997; Eckstein et al. 2009). To understand this point, it is useful to consider how an ideal observer should update current beliefs about whether a stimulus occurred on the basis of new sensory information:

$$p(H_i \mid d) = \frac{p(d \mid H_i)p(H_i)}{p(d)}$$

Thus, beliefs that a stimulus occurred $p(H_i|d)$ should reflect both the sensory evidence $p(d|H_i)$ concerning its presence or absence and its prior probability of occurrence

$p(H_i)$. Now consider an observer detecting whether a target signal occurred in one of n mutually independent locations (where the cue predicts the location of the target but not the probability of the signal being present per se). Following Eckstein (Eckstein et al. 2009), the combined probability of occurrence across location is thus:

$$p(H_i \mid d) = \frac{p(H_i)\sum_{n=1}^{N} p(d \mid H_i)p(k_i)}{P(d)}$$

where $p(k_i)$ is the probability that the signal will occur at the kth of n locations. Intuitively, thus, when attentional cues indicate that a target is more likely to occur at location k than location m, i.e. where $p(k_i) > p(\neg k_i)$, the sensory evidence at location k will have more influence in the final choice than that at location $\neg k$. Thus, where $p(k_i) = 0.8$, and $p(\neg k_i) = 0.2$, as is the case in the classic Posner experiments, even when $p(d|H_i)$ is high at location $\neg k$ because of noise-driven fluctuations, it will nevertheless be unlikely to perturb the decision, because the evidence at location k carries four times more weight in the eventual choice. Therefore, in the presence of noise, the performance of a Bayesian ideal observer under asymmetric cueing conditions should be superior to that during symmetric (or neutral) conditions, simply because the cue denotes which information is most relevant to the decision—or conversely, which locations it is safe for the observer to ignore. One interesting feature of this decision-theoretic proposal is that it obviates the key component of most models of attention, i.e. that attention is required because perceptual processing is capacity-limited and hence only a subset of the information arriving at the receptors can be processed at any one time. Rather, the ideal observer framework implies that performance is limited by noise rather than capacity: even an agent with limitless capacity would show cueing benefits, because the cues provide advance information about the relevance (and thus, optimal weighting) of the sensory input to the perceptual decision. Empirically observed departures from optimality might thus reflect a failure to weight information appropriately (e.g. base-rate neglect), rather than an upper bound on the information that can be processed in a given time period (Beck et al. 2012).

Sensory facilitation vs. uncertainty reduction

As the number of to-be-sampled locations increases, the spatial uncertainty associated with the judgement grows. Thus, the ideal observer framework predicts that the benefit of cueing will increase lawfully with the number of distractor locations, a finding that is supported by empirical evidence (Shaw 1984; Foley 1998). Moreover, at least in the presence of a single distractor, attentional cueing effects are reduced when the target location is made salient by mounting the target on a high-contrast 'pedestal', a patch of background that differs saliently in luminance from the rest of the screen (Foley 1998), or other markers (e.g. 'fiducial' crosses) that radically reduce uncertainty about which is the relevant target location (Gould et al. 2007). Conversely, attentional cueing effects are more pronounced when the task is rendered more challenging, such as reducing discriminability (Cohn 1981; Pelli 1985; Carrasco et al. 2000), or imposing a post-stimulus mask (Smith 2000; Smith et al. 2004). These results demonstrate that cueing confers maximal benefit in situations where uncertainty about which information is most relevant for choice is greatest, as the ideal observer framework predicts it should (Eckstein et al. 2009).

Nevertheless, despite the support for the ideal observer framework provided by these observations, many researchers now agree that attentional cueing effects cannot be attributed to uncertainty reduction alone, but result from a mixture of sensory facilitation and noise reduction. Firstly, even the earliest studies demonstrating that cueing effects were greater under increased spatial uncertainty reported residual benefits, over and above that predicted by purely statistical models, particularly in tasks with relatively complex stimuli such as letter discrimination (Shaw 1984). Secondly, subsequent testing has revealed that even when great care is taken to remove all possible sources of uncertainty, by removing masks, and maintaining performance at high levels, there is still a net benefit to an advance spatial cue (Carrasco et al. 2000). This has been shown even for low-level tasks, such as luminance increment detection, which were previously assumed to be purely automatic (Muller and Humphreys 1991). Other behavioural data also favour sensory facilitation as a necessary explanation for cueing benefits: one particularly convincing demonstration comes from a manipulation in which increased contrast actually has a detrimental effect on performance, and corresponding reductions in sensitivity in human observers were observed under attention (Yeshurun and Carrasco 1998). Thirdly, imposition of a concurrent secondary, attention-demanding task increases thresholds for visual discrimination, as predicted by models in which perception is limited by capacity limitations, but not by ideal observer models, in which perception is limited by external noise alone (Lee et al. 1997). An invaluable summary of this debate can be found in a comprehensive review article by Carrasco (Carrasco 2011).

Finally, and perhaps most decisively, neural recordings have demonstrated unequivocally that neuronal responses in the extrastriate visual cortex, and possibly also in primary visual cortex, are modulated by attention (Reynolds and Chelazzi 2004). Although the form of this modulation is the topic of ongoing debate, there is now little doubt that the responses of neurons that are sensitive to the cued feature and location are either amplified (Reynolds et al. 2000) or sharpened (McAdams and Maunsell 1999a, 1999b) by advance cues. Moreover, this facilitation occurs even to a single stimulus presented in isolation (Ito and Gilbert 1999). It is hard to reconcile these findings with the view that attention changes the relevant (synaptic) weight which each neuron carries in a later decision stage as implied by ideal observer models (although see Eckstein et al. 2009 for an insightful review of this topic). Together, these findings suggest that despite the elegance and parsimony of the ideal observer framework, the benefits of attentional cueing seem to go beyond the reduction in uncertainty proposed by ideal observer models. Empirical evidence favours the view that attention has evolved to deal with both external noise and capacity limitations in visual perception.

SERIAL SAMPLING MODELS

Signal detection theory provides a useful explanatory framework for considering the influence of attention on perceptual judgement, but it has a number of important limitations. One of the most conspicuous of these is that it treats evidence gathering as an instantaneous, single-step process, thus precluding predictions about the timing of the decision process. An alternative class of model assumes that several noisy samples of evidence are collected in series and *integrated* in some way, leading to an optimization of the signal-to-noise ratio as the noise is averaged out (Wald and Wolfowitz 1949). Many variants of this class of 'serial sampling' model have been proposed, but in the simplest, samples are often integrated by addition ('accumulation'). Here, we describe one popular variant known as the 'drift-diffusion model' (Fig. 1b):

$$DV_t = DV_{t-1} + \delta + n(0, \sigma)$$

where the DV at time t is incremented by a quantity δ encoding the rate (or gain) of evidence accumulation and n (zero-mean Gaussian noise). Rather than being based on a single sample, choices reflect the integrated tally of evidence. For speeded judgements, a stopping rule is required, that dictates when sufficient evidence has been accumulated for action to be selected. In most models, this takes the form of a criterial level (or 'bound', θ), such that for unterminated choices $\theta_1 < DV < \theta_2$.

This class of model has the virtue of being able to predict both choice accuracy, as the probability that the (correct) bound will be breached, and choice latency (RT), as the number of samples required to cross the bound. Empirical evidence indicates that the drift-diffusion model does so very well for a wide range of choice behaviours, from psychophysical judgements (Smith et al. 2004) to lexical decisions (Ratcliff et al. 2004), predicting a number of features of mental chronometry, including the rightward skew of reaction time distributions, the trade-off between speed and accuracy, and, in more sophisticated incarnations, the relative RT of correct and error trials (Ratcliff and McKoon 2008).

Attention and serial sampling models

As discussed above, whether attention confers a benefit on detection sensitivity for well-earmarked stimuli in uncluttered arrays has been a topic of intense debate. This contrasts sharply with the influence of attention on reaction times, for which cueing benefits first described by Posner are extremely well replicated and entirely uncontroversial. Under the serial sampling framework, reduced decision latencies without a corresponding sensitivity benefit can be explained by a change in the decision bound, θ, leading to early proposals that attentional cueing effect can be accounted for by a change in speed–accuracy trade-off (Sperling and Dosher 1986). This proposal is akin to those theories described above suggesting that attention shifts the decision criterion under

SDT. However, where consistent cueing benefits to accuracy *and* RT are observed—as is often the case—under serial sampling models this can only be accounted for with an increase in drift rate (or reduction in noise), not a change in the bound. Moreover, any simple account will struggle to explain the full range of experimental manipulations over which cueing benefits to performance are (or are not) observed, for example the fact that such benefits are greatest when targets are backward masked and reduced when pedestals or other signals reduce spatial uncertainty (Smith 2000). Accounting for the effects of attention on both RTs and performance under masked and unmasked conditions requires a more sophisticated theory, which incorporates both perceptual processing of the stimulus and its continued integration of information beyond stimulus onset.

One such theory is provided by Smith and Ratcliff (Smith and Ratcliff 2009), building upon a number of key empirical studies that have carefully charted the conditions under which attentional benefits to performance are most likely to be found (Smith 2000; Smith et al. 2004; Gould et al. 2007). In their model, the early stages of which share some features with the template models described below, incoming information is nonlinearly transformed and passed into an iconic buffer or visual short-term memory (VSTM) store, which in turn controls the momentary (time-inhomogeneous) drift δ of the decision variable over serial samples. Attention controls the gain on the passage of information to VSTM, such that the drift rates for attended and unattended stimuli diverge early but reach a common asymptote. This ensures that when the passage of information into VSTM is interrupted early, by a backward mask, drift rates diverge strongly for attended and unattended conditions, leading to benefits to both accuracy and RT. However, when no masks are presented, the drift rates continue to grow in parallel for both attended and unattended conditions, leading to a benefit to RT but not accuracy. This model has the virtue of being able to account for the effect of manipulations of the visual display and spatial attention on choices and their latencies.

TEMPLATE MODELS

Both signal detection theory and serial sampling models focus on the comparison of evidence to a decision criterion or bound. However, most offer a relatively simplistic picture of how the input signal to the decision process ('evidence') is computed. Fortunately, many years of research in psychophysics and neuroscience have provided a converging mathematical and biological framework for understanding how simple transformations occur in early visual processing (Hubel and Wiesel 1959; DeValois and DeValois 1988). We summarize models that have drawn upon this framework to chart the steps occurring prior to a decision under the rubric 'template models'; the best-known of these is probably the 'perceptual template model' of Lu and Dosher (Lu and Dosher 2008) although other related models have been proposed (Pelli and Farell 1999).

Consider, for example, the task described above in which an observer is required to decide whether a vertically oriented grating is present or absent at either of two spatial locations. Neurons in the primary visual cortex are well known to have receptive fields that are sensitive to the orientation and spatial frequency of the information in their receptive fields, allowing us to think of them as Gabor filters or 'templates' with a given preferred orientation (for simplicity, we consider only tilt, and not frequency). The template, T, corresponds to the to-be-detected signal (e.g. a vertically tilted Gabor) corrupted by some Gaussian noise with a mean of zero and a standard deviation of sigma $n(0,\sigma)$. The evidence $E(S|T)$ for the signal at a given location, i, given this stimulus (assuming fixed phase) and template T is thus computed by

$$E(S|T) = \lambda[S \bullet T]$$

where $\bullet$ is the cross-correlation operator and $\lambda[.]$ signifies a nonlinear transformation (see below) (Naka and Rushton 1966) (see appendix).

Attention and template models

Now, consider the influence of an advance cue that directs attention into the receptive field of the neuron. Three broad theories have been proposed for how attention might influence processing at the input stage (see Fig. 2 and appendix).

According to *response gain* models, attention serves to multiply the response of the neuron by a scaling factor, w, where w > 1:

$$E(S|T)_i = E(S|T) \times w$$

According to *contrast gain* models, attention acts earlier, boosting signal processing in a manner that is equivalent to increasing the contrast on the stimulus itself. Mathematically, this is indistinguishable from increasing the contrast of the template at the attended location, T_i, by an additive factor, w, where w > 1:

$$T_i = T + (w - 1)$$

A final mechanism by which attention could facilitate responding is by *noise reduction*, i.e. reducing the variability in the template T across the neuronal population (or across trials). This is implemented by reducing the template noise σ by a scaling factor w, where w>1:

$$\sigma_i = \sigma / w$$

$$T_i = T + N(0, \sigma_i)$$

These models all predict an enhancement of detection sensitivity at the attended location, although their influence on the psychometric function that maps discrimination performance on to stimulus contrast is not identical (Fig. 29.2). Simulations show that whereas both response gain and contrast gain predict a leftward shift in the psychometric function (that is, less stimulus energy is required to elicit detection under attended

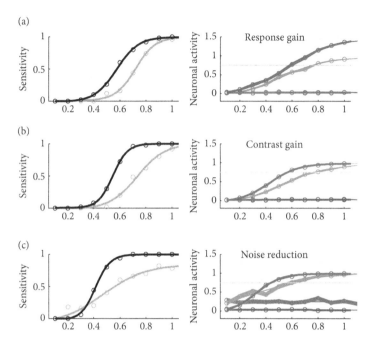

FIGURE 29.2 Simulations of the influence of attention on detection performance (left panels) and neuronal activity (right panels) under response gain (a), contrast gain (b), and noise reduction (c) models. See appendix for detailed description of the models. Left panels: detection sensitivity (hit rate minus false alarm rate) plotted as a function of signal contrast for attended (black dots) and unattended (grey dots) conditions. Line shows best-fitting sigmoidal fit. Right panels: simulated neuronal activity as a function of signal contrast for signal present trials (blue dots) and signal absent trials (red dots). Darker traces are attended conditions; lighter are unattended. Shaded section shows the standard error of the mean at each point; blue and red curves are best-fitting sigmoidal fits. The grey line shows the simulated detection threshold for calculating sensitivity (see appendix).

than unattended conditions), noise reduction predicts that attention will have greater influence at higher levels of signal contrast, but confer relatively little benefit on low contrast stimuli, where performance is limited by the energy in the stimulus and not by noise in perceptual or decision processes (see Fig. 29.2 and appendix).

These mechanisms of attention also predict a modulation of neural responses in the visual cortex by attention, but they do so in different ways (see Fig. 2). Consider first the effect on the contrast response function (CRF), that is, the function that describes how the neuronal response grows with increasing stimulus contrast. Empirically, and independent of attention, the CRF is nonlinear, presumably because neurons are maximally sensitive to stimulation of a particular intensity, with responses saturating at intensities that deviate substantially from their preferred gain range (Naka and Rushton 1966), or because a neuron's activity is normalized by that of its neighbours (Heeger 1993; Boynton 2009; Reynolds and Heeger 2009). Both of these accounts predict that the CRF is roughly sigmoidal (Fig. 29.2). Response gain models predict that under attended conditions, the response at each contrast level will be multiplied by a constant scaling factor; naturally, this enhances responses in the upper portion of the CRF (to high contrast stimuli) to a larger degree than in the lower portion (to low contrast stimuli) (Fig. 29.2a). However, contrast gain models make a different prediction—they suggest that the CRF will be shifted leftwards by attention; an equivalent response is predicted from a lower level of contrast (Fig. 29.2b). By contrast, reducing decision noise, by simply lowering the variability on the decision template T, has an effect on the CRF that depends on external noise; but performance can be enhanced without a necessary change in average neuronal activity (Fig. 2c).

The divergent predictions of these models have allowed researchers to use empirical data from single-cell recordings (Williford and Maunsell 2006) and (Boynton 2009; Herrmann et al. 2010) to arbitrate among these computational accounts of how attention influences sensory processes. Over the past 10 years, this has given rise to a rich empirical and theoretical literature, the details of which are beyond the scope of this chapter, but which is described comprehensively elsewhere (Reynolds and Chelazzi 2004; Boynton 2005; Maunsell and Treue 2006). In summary, however, recordings from extrastriate cortex have found evidence for all three attentional mechanisms. One recent proposal, known as the *normalization model*, proposes that the class of gain control depends on the relevant influence of attention on a neuron's response (stimulus drive) and the normalizing influence of its neighbours (suppressive drive). Specifically, contrast gain effects emerge when attention enhances both the stimulus and the normalization ('suppressive drive') in concert, for example where the stimulus is large and the attention field (in space and/or feature space) is small; but response gain can emerge when the attention field is smaller than the stimulus, because suppressive drive is unaffected by attention. This model unites contrast gain and response gain theories of attention in a single framework (Reynolds and Heeger 2009) and is supported by behavioural and neural evidence (Herrmann et al. 2010).

To summarize the arguments set forth thus far: there is a broad consensus among researchers that the computations underlying (visual) perceptual decision-making are capacity-limited, and that attention allows us to allocate resources in such a way that attended (or cued) locations receive preferential processing. The facilitatory effects of attention might act by boosting inputs (contrast gain), enhancing activity (response gain), or decreasing neuronal variability (noise reduction), and behavioural and neural evidence exists for all of these mechanisms. Next we turn to the question of how exactly these mechanisms contribute to the wider problem of interpreting the sensory world around us.

PREDICTIVE PERCEPTION

Thus far, we have considered attention as a mechanism by which information relevant to a perceptual decision is filtered or weighted, in the service of providing the observer with the most efficient and accurate interpretation of the local sensory environment. An organism struggling to negotiate a complex world can thus focus on that portion of the information which is key for survival—for example, an animal in the wild might elaborate preferentially those perceptual codes that pertain to likely sources of nourishment or that herald impending danger. However, there is another potentially orthogonal source of information upon which observers might capitalize in order to alleviate the computational burden of visual processing and optimize behaviour. Outside of the controlled conditions offered by laboratory experiments, perceptual events tend to differ in terms of their base rates of occurrence, or their conditional likelihood given the recent stimulation history. In other words, statistical information about the frequencies or probabilities of occurrence of one percept over another offers anticipatory information that is potentially complementary to that provided by 'attentional' cues signalling the relevance of the forthcoming information.

Prediction and perceptual inference

Items that occur more frequently in a given environment are recognized more readily. This idea motivates an influential body of work concerned with scene perception and object recognition, which has long demonstrated that objects placed in a congruent scene (e.g. a toaster in a kitchen) are detected more rapidly and more accurately, whereas those placed in an incongruent context (e.g. a sofa on the beach) delay recognition or provoke misperceptions (Bar 2004). More formally, systematic dependencies among features and objects ensue naturally from the generative model that expresses the causal structure of the world, such that the occurrence of a given sensory feature provides contextual information relevant to interpreting nearby parts of the scene. For example, the presence of a linear contour in a visual scene might predict its continuation beyond an occluding object, or the presence of certain colours in a given scene (e.g. green in one part of a forest scene) might lead one to predict their occurrence elsewhere in the scene. In laboratory-based settings, an investigation of the influence of base rates of occurrence of stimuli on decision-making was an early topic of research by the pioneers of SDT, who rapidly discovered that elevated frequencies of signal occurrence increase an observer's bias to interpret a noisy stimulus as containing a signal (increased bias) but had no impact on overall detection sensitivity, i.e. the observer's ability to distinguish signal from noise (Green and Swets 1966). Under the framework of signal detection theory and serial sampling models, this finding suggests that expectation that a signal will occur leads to a change in the decision criterion (or bound), with a more 'liberal' criterion adopted when signals occur frequently (or a tighter bound), but no change in the overall encoding distributions (although for an alternative account, see Balakrishnan 1999).

However, the notion that observers' expectations about signal occurrence influence only the decision criterion, rather than affecting an earlier, perceptual stage, seems to be at odds with a large body of work demonstrating that neural signals in sensory cortices are sensitive to whether a signal occurs rarely or frequently. The occurrence of 'mismatch' signals in event-related potential (ERP) studies at early latencies (Näätänen et al. 1987) with sources in the relevant visual or auditory cortices (Baldeweg et al. 2006) and corresponding sensory activations in fMRI studies (Opitz et al. 1999) come together to suggest that signals that are unexpected are encoded differently from those that are expected even at the very earliest stages of processing. Indeed, an alternative way to think about the influence of probabilistic context on detection and recognition is as the product of backwards-flowing signals that convey top-down information from higher association cortices to the sensory levels below. According to one class of theory (Grossberg 1988; Mumford 1992; Friston 2005), such signals could act to constrain the set of possible interpretations of bottom-up sensory information, biasing perceptual inference towards those alternatives that are most likely given the context. This would provide a computationally efficient mechanism for the brain to capitalize on contextual information—from the recent past or adjacent space—to interpret the sensory world appropriately.

However, despite the intuitive appeal of this account, it leaves a number of thorny issues unresolved. One key question is why stimuli that are attended garner relatively increased neural responses, whereas responses evoked by stimuli that are expected tend to be reduced in amplitude (Summerfield and Egner 2009). One theory, known as *predictive coding*, that can account for this phenomenon is described in the next section.

PREDICTIVE CODING

Predictive coding proposes that perception is a natural consequence of building and refining (and inverting) a generative model of the causes of sensation. The encoding of such a model means that rather than simply forming a hierarchy of passive feature detectors, the sensory cortices explicitly predict which is likely to occur in the external world, conditioned both on past experience and the present context. Predictions are tuned online during perception by 'error' signals encoding the mismatch between expected and observed perceptual information, as well as by perceptual outcomes over the longer term. According to computational implementations of this scheme (Friston 2005), these prediction and error signals are reflected in the responses of distinct neurons at each stage of the visual hierarchy, with some neurons ('prediction' or 'representation' neurons) evolving 'predictive fields' that respond when a particular class of stimulus is likely to occur, and others ('error neurons') signalling the extent to which incoming sensory information diverges from these predictions, both in a spatially bounded fashion. Prediction neurons at each stage of the visual hierarchy project backwards to lower levels, allowing them to 'explain away' incoming sensory information that is consistent with perceptual hypotheses (Fig. 29.3). By contrast, error signals are fed forward, permitting online adjustment of predictions. This scheme affords a natural implementation of perception as an iterative Bayesian inference process, with the beliefs about the causes

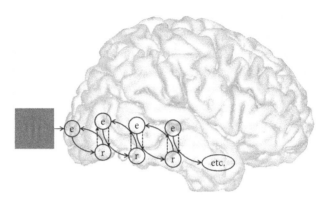

FIGURE 29.3 Predictive coding in visual perceptual inference. Each region in the visual hierarchy passes feedback predictions concerning forthcoming sensory states to the next lower level, and feedforward prediction error signals (the mismatch between the predicted and actual inputs) on to next higher-level regions, where predictions are updated accordingly. This message passing and reconciliation of expectations and prediction error is held to involve two distinct computational units at each level of the hierarchy, representational (r) or prediction units, and error (e) units. Extrinsic connections between levels are shown as solid arrows, and intrinsic (within-level) interactions via dotted line arrows.

of sensation (priors) adjusted by error signals (likelihoods) to form a new (posterior) belief, which in turn serves as a prior in the next cycle. Under this account, thus, perceptual inference does not merely depend on the product of incoming information with a to-be-detected template, as in the models outlined above, but instead on the gradual adjustment of predictions via recurrent interactions between adjacent levels of the sensory hierarchy. Moreover, sensory responses do not uniquely index the representational properties of the external world, but form part of an economy of expectation and surprise by which we actively predict and interpret our local environment.

Predictive coding offers a unifying framework for understanding a diverse range of well-established empirical phenomena. For example, the well-described susceptibility of neurons to 'extra-retinal' influences, i.e. to information falling beyond their classically defined receptive field (RF), can be explained as a consequence of backwards-flowing contextual information from neurons in subsequent processing stages with larger zones of influence (Angelucci et al. 2002). The theory offers a sensible account of how such higher information is used at the lower level: to facilitate those interpretations that are consistent with the gestalt picture emerging at the higher levels of processing. For example, the sensitivity of V1 responses to an oriented grating is facilitated when it is co-linear with flanking gratings, even when the latter are spaced such that they fall outside the classical RF (Polat and Sagi 1994). Other well-described effects, such as neural adaptation or *repetition suppression* can be seen at least in part as a consequence of the reduction in surprise that occurs when a recently or frequently occurring stimulus is expected (Grill-Spector et al. 2006). Finally, the theory offers an explanation for the brain's vigorous response to violations of expectation, which are prominent in scalp-evoked potentials such as the mismatch negativity and P300 (Näätänen et al. 1987; Baldeweg et al. 2006; Mars et al. 2008).

The theory also makes novel and testable predictions, some of which have been verified empirically. Here, we cite just a few. Firstly, it suggests that single neuronal responses will be modulated by the probability of occurrence of a stimulus, a finding recently confirmed in the temporal cortex of the non-human primate (Meyer and Olson 2011). Secondly, it predicts that electrophysiological responses to sensory violation will depend on top-down inputs, a finding that draws support from analyses of effective connectivity data from magnetoencephalographic (MEG) recordings (Garrido et al. 2008). Thirdly, the theory correctly predicts that disordered visual information (e.g. line fragments that do not combine to form a coherent shape) should lead to neural activity increases at early processing stages (e.g. V1) but decreases at later stages (e.g. lateral occipital complex, LOC), whereas ordered visual information (e.g. lines that are assembled to produce the coherent shapes to which higher visual neurons are sensitive) should show the reverse pattern (Murray et al. 2002), as the spatial context provided by the gestalt 'explains away' the incoming information. Fourthly, it predicts that the neural response to repetition should be tempered according to the likelihood of encountering stimulus repetitions, because error signals will depend on how surprising a repetition is; this has been confirmed by a number of fMRI, EEG, and MEG studies (Summerfield et al. 2008, 2011; Todorovic et al. 2011; Larsson and Smith 2012), although not in single-unit recordings (Kaliukhovich and Vogels 2011). Fifthly, it predicts that information about an image that has had a portion removed will be available even in the retinotopic location corresponding to the removed portion, owing to backwards-flowing predictions about what 'should' be present there (Smith and Muckli 2010). Finally, it predicts that neural responses to expectation and surprise should be intermingled in sensory regions, should be stable over time, and differ with respect to their connectivity and latency of responding. Multivariate analyses of fMRI data have recently confirmed the latter two predictions (de Gardelle et al. 2012). Predictive coding also offers an explanatory framework for understanding observed features of the microcircuitry of the sensory cortices, and in particular the finding that backward connections tend to be inhibitory (Olsen et al. 2012), consistent with their role in 'explaining away' predictions and suppressing prediction errors (Bastos et al. 2012).

Predictive coding and attention

In the preceding sections, we summarized research that has addressed how cues that direct attention to a stimulus feature or location in space influence the computational and neural mechanisms underlying visual perception. We focused on the specific case in which an observer is required to make inferences about the identity of a visual stimulus, for example a tilted Gabor patch, at a cued or uncued location. In the bulk of experimental work making up the literature, such as in the Posner task, the advance cue provides information about which location is relevant for behaviour by signalling the overall probability that the signal will occur there. In other words, the cues provide simultaneous (and confounded) information about the probability of occurrence of a signal, and its relevance (Summerfield and Egner 2009). In many cases, it is true that information about probability and relevance are closely related: for example, when searching for lost keys, one might want to begin by looking in those locations where they are most frequently found—in other words, sensory information is relevant to the task by dint of the probabilistic structure of the world. However, in many other circumstances the probability and relevance information provided by a cue are orthogonal. For example, different auditory cues might signal the arrival of either a highly dangerous or relatively innocuous predator; the call of the dangerous predator is more relevant for survival, and thus more predictive of the decision to take evasive action. However, one might also assume that different species of predator are sighted relatively rarely or quite frequently: thus, the cue also provides information about the statistical likelihood that a predator is nearby. Cues thus provide independent information about the *probability* of occurrence of a coming event, and the *relevance* of that event once it arrives. Indeed, more generally, even information that is irrelevant for the goal at hand can be expected, or unexpected, as demonstrated by empirical work showing that we are sensitive to expectancies (and their violation) even when attention is diverted elsewhere (Turk-Browne et al. 2009, 2010).

A key question emerging from the intuition that *probability* (fostering expectations) and *relevance* (driving attention) are potentially orthogonal sources of top-down influence on perception is whether their influences are empirically dissociable and, if so, at which stage attention and expectation might intervene during processing. Within the framework provided by predictive coding, at least two possibilities suggest themselves. Firstly, attention might act to strengthen predictions about what is likely to occur. In other words, attention might boost our expectation that an anticipated stimulus, such as a Gabor patch, will be present, facilitating neural signals and behaviour when that stimulus arrives. Under the computational framework provided by template models (outlined above) this could be consistent with a facilitation of the 'template' or to-be-detected stimulus, with consequent effects on perception that are described by a contrast gain model (cf. Fig. 29.2). Alternatively, in Bayesian terms, one can think of attention here as acting as a Bayesian filter on incoming information, sharpening the prior to encompass only those spatial locations where relevant information is likely to occur. For example, in the cueing task, one could implement an attentional 'spotlight' as a prior with zeros at locations outside the focus of attention (Dayan and Zemel 1999; Yu and Dayan 2004). Another recent proposal that draws upon a Bayesian framework begins with the idea that the true posterior over all possible interpretations of complex sensory information is too large to be computationally tractable, and the inference problem is most likely solved by factorization, i.e. matching of predictions and evidence over local portions of the posterior (e.g. a given feature or dimension of the input). Attention can here be conceived as a mechanism that allows local optimization of the matching between prior and evidence (Whiteley and Sahani 2012). All of these schemes are broadly consistent with the classical framework for investigating cueing effects, by which attention is diverted to those locations where it is most probable that a stimulus will occur, and the influences of attention and expectation on perception are broadly aligned.

However, an alternative is that attention might act to boost prediction error signals that occur when sensory information is unexpected (Feldman and Friston 2010). In other words, consistent with the theoretically dissociable information provided by cues for probability and relevance, expectation and attention may have complementary influences on perception, with expectations furnishing a prior belief about what is most likely in the given environment, and attention influencing the rate at which predictions are adjusted to reflect the true state of the world. One specific proposal is that the *precision* (inverse variability) of the error signal determines how potently it affects top-down predictions, such that more reliable error signals have greater impact on perception. This scheme provides a natural mechanism for attention to intervene, by sharpening prediction error signals, thereby leading to a more effective adjustment of predictions by bottom-up information (Feldman and Friston 2010).

Empirical evidence for dissociable influences of expectation and attention

Empirical investigation of the respective influences of expectation and attention on perceptual choice is in its infancy, but has thus far been supportive of the notion that the two have distinct effects. A number of key principles defining these distinctions are rapidly becoming established. The first, alluded to above and in accordance with the notion of 'explaining away', is the phenomenon of *expectation suppression*, whereby, contrary to the generally facilitatory effects of attention on neural signals for perception, expected stimuli elicit lower-amplitude evoked neural signals than unexpected stimuli (although see Spratling 2008 for an account that reconciles these effects in a single model). It has been known for some time that specific brain potentials accompany the mismatch that occurs when a rare stimulus intervenes in a sequence of frequent 'standard' stimuli (Näätänen et al. 1987), but these *oddball* paradigms often confound expectation with the global rarity or novelty of the mismatching stimulus. In a more targeted exploration of expectation suppression, Egner and colleagues (Egner et al. 2010) demonstrated that when a predictive cue signals which of two classes of visual stimulus—a face or a building—was more likely to occur 500 ms later, the evoked blood oxygen level dependent (BOLD) response in face-responsive extrastriate regions (the fusiform face area or FFA) was reduced for expected relative to unexpected faces, with similar results for buildings in scene-responsive regions. Other studies have suggested that repetition suppression (RS) may be in part driven by expectation suppression, as observers draw upon the auto-correlated structure of sensory signals to predict that currently available information will continue to be present in the near future: indeed, RS is sensitive to the proportion of repetitions in the recent history, suggesting that it is at least in part modulated by expectation. Todorovic et al. (2011) used MEG to examine the time-course of repetition suppression and expectation suppression in a design in which a repeated stimulus was either expected or unexpected, and were able to show that whereas repetition suppression in the auditory domain is first indexed by neural signals that onset at about 50 ms post-stimulus, the influence of expectation suppression is felt later, at approximately 100 ms. These results contrast sharply with the well-studied effect of feature-based attention, whereby BOLD signals are enhanced in those extrastriate regions that preferentially process information associated with the relevant class of stimulus (Corbetta et al. 1990).

Importantly for the current argument, the interaction between expectation suppression and attention was explored using functional neuroimaging in a study by Kok et al., who adapted a conventional attentional cueing task in which advance cues dictated which of two spatial locations (left or right) was relevant for a subsequent orientation discrimination task; participants were instructed to ignore gratings occurring on the uncued side (Kok et al. 2012). Critically, orthogonal blockwise cues indicated whether stimuli were more likely to appear on the left or right of the screen, allowing the authors to plot BOLD responses in retinotopically mapped visual regions to stimuli that were expected or unexpected, on the attended and unattended side of the screen, in a fully orthogonalized fashion. When gratings were unattended, expectation suppression was observed as in previous studies, with expected gratings eliciting a lower overall BOLD response in early visual regions than unexpected gratings. However, the *reverse* pattern of results was obtained for gratings that were cued as relevant and required a discrimination response: expected stimuli elicited a larger BOLD response than unexpected stimuli.

At first, this finding might appear to support the view that attention heightens (or sharpens) predictions, rather than prediction errors, because attention influenced only the height of the BOLD response associated with the expected, rather than the unexpected, stimulus. However, the authors offer a different explanation: the 'explaining away' of expected information that occurs in the unattended condition (leading to an expected > unexpected profile in the visual cortex) is *reversed* in the attended condition because attention acts to enhance prediction errors at the attended side of space. This explanation is appealing, but leaves open the question of why attention boosts prediction errors selectively for expected signals and not for unexpected signals—i.e. why there is such a strong interaction between expectation and attention.

In a second fMRI study, the same authors asked whether expectation suppression is accompanied by a sharpening of the population response measured at the level of multivariate patterns of responses across voxels (Kok et al. 2012). Importantly, they found that it was: expectation decreased the overall mean BOLD response in stimulus-selective regions, but enhanced the consistency of the overall pattern of V1 activity, thereby allowing a multivariate classifier to 'decode' more effectively the expected than the unexpected orientation. Critically, when the authors subdivided voxels (according to their mean response) into those that preferred the expected stimulus and those that preferred alternative orientations, expectation suppression was strongest for the non-stimulus-selective voxels, suggesting that any 'explaining away' in expectation suppression acts mainly on those voxels that might respond to distracting information, rather than to the stimulus itself. In other words, expectation suppression acts to sharpen predictions, rather than increase the precision of prediction errors. Together, these two studies provide some of the first empirical evidence for the view that expectation and attention have distinct influences on the neural correlates of visual perception, with attention possibly acting to sharpen prediction errors, and expectation enhancing the strength of predictions.

In a parallel line of experimentation, Wyart et al. (Wyart et al. 2012) investigated the computational mechanisms by which expectation and attention modulate perceptual decisions, employing a novel cueing paradigm in which to-be-detected gratings could occur (or not) independently in each of two lateralized placeholders. A post-stimulus cue indicated at which of the two placeholders the detection judgement was required to be made. Two advance cues offered distinct information about the probability and relevance of the signals. Firstly, a *relevance* cue dictated which of the two placeholders was more likely to be probed post hoc. Secondly, a probability cue revealed in which of the two placeholders a grating was likely to occur. Importantly, these two advance cues offered entirely orthogonal information: the probability cue provided observers with statistical information about what was likely to occur, but no information about how relevant each signal was for behaviour. By contrast, the relevance cue offered no hint as to what was to occur, but predicted which decision the observer was likely to have to make following the stimulus presentation.

Using a reverse-correlation technique, Wyart and colleagues observed that both probability and relevance signals facilitated detection sensitivity, with more relevant and more probable gratings distinguished better from noise. Critically, however, the reverse correlation approach allowed the authors to calculate separate estimates of sensitivity for those trials with a signal present (i.e. high energy) and those with a signal absent (low energy). This permitted the observation that whereas relevance cues conferred the most benefit when energy was strong, probability cues were most effective at low energy levels. This is informative because under the template model framework described above, contrast gain models (in which attention acts as if it boosts sensory inputs) predict an enhancement that is most beneficial when those input signals are weak, whereas noise reduction models confer the greatest benefit when energy is greatest, i.e. when performance is limited by the presence of noise and not the paucity of input. One appealing interpretation of these data, thus, is that relevance cues (i.e. attention) reduce internal noise (by enhancing the precision of error signals), whereas probability cues (i.e. expectation) boost inputs (by decreasing the noise on the template, i.e. by sharpening predictions). This is consistent with the view that attention increases the precision of the error signals on which perception is based (Wyart et al. 2012).

Conclusions

In this chapter, we have summarized models that describe the mechanisms by which we make judgements about visual stimuli, and reviewed different accounts of how attention might intervene to bias or facilitate these judgements. Our review encompasses both classic models of the choice process, such as signal detection theory and serial sampling models, and 'template' models that draw upon the psychophysical and neurobiological mechanisms that occur in early vision to provide a more detailed description of the nature of sensory evidence in the choice process. We have also discussed the approach offered by normative (ideal observer) models, which typically provide less detail about the transformations that sensory information undergoes during perceptual judgement, but seek to explain perception as an optimal process limited only by noise in the external world. Finally, we describe more recent, 'predictive' approaches to understanding perceptual decisions that suggest that inference about the local environment depends on a generative model of the causes of sensation.

The latter class of model, known broadly as 'predictive coding', raises the interesting question of whether contextual information about (i) which sensory events are likely to occur ('expectation'), and (ii) how relevant these events might be for the current task or goal ('attention') have biologically or computationally distinct influences on perception. We conclude that currently, there exists preliminary evidence for the view that expectation and attention act via separate mechanisms. However, under the framework of predictive coding, our analysis does not provide strong evidence that allows us to arbitrate between the views that attention strengthens predictions (Dayan and Zemel 1999), or enhances error signalling (Feldman and Friston 2010). In part, the difficulty in separating these accounts might arise from the fact that if perceptual inference relies on reciprocal interactions between top-down and bottom-up signalling, then there will be a complex, nonlinear interdependence between prediction and error signal that makes it hard to pinpoint where the influence of attention is felt. Nevertheless, there is strong circumstantial evidence that attention and expectation interact (Kok et al. 2012) and may facilitate detection sensitivity via complementary mechanisms, with expectation acting earlier (Wyart et al. 2012).

One firm conclusion that we do draw, however, is that it will probably benefit researchers designing attentional cueing experiments such as those described above to consider whether their cues offer information about the probability or relevance of forthcoming signals, or both. For example, above we allude to (but do not discuss in detail) a debate amongst researchers as to whether advance cues benefit perception via a response gain or a contrast gain mechanism (Williford and Maunsell 2006; Reynolds and Heeger 2009). The results of Wyart et al. (Wyart et al. 2012) suggest that where attention and expectation are confounded, both mechanisms may be in operation, potentially clouding the debate about the specific role of each mechanism. Experiments offering fully orthogonal information about probability and relevance are required to further address this question, in particular at the biological level. We hope that researchers involved in making neural recordings, in particular those working with single-cell recordings in awake behaving animals, will be inspired to address these questions in future research.

References

Angelucci, A., Levitt, J. B., Walton, E. J., Hupe, J. M., Bullier, J., and Lund, J. S. (2002). Circuits for local and global signal integration in primary visual cortex. *Journal of Neuroscience* 22(19): 8633–8646.

Balakrishnan, J. D. (1999). Decision processes in discrimination: Fundamental misrepresentations of signal detection theory. *Journal of Experimental Psychology: Human Perception and Performance* 25(5): 1189–1206.

Baldeweg, T., Wong, D. and Stephan, K. E. (2006). Nicotinic modulation of human auditory sensory memory: Evidence from mismatch negativity potentials. *International Journal of Psychophysiology* 59(1): 49–58.

Bar, M. (2004). Visual objects in context. *Nature Reviews Neuroscience* 5(8): 617–629.

Bashinski, H. S. and Bacharach, V. R. (1980). Enhancement of perceptual sensitivity as the result of selectively attending to spatial locations. *Perception & Psychophysics* 28(3): 241–248.

Bastos, A. M., Usrey, W. M., Adams, R. A., Mangun, G. R., Fries, P., and Friston, K. J. (2012). Canonical microcircuits for predictive coding. *Neuron* 76(4): 695–711.

Beck, J. M., Ma, W. J., Pitkow, X., Latham, P. E., and Pouget, A. (2012). Not noisy, just wrong: The role of suboptimal inference in behavioral variability. *Neuron* 74(1): 30–39.

Bogacz, R., Brown, E., Moehlis, J., Holmes, P., and Cohen, J. D. (2006). The physics of optimal decision making: A formal analysis of models of performance in two-alternative forced-choice tasks. *Psychological Review* 113(4): 700–765.

Boynton, G. M. (2005). Attention and visual perception. *Current Opinion in Neurobiology* 15(4): 465–469.

Boynton, G. M. (2009). A framework for describing the effects of attention on visual responses. *Vision Research* 49(10): 1129–1143.

Broadbent, D. E. (1958). *Perception and Communication*. Elmsford, N.Y.: Pergamon Press.

Bundesen, C. (1990). A theory of visual attention. *Psychological Review* 97(4): 523–547.

Carrasco, M. (2011). Visual attention: The past 25 years. *Vision Research* 51(13): 1484–1525.

Carrasco, M., Penpeci-Talgar, C., and Eckstein, M. (2000). Spatial covert attention increases contrast sensitivity across the CSF: Support for signal enhancement. *Vision Research* 40(10–12): 1203–1215.

Cavanagh, P. and Alvarez, G. A. (2005). Tracking multiple targets with multifocal attention. *Trends in Cognitive Sciences* 9(7): 349–354.

Clark, A. (2013). Whatever next? Predictive brains, situated agents, and the future of cognitive science. *Behavioral and Brain Sciences* 36(3): 181–204

Cohn, T. E. (1981). Absolute threshold: Analysis in terms of uncertainty. *Journal of the Optical Society of America* 71(6): 783–785.

Corbetta, M., Miezin, F. M., Dobmeyer, S., Shulman, G. L., and Petersen, S. E. (1990). Attentional modulation of neural processing of shape, color, and velocity in humans. *Science* 248(4962): 1556–1559.

Dayan, P. and Zemel, R. (1999). Statistical models and sensory attention. Paper presented to the Ninth International Conference on Artificial Neural Networks, London.

de Gardelle, V., Waszczuk, M., Egner, T., and Summerfield, C. (2012). Concurrent repetition enhancement and suppression responses in extrastriate visual cortex. *Cerebral Cortex*. doi: 10.1093/cercor/bhs211.

Deco, G., Rolls, E. T., Albantakis, L., and Romo, R. (2013). Brain mechanisms for perceptual and reward-related decision-making. *Progress in Neurobiology* 103: 194–213.

Desimone, R. and Duncan, J. (1995). Neural mechanisms of selective visual attention. *Annual Review of Neuroscience* 18: 193–222.

DeValois, R. L. and DeValois, K. K. (1988). *Spatial Vision*. New York: Oxford University Press.

Downing, C. J. (1988). Expectancy and visual-spatial attention: Effects on perceptual quality. *Journal of Experimental Psychology: Human Perception and Performance* 14(2): 188–202.

Eckstein, M. P., Peterson, M. F., Pham, B. T., and Droll, J. A. (2009). Statistical decision theory to relate neurons to behavior in the study of covert visual attention. *Vision Research* 49(10): 1097–1128.

Egner, T., Monti, J. M. and Summerfield, C. (2010). Expectation and surprise determine neural population responses in the ventral visual stream. *Journal of Neuroscience* 30(49):16601–16608.

Feldman, H. and Friston, K. J. (2010). Attention, uncertainty, and free-energy. *Frontiers in Human Neuroscience* 4: 215.

Foley, J. M. S. W. (1998). Spatial attention: Effect of position uncertainty and number of distractor patterns on the threshold-versus-contrast function for contrast discrimination. *Journal of the Optical Society of America A: Optics, Image Science, and Vision* 15: 1036–1047.

Friston, K. (2005). A theory of cortical responses. *Philosophical Transactions of the Royal Society B: Biological Sciences* 360(1456): 815–836.

Garrido, M. I., Friston, K. J., Kiebel, S. J., Stephan, K. E., Baldeweg, T., and Kilner, J. M. (2008). The functional anatomy of the MMN: A DCM study of the roving paradigm. *NeuroImage* 42(2): 936–944.

Gigerenzer, G. and Gaissmaier, W. (2011). Heuristic decision making. *Annual Review of Psychology* 62: 451–482.

Glimcher, P. W., Dorris, M. C., and Bayer, H. M. (2005). Physiological utility theory and the neuroeconomics of choice. *Games and Economic Behavior* 52(2): 213–256.

Gold, J. I. and Shadlen, M. N. (2007). The neural basis of decision making. *Annual Review of Neuroscience* 30: 535–574.

Gould, I. C., Wolfgang, B. J., and Smith, P. L. (2007). Spatial uncertainty explains exogenous and endogenous attentional cuing effects in visual signal detection. *Journal of Vision* 7(13): 4 1–17.

Green, D. M. and Swets, J. A. (1966). *Signal Detection Theory and Psychophysics*. New York: Wiley.

Gregory, R. L. (1980). Perceptions as hypotheses. *Philosophical Transactions of the Royal Society B: Biological Sciences* 290(1038): 181–197.

Grill-Spector, K., Henson, R., and Martin, A. (2006). Repetition and the brain: Neural models of stimulus-specific effects. *Trends in Cognitive Sciences* 10(1): 14–23.

Grossberg, S. (1988). Nonlinear neural networks: Principles, mechanisms, architectures. *Neural Networks* 1: 17–61.

Hawkins, H. L., Hillyard, S. A., Luck, S. J., Mouloua, M., Downing, C. J., and Woodward, D. P. (1990). Visual attention modulates signal detectability. *Journal of Experimental Psychology: Human Perception and Performance* 16(4): 802–811.

Heeger, D. J. (1993). Modeling simple-cell direction selectivity with normalized, half-squared, linear operators. *Journal of Neurophysiology* 70(5): 1885–1898.

Helmholtz, H. von (1896). *Handbuch der Physiologischen Optik, Dritter Abschnitt*. Hamburg: Voss.

Helmholtz, H. von (1909). *Treatise on Physiological Optics*, vol. 3, 3rd edn. Hamburg: Voss.

Herrmann, K., Montaser-Kouhsari, L., Carrasco, M., and Heeger, D. J. (2010). When size matters: attention affects performance by contrast or response gain. *Nature Neuroscience* 13(12): 1554–1559.

Hubel, D. H. and Wiesel, T. N. (1959). Receptive fields of single neurones in the cat's striate cortex. *Journal of Physiology* 148: 574–591.

Ito, M. and Gilbert, C. D. (1999). Attention modulates contextual influences in the primary visual cortex of alert monkeys. *Neuron* 22(3): 593–604.

Kahneman, D., Slovic, P., and Tversky, A. (1982). *Judgment Under Uncertainty: Heuristics and Biases.* New York: Cambridge University Press.

Kahneman, D. and Tversky, A. (1979). Prospect theory: An analysis of decision under risk. *Econometrica* 47(2): 263–291.

Kaliukhovich, D. A. and Vogels, R. (2011). Stimulus repetition probability does not affect repetition suppression in macaque inferior temporal cortex. *Cerebral Cortex* 21(7): 1547–1558.

Kok, P., Rahnev, D., Jehee, J. F., Lau, H. C., and de Lange, F. P. (2012). Attention reverses the effect of prediction in silencing sensory signals. *Cerebral Cortex* 22(9): 2197–2206.

Larsson, J. and Smith, A. T. (2012). fMRI repetition suppression: Neuronal adaptation or stimulus expectation? *Cerebral Cortex* 22(3): 567–576.

Lee, D. K., Koch, C., and Braun, J. (1997). Spatial vision thresholds in the near absence of attention. *Vision Research* 37(17): 2409–2418.

Lu, Z. L. and Dosher, B. A. (2008). Characterizing observers using external noise and observer models: Assessing internal representations with external noise. *Psychological Review* 115(1): 44–82.

McAdams, C. J. and Maunsell, J. H. (1999a). Effects of attention on orientation-tuning functions of single neurons in macaque cortical area V4. *Journal of Neuroscience* 19(1): 431–441.

McAdams, C. J. and Maunsell, J. H. (1999b). Effects of attention on the reliability of individual neurons in monkey visual cortex. *Neuron* 23(4): 765–773.

Mars, R. B., Debener, S., Gladwin, T. E., Harrison, L. M., Haggard, P., Rothwell, J. C., and Bestmann, S. (2008). Trial-by-trial fluctuations in the event-related electroencephalogram reflect dynamic changes in the degree of surprise. *Journal of Neuroscience* 28(47): 12539–12545.

Maunsell, J. H. and Treue, S. (2006). Feature-based attention in visual cortex. *Trends in Neurosciences* 29(6): 317–322.

Meyer, T. and Olson, C. R. (2011). Statistical learning of visual transitions in monkey inferotemporal cortex. *Proceedings of the National Academy of Sciences USA* 108(48): 19401–19406.

Muller, H. J. and Humphreys, G. W. (1991). Luminance-increment detection: Capacity-limited or not? *Journal of Experimental Psychology: Human Perception and Performance* 17(1): 107–124.

Mumford, D. (1992). On the computational architecture of the neocortex. II: The role of cortico-cortical loops. *Biological Cybernetics* 66(3): 241–251.

Murray, S. O., Kersten, D., Olshausen, B. A., Schrater, P., and Woods, D. L. (2002). Shape perception reduces activity in human primary visual cortex. *Proceedings of the National Academy of Sciences USA* 99(23): 15164–15169.

Näätänen, R., Paavilainen, P., Alho, K., Reinikainen, K., and Sams, M. (1987). The mismatch negativity to intensity changes in an auditory stimulus sequence. *Electroencephalography and Clinical Neurophysiology: Supplement* 40: 125–131.

Naka, K. I. and Rushton, W. A. (1966). S-potentials from luminosity units in the retina of fish (Cyprinidae). *Journal of Physiology* 185(3): 587–599.

Neisser, U. (1967). *Cognitive Psychology.* New York: Appleton-Century-Crofts.

Olsen, S. R., Bortone, D. S., Adesnik, H., and Scanziani, M. (2012). Gain control by layer six in cortical circuits of vision. *Nature* 483(7387): 47–52.

Opitz, B., Mecklinger, A., Von Cramon, D. Y., and Kruggel, F. (1999). Combining electrophysiological and hemodynamic measures of the auditory oddball. *Psychophysiology* 36(1): 142–147.

Pelli, D. G. (1985). Uncertainty explains many aspects of visual contrast detection and discrimination. *Journal of the Optical Society of America A: Optics, Image Science, and Vision* 2(9): 1508–1532.

Pelli, D. G. and Farell, B. (1999). Why use noise? *Journal of the Optical Society of America A: Optics, Image Science, and Vision* 16(3): 647–653.

Polat, U. and Sagi, D. (1994). Spatial interactions in human vision: From near to far via experience-dependent cascades of connections. *Proceedings of the National Academy of Sciences USA* 91(4): 1206–1209.

Posner, M. I. and Petersen, S. E. (1990). The attention system of the human brain. *Annual Review of Neuroscience* 13: 25–42.

Posner, M. I., Snyder, C. R., and Davidson, B. J. (1980). Attention and the detection of signals. *Journal of Experimental Psychology* 109(2): 160–174.

Ratcliff, R., Gomez, P., and McKoon, G. (2004). A diffusion model account of the lexical decision task. *Psychological Review* 111(1): 159–182.

Ratcliff, R. and McKoon, G. (2008). The diffusion decision model: Theory and data for two-choice decision tasks. *Neural Computation* 20(4): 873–922.

Rensink, R. A. (2002). Change detection. *Annual Review of Psychology* 53: 245–277.

Reynolds, J. H. and Chelazzi, L. (2004). Attentional modulation of visual processing. *Annual Review of Neuroscience* 27: 611–647.

Reynolds, J. H. and Heeger, D. J. (2009). The normalization model of attention. *Neuron* 61(2): 168–185.

Reynolds, J. H., Pasternak, T., and Desimone, R. (2000). Attention increases sensitivity of V4 neurons. *Neuron* 26(3): 703–714.

Shaw, M. L. (1980). Identifying attentional and decision-making components in information processing. In R. S. Nickerson (ed.), *Attention and Performance* (vol. 8, pp. 277–296). Hillsdale, N.J.: Lawrence Erlbaum Associates.

Shaw, M. L. (1984). Division of attention among spatial locations: A fundamental difference between detection of letters and detection of luminance increments. In H. Bouma and D. G. Bouwhuis (eds.), *Attention and Performance* (vol. 10, pp. 109–121). Hillsdale, N.J.: Lawrence Erlbaum Associates.

Smith, F. W. and Muckli, L. (2010). Nonstimulated early visual areas carry information about surrounding context. *Proceedings of the National Academy of Sciences USA* 107(46): 20099–20103.

Smith, P. L. (2000). Attention and luminance detection: Effects of cues, masks, and pedestals. *Journal of Experimental Psychology: Human Perception and Performance* 26(4): 1401–1420.

Smith, P. L. and Ratcliff, R. (2009). An integrated theory of attention and decision making in visual signal detection. *Psychological Review* 116(2): 283–317.

Smith, P. L., Ratcliff, R., and Wolfgang, B. J. (2004). Attention orienting and the time course of perceptual decisions: Response time distributions with masked and unmasked displays. *Vision Research* 44(12): 1297–1320.

Sperling, G. and Dosher, B. A. (1986). Strategy and optimization in human information processing. In K. R. Boff, L. Kaufman, and J. P. Thomas (eds.), *Handbook of Perception and Human Performance* (pp. 1–65). New York: Wiley.

Spratling, M. W. (2008). Reconciling predictive coding and biased competition models of cortical function. *Frontiers in Computational Neuroscience* 2(4). doi: 10.3389/neuro.10.004.2008.

Summerfield, C. and Egner, T. (2009). Expectation (and attention) in visual cognition. *Trends in Cognitive Sciences* 13(9): 403–409.

Summerfield, C., Trittschuh, E. H., Monti, J. M., Mesulam, M. M., and Egner, T. (2008). Neural repetition suppression reflects fulfilled perceptual expectations. *Nature Neuroscience* 11(9): 1004–1006.

Summerfield, C., Wyart, V., Johnen, V. M., and de Gardelle, V. (2011). Human scalp electro-encephalography reveals that repetition suppression varies with expectation. *Frontiers in Human Neuroscience* 5(67). doi: 10.3389/fnhum.2011.00067.

Todorovic, A., van Ede, F., Maris, E., and de Lange, F. P. (2011). Prior expectation mediates neural adaptation to repeated sounds in the auditory cortex: An MEG study. *Journal of Neuroscience* 31(25): 9118–9123.

Treisman, A. M. and Gelade, G. (1980). A feature-integration theory of attention. *Cognitive Psychology* 12(1): 97–136.

Tsotsos, J. K. (1997). Limited capacity of any realizable perceptual system is a sufficient reason for attentive behavior. *Consciousness and Cognition* 6(2–3): 429–436.

Turk-Browne, N. B., Scholl, B. J., Chun, M. M., and Johnson, M. K. (2009). Neural evidence of statistical learning: Efficient detection of visual regularities without awareness. *Journal of Cognitive Neuroscience* 21(10): 1934–1945.

Turk-Browne, N. B., Scholl, B. J., Johnson, M. K., and Chun, M. M. (2010). Implicit perceptual anticipation triggered by statistical learning. *Journal of Neuroscience* 30(33): 11177–11187.

Wald, A. and Wolfowitz, J. (1949). Bayes solutions of sequential decision problems. *Proceedings of the National Academy of Sciences USA* 35(2): 99–102.

Whiteley, L. and Sahani, M. (2012). Attention in a Bayesian framework. *Frontiers in Human Neuroscience* 6(100). doi: 10.3389/fnhum.2012.00100.

Williford, T. and Maunsell, J. H. (2006). Effects of spatial attention on contrast response functions in macaque area V4. *Journal of Neurophysiology* 96(1): 40–54.

Wolfe, J. M. (2010). Visual search. *Current Biology* 20: R346–R349.

Wyart, V., Nobre, A. C., and Summerfield, C. (2012). Dissociable prior influences of signal probability and relevance on visual contrast sensitivity. *Proceedings of the National Academy of Sciences USA* 109(9): 3593–3598.

Yeshurun, Y. and Carrasco, M. (1998). Attention improves or impairs visual performance by enhancing spatial resolution. *Nature* 396(6706): 72–75.

Yu, A. and Dayan, P. (2004). Inference, attention, and decision in a Bayesian neural architecture. *Advances in Neural Information Processing Systems* 16: 1577–1584.

APPENDIX

We simulated performance on a detection task in which oriented Gabors could occur at attended or unattended locations. Our model calculated simulated neuronal responses Y^+ on signal present trials according to the following equation:

$$Y^+ = \lambda \left[\left(S_c + N_S \right) \bullet \left(T_d + N_T \right) \right] \gamma$$

where S_c is a Gabor patch of contrast c {0.1,0.2,0.3…1}, T is a template (to-be-detected Gabor of the same orientation) of contrast d, and N_S and N_T are zero-mean Gaussian noise of standard deviation σ_S (external, or stimulus noise) and σ_T (internal, or template noise) respectively. γ is a factor by which the entire response is multiplied. The transformation $\lambda[.]$ is a sigmoidal squashing function of the following form (Naka and Rushton 1966):

$$\lambda[W] = \begin{cases} \dfrac{uW^N}{s^N + W^N} \\ 0 \end{cases}$$

For all models, we assumed that external noise σ_S was fixed at 0.01, and the parameters of the Naka–Rushton function were $u = 1$, $N = 5$, and $s = 0.01$.

To simulate the influence of attention as response gain control (panels A), we fixed $d = 0.5$ and $\sigma_T = 0.001$, and varied γ at 1 (unattended, light blue lines) and 1.5 (attended, darker lines). To simulate the influence of attention as contrast gain control (panels B), we fixed σ_T at 0.001 and γ at 1 and varied d at 0.5 (unattended, light blue lines) and 0.8 (attended, dark blue lines). To simulate the influence of attention as noise reduction (panels C), we set $\gamma = 1$ and $d = 1$ and varied σ_T at 0.005 (unattended, light blue lines) and 0.001 (attended, dark blue lines). As a control, we also calculated Y^-, the value on simulated signal absent trials:

$$Y^- = \lambda\left[\left(N_S\right) \bullet \left(T_d + N_T\right)\right]\gamma$$

In Fig. 29.2, lines show values of Y^+ (blue) and Y^- (red) in attended and unattended conditions as a function of stimulus contrast, c.

We calculated simulated sensitivity across the 100 trials by imposing a threshold on Y at 0.75 (grey line, right hand plots). Y^+ trials were thus deemed a hit if $Y^+ > 0.75$, or a miss if $Y^+ < 0.75$; Y^- trials were deemed a false alarm if $Y^- > 0.75$, or a correct rejection if $Y^- < 0.75$. This allowed us to calculate sensitivity as a function of c for attended (darker lines) and unattended (lighter lines), plotted here as hit rate–false alarm rate.

CHAPTER 30

ATTENTION AND ACTION

HEINER DEUBEL

INTRODUCTION

Our visual world contains far too many things for them to be processed all together, and among this wealth of information attention enables us to select relevant objects and locations over less important ones. In the classic view of attention (Broadbent 1958; Posner 1980), the purpose of attention is to choose which of these stimuli would gain access to awareness and which would not. Indeed, it has been proposed for the visual system that most of the retinal input is filtered out (Ullman 1984), and only a very limited amount of the available information is processed to the level of conscious representations, accompanied by object recognition and the encoding into working memory. This type of selection has been termed 'selection-for-perception'.

Starting in the 1980s, researchers began to point towards another important function of visual attention, related to the control of goal-directed movements (Allport 1987; Neumann 1987). Consider a seemingly simple task like taking a banana out of a basket of fruit. How can the hand grasp the particular fruit without being distracted by the other objects? Obviously, a mechanism is required that selectively provides the spatial information of the target object for the grasp (i.e. its location, size, orientation, etc.), while filtering out this information for the other objects that may compete for the action. Allport (1987) and Neumann (1987) proposed that visual attention is also central to this kind of selection, which they termed 'selection-for-action'.

This chapter will discuss the role of visual attention in preparation and control of goal-directed actions, and specifically in the attentional selection of action goals. The focus will be on attention in the visual modality, and the motor actions that are arguably most relevant to us, namely eye movements, manual reaching, and grasping. The review will be limited to some of the (many) behavioural studies that have been carried out with healthy human subjects and non-human primates, while the neurophysiology and neuropsychology of attention and its relation to action are presented in other chapters of this handbook.

THEORIES OF 'SELECTION-FOR-ACTION'

Several theories and models have been proposed to address specifically the relationship between action and attention. The most influential work in this context has probably been the *premotor theory* of Rizzolatti and colleagues. In its original form (Rizzolatti et al. 1987), the theory proposed that shifts of visual attention are a consequence of the preparation of an eye movement to a particular location in space. Accordingly, a central prediction of the theory is that attention shifts cannot occur without the concurrent preparation of a spatially congruent eye movement. The preparation of the saccade produces a processing advantage for stimuli at the location of the saccade goal, resulting in a spatially selective enhancement of visual processing. Whether the saccade is actually performed, depends on a go-signal for releasing the oculomotor system into execution. In a later version, the theory was expanded to other types of motor actions (Rizzolatti et al. 1994), stating the existence of distinct, effector-specific maps ('spatial pragmatic maps') that become active when a movement is prepared. As the theory's central idea, Rizzolatti and colleagues postulated a tight functional coupling between movement preparation and attention, stating 'the system that controls action is the same system that controls spatial attention' (Rizzolatti et al. 1994: 256).

A second prominent theory that accounts for the link between attention and action is the *visual attention model* (VAM) proposed by Schneider (1995). It postulates a unitary mechanism which is responsible for selection in separate, parallel pathways in the brain: 'selection-for-perception' in the ventral pathway and 'selection-for-action' in the dorsal pathway. Critically, a common target object for perception in the ventral stream and action generation in the dorsal stream is selected by task-based feedback signals from higher level visual areas to primary visual cortex (V1). At the behavioural level, VAM predicts that the preparation of a motor action will bind processing in the perceptual system to the location of the movement target, boosting visual performance at that location. It also assumes that higher-level processing in the dorsal and ventral streams is capacity-limited, that is, it can occur for only one object at a time, resulting in a single focus of attention at the target location. Recently, VAM has been linked to Bundesen's (1990) *theory of visual attention* for a computer vision model of task-based control of 'where-to-look-next' (Wischnewski et al. 2010). In contrast to the original version of VAM, selection is now assumed to be coordinated not in V1 but in attentional priority maps such as supposed in the lateral intraparietal (LIP) region (e.g. Bisley and Goldberg, 2010).

Both the premotor theory and VAM predict that visual attention shifts to the saccade goal when an eye movement is prepared. However, there is an important difference between the theories: while the premotor theory claims that attention is a necessary and immediate *consequence* of oculomotor programming, VAM postulates that attentional selection signals originate in brain areas involved in target feature processing (e.g. in inferior temporal (IT) cortex) and propagate from there via V1 to motor-related areas in the dorsal stream (e.g. LIP). In this sense, the allocation of visual attention in perception and saccade preparation are conceptualized in VAM as distinct but coupled processes. This is compatible with recent observations from neurophysiology indicating that the activity of a particular class of neurons in the frontal eye fields results in selective visual attention, but not in motor preparation (e.g. Schafer and Moore 2011).

The *biased competition* theory of visual attention (Desimone and Duncan 1995) also speaks to the relation of attention and action, but its main focus is to provide a general framework of how attention emerges in the brain. Its basic assumptions are that processing of visual input is competitive at many levels in the brain, and that this competition is biased to favour inputs that match task requirements. Thus, selective attention and action selection may just be two facets of the same biased competition occurring throughout visuomotor processing areas (Duncan 2006; Cisek 2007).

ATTENTION AND EYE MOVEMENTS

Saccade preparation and attention are closely coupled

Saccadic eye movements are used to bring interesting aspects of the world around us onto the retinal locus of our most accurate visual perception, the fovea. But since natural scenes contain far too many potential saccade targets, a mechanism for sequential selection of targets to be preferentially foveated is required, a function known to be fulfilled by visual attention. Psychophysical investigations demonstrating a close link between attention and oculomotor programming are now abundant. The majority of this research has used dual-task paradigms in which participants were planning a saccade to a target, while the spatial allocation of attention was measured in a secondary perceptual task. Historically, the first systematic studies of this kind were done in 1980, independently by Raymond Klein and Roger Remington. Klein (1980) used a manual reaction time task, reasoning that planning a saccade to a region in space should reduce manual response times to a visual probe appearing in this region. He did not find such a facilitation and concluded that saccade preparation and attention shifts are based on independent processes. However, reaction times were extraordinarily long in his study, pointing to potential methodological problems. Indeed, Klein's task required participants to perform two speeded responses, a saccade and a manual key press, in close temporal vicinity. A number of later studies (most notably, Pashler et al. 1993) have demonstrated that manual reactions are delayed if required shortly after saccades (for a recent review see Huestegge 2011). Recent evidence suggests that these bottleneck effects acting on the reaction time of the second of two motor responses, also denoted as 'psychological refractory period', result from post-attentional processing stages, probably at the level of response selection (Jonikaitis et al. 2010). One may infer that paradigms that use *non-speeded* responses as measures for attention allocation (such as non-speeded discrimination tasks) might be favourable for studying the relation of attention and action preparation.

Remington (1980) asked subjects to detect a brief luminance increment before the saccade. He found that detection was equally likely at the saccade goal as at other locations, and argued against a strong link between saccades and attention. However, his data also showed that saccadic latencies were prolonged when the luminance increment occurred at a location different from the saccade target, reflecting some effect of the attentional manipulation on the saccadic response. Shepherd et al. (1986) eliminated some of the methodological problems of these early studies. They also used a speeded detection task in which a central arrow cued observers to make a saccade to the left or right. Shortly before the saccade a flash was presented either at the saccade target or at the opposite location. Manual reaction times to the flash were indeed shorter when it was presented at the side of the saccade target, even when the flash was more likely to appear at the opposite location. From this finding Shepherd et al. (1986) concluded that it is not possible to make an eye movement without a preceding shift of attention to the saccade target.

The most convincing evidence for a close coupling of attention and saccade preparation has resulted from a number of investigations that applied a dual task paradigm in which *perceptual identification* rather than saccadic or manual reaction times was used as a measure of attentional deployment. Hoffman and Subramaniam (1995) asked participants to saccade to a specified location and to detect a target letter presented at one of four possible locations well before the eye movement. Performance was best when the letter was presented at the saccade target location as compared to non-congruent conditions. In a particularly important study, Kowler et al. (1995) also combined a letter identification task with an eye movement task. Participants were presented with a display consisting of a circular display of eight pre-masks. They were asked to make a saccade from the central fixation to one of these items, upon the appearance of a central arrow cue. Simultaneously with cue onset, the masks changed into letters which were again masked after 200 ms. Kowler and co-workers found that the accuracy to report a letter was considerably higher at the saccade target location, demonstrating that the preparation of a saccade facilitated perceptual discrimination at the saccade target location. In a second, 'fixed report' experiment, participants were asked always to report the letter presented at the same, fixed location during a block of trials, while preparing saccades according to the variable arrow cue. An important result of this experiment was that participants now could, to some degree, also report letters that were not presented at the saccade target, but only at the expense of prolonged saccade latencies. Also, saccadic landing positions became less precise if more attentional effort was devoted to the remote perceptual location.

In the study by Deubel and Schneider (1996) participants also had to perform a dual task, identifying a perceptual discrimination target while preparing a saccadic eye movement. They were initially presented with a string-like horizontal array of mask characters, with five characters located to the left and five to the right of the fixation point. The central three of these masks on each side were marked by different colours. A central arrow was then presented, whose colour indicated one of the peripheral items as the goal for the upcoming saccade. The saccade had to be elicited upon the offset of the central arrow. Shortly after cue removal but before the saccade, a discrimination letter consisting of a digital 'E' or '3' appeared at one of the mask locations in the string, while the other mask elements were replaced by distractors. This critical display was presented for 120 ms, until all characters were removed, still before saccade onset. During the experiment, the spatial relationship between the saccade target and the location of the discrimination stimulus was systematically varied. The results yielded very good discrimination performance in the conditions where saccade target and discrimination target coincided, while performance was at or close to chance at the adjacent, non-target locations. This held even in a second experiment (Deubel and Schneider 1996: Exp. 2) in which participants knew in advance the location of the discrimination target. The authors therefore argued that it is not possible to voluntarily shift attention away to a location of interest while preparing a saccade to a separate location in space, concluding that 'the coupling of visual attention and saccade target selection is obligatory' (Deubel and Schneider 1996: 1835). The degree of spatial selectivity of attentional focusing demonstrated in these experiments is remarkable, given the fact that target and non-targets were separated by only 1 degree, appearing at 5 degrees in the visual periphery. According to Deubel and Schneider (1996), this indicates an object-specific allocation of attention, such that only the selected object can be recognized (LaBerge and Brown 1989; Schneider 1995).

A considerable number of follow-up studies have found converging evidence for the mandatory allocation of visual attention at the saccade goal during the preparation of the eye movement, under a variety of different experimental settings (e.g. McPeek et al. 1999; Godijn and Pratt 2002; Godijn and Theeuwes 2003; Castet et al. 2006; Deubel and Schneider 2003; Deubel 2008; Baldauf and Deubel 2008a; Tibber et al. 2009; Filali-Sadouk et al. 2010). There is also some evidence that saccade preparation has similar, spatially selective attentional effects on the processing of auditory (Rorden and Driver 1999) and tactile stimuli (Rorden et al. 2002; Juravle and Deubel 2009). In summary, the conjecture that the preparation of a saccade is tightly linked to the allocation of attention at the saccade target has become firmly established.

Time course of presaccadic attention shifts

Given the tight link between attention and saccade target selection, questions arise as to the precise temporal dynamics of this coupling. When exactly does attention move to the saccade target, how long does the attention shift take, and how strictly is the time of the attention shift linked to the onset of the saccade? Only a few empirical studies have directly addressed these issues. Doré-Mazars et al. (2004) let participants saccade to a string of letters and detect a letter change that occurred at various times before saccade onset. They found that perceptual performance was best at the saccade target location only if the target letter was displayed 50 ms before saccade onset. This suggests that the attention focus is allocated on the saccade target only very shortly before the saccade, when the motor programme is ready to be executed, while for earlier temporal intervals attention allocation and saccade target may be dissociated. In contrast, Castet et al. (2006; see also Montagnini and Castet 2007) reported that the discrimination of a Gabor patch displayed at various times before the saccade improved gradually over a period of 150–200 ms before saccade onset, and attentional deployment appeared to be more closely related to the onset of the saccade cue than to saccade onset. Deubel (2008) studied the attentional dynamics in a task in which a discrimination target was briefly presented among distractors, either at the saccade goal or at a spatially separate, pre-cued location, and at variable times before the saccade. Interestingly, his results showed that the temporal dynamics of attentional allocation varied with the experimental conditions—attention shifted to the saccade target early or late during saccade preparation, depending on the task. In parallel to the deployment of attentional resources at the saccade target, attention was disengaged from other task-relevant locations in the visual field, indicating that attentional resources cannot be voluntarily distributed to locations other than the saccade target. The results estimated the duration of the presaccadic attention shifts to be in the range of 50–150 ms. Importantly, while the time of the attention shift to the saccade goal varied with the task, attention in all these conditions was allocated to the eye movement target just before saccade execution. Recent studies have since confirmed this temporal co-variation between the dynamics of the presaccadic attention shift and the time of saccade onset (Filali-Sadouk et al. 2010; Jonikaitis and Deubel 2011).

Can attention allocation and saccade preparation be dissociated, and to what degree?

While the close coupling of attention and saccade preparation seems to constitute the default mode of visuomotor processing before eye movement, the question arises whether there are circumstances under which both can be dissociated. A number of studies suggest that there is indeed some capability to allocate attentional resources at locations separate from the saccade goal, but it seems that the degree to which attention can be withdrawn from the saccade target is rather limited. Kowler et al. (1995) first illustrated this fact through representing their data in the form of an 'attentional operating characteristic' (AOC) curve, which represents the trade-off between the latency of the saccadic response and the perceptual performance in the letter identification task. These AOC curves made obvious that response speed was traded for visual performance: saccadic latencies were longer when more emphasis was given to the perceptual task. However, the curves also showed that—under no condition—could the perceptual and the motor task be done without interference. These findings have found further support in more recent investigations (Tibber et al. 2009).

Along similar lines, Montagnini and Castet (2007) reported that attentional resources could voluntarily be directed away from the saccade target, at least under conditions that support the distribution of attention among two locations. In their task, participants were strongly encouraged to attend away from the saccade target by presenting the perceptual target in most cases opposite to the direction of the saccade, simultaneously with the onset of the saccade cue. This probability manipulation resulted in a strong improvement to discriminate the test stimulus at the location opposite to the saccade, without marked costs in saccadic latency, demonstrating that it is possible to divert an independent component of visual attention away from the saccade target. Nevertheless, perceptual performance was still superior at the saccade target location.

The experiments described above were all performed under conditions where saccades were elicited endogenously, with central cues indicating the saccade target. The question arises whether sudden peripheral stimulus onsets that are supposed to capture attention automatically, would result in a disengagement of attention for the saccade target, while the saccade would still be prepared. Indeed, sudden visual transients in a scene were found to attract involuntary saccades, as demonstrated in the prominent 'oculomotor capture' paradigm developed by Theeuwes et al. (1998). A modified version of the oculomotor capture paradigm was used in a study by Peterson et al. (2004) that looked specifically at the question whether *involuntary* saccades as elicited by sudden visual onsets are also accompanied by a deployment of attention to the saccade target. In each trial, participants first fixated in the centre of a circular array of six white circles that contained figure-8 pre-masks. Five of the six circles then turned red and the participants had to quickly saccade to the single circle that remained white. Simultaneously, the pre-masks briefly changed into letters, and participants had to later report the letter presented within the target circle. Importantly, an additional circle was also presented at a previously unoccupied location, representing a sudden onset in the display. Although this onset was completely irrelevant to the task, observers frequently made an involuntary saccade to this stimulus, which was then quickly followed by another saccade to the instructed target (the white circle). Using a measure based on response compatibility, the authors concluded that when an involuntary saccade is made, attention first goes to the sudden onset location (the goal of the unintended saccade). Thus, it seems that reflexive saccadic eye movements are also preceded by shifts of covert attention. Interestingly, their results also suggest that attention then quickly switched to the intended location, with the eye following this attentional double-step pattern a short time later. While Peterson et al. favoured such a sequential model, it seems that their data can also be explained by a parallel allocation of attention to both the intended and the unintended stimulus locations. It should be noted that there are also some conflicting reports suggesting that reflexive, unintended saccades that occur in an antisaccade task may *not* be preceded by attention shifts (Mokler and Fischer 1999; Mokler and Deubel 2000).

Schneider and Deubel (2002) also studied the effect of onset cues on presaccadic attention. In an experimental paradigm modified from Deubel and Schneider (1996) observers had to identify a letter briefly presented before the saccade within bilateral letter strings. In the first two of their experiments, a peripheral onset (two lines appearing above and below one of the letters) cued the location to which the saccade had to be directed. Perceptual performance was always superior at the saccade target location. Even when participants were informed about the location of the discrimination target, they could only identify the letter if it was also the target of the eye movement. This replicated the basic findings of Deubel and Schneider (1996) for exogenously triggered saccades. In a third experiment the location of the discrimination stimulus was again kept constant, while participants had either to saccade to a peripheral onset cue or to ignore it while fixating. The results showed that an onset cue per se did not necessarily attract attention, but a peripheral cue that was also the target of the saccade always bound attention. This implies that the coupling of attention and saccade preparation observed for onset targets is mainly due to the function of the stimulus as a target for the saccade. So, it seems that the coupling between saccade target selection and perceptual selection is obligatory for stimulus-driven saccades as well.

Another possible factor determining how much processing resources are moved away from the saccade target is the difficulty of the tasks involved. Wilder et al. (2009) studied attention to action-irrelevant Gabor probes during the pauses between saccades performed in three 'real-world' tasks, namely counting dots, pointing to dots, or simply looking at the dots. They report that perceptual performance at movement-irrelevant locations suffered most for the counting task, but considerably less for pointing or just looking. On the one hand, these results confirm that even for these more natural situations, attention is required to control the saccades. On the other hand, as the authors also emphasize, it seems that the attentional demands for saccades may be less than those required for some demanding cognitive tasks such as counting.

Altogether, the investigations that have focused on the distribution of perceptual capabilities (mostly, visual discrimination) before saccades have indeed revealed some capability in subjects to divert their attention away from the saccade target. However, under all the different experimental variations used in these studies, it has consistently been found that there is superior perceptual performance at the saccade target location during eye movement preparation. This suggests that when a saccade is planned, saccade target selection is the major determinant for attention distribution, summoning most of the attentional resources at the target location.

It should be noted that there are a few reports which have argued for a complete independence of attention control and saccade preparation (Hunt and Kingstone 2003a, 2003b; Belopolsky and Theeuwes 2009). While most of the previously described studies have used non-speeded perceptual tasks, they used manual or saccadic reaction times to measure attentional allocation. Further studies are necessary to systematically investigate differences and similarities in attention during discrimination and speeded detection tasks. As Prinzmetal et al. (2005) pointed out, it is possible that non-speeded discrimination tasks and reaction time tasks measure different types of attention. While discrimination tasks mainly involve top-down attention, reaction time tasks may involve a combination of top-down and bottom-up attention.

Effect of attention on saccade trajectories

Attentional manipulations have effects on the trajectories of saccades. Sheliga et al. (1994, 1995) showed that directing covert attention to a location in space while planning a saccade to another target leads to a deviation of the saccade trajectory away from the attended location. This finding was seen as providing important evidence in favour of the premotor theory of Rizzolatti et al. (1994). According to the theory, the trajectory deviations result from the competition between the two potential saccade target locations. In case of a target and an attended distractor two saccades are being programmed in parallel which causes the neural populations corresponding to the stimuli to interfere. In order to saccade successfully to the target, the irrelevant saccade programme has to be inhibited, shifting the resulting initial saccade vector such that curved trajectories appear. A considerable number of studies have since investigated the conditions under which saccade trajectories deviate away or towards locations in the visual field. They have demonstrated that trajectory deviations provide valuable measures of mechanisms of saccadic programming, but also insights into how attention and other cognitive factors interfere with oculomotor programming. For a recent, comprehensive review on the causes and implications of saccade trajectory deviations, see van der Stigchel (2010).

Attention for initiating and maintaining smooth pursuit

Smooth pursuit eye movements are used by humans and non-human primates to stabilize a moving object of interest on or near the fovea, and they help to keep the environment stable during self-motion. The major input to the smooth pursuit system is retinal image motion, i.e. the motion of the target with respect to the eye. When there is only one moving object in the visual field, the smooth pursuit system acts like a visuomotor reflex that matches eye velocity to stimulus velocity. However, when there is more than one moving stimulus present, primates can easily select which target to track. This was already demonstrated in a classic study by Ter Braak and Buis (1970), showing that participants can choose to pursue one out of two interleaved patterns of moving stripes. A considerable number of investigations have since suggested that the selection of targets for pursuit eye movements is related to the allocation of visual attention. Broadly, these studies can be separated into two categories. The first group of studies has addressed the question how targets are selected for the *initiation* of pursuit. Typically, participants (humans or monkeys) in these studies had to choose between two simultaneously presented objects that moved in different directions. The second group of studies has focused on the steady-state phase of pursuit, in which visual feedback about target velocity and position is used to maintain pursuit velocity.

Without any cues about which target to track, the initial response of the smooth pursuit system to two identical targets that move in different directions approximates a vector average of the responses that each target would have evoked alone (Lisberger and Ferrera 1997). However, obligatory vector averaging would prevent participants from being able to precisely follow a stimulus in the presence of competing distractors. Therefore, an obvious function of attention to one specific stimulus could be to overcome the effect of averaging, by weighting the conflicting stimuli according to their behavioural relevance. Indeed, when cues about the target to be tracked are provided, the initial pursuit response is found to be biased towards the cued stimulus, showing that target selection is affected by attention (Ferrera 2000). In one of their experiments, Garbutt and Lisberger (2006) pre-cued human subjects about the direction of motion of the target they would have to track while a distractor was moving in a different direction. This created a strong bias in the initial open-loop phase of the pursuit response to track the cued stimulus, demonstrating that target choice in smooth pursuit can be based on stimulus features such as motion direction. In a recent study, Souto and Kerzel (2011) used a dual-task paradigm in which human observers were explicitly asked to track a designated pursuit target moving in one direction while they had to make a perceptual judgement on a perceptual target moving in the opposite direction. The perceptual target was briefly presented before the eye started to move, i.e. during pursuit initiation, and the priority assigned to the perceptual and to the pursuit task was varied by instruction. The results showed that pursuit performance was traded for perceptual performance. In particular, when priority was given to the perceptual task, the pursuit latencies were strongly delayed, and participants frequently pursued the perceptual target. Taken together, these studies demonstrate that when an oculomotor choice has to be made during pursuit initiation, successful pursuit of the designated stimulus depends on attentional selection of the target.

Attention also plays an important role during pursuit maintenance. For instance, ongoing attention-demanding secondary tasks have been shown to impair pursuit (Hutton and Tegally 2005). Khurana and Kowler (1987) demonstrated in a visual search task that targets were found more quickly when they were among the pursuit stimuli than among the background stimuli, and suggested that smooth pursuit eye movements and perception share the same selective mechanism. Kerzel et al. (2008) showed that the mere presence of a (task-irrelevant) distractor has only minor influence on ongoing pursuit, but it strongly affects pursuit once it is attended and its motion conflicts with that of the target motion. Along similar lines, Spering et al. (2006) made participants follow a continuously moving stimulus. At a particular point during pursuit, a distractor stimulus split off from the moving target and moved in a different, unpredictable direction. Results yield strong interference effects of the distractor, as reflected in a slowing down and a vertical deviation of ocular pursuit shortly after distractor appearance. However, this vector averaging of target and distractor motion was reduced if participants had advance knowledge of the to-be-selected target, suggesting that top-down signals can modulate vector averaging.

While the previously described studies have looked at the effects of attentional manipulations on smooth pursuit parameters, a number of recent investigations have tried to determine the spatial distribution of attention during pursuit directly, by measuring perceptual discrimination performance or reaction times for stimuli presented at various locations around the pursued target. Where precisely in space is attention when moving objects are being tracked? Ocular pursuit has predictive components, which may require attention to anticipate the trajectory of stimulus motion and to focus ahead of the moving target. In an early study on this issue, van Donkelaar and Drew (2002) measured manual reaction times to probe onsets and indeed found that reaction times were lower to probes shortly ahead of the pursuit target, as compared to probes presented in the opposite direction or further ahead. This is well in line with a recent study by Khan et al. (2010) who used both saccadic and manual reaction times to flashed stimuli as measures of attentional allocation. These stimuli could be presented at various locations in two-dimensional space while participants were pursuing the moving target. The authors found that both saccadic and manual reaction times were shorter in the entire half of the visual field ahead of pursuit as compared to behind pursuit, and propose that attention is by default 'broadly' allocated ahead the line of sight during smooth pursuit eye movements. However, this conclusion is in seeming conflict with the results of another recent study which used perceptual discrimination as a measure of attention allocation (Lovejoy et al. 2009). These authors adopted a discrimination paradigm similar to Deubel and Schneider (1996). Participants tracked a horizontal string of characters that briefly changed into distractors and a critical character ('E' or '3') which had to be reported in a 2AFC task. Discrimination performance as determined for the various locations at or around the pursuit target suggested that the focus of attention was centred on the tracked target, without appreciable lead or lag. It is as yet unclear why these different experimental paradigms yield partly conflicting results. Khan et al. (2010) speculate that the differences may be explained by different task demands: while the mere pursuing of a single target may not require much attention and hence attention can be deployed ahead, challenging tasks such as those in the Lovejoy et al. study may require more attention at the pursuit target. Obviously, further studies are necessary to clarify this issue.

To track moving targets, primates use a combination of smooth pursuit and saccadic eye movements. So, is the attention system for pursuit target selection the same as that for the selection of saccade targets? A number of investigations have suggested that this may indeed be the case. In particular, Krauzlis and colleagues have provided strong behavioural and physiological evidence for an attention-related target selection mechanism that is shared between saccades and smooth pursuit (e.g. Krauzlis 2004; Liston and Krauzlis 2003, 2005; Madelain et al. 2005). A recent study (Case and Ferrera 2007) presented monkeys with two moving targets and a task that gave them a high degree of flexibility to pursue one target and then saccade to the other. Yet this separation of saccade and pursuit target selection rarely occurred. On most occasions, the saccade was directed to the target that was selected for initial pursuit, and smooth pursuit was driven, before and after the saccade, by the target of the saccade. The authors propose a model in which a shared target selection signal is simultaneously available to both the saccade and the pursuit system, guiding the interplay between both systems.

In summary, similar to the case for saccadic eye movements, ocular smooth pursuit and visual attention are closely intertwined. Attention is necessary to select to-be-pursued targets out of competing stimuli. When a target is selected for pursuit, attention is deployed to this stimulus, enhancing perceptual processing at the target location. On the other hand, distracting attention away from the pursuit target deteriorates smooth pursuit.

ATTENTION AND MANUAL REACHING

In contrast to the abundant research on the coupling between attention and eye movements, considerably less experimental work has been done on attention in manual actions such as reaching. Among the pioneers were Tipper and colleagues (e.g. Tipper et al. 1992, 1998). In their seminal research on 'negative priming', they investigated the role of visual attention for manual reaching in an interference paradigm. Participants reached, as quickly as possible, from a starting position to one of nine locations cued by a red target light, while they ignored a yellow distractor button that appeared simultaneously with the target. The task-irrelevant distractors led to a marked slowing of reaction times to initiate the pointing movement when they were presented near the hand or between the start and the target location of the movement, regardless of movement direction. Also, distractors beyond the target location did not influence the response latency. It is important to note that these configuration-dependent effects on attention did not occur when verbal responses were required instead of manual pointing, which emphasizes the action-specificity of the effect. Tipper et al. (1992) argued that their findings reflect 'action-centred attention', because the locations close to the effector and the movement goal were most relevant for the amount of interference.

The first direct indication for the spatially selective allocation of perceptual resources to reaching goals was provided by Deubel et al. (1998). They used a paradigm similar to Deubel and Schneider (1996). Participants were cued to point with the right index finger to one particular object in an array of objects arranged horizontally, left and right of a central fixation. Before movement onset, a discrimination probe was briefly presented among the distractors. The results showed that when the probe was presented at the location to where a movement had been programmed, discrimination performance was considerably better than when it was presented at one of the other, movement-irrelevant locations. Even when the probe was presented at a predictable location on each trial, perceptual performance was superior when the pointing movement was made to the object containing the probe rather than when it was made to any other object. Qualitatively, the results were amazingly similar to those found previously for saccadic eye movements in the analogous paradigm (Deubel and Schneider 1996). Deubel et al. (1998) took these findings as evidence that attention shifts to the movement goal before the onset of the reach movement, just as it does before saccades. Again, this coupling between movement planning and attention seems to be obligatory: participants can hardly attend away from the goal location to the probe location, even if this location is predictable. Several follow-up studies have since confirmed the close coupling between reach planning and selective attention, both in behavioural studies (Baldauf et al. 2006) and in electrophysiological investigations (e.g. Eimer et al. 2005, 2006; Baldauf and Deubel, 2009; Gherri and Eimer 2010).

While these findings demonstrate that action and attention are coupled also for the case of manual pointing, they do not specify whether the selective processing occurs at the *location* to which the reach is directed, or whether attentional selection occurs for the *object* to which the action is made. This question was addressed by Linnell et al. (2005) who showed that object-based attention that occurs under a simple viewing condition is disrupted by the planning of a reaching movement to a part of the object, leading to a single, location-specific focus of attention at the reach target. This suggests that the planning of a goal-directed action can modulate object-based attention, emphasizing the selection of spatial locations at the expense of object-based selection.

ATTENTION AND GRASPING

Visuomotor processing for the control of grasping is certainly more challenging than that for reaching. It is not just the transport of the hand to an appropriate location that has to be controlled, but also the hand orientation when approaching the object, as well as hand aperture and placement of individual fingers on the object. Moreover, the grasp forces applied initially to the object anticipate the weight of the object. Visual attention has turned out to be an important factor also for this type of motor action.

Despite the obvious importance of grasping for primates to interact with their environment, relatively few investigations have studied selective processing during grasp preparation. The majority of these studies have looked at *overt* attention during grasping and manipulating objects. Johansson and colleagues were among the first to thoroughly study eye fixation behaviour during grasping (Johansson et al. 2001). Participants were asked to grasp a bar and use it to press a target switch. Additionally, on some occasions, obstacles had to be avoided. The results revealed that people always looked at the positions at with they were about to make contact, such as the grasp location of the bar and the target switch. Interestingly, they also frequently fixated locations they had to avoid, such as the obstacles. This anticipatory behaviour of eye gaze is well in line with studies by Mary Hayhoe and Michael Land on gaze behaviour in natural tasks such as making tea and sandwiches (e.g. Hayhoe 2000; Land and Hayhoe 2001). In striking demonstrations, they showed that people prepare their hand movements several steps ahead by means of look-ahead fixations to the action-relevant items. A particularly interesting study in this context was recently presented by Brouwer et al. (2009) who studied participants' fixation locations when they were about to grasp flat shapes. The objects were arranged such that the contact positions of index finger and thumb were both visible. Brouwer at al. found that the initial saccade directed from a peripheral location to the object aimed at its centre of gravity, but later saccades tended to shift gaze location more towards the location where the index finger would make contact with the object. This contrasted with a no-grasping control condition where the gaze stayed close to the object's centre of gravity. These findings suggest that during grasping, fixation strategies are modulated by the intended action; overt selection thus supports the selective processing of the information that is critical for the grasp, such as the future contact locations of the fingers.

The first systematic study on the role of *covert* attention in grasping was performed by Castiello (1996). In one of his experiments, subjects had to grasp an apple as their primary task. On some occasions, a secondary, attention-demanding task was required that involved the observation of another object (either another apple or a small berry). Castiello reported specific interference effects of the secondary task on the kinematics of the grasping movement. For example, when the distractor was the small berry, the maximum aperture of the grasping hand was smaller than in trials with larger or without distractor. This suggests that otherwise task-irrelevant spatial parameters of attended objects are automatically integrated into the kinematic properties of the resulting grasp.

Schiegg et al. (2003) studied the spatial allocation of attention during grasp preparation directly, in a perceptual discrimination paradigm. Participants were asked to grasp a wooden, cross-like object with either the right or the left hand. When the right hand was used, the thumb aimed at the lower left branch end of the object, and the index finger aimed at the upper right end. When the left hand was used, upper left end and lower right end were touched by index finger and thumb. During preparation of the grasp, visual probe stimuli ('E' or '3') were briefly presented among distractors, close to the to-be-grasped object. The results revealed superior perceptual performance in those cases where the discrimination stimuli were presented at one of the locations to which thumb or index finger were aimed in the actual trial, as compared to the action-irrelevant locations. Moreover, even when participants were informed about the location at which the discrimination stimulus would appear, they could hardly attend to that location if they had to prepare a grasp directed to other areas of the very same object. This was taken as evidence that the coupling of grasp preparation and attention allocation is obligatory. Just as the previously discussed results for manual pointing, these findings suggest that attention allocation is a necessary element of grasp planning, and likely related to the spatial selection of grasp points.

Visual attention is also involved in the control of the kinematics of the manipulation component, i.e. of the opening and closing of the hand to be appropriate for the object size. Hesse and Deubel (2011) recently asked whether and how a secondary task that withdraws attentional resources from the to-be-grasped object would interfere with grasp preparation and execution. Participants had to detect a target digit in a rapid serial visual presentation of digits while they performed a grasping movement to a spatially separate object. As expected from findings as discussed above, participants showed a considerable drop of perceptual performance in the dual-task situation, as compared to an observation-only condition. More importantly, however, the concurrent perceptual task also resulted in a less efficient adaptation of grip aperture to the size of the to-be-grasped object in an early phase of the movement, while movement time and maximum grip aperture were unaffected. These findings demonstrate that there are prominent dual-task costs when a grasping movement and an attention-demanding perceptual task are performed together: When a concurrent grasping task is required, attentional resources are withdrawn from the perceptual discrimination task. Conversely, when attentional resources are allocated to the perceptual task, efficiency of the grasping movement suffers. This shows that in grasping, beyond the mere selection of grasp locations, visual attention is needed for a precise adjustment of the hand aperture to object size when approaching the object.

Other research related to grasping has addressed the question whether planning goal-directed actions also engage *feature-based* attentional mechanisms. Craighero et al. (1999) demonstrated that the preparation to grasp a bar of a certain orientation facilitated perceptual processing of bars of the same orientation. In an elegant study, Bekkering and Neggers (2002) investigated the effect of action intentions on overt attention. Participants searched for targets with a defined orientation and colour among a set of distractor objects. The task was either to point to or to grasp the target. The results showed that participants made more fixations on objects that shared their orientation with the search target, but, importantly, this was more pronounced before they initiated grasping responses than before pointing. Thus, the required action affected how perceptual features were 'weighted' for attention; object orientation being relevant for grasping was weighted more before grasping than before pointing. Along a similar line, Fischer and Hoellen (2004) compared visual selectivity related to simple finger lifting, pointing, and grasping in a reaction time task. They found that reaction times and movement times showed more space-based attention for pointing than for finger lifting, and more object-based attention for grasping than for pointing. Recently, Gutteling et al. (2011) used a change detection task in which participants were asked either to grasp or point to a bar that could slightly change its orientation during the preparation of the action. Results showed increased sensitivity to orientation changes when the bar had to be grasped, as compared to pointing. In contrast, when the change involved luminance, a feature not relevant for grasping, no sensitivity differences were observed. Taken together, these intriguing findings support the view that the selectivity for visual features during action preparation is tuned to specific motor intentions, enhancing the processing of those visual features that are important for the planning of the movement.

Attentional Landscapes for the Preparation of Goal-directed Actions

Obviously, effectors like the eye or the hand can only be directed to one object at a time. The studies discussed previously have accordingly looked at how attention is involved in goal-directed movements that are directed to single objects. However, many goal-directed actions that we plan and perform in natural contexts are more complex in the sense that their preparation requires us to consider more than just a single item or location. For example, when we intend to open a bottle of beer we may first take the opener and only then move on to grasp the bottle. The question arises whether the covert, attention-mediated selection of the movement goals also follows this sequential regime, such that the second movement target (the bottle) would only be selected after the completion of the first movement (picking up the opener). Alternatively, the selection of the second movement target may have begun before the first movement started, or both movement targets may even have been selected in parallel. Likewise, when we grasp an object with two or more fingers, the precise locations where the fingers will touch the object are of relevance for the grasp and may all be selected even before the onset of the movement. Finally, goal-directed actions such as reaching and grasping in natural scenes often require avoiding obstacles. At some point in time during movement preparation, obstacle position and spatial spread-out have to be computed in order to guide the hand effectively around it. Recent investigations have only begun to study the distribution of attention in these more complex situations, with a number of surprising findings. They seem to suggest that action-related attention should be conceptualized as a complex spatiotemporal distribution of attentional resources, reflecting the requirements of the planned motor task.

When actions are planned that consist of a rapid sequence of several movement segments, the processing of future movement goals already starts before the onset of the initial movement. This was indicated already in a number of earlier studies that found effects of the length of the planned sequence on the reaction time of the initial movement, for manual action sequences (Henry and Rogers 1960) as well as for sequences of saccades (Inhoff 1986; Zingale and Kowler 1987). Lajoie and Franks (1997) studied the influence of task complexity on aiming tasks in which participants made sequential manual movements to two circular targets and found that the kinematics of the initial movement segment depended on the difficulty of the second segment. Ricker et al. (1999) also asked participants to make fast sequential aiming movements to two targets. They reported that when the size of the second target increased, peak velocity of the initial movement became higher. All this evidence suggested that the planning of the second movement occurred already before or during the execution of the initial movement, and accordingly implied that more than one target may be attended during the initial movement planning.

Direct evidence for this conjecture came from later dual-task studies in which participants were required to plan sequences of multiple saccades. Godijn and Theeuwes (2003) studied attention in sequences of two speeded saccades to designated targets. In one of their experiments, a circular array of eight grey discs was initially presented. Six of the discs then turned red, and the subject was asked to perform a sequence of saccades to the two remaining grey discs as quickly as possible in a self-determined order. In another experiment the first and the second saccade targets were indicated with central arrow cues. The secondary task was a forced-choice letter discrimination task. The results showed that discrimination performance was superior for letters presented at any of the saccade goals as compared to the no-saccade locations, indicating that during planning of the saccade sequence, attention is allocated to both movement goals. Moreover, using a letter matching task in which two critical letters were presented simultaneously, Godijn and Theeuwes (2003) provided evidence in favour of a parallel model of attentional selection in which attention is deployed to both the first and the second saccade target simultaneously rather than sequentially.

This initial demonstration of multiple foci of attention occurring during the planning of action sequences was corroborated in a study by Baldauf and Deubel (2008a; see also Rolfs et al. 2011), which also used a dual-task paradigm in which characters had to be discriminated along with preparation and execution of the saccade sequence (see Fig. 30.1a, b). Moreover, these authors extended the findings of Godijn and Theeuwes by showing that items located at intermediate positions between the first and the second movement goal are *not* attended, which argues for a spatially highly selective focusing of perceptual capabilities. Finally, the data showed that when triple saccade sequences were prepared, perceptual processing of even the third out of three subsequent movement goals was enhanced. In another series of investigations, Baldauf and colleagues addressed the spatial deployment of attention during the preparation of sequential manual reaching movements (Baldauf et al. 2006;Baldauf and Deubel 2009; Baldauf 2011). The findings were strikingly similar to those for saccade sequences; when rapid sequences of two or three reaches were planned, attention was deployed simultaneously to all movement-relevant goals involved in the intended action, while intermediate locations were not attended. Interestingly, perceptual performance reflected the sequential properties of the planned sequence, being best at the first target location and deteriorating at the second and third movement goal.

However, there are also reports conflicting with the previously described findings. In two studies, Gersch et al. (2004, 2009) asked participants to perform self-initiated saccade sequences along predefined pathways and reported that attention (assessed by an orientation discrimination task) was essentially limited to the goal of the next saccade, but rarely spread beyond to targets further ahead. Methodological differences between the various studies can possibly account for these discrepancies. So, in the tasks by Godijn and Theeuwes (2003) and by Baldauf and colleagues saccades were elicited by a central arrow cue which had to be encoded, interpreted, and converted into a representation of a motor sequence. In contrast, Gersch and colleagues measured attention during the ongoing saccade sequence, without any cueing component. Another important difference concerns the timing requirements of the motor tasks. While in the studies of Gersch et al. participants could perform the saccade sequences at their own, comfortable pace, Godijn and Theeuwes and Baldauf and colleagues instructed the participants to perform the sequence as fast as possible. This may turn out to be critical, given the recent finding of Baldauf (2011) that the allocation of attention to more than just the immediate movement goal critically depends on the speed of the planned movement sequence. For sequential reaching movements, he showed that with longer inter-reach delays less attention is deployed to the subsequent goals. This seems to indicate that

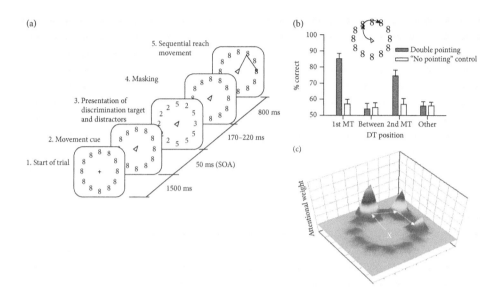

FIGURE 30.1 (a) Dual-task paradigm combining a perceptual letter discrimination task with a sequential reaching task. Participants fixate in the centre of a circular array of distractors (consisting of digital-'8'), with the index finger at the fixation cross. Upon the appearance of the central arrow, they have to perform a fast sequential reaching movement to the indicated item and then further on to next-but-one item in the clockwise direction. Well before the onset of this movement sequence, distractors change into digital-'5' or '2', while at one location the critical discrimination letter (digital-'E' or '3') is briefly presented. This critical display is then masked. (b) Black bars: Discrimination performance in the two-alternative forced choice task is best at the initial target position and lower but still far above chance for the second movement target. Performance is at chance for the position intermediate to both targets, and for the movement-irrelevant locations. Open bars indicate discrimination performance in a control experiment without pointing. Replotted with permission from Baldauf et al. (2006). (c) Schematic illustration of a hypothetical 'attentional landscape', resulting from the planning of a triple reach sequence. The peaks of activation represent the intended target locations of the planned sequence.

future movement goals are attended only if they are integrated into a motor chunk of consecutive movement elements that can be performed quickly and fluently.

Conditions where two *different* effectors are aimed simultaneously at spatially separate locations also seem to involve multiple foci of attention during action preparation. Baldauf and Deubel (2008b) asked participants to execute bimanual reaching movements directed to two separate parts of a wooden object, while attention was assessed with a letter discrimination task. Again, the experimental results revealed that both movement-relevant locations were attended, and they also provided evidence for a parallel rather than sequential allocation of attention to both spatial goals during movement preparation. Along a similar line, Jonikaitis and Deubel (2011) recently measured the time course of attention allocation in tasks that involved simultaneous or asynchronous eye and hand movements to spatially separate locations. Perceptual performance in the perceptual task was significantly better at both the target of the eye saccade and the target of the manual reach, as compared to the movement-irrelevant locations. Also, the results showed that attentional deployment occurred temporally in parallel at both target locations when simultaneous eye–hand movements were required. Finally, under conditions where one of the movements (the saccade) was delayed, attention moved accordingly later to the saccade target during the preparation period, without affecting the attention deployment at the hand movement target. The latter result is particularly striking, since it implies that attentional resources are allocated independently to the targets of eye and hand movements, suggesting separate attention-related target selection mechanisms for these two effector systems. Multiple foci of attention are also evidenced when participants use tools to reach to targets (Collins et al. 2008). Finally, when an object is to be grasped with two fingers, attention again seems to split and focus at the two locations where the fingers will touch the object (Gilster and Deubel 2011).

Taken together, the findings reviewed in the previous paragraph demonstrate that the planning of movements which require accounting for more than just a single target location involves the concurrent deployment of attentional resources to multiple locations, rather than the sequential processing of locations and features by a serial mechanism. Thus, it seems that under such conditions selection-for-action enacts the formation of an 'attentional landscape' (for an illustration, see Fig. 30.1c) which tags all those locations in the visual layout that are relevant for the movement plan (for a recent review on this issue, see Baldauf and Deubel 2010). Within this landscape, each region of activity represents the location of a potential target for attention and action. This is consistent with the view developed from neurophysiological findings that, in order to select objects as action targets, the visuomotor system generates maps that encode the behavioural priority of the relevant stimuli in the scene (e.g. Bisley and Goldberg 2010).

ATTENTION IS AFFECTED BY THE ACTION AFFORDANCES OF OBJECTS

So far, this review has focused mainly on the processes involved in selecting the locations and stimuli for various goal-directed actions, and on how selective processing is influenced by the intended action. However, it seems that attention is also *guided* by the perceived 'action affordances' of objects. In a set of striking experiments, Handy et al. (2003) demonstrated that graspable objects are able to draw visual attention to their location, once the motor affordance of the object is recognized. Participants viewed a line drawing of either a tool or a non-tool. Using the amplitude of P1 of the event-related potentials as a measure of attention allocation, the authors showed that spatial attention was systematically drawn to the tools (given that they appeared in the right hemisphere), but only when tool presentation also activated dorsal premotor and prefrontal regions. This seemed to occur automatically, even if the object was irrelevant to the current behavioural task. Along a similar vein, Symes et al. (2008) recently demonstrated in a change detection task that preparing a certain hand grasp (a whole hand power grasp or a pinch precision grasp) biased selective attention to objects with congruent features. Further evidence for this kind of interaction between attention and action affordances comes from a number of neuropsychological studies (for a recent review, see Humphreys et al. 2010). Taken together, the findings suggest that selective attention is automatically guided to action-relevant locations. The perceptual priority given to the action-relevant aspects of the visual input is probably functionally important for selecting the appropriate actions and the appropriate action parameters to interact with the object.

CONCLUSIONS

Overall, the reviewed research provides much support for theories of visual selection that assume a strong relationship between action preparation and attention. The studies show, for both saccadic and manual movements, that visual attention is necessarily focused on the movement target and can hardly be withdrawn before the onset of the movement. Also, shifts of attention and movement onsets are temporally closely related. This suggests that attention is functional for the selection of spatial locations which constitute action goals. The close relationship between visual selection and action planning is further emphasized under conditions in which several, spatially separate locations have to be considered in the movement plan. Perceptual priorities are then distributed in the visual field according to the requirements of the intended action, reflected in multiple, spatially separate foci of attention. However, the intended action not only determines *where* perceptual resources are allocated, but also *what* is selected. Activation of an object-specific motor programme (like a grasp to an oriented bar) has strong influence on how different object properties are weighted in this selection. That is, movement intentions guide visual selection by giving priority to the visual processing of those visual features and object parts that are relevant for the intended action.

REFERENCES

Allport, D. A. (1987). Selection for action: Some behavioral and neurophysiological considerations of attention and action. In H. Heuer and A. F. Sanders (eds.), *Perspectives on Perception and Action* (pp. 395–419). Hillsdale, N.J.: Lawrence Erlbaum Associates.

Baldauf, D. (2011). Chunking movements into sequence: The visual pre-selection of subsequent goals. *Neuropsychologia* 49(5): 1383–1387.

Baldauf, D. and Deubel, H. (2008a). Properties of attentional selection during the preparation of sequential saccades. *Experimental Brain Research* 184(3): 411–425.

Baldauf, D. and Deubel, H. (2008b). Visual attention during the preparation of bimanual movements. *Vision Research* 48(4): 549–563.

Baldauf, D. and Deubel, H. (2009). Attentional selection of multiple goal positions before rapid hand movement sequences: An event-related potential study. *Journal of Cognitive Neuroscience* 21(1): 18–29.

Baldauf, D. and Deubel, H. (2010). Attentional landscapes in reaching and grasping. *Vision Research* 50(11): 999–1013.

Baldauf, D., Wolf, M., and Deubel, H. (2006). Deployment of visual attention before sequences of goal-directed hand movements. *Vision Research* 46(26): 4355–4374.

Bekkering, H. and Neggers, S. F. W. (2002). Visual search is modulated by action intentions. *Psychological Science* 13(4): 370–374.

Belopolsky, A. V. and Theeuwes, J. (2009). When are attention and saccade preparation dissociated? *Psychological Science* 20(11): 1340–1347.

Bisley, J. W. and Goldberg, M. E. (2003). Neuronal activity in the lateral intraparietal area and spatial attention. *Science* 299: 81–86.

Bisley J. W. and Goldberg M. E. (2010). Attention, intention, and priority in the parietal lobe. *Annual Review of Neuroscience* 33: 1–21. doi: 10.1146/annurev-neuro-060909-152823.

Broadbent, D. E. (1958). *Perception and Communication*. New York: Pergamon.

Brouwer, A. M., Franz, V. H., and Gegenfurtner, K. R. (2009). Differences in fixations between grasping and viewing objects. *Journal of Vision* 9(1): 18.1–24.

Bundesen, C. (1990). A theory of visual attention. *Psychological Review* 97(4): 523–547.

Case, G. R. and Ferrera, V. P. (2007). Coordination of smooth pursuit and saccade target selection in monkeys. *Journal of Neurophysiology* 98(4): 2206–2214.

Castet, E., Jeanjean, S., Montagnini, A., and Masson, G. M. (2006). Dynamics of attentional deployment during saccadic programming. *Journal of Vision* 6(3): 196–212.

Castiello, U. (1996). Grasping a fruit: Selection for action. *Journal of Experimental Psychology: Human Perception and Performance* 22(3): 582–603.

Cisek, P. (2007). Cortical mechanisms of action selection: The affordance competition hypothesis. *Philosophical Transactions of the Royal Society B: Biological Sciences* 362(1485): 1585–1599.

Collins, T., Schicke, T., and Roder, B. (2008). Action goal selection and motor planning can be dissociated by tool use. *Cognition* 109(3): 363–371.

Craighero, L., Fadiga, L., Rizzolatti, G., and Umiltà, C. (1999). Action for perception: A motor-visual attentional effect. *Journal of Experimental Psychology: Human Perception and Performance* 25(6): 1673–1692.

Desimone, R. and Duncan, J. (1995). Neural mechanisms of selective visual-attention. *Annual Review of Neuroscience* 18: 193–222.

Deubel, H. (2008). The time course of presaccadic attention shifts. *Psychological Research* 72(6): 630–640.

Deubel, H. and Schneider, W. X. (1996). Saccade target selection and object recognition: Evidence for a common attentional mechanism. *Vision Research* 36(12): 1827–1837.

Deubel, H. and Schneider, W. X. (2003). Delayed saccades, but not delayed manual aiming movements, require visual attention shifts. *Annals of the New York Academy of Sciences* 1004: 289–296.

Deubel, H., Schneider, W. X., and Paprotta, I. (1998). Selective dorsal and ventral processing: Evidence for a common attentional mechanism in reaching and perception. *Visual Cognition* 5(1–2): 81–107.

Doré-Mazars, K., Pouget, P., and Beauvillain, C. (2004). Attentional selection during preparation of eye movements. *Psychological Research* 69(1–2): 67–76.

Duncan, J. (2006). EPS Mid-Career Award 2004—Brain mechanisms of attention. *Quarterly Journal of Experimental Psychology* 59(1): 2–27.

Eimer, M., Forster, B., Van Velzen, J., and Prabhu, G. (2005). Covert manual response preparation triggers attentional shifts: ERP evidence for the premotor theory of attention. *Neuropsychologia* 43(6): 957–966.

Eimer, M., Van Velzen, J., Gherri, E., and Press, C. (2006). Manual response preparation and saccade programming are linked to attention shifts: ERP evidence for covert attentional orienting and spatially specific modulations of visual processing. *Brain Research* 1105: 7–19.

Ferrera, V. P. (2000). Task-dependent modulation of the sensorimotor transformation for smooth pursuit eye movements. *Journal of Neurophysiology* 84(6): 2725–2738.

Filali-Sadouk, N., Castet, E., Olivier, E., and Zenon, A. (2010). Similar effect of cueing conditions on attentional and saccadic temporal dynamics. *Journal of Vision* 10(4): 21.1–13.

Fischer, M. H. and Hoellen, N. (2004). Space- and object-based attention depend on motor intention. *Journal of General Psychology* 131(4): 365–377.

Garbutt, S. and Lisberger, S. G. (2006). Directional cuing of target choice in human smooth pursuit eye movements. *Journal of Neuroscience* 26(48): 12479–12486.

Gersch, T. M., Kowler, E., and Dosher, B. (2004). Dynamic allocation of visual attention during the execution of sequences of saccades. *Vision Research* 44(12): 1469–1483.

Gersch, T. M., Kowler, E., Schnitzer, B. S., and Dosher, B. A. (2009). Attention during sequences of saccades along marked and memorized paths. *Vision Research* 49(10): 1256–1266.

Gherri, E. and Eimer, M. (2010). Manual response preparation disrupts spatial attention: An electrophysiological investigation of links between action and attention. *Neuropsychologia* 48(4): 961–969.

Gilster, R. and Deubel, H. (2011). Divided attention to grasp-relevant locations. *Perception* 40 (Suppl.): 12. doi: 10.1068/v110317.

Godijn, R. and Pratt, J. (2002). Endogenous saccades are preceded by shifts of visual attention: Evidence from cross-saccadic priming effects. *Acta Psychologica (Amsterdam)* 110(1): 83–102.

Godijn, R. and Theeuwes, J. (2003). Parallel allocation of attention prior to the execution of saccade sequences. *Journal of Experimental Psychology: Human Perception and Performance* 29(5): 882–896.

Gutteling, T. P., Kenemans, J. L., and Neggers, S. F. W. (2011). Grasping preparation enhances orientation change detection. *PLoS One* 6(3). doi: 10.1371/journal.pone.0017675.

Handy, T. C., Grafton, S. T., Shroff, N. M., Ketay, S., and Gazzaniga, M. S. (2003). Graspable objects grab attention when the potential for action is recognized. *Nature Neuroscience* 6(4): 421–427.

Hayhoe, M. (2000). Vision using routines: A functional account of vision. *Visual Cognition* 7(1–3): 43–64.

Henry, F. M. and Rogers, D. E. (1960). Increased response latency for complicated movements and a 'memory drum' theory of neuromotor action. *Research Quarterly* 31: 448–458.

Hesse, C. and Deubel, H. (2011). Efficient grasping requires attentional resources. *Vision Research* 51(11): 1223–1231.

Hoffman, J. E. and Subramaniam, B. (1995). The role of visual attention in saccadic eye movements. *Perception & Psychophysics* 57(6): 787–795.

Huestegge, L. (2011). The role of saccades in multitasking: Towards an output-related view of eye movements. *Psychological Research* 75(6): 452–465.

Humphreys, G. W., Yoon, E. Y., Kumar, S., Lestou, V., Kitadono, K., Roberts, K. L., and Riddoch, M. J. (2010). The interaction of attention and action: From seeing action to acting on perception. *British Journal of Psychology* 101(2): 185–206.

Hunt, A. R. and Kingstone, A. (2003a). Covert and overt voluntary attention: Linked or independent? *Cognitive Brain Research* 18(1): 102–105.

Hunt, A. R. and Kingstone, A. (2003b). Inhibition of return: Dissociating attentional and oculomotor components. *Journal of Experimental Psychology: Human Perception and Performance* 29(5): 1068–1074.

Hutton, S. B. and Tegally, D. (2005). The effects of dividing attention on smooth pursuit eye tracking. *Experimental Brain Research* 163(3): 306–313.

Inhoff, A. W. (1986). Attentional orienting precedes conscious identification. *Behavioral and Brain Sciences* 9(1): 35–35.

Johansson, R. S., Westling, G. R., Backstrom, A., and Flanagan, J. R. (2001). Eye–hand coordination in object manipulation. *Journal of Neuroscience* 21(17): 6917–6932.

Jonikaitis, D. and Deubel, H. (2011). Independent allocation of attention to eye and hand targets in coordinated eye–hand movements. *Psychological Science* 22(3): 339–347.

Jonikaitis, D., Schubert, T., and Deubel, H. (2010). Preparing coordinated eye and hand movements: Dual-task costs are not attentional. *Journal of Vision* 10(14): 23. doi: 10.1167/10.14.23.

Juravle, G. and Deubel, H. (2009). Action preparation enhances the processing of tactile targets. *Experimental Brain Research* 198(2–3): 301–311.

Kerzel, D., Souto, D., and Ziegler, N. E. (2008). Effects of attention shifts to stationary objects during steady-state smooth pursuit eye movements. *Vision Research* 48(7): 958–969.

Khan, A. Z., Lefevre, P., Heinen, S. J., and Blohm, G. (2010). The default allocation of attention is broadly ahead of smooth pursuit. *Journal of Vision* 10(13): 7. doi: 10.1167/10.13.7.

Khurana, B. and Kowler, E. (1987). Shared attentional control of smooth eye-movement and perception. *Vision Research* 27(9): 1603–1618.

Klein, R. (1980). Does oculomotor readiness mediate cognitive control of visual attention? In R. Nickerson (ed.), *Attention and Performance* (vol. 8, pp. 259–276). Hillsdale, N.J.: Lawrence Erlbaum Associates.

Kowler, E., Anderson, E., Dosher, B., and Blaser, E. (1995). The role of attention in the programming of saccades. *Vision Research* 35(13): 1897–1916.

Krauzlis, R. J. (2004). Recasting the smooth pursuit eye movement system. *Journal of Neurophysiology* 91(2): 591–603.

LaBerge, D. and Brown, V. (1989). Theory of attentional operations in shape identification. *Psychological Review* 96(1): 101–124.

Lajoie, J. M. and Franks, I. M. (1997). Response programming as a function of accuracy and complexity: Evidence from latency and kinematic measures. *Human Movement Science* 16(4): 485–505.

Land, M. F. and Hayhoe, M. (2001). In what ways do eye movements contribute to everyday activities? *Vision Research* 41(25–26): 3559–3565.

Linnell, K. J., Humphreys, G. W., McIntyre, D. B., Laitinen, S., and Wing, A. M. (2005). Action modulates object-based selection. *Vision Research* 45(17): 2268–2286.

Lisberger, S. G. and Ferrera, V. P. (1997). Vector averaging for smooth pursuit eye movements initiated by two moving targets in monkeys. *Journal of Neuroscience* 17(19): 7490–7502.

Liston, D. and Krauzlis, R. J. (2003). Shared response preparation for pursuit and saccadic eye movements. *Journal of Neuroscience* 23(36): 11305–11314.

Liston, D. and Krauzlis, R. J. (2005). Shared decision signal explains performance and timing of pursuit and saccadic eye movements. *Journal of Vision* 5(9): 678–689.

Lovejoy, L. P., Fowler, G. A., and Krauzlis, R. J. (2009). Spatial allocation of attention during smooth pursuit eye movements. *Vision Research* 49(10): 1275–1285.

McPeek, R. M., Maljkovic, V., and Nakayama, K. (1999). Saccades require focal attention and are facilitated by a short-term memory system. *Vision Research* 39(8): 1555–1566.

Madelain, L., Krauzlis, R. J., and Wallman, J. (2005). Spatial deployment of attention influences both saccadic and pursuit tracking. *Vision Research* 45(20): 2685–2703.

Mokler, A. and Fischer, B. (1999). The recognition and correction of involuntary prosaccades in an antisaccade task. *Experimental Brain Research* 125(4): 511–516.

Mokler, A. and Deubel, H. (2000). Unattended saccades can be executed without presaccadic attention shifts. *Perception* 29 (Suppl.): 54.

Montagnini, A. and Castet, E. (2007). Spatiotemporal dynamics of visual attention during saccade preparation: Independence and coupling between attention and movement planning. *Journal of Vision* 7(14): 8.1–16.

Neumann, O. (1987). Beyond capacity: A functional view of attention. In H. Heuer and A. F. Sanders (eds.), *Perspectives on Perception and Action* (pp. 361–394). Hillsdale, N.J.: Lawrence Erlbaum Associates.

Pashler, H., Carrier, M., and Hoffman, J. (1993). Saccadic eye movements and dual-task interference. *Quarterly Journal of Experimental Psychology A: Human Experimental Psychology* 46(1): 51–82.

Peterson, M. S., Kramer, A. F., and Irwin, D. E. (2004). Covert shifts of attention precede involuntary eye movements. *Perception & Psychophysics* 66(3): 398–405.

Posner, M. I. (1980). Orienting of attention. *Quarterly Journal of Experimental Psychology* 32(1): 3–25.

Prinzmetal, W., McCool, C., and Park, S. (2005). Attention: Reaction time and accuracy reveal different mechanisms. *Journal of Experimental Psychology: General* 134(1): 73–92.

Remington, R. W. (1980). Attention and saccadic eye movements. *Journal of Experimental Psychology: Human Perception and Performance* 6(4): 726–744.

Ricker, K. L., Elliott, D., Lyons, J., Gauldie, D., Chua, R., and Byblow, W. (1999). The utilization of visual information in the control of rapid sequential aiming movements. *Acta Psychologica* 103(1–2): 103–123.

Rizzolatti, G., Riggio, L., Dascola, I., and Umiltà, C. (1987). Reorienting attention across the horizontal and vertical meridians: Evidence in favor of a premotor theory of attention. *Neuropsychologia* 25(1A): 31–40.

Rizzolatti, G., Riggio, L., and Sheliga, B. M. (1994). Space and selective attention. In C. Umiltà and M. Moscovitch (eds.), *Attention and Performance: Conscious and Nonconscious Information Processing* (vol. 15, pp. 231–265). Cambridge, Mass.: MIT Press.

Rolfs, M., Jonikaitis, D., Deubel, H., and Cavanagh, P. (2011). Predictive remapping of attention across eye movements. *Nature Neuroscience* 14(2): 252–256.

Rorden, C. and Driver, J. (1999). Does auditory attention shift in the direction of an upcoming saccade? *Neuropsychologia* 37(3): 357–377.

Rorden, C., Greene, K., Sasine, G. M., and Baylis, G. C. (2002). Enhanced tactile performance at the destination of an upcoming saccade. *Current Biology* 12(16): 1429–1434.

Schafer, R. J. and Moore, T. (2011). Selective attention from voluntary control of neurons in prefrontal cortex. *Science* 332(6037): 1568–1571.

Schiegg, A., Deubel, H., and Schneider, W. X. (2003). Attentional selection during preparation of prehension movements. *Visual Cognition* 10(4): 409–431.

Schneider, W. X. (1995). VAM: A neuro-cognitive model for attention control of segmentation, object recognition and space-based motor action. *Visual Cognition* 2(2–3): 331–374.

Schneider, W. X. and Deubel, H. (2002). Selection-for-perception and selection-for-spatial-motor-action are coupled by visual attention: A review of recent findings and new evidence from stimulus-driven saccade control. In W. Prinz and B. Hommel (eds.), *Attention and Performance: Common Mechanisms in Perception and Action* (vol. 19, pp. 609–627). Oxford: Oxford University Press.

Sheliga, B. M., Riggio, L., Craighero, L., and Rizzolatti, G. (1995). Spatial attention-determined modifications in saccade trajectories. *NeuroReport* 6(3): 585–588.

Sheliga, B. M., Riggio, L., and Rizzolatti, G. (1994). Orienting of attention and eye-movements. *Experimental Brain Research* 98(3): 507–522.

Shepherd, M., Findlay, J. F., and Hockey, R. J. (1986). The relationship between eye movements and spatial attention. *Quarterly Journal of Experimental Psychology A: Human Experimental Psychology* 38(3): 475–491.

Souto, D. and Kerzel, D. (2011). Attentional constraints on target selection for smooth pursuit eye movements. *Vision Research* 51(1): 13–20.

Spering, M., Gegenfurtner, K. R., and Kerzel, D. (2006). Distractor interference during smooth pursuit eye movements. *Journal of Experimental Psychology: Human Perception and Performance* 32(5): 1136–1154.

Symes, E., Tucker, M., Ellis, R., Vainio, L., and Ottoboni, G. (2008). Grasp preparation improves change detection for congruent objects. *Journal of Experimental Psychology: Human Perception and Performance* 34(4): 854–871.

Ter Braak, J. W. and Buis, C. (1970). Optokinetic nystagmus and attention. *International Journal of Neurology* 8(1): 34–42.

Theeuwes, J., Kramer, A. F., Hahn, S., and Irwin, D. E. (1998). Our eyes do not always go where we want them to go: Capture of the eyes by new objects. *Psychological Science* 9(5): 379–385.

Tibber, M. S., Grant, S., and Morgan, M. J. (2009). Oculomotor responses and visuospatial perceptual judgments compete for common limited resources. *Journal of Vision* 9(12): 21.1–13.

Tipper, S. P., Howard, L. A., and Houghton, G. (1998). Action-based mechanisms of attention. *Philosophical Transactions of the Royal Society of London B: Biological Sciences* 353(1373): 1385–1393.

Tipper, S. P., Lortie, C., and Baylis, G. C. (1992). Selective reaching: Evidence for action-centered attention. *Journal of Experimental Psychology: Human Perception and Performance* 18(4): 891–905.

Ullman, S. (1984). Visual routines. *Cognition* 18(1–3): 97–159.

Van der Stigchel, S. (2010). Recent advances in the study of saccade trajectory deviations. *Vision Research* 50(17): 1619–1627.

Van Donkelaar, P. and Drew, A. S. (2002). The allocation of attention during smooth pursuit eye movements. *Progress in Brain Research* 140: 267–277.

Wilder, J. D., Kowler, E., Schnitzer, B. S., Gersch, T. M., and Dosher, B. A. (2009). Attention during active visual tasks: Counting, pointing, or simply looking. *Vision Research* 49(9): 1017–1031.

Wischnewski, M., Belardinelli, A., and Schneider, W. X. (2010). Where to look next? Combining static and dynamic proto-objects in a TVA-based model of visual attention. *Cognitive Computation* 2: 326–343.

Zingale, C. M. and Kowler, E. (1987). Planning sequences of saccades. *Vision Research* 27(8): 1327–1341.

PART F

ATTENTION-RELATED DISORDERS

CHAPTER 31

DEVELOPMENTAL DISORDERS: A WINDOW ONTO ATTENTION DYNAMICS

GAIA SCERIF AND RACHEL WU

INTRODUCTION: WHY STUDY ATTENTION DISORDERS OVER DEVELOPMENT?

NEUROCOGNITIVE models of attentional processes have long been informed by the breakdown of those functions following cases of brain damage acquired in adulthood, as in the case of hemispatial neglect and Balint's syndrome (e.g. Egly, Driver, and Rafal 1994; Husain, Shapiro, Martin, and Kennard 1997; Ladavas, Petronio, and Umiltá 1990; Mesulam 1981; Mort et al. 2003; Robertson, Treisman, Friedman-Hill, and Grabowecky 1997; Vallar and Perani 1986). Are developmental disorders with clearly defined genetic or systems neuroscience abnormalities equally useful for attention researchers? At the *cognitive level*, given that attention modulates interactions with the environment, memory, and learning, studying attention disorders in adults is a window on to the consequences of poor attention on these other cognitive processes. In a complementary fashion, studying developmental disorders allows us to understand how attention and these processes interact to produce cascading effects across developmental time. At a *systems neuroscience level*, developmental disorders with effects on attention can reveal the systems and networks necessary to attain adults' efficient attentional processes. At the level of *cellular neuroscience and functional genomics*, disorders whose genetic aetiology is known may provide inroads into cellular pathways and protein networks leading to attentional deficits across development.

The promise of insights into attention offered by neurodevelopmental disorders comes precisely from the differences from cases of adult brain damage. Distinctions between the two have been discussed extensively outside of the field of attention (Bishop 1997; Karmiloff-Smith 1998; Scerif and Karmiloff-Smith 2005). First and foremost, developmental disorders affect neurocognitive functioning before the adult end-state is attained, highlighting the importance of investigating empirically the early developmental trajectories and changing profiles of each condition, rather than assuming a priori that the cognitive profile in adults is representative of earlier abilities (Karmiloff-Smith 1998; Karmiloff-Smith 2007a, 2009; Karmiloff-Smith, Scerif, and Ansari 2003; Karmiloff-Smith, Scerif, and Thomas 2002; Thomas and Karmiloff-Smith 2002). Furthermore, unlike adult neuropsychological cases, developmental disorders are very often characterized not just by dissociations of function, but also by striking associations of impairments over time (Bishop 1997, 2006; Karmiloff-Smith et al. 2003). In the context of attention research in particular, if attention operates as a set of biases on information processing, learning, and memory, investigating the cascading effects of attention deficits on other processes over developmental time at the cognitive, systems neuroscience, and genetic levels has the potential to uncover a deeper understanding of attentional processes and their role for other developing functions.

Here, we draw from examples of attentional deficits across two classes of developmental disorders: functionally defined and genetically defined conditions. Functionally defined disorders of attention, such as attention deficit/hyperactivity disorder (ADHD), with clear abnormalities in frontostriatal, mesocorticolimbic circuits, and pharmacological response to dopaminergic reuptake inhibitors, have attracted much interest in cognitive neuroscience. Genetically defined disorders associated with attentional deficits have offered complementary information into low-level mechanisms of attention development because of their known genetic origin and relatively well understood impact on molecular and cellular neurophysiology. We focus on two such disorders, fragile X syndrome (FXS) and Williams syndrome (WS), as the high incidence of behavioural hyperactivity and inattention in both groups, combined with distinct neurocognitive attentional profiles from infancy, clearly illustrates that there can be multiple pathways to symptoms of ADHD. Both the functionally and genetically defined disorders paint a complex picture of attentional deficits and their neural correlates over developmental time. We conclude by offering an experimental approach and new data that capitalize upon these complexities. This emerging field studies the interactions between attention and learning in typical development and will allow for a better understanding of atypically developing systems.

FUNCTIONALLY DEFINED ATTENTION DISORDERS: ATTENTION DEFICIT/ HYPERACTIVITY DISORDER

ADHD is one of the most common neurodevelopmental disorders, affecting 3–5% of children worldwide (Faraone, Sergeant, Gillberg, and Biederman 2003; Polanczyk, de

Lima, Horta, Biederman, and Rohde 2007), and is characterized by pervasive behavioural symptoms of hyperactivity, impulsivity, and inattention (DSM-IV, American Psychiatric Association 1994). These difficulties impact everyday functioning from childhood and persist into adulthood for a large proportion of affected individuals (Barkley, Fischer, Smallish, and Fletcher 2002; Biederman 2005; Kessler et al. 2006). Stimulant medications that increase the availability of synaptic dopamine, such as methylphenidate and dexamphetamine, are effective in reducing symptoms for the vast majority of cases (Volkow and Swanson 2003; Volkow, Wang, Fowler, and Ding 2005). Current theories of ADHD explain the core symptoms either in terms of an underlying cognitive deficit (centred on response inhibition and executive dysfunctions) or a motivational style (delay aversion, reward dysfunction, and state regulation hypotheses). Therefore, understanding the mechanisms underpinning ADHD can inform the extent to which behavioural and attentional control are dependent on executive and motivational processes, as well as their independence and interactions. Beyond cognitive models, studying the neural systems involved in ADHD, response to stimulants, and genetics can shed light on the neural bases of attentional processes and their modulation by motivation/reward value at complementary levels of description.

Cognitive underpinnings

One of the leading accounts of the disorder proposes that a fundamental deficit in inhibitory control mechanisms lies at the core of the cognitive symptoms of ADHD (Barkley 1997). However, the finding of executive-inhibitory deficits in ADHD is inconsistent (Kuntsi, Oosterlaan, and Stevenson 2001; Scheres, Oosterlaan, and Sergeant 2001a). Meta-analyses of executive functioning in ADHD questioned the suggestion that the disorder's symptoms arise solely from executive dysfunction (Willcutt, Doyle, Nigg, Faraone, and Pennington 2005). Willcutt et al. (2005) found differences between individuals with ADHD and healthy controls on performance in multiple executive functioning tasks, with the largest effects sizes for response inhibition, vigilance, planning, and working memory. However, effect sizes were smaller than would be expected if the tasks were tapping a major cause of the disorder, as the range of differences between ADHD cases and controls on the executive functioning tasks was much smaller than that for ADHD symptoms. They concluded that while executive functioning weaknesses are significantly associated with ADHD, these deficits are not the single cause of the disorder in all individuals, but rather that executive dysfunction is one of several deficits that comprise the condition. Indeed, only 10% of children in Willcutt et al.'s (2005) meta-analysis showed weakness across all five domains, and 21% of the children with ADHD were unimpaired on all five measures. This heterogeneity is not entirely unexpected, given that the diagnosis of ADHD, defined entirely at the behavioural level, may subsume multiple aetiologic subtypes at the neurocognitive level, of which the group of children with clear executive deficits may be one (Nigg, Willcutt, Doyle, and Sonuga-Barke 2005).

Furthermore, inhibitory deficits on cognitive tasks are typically characterized by a high degree of within-subject variability in performance in ADHD children (Castellanos et al. 2005; Castellanos and Tannock 2002; Leth-Steensen, Elbaz, and Douglas 2000). This fits with the observation that ADHD children perform poorly on boring or monotonous tasks requiring sustained mental effort in situations with low levels of environmental stimulation, but that their performance can be improved by novelty or positive feedback (Luman, Oosterlaan, and Sergeant 2005). In line with these findings, an alternative 'motivational' account of ADHD has emphasized abnormal sensitivity to reward and motivational style (Douglas 1999; Sagvolden, Aase, Zeiner, and Berger 1998; Sagvolden, Johansen, Aase, and Russell 2005; Sonuga-Barke 2002). In one incarnation of this account, executive and motivational deficits are construed as independent. Sonuga-Barke (2002, 2005) proposed a 'dual pathway' model with two distinct sub-types of ADHD reflecting separate executive-inhibitory and motivational systems. In this model, delay aversion and an altered reward gradient is related to dysfunction of mesolimbic dopaminergic pathways, while poor executive-inhibitory control is related to dysfunction of right lateralized cortico-striatal dopaminergic loop. Other accounts of ADHD instead propose that executive deficits are secondary to motivational difficulties. For example, abnormalities of state-regulation, allocation of effort, and cognitive activation in ADHD would underpin cognitive attentional deficits (Sergeant 2000; Sergeant, Geurts, Huijbregts, Scheres, and Oosterlaan 2003). A complementary account of the core symptoms focuses on how deficits in reinforcement learning could drive the development of poor executive control (Sagvolden et al. 2005). Solanto et al. (2001) argued for the relative independence of executive-inhibition and motivational processes by showing that performance on the Stop Signal Task (SST) and Choice-Delay Task were not significantly correlated and predict ADHD better when used in combination than in isolation.

A test of the independence of these pathways is whether inhibitory deficits in ADHD can be improved or even abolished in the presence of motivational incentives. Slusarek, Velling, Bunk, and Eggers (2001) assessed children with ADHD, children with anxiety/depression and conduct or oppositional defiant disorders, and typically developing children, all of whom completed a Stop Signal Task under different levels of extrinsic incentives, provided by points in a game setting. In a high-incentive condition, children with ADHD were able to perform the task as well as other children, suggesting that they require greater external incentives (rewards) to obtain the same level of inhibitory control performance as typically developing children. However, other studies have failed to detect a differential effect of reward on inhibitory performance in ADHD children across a variety of tasks (Scheres, Oosterlaan, and Sergeant 2001b) or suggest independence of executive and motivational inhibitory systems in ADHD (Crone, Jennings, and Van der Molen 2003). The inconsistencies can be at least in part accommodated by the suggestion that task demands are critical in determining task engagement and the salience of reward or inhibitory demands, even for typically developing children (Liddle et al. 2009). This could account for why, under some conditions, children with ADHD are affected by rewards, and under others they are not. In addition, a further dimension that has not been empirically studied in this regard is the extent to which younger individuals with ADHD may be more sensitive to extrinsic motivation compared to older individuals, resulting in mixed or null effects when samples span a broad age range. Investigating the neural bases of the independence and interactions between inhibitory, motivational, and learning deficits has been critical in elucidating their independence and interactions.

Systems neuroscience

ADHD is associated with both functional and structural abnormalities of a distributed right lateralized corticostriatal network implicated in inhibitory control. Early reports of localized structural abnormalities (Filipek et al. 1997; Giedd et al. 1994) have been complemented by large-scale studies of cortical development in children and adolescents with ADHD (Shaw et al. 2007). These suggest a marked delay in ADHD in typical cortical thickness throughout most of the cerebrum, but most prominently in prefrontal regions. Both gross abnormalities and localized differences in cortical thickness, particularly in areas functionally implicated in cognitive control have been replicated across studies of both children and adults with ADHD (Batty et al. 2010; Makris et al. 2007; Seidman et al. 2006, 2011), together with abnormal connectivity in frontal and cerebellar white matter (Liston, Cohen, Teslovich, Levenson, and Casey 2011; Makris et al. 2008). Longitudinal studies of these abnormalities have also highlighted how differences across patients with ADHD in prefrontal cortical thickness predict later clinical outcome (Shaw et al. 2006).

Functional abnormalities of control related circuits are well established in ADHD (Castellanos et al. 1996; Durston et al. 2003; Rubia et al. 1999). For example, fMRI studies using the SST in ADHD adolescents (Rubia et al. 1999) and the Go/No Go task in children with ADHD (Durston et al. 2003) showed reduced activation of inferior prefrontal cortex and caudate nucleus compared to healthy age-matched controls (Rubia et al. 1999), as well as a failure to activate frontostriatal regions in the same manner as typically developing children (Durston et al. 2003). In addition to these localized differences, recent approaches have focused on altered connectivity distributed across cortical and subcortical areas implicated in ADHD (Castellanos et al. 2008; Konrad and Eickhoff 2010), both while performing active tasks (Peterson et al. 2009) and at rest (Fair et al. 2010). Within this framework, ADHD research has highlighted in particular abnormalities in activity of the default mode network (DMN). The DMN is a network of brain regions that is associated with task-irrelevant processes, or 'mind wandering' (Fox et al. 2005; Greicius, Krasnow, Reiss, and Menon 2003). It is active during rest, with activity decreasing when actively engaging in a task. Stronger deactivation is associated with increased task difficulty, and persistent DMN activity during tasks is associated with decreased performance. The hypothesis that DMN activity fails to decrease when individuals with ADHD engage in tasks, interfering with task performance (Sonuga-Barke and Castellanos 2007) has thus far been supported (Liddle et al.

2011; Peterson et al. 2009). For example, Peterson and colleagues found that, when off stimulant medication, children and adolescents with ADHD were unable to suppress default-mode activity to the same degree as control children when performing a Stroop task. In contrast, medication normalized their suppression of DMN, suggesting that stimulant-induced improvements in task engagement could be mediated by a greater ability to suppress mind-wandering.

In addition to functional imaging data, temporal dynamics as revealed by multiple electrophysiological studies suggest that children with ADHD differ from controls at multiple time-points in the information processing cascade leading to the inhibition of a response or when resolving conflict (Brandeis et al. 1998; Dimoska, Johnstone, Barry, and Clarke 2003; Liotti, Pliszka, Perez, Kothmann, and Woldorff 2005; Liotti et al. 2007; Pliszka, Liotti, and Woldorff 2000). Amongst the first event-related potential (ERP) findings in the context of inhibitory control in ADHD, children with ADHD displayed a reduced N2 over the right prefrontal area in tasks requiring response inhibition and executive control (Pliszka et al. 2000). Two other ERP components associated with the Stop Signal also differentiate children with ADHD and controls. In controls, the ERP evoked by the stop signal differs for successful compared to failed inhibitions, with greater amplitude of a positive wave peaking around 320 msec over the anterior medial frontal scalp (P3a). Such success-related P3a activity was significantly reduced in the ADHD group (Liotti et al. 2005; Overtoom et al. 2002). In addition, the error-related negativity (ERN), a sharp negative wave that is present selectively on error trials in choice reaction time experiments, was also markedly reduced in the ADHD group (Liotti et al. 2005). Scalp distributions of the group differences in P3a and ERN are consistent with a reduction of activity of sources in dorsal anterior cingulate cortex, also documented by functional MRI (fMRI) data. These differences have now been extensively replicated and some are long lasting. For example, abnormalities in P3 responses when performing on simple response inhibition tasks persist in adults with ADHD, even when inhibitory performance and other ERP components N2 appear to have normalized (Wiersema, van der Meere, and Roeyers 2005).

Motivated by criticisms of executive dysfunctions as the single core deficit in ADHD (Castellanos, Sonuga-Barke, Milham, and Tannock 2006; Castellanos and Tannock 2002), functional imaging and electrophysiological data have begun to address the extent to which individuals with ADHD differ in their recruitment of reward-related circuitry. These data support an abnormality in circuits normally implicated in the anticipation of rewards, as well as those involved in inhibitory processes (Plichta et al. 2009; Scheres, Milham, Knutson, and Castellanos 2007; Stroehle et al. 2008; Volkow et al. 2010; Volkow et al. 2011). For example, Volkow et al. (2011) found that individual differences in motivation, measured by Achievement scale on the Multidimensional Personality Questionnaire were significantly correlated with D2/D3 receptors in the nucleus accumbens and midbrain, and dopamine transporter availability in the accumbens in ADHD participants, but not in controls. In addition, just as in the context of functional imaging studies of ADHD in general, work on motivation and reward processing in ADHD has gradually shifted from localized areas to networks implicated in the disorder. Tomasi and Volkow (2012) compared functional connectivity of two large samples of children with ADHD and typically developing control children. Children with ADHD had lower connectivity in the regions of the dorsal attention (superior parietal cortex) and default-mode (precuneus) networks and higher connectivity in reward-motivation regions (ventral striatum and orbitofrontal cortex) than control subjects. In ADHD children, the orbitofrontal cortex also had higher connectivity with reward-motivation regions (striatum and anterior cingulate) and lower connectivity with superior parietal cortex. These findings therefore suggest impaired interactions between control and reward pathways in ADHD that might underlie attention and motivation deficits characteristic of the condition.

In addition, electrophysiological markers indicate that the temporal dynamics of cognitive processes are modified by motivational incentives in children with ADHD. Van Meel, Heslenfeld, Oosterlaan, Luman, and Sergeant (2011) used a time production paradigm that required participants to press a button when they thought a one-second interval had elapsed, under three different reinforcement contingency conditions: reward, punishment, or feedback only. In control children, as expected given previous studies, the feedback-related negativity (FRN) was elicited by negative feedback in the reward condition, but by positive feedback in the punishment condition. In contrast, for children with ADHD reward and punishment did not modulate the FRN. Furthermore, ERP markers of executive and inhibitory control are also directly modulated by motivational incentives. Groom et al. (2010) found that, for both children with ADHD and controls, motivational incentives and stimulant medication resulted in increased amplitude of N2 and P3 components of stimulus-locked ERPs in a Go/No Go task. Some of the reported effects are independent of methylphenidate (MPH) treatment, whereas others rely on their interaction, with for example the ERN normalizing to the levels of controls in children with ADHD, but only when on medication, and under high motivational incentives (Groom et al. 2013). Functional and structural effects clearly implicate an imbalance of dopaminergic neuromodulation in ADHD, a suggestion that is supported, but also complicated, by the psychopharmacology and genetics of the disorder.

Psychopharmacology and genetics

The involvement of striatal circuits in ADHD is heavily supported by the fact that MPH, a dopamine reuptake inhibitor, alleviates symptoms of the disorder in the majority of affected cases. Volkow and colleagues demonstrated that therapeutic doses of MPH are linked to increased availability of dopamine in the striatum (Volkow, Fowler, Wang, Ding, and Gatley 2002; Volkow et al. 2001, 2005, 2012). MPH increases the saliency and interest of a task by increasing dopamine levels and the increase in dopamine appears context dependent with greater dopamine release associated with salient tasks (Volkow et al. 2004). This suggests significant interaction between stimulant medication effects and context (e.g. reward contingencies) with stimulants potentially acting to increase the strength of rewards and incentives for ADHD children. Indeed, MPH reduces inhibitory deficits and their neural markers in ADHD seen on the Go/No Go task (Vaidya et al. 1998) and SST (Aron, Dowson, Sahakian, and Robbins 2003). These effects are at least in part dependent on similar circuits to those upon which motivational incentives have an effect: Liddle et al. (2011) showed that MPH treatment and rewards can operate in concert to normalize specific types of functional activity (suppression of DMN) in children and adolescents with ADHD engaged in inhibitory control.

Consistent with the psychopharmacology of the condition, early molecular genetic studies in ADHD patients focused on candidate genes implicated in the efficiency of dopaminergic transmission, as well as serotonergic ones (Faraone et al. 2005; Murphy, Lerner, Rudnick, and Lesch 2004). Dissecting dopamine and serotonin pathways identified seven gene polymorphisms which confer susceptibility to ADHD (*DRD4, DRD5, DAT1 [SLC6A3], DBH, HTT [SLC6A4], HTR1B, and SNAP25*). These associations were based on pooled odds ratios (OR) across at least three studies for each gene. The ORs for these associations were relatively small (1.18–1.46), providing evidence for the idea that genetic vulnerability to ADHD is mediated by many genes of small effect (Faraone et al. 2005). For example, amongst the most consistent findings were the association with polymorphisms in a 40 base pair variable tandem nucleotide repeat in the 3′ untranslated region of the human dopamine transporter (*DAT1*) gene. The dopamine transporter is responsible for reuptake of dopamine from the synapse and is predominantly expressed in the striatum. A particular variant of *DAT*, the 10-repeat allele of *DAT1*, has been associated with increased expression of the transporter (Mill, Asherson, Browes, D'Souza, and Craig 2002) which is consistent with dopaminergic hypofunction in the striatum in ADHD. This is also consistent with a modulatory role of DAT1 on functional brain abnormalities, both in the context of magnetic resonance imaging (Durston et al. 2008) and EEG (Althaus et al. 2010).

However, the role of specific genes in conferring risk for ADHD is by no means simple: variants of *DAT1* also increase the risk of ADHD persisting into adulthood, but intriguingly these variants are not the ones that confer risk in childhood, suggesting the need to think about these relationships developmentally, and that *DAT1* might have a modulatory, rather than causative role in ADHD (Franke et al. 2010). Furthermore, recent work from genome-wide association studies of ADHD has revised considerably perspectives on key genes associated with ADHD (Franke, Neale, and Faraone 2009). Rather than the usual suspects emerging as significantly associated with ADHD risk, as the literature on candidate genes would suggest, genes involved in setting up neurodevelopmental networks for neurite outgrowth seem to be more prominent (Poelmans, Pauls, Buitelaar, and Franke 2011). Furthermore, epigenetic factors also play a role in ADHD risk, modulating any effects of genes such as the candidates discussed above. For example, Thapar and colleagues found that risk for conduct disorder in ADHD is mediated by early adverse factors such as maternal smoking or very low birth weight (Langley et al. 2008).

The cognitive neuroscience of ADHD: Concluding remarks

Despite great advances in understanding the neurocognitive mechanisms underpinning ADHD hyperactivity and inattention in the context of inhibitory control and reward processing, multiple complexities remain. First, although ADHD is a neurodevelopmental disorder, fewer studies focus on understanding the developmental course of the condition from early childhood (Sonuga-Barke, Auerbach, Campbell, Daley, and Thompson 2005; Sonuga-Barke, Dalen, Daley, and Remington 2002), although much recent work focuses on the presentation of ADHD in adults (Kessler et al. 2005, 2006). Research on changes not only in symptomatology, but also in underlying cognitive difficulties over developmental time has lagged behind the work on understanding ADHD at discrete time-points, such as childhood, adolescence, or adulthood.

Much of the research demonstrating the need for a developmental perspective in ADHD focuses on changes or stability in behavioural symptoms over time, and persistence of ADHD diagnosis (Barkley et al. 2002). Indeed, while a large proportion of childhood ADHD sufferers continue to meet diagnostic criteria for ADHD in adulthood, the majority do recover from their ADHD (Biederman et al. 1996a; Kessler et al. 2005). Are these individuals developing compensatory mechanisms that allow them to overcome their cognitive deficits? If so, what are the neurocognitive correlates for these compensatory mechanisms? Longitudinal data from large cohorts of children with ADHD support the notion of change in symptomatology over developmental time, even for children who continue to meet diagnostic criteria for the disorder (Biederman et al. 1996b). Even less studied are the interactions of attentional difficulties in ADHD with other developing domains of cognition, such as social cognition.

Following changes over developmental time is a challenge in the context of a condition like ADHD, as a formal diagnosis is achieved during the school years, but not earlier (see examples of approaches to this question by using 'at-risk' populations, Auerbach et al. 2005). Studying genetic disorders diagnosed much earlier in life and at high risk for inattention and hyperactivity, however, provides a route into early predictors of attention difficulties. We will review two such genetic disorders in the following section.

GENETICALLY DEFINED DISORDERS: MULTIPLE ROUTES TO HIGH RISK OF ADHD

A number of advantages render genetic disorders an ideal platform to enlighten links between genes, brain development, and attentional control. First, unlike functionally defined disorders (e.g. ADHD), they are associated with a single aetiology. Therefore, attention difficulties associated with genetic disorders pose a forward (albeit complex) problem as opposed to an inverse problem with multiple possible causes. Furthermore, given the well-defined genetic underpinnings, neural mechanisms can be and have been investigated though constrained animal models. Systems neuroscience studies can also be further constrained by a clearer understanding of the precise causative factors involved. At a cognitive level, diagnoses from infancy offer the potential to examine developmental trajectories earlier than disorders diagnosed later in childhood. This in turn allows tracing cascading effects of early attentional difficulties onto multiple distinct cognitive outcomes from very early in development (Karmiloff-Smith 2007a), contrasting disorders with distinct aetiologies but similar attentional outcomes (Scerif and Steele 2011) and identifying early precursors of later behavioural manifestations like ADHD (Scerif et al. 2012). The ability to build specific models of the causative dysfunction clarifies relationships across levels of description, from the genetic, to the systems neuroscience and cognitive level.

Here, we focus on two increasingly studied genetic disorders that share all of these advantages, WS and FXS, because of the high incidence of hyperactivity and inattention from very early in childhood. WS has attracted much interest by both geneticists and cognitive neuroscientists despite its relatively low prevalence (1 in 7500; Stromme, Bjornstad, and Ramstad 2002) because of a strikingly uneven cognitive profile, with relative strengths in language, a highly/hyper sociable nature in the context of low IQ, and extremely poor visuo-spatial cognition (see Karmiloff-Smith 2007b; Mervis and John 2010; Meyer-Lindenberg, Mervis, and Berman 2006, for the broader cognitive profile). FXS is the most common cause of genetically inherited learning disability, with a prevalence of 1 in approximately 2400 individuals (Hagerman 2008). Profound attentional and social cognition difficulties, all more severe than expected given the overall low IQ and developmental delay, characterize the cognitive profile of the syndrome (see Cornish, Turk, and Hagerman 2008; Cornish et al. 2004; Hagerman, Ono, and Hagerman 2005, for reviews of the broader cognitive phenotype).

Studies of the attentional profile in WS are rarer than those on other aspects of cognition in the syndrome, but they converge on weaknesses in attentional control over and above what would be expected given low intellectual ability, and a behavioural phenotype that resembles closely that of individuals with ADHD (Rhodes, Riby, Matthews, and Coghill 2011). Indeed, very high rates of inattention and hyperactivity are reported in children and adolescents with WS (Cornish et al. 2012b; Rhodes, Riby, Park, Fraser, and Campbell 2010). Similarly high rates of ADHD are also reported for individuals affected by FXS, both in North America and the UK (Sullivan et al. 2006; Cornish et al. 2012a). Therefore, WS and FXS provide well-defined models in which to study how known genetic modifications impact brain development and are associated with severe attentional difficulties and their potential impact on other cognitive domains. Despite the high shared risk for ADHD, individuals with WS or FXS differ at multiple levels, both in terms of brain functioning, development, and detailed attentional profiles. We explore these levels in the following sections, starting from molecular genetics and psychopharmacology, and moving to the systems neuroscience and cognitive under-pinnings of attention difficulties.

Genetics and psychopharmacology

Williams syndrome results from a heterozygous deletion of approximately 28 genes on chromosome 7 (Donnai and Karmiloff-Smith 2000; Morris 2010). Some of these genes were put forward as drivers of abnormal brain structure and function in individuals with WS. For example, *LIMK1* first was proposed as a key gene associated with the visuo-spatial difficulties in the disorder at the cognitive level, and for the clear abnormalities of pari-etal cortices in WS (Frangiskakis et al. 1996). The unique role of LIMK1 in accounting for these differences, however, has been questioned (Tassabehji et al. 1999) because deletions of *LIMK1* alone are not associated with the WS profile of visuo-spatial difficulties (Gray, Karmiloff-Smith, Funnell, and Tassabehji 2006), suggesting a more complex picture of the mapping between genes in the critical region of chromosome 7 and the WS cognitive pro-file. Recent work on small deletions in the critical region implicated in WS reveals that it is the haploinsufficiency of four specific genes at the telomeric end of the deletion that appears to give rise to more specific vulnerabilities for cognitive functions in WS (Dai et al. 2009).

FXS is caused by the silencing of a single gene on the X chromosome, fragile X men-tal retardation 1, *FMR1*, and, in boys with the condition, near complete absence of its associated protein product, fragile X mental retardation protein, FMRP (Verkerk et al. 1991). FMRP is a key player in translational regulation of activity-dependent changes engendered by metabotropic glutamatergic receptors (Bagni and Greenough 2005; Bear, Huber, and Warren 2004). The causative mutation affects dendritic spine morphology (Bagni and Greenough 2005) and results in cascading effects on the regulation of intrin-sic (D'Hulst et al. 2006) and extrinsic neurotransmitter systems (monoamines, Wang et al. 2008) that are critical to the regulation of frontoparietal and frontostriatal circuits.

Psychopharmacological treatments in both cases bridge these distinct mecha-nisms. In WS, a number of studies suggest responsiveness to MPH treatment (Bawden, MacDonald, and Shea 1997; Green et al. 2012). In FXS treatment has been highly var-ied, but ameliorating the symptoms of hyperactivity and inattention has involved stimu-lant treatment from very early in development (Roberts et al. 2011). At the same time, accumulating knowledge on the glutamatergic and GABA-ergic downstream effects of FMR1 silencing has meant more precise targeting of these mechanisms (D'Hulst and Kooy 2007; McBride et al. 2005).

Systems neuroscience

The functioning of the dorsal stream in WS is compromised (Atkinson and Braddick 2011; Atkinson et al. 2003; Braddick, Atkinson, and Wattam-Bell 2003; Meyer-Lindenberg et al. 2004). In the context of FXS, evidence suggests that FMRP is more strongly expressed in magnocellular than parvocellular neurons of the lateral geniculate nucleus (Kogan et al. 2004), and that this in turn has a differentially greater effect on the functioning and development of the dorsal stream, including parietal cortex (Farzin and Rivera 2010; Farzin, Whitney, Hagerman, and Rivera 2008; Kogan et al. 2004). These findings converge on the suggestion of dorsal stream vulnerability in FXS, just as in WS, and distinct but converging molecular pathways leading to dorsal stream abnormalities (Walter, Mazaika, and Reiss 2009). Frontostriatal dysfunctions have also been replicated for both disorders: Mobbs et al. (2007) found that WS participants demonstrated significantly reduced activity in the striatum, dorsolateral prefrontal, and dorsal anterior cingulate cortices, when required to inhibit responses in a Go/No Go task. Individuals with fragile X syndrome also recruit these circuits to a lesser extent than controls (Hoeft et al. 2007).

Unfortunately, because of difficulties in dealing with the scanning environment, many of these studies only included very high functioning or older participants with either syndrome, rather than representing the full population of affected individuals, with the consequence that at least some of the activation differences between affected individuals and typically developing controls may be targeting compensatory mechanisms. For example, Hoeft et al. (2007) found that adolescents with FXS recruited increased VLPFC activation compared to control groups and this activity was positively correlated with task performance only in FXS. A small number of recent structural imaging studies have instead targeted younger and less able individuals with fragile X syndrome as young as 1–3 years of age (Haas et al. 2009; Hoeft et al. 2010; Hoeft et al. 2008, 2011), illustrating the benefits of a developmental perspective that is currently not available to cognitive neuroscientists working with ADHD because of the later childhood diagnosis.

The temporal dynamics of attentional control in FXS and WS also show abnormalities at multiple time-points in processing. Van der Molen et al. (2012b) assessed men with FXS and age-matched control participants on a standard oddball task in both auditory and visual modalities. N1 and N2b ERP components were significantly enhanced in FXS men to both auditory and visual stimuli, whereas the P3b to auditory stimuli was significantly reduced relative to visual stimuli. These modality differences were also related to a greater number of errors with auditory compared to visual stimuli. Relative weaknesses in the auditory modality also emerged in a study of auditory change detection (Van der Molen et al. 2012a). N1 and P2, sensory evoked potentials, were significantly enhanced in FXS compared to age-matched control participants, a finding consistent with an early auditory MEG study of FXS (Rojas et al. 2001). In addition, the N1 to standard tones failed to show long-term habituation to stimulus repetition in FXS. Furthermore, both mismatch negativity and P3a, reflecting automatic change detection and the involuntary switch of attention, respectively, were attenuated in FXS males. These findings as a whole suggest abnormalities that span early sensory processing as well as attentional selection mechanisms, and that are greater in the auditory compared to the visual modality for men with FXS. Similar EEG studies targeting attentional processing in WS are currently lacking, but may be spurred in future by the similarities in profile to ADHD (Rhodes et al. 2011).

While WS and FXS share similarities in the systems neuroscience of their difficulties, these arise through distinct pathways at the genetic and molecular level, and result in broader cognitive profiles that are clearly different from each other. This in turn highlights how the interactions with the remainder of the cognitive system may result in both associations and dissociations across syndromes. In the next section, we detail these complexities in the context of attentional profiles.

Cognitive underpinnings of attention difficulties in WS and FXS

As reviewed by Posner and colleagues (Posner, Rothbart and Rueda (chapter 19), this volume), models of attention in typically developing infants and children construe attention as a set of related, but distinguishable processes, or 'varieties of attention': selective attention involved in visuo-spatial orienting attention, transient alerting and sustained processes maintaining attention over time, and executive attention responsible for the resolution of stimulus–response conflict, although the way in which these processes cluster may change over developmental time (Steele et al. 2012).

Are there similarities and differences across these attentional processes in individuals with FXS and WS, given their shared high risk for ADHD? We have detailed these further elsewhere (Scerif and Steele 2011), but here we draw overarching themes on the literature on attentional profiles in WS and FXS. A first consideration is that, although the neurobiology of the two disorders offers a clear rationale for comparing in detail the attentional profiles in WS and FXS, very few studies have gathered data contrasting the two groups directly. More commonly, they are compared to individuals with another neurodevelopmental disorder, Down's syndrome (DS), or simply typically developing individuals matched in either chronological age (CA) or ability level (mental age, MA). All of these approaches have strengths and weaknesses: the comparison with DS takes into account lower intellectual functioning, but this syndrome is characterized not by a flat cognitive profile outside the context of attention, with strengths and weaknesses that differ from those experienced by individuals with WS/FXS, complicating an interpretation of the attentional difficulties. The comparison with younger typically developing individuals (MA controls) is also problematic, because the choice of reference/ability measure can accentuate or decrease differences (e.g. Thomas et al. 2009).

The few direct comparisons highlight clear cognitive differences across the two syndromes, despite similar ADHD-like symptoms. Starting from infancy, atypical attentional orienting and control of eye-movements in infants and toddlers with WS or FXS were targeted in an experiment designed to investigate children's ability to inhibit orienting to a suddenly presented but boring peripheral stimulus, and orient faster towards another peripheral stimulus that is more exciting and rewarding. Young children with FXS showed difficulties inhibiting looks towards the sudden boring peripheral stimuli (Scerif et al. 2005), an executive failure that is consistent with other findings from young children in this group. In contrast, toddlers with WS tested with the same paradigm struggled to orient peripherally at all, remaining fixated on the central stimulus (Cornish, Scerif, and Karmiloff-Smith 2007), a pattern that is consistent with findings obtained in other oculomotor control and orienting paradigms for children with WS (Atkinson et al. 2003; Brown et al. 2003). Furthermore, when covert orienting skills were assessed, these two groups of young children differed (Cornish et al. 2007). In an adaptation of the Posner cueing paradigm, peripheral cue preceded the appearance of an interesting visual stimulus either at its location, validly cueing the target location, or was presented at a different location, requiring children to disengage from the cued location to orient to the target. Toddlers with WS were significantly slower in deploying this disengagement process than toddlers with FXS, suggesting subtle differences in both covert and overt orienting of attention.

Moving on to slightly older children, Scerif, Cornish, Wilding, Driver, and Karmiloff-Smith (2004) examined attentional abilities of children with WS or FXS and typically developing children under 4 years of age using a visual search task presented on a touchscreen computer. The task required them to find targets marked by big circles amongst distractor circles, whose perceptual similarity (size) to the targets varied. Even though the two atypical groups did not differ from typically developing controls in terms of search speed, both groups made significantly more errors on the task. The WS group made significantly more touches to distractors, whereas the children with FXS made more perseverative errors (see also Scerif, Cornish, Wilding, Driver, and Karmiloff-Smith 2007, for a replication with distinct target-distractor parameters). Therefore, the study highlighted common deficits in selective attention in children with FXS and WS, who produced more errors of all kinds than typically developing children, but found, respectively, response control and appropriate stimulus selection relatively more challenging. This brief review exhausts direct comparisons across the two syndromes, and highlights the need for further studies in this context.

A second emerging theme from the extant literature, in addition to the differences *across syndromes*, is the change in attentional strengths and weaknesses *within each syndrome* over developmental time. In the case of FXS, Cornish, Munir, and Cross (2001) asked adults with DS and FXS to perform on tests of sustained and selective attention, as well as executive control. Both groups showed deficits relative to MA matched controls in executive control, but the FXS group were significantly less impaired than the DS group on the selective attention test, whereas they performed much more poorly for all other measures. In contrast, employing comparable measures with children and adolescents with FXS or DS aged between 7 and 15, Munir, Cornish, and Wilding (2000) found that children with both DS and FXS displayed significant impairments in relation to a control group of typically developing children, but, contrary to the adult pattern, the DS group performed better than the FXS group on selective attention. Similarities with the adult profile also emerged, with overall weaknesses by children and adolescents with FXS on sustained, divided attention, and inhibition tasks. Therefore, both stable and changing deficits seem to characterize the attentional profile of FXS from childhood into adulthood.

For WS, Steele, Brown, and Scerif (2012) compared sustained, selective, and executive attention in younger children with either WS or DS aged 4 to 8 years of age. When the two atypically developing groups were compared to each other and to the MA matched typically developing group, the WS group displayed a relative strength in sustained attention, while children with DS performed similarly to the MA matched typically developing group. However, children with WS made significantly more commission errors on a continuous performance task, a measure that is generally interpreted as an index of poor executive attentional control. As a whole, therefore, profiles for young children with WS reveal relative strengths in sustaining attention and a weakness in executive attention that are both consistent with other studies including older children and adolescents with WS (Rhodes et al. 2010). In essence, then, stable and changing patterns need to be assessed over developmental time, rather than assumed a priori, for both syndromes. Of course, at least in part changes may depend on the use of distinct measures across age groups and studies, and may be complicated by individual differences across samples. Ideally, then, patterns of stability and change should be studied longitudinally, but very few studies have attempted this in the context of attention in FXS or WS. Cornish et al. (2013b), used experimental measures of attentional control in a longitudinal study of boys with FXS aged between 3 and 10 years of age when first assessed. Although the gap between older boys with FXS and typically developing peers seemed to widen, when individual children were followed over time they improved significantly, highlighting how cross-sectional trajectories drawn across different individuals can mislead into predicting developmental plateaux.

Beyond changes over developmental time, a third source of complexity in the context of attention in WS and FXS are the interactions of attentional processes with strengths and weaknesses *outside* the domain of attention. For example, Atkinson et al. (2003) employed a range of tasks to measure different aspects of visual processing and attention in individuals with WS aged 4 to 15 years. Children with WS struggled with a detour box reaching task, as well as a counterpointing task, both designed to require inhibition and control of prepotent responses. However, they showed no marked impairment compared to a control group of typically developing children on the Day–Night Stroop task (Gerstadt et al. 1994), most likely because verbal responses are required for the Day–Night task, whereas visuo-spatial motor responses are required for the other two tasks. Children and adolescents with WS therefore do show impairments in attentional and executive tasks, but this is particularly evident in the domain of visuo-spatial processing, an area where people with WS are known to be profoundly impaired (Meyer-Lindenberg et al. 2006). This study underscores the importance of placing executive attention in the context of other developing strengths and weaknesses for children and adolescents with WS. In the context of FXS, it is also clear that overall weaknesses in attention operate differently depending on specific characteristics of the to-be-attended stimuli: complementing ERP and behavioural data in adults with FXS (Van der Molen et al. 2012a, 2012b), Scerif et al. (2012) found that young boys with FXS show relatively greater impairments in attending to simple auditory, compared to visual, stimuli. Furthermore, attention to stimuli in the two modalities related differentially to functional outcomes: auditory attention predicted later autistic symptomatology in boys with the disorder, whereas visual attention predicted concurrent and later ADHD symptoms as reported by teachers (Cornish et al. 2013b).

Genetic disorders and attention: Concluding remarks

To summarize, a rather complex pattern emerges when studying attention difficulties in genetic disorders. First, cross-syndrome comparisons underscore both similarities and differences across genetic disorders that share ADHD-like profiles. For example, despite common behavioural difficulties and dorsal stream vulnerability, toddlers and children with WS and FXS differ in how they orient their attention (Scerif et al. 2004, 2005; Cornish et al. 2007). Second, within-syndrome strengths and weaknesses do not necessarily remain stable. In individuals with FXS, weaknesses in executive attention, selective attention (e.g. Munir et al. 2000; Scerif et al. 2004, 2007; Wilding et al. 2002), and even simple attentional control of eye-movements (Scerif et al. 2005) are evident in early childhood. Yet, selective attention difficulties in adults with FXS seem to be resolved (Cornish et al. 2001), and tracking attention longitudinally shows improvements for some but not all functions (Cornish et al. forthcoming a). At the neural level, then, rather than understanding static and localized effects such as those that can affect modularized functions in the adult brain, genetic disorders call for the study of much more distributed neural pathways that are likely to change dynamically over time. Finally, for these genetic disorders interactions across domains of relative strengths and weaknesses can lead to a complex pattern of 'poor' performance or compensation (e.g. Atkinson et al. 2003) or of relative weaknesses when dealing with certain stimuli (e.g. auditory vs. visual stimuli, Van der Molen et al. 2012a; Scerif et al. 2012). In turn, these changing relationships suggest that the neurobiology of attention deficits in genetic disorders cannot be understood without taking into consideration the broader and developing neurocognitive landscape. These interactions lead to the need to further understand how attentional processes shape and are shaped by other developing aspects of cognition through memory and learning, which we explore in the next section.

WHY ARE ATYPICALLY DEVELOPING ATTENTIONAL PROFILES SO COMPLEX? ATTENTION DYNAMICS

A critical difference between developmental disorders and adult brain damage depends on the tight coupling between attention and learning: learning is enabled and facilitated by attentional selection, and attentional selection builds on previously learned knowledge. For example, studies with adults have shown that appropriate attentional selection can help filter distractors to learn about targets (e.g. Hillyard, Hink, Schwent, and Picton 1973) and that learned knowledge about targets and distractors allows more efficient target selection among distractors (e.g. Chun and Jiang 1999; Kruschke 2011; Mazza, Turatto, Umiltá, and Eimer 2007). While an adult patient with neglect, for example, will have already deployed attention previously to learn about the fundamentals in the environment (e.g. social interactions, object probabilities, language), young children with attention disorders tackle these tasks differently from the outset. Accounting for the relationship between attention and learning across domains is therefore critical for understanding developmental disorders. This is because difficulties with selecting relevant information, ignoring distractions, and maintaining newly processed information and task goals in mind can all exacerbate atypical ways of dealing with specific learning materials and everyday situations.

What is the current state of the evidence for changes in attention and learning dynamics at multiple levels for developmental disorders? In the case of ADHD, attentional difficulties (and their downstream effects) have been suggested to depend on motivational and reinforcement learning deficits (Sagvolden et al. 2005). In addition to these, longitudinal studies have highlighted effects of ADHD on learning in the context of literacy and numeracy (Massetti et al. 2008; McGee, Prior, Williams, Smart, and Sanson 2002). The relevant work on genetic disorders is only in its infancy, as few longitudinal studies have asked whether, and if so, how, specific attentional processes constrain learning about the environment. Recent findings suggest that individual differences in early attentional processes across children with the disorder have been found to predict outcomes in the classroom (Cornish et al. 2012a; Scerif et al. 2012). In WS, similar behavioural markers of attention difficulties do not predict later literacy and numeracy development, whereas they do in the case of Down's syndrome (Cornish et al. 2012b; Steele et al. 2012), highlighting the complexities and specificity to each disorder of atypical interactions between attention and learning. These data are highly suggestive, but correlational in nature and therefore underscore the need to test more directly how poor learning outcomes (e.g. poor numeracy or poor learning from peers in the classroom) originate from very different cognitive routes. Understanding these routes requires clear models of the interplay between attention and learning in typical development.

Attention and learning interplay over development

The interplay between attention and learning is especially important for young human learners, because they must actively select what and how to attend for further learning. While expert learners can exploit the environment using previously acquired knowledge, naïve learners are confronted with exploring a complex learning environment that is filled with ambiguity. In ambiguous and uncertain environments, selective attention is critical for learning (e.g. Dayan, Kakade, and Montague 2000; Kruschke 2011).

There is an emerging literature investigating the fundamental link between attention and learning throughout development. This work addresses critical issues such as optimal learning parameters for typical cognitive development, as well as for developmental disorders. Recent advances in methodologies (e.g. eye-tracking) allow for paradigms to address real-time attention–learning issues in more ecologically valid environments with noise and distraction, as well as in younger age groups (e.g. Amso and Johnson 2006; Ross-Sheehy, Oakes, and Luck 2011; Wu and Kirkham 2010). This work on typical development reveals bidirectional relations between attention and other developing domains. Issues in this emerging literature that cannot be addressed within the separate attention and learning fields are: (1) understanding how young learners use the information they acquire, how a bias to select particular types of information is useful for young learners; (2) the cascading effects of attention–learning dynamics; and (3) the mechanisms supporting optimal dynamics of learning and attentional selection. For example, early attentional biases mediate learning for infants who may not know what to learn at a given moment (Gliga and Csibra 2009; Houston-Price, Plunkett, and Duffy 2006; Kidd, Piantadosi, and Aslin 2010; Leekam, Solomon, and Teoh 2010; Wu, Gopnik, Richardson, and Kirkham 2011; Wu and Kirkham 2010; Yoon, Johnson, and Csibra 2008). Eight-month-old infants will attend to the most learnable events (Kidd et al. 2012), and the amount of noise and attentional capture in an environment will mediate what infants learn (e.g. Tummeltshammer and Kirkham 2013). Kidd et al. (2012) found that 7- to 8-month-old infants looked more at visual events that were semi-predictable in appearance, and were more likely to look away when presented with deterministic or random events. This finding suggests that by this age, infants are capable of regulating their information intake via selective attention. Tummeltshammer and Kirkham (2013) found that, without distraction, the same age infants attend to and learn semi-predictable events. With distraction, however, infants tend to learn deterministic events. Taken together, these studies show that infants' attention (defined by where infants look) is mediated by the variability of the input and the surrounding environment, which have a knock-on effect on what infants subsequently learn. Implications for atypically developing infants remain to be studied, but an empirical prediction arising out of these data is that infants who are more vulnerable to distraction than typically developing individuals may shift to learning about different kinds of events in their environment.

Learning from attention-directing cues is another context for studying the interaction between selective attention and learning efficacy. In a distraction-filled environment, visual spatial attention cues can highlight events in a particular location and facilitate the processing of those events. Cues can either attract attention (bright flashing lights, big moving objects) or shift attention from themselves to another location (learned attention cues: eye gaze, arrows). Wu and Kirkham (2010) found that while 8-month-old infants' attention was captured equally well by both social and non-social cues, social objects (faces) shaped the likelihood of learning, and that following social cues provided them with an optimal strategy for learning despite the presence of distractions. When cued by a turning face, infants correctly anticipated the appearance of an upcoming audiovisual event, but when cued by a flashing square, infants only remembered the location of the cues regardless of the multimodal information. Wu, Kirkham,

Swan, and Gliga (2011) also found that initial exposure to familiar social cues can elicit and maintain specific learning from novel attention-orienting cues in 9-month-olds. The findings from Wu et al. (2011) provide an important first step towards elucidating an emerging ability to use familiar attention cues to support, enhance, and mediate learning about unfamiliar cues, going beyond documenting which cues guide attention and learning during infancy to proposing a mechanism for how this cascading learning effect occurs. Infants who may not attend to faces or other attention-directing cues are therefore at risk for learning fewer or about different events in their environment. Some evidence for this comes from study on attention and social cognition in infants at high risk for later developmental disorders, such as autistic spectrum disorder (Elsabbagh et al. 2012), but has not as yet been fully explored in young children at high risk for ADHD, or children with the genetic disorders discussed here. An open question, for both typically developing children and children with developmental disorders, centres around the precise neurocognitive mechanisms by which attention modulates learning and is in turn influenced by learned information. Work on both short-term and long-term memory has offered insights into this interaction in adults, and is beginning to influence developmental work.

Studying attention and learning via memory?

Introducing the issue of how attentional profiles might relate to learning over time requires investigations into the interplay of attention and learning with memory. This is because attentional control impacts the initial filtering, coordination, and rehearsal of to-be-remembered materials in working memory for further processing into long-term memory and learning, both for adults and children (Alloway, Gathercole, Willis, and Adams 2004; Baddeley 1996). As reviewed in this volume (Kuhl and Chun (chapter 28); see also Chun, Golomb, and Turk-Browne 2011; Chun and Johnson 2011), especially in the context of visual material, attentional control in adults biases perceptual representations in function of visual working memory and its maintenance (Astle, Nobre, and Scerif 2009; Astle, Scerif, Kuo, and Nobre 2009; Fukuda and Vogel 2009; Griffin and Nobre 2003; Kuo, Rao, Lepsien, and Nobre 2009; McNab and Klingberg 2008), but the relationship between attentional control and memory is bidirectional, because information in short-term and long-term memory also influences how attention is deployed (Chun and Jiang 1999; Scerif, Worden, Davidson, Seiger, and Casey 2006; Summerfield, Lepsien, Gitelman, Mesulam, and Nobre 2006).

Much of this work has been carried out in adults, but attentional control in function of memory and learning is challenged over early childhood by the continuous requirement to select, encode, and maintain novel information, suggesting that the attention–memory interplay literature can be informed by developmental studies (Astle and Scerif 2011). Indeed, there is mounting evidence that, in a classroom setting, attentional control predicts the efficiency of learning new information, and in turn academic achievement (e.g. Gathercole and Pickering 2000). Attentional control abilities, for example, distinguish low and high mathematics ability in school-aged children (Bull and Scerif 2001) and individual differences in attentional skills predict preschoolers' later academic outcomes, especially in the context of mathematical cognition (Bull, Espy, and Wiebe 2008; Steele et al. 2012b). Individual differences in the ability to orient attention to internal representations predict working memory capacity in young children (Astle, Nobre, and Scerif 2012; Shimi et al. forthcoming). As discussed earlier, implications for atypically developing children are also emerging: early attentional control predicts learning about basic literacy and numeracy in some but not all children with genetic disorders (Steele et al. 2012a).

At the neural level, preliminary EEG data from 10- and 11-year-olds also suggest that attentional orienting cues directing children to select information held in memory result in the modulation of similar EEG components that are modulated by attentional selection of incoming perceptual input (Shimi, Kuo, Astle, Nobre and Scerif, submitted), a finding that is consistent with extensive adult data, and suggests that similar attentional processes modulate mnemonic representations for further retention in children and adults. We can take the interactions among attention, learning, and memory one step further. Since knowing what to look for (i.e. using top-down selection) requires using previously learned information to select current information, the precision of an attentional template—representations that are stored in visual working memory and specify the physical features of a relevant target object (e.g. Desimone and Duncan 1995; Olivers, Peters, Houtkamp, and Roelfsema 2011)—can be a measure of having learned what is relevant and is to be selected in a distraction-filled or ambiguous environment (e.g. Amso and Johnson 2006; Wu, Scerif, Aslin, Smith, Nako, and Eimer 2013). These neural markers of attention in function of memory and learning could prove very useful in understanding how the three factors operate differently in children with developmental disorders, but have not yet been pursued by developmental cognitive neuroscientists. We now turn to this and other future directions for the field.

ATTENTION AND DEVELOPMENTAL DISORDERS: FUTURE DIRECTIONS

Attention researchers working with adults can perhaps afford to be agnostic, to some degree, about the modularity and independence of attention functions, even though it is becoming increasingly of interest to attention researchers how attention interacts with memory and learning. Researchers interested in developmental disorders cannot avoid the interactions, and developmental dynamics therefore become critical. If attentional networks were modular in nature, we may expect effects that impact single functions and do so throughout developmental time, but this does not seem to be the case. Attentional control seems particularly vulnerable across genetic disorders, but commonalities and differences across disorders reveal highly dynamic profiles when charted developmentally. Interactions between attention and other developing strengths and weaknesses reinforce the point that attention deficits in a developmental context are not selective and circumscribed. Emerging work on ADHD has addressed the question of whether executive deficits are the single core cognitive dysfunction in this condition, or are modulated flexibly by atypical reward processing and response to motivational incentives. The evidence points away from ADHD as simply a dysexecutive disorder, and towards the suggestion that changes in reinforcement learning also play a role in the difficulties experienced by children and adolescents with the disorder.

Independent and interacting processes need to be increasingly studied at multiple levels of description, from genetics to systems neuroscience and cognition, in order to advance our understanding of the role played by attention deficits in other developing functions, and in turn their influence on efficient attentional control itself. Exciting future directions for functionally and genetically defined developmental disorders of attention can take this interdisciplinary endeavour further by studying the malleability of attentional networks through intervention (mirroring environmental effects reported by Posner and, Rothbart, and Rueda, this volume). At the neural level, testing the effects of controlled environmental intervention on attention-related neural circuits will assess the limits of their plasticity and, in genetic disorders, the interplay between genetic factors and environmental input on shaping attention. At a cognitive level, there are two distinct effects of attentional deficits that have implications for training paradigms: deficits in deciding *what* to learn and deficits in deciding *how* to learn. On one hand, knowing what to learn involves selecting appropriate targets and ignoring distractors, which can involve learning from cues described earlier. On the other hand, deficits in knowing how to learn involve inadequate sustained attention once targets have been selected (e.g. Posner, Rothbart, and Rueda (chapter 19), this volume). Modifying sustained attention and executive function processes may have an effect on how children learn, while training selective attention can modify what they learn (see Diamond et al. 2007; Rueda et al. 2005; Klingberg 2010). Changing what is learned and how things are learned will have an effect on later deployment of attention, which then will have a knock-on effect on later learning, and so on. Future research that systematically investigates the optimal parameters for the dynamics of attention and learning in naïve learners will indicate signatures of useful attentional deployment (based on multiple factors) for successful learning among distraction.

Given the evidence of the interplay between attention and learning in typical development, attentional deficits need to be considered more dynamically in terms of their interactions with other developing processes. Studying developmental disorders in comparison with typical development would inform the direct link between an attentional deficit and cascading effects to learning and memory difficulties. In this chapter, we considered how going beyond the study of attentional processes in isolation, and therefore investigating their relationships with memory and learning, will provide critical information about optimal attentional strategies for different types of learners. Investigating these relationships will yield insight into the emergence and use of efficient and flexible cognitive abilities.

Acknowledgements

The authors are grateful to colleagues who have contributed to the ideas presented in this chapter. Maddie Groom, Elizabeth Liddle, Martin Batty, Peter Liddle, Mario Liotti, and Chris Hollis are responsible for much of the exciting work on ADHD reported here. Kim Cornish and Annette Karmiloff-Smith continue to shape the field on genetic disorders, while Duncan Astle and Andria Shimi contributed extensively to thinking about attention, memory, and typical development.

References

Alloway, T. P., Gathercole, S. E., Willis, C., and Adams, A. M. (2004). A structural analysis of working memory and related cognitive skills in young children. *Journal of Experimental Child Psychology* 87(2): 85–106.

Althaus, M., Groen, Y., Wijers, A. A., Minderaa, R. B., Kema, I. P., Dijck, J. D. A., and Hoekstra, P. J. (2010). Variants of the SLC6A3 (DAT1) polymorphism affect performance monitoring-related cortical evoked potentials that are associated with ADHD. *Biological Psychology* 85(1): 19–32.

American Psychiatric Association (1994). *Diagnostic and Statistical Manual of Mental Health Disorders* (4th edn.). Washington, D.C.: APA.

Amso, D. and Johnson, S. P. (2006). Learning by selection: Visual search and object perception in young infants. *Developmental Psychology* 42(6): 1236–1245.

Aron, A. R., Dowson, J. H., Sahakian, B. J., and Robbins, T. W. (2003). Methylphenidate improves response inhibition in adults with attention-deficit/hyperactivity disorder. *Biological Psychiatry* 54(12): 1465–1468.

Astle, D. E., Nobre, A. C., and Scerif, G. (2009). Applying an attentional set to perceived and remembered features. *PLoS One* 4(10).

Astle, D. E., Nobre, A. C., and Scerif, G. (2012). Attentional control constrains visual short-term memory: Insights from developmental and individual differences. *Quarterly Journal of Experimental Psychology* 65(2): 277–294.

Astle, D. E. and Scerif, G. (2011). Interactions between attention and visual short-term memory (VSTM): What can be learnt from individual and developmental differences? *Neuropsychologia* 49(6): 1435–1445.

Astle, D. E., Scerif, G., Kuo, B. C., and Nobre, A. C. (2009). Spatial selection of features within perceived and remembered objects. *Frontiers in Human Neuroscience* 3. doi: 10.3389/neuro.09.006.2009.

Atkinson, J. and Braddick, O. (2011). From genes to brain development to phenotypic behavior: 'Dorsal-stream vulnerability' in relation to spatial cognition, attention, and planning of actions in Williams syndrome (WS) and other developmental disorders. *Progress in Brain Research* 189: 261–283.

Atkinson, J., Braddick, O., Anker, S., Curran, W., Andrew, R., Wattam-Bell, J., and Braddick, F. (2003). Neurobiological models of visuospatial cognition in children with Williams syndrome: Measures of dorsal-stream and frontal function. *Developmental Neuropsychology* 23(1–2): 139–172.

Auerbach, J. G., Landau, R., Berger, A., Arbelle, S., Faroy, M., and Karplus, M. (2005). Neonatal behavior of infants at familial risk for ADHD. *Infant Behavior and Development* 28(2): 220–224.

Baddeley, A. (1996). Exploring the central executive. *Quarterly Journal of Experimental Psychology Section A: Human Experimental Psychology* 49(1): 5–28.

Bagni, C. and Greenough, W. T. (2005). From mRNP trafficking to spine dysmorphogenesis: The roots of fragile X syndrome. *Nature Reviews Neuroscience* 6(5): 376–387.

Barkley, R. A. (1997). Behavioral inhibition, sustained attention, and executive functions: Constructing a unifying theory of ADHD. *Psychological Bulletin* 121(1): 65–94.

Barkley, R. A., Fischer, M., Smallish, L., and Fletcher, K. (2002). The persistence of attention-deficit/hyperactivity disorder into young adulthood as a function of reporting source and definition of disorder. *Journal of Abnormal Psychology* 111(2): 279–289.

Batty, M. J., Liddle, E. B., Pitiot, A., Toro, R., Groom, M. J., Scerif, G., Liotti, M., Liddle, P. F., Paus, T., and Hollis, C. (2010). Cortical gray matter in attention-deficit/hyperactivity disorder: A structural magnetic resonance imaging study. *Journal of the American Academy of Child and Adolescent Psychiatry* 49(3): 229–238.

Bawden, H. N., MacDonald, G., and Shea, S. (1997). Treatment of children with Williams syndrome with methylphenidate. *Journal of Child Neurology* 12(4): 248–252.

Bear, M. F., Huber, K. M., and Warren, S. T. (2004). The mGluR theory of fragile X mental retardation. *Trends in Neurosciences* 27(7): 370–377.

Biederman, J. (2005). Attention-deficit/hyperactivity disorder: A selective overview. *Biological Psychiatry* 57(11): 1215–1220.

Biederman, J., Faraone, S., Milberger, S., Curtis, S., Chen, L., Marrs, A., et al. (1996a). Predictors of persistence and remission of ADHD into adolescence: Results from a four-year prospective follow-up study. *Journal of the American Academy of Child and Adolescent Psychiatry* 35(3): 343–351.

Biederman, J., Faraone, S., Milberger, S., Guite, J., Mick, E., Chen, L., et al. (1996b). A prospective 4-year follow-up study of attention-deficit hyperactivity and related disorders. *Archives of General Psychiatry* 53(5): 437–446.

Bishop, D. V. M. (1997). Cognitive neuropsychology and developmental disorders: Uncomfortable bedfellows. *Quarterly Journal of Experimental Psychology Section A: Human Experimental Psychology* 50(4): 899–923.

Bishop, D. V. M. (2006). Developmental cognitive genetics: How psychology can inform genetics. *Quarterly Journal of Experimental Psychology* 59(7): 1153–1168.

Braddick, O., Atkinson, J., and Wattam-Bell, J. (2003). Normal and anomalous development of visual motion processing: motion coherence and 'dorsal-stream vulnerability'. *Neuropsychologia* 41(13): 1769–1784.

Brandeis, D., van Leeuwen, T. H., Rubia, K., Vitacco, D., Steger, J., Pascual-Marqui, R. D., and Steinhausen, H. C. (1998). Neuroelectric mapping reveals precursor of stop failures in children with attention deficits. *Behavioural Brain Research* 94(1): 111–125.

Brown, J. H., Johnson, M. H., Paterson, S. J., Gilmore, R., Longhi, E., and Karmiloff-Smith, A. (2003). Spatial representation and attention in toddlers with Williams syndrome and Down syndrome. *Neuropsychologia* 41(8): 1037–1046.

Bull, R., Espy, K. A., and Wiebe, S. A. (2008). Short-term memory, working memory, and executive functioning in preschoolers: Longitudinal predictors of mathematical achievement at age 7 years. *Developmental Neuropsychology* 33(3): 205–228.

Bull, R. and Scerif, G. (2001). Executive functioning as a predictor of children's mathematics ability: Inhibition, switching, and working memory. *Developmental Neuropsychology* 19(3): 273–293.

Castellanos, F. X., Giedd, J. N., Marsh, W. L., Hamburger, S. D., Vaituzis, A. C., Dickstein, D. P., et al. (1996). Quantitative brain magnetic resonance imaging in attention-deficit hyperactivity disorder. *Archives of General Psychiatry* 53(7): 607–616.

Castellanos, F. X., Margulies, D. S., Kelly, C., Uddin, L. Q., Ghaffari, M., Kirsch, A., et al. (2008). Cingulate-precuneus interactions: A new locus of dysfunction in adult attention-deficit/hyperactivity disorder. *Biological Psychiatry* 63(3): 332–337.

Castellanos, F. X., Sonuga-Barke, E. J. S., Milham, M. P., and Tannock, R. (2006). Characterizing cognition in ADHD: Beyond executive dysfunction. *Trends in Cognitive Sciences* 10(3): 117–123.

Castellanos, F. X., Sonuga-Barke, E. J. S., Scheres, A., Di Martino, A., Hyde, C., and Walters, J. R. (2005). Varieties of attention-deficit/hyperactivity disorder-related intra-individual variability. *Biological Psychiatry* 57(11): 1416–1423.

Castellanos, F. X. and Tannock, R. (2002). Neuroscience of attention-deficit/hyperactivity disorder: The search for endophenotypes. *Nature Reviews Neuroscience* 3(8): 617–628.

Chun, M. M., Golomb, J. D., and Turk-Browne, N. B. (2011). A taxonomy of external and internal attention. In S. T. Fiske (ed.), *Annual Review of Psychology* 62 (pp. 73–101). Palo Alto, Calif.: Annual Reviews.

Chun, M. M. and Jiang, Y. H. (1999). Top-down attentional guidance based on implicit learning of visual covariation. *Psychological Science* 10(4): 360–365.

Chun, M. M. and Johnson, M. K. (2011). Memory: Enduring traces of perceptual and reflective attention. *Neuron* 72(4): 520–535.

Cornish, K., Cole, V., Longhi, E., Karmiloff-Smith, A., and Scerif, G. (2012a). Does attention constrain developmental trajectories in fragile X syndrome? A 3-year prospective longitudinal study. *American Journal on Intellectual and Developmental Disabilities* 117(2): 103–120. doi: 10.1352/1944-7558-117.2.103.

Cornish, K., Cole, V., Longhi, E., Karmiloff-Smith, A., and Scerif, G. (2013b). Mapping developmental trajectories of attention and working memory in fragile X syndrome: Developmental freeze or developmental change? *Development and Psychopathology* 25(2): 365–376. doi: 10.1017/S0954579412001113.

Cornish, K. M., Munir, F., and Cross, G. (2001). Differential impact of the FMR-1 full mutation on memory and attention functioning: A neuropsychological perspective. *Journal of Cognitive Neuroscience* 13(1): 144–150.

Cornish, K., Scerif, G., and Karmiloff-Smith, A. (2007). Tracing syndrome-specific trajectories of attention across the lifespan. *Cortex* 43(6): 672–685.

Cornish, K., Steele, A., Monteiro, C., Karmiloff-Smith, A., and Scerif, G. (2012b). Attention deficits predict phenotypic outcomes in syndrome-specific and domain-specific ways. *Frontiers in Psychology* 3: 227. doi: 10.3389/fpsyg.2012.00227.

Cornish, K., Turk, J., and Hagerman, R. (2008). The fragile X continuum: New advances and perspectives. *Journal of Intellectual Disability Research* 52: 469–482.

Cornish, K. M., Turk, J., Wilding, J., Sudhalter, V., Munir, F., Kooy, F., and Hagerman, R. (2004). Annotation: Deconstructing the attention deficit in fragile X syndrome: A developmental neuropsychological approach. *Journal of Child Psychology and Psychiatry* 45(6): 1042–1053.

Crone, E. A., Jennings, J. R., and Van der Molen, M. W. (2003). Sensitivity to interference and response contingencies in attention-deficit/hyperactivity disorder. *Journal of Child Psychology and Psychiatry and Allied Disciplines* 44(2): 214–226.

Dai, L., Bellugi, U., Chen, X. N., Pulst-Korenberg, A. M., Jarvinen-Pasley, A., Tirosh-Wagner, T., et al. (2009). Is it Williams syndrome? GTF2IRD1 implicated in visual-spatial construction and GTF2I in sociability revealed by high resolution arrays. *American Journal of Medical Genetics Part A 149A*(3): 302–314.

Dayan, P., Kakade, S., and Montague, P. R. (2000). Learning and selective attention. *Nature Neuroscience 3 Supplement*: 1218–1223.

Desimone, R. and Duncan, J. (1995). Neural mechanisms of selective visual-attention. *Annual Review of Neuroscience 18*: 193–222.

D'Hulst, C., De Geest, N., Reeve, S. P., Van Dam, D., De Deyn, P. P., Hassan, B. A., and Kooy, R. F. (2006). Decreased expression of the GABA(A) receptor in fragile X syndrome. *Brain Research 1121*: 238–245.

D'Hulst, C. and Kooy, R. F. (2007). The GABA(A) receptor: A novel target for treatment of fragile X? *Trends in Neurosciences 30*(8): 425–431.

Diamond, A., Barnett, W. S., Thomas, J., and Munro, S. (2007). The early years: Preschool program improves cognitive control. *Science 318*(5855): 1387–1388.

Dimoska, A., Johnstone, S. J., Barry, R. J., and Clarke, A. R. (2003). Inhibitory motor control in children with attention-deficit/hyperactivity disorder: Event-related potentials in the stop-signal paradigm. *Biological Psychiatry 54*(12): 1345–1354.

Donnai, D. and Karmiloff-Smith, A. (2000). Williams syndrome: From genotype through to the cognitive phenotype. *American Journal of Medical Genetics 97*(2): 164–171.

Douglas, V. I. (1999). Cognitive control processes in attention deficit/ hyperactivity disorder. In H. C. Quay and A. E. Hogan (eds.), *Handbook of Disruptive Behaviour Disorders* (pp. 105–138). New York: Plenum Press.

Durston, S., Fossella, J. A., Mulder, M. J., Casey, B. J., Ziermans, T. B., Vessaz, M. N., and van Engeland, H. (2008). Dopamine transporter genotype conveys familial risk of attention-deficit/hyperactivity disorder through striatal activation. *Journal of the American Academy of Child and Adolescent Psychiatry 47*(1): 61–67.

Durston, S., Tottenham, N. T., Thomas, K. M., Davidson, M. C., Eigsti, I. M., Yang, Y. H., et al. (2003). Differential patterns of striatal activation in young children with and without ADHD. *Biological Psychiatry 53*(10): 871–878.

Egly, R., Driver, J., and Rafal, R. D. (1994). Shifting visual-attention between objects and locations: Evidence from normal and parietal lesion subjects. *Journal of Experimental Psychology: General 123*(2): 161–177.

Elsabbagh, M., Mercure, E., Hudry, K., Chandler, S., Pasco, G., Charman, T., Pickles, A., Baron-Cohen, S., Bolton, P., and Johnson, M. H. (the BASIS Team) (2012). Infant neural sensitivity to dynamic eye gaze is associated with later emerging autism. *Current Biology 22*(4): 338–342.

Fair, D. A., Posner, J., Nagel, B. J., Bathula, D., Dias, T. G. C., Mills, K. L., et al. (2010). Atypical default network connectivity in youth with attention-deficit/hyperactivity disorder. *Biological Psychiatry 68*(12): 1084–1091.

Faraone, S. V., Perlis, R. H., Doyle, A. E., Smoller, J. W., Goralnick, J. J., Holmgren, M. A., and Sklar, P. (2005). Molecular genetics of attention-deficit/hyperactivity disorder. *Biological Psychiatry 57*(11): 1313–1323.

Faraone, S. V., Sergeant, J., Gillberg, C., and Biederman, J. (2003). The worldwide prevalence of ADHD: Is it an American condition? *World Psychiatry: Official Journal of the World Psychiatric Association (WPA) 2*(2): 104–113.

Farzin, F. and Rivera, S. M. (2010). Dynamic object representations in infants with and without fragile X syndrome. *Frontiers in Human Neuroscience 4*. doi: 12 10.3389/neuro.09.012.2010.

Farzin, F., Whitney, D., Hagerman, R. J., and Rivera, S. M. (2008). Contrast detection in infants with fragile X syndrome. *Vision Research 48*(13): 1471–1478.

Filipek, P. A., Semrud-Clikeman, M., Steingard, R. J., Renshaw, P. F., Kennedy, D. N., and Biederman, J. (1997). Volumetric MRI analysis comparing subjects having attention-deficit hyperactivity disorder with normal controls. *Neurology 48*(3): 589–601.

Fox, M. D., Snyder, A. Z., Vincent, J. L., Corbetta, M., Van Essen, D. C., and Raichle, M. E. (2005). The human brain is intrinsically organized into dynamic, anticorrelated functional networks. *Proceedings of the National Academy of Sciences USA 102*(27): 9673–9678.

Frangiskakis, J. M., Ewart, A. K., Morris, C. A., Mervis, C. B., Bertrand, J., Robinson, B. F., et al. (1996). LIM-kinase1 hemizygosity implicated in impaired visuospatial constructive cognition. *Cell 86*(1): 59–69.

Franke, B., Neale, B. M., and Faraone, S. V. (2009). Genome-wide association studies in ADHD. *Human Genetics 126*(1): 13–50.

Franke, B., Vasquez, A. A., Johansson, S., Hoogman, M., Romanos, J., Boreatti-Huemmer, A., et al. (2010). Multicenter analysis of the SLC6A3/DAT1 VNTR haplotype in persistent ADHD suggests differential involvement of the gene in childhood and persistent ADHD. *Neuropsychopharmacology 35*(3): 656–664.

Fukuda, K. and Vogel, E. K. (2009). Human variation in overriding attentional capture. *Journal of Neuroscience 29*(27): 8726–8733.

Gathercole, S. E. and Pickering, S. J. (2000). Working memory deficits in children with low achievements in the national curriculum at 7 years of age. *British Journal of Educational Psychology 70*(2), 177–194.

Giedd, J. N., Castellanos, F. X., Casey, B. J., Kozuch, P., King, A. C., Hamburger, S. D., and Rapoport, J. L. (1994). Quantitative morphology of the corpus-callosum in attention-deficit hyperactivity disorder. *American Journal of Psychiatry 151*(5): 665–669.

Gliga, T. and Csibra, G. (2009). One-year-old infants appreciate the referential nature of deictic gestures and words. *Psychological Science 20*(3): 347–353.

Gray, V., Karmiloff-Smith, A., Funnell, E., and Tassabehji, M. (2006). In-depth analysis of spatial cognition in Williams syndrome: A critical assessment of the role of the LIMK1 gene. *Neuropsychologia 44*(5): 679–685.

Green, T., Avda, S., Dotan, I., Zarchi, O., Basel-Vanagaite, L., Zalsman, G., et al. (2012). Phenotypic psychiatric characterization of children with Williams syndrome and response of those with ADHD to methylphenidate treatment. *American Journal of Medical Genetics Part B: Neuropsychiatric Genetics 159B*(1): 13–20.

Greicius, M. D., Krasnow, B., Reiss, A. L., and Menon, V. (2003). Functional connectivity in the resting brain: A network analysis of the default mode hypothesis. *Proceedings of the National Academy of Sciences USA 100*(1): 253–258.

Griffin, I. C. and Nobre, A. C. (2003). Orienting attention to locations in internal representations. *Journal of Cognitive Neuroscience 15*(8): 1176–1194.

Groom, M. J., Scerif, G., Liddle, P. F., Batty, M. J., Liddle, E. B., Roberts, K. L., et al. (2010). Effects of motivation and medication on electrophysiological markers of response inhibition in children with attention-deficit/hyperactivity disorder. *Biological Psychiatry 67*(7): 624–631.

Groom, M. J., Liddle, E. B., Scerif, G., Liddle, P. F., Batty, M. J., Liotti, M., and Hollis, C. P. (2013). Motivational incentives and methylphenidate enhance electrophysiological correlates of error monitoring in children with attention deficit/hyperactivity disorder. *Journal of Child Psychology and Psychiatry 54*(8): 836–845. doi: 10.1111/jcpp.12069.

Haas, B. W., Barnea-Goraly, N., Lightbody, A. A., Patnaik, S. S., Hoeft, F., Hazlett, H., et al. (2009). Early white-matter abnormalities of the ventral frontostriatal pathway in fragile X syndrome. *Developmental Medicine and Child Neurology* 51(8): 593–599.

Hagerman, P. J. (2008). The fragile X prevalence paradox. *Journal of Medical Genetics* 45(8): 498–499.

Hagerman, R. J., Ono, M. Y., and Hagerman, P. J. (2005). Recent advances in fragile X: A model for autism and neurodegeneration. *Current Opinion in Psychiatry* 18(5): 490–496.

Hillyard, S. A., Hink, R. F., Schwent, V. L., and Picton, T. W. (1973). Electrical signs of selective attention in human brain. *Science* 182(4108): 177–180.

Hoeft, F., Carter, J. C., Lightbody, A. A., Hazlett, H. C., Piven, J., and Reiss, A. L. (2010). Region-specific alterations in brain development in one- to three-year-old boys with fragile X syndrome. *Proceedings of the National Academy of Sciences USA* 107(20): 9335–9339.

Hoeft, F., Hernandez, A., Parthasarathy, S., Watson, C. L., Hall, S. S., and Reiss, A. L. (2007). Fronto-striatal dysfunction and potential compensatory mechanisms in male adolescents with fragile X syndrome. *Human Brain Mapping* 28(6): 543–554.

Hoeft, F., Lightbody, A. A., Hazlett, H. C., Patnaik, S., Piven, J., and Reiss, A. L. (2008). Morphometric spatial patterns differentiating boys with fragile X syndrome, typically developing boys, and developmentally delayed boys aged 1 to 3 years. *Archives of General Psychiatry* 65(9): 1087–1097.

Hoeft, F., Walter, E., Lightbody, A. A., Hazlett, H. C., Chang, C., Piven, J., and Reiss, A. L. (2011). Neuroanatomical differences in toddler boys with fragile X syndrome and idiopathic autism. *Archives of General Psychiatry* 68(3): 295–305.

Houston-Price, C., Plunkett, K., and Duffy, H. (2006). The use of social and salience cues in early word learning. *Journal of Experimental Child Psychology* 95(1): 27–55.

Husain, M., Shapiro, K., Martin, J., and Kennard, C. (1997). Abnormal temporal dynamics of visual attention in spatial neglect patients. *Nature* 385(6612): 154–156.

Karmiloff-Smith, A. (1998). Development itself is the key to understanding developmental disorders. *Trends in Cognitive Sciences* 2(10): 389–398.

Karmiloff-Smith, A. (2007a). Atypical epigenesis. *Developmental Science* 10(1): 84–88.

Karmiloff-Smith, A. (2007b). Williams syndrome. *Current Biology* 17(24): R1035–R1036.

Karmiloff-Smith, A. (2009). Nativism versus neuroconstructivism: Rethinking the study of developmental disorders. *Developmental Psychology* 45(1): 56–63.

Karmiloff-Smith, A., Scerif, G., and Ansari, D. (2003). Double dissociations in developmental disorders? Theoretically misconceived, empirically dubious. *Cortex* 39(1): 161–163.

Karmiloff-Smith, A., Scerif, G., and Thomas, M. (2002). Different approaches to relating genotype to phenotype in developmental disorders. *Developmental Psychobiology* 40(3): 311–322.

Kessler, R. C., Adler, L., Barkley, R., Biederman, J., Conners, C. K., Demler, O., et al. (2006). The prevalence and correlates of adult ADHD in the United States: Results from the National Comorbidity Survey Replication. *American Journal of Psychiatry* 163(4): 716–723.

Kessler, R. C., Adler, L. A., Barkley, R., Biederman, J., Conners, C. K., Faraone, S. V., et al. (2005). Patterns and predictors of attention-deficit/hyperactivity disorder persistence into adulthood: Results from the National Comorbidity Survey Replication. *Biological Psychiatry* 57(11): 1442–1451.

Kidd, C., Piantadosi, S. T., and Aslin, R. N. (2012). The Goldilocks Effect: Human infants allocate attention to visual sequences that are neither too simple nor too complex. *PLoS One* 7(5): e36399.

Kidd, C., Piantadosi, S. T., and Aslin, R. N. (2010). The Goldilocks effect: Infants' preference for visual stimuli that are neither too predictable nor too surprising. In S. Ohlsson and R. Catrambone (eds.), *Proceedings of the 32nd Annual Conference of the Cognitive Science Society* (pp. 2476–2481). Austin, Tex.: Cognitive Science Society.

Klingberg, T. (2010). Training and plasticity of working memory. *Trends in Cognitive Sciences* 14(7): 317–324.

Kogan, C. S., Boutet, I., Cornish, K., Zangenehpour, S., Mullen, K. T., Holden, J. J. A., et al. (2004). Differential impact of the FMR1 gene on visual processing in fragile X syndrome. *Brain* 127: 591–601.

Konrad, K. and Eickhoff, S. B. (2010). Is the ADHD brain wired differently? A review on structural and functional connectivity in attention deficit hyperactivity disorder. *Human Brain Mapping* 31(6): 904–916.

Kruschke, J. K. (2011). Six Models of attentional learning. In E. M. Pothos and A. J. Wills (eds.), *Formal Approaches in Categorization* (pp. 120–152). Cambridge: Academic.

Kuntsi, J., Oosterlaan, J., and Stevenson, J. (2001). Psychological mechanisms in hyperactivity. I: Response inhibition deficit, working memory impairment, delay aversion, or something else? *Journal of Child Psychology and Psychiatry* 42(2): 199–210.

Kuo, B. C., Rao, A., Lepsien, J., and Nobre, A. C. (2009). Searching for targets within the spatial layout of visual short-term memory. *Journal of Neuroscience* 29(25): 8032–8038.

Ladavas, E., Petronio, A., and Umiltá, C. (1990). The deployment of visual-attention in the intact field of hemineglect patients. *Cortex* 26(3): 307–317.

Langley, K., Turic, D., Rice, F., Holmans, P., van den Bree, M. B. M., Craddock, N., et al. (2008). Testing for gene × environment interaction effects in attention deficit hyperactivity disorder and associated antisocial behavior. *American Journal of Medical Genetics Part B: Neuropsychiatric Genetics* 147B(1): 49–53.

Leekam, S. R., Solomon, T. L., and Teoh, Y. S. (2010). Adults' social cues facilitate young children's use of signs and symbols. *Developmental Science* 13(1): 108–119.

Leth-Steensen, C., Elbaz, Z. K., and Douglas, V. I. (2000). Mean response times, variability, and skew in the responding of ADHD children: A response time distributional approach. *Acta Psychologica* 104(2): 167–190.

Liddle, E. B., Hollis, C., Batty, M. J., Groom, M. J., Totman, J. J., Liotti, M., et al. (2011). Task-related default mode network modulation and inhibitory control in ADHD: Effects of motivation and methylphenidate. *Journal of Child Psychology and Psychiatry* 52(7): 761–771.

Liddle, E. B., Scerif, G., Hollis, C. P., Batty, M. J., Groom, M. J., Liotti, M., and Liddle, P. F. (2009). Looking before you leap: A theory of motivated control of action. *Cognition* 112(1): 141–158.

Liotti, M., Pliszka, S. R., Perez, R., Kothmann, D., and Woldorff, M. G. (2005). Abnormal brain activity related to performance monitoring and error detection in children with ADHD. *Cortex* 41(3): 377–388.

Liotti, M., Pliszka, S. R., Perez, R. I. I. I., Luus, B., Glahn, D., and Semrud-Clikeman, M. (2007). Electrophysiological correlates of response inhibition in children and adolescents with ADHD: Influence of gender, age, and previous treatment history. *Psychophysiology* 44(6): 936–948.

Liston, C., Cohen, M. M., Teslovich, T., Levenson, D., and Casey, B. J. (2011). Atypical prefrontal connectivity in attention-deficit/hyperactivity disorder: Pathway to disease or pathological end point? *Biological Psychiatry* 69(12): 1168–1177.

Luman, M., Oosterlaan, J., and Sergeant, J. A. (2005). The impact of reinforcement contingencies on AD/HD: A review and theoretical appraisa3. *Clinical Psychology Review* 25(2): 183–213.

McBride, S. M. J., Choi, C. H., Wang, Y., Liebelt, D., Braunstein, E., Ferreiro, D., et al. (2005). Pharmacological rescue of synaptic plasticity, courtship behavior, and mushroom body defects in a Drosophila model of fragile X syndrome. *Neuron* 45(5): 753–764.

McGee, R., Prior, M., Williams, S., Smart, D., and Sanson, A. (2002). The long-term significance of teacher-rated hyperactivity and reading ability in childhood: Findings from two longitudinal studies. *Journal of Child Psychology and Psychiatry and Allied Disciplines* 43(8): 1004–1017.

McNab, F. and Klingberg, T. (2008). Prefrontal cortex and basal ganglia control access to working memory. *Nature Neuroscience* 11(1): 103–107.

Makris, N., Biederman, J., Valera, E. M., Bush, G., Kaiser, J., Kennedy, D. N., et al. (2007). Cortical thinning of the attention and executive function networks in adults with attention-deficit/hyperactivity disorder. *Cerebral Cortex* 17(6): 1364–1375.

Makris, N., Buka, S. L., Biederman, J., Papadimitriou, G. M., Hodge, S. M., Valera, E. M., et al. (2008). Attention and executive systems abnormalities in adults with childhood ADHD: A DT-MRI study of connections. *Cerebral Cortex* 18(5): 1210–1220.

Massetti, G. M., Lahey, B. B., Pelham, W. E., Loney, J., Ehrhardt, A., Lee, S. S., and Kipp, H. (2008). Academic achievement over 8 years among children who met modified criteria for attention-deficit/hyperactivity disorder at 4–6 years of age. *Journal of Abnormal Child Psychology* 36(3): 399–410.

Mazza, V., Turatto, M., Umiltá, C., and Eimer, M. (2007). Attentional selection and identification of visual objects are reflected by distinct electrophysiological responses. *Experimental Brain Research* 181(3): 531–536.

Mervis, C. B. and John, A. E. (2010). Cognitive and behavioral characteristics of children with Williams syndrome: Implications for intervention approaches. *American Journal of Medical Genetics Part C: Seminars in Medical Genetics* 154C(2): 229–248.

Mesulam, M. M. (1981). A cortical network for directed attention and unilateral neglect. *Annals of Neurology* 10(4): 309–325.

Meyer-Lindenberg, A., Kohn, P., Mervis, C. B., Kippenhan, J. S., Olsen, R. K., Morris, C. A., and Berman, K. F. (2004). Neural basis of genetically determined visuospatial construction deficit in Williams syndrome. *Neuron* 43(5): 623–631.

Meyer-Lindenberg, A., Mervis, C. B., and Berman, K. F. (2006). Neural mechanisms in Williams syndrome: A unique window to genetic influences on cognition and behaviour. *Nature Reviews Neuroscience* 7(5): 380–393.

Mill, J., Asherson, P., Browes, C., D'Souza, U., and Craig, I. (2002). Expression of the dopamine transporter gene is regulated by the 3′ UTR VNTR: Evidence from brain and lymphocytes using quantitative RT-PCR. *American Journal of Medical Genetics* 114(8): 975–979.

Mobbs, D., Eckert, M. A., Mills, D., Korenberg, J., Bellugi, U., Galaburda, A. M., and Reiss, A. L. (2007). Frontostriatal dysfunction in Williams syndrome. *Biological Psychiatry* 62(3): 256–261.

Morris, C. A. (2010). The behavioral phenotype of Williams syndrome: A recognizable pattern of neurodevelopment. *American Journal of Medical Genetics Part C: Seminars in Medical Genetics* 154C(4): 427–431.

Mort, D. J., Malhotra, P., Mannan, S. K., Rorden, C., Pambakian, A., Kennard, C., and Husain, M. (2003). The anatomy of visual neglect. *Brain* 126: 1986–1997.

Munir, F., Cornish, K. M., and Wilding, J. (2000). A neuropsychological profile of attention deficits in young males with fragile X syndrome. *Neuropsychologia* 38(9): 1261–1270.

Murphy, D. L., Lerner, A., Rudnick, G., and Lesch, K. P. (2004). Serotonin transporter: Gene, genetic disorders, and pharmacogenetics. *Molecular Interventions* 4(2): 109–123.

Nigg, J. T., Willcutt, E. G., Doyle, A. E., and Sonuga-Barke, E. J. S. (2005). Causal heterogeneity in attention-deficit/hyperactivity disorder: Do we need neuropsychologically impaired subtypes? *Biological Psychiatry 57*(11): 1224–1230.

Olivers, C. N. L., Peters, J., Houtkamp, R., and Roelfsema, P. R. (2011). Different states in visual working memory: When it guides attention and when it does not. *Trends in Cognitive Sciences 15*(7): 327–334.

Overtoom, C. C. E., Kenemans, J. L., Verbaten, M. N., Kemmer, C., Van der Molen, M. W., van Engeland, H., et al. (2002). Inhibition in children with attention-deficit/hyperactivity disorder: A psychophysiological study of the stop task. *Biological Psychiatry 51*(8): 668–676.

Peterson, B. S., Potenza, M. N., Wang, Z., Zhu, H., Martin, A., Marsh, R., et al. (2009). An fMRI study of the effects of psychostimulants on default-mode processing during Stroop task performance in youths with ADHD. *American Journal of Psychiatry 166*(11): 1286–1294.

Plichta, M. M., Vasic, N., Wolf, R. C., Lesch, K.-P., Brummer, D., Jacob, C., et al. (2009). Neural hyporesponsiveness and hyperresponsiveness during immediate and delayed reward processing in adult attention-deficit/hyperactivity disorder. *Biological Psychiatry 65*(1): 7–14.

Pliszka, S. R., Liotti, M., and Woldorff, M. G. (2000). Inhibitory control in children with attention-deficit/hyperactivity disorder: Event-related potentials identify the processing component and timing of an impaired right-frontal response-inhibition mechanism. *Biological Psychiatry 48*(3): 238–246.

Poelmans, G., Pauls, D. L., Buitelaar, J. K., and Franke, B. (2011). Integrated genome-wide association study findings: Identification of a neurodevelopmental network for attention deficit hyperactivity disorder. *American Journal of Psychiatry 168*(4): 365–377.

Polanczyk, G., de Lima, M. S., Horta, B. L., Biederman, J., and Rohde, L. A. (2007). The worldwide prevalence of ADHD: A systematic review and metaregression analysis. *American Journal of Psychiatry 164*(6): 942–948.

Rhodes, S. M., Riby, D. M., Matthews, K., and Coghill, D. R. (2011). Attention-deficit/hyperactivity disorder and Williams syndrome: Shared behavioral and neuropsychological profiles. *Journal of Clinical and Experimental Neuropsychology 33*(1): 147–156.

Rhodes, S. M., Riby, D. M., Park, J., Fraser, E., and Campbell, L. E. (2010). Executive neuropsychological functioning in individuals with Williams syndrome. *Neuropsychologia 48*(5): 1216–1226.

Roberts, J. E., Miranda, M., Boccia, M., Janes, H., Tonnsen, B. L., and Hatton, D. D. (2011). Treatment effects of stimulant medication in young boys with fragile X syndrome. *Journal of Neurodevelopmental Disorders 3*(3): 175–184.

Robertson, L., Treisman, A., Friedman-Hill, S., and Grabowecky, M. (1997). The interaction of spatial and object pathways: Evidence from Balint's syndrome. *Journal of Cognitive Neuroscience 9*(3): 295–317.

Rojas, D. C., Benkers, T. L., Rogers, S. J., Teale, P. D., Reite, M. L., and Hagerman, R. J. (2001). Auditory evoked magnetic fields in adults with fragile X syndrome. *NeuroReport 12*(11): 2573–2576.

Ross-Sheehy, S., Oakes, L. M., and Luck, S. J. (2011). Exogenous attention influences visual short-term memory in infants. *Developmental Science. 14*(3): 490–501. doi: 10.1111/j.1467-768 7.2010.00992.x. Epub 2010 Sep 6.

Rubia, K., Overmeyer, S., Taylor, E., Brammer, M., Williams, S. C. R., Simmons, A., and Bullmore, E. T. (1999). Hypofrontality in attention deficit hyperactivity disorder during higher-order motor control: A study with functional MRI. *American Journal of Psychiatry 156*(6): 891–896.

Rueda, M. R., Rothbart, M. K., McCandliss, B. D., Saccomanno, L., and Posner, M. I. (2005). Training, maturation, and genetic influences on the development of executive attention. *Proceedings of the National Academy of Sciences USA* 102(41): 14931–14936.

Sagvolden, T., Aase, H., Zeiner, P., and Berger, D. (1998). Altered reinforcement mechanisms in attention-deficit/hyperactivity disorder. *Behavioural Brain Research* 94(1): 61–71.

Sagvolden, T., Johansen, E. B., Aase, H., and Russell, V. A. (2005). A dynamic developmental theory of attention-deficit/hyperactivity disorder (ADHD) predominantly hyperactive/impulsive and combined subtypes. *Behavioral and Brain Sciences* 28(3): 397–419.

Scerif, G., Cornish, K., Wilding, J., Driver, J., and Karmiloff-Smith, A. (2004). Visual search in typically developing toddlers and toddlers with fragile X or Williams syndrome. *Developmental Science* 7(1): 116–130.

Scerif, G., Cornish, K., Wilding, J., Driver, J., and Karmiloff-Smith, A. (2007). Delineation of early attentional control difficulties in fragile X syndrome: Focus on neurocomputational changes. *Neuropsychologia* 45(8): 1889–1898.

Scerif, G., and Karmiloff-Smith, A. (2005). The dawn of cognitive genetics? Crucial developmental caveats. *Trends in Cognitive Sciences* 9(3): 126–135.

Scerif, G., Karmiloff-Smith, A., Campos, R., Elsabbagh, M., Driver, J., and Cornish, K. (2005). To look or not to look? Typical and atypical development of oculomotor control. *Journal of Cognitive Neuroscience* 17(4): 591–604.

Scerif, G., Longhi, E., Cole, V., Karmiloff-Smith, A., and Cornish, K. (2012). Attention across modalities as a longitudinal predictor of early outcomes: The case of fragile X syndrome. *Journal of Child Psychology and Psychiatry and Allied Disciplines* 53(6): 641–650.

Scerif, G. and Steele, A. (2011). Neurocognitive development of attention across genetic syndromes: Inspecting a disorder's dynamics through the lens of another. *Progress in Brain Research* 189: 285–301.

Scerif, G., Worden, M. S., Davidson, M., Seiger, L., and Casey, B. J. (2006). Context modulates early stimulus processing when resolving stimulus–response conflict. *Journal of Cognitive Neuroscience* 18(5): 781–792.

Scheres, A., Milham, M. P., Knutson, B., and Castellanos, F. X. (2007). Ventral striatal hyporesponsiveness during reward anticipation in attention-deficit/hyperactivity disorder. *Biological Psychiatry* 61(5): 720–724.

Scheres, A., Oosterlaan, J., and Sergeant, J. A. (2001a). Response execution and inhibition in children with AD/HD and other disruptive disorders: The role of behavioural activation. *Journal of Child Psychology and Psychiatry and Allied Disciplines* 42(3): 347–357.

Scheres, A., Oosterlaan, J., and Sergeant, J. A. (2001b). Response inhibition in children with DSM-IV subtypes of AD/HD and related disruptive disorders: The role of reward. *Child Neuropsychology* 7(3): 172–189.

Seidman, L. J., Biederman, J., Liang, L., Valera, E. M., Monuteaux, M. C., Brown, A., et al. (2011). Gray matter alterations in adults with attention-deficit/hyperactivity disorder identified by voxel based morphometry. *Biological Psychiatry* 69(9): 857–866.

Seidman, L. J., Valera, E. M., Makris, N., Monuteaux, M. C., Boriel, D. L., Kelkar, K., et al. (2006). Dorsolateral prefrontal and anterior cingulate cortex volumetric abnormalities in adults with attention-deficit/hyperactivity disorder identified by magnetic resonance imaging. *Biological Psychiatry* 60(10): 1071–1080.

Sergeant, J. (2000). The cognitive-energetic model: An empirical approach to attention-deficit hyperactivity disorder. *Neuroscience and Biobehavioral Reviews* 24(1): 7–12.

Sergeant, J. A., Geurts, H., Huijbregts, S., Scheres, A., and Oosterlaan, J. (2003). The top and the bottom of ADHD: A neuropsychological perspective. *Neuroscience and Biobehavioral Reviews* 27(7): 583–592.

Shaw, P., Eckstrand, K., Sharp, W., Blumenthal, J., Lerch, J. P., Greenstein, D., et al. (2007). Attention-deficit/hyperactivity disorder is characterized by a delay in cortical maturation. *Proceedings of the National Academy of Sciences USA* 104(49): 19649–19654.

Shaw, P., Lerch, J., Greenstein, D., Sharp, W., Clasen, L., Evans, A., et al. (2006). Longitudinal mapping of cortical thickness and clinical outcome in children and adolescents with attention-deficit/hyperactivity disorder. *Archives of General Psychiatry* 63(5): 540–549.

Shimi, A., Kuo, B.-C., Astle, D., Nobre, A. C., and Scerif, G. (submitted). Orienting attention to VSTM: ERP correlates of developmental and individual differences.

Shimi, A., Nobre, A. C., Astle, D., and Scerif, G. (forthcoming). Orienting attention within visual short-term memory: Development and mechanisms. *Child Development*.

Slusarek, M., Velling, S., Bunk, D., and Eggers, C. (2001). Motivational effects on inhibitory control in children with ADHD. *Journal of the American Academy of Child and Adolescent Psychiatry* 40(3): 355–363.

Solanto, M. V., Abikoff, H., Sonuga-Barke, E., Schachar, R., Logan, G. D., Wigal, T., et al. (2001). The ecological validity of delay aversion and response inhibition as measures of impulsivity in AD/HD: A supplement to the NIMH multimodal treatment study of AD/HD. *Journal of Abnormal Child Psychology* 29(3): 215–228.

Sonuga-Barke, E. J. S. (2002). Psychological heterogeneity in AD/HD: A dual pathway model of behaviour and cognition. *Behavioural Brain Research* 130(1-2): 29–36.

Sonuga-Barke, E. J. S. (2005). Causal models of attention-deficit/hyperactivity disorder: From common simple deficits to multiple developmental pathways. *Biological Psychiatry* 57(11): 1231–1238.

Sonuga-Barke, E. J. S., Auerbach, J., Campbell, S. B., Daley, D., and Thompson, M. (2005). Varieties of preschool hyperactivity: Multiple pathways from risk to disorder. *Developmental Science* 8(2): 141–150.

Sonuga-Barke, E. J. S. and Castellanos, F. X. (2007). Spontaneous attentional fluctuations in impaired states and pathological conditions: A neurobiological hypothesis. *Neuroscience & Biobehavioral Reviews* 31(7): 977–986.

Sonuga-Barke, E. J. S., Dalen, L., Daley, D., and Remington, B. (2002). Are planning, working memory, and inhibition associated with individual differences in preschool ADHD symptoms? *Developmental Neuropsychology* 21(3): 255–272.

Steele, A., Brown, J., and Scerif, G. (2012a). Integrating general and specific developmental processes: Cross-syndrome, cross-domain dynamics. In E. K. Farran and A. Karmiloff-Smith (eds.). *Neurodevelopmental Disorders across the Lifespan: A Neuroconstructivist Approach* (pp. 339–362). Oxford: Oxford University Press.

Steele, A., Karmiloff-Smith, A., Cornish, K. M. and Scerif, G. (2012b). The multiple sub-functions of attention: Differential developmental gateways to literacy and numeracy. *Child Development.* 83(6): 2028–2041. doi: 10.1111/j.1467-8624.2012.01809.x. Epub 2012 Jul 13.

Stroehle, A., Stoy, M., Wrase, J., Schwarzer, S., Schlagenhauf, F., Huss, M., et al. (2008). Reward anticipation and outcomes in adult males with attention-deficit/hyperactivity disorder. *NeuroImage* 39(3): 966–972.

Stromme, P., Bjornstad, P. G., and Ramstad, K. (2002). Prevalence estimation of Williams syndrome. *Journal of Child Neurology* 17(4): 269–271.

Sullivan, K., Hatton, D., Hammer, J., Sideris, J., Hooper, S., Ornstein, P., and Bailey, D., Jr. (2006). ADHD symptoms in children with FXS. *American Journal of Medical Genetics Part A 140A*(21): 2275–2288.

Summerfield, J. J., Lepsien, J., Gitelman, D. R., Mesulam, M. M., and Nobre, A. C. (2006). Orienting attention based on long-term memory experience. *Neuron 49*(6): 905–916.

Tassabehji, M., Metcalfe, K., Karmiloff-Smith, A., Carette, M. J., Grant, J., Dennis, N., et al. (1999). Williams syndrome: Use of chromosomal microdeletions as a tool to dissect cognitive and physical phenotypes. *American Journal of Human Genetics 64*(1): 118–125.

Thomas, M. and Karmiloff-Smith, A. (2002). Are developmental disorders like cases of adult brain damage? Implications from connectionist modelling. *Behavioral and Brain Sciences 25*(6): 727–750.

Thomas, M. S., Annaz, D., Ansari, D., Scerif, G., Jarrold, C., and Karmiloff-Smith, A. (2009). Using developmental trajectories to understand developmental disorders. *Journal of Speech, Language, and Hearing Research 52*(2): 336–358.

Tummeltshammer, K. S. and Kirkham, N. Z. (2013). Learning to look: Statistical variation and noise guide infants' eye movements. *Developmental Science*. doi: 10.1111/desc.12064.

Tomasi, D. and Volkow, N. D. (2012). Abnormal functional connectivity in children with attention-deficit/hyperactivity disorder. *Biological Psychiatry 71*(5): 443–450.

Vaidya, C. J., Austin, G., Kirkorian, G., Ridlehuber, H. W., Desmond, J. E., Glover, G. H., and Gabrieli, J. D. E. (1998). Selective effects of methylphenidate in attention deficit hyperactivity disorder: A functional magnetic resonance study. *Proceedings of the National Academy of Sciences USA 95*(24): 14494–14499.

Vallar, G. and Perani, D. (1986). The anatomy of unilateral neglect after right-hemisphere stroke lesions: A clinical CT-scan correlation study in man. *Neuropsychologia 24*(5): 609–622.

Van der Molen, M. J., Van der Molen, M. W., Ridderinkhof, K. R., Hamel, B. C., Curfs, L. M., and Ramakers, G. J. (2012a). Auditory change detection in fragile X syndrome males: A brain potential study. *Clinical Neurophysiology 123*(7): 1309–1318.

Van der Molen, M. J., Van der Molen, M. W., Ridderinkhof, K. R., Hamel, B. C., Curfs, L. M., and Ramakers, G. J. (2012b). Auditory and visual cortical activity during selective attention in fragile X syndrome: A cascade of processing deficiencies. *Clinical Neurophysiology 123*(4): 720–9.

van Meel, C. S., Heslenfeld, D. J., Oosterlaan, J., Luman, M., and Sergeant, J. A. (2011). ERPs associated with monitoring and evaluation of monetary reward and punishment in children with ADHD. *Journal of Child Psychology and Psychiatry 52*(9): 942–953.

Verkerk, A., Pieretti, M., Sutcliffe, J. S., Fu, Y. H., Kuhl, D. P. A., Pizzuti, A., et al. (1991). Identification of a gene (FMR-1) containing a CGG repeat coincident with a breakpoint cluster region exhibiting length variation in fragile-X syndrome. *Cell 65*(5): 905–914.

Volkow, N. D., Fowler, J. S., Wang, G., Ding, Y., and Gatley, S. J. (2002). Mechanism of action of methylphenidate: Insights from PET imaging studies. *Journal of Attention Disorders 6 Supplement 1*: S31–S43.

Volkow, N. D. and Swanson, J. M. (2003). Variables that affect the clinical use and abuse of methylphenidate in the treatment of ADHD. *American Journal of Psychiatry 160*(11): 1909–1918.

Volkow, N. D., Wang, G. J., Fowler, J. S., and Ding, Y. S. (2005). Imaging the effect of methylphenidate on brain dopamine: New model on its therapeutic actions for attention-deficit/hyperactivity disorder. *Biological Psychiatry 57*(11): 1410–1415.

Volkow, N. D., Wang, G., Fowler, J. S., Logan, J., Gerasimov, M., Maynard, L., et al. (2001). Therapeutic doses of oral methylphenidate significantly increase extracellular dopamine in the human brain. *Journal of Neuroscience: The Official Journal of the Society for Neuroscience* 21(2): RC121.

Volkow, N. D., Wang, G. J., Fowler, J. S., Telang, F., Maynard, L., Logan, J., et al. (2004). Evidence that methylphenidate enhances the saliency of a mathematical task by increasing dopamine in the human brain. *American Journal of Psychiatry* 161(7): 1173–1180.

Volkow, N. D., Wang, G.-J., Kollins, S., Wigal, T., Newcorn, J., Telang, F., et al. (2010). Dopamine's role in ADHD symptoms: Beyond an attention deficit. *Biological Psychiatry* 67(9): 96S–96S.

Volkow, N. D., Wang, G. J., Newcorn, J. H., Kollins, S. H., Wigal, T. L., Telang, F., et al. (2011). Motivation deficit in ADHD is associated with dysfunction of the dopamine reward pathway. *Molecular Psychiatry* 16(11): 1147–1154.

Volkow, N. D., Wang, G.-J., Tomasi, D., Kollins, S. H., Wigal, T. L., Newcorn, J. H., et al. (2012). Methylphenidate-elicited dopamine increases in ventral striatum are associated with long-term symptom improvement in adults with attention deficit hyperactivity disorder. *Journal of Neuroscience* 32(3): 841–849.

Walter, E., Mazaika, P. K., and Reiss, A. L. (2009). Insights into brain development from neurogenetic syndromes: Evidence from fragile X syndrome, Williams syndrome, Turner syndrome and velocardiofacial syndrome. *Neuroscience* 164(1): 257–271.

Wang, H., Wu, L.-J., Kim, S. S., Lee, F. J. S., Gong, B., Toyoda, H., et al. (2008). FMRP acts as a key messenger for dopamine modulation in the forebrain. *Neuron* 59(4): 634–647.

Wiersema, J. R., van der Meere, J. J., and Roeyers, H. (2005). ERP correlates of impaired error monitoring in children with ADHD. *Journal of Neural Transmission* 112(10): 1417–1430.

Wilding, J., Cornish, K., and Munir, F. (2002). Further delineation of the executive deficit in males with fragile-X syndrome. *Neuropsychologia, 40*(8), 1343–1349.

Willcutt, E. G., Doyle, A. E., Nigg, J. T., Faraone, S. V., and Pennington, B. F. (2005). Validity of the executive function theory of attention-deficit/hyperactivity disorder: A meta-analytic review. *Biological Psychiatry* 57(11): 1336–1346.

Wu, R., Gopnik, A., Richardson, D. C., and Kirkham, N. Z. (2011). Infants learn about objects from statistics and people. *Developmental Psychology* 47(5): 1220–1229.

Wu, R. and Kirkham, N. Z. (2010). No two cues are alike: Depth of learning during infancy is dependent on what orients attention. *Journal of Experimental Child Psychology* 107(2): 118–136.

Wu, R., Kirkham, N. Z., Swan, K. A., and Gliga, T. (2011). Social signals scaffold learning from novel cues during infancy. *European Perspectives on Cognitive Science*.

Wu, R., Scerif, G., Aslin, R. N., Smith, T. J., Nako, R., and Eimer, M. (2013). Searching for Something Familiar or Novel: Top–Down Attentional Selection of Specific Items or Object Categories. *Journal of Cognitive Neuroscience* 25(5), 719–729.

Yoon, J. M., Johnson, M. H., and Csibra, G. (2008). Communication-induced memory biases in preverbal infants. *Proceedings of the National Academy of Sciences USA* 105(36): 13690–13695.

CHAPTER 32

ATTENTION AND AGEING

THEODORE P. ZANTO AND ADAM GAZZALEY

INTRODUCTION

THE term 'attention' has been part of the English language for centuries, and the 'state of giving heed' has been recognized across cultures for millennia. The ubiquitous nature of this phenomenon has led to the notion that '[o]n attention itself, it is needless to discourse at length; its nature and conditions are familiar to every thoughtful student' (Munsell 1873: 11), and more succinctly, 'everyone knows what attention is' (James 1890, vol. 1: 403). Yet James (1890) discusses different types of attention, just as other chapters in this volume show that attention is more multifaceted than is appreciated in common parlance. Thus, attention is a set of cognitive processes, and transcends a single definition or overarching theory (Parasuraman 1998). The goal of this chapter is to review the various aspects of attention in the context of how they change in normal ageing.

There are several critical reviews on ageing and attention (e.g. Hartley 1992; Kok 2000; McDowd and Shaw 2000; Rogers 2000), some within the last few years (Madden 2007; Kramer and Madden 2008; Drag and Bieliauskas 2010). However, as mentioned, there are many aspects of attention and thus many ways to consider how attention may be affected by ageing. Here, we will attempt to summarize and present a broad overview of the current state of attention and ageing research. The chapter is organized according to the following categories of attention: selective attention, sustained attention, divided attention, task-switching, and attentional capture. The final section will provide an overview of several current theories on cognitive ageing and specifically how they pertain to attention. Although the term 'attention' can be ambiguous, we will attempt to use it in context of specific processes with the understanding that lines drawn in the sand are influenced by the ocean's tide. Throughout this chapter, several questions are revisited: Does ageing impact this particular aspect of attention? If so, what are the sources of attentional decline? Do deficits in performance reflect true changes in attention or are they a manifestation of other age-related changes, such as alterations in sensory or perceptual abilities, memory, or processing speed?

SELECTIVE ATTENTION

Selective attention refers to goal-directed focus on task-relevant information while ignoring other irrelevant information. This section is subdivided according to the type of information that is selectively attended/ignored: spatial location, features, objects, intermodal information, time, and internally based items.

Spatial

Spatial selective attention refers to allocating attention to one location while ignoring another. One of the most commonly used paradigms to assess spatial selective attention utilizes a central or a peripheral cue to indicate where a target will subsequently appear. The response-time difference between validly cued and invalid, neutral, or uncued targets serves to measure attentional orienting processes (Posner 1980). Whereas peripheral cues are thought to provoke reflexive shifts in spatial attention, central cues invoke both volitional and reflexive orienting (Ristic and Kingstone 2006; Olk et al. 2008). There has been an accumulation of evidence indicating that cue-based facilitation of attentional shift to a location is preserved in ageing (Nissen and Corkin 1985; Hartley et al. 1990; Gottlob and Madden 1998), regardless of whether the cue attracts attention automatically or wilfully (Tales et al. 2002). However, age-related declines in central cueing may be observed by diminishing the saliency of the cue, although this has been attributed to deficient sensory mechanisms in older adults and not to a decline in attentional shifting (Folk and Hoyer 1992). Thus, top-down control of spatial orienting may indeed be preserved in ageing. This is supported by neural evidence of the cue validity effect on the event-related potential (ERP) amplitude being unaffected by ageing, although older adults exhibited delayed early ERP components following target stimuli (i.e. P1, N1, Nd1), suggesting a decline in early sensory (bottom-up) processes (Yamaguchi et al. 1995; Curran et al. 2001; Lorenzo-Lopez et al. 2002). Related to this, there is evidence of additional recruitment of frontal (top-down) resources in older adults during a cued spatial selective attention task (Talsma et al. 2006), suggesting that top-down processes may compensate for declines in bottom-up function in order to retain performance.

Interestingly, younger adults show a leftward bias in visual-spatial tasks that dissipates in older adults (Barrett and Craver-Lemley 2008), potentially due to more distributed neural processing in ageing (Cabeza 2002). Along these lines, recent research has shown an age-related decline when attention is cued to the left visual field (Nagamatsu et al. 2011), suggesting that previous spatial cueing research may be oversimplified when averaging data from both visual fields. Furthermore, the age-based deficit observed in the left visual field may be attributed to both sensory (delayed P1 of the ERP) and attentional processes (reduced anterior directing attentional negativity) (Nagamatsu et al. 2011). Incidentally, older adults with diminished attentional enhancement of the left visual field are more likely to experience a fall (Nagamatsu et al. 2009). Taken together, cueing paradigms have historically shown that volitional shifts in spatial attention are preserved in older adults as long as bottom-up declines in sensory processes are controlled for, yet attentional declines specific to the left visual field may occur in normal ageing. Additional research is required to verify these recent findings.

Another way to assess spatial attention in the visual domain is through search tasks that require identifying a target in the presence of multiple non-target (distractor) items. The measure of search efficiency typically relies on response time (RT) for target detection. When the target differs from distractors in a particular feature (e.g. size, colour, shape), detection is highly efficient, as the target appears to 'pop-out' due to bottom-up influences that capture attention automatically. However, visual search becomes less efficient when the target shares some feature with the distractors, and this efficiency is also contingent on the number of distractors in the visual field (display size). Thus, top-down influences such as prior knowledge of the differences between the target and distractor are thought to play a prominent role in search detection when task difficulty increases via featural similarity and display size. When targets share similar features to the distractors (i.e. non-singletons), older adults are slower and less accurate in detecting non-singleton targets (McDowd and Shaw 2000; Hommel et al. 2004; Madden and Whiting 2004). However, it is unclear whether this reflects diminished top-down processes or is due to compensatory mechanisms being over-taxed in older adults so that they can no longer adjust for deficient bottom-up processes. Indeed, there are numerous age-related declines in sensory and perceptual processes that may contribute to slower and less accurate visual search (Schneider and Pichora-Fuller 2000; Salthouse and Madden 2007), and as such, additional reliance on top-down mechanisms in older adults may be necessary to compensate for a decline in bottom-up processes. Thus, more research will be required to control for age-related differences in bottom-up sensory processes in order to assess whether top-down attentional processes for visual search are retained in ageing.

Although the vast majority of ageing research in spatial selective attention has focused on the visual domain, there is some evidence for an age-related decline in spatial selective attention in the auditory domain. Although both younger and older groups demonstrated comparable benefits from a priori knowledge of a target sentence source (Singh et al. 2008), older adults exhibit a deficit in identifying target sentences in the presence of distractors that are presented from spatially distinct locations (Duquesnoy 1983; Singh et al. 2008). These results suggest an age-based decline in filtering auditory distraction from distinct spatial locations. Indeed, a binaural auditory cued attention task has identified ageing differences in ERP measures to cues and targets which was interpreted as signatures of an age-related decline in attentional regulation (Bennett et al. 2004). Again, it is possible that age-related differences in auditory spatial attention may be attributed to declines in sensory processing, such as sound segregation. In either case, ageing research on spatial selective attention in the auditory domain is limited and additional research is required to fully assess whether top-down attentional declines are present.

Overall, research in spatial selective attention suggests that once age-based general slowing and declines in bottom-up sensory processes are accounted for, this ability is largely preserved in ageing. However, a specific attentional decline to the left visual field may be present. Also, there exists the possibility that studies of spatial attention have not been challenging enough, and if the demands were increased, age-related effects may be apparent. For example, age-related changes in visual search appear when task difficulty is increased. Future research must delineate whether this represents a decline in top-down processes or a limitation in compensatory top-down processes to overcome bottom-up deficits.

Feature-based

Selective attention to features typically refers to attending and ignoring elementary parts of a stimulus, such as colour or shape, or analogously, a tone in an auditory environment. A common paradigm used to assess feature selectivity and interference control is known as the Stroop task (Stroop 1935). Participants are required to report the colour of a word and not the word itself, which is the name of a different colour. For example, the word 'red' in blue ink would require a participant to say 'blue' and withhold the reflexive response to read and say the word 'red'. In general, older adults are slower than younger adults during the Stroop task (e.g. Comalli et al. 1962; Cohn et al. 1984; Klein et al. 1997), indicating a decline in interference control. Interestingly, an auditory version of the Stroop task shows similar age-related declines (Sommers and Danielson 1999; Sommers and Huff 2003). However, it has been argued that the Stroop task does not reflect a decline in selective attention per se, but rather, may reflect basic (or central) processing speed differences (Salthouse and Meinz 1995; Earles et al. 1997; Verhaeghen and Cerella 2002). Yet others have attempted to account for generalized slowing and suggest an age-related decline in selective attention remains present (Hartley 1993; Spieler et al. 1996). Although more empirical and theoretical work may be required to resolve this conflict (McDowd and Shaw 2000), here, we will review other paradigms to assess age-related differences in feature-based selective attention.

Another common paradigm used to assess selective attention is negative priming, in which the target stimulus is either novel (control) or has been presented in the preceding trial as a distractor. The slowing in response times to targets that were previously used as a distractor measures the amount the distractor was inhibited and is referred to as negative priming. Younger adults display negative priming effects to visual features, which may be observed electrophysiologically as changes in early ERP signatures of feature processing (Nobre et al. 2006). However, there is conflicting evidence as to how the negative priming task affects older adults' ability to inhibit irrelevant features. Whereas early reports suggested an age-related decline in inhibition (Hasher et al. 1991; Tipper 1991; Connelly and Hasher 1993), subsequent research has concluded age-equivalence in feature-based negative priming effects (Sullivan et al. 1995; Schooler et al. 1997; Simone and McCormick 1999). Thus, it is unclear whether older adults exhibit differences in inhibitory control during negative priming tasks for visual features. Interestingly, meta-analyses on negative priming tasks (not just for visual features) also disagree whether age-based inhibition differences exist. Although the meta-analyses agree that both younger and older adults display negative priming effects, one meta-analysis of 21 studies suggested older adults exhibited less of an effect (Verhaeghen and De Meersman 1998) whereas a later meta-analysis of 36 studies found no age differences (Gamboz et al. 2002). Due to this ambiguity, negative priming tasks for objects will not be discussed in the object-based selective attention section. We will turn to other ageing research on feature selection for more definite answers.

In a recent delayed recognition task for colour and motion features, older adults were observed to respond slower to features at the time of the memory probe, even after correcting for age-related declines in perceptual processing and general response slowing (Zanto et al. 2010b). Furthermore, ERP data indicated age-equivalence in early perceptual processes (at the P1), but older adults exhibited reduced amplitudes and processing delays at the stage of feature selection (selection negativity), which predicted subsequent response times. Although the behavioural responses assessed working memory performance, these results are similar to a previous discrimination task that reported an age-related decline in feature selective attention performance concomitant with a decrease in neural measures of feature selection (selection negativity) (Kenemans et al. 1995). A more recent report has corroborated these findings, such that when instructed to detect coherent motion from one of two superimposed random dot kinematograms (RDKs) that differ by colour, older adults perform equivalently to younger adults in motion detection, but are less reliable in discriminating the target from distractor motion (Quigley et al. 2010). Furthermore, Quigley and colleagues (2010) show that electroencephalography (EEG) frequency tagging of the steady-state visual evoked potential (SSVEP) was present in both age groups, but only modulated by attention in the young adults. This indicates that older adults exhibit declines in the attentional modulation of feature processing, which may not be attributed to sensory declines. Taken together, recent data indicate that age-related declines in feature-based selective attention may be manifest via reduced selectivity as well as processing speed delays.

Overall, there is much conflicting evidence on the effects of ageing in feature-based selective attention. Additional empirical or theoretical work will be required to account for these discrepancies. However, the current state of research would indicate that older adults exhibit a decline in visual attention to features based on processing speed delays and deficient neural modulation during feature selection. Additional research will be required to ascertain ageing differences in auditory-based feature selection.

Object-based

Everyday visual items consist of objects that may differ in component features such as colour or shape. However, the visual system can process objects holistically, based on integrated features and not individual parts (Egly et al. 1994; Rodriguez et al. 2002). The

Flanker task (Eriksen and Eriksen 1974) has been a popular method to assess age-related differences in object-based selective attention. The task entails responding to a central object (e.g. letter or arrow) that is flanked by either congruent (e.g. >>>) or incongruent (e.g. <><) objects. The response-time difference between congruent and incongruent trials measures interference control. Although some research has indicated that older adults are more negatively impacted by incongruent distraction (Zeef and Kok 1993; Zeef et al. 1996; Colcombe et al. 2005), some researchers have observed no differences in ageing (Kramer et al. 1994; Falkenstein et al. 2001; Fernandez-Duque and Black 2006; Kamijo et al. 2009), and others have suggested younger adults are more negatively affected by flanker interference (Wright and Elias 1979; Madden and Gottlob 1997; Mathewson et al. 2005). As can be seen, flanker effects are highly variable, potentially due to variable proximity between the target and flankers and the nature of the objects. Age-related declines in flanker interference are lessened by increasing the target-flanker distance (Cerella 1985; Zeef et al. 1996), which has been attributed to peripheral acuity changes in older adults (Cerella 1985). This suggests that age-related declines in the Flanker task may be due to sensory deficits and not object-based selective attention. However, recent neuroimaging research has shown older adults display decreased prefrontal cortical activity concomitant with declines in flanker interference relative to younger adults (Colcombe et al. 2005; Samanez-Larkin et al. 2009), indicating selective attention mechanisms may be affected in ageing. Taken together, both bottom-up and top-down attentional mechanisms may drive ageing differences in the Flanker task. However, the results are mixed as to whether an age-related difference actually exists. Thus, additional paradigms will be reviewed to assess object-based selective attention changes in normal adults.

In delayed-recognition working memory tasks for faces and scenes, older adults exhibit diminished object recognition accuracy accompanied by a selective decline in suppressing the processing of irrelevant objects at multiple stages, as assessed using functional magnetic resonance imaging (fMRI) (Gazzaley et al. 2005) and comparing the amplitude and latency of ERP components (P1, N1, P3) (Gazzaley et al. 2008; Clapp and Gazzaley 2012). These ageing differences may be due to deficient prefrontal control mechanisms modulating activity at sensory cortices specific for the object category (Gazzaley et al., 2005, 2007), which include deficits in the modulation of sensory cortical activity prior to object onset, along with accompanying deficiencies in prefrontal–visual cortical functional connectivity, thus alluding to an age-related impairment in anticipatory processes (see temporal attention section for another example) (Bollinger et al., 2010, 2011). As such, an age-based suppression deficit exists even if older adults can predict the onset of the irrelevant object (Zanto et al. 2010a). Although the behavioural measure from these tasks was working memory performance, the age-related suppression deficit predicts subsequent memory accuracy indicating the source of the deficit is attentional in nature (Gazzaley et al. 2005). Interestingly, older adults' ability to suppress irrelevant objects is not abolished, rather it is limited exclusively to later processing stages (> 500 ms) (Gazzaley et al. 2008). It should be noted that this suppression deficit in ageing to faces was not replicated in a recent face–letter delayed recognition task (Deiber et al. 2010), which seems likely due to differences in task demands. It has been shown that as task demands increase, neural measures of attended stimuli are enhanced while ignored stimuli are more suppressed (Rees et al. 1997; Handy et al. 2001; Rorden et al. 2008). Deiber et al. (2010) reported age-equivalence during letter recognition, but ceiling level accuracy scores for both age groups were observed. Thus, suppressing irrelevant face stimuli during the letter task may not have been necessary. Furthermore, Deiber et al. (2010) report an age-related decline in face recognition accuracy along with a suppression deficit (at the N170) to irrelevant letters, suggesting ageing differences in suppressing irrelevant information may become apparent in more difficult tasks. Additional recent research has lent support to the hypothesis that older adults exhibit declines in object-based selective attention exclusively under increased task demands (Schmitz et al. 2010). Taken together, it appears that older adults exhibit a deficit in visual selective attention specifically for ignoring irrelevant objects when the task is sufficiently challenging.

In the auditory domain, words may be considered objects because the individual letters (i.e. features) are not processed individually. There is a long history documenting a decrement in older adults' ability to understand speech in the presence of competing speech or distracting sounds (Carhart and Tillman 1970; Duquesnoy 1983; Li et al. 2004; Kim et al. 2007). This decline has been attributed to a combination of reduced auditory capabilities and slowed speed of processing in older adults (Van Rooij and Plomp 1991; Tun and Wingfield 1999). Interestingly, older adults may exhibit declines in auditory selective attention when the source of distraction is uncertain (Humes et al. 2006) and show an additional decline in attending to speech when the distracting speech is meaningful (Tun et al. 2002; Rossi-Katz and Arehart 2009), suggesting an influence of age-related changes in top-down processes. Furthermore, older adults exhibit deficits during selective dichotic listening (attend to one ear, ignore the other) (Gootjes et al. 2004; Hommet et al. 2010), which is exacerbated in the left ear (Alden et al. 1997; Hallgren et al. 2001), similar to the aforementioned age-based left hemifield declines in spatial selective attention for the visual domain. However, in recent studies assessing energetic (bottom-up, peripheral) and informational (top-down, cognitive) masking, the impact of meaningful distracting speech was age-equivalent (Helfer and Freyman 2008; Agus et al. 2009). Therefore, although bottom-up sensory processing may account for some deficiencies in selective attention to speech in the elderly, attentional declines in ageing may be present.

Overall, there is much conflicting evidence on the effects of ageing in object-based selective attention, similar to the accounts of feature-based selective attention using the Stroop and negative priming tasks. Additional empirical or theoretical work will be required to account for these discrepancies. It seems plausible that conflicting evidence in both the auditory and visual domain may stem from variable task difficulty. This should be addressed in future research. Nonetheless, the current state of research would indicate that older adults exhibit a decline in auditory object-based selective attention due (at least in part) to deficient bottom-up sensory processes, whereas visual deficits are exclusive to ignoring distraction when the task is difficult. However, as noted for spatial attention (visual search), a distinction must be made to determine whether increased task difficulty reflects deficient top-down mechanisms as the basis or not enough top-down compensation to overcome bottom-up declines in ageing.

Intermodal

The previous sections on selective attention reviewed studies where the attended and ignored stimuli were in the same modality. Although age-related declines in unimodal selective attention were reported, research in intermodal selective attention tends to indicate older adults retain their abilities to ignore distraction in a different modality. For example, both younger and older adults are equally affected by irrelevant background speech during a visual serial recall task (e.g. digits) (Beaman 2005; Bell and Buchner 2007), regardless of the type or intensity of the auditory distraction (Rouleau and Belleville 1996; Belleville et al. 2003). Furthermore, age-equivalence is retained on different visual tasks in the setting of auditory distraction, such as feature detection (Talsma et al., 2006: Experiment 2), verbal learning (Meijer et al. 2006), and star counting (Van Gerven et al. 2007). Although it is less explored, auditory selective attention also exhibits age-equivalence when distracting stimuli are in the visual modality. During auditory detection (Campbell et al. 2010), auditory word–pair memory tasks (Einstein et al. 2002), or auditory localization and categorization (Hugenschmidt et al. 2009), both younger and older adults were impacted by visual distraction to the same degree. Interestingly, performance may be enhanced with intermodal distraction and older adults may benefit more from multisensory information during detection (Peiffer et al. 2007; Diederich et al. 2008) and discrimination (Laurienti et al. 2006) tasks. Taken together, older adults appear unimpaired by distracting stimuli in a modality distinct from what is attended.

Neuroimaging data have lent some support to these intermodal findings in that both younger and older adults equally enhance neural activity in the sensory cortex of the attended modality while equally suppressing neural activity in the sensory cortex of the ignored modality (Peiffer et al. 2009). However, others have demonstrated an increased response in older adults' sensory cortex of the ignored modality along with increased prefrontal cortical activity (Townsend et al. 2006). Given that older adults did not display behavioural performance declines to the distracting stimuli, this suggests that age-related declines in suppressing irrelevant information may be compensated by recruiting additional attentional resources.

Recent research has used an auditory and visual n-back task with intermodal distraction to directly assess intermodal selective attention and ageing (Guerreiro and Van Gerven 2011). Interestingly, neither age group was negatively impacted by auditory distraction during the visual n-back task, while both age groups were affected by the visual distraction during the auditory n-back task. Importantly, older adults displayed a disproportionately larger impact from visual distraction. These results indicate that age-related distraction is modality-dependent such that suppressing intermodal auditory distraction is relatively preserved whereas intermodal visual distractibility is impaired in normal ageing. The age-related decline to visual distraction during an auditory task is in contrast to results discussed above. However, very little ageing research has been conducted on this type of intermodal selective attention and so additional work must be done to explain these conflicting results.

In an impressive meta-analysis of 231 ageing experiments, Guerreiro et al. (2010) suggest that distraction in ageing is more likely to be observed in unimodal than intermodal paradigms, as well as when distraction is in the visual domain rather than auditory. Although conflicting results were observed, their conclusions were drawn based on the likelihood of occurrence. Additionally, they recognize the lack of intermodal paradigms for auditory attention with visual distraction, which may help resolve certain conflicts. Furthermore, it should be noted that this meta-analysis was not exclusive to selective attention paradigms, but incorporated many tasks that assess attentional capture (see below). Nonetheless, the current state of research on selective attention generally indicates that intermodal distraction is less impacted in ageing than unimodal distraction.

Temporal

Attention may be allocated to specific points in time to optimize behavioural performance by forming expectations for the onset of an impending stimulus (Woodrow 1914). These expectations engage neural networks that encompass frontal, parietal, premotor, and sensory areas (Coull and Nobre 1998; Nobre et al. 2007). Electrophysiologically, posterior alpha and the contingent negative variation (CNV) may be enhanced prior to the expected stimulus (Miniussi et al. 1999; Praamstra et al. 2006) and the magnitude of this priming predicts subsequent perceptual processing and behavioural performance (Hillyard 1969; Ergenoglu et al. 2004; Hanslmayr et al. 2007). Interestingly, it has recently been shown that older adults do not utilize temporal cues to effectively allocate attentional processes in time, as compared to younger adults (Zanto et al. 2011). This was reflected by a lack of performance benefits and decreased neural signatures of expectation (CNV, alpha activity) when older participants were cued to when a target would appear. Importantly, Zanto and colleagues (2011) demonstrated that this age-based decline in allocating attention in time occurs for several types of tasks that vary in complexity, from simple detection to more complex discrimination and go/no-go tasks. Furthermore, Zanto and colleagues (2010a) also showed that older adults do not use temporal cues to enhance performance during a delayed working memory task. Together, these results indicate age-related declines in temporal based (anticipatory) attentional processes may be observed regardless of task difficulty. Recent neuroimaging research on expectation processes suggests that age-related declines in anticipation may stem from prefrontal cortex failing to prime sensory regions specific to the expected stimulus category (Bollinger et al. 2011).

In terms of timing abilities in general, older adults show greater variability in judging a timed interval (Block et al. 1998; Wild-Wall et al. 2009), less accuracy in producing intervals (Bherer et al. 2007; Gooch et al. 2009), and require slower tapping rates when producing syncopated movements (Stegemoller et al. 2009). Furthermore, older adults display deficits in the temporal ordering of sequential stimuli, which is contingent on individual speed of fluid reasoning, short-term memory, and attention (Ulbrich et al. 2009). Although it could be argued that timing abilities in older adults decline due to deficient automatic internal timing mechanisms, attention is thought to play an important role in timing tasks (Fortin 2003) and age-related declines in interval timing have been attributed to a reduction in attentional resources (reviewed in Lustig 2003; Balci et al. 2009). Neuroimaging data have supported this notion in that the source of age-based timing variability may stem from deficits in fronto-parietal attentional networks (Gunstad et al. 2006; Vallesi et al. 2009). Neurochemically, age-related timing deficits may reflect deficient dopaminergic and cholinergic inputs to time processing regions of the forebrain (Strong 1988; Wenk et al. 1989; Sarter and Bruno 2004), which may disrupt the encoding of temporal markers that help assess duration (Balci et al. 2009). Taken together, these results indicate that timing mechanisms are impacted as a result of attentional decline in normal ageing.

Overall, results from research on selective attention to time in older adults are fairly straightforward. Older adults exhibit declines in both expectation processes and timing functions that may be attributed to deficient fronto-parietal neural networks subserving attention. However, further research is required to determine whether the decrement in timing mechanisms is directly related to an age-related decline in temporal expectation processes.

Internal

Internal attention refers to the focusing of attention on representations that are not present in the environment via refreshing working memory traces, recalling long-term memory, or self-generation, as in mental imagery. To assess internal selective attention, researchers have used measures of mental imagery performance. Older adults exhibit declines in image rotation and activation (accessing stored visual memory) while they retain the ability to compose (generating shapes) and scan visual mental images (Dror and Kosslyn 1994). Indeed, more recent research has confirmed that ageing selectively affects different aspects of imagery processes (De Beni et al. 2007). In a study assessing age differences in active and passive visual imagery, older adults exhibited declines in an imagery-based jigsaw puzzle (active), whereas no age differences were observed in composing visual mental images (passive) (Vecchi and Cornoldi 1999), similar to previous reports. In a different set of tasks designed to explore imagery and ageing, Craik and Dirkx (1992) report age-related declines in the clock test (determine angle of clock hands), the Brooks letter test (give walking direction around the outside edge of a letter), as well as the east–west test (receive walking directions (e.g. right, left, right, back) and report direction they face (e.g. north)). The age-related decline in image activation has been attributed to inhibitory mechanisms, speed of processing, and working memory (Bruyer and Scailquin 2000). Interestingly, although older adults may not perform as well as younger adults on imagery performance, prior occupational experience may reduce this discrepancy when the profession requires imagery-based attentional allocation (e.g. graphic designers) (Lindenberger et al. 1992).

Neuroimaging data have shown that visual imagery elicits neural activity in sensory cortical regions specific for the imagined item (e.g. FFA for faces, V5 for motion) (Kosslyn et al. 1999; O'Craven and Kanwisher 2000). This imagery-evoked activity in sensory cortex is thought to be under top-down attentional influences from the prefrontal cortex (Kosslyn et al. 1997) via functional connectivity (Mechelli et al. 2004). It has been suggested that age-related declines in mental imagery may stem from shrinkage of the prefrontal cortex (Raz et al. 1999). Indeed, recent research has shown an age-related decline in the selectivity of representations during imagery as well as changes in selectivity of prefrontal networks functionally connected to visual cortical regions involved in imagery (Kalkstein et al. 2011). These data indicate that age-related declines in mental imagery may stem from a loss of neural selectivity for imagined items in fronto-posterior networks.

It could be argued that many mental imagery tasks involve assessing memory and other executive functions in addition to internal selective attention. Another means to evaluate internal selective attention is via measuring activity of brain regions in a 'default network' that is preferentially active during self-referential thoughts (Gusnard et al. 2001) and mind wandering (Mason et al. 2007). This network consists largely of cortical midline structures such as the medial prefrontal cortex, anterior cingulate, and posterior cingulate cortex (Northoff et al. 2006). Of current interest, older adults display declines in activity (Koch et al. 2010) and connectivity (Grady et al. 2010) within the default mode network. Furthermore, older adults do not disengage the default network during cognitive tasks as much as younger adults (Lustig et al. 2003), and these age-based differences become more pronounced with increased task difficulty, which enhances the magnitude of this deactivation in younger (but not older) adults (Persson et al. 2007). Moreover, decreased default mode activity during rest predicts declines in attention, processing speed, and executive function in ageing (Damoiseaux et al. 2008) as well as decreased memory performance (Sambataro et al. 2010).

Overall, the current data support the notion of an age-related decline in internally based selective attention due to impaired prefrontal attentional control. However, some mental imagery tasks may be preserved in age, such as composing and scanning mental images. Nonetheless, additional research will be required to fully dissociate attentional from memory and other executive functions that may underlie the observed ageing deficits.

Summary of selective attention in ageing

Although a general slowing of information processing (Salthouse 2000; Glisky 2007), as well as declines in bottom-up sensory processes may account for many age-related changes, deficits in selective attention do appear to exist in several domains: feature selection, object-based attention, temporal attention, and some imagery abilities. Furthermore, age-related declines in spatial search appear to be attributable to deficits in selective attention, yet it is unclear whether this reflects deficient top-down mechanisms or insufficient compensation to overcome bottom-up declines. However, there is accumulating evidence that the ability to orient attention in space, ignore intermodal distraction, and execute other imagery tasks appears to be relatively unaffected by age. Additional research is required to assess whether deficits become apparent in these aspects of attention if task difficulty is increased, as well as fully delineate declines in selective attention from other cognitive processes and bottom-up effects.

SUSTAINED ATTENTION

Sustained attention refers to the ability to maintain vigilance over time and is considered a basic attentional process (Drag and Bieliauskas 2010). Two reviews on sustained attention and ageing both report conflicting results within the literature, hindering a definitive conclusion (Davies and Parasuraman 1982; Giambra 1993). Recent research has shown that older adults perform comparably to younger adults on a classic test of sustained attention, the sustained attention to response task (SART), which requires a response to standard digits (e.g. 1–9; GO trials) and withholding a response when a rare digit appears (e.g. 3; NOGO trials) (Carriere et al. 2010). Similar results have been observed using the same basic task, except requiring responses only for rare targets (Berardi et al. 2001). However, it has been suggested that sustained attention is retained in adults aged 50–69 years but that deficits appear in adults older than 70 years of age (Filley and Cullum 1994). The aforementioned SART studies reported age-equivalence assessed only in older adults in the younger age category (i.e. 50–69 years). Indeed, changes in visual sustained attention appear as a function of age and are most prevalent in the more advanced age groups (Parasuraman and Giambra 1991; Mani et al. 2005). Interestingly, older adults that are not physically fit tend to display the largest decline in sustained attentional processes (Bunce et al. 1993), although this fitness-based attention deficit in ageing may be related (at least in part) to slowed processing speed (Bunce et al. 1996).

Using Parasuraman and Giambra's (1991) 30-minute target detection paradigm with a large sample size (~400 subjects), Giambra (1997) did not replicate their previous findings, but rather showed a modest ageing effect when non-sustained attentional aspects were minimized. Furthermore, ageing differences in sustained attention have been reported under increased perceptual demands, while age-equivalence may be observed with decreased task difficulty (Parasuraman et al. 1989; Mouloua and Parasuraman 1995). Thus, conflicting reports of an age-related decline in sustained attention may be attributed to differences in task difficulty, age and fitness of the subjects being assessed, or other non-sustained attentional processes.

Neuroimaging data from older adults have indicated a fronto-parietal network of regions recruited during a sustained attention task (Johannsen et al. 1997). During an auditory delayed-match-to-sample task, older adults' working memory performance is impaired by the presence an auditory distraction during the delay at long (i.e. > 9 sec) but not short (i.e. < 9 sec) intervals (Chao and Knight 1997). This suggests an age-related decline in sustained attention in the auditory domain, although this is difficult to distinguish from a decline in maintaining information in working memory and/or an inhibition deficit. Electrophysiologically, older adults (unlike younger) did not suppress activity in the primary auditory cortex to distracting tones during long delays (measured by Pa of the mid-latency auditory evoked potential), which predicted declines in behavioural measures of frontal lobe functioning (Wisconsin card sorting test). Furthermore, an age-based deficit was observed in prefrontal cortex function (less sustained frontal negativity). Thus, declines in sustained attention may result from the prefrontal cortex failing to suppress distraction-related neural processing in sensory cortex over time.

Overall, little research has been conducted to directly assess sustained attention abilities in older adults. Currently, it appears that sustained attention abilities are affected in ageing, although it may be contingent on task difficulty and the onset of this decline may be years later than other forms of attentional deficits. Nonetheless, additional research will be required to confirm the presence of an age-based change in sustained attention that is distinct from other non-sustained attentional processes and generalized slowing.

DIVIDED ATTENTION

Divided attention tasks require participants to perform two or more tasks or process two or more sources of information concurrently. To assess the cost of dividing attention, performance under dual task conditions are often compared to performance when the tasks are performed separately. Here, we will discuss three types of divided attention in ageing: (1) multistream (allocating attention to multiple pieces of information in the same modality), (2) multimodal (allocating attention to multiple pieces of information in different modalities), and (3) multitasking (performing multiple tasks simultaneously).

Multistream

Multistream divided attention refers to attention that is oriented towards multiple items that are simultaneously presented in the same modality with one task goal. Older adults perform equivalently to younger adults in the ability to divide attention across a visual display requiring multiple target detection (Somberg and Salthouse 1982) or target comparison (Hahn and Kramer 1995). However, if both letters and numbers are utilized as targets, an age-related decline in performance is observed with increasing task difficulty (Salthouse et al. 1984), which may explain the conflicting results. Similarly, when tracking multiple objects in the visual domain, older adults become less accurate with an increasing number of tracked items (Tsang and Shaner 1998; Trick et al. 2005). Additionally, these age-related deficits increase with a longer duration of tracking or increased rate of motion (Sekuler et al. 2008). Importantly, Sekuler et al. (2008) provide evidence that these changes in multistream tracking are not due to an age-related deficit in working memory capacity.

In the auditory domain, older adults also exhibit declines in attending to multiple auditory streams (Wild-Wall and Falkenstein 2010), which is more prominent with increased task difficulty (Wilson and Jaffe 1996). Moreover, these declines may not be fully attributed to bottom-up deficits in auditory processing (Humes et al. 2006). Interestingly, both younger and older adults exhibit a right ear advantage during dichotic listening; however, there is a selective decline in the abilities of older adults to attend to their left ear during these divided attention tasks (Johnson et al. 1979; Martin and Jerger 2005; Andersson et al. 2008). Although white-matter hyperintensities are thought to play a role in this asymmetry (Gootjes et al. 2007), it more likely reflects a breakdown in fronto-parietal attentional networks that subserve inhibitory control (i.e. discriminate between lexical competitors) and disengagement processes (Sommers 1996; Bouma and Gootjes 2011). These results are similar to those reporting a deficit in orienting attention to the left visual field, which would suggest general declines in the right hemisphere of the aged brain.

Taken together, age-related declines in multistream divided attention are apparent with sufficient task difficulty. Interestingly, both younger and older adults are equally affected by distracting stimuli in the unattended visual field during visual tracking (Stormer et al. 2011). This provides additional evidence that certain aspects of spatial selective attention are retained in normal ageing, and of current interest, indicates that declines in divided spatial attention may not be attributed to deficits in spatial selective attention, although both forms of attention may be susceptible to some left hemifield neglect.

Multimodal

Multimodal divided attention refers to attention that is oriented towards multiple items that are simultaneously presented in different modalities, but the task remains the same. In an audio-visual detection task, an age-related decline in performance was exhibited when attention was divided across modalities, but interestingly diminished following a 10-week aerobic exercise regimen (Hawkins et al. 1992). This benefit was observed only during multimodal divided attention (not focused attention to a single modality), indicating that enhanced cerebrovascular function may increase attentional capacity, but not efficiency in terms of speed. Similar research on the effects of aerobic exercise and ageing during multimodal divided attention did not observe such benefits of exercise (Madden et al. 1989). However, Hawkins et al. (1992) assessed divided attention via two simultaneous discrimination tasks with each trial presented in rapid succession, whereas Madden et al. (1989) implemented a self-paced dual task (multitasking; see next section) with a priority for one task over the other. Thus, aerobic-related improvements in older adults' multimodal divided attention may be observed when it is under high demand, similar to how age-related declines are most prominent with increased task difficulty.

Multitasking

Although multitasking can include multistream or multimodal divided attention, it is typically more cognitively demanding, as it requires attention to be allocated to multiple task goals as well as several stimuli. When attending to both auditory and visual stimuli with different task goals (e.g. detect auditory words denoting living things while categorizing visually displayed alphanumeric characters), older adults' performance declines with increasing difficulty (multimodal multitasking) (McDowd and Craik 1988), similar to reports from multistream divided attention research (Salthouse et al. 1984). Additionally, recent research using visual multistream multitasking has provided evidence of an age-related decline in dividing attention across detection and identification tasks (Mapstone et al. 2008), mental image rotation (Plankin task) and tracking, as well as memory recognition (Sternberg task) and tracking (Tsang and Shaner 1998). Tsang and Shaner (1998) attributed this divided attention deficit in ageing to reduced processing efficiency, which could be attributed to generalized slowing, and not a decline specific to the attentional domain. Similarly, data from psychological refractory period experiments indicate that older (relative to younger) adults are slower to respond to a second task when the stimulus onset asynchrony between tasks decreases (Allen et al. 1998; Glass et al. 2000). This provides additional evidence that generalized slowing may account for some age-related changes in multitasking.

In the auditory domain, older adults exhibit declines comparable to younger adults in multistream multitasking, such as with competing speech signals during concurrent target detection and voice counting tasks (Helfer et al. 2010). However, age-related declines became apparent when the task became more complex via informational masking as well as spatial segregation of the sound sources. This indicates that in addition to generalized slowing, attentional resources may also contribute to age-based deficits in multitasking. Importantly, a meta-analysis of multitasking in ageing has suggested that once generalized slowing is accounted for, an additional decline persists in older adults (Verhaeghen et al. 2003), which extends earlier sentiments from another review on age-based reductions in multitasking abilities (Kramer and Larish 1996). Thus, age-based differences in multitasking may not be solely attributed to generalized slowing, but to declines in attentional mechanisms as well. Moreover, it should be noted that some declines in multitasking may also be attributed to task-switching (Hartley and Little 1999) or task coordination strategy (Glass et al. 2000). Given the complexity of multitasking, it is not surprising that multiple cognitive sources may underlie an age-based decline during divided attention tasks.

Whereas standing and walking are often considered automatic motor activity with negligible cognitive requirements, previous research has indicated that they utilize spatial attention resources (Kerr et al. 1985) from fronto-posterior neural networks (Malouin et al. 2003). As such, performing a cognitive task while standing or walking may be considered multitasking. Indeed, similar to other forms of multitasking, older adults exhibit a decline in postural control and gait when performing a variety of cognitive tasks and these declines are contingent on the type and complexity of the task (reviewed in Woollacott and Shumway-Cook 2002). Berger and Bernard-Demanze (2011) suggest that older adults prioritize posture stability whereas younger adults incorporate a 'cognition first' principle during multitasking. A recent review on attention and gait has indicated that older adults may reduce gait speed or decrease response times to the cognitive task in order to retain gait stability (Yogev-Seligmann et al. 2008). Similarly, during a mobile phone conversation, older adults require more time to cross a street relative to younger adults, suggesting impairments in cognitive planning processes and divided attention (Neider et al. 2011). Together, these results indicate that age-related declines in attention may not only result in reduced cognitive performance, but may increase the risk for falling and personal injury (Sheridan and Hausdorff 2007).

In a recent multistream multitask study requiring tracking and target detection, older adults exhibited a decline in dual-task performance that was more pronounced when a motor response was required while multitasking (Wild-Wall et al. 2011). This result corroborates data from posture and gait multitasking experiments to suggest that motor activity usurps attentional resources, which has strong implications for driving performance in the elderly (Keskinen et al. 1998; Hahn et al. 2010). Neurally, Wild-Wall et al. (2011) provide electrophysiological evidence that older adults recruit additional processing resources during multitasking as indexed by an enhanced CNV. Moreover, this additional neural recruitment in older adults may reflect fronto-parietal compensatory mechanisms in order to retain multitasking abilities (Fernandes et al. 2006; Hartley et al. 2011).

In a recent experiment, older adults displayed a working memory performance deficit relative to younger adults when presented with distracting information (Clapp and Gazzaley 2012), similar to previous reports of a suppression deficit for object-based selective attention. Of current interest, Clapp and Gazzaley (2012) also showed that older adults exhibited an even greater working memory performance decline relative to younger adults when multitasking was required, i.e. discrimination task during the working memory maintenance period. Moreover, using the N170 latency of the ERP as an indicator of visual attention, age-based decrements in selective attention and multitasking in the setting of a working memory task arise from different attentional processing stages: selective attention differences (i.e. distractibility) are driven by over-allocation of attention to distractors in early visual processing stages, whereas multitasking declines are not due to excessive attention by older adults to the secondary task/stimuli, but rather arise from age-related changes at other processing stages. In support of this finding, fMRI data confirmed that older adults do not allocate more attention to interrupting stimuli during a working memory maintenance period than younger adults. Task-based functional connectivity analysis extended the finding by revealing that older adults fail to disengage neural networks associated with the inter-rupting task and fail to re-establish functional connections of the neural networks sub-serving the initial memory task (Clapp et al. 2011).

Fortunately, there is evidence that age-related declines in multitasking are not abso-lute. Tsang and Shaner (1998) reported that previous occupation lessened the impact of multitasking in older adults when the task was domain-specific to prior experience. Moreover, dual-task training can help alleviate some age-related declines in multitask-ing by enhancing attentional control (Bherer et al. 2005, 2006), which can generalize to new task combinations and stimuli (Bherer et al. 2008). Furthermore, multitasking training may improve multiple cognitive domains that invoke attentional processes such as task-switching, working memory, and reasoning (Basak et al. 2008). These improve-ments via training have been linked to neural plasticity in older adults' prefrontal cortex to yield more asymmetric activations similar to younger adults (Erickson et al. 2007).

Summary of divided attention in ageing

In general, divided attention tasks yield significant age-related declines in performance, particularly when tasks are complex. It is possible that the division of attention may sim-ply act to increase the overall complexity of the task, which necessitates the involvement of more mental operations. These findings are typically explained in terms of declining processing resources in normal ageing, which are over-extended in older adults when attention must be divided between two or more sources (Glisky 2007). Importantly, declines in attentional processes may increase the risk in older adults for personal injury when performing a cognitive task while they are executing motor behaviours such as walking or driving.

TASK-SWITCHING

Similar to divided attention, task-switching is the ability to switch rapidly among different skills, tasks, or cognitive sets. Older adults' performance is slower than younger adults when attention must be switched from one task to another, requiring a global change of the cognitive set, and less so (if at all) during local task-switching (where both mental task sets are active) (Mayr and Liebscher 2001; Verhaeghen and Cerella 2002; Wasylyshyn et al. 2011). It has been suggested that age-based changes in task-switching may be due to perceptual processing slow-ing (Salthouse et al. 2000). Recently, it has been argued that age-related deficits in task-switching occur at the stage of maintaining representations outside the focus of attention, whereas age-equivalence may be observed when switching represen-tations into and out of the focus of attention (Dorbath and Titz 2011). However, this more likely reflects age-equivalence during local task-switching. Although age-related declines in memory may account for some task-switching effects (Kramer et al. 1999a; Kray and Lindenberger 2000), global task-switching deficits in ageing may also be attributed to attentional changes as they may be observed in the absence of a memory component (e.g. Cepeda et al. 2001; Kray et al. 2002). Furthermore, research has shown that older adults may minimize task-switching declines when the need to switch tasks is predictable (Mayr and Kliegl 2000; Kray 2006; Coubard et al. 2011). Together, this may be interpreted as providing evidence for general slowing in older adults and/or an inability to disengage attention from one task and refocus attention on another task (Hartley and Little 1999; Clapp et al. 2011).

Interestingly, during a rapid sequential audio-to-visual detection task, an age-related decline in attentional switching performance was reduced following a 10-week aerobic exercise regimen (Hawkins et al. 1992). This benefit was only observed when switching between modalities (not the within modality task), indicating that enhanced cerebro-vascular function may increase attentional orienting, but not a general increase in detection speed efficiency. However, in a recent training study specific for task-switching, older adults do not benefit as much as younger adults suggesting trainability for switching is reduced in older adults (Dorbath et al. 2011).

Task-switching is thought to rely on control processes related to executive functioning. It has been associated with activity in areas subserving attention such as prefrontal (Rushworth et al. 2002) and parietal (Kimberg et al. 2000) cortex, particularly in the left hemisphere of the prefrontal cortex (Rogers et al. 1998; Braver et al. 2003). Age-related declines in task-switching have been attributed to decreased functional connectivity in fronto-parietal neural networks (Madden et al. 2010). Moreover, older adults display decreased fronto-central slow waves of the EEG, which may index declines in the maintenance of task-set information (Adrover-Roig and Barcelo 2010) or a failure to fully implement the task set (West and Travers 2008). However, frontal declines have also been observed during local task-switching without an age-based switching cost (Hampshire et al. 2008). Despite recent reports of decreased frontal activity in older adults during task-switching, when switching between a discrete processing task and an ongoing working memory task, high performing younger adults do not utilize prefrontal regions, whereas older adults and low performing younger adults recruit prefrontal regions (Smith et al. 2001). Similar to other aspects of attentional decline, older adults may recruit additional frontal regions to potentially offset age-based deficits in task-switching (DiGirolamo et al. 2001; Goffaux et al. 2008).

Overall, age-related declines may be observed when switching between tasks that require a global shift in the cognitive set. However, age-equivalence is often observed when both task sets are actively maintained or well practised (Bojko et al. 2004). Older adults may exhibit additional neural activity in the prefrontal cortex to retain performance abilities, but these compensatory mechanisms are insufficient for more dramatic shifts in attention, as in global task-switching. Although exercise and cognitive training may alleviate some of these switching declines, training may not be as effective in ageing as in youth.

ATTENTIONAL CAPTURE

Here, we refer to attentional capture as the automatic or reflexive orienting of attention due to a (often unexpected) stimulus. Top-down attentional processes may minimize or inhibit stimulus-driven attentional capture (e.g. Bacon and Egeth 1994) and the ability to do so is arguably the most experimentally tested phenomena in attention and ageing research. One of the most basic assessments of attentional capture is the Simon task, where a single item is presented in one of two locations (left or right) and participants must respond with a left or right key press that is contingent on the stimulus location or feature. Response times (RTs) are speeded when the stimulus and response location are congruent (e.g. both on the right) relative to incongruent trials (i.e. when response must be on the opposite side relative to stimulus location), and this result is observed regardless of whether participants respond to spatial (Simon 1969) or non-spatial features of the stimulus (Craft and Simon 1970), whether the stimulus is auditory, visual, or somatosensory (Simon et al. 1971; Hasbroucq and Guiard 1992), or whether the participant responds with their hand, foot, or eyes (Leuthold and Schroter 2006). The difference in RTs between congruent and incongruent trials serves to measure inhibitory control of the prepotent stimulus–response mapping.

During the Simon task, older adults exhibit a disproportionately larger impairment in RT on incongruent trials compared to younger adults in both auditory and visual domains (Pick and Proctor 1999; Juncos-Rabadan et al. 2008; Vu and Proctor 2008), even after correcting for general slowing in the older population (Van der Lubbe and Verleger 2002; Castel et al. 2007). However, bilingual older adults show less of a decline than monolingual older adults during both a simple and complex (i.e. requiring working memory) Simon task (Bialystok et al. 2004), suggesting that inhibitory control of the prepotent response is better retained in age when linguistic control of multiple languages is utilized across the lifespan. However, this advantage was only replicated during the simple Simon task, and not when the task difficulty is increased by an additional working memory component (Rosselli and Salvatierra 2011). Interestingly, the age-related decline during the Simon task may be eliminated by introducing a third 'no-go' option that requires participants to respond left, right, or withhold the response (Kawai and Kubo-Kawai 2010). Although it is unclear how response inhibition interacts with the prepotent stimulus–response mapping, this finding suggests a dissociation between these processes that may be differentially affected by normal ageing.

EEG data during the Simon task have shown age-related differences in the relationship between the amplitudes of the posterior contralateral negativity (i.e. N2pc) and the early lateralized readiness potential (Van der Lubbe and Verleger 2002). These data indicate that neural network activity between posterior and motor cortex may be affected by age, which results in a decline of inhibitory processes that control visuomotor transmission. Source localization of magnetoencephalography (MEG) during the Simon task indicates that the advantage observed in bilingual adults stems from increased reliance on left hemisphere fronto-temporal regions suggesting systematic changes in frontal executive functions (Bialystok et al. 2005). Thus, research from the Simon task shows an age-related decline in inhibiting the prepotent response, which may be partially retained in bilingual older adults so long as task difficulty remains minimal.

Although older adults display declines in the Simon task to irrelevant spatial information, no such declines are observed in an accessory-stimulus version of the Simon task (Simon and Pouraghabagher 1978; Proctor et al. 2005). In these experiments, participants made left or right button responses based on a relevant visual stimulus presented centrally which was accompanied by an irrelevant auditory tone to the left or right ear. These results suggest that age-related differences elicited by the Simon task may be driven by single stimuli that convey more than one type of information which overload processing resources, while older adults retain their ability to ignore spatial information from another modality. These findings are similar to the age-equivalence reported during intermodal selective attention paradigms.

Similar to the Simon task, peripheral cues reflexively orient attention to the cued location. Although spatial cueing paradigms do not typically elicit age-related differences in reflexive (peripherally cued) or volitional (centrally cued) attention, several exceptions have been noted. Older adults do not benefit as much as younger adults to central cues when a peripheral cue is presented simultaneously (Brodeur and Enns 1997) or in rapid succession (Iarocci et al. 2009). This suggests that control over attentional capture declines in normal ageing. Furthermore, although the time course of cued facilitation is comparable between younger and older adults following central cues (Folk and Hoyer 1992; Lincourt et al. 1997), age-related differences are evident during peripheral cueing paradigms such that older adults exhibit prolonged facilitation at short cue-target intervals (e.g. 50–200 ms) and a delayed inhibition of return (slowed RT to cued location after attention shifts back from periphery to centre) at longer intervals (Brodeur and Enns 1997; Lincourt et al. 1997; Castel et al. 2003), even after correcting for age-related slowing (McLaughlin et al. 2010). This suggests that older adults have greater difficulty disengaging from spatial cues that reflexively orient attention (Castel et al. 2003; Langley et al. 2011). ERP data have supported this notion by showing an age-related absence of an N2 (reflecting control or inhibition) following a peripheral (reflexive) cue and instead displaying a P3b (reflecting processing of information) (Wascher et al. 2011).

During visual search paradigms, if a target differs from distractors in a particular feature (e.g. size, colour, shape), detection is highly efficient, as the target appears to 'pop-out' due to bottom-up influences that capture attention automatically. When older adults are presented with targets whose features differ from distractors (singleton), age-equivalence may be observed when ignoring a singleton distractor (Theeuwes et al. 1998; Kramer et al. 1999b; Colcombe et al. 2003). Yet others have shown an age-related decline when attempting to inhibit an irrelevant singleton (Pratt and Bellomo 1999: Experiment 3; Whiting et al. 2005) and are slower to disengage once attention has been captured (Juola et al. 2000). These conflicting results may be due to differences in the singleton used (Pratt and Bellomo 1999) or task difficulty, as older adults show greater declines in ignoring distraction when the singleton is more salient (Kramer et al.

2000). Interestingly, a general age-based RT slowing to target singletons is observed that is not contingent on display size (Plude and Doussard-Roosevelt 1989; Whiting et al. 2005). This indicates that although perceptual processing and/or motor execution mechanisms are slowed in older adults, there is some preservation of bottom-up processes that facilitate highly efficient search.

Whereas detection of target singletons may be driven by bottom-up processes, top-down knowledge of the target feature may help to reduce or eliminate the effects of distraction (Leber and Egeth 2006). Indeed, older adults may display similar benefits as younger adults in utilizing top-down processes to enhance the detection of target singletons (Madden et al. 2004; Whiting et al. 2005; Costello et al. 2010), suggesting some control of attentional capture is retained in ageing. However, when the task requires greater attentional demand, older adults do not benefit as much as younger adults in utilizing top-down processes against attentional capture (Whiting et al. 2007). Moreover, when features of a target singleton or distractors vary on a trial-to-trial basis, older adults do not benefit as much as younger adults from prior knowledge of the target (Madden et al. 2005, 2007a). This may be due to age-related declines in switching their cognitive set (see section on task-switching), or potentially indicating that older adults may rely more heavily on top-down attention to target features in order to compensate for slowed bottom-up processes.

Neuroimaging research has lent some support for this top-down hypothesis, indicating that older adults utilize prefrontal cortical regions during target singleton detection whereas younger adults recruit posterior visual processing areas (Madden et al. 2007b). However, others have shown a similar age-based shift in posterior to frontal recruitment in singleton detection concomitant with age-related declines in accuracy, suggesting these attentional processes are vulnerable in ageing (Lorenzo-Lopez et al. 2008b). Furthermore, the N2pc of the ERP (a neural correlate of target selection) is attenuated and slowed in older adults during singleton detection, which may indicate a reduction in attentional resources in normal ageing that occurs later than the capture of attention per se (Lorenzo-Lopez et al. 2008a).

Another popular method to assess attentional capture is through oddball tasks where a standard stimulus is presented many times and infrequent oddball (target) stimuli occur randomly throughout the task to capture attention. In general, older adults exhibit reduced ERPs (mismatch negativity, P3, N400) to oddball stimuli in both the auditory and visual modalities (reviewed in Kok 2000). This was interpreted as a decline in the efficiency of detecting deviant stimuli from common background information. During a bi-field visual selective attention task where participants were required to detect infrequent targets (oddballs) in one hemifield (and ignore the other hemifield), older adults retained detection accuracy, but committed more false alarms than younger adults (Solbakk et al. 2008). False alarms were observed primarily in the attended hemifield, so age-related differences in this task may be due to difficulties in stimulus discrimination and/or inhibitory control of erroneous responses. Interestingly, the extent of neural activations measured by fMRI predicted behavioural performance in both groups; however, the locus of this activity differed such that younger adults utilized posterior regions whereas older adults relied on frontal areas. These results are similar to target singleton search paradigms in that older adults shift processing resources from relatively automatic posterior regions to more controlled functioning via frontal areas.

Overall, these results indicate that older adults show deficits in suppressing reflexive attentional capture as well as difficulty disengaging their attentional resources once it has been captured. Although some aspects of capture may be retained in age, top-down control of these prepotent responses tends to decline with increasing task difficulty. Moreover, older adults rely more heavily on prefrontal neural regions during control of attentional capture. Future research will be required to assess whether this reflects deficient top-down processes or insufficient compensatory mechanisms to account for declines in bottom-up processing.

THEORIES OF COGNITIVE AGEING

Although many theories on cognitive ageing focus on changes in multiple cognitive domains, they provide an important framework by which alterations in attention as we age may be understood. One of the most common findings in ageing research is that older adults are slower to respond to target stimuli. Additionally, as discussed above, there are also age-related delays in neural processing. These measures of slowing may not be attributed to any specific type of processing delay such as sensory or higher functions, but rather, appear pervasive throughout all stages of cognitive performance (Salthouse 1985; Birren and Fisher 1995; Salthouse 1996). Indeed, this slowing may be associated with age-based decline in the structural integrity of white-matter tracts (Rabbitt et al. 2007a; Turken et al. 2008) as well as loss of brain volume (Rabbitt et al. 2007b). As such, it has been proposed that age-related cognitive differences are due to a generalized slowing that results in less computational processing being completed in a set amount of time, which leads to less available information for higher-level functions (Salthouse 1996; Salthouse and Madden 2007). Importantly, as mentioned throughout this chapter, many examples of attentional decline may be accounted for by generalized slowing. Yet even after controlling for generalized slowing, age-related declines in attention persist, such as during inhibitory control.

Age-related declines in memory have been attributed to deficient inhibition processes that influence multiple cognitive functions (Hasher and Zacks 1988; Hasher et al. 1999). In this framework, working memory serves as the focus of attention, while inhibitory processes act as a central control mechanism to deny irrelevant information access, delete no longer relevant information, and restrain prepotent responses (Hasher et al. 2007). The inhibitory deficit view has been able to explain a wide array of age-related cognitive decline such as that documented in working memory (attentional focus), learning, and comprehension. Recent research has provided evidence linking age-related inhibitory deficits with processing speed declines, such that ERP latencies that index age-based slowing were altered in a manner selective to the suppression of irrelevant information (Gazzaley et al. 2008). Thus, measures of neural processing speed and inhibition were shown to interact during early stages of visual processing and neural slowing may result in a failure to suppress irrelevant information leading to a working memory impairment.

A load theory proposed by Lavie and colleagues (Lavie and Tsal 1994; Lavie et al. 2004) suggests that ignoring irrelevant information only becomes necessary once attentional demands to relevant items reach a capacity limit. Thus, load theory agrees with the inhibitory view in attributing a source of an age-based decline in selective attention to ignoring distraction (Maylor and Lavie 1998). Interestingly, it was proposed that increased perceptual load and increased cognitive load (e.g. working memory, task-switching) have opposing effects on how distracting information is processed such that low perceptual load or high cognitive load result in increased distraction by irrelevant items (Lavie et al. 2004). Thus, under load theory, age-related declines in selective attention may be attributed to both perceptual and cognitive load capacity limitations. Yet others have suggested that age differences in selective attention may not be fully attributable to capacity limitations (Madden and Langley 2003; Kramer and Madden 2008).

Another theory attributes frontal lobe impairment to age-related declines in inhibition processes (Dempster 1992). This work was later expanded to relate prefrontal cortex dysfunction to an array of cognitive deficits, such as impairments in prospective memory, retrospective memory, interference control, and inhibiting prepotent responses (West 1996). This frontal lobe hypothesis has been successful in describing age-based changes during multiple task paradigms due to the role of the frontal lobe in executive functions. Thus, the frontal lobe hypothesis predicts increased distractibility in older adults because age-related declines in memory and attention to the task structure result in deficient selectivity for a target (Wecker et al. 2000; West and Bowry 2005). Indeed, much research has attributed attentional decline in ageing to changes in the prefrontal cortex and as such, many subsequent theories have been formed.

The use of context has been suggested to be a fundamental mechanism that changes in age, which results in attentional differences (Braver et al. 2001; Braver and Barch 2002). Here, context refers to the internal representations of task-relevant information that biases neural pathways responsible for task performance. Simulations of the context model have accurately predicted age-related changes in response times and inhibitory control (Braver et al. 2001), and can account for data that are not easily accommodated by load theory or generalized slowing. For example, Braver et al. (2001) utilized the AX-CPT task that requires a response to a probe (X) only if it follows a specific cue (A), and to withhold responses otherwise. During the task, older adults displayed higher false alarms (X preceded by the wrong cue) as well as increased correct rejections (withhold response to non-X probes cued by A), suggesting that older adults did not properly utilize the contextual cue information. This model may also help explain age-related declines in utilizing predictive cues to form expectations that may otherwise enhance behavioural performance (see section on temporal attention). Neurally, this model attributes contextual control to the dorsolateral prefrontal cortex and postulates that declines in context processing stem from impairment of a gating mechanism that is mediated by dopaminergic projections to that brain region. Due to the incorporation of the prefrontal cortex in explaining cognitive decline, the context model is compatible with the frontal lobe hypothesis (West and Schwarb 2006) and extends its basic tenets to a specific neuromodulatory mechanism.

Although neuroimaging research provides support for the frontal lobe hypothesis, additional subtleties have been observed. As mentioned throughout this chapter, older adults appear to utilize additional prefrontal cortical regions to compensate for declines in attentional processes. During various tasks, younger adults often utilize lateral prefrontal cortical regions, whereas older adults recruit an additional contralateral homologue in order to retain performance abilities (Reuter-Lorenz et al. 2000; Rypma and D'Esposito 2000). These findings form the basis of the hemispheric asymmetry reduction in older adults (HAROLD) model and this asymmetry reduction in ageing has been observed in the domains of working memory, episodic memory, perceptual processes, and inhibitory control (Cabeza 2002; Daselaar and Cabeza 2005). Interestingly, some research indicates that asymmetry reduction is further pronounced in more advanced years (75–80 years of age) than in earlier elder years (60–70 years of age). This could indicate that asymmetry reduction may serve as a marker for some forms of neuro-cognitive decline. However, it should be noted that not all neural recruitment in older adults can be considered compensatory. Within-group analysis has shown that older adults with bilateral activity may perform worse than older adults with more unilateral activity, and that only certain contralateral homologues may be compensatory based on interhemispheric connectivity (Colcombe et al. 2005). Nonetheless, the HAROLD model is largely based on research in the memory domain and additional research will be required to ascertain its significance for attentional processes in ageing aside from inhibitory control.

Although neuroimaging research has indicated that older adults rely on more prefrontal cortical areas during attention-demanding tasks, this does not always reflect an asymmetry reduction as younger adults may utilize posterior occipito-temporal regions in lieu of frontal cortical function (Grady et al. 1994; Madden et al. 2002; Cabeza et al. 2004). This posterior to anterior shift in ageing (PASA) observation is thought to represent compensatory mechanisms in older adults, and not merely a reflection of task difficulty (Davis et al. 2008). Importantly, Davis et al. (2008) also demonstrate the generalizability of PASA to posterior cortical deactivations, suggesting that ageing results in a global shift in brain function that is not exclusive to the prefrontal cortex. However, ageing differences are most prominent under increased attentional demand and PASA does not appear to be contingent on task difficulty. Thus, additional concepts must be incorporated to account for these discrepancies.

The compensation-related utilization of neural circuits hypothesis (or CRUNCH) has attempted to account for age-related changes as a function of task difficulty, as well as incorporate why prefrontal neural recruitment may not always be compensatory (Reuter-Lorenz and Lustig 2005; Reuter-Lorenz and Cappell 2008). This hypothesis suggests that age-related neural compensation is effective with low task demands, but that age-related declines in performance become apparent with increasing task difficulty as a resource limit is reached. This is effectively similar to load theory in attributing cognitive load limitations to declines observed in ageing. Yet, CRUNCH incorporates differential neural activity profiles in ageing and provides a means to regain or retain functionality in ageing through interventions such as cognitive training or exercise (Reuter-Lorenz and Mikels 2006). These interventions may serve to enhance compensatory potential by increasing available cognitive resources (Stern et al. 2005).

Along similar lines, the scaffolding theory of ageing and cognition (STAC) invokes plasticity as a central mechanism by which detrimental effects of ageing may be minimized (Park and Reuter-Lorenz 2009). Scaffolding refers to the neural dynamics that occur in response to challenge and is a normal and adaptive process that is present throughout the lifespan. The central tenet of STAC is that in response to ageing, older adults may form new scaffolds or recruit previously established scaffolds that formed during early development or new learning. Due to age-related cortical shrinkage, white matter degradation, and dopamine depletion, scaffolding acts particularly in the prefrontal cortex to support cognitive function in response to neural declines. Although scaffolding is thought to be more prevalent in older adults due to increased challenge with lower task demands, scaffolding in older adults is less plastic and may be less efficient than in younger adults. This age-related loss in scaffolding quality and efficiency may result in cognitive performance deficits, especially with increased task difficulty. As such, STAC is compatible with other theories that posit age-related deficiencies stem from limited cognitive resources and predicts that scaffolding cannot compensate for cognitive processes that exceed available resources during high task demands. STAC incorporates many strengths of the previously mentioned theories on cognitive ageing, yet it is a more recent theory and only time will tell whether the scaffolding theory will withstand the pressure of future scientific scrutiny.

Whereas PASA, CRUNCH, and STAC each may incorporate age-based changes within any region of the cortex, the focus is generally on the prefrontal cortex. Although hypotheses based on frontal lobe dysfunction have had great success in explaining many age-related declines in cognition, West (1996) acknowledges that other neural regions may be diminished in ageing that could account for what frontal lobe-based hypotheses cannot. Indeed, attentional processes are distributed among frontal and posterior neural networks (e.g. Corbetta and Shulman 2002) and age-related changes are most likely widespread throughout the brain (Salthouse et al. 1996a). Thus, more generalized neuropsychologically based approaches may be required.

The cognitive reserve hypothesis stems from the repeated observation that the amount of brain pathology or damage does not necessarily relate to the clinical manifestation of the damage (Stern 2002). This hypothesis forms an important distinction between reserves and compensation. Essentially, cognitive reserve refers to the ability to maximize normal performance whereas compensation is the attempt to maximize performance following brain damage by recruiting neural regions that would not otherwise be involved in the task. Importantly, indices of cognitive reserve have been positively associated with cognitive performance in multiple domains including attention and memory (e.g. Corral et al. 2006). Notably, the cognitive reserve hypothesis is compatible with other theories invoking capacity limits and compensatory measures, yet it retains some generalizability to differentially address age-related changes in cognitive reserves and compensatory mechanisms.

Arguably, the most generalizable neural model for cognitive ageing suggests that neural noise throughout the brain may account for age-related declines in various cognitive tasks (Crossman and Szafran 1956; Welford 1981). As a formalized model, Li and colleagues (Li et al. 2001; Li 2005) propose the dopaminergic system modulates the neural signal to noise ratio, which is decreased (increased noise) in older adults. Although the neural noise, context, and scaffolding models incorporate dopaminergic processes as a source of age-based decline, the neural noise model is not specific to the prefrontal cortex, nor does it invoke the use of context. Yet, similar to other models, it incorporates generalized slowing that is consistently observed throughout the ageing literature. In the neural noise model, a decreased signal to noise ratio may lead to slowing at information processing stages in order to properly evaluate perceptual representations. Single-cell recordings in animals as well as human neuroimaging have supported this hypothesis to show that the aged brain yields broader tuning curves and less precision of attribute- and category-specific coding in posterior cortices (reviewed in Reuter-Lorenz and Lustig 2005). Importantly, variability in measures of visual and auditory function strongly relate to age-based variance on cognitive assessments such as reasoning, fluency, memory, knowledge, and speed (Lindenberger and Baltes 1994; Salthouse et al. 1996b; Baltes and Lindenberger 1997). Of current interest, some research has indicated that certain attentional processes may serve to reduce neural noise in older adults with a disproportional improvement in performance relative to younger adults (Allen et al. 1992; Bucur et al. 2005). Thus, additional research will be required to fully ascertain the role of attention and neural noise in ageing.

From the viewpoint of attention deficits being an underlying factor in the widespread impairment associated with cognitive ageing, emerging evidence based on neural data shows consistent deficits in top-down modulation in older adults (Gazzaley 2012). Top-down modulation, defined as the modulation of neural activity in neurons of sensory or motor areas based on an individual's goals, involves the enhancement of task-relevant representations and/or suppression for task-irrelevant representations. Top-down modulation can occur, both when stimuli are present in the environment, and when stimuli are absent and representations are generated solely based on goals. It thus serves a critical role at the crossroads of perception, attention, and memory abilities (Gazzaley 2011; Gazzaley and Nobre 2012). As discussed throughout this chapter, it is becoming evident that healthy older adults exhibit a top-down modulation deficit both when stimuli are present (e.g. perceptual discrimination, memory encoding) and when stimuli are absent from the environment (e.g. working memory maintenance, memory retrieval, mental imagery, and stimulus expectation, both for object-category and timing). Importantly, these neural deficits are associated with broad performance deficits (e.g. working memory, episodic memory, and perception). Top-down modulation may serve to alter internal signal to noise ratios in a manner posited by neural noise theories. Furthermore, it should be noted that many examples of age-related declines in top-down modulation are associated specifically with a failure to suppress neural activity to irrelevant information, which has been suggested to act as a neural basis that links theories on inhibition and processing speed (Gazzaley et al. 2008). Consistent with other theories of cognitive ageing, it has been proposed that age-related changes in top-down modulation are mediated by alterations in fronto-posterior neural networks. Thus, age-related deficits in top-down modulation may play a key role in why older adults exhibit widespread cognitive decline.

Overall, there are many theories on the basis of cognitive ageing as it relates to attentional processes. Although no one theory may account for the plethora of age-related changes observed in the literature, many of the most common aspects of attention and ageing have been taken into account. Specifically, current theories have incorporated generalized slowing, reduced inhibitory processes, the retention of performance abilities, as well as declines in performance with increased task difficulty. Current theories on attention and ageing are often successful because they incorporate the strengths of previous theories. Although each theory has had success in attributing some cognitive declines to one deficient mechanism, age-related changes appear to be multidimensional and, as such, theories on cognitive ageing should be as well. Thus, future theories should continue to capitalize on the strengths of current models and attempt to further integrate the vast array of cognitive changes in ageing.

CONCLUSION

The currently available research on attention and ageing is vast and complex with many conflicting reports. However, this literature may be simplified, and some discrepant evidence may be consolidated, by accounting for the heterogeneity of the ageing population, as well as the many various forms of attentional processes. Here, we addressed attention as it pertains to normal ageing. However, it should be noted that what we consider 'normal' ageing might not be very normal in terms of historical human life expectancy, or overall population norms. Nonetheless, older adults without clinically indentified pathology display great heterogeneity in performance during attention-demanding tasks, such that some older adults exhibit pronounced decline whereas others perform on a par with younger adults. It is not clear that all aspects of attention are affected by ageing, especially once changes in bottom-up sensory deficits or generalized slowing are taken into account. Namely, older adults often retain the ability to orient attention to a spatial location, ignore intermodal distraction, scan mental images, and perform local task-switching. However, it still remains to be seen whether deficits in these abilities are evident when task demands are increased. What has emerged from the literature is that age-based declines have been reported during many tasks with low cognitive demands on selective attention, divided attention, sustained attention, global task-switching, and controlling attentional capture.

Compensatory mechanisms, particularly in the prefrontal cortex, are thought to help retain certain performance abilities in ageing. However, it is unclear which processes are in need of compensation. A likely candidate is that bottom-up sensory processes decline in ageing due to reduced neural specialization (Park et al. 2004), which may affect multiple cognitive domains (Baltes and Lindenberger 1997). Therefore, additional attentional processes may be recruited via enhanced frontal cortical activity to discriminate between different perceptual representations. Yet as task difficulty increases, age-related declines in attention become more prominent. This suggests that as task difficulty increases, either neural recruitment is insufficient to compensate for declines in bottom-up processes, or older adults have declines in their top-down attentional mechanisms, such as capacity limitations or inefficient context processing. Thus, additional research will be required to fully understand the nature of compensatory recruitment.

Fortunately, the older brain retains plasticity abilities and as such, cognitive training and exercise may help reduce negative effects of age on attention. Interestingly, several studies have indicated how prior occupation may benefit older adults in attentional abilities that are specific to their previous line of work. This implies that personal experiences throughout the lifespan may help dictate how well attentional abilities are retained in later stages of life. Therefore, there is no need to wait for a noticeable decline in attention to begin cognitive training and/or exercising. It seems we are all fighting against the clock and it is time to pay attention.

REFERENCES

Adrover-Roig, D. and Barcelo. F (2010). Individual differences in aging and cognitive control modulate the neural indexes of context updating and maintenance during task-switching. *Cortex* 46: 434–450.

Agus, T. R., Akeroyd, M. A., Gatehouse, S., and Warden D. (2009). Informational masking in young and elderly listeners for speech masked by simultaneous speech and noise. *Journal of the Acoustical Society of America* 126: 1926–1940.

Alden, J. D., Harrison, D. W., Snyder, K. A., and Everhart, D. E. (1997). Age differences in intention to left and right hemispace using a dichotic listening paradigm. *Neuropsychiatry, Neuropsychology, and Behavioral Neurology* 10: 239–242.

Allen, P. A., Madden, D. J., Groth, K. E., and Crozier, L. C. (1992). Impact of age, redundancy, and perceptual noise on visual-search. *Journal of Gerontology* 47: P69–P74.

Allen, P. A., Smith, A. F., Vires-Collins, H., and Sperry, S. (1998). The psychological refractory period: Evidence for age differences in attentional time-sharing. *Psychology and Aging* 13: 218–229.

Andersson, M., Reinvang, I., Wehling, E., Hugdahl, K., and Lundervold, A. J. (2008). A dichotic listening study of attention control in older adults. *Scandinavian Journal of Psychology* 49: 299–304.

Bacon, W. F. and Egeth, H. E. (1994). Overriding stimulus-driven attentional capture. *Perception & Psychophysics* 55: 485–496.

Balci, F., Meck, W. H., Moore, H., and Brunner, D. (2009). Timing deficits in aging and neuropathology. In J. L. Bizon and A. Woods (eds.), *Animal Models of Human Cognitive Aging* (pp. 161–201). Totowa, N.J.: Humana Press.

Baltes, P. B. and Lindenberger, U. (1997). Emergence of a powerful connection between sensory and cognitive functions across the adult life span: A new window to the study of cognitive aging? *Psychology and Aging* 12: 12–21.

Barrett, A. M. and Craver-Lemley, C. E. (2008). Is it what you see, or how you say it? Spatial bias in young and aged subjects. *Journal of the International Neuropsychological Society* 14: 562–570.

Basak, C., Boot, W. R., Voss, M. W., and Kramer, A. F. (2008). Can training in a real-time strategy video game attenuate cognitive decline in older adults? *Psychology and Aging* 23: 765–777.

Beaman, C. P. (2005). Irrelevant sound effects amongst younger and older adults: Objective findings and subjective insights. *European Journal of Cognitive Psychology* 17: 241–265.

Bell, R. and Buchner, A. (2007). Equivalent irrelevant-sound effects for old and young adults. *Memory & Cognition* 35: 352–364.

Belleville, S., Rouleau, N., Van der Linden, M., and Collette, F. (2003). Effect of manipulation and irrelevant noise on working memory capacity of patients with Alzheimer's dementia. *Neuropsychology* 17: 69–81.

Bennett, I. J., Golob, E. J., and Starr, A. (2004). Age-related differences in auditory event-related potentials during a cued attention task. *Clinical Neurophysiology* 115: 2602–2615.

Berardi, A., Parasuraman, R., and Haxby, J. V. (2001). Overall vigilance and sustained attention decrements in healthy aging. *Experimental Aging Research* 27: 19–39.

Berger, L. and Bernard-Demanze, L. (2011). Age-related effects of a memorizing spatial task in the adults and elderly postural control. *Gait & Posture* 33: 300–302.

Bherer, L., Desjardins, S., and Fortin, C. (2007). Age-related differences in timing with breaks. *Psychology and Aging* 22: 398–403.

Bherer, L., Kramer, A. F., and Peterson, M. S. (2008). Transfer effects in task-set cost and dual-task cost after dual-task training in older and younger adults: Further evidence for cognitive plasticity in attentional control in late adulthood. *Experimental Aging Research* 34: 188–219.

Bherer, L., Kramer, A. F., Peterson, M. S., Colcombe, S., Erickson, K., and Becic, E. (2005). Training effects on dual-task performance: Are there age-related differences in plasticity of attentional control? *Psychology and Aging* 20: 695–709.

Bherer, L., Kramer, A. F., Peterson, M. S., Colcombe, S., Erickson, K., and Becic, E. (2006). Testing the limits of cognitive plasticity in older adults: Application to attentional control. *Acta Psychologica* 123: 261–278.

Bialystok, E., Craik, F. I. M., Grady, C., Chau, W., Ishii, R., Gunji, A., and Pantev, C. (2005). Effect of bilingualism on cognitive control in the Simon task: Evidence from MEG. *NeuroImage* 24: 40–49.

Bialystok, E., Craik, F. I. M., Klein, R., and Viswanathan, M. (2004). Bilingualism, aging, and cognitive control: Evidence from the Simon task. *Psychology and Aging* 19: 290–303.

Birren, J. E. and Fisher, L. M. (1995). Aging and speed of behaviour: Possible consequences for psychological functioning. *Annual Review of Psychology* 46: 329–353.

Block, R. A., Zakay, D., and Hancock, P. A. (1998). Human aging and duration judgments: A meta-analytic review. *Psychology and Aging* 13: 584–596.

Bojko, A., Kramer, A. F., and Peterson, M. S. (2004). Age equivalence in switch costs for prosaccade and antisaccade tasks. *Psychology and Aging* 19: 226–234.

Bollinger, J., Rubens, M. T., Masangkay, E., and Gazzaley, A. (2011). An expectation-based memory deficit in aging. *Neuropsychologia* 49: 1466–1475.

Bollinger, J., Rubens, M. T., Zanto, T. P., and Gazzaley, A. (2010). Expectation-driven changes in cortical functional connectivity influence working-memory and long-term memory performance. *Journal of Neuroscience* 30: 14399–14410.

Bouma, A. and Gootjes, L. (2011). Effects of attention on dichotic listening in elderly and patients with dementia of the Alzheimer type. *Brain and Cognition 76*: 286–293.

Braver, T. S. and Barch, D. M. (2002). A theory of cognitive control, aging cognition, and neuromodulation. *Neuroscience and Biobehavioral Reviews 26*: 809–817.

Braver, T. S., Barch, D. M., Keys, B. A., Carter, C. S., Cohen, J. D., Kaye, J. A., Janowsky, J. S., Taylor, S. F., Yesavage, J. A., Mumenthaler, M. S., Jagust, W. J., and Reed, B. R. (2001). Context processing in older adults: Evidence for a theory relating cognitive control to neurobiology in healthy aging. *Journal of Experimental Psychology: General 130*: 746–763.

Braver, T. S., Reynolds, J. R., and Donaldson, D. I. (2003). Neural mechanisms of transient and sustained cognitive control during task switching. *Neuron 39*: 713–726.

Brodeur, D. A. and Enns, J. T. (1997). Covert visual orienting across the lifespan. *Canadian Journal of Experimental Psychology/Revue Canadienne de Psychologie Experimentale 51*: 20–35.

Bruyer, R. and Scailquin, J. C. (2000). Effects of aging on the generation of mental images. *Experimental Aging Research 26*: 337–351.

Bucur, B., Madden, D. J., and Allen, P. A. (2005). Age-related differences in the processing of redundant visual dimensions. *Psychology and Aging 20*: 435–446.

Bunce, D. J., Barrowclough, A., and Morris, I. (1996). The moderating influence of physical fitness on age gradients in vigilance and serial choice responding tasks. *Psychology and Aging 11*: 671–682.

Bunce D. J., Warr, P. B., and Cochrane, T. (1993). Blocks in choice responding as a function of age and physical-fitness. *Psychology and Aging 8*: 26–33.

Cabeza, R. (2002). Hemispheric asymmetry reduction in older adults: The HAROLD model. *Psychology and Aging 17*: 85–100.

Cabeza, R., Daselaar, S. M., Dolcos, F., Prince, S. E., Budde, M., and Nyberg, L. (2004). Task-independent and task-specific age effects on brain activity during working memory, visual attention and episodic retrieval. *Cerebral Cortex 14*: 364–375.

Campbell, K. L., Al-Aidroos, N., Fatt, R., Pratt, J., and Hasher, L. (2010). The effects of multisensory targets on saccadic trajectory deviations: Eliminating age differences. *Experimental Brain Research 201*: 385–392.

Carhart, R. and Tillman, T. W. (1970). Interaction of competing speech signals with hearing losses. *Archives of Otolaryngology 91*: 273–279.

Carriere, J. S.A., Cheyne, J. A., Solman, G. J. F., and Smilek, D. (2010). Age trends for failures of sustained attention. *Psychology and Aging 25*: 569–574.

Castel, A. D., Balota, D. A., Hutchison, K. A., Logan, J. M., and Yap, M. J. (2007). Spatial attention and response control in healthy younger and older adults and individuals with Alzheimer's disease: Evidence for disproportionate selection impairments in the Simon task. *Neuropsychology 21*: 170–182.

Castel, A. D., Chasteen, A. L., Scialfa, C. T., and Pratt, J. (2003). Adult age differences in the time course of inhibition of return. *Journals of Gerontology B: Psychological Sciences and Social Sciences 58*: P256–P259.

Cepeda, N. J., Kramer, A. F., and de Sather, J. C. M. G. (2001). Changes in executive control across the life span: Examination of task-switching performance. *Developmental Psychology 37*: 715–730.

Cerella, J. (1985). Age-related decline in extrafoveal letter perception. *Journal of Gerontology 40*: 727–736.

Chao, L. L. and Knight, R. T. (1997). Prefrontal deficits in attention and inhibitory control with aging. *Cerebral Cortex 7*: 63–69.

Clapp, W. C. and Gazzaley, A. (2012). Distinct mechanisms for the impact of distraction and interruption on working memory in aging. *Neurobiology of Aging 33*: 134–148.

Clapp, W. C., Rubens, M. T., Sabharwal, J., and Gazzaley, A. (2011). Deficit in switching between functional brain networks underlies the impact of multitasking on working memory in older adults. *Proceedings of the National Academy of Sciences USA 108*(17): 7212–7217.

Cohn, N. B., Dustman, R. E., and Bradford, D. C. (1984). Age-related decrements in Stroop color test-performance. *Journal of Clinical Psychology 40*: 1244–1250.

Colcombe, S. J., Kramer, A. F., Erickson, K. I., and Scalf, P. (2005). The implications of cortical recruitment and brain morphology for individual differences in inhibitory function in aging humans. *Psychology and Aging 20*: 363–375.

Colcombe, A. M., Kramer, A. F., Irwin, D. E., Peterson, M. S., Colcombe, S., and Hahn, S. (2003). Age-related effects of attentional and oculomotor capture by onsets and color singletons as a function of experience. *Acta Psychologica 113*: 205–225.

Comalli, P. E., Wapner, S., and Werner, H. (1962). Interference effects of Stroop color-word test on childhood, adulthood, and aging. *Journal of Genetic Psychology 100*: 47–53.

Connelly, S. L. and Hasher, L. (1993). Aging and the inhibition of spatial location. *Journal of Experimental Psychology: Human Perception and Performance 19*: 1238–1250.

Corbetta, M. and Shulman, G. L. (2002). Control of goal-directed and stimulus-driven attention in the brain. *Nature Reviews Neuroscience 3*: 201–215.

Corral, M., Rodriguez, M., Amenedo, E., Sanchez, J. L., and Diaz, F. (2006). Cognitive reserve, age, and neuropsychological performance in healthy participants. *Developmental Neuropsychology 29*: 479–491.

Costello, M. C., Madden, D. J., Shepler, A. M., Mitroff, S. R., and Leber, A. B. (2010). Age-related preservation of top-down control over distraction in visual search. *Experimental Aging Research 36*: 249–272.

Coubard, O. A., Ferrufino, L., Boura, M., Gripon, A., Renaud, M., and Bherer, L. (2011). Attentional control in normal aging and Alzheimer's disease. *Neuropsychology 25*: 353–367.

Coull, J. T. and Nobre, A. C. (1998). Where and when to pay attention: The neural systems for directing attention to spatial locations and to time intervals as revealed by both PET and fMRI. *Journal of Neuroscience 18*: 7426–7435.

Craft, J. L. and Simon, J. R. (1970). Processing symbolic information from a visual display: Interference from an irrelevant directional cue. *Journal of Experimental Psychology 83*: 415.

Craik, F. I. M. and Dirkx, E. (1992). Age-related differences in 3 tests of visual-imagery. *Psychology and Aging 7*: 661–665.

Crossman, E. R. and Szafran, J. (1956). Changes in age with the speed of information-intake and discrimination. *Experientia Supplementum 4*: 128–134.

Curran, T., Hills, A., Patterson, M. B., and Strauss, M. E. (2001). Effects of aging on visuospatial attention: An ERP study. *Neuropsychologia 39*: 288–301.

Damoiseaux, J. S., Beckmann, C. F., Arigita, E. J. S., Barkhof, F., Scheltens, P., Stam, C. J., Smith, S. M., and Rombouts, S. (2008). Reduced resting-state brain activity in the 'default network' in normal aging. *Cerebral Cortex 18*: 1856–1864.

Daselaar, S. and Cabeza, R. (2005). Age-related changes in hemispheric organization. In R. Cabeza, L. Nyberg, and D. Park (eds.), *Cognitive Neuroscience of Aging: Linking Cognitive and Cerebral Aging* (pp. 325–353). New York: Oxford University Press.

Davies, D. R. and Parasuraman, R. (1982). *The Psychology of Vigilance*. London: Academic Press.

Davis, S. W., Dennis, N. A., Daselaar, S. M., Fleck, M. S., and Cabeza, R. (2008). Que PASA? The posterior–anterior shift in aging. *Cerebral Cortex 18*: 1201–1209.

De Beni, R., Pazzaglia, F., and Gardini, S. (2007). The generation and maintenance of visual mental images: Evidence from image type and aging. *Brain and Cognition 63*: 271–278.

Deiber, M. P., Rodriguez, C., Jaques, D., Missonnier, P., Emch, J., Millet, P., Gold, G., Giannakopoulos, P., and Ibanez, V. (2010). Aging effects on selective attention-related electroencephalographic patterns during face encoding. *Neuroscience 171*: 173–186.

Dempster, F. N. (1992). The rise and fall of the inhibitory mechanism: Toward a unified theory of cognitive development and aging. *Developmental Review 12*: 45–75.

Diederich, A., Colonius, H., and Schomburg, A. (2008). Assessing age-related multisensory enhancement with the time-window-of-integration model. *Neuropsychologia 46*: 2556–2562.

DiGirolamo, G. J., Kramer, A. F., Barad, V., Cepeda, N. J., Weissman, D. H., Milham, M. P., Wszalek, T. M., Cohen, N. J., Banich, M. T., Webb, A., Belopolsky, A. V., and McAuley, E. (2001). General and task-specific frontal lobe recruitment in older adults during executive processes: A fMRI investigation of task-switching. *NeuroReport 12*: 2065–2071.

Dorbath, L., Hasselhorn, M., and Titz, C. (2011). Aging and executive functioning: A training study on focus-switching. *Frontiers in Psychology 2*: 257. doi: 10.3389/fpsyg.2011.00257.

Dorbath, L. and Titz, C. (2011). Dissociable age effects in focus-switching: Out of sight, out of mind. *GeroPsych 24*: 103–109.

Drag, L. L. and Bieliauskas, L. A. (2010). Contemporary review 2009: Cognitive aging. *Journal of Geriatric Psychiatry and Neurology 23*: 75–93.

Dror, I. E. and Kosslyn, S. M. (1994). Mental imagery and aging. *Psychology and Aging 9*: 90–102.

Duquesnoy, A. J. (1983). Effect of single interfering noise or speech source upon the binaural sentence intelligibility of aged persons. *Journal of the Acoustical Society of America 74*: 739–743.

Earles, J. L., Connor, L. T., Frieske, D., Park, D. C., Smith, A. D., and Zwahr, M. (1997). Age differences in inhibition: Possible causes and consequences. *Aging, Neuropsychology and Cognition 4*: 45–57.

Egly, R., Driver, J., and Rafal, R. D. (1994). Shifting visual-attention between objects and locations: Evidence from normal and parietal lesion subjects. *Journal of Experimental Psychology: General 123*: 161–177.

Einstein, G. O., Earles, J. L., and Collins, H. M. (2002). Gaze aversion: Spared inhibition for visual distraction in older adults. *Journals of Gerontology B: Psychological Sciences and Social Sciences 57*: P65–P73.

Ergenoglu, T., Demiralp, T., Bayraktaroglu, Z., Ergen, M., Beydagi, H., and Uresin, Y. (2004). Alpha rhythm of the EEG modulates visual detection performance in humans. *Cognitive Brain Research 20*: 376–383.

Erickson, K. I., Colcombe, S. J., Wadhwa, R., Bherer, L., Peterson, M. S., Scalf, P. E., Kim, J. S., Alvarado, M., and Kramer, A. F. (2007). Training-induced plasticity in older adults: Effects of training on hemispheric asymmetry. *Neurobiology of Aging 28*: 272–283.

Eriksen, B. A. and Eriksen, C. W. (1974). Effects of noise letters upon identification of a target letter in a nonsearch task. *Perception & Psychophysics 16*: 143–149.

Falkenstein, M., Hoormann, J., and Hohnsbein, J. (2001). Changes of error-related ERPs with age. *Experimental Brain Research 138*: 258–262.

Fernandes, M. A., Pacurar, A., Moscovitch, M., and Grady, C. (2006). Neural correlates of auditory recognition under full and divided attention in younger and older adults. *Neuropsychologia 44*: 2452–2464.

Fernandez-Duque, D. and Black, S. E. (2006). Attentional networks in normal aging and Alzheimer's disease. *Neuropsychology 20*: 133–143.

Filley, C. M. and Cullum, C. M. (1994). Attention and vigilance functions in normal aging. *Applied Neuropsychology 1*: 29–32.

Folk, C. L. and Hoyer, W. J. (1992). Aging and shifts of visual spatial attention. *Psychology and Aging 7*: 453–465.

Fortin, C. (2003). Attentional time-sharing in interval timing. In W. H. Meck (ed.), *Functional and Neural Mechanisms of Interval Timing* (pp. 235–259). Boca Raton, Fla.: CRC Press.

Gamboz, N., Russo, R., and Fox, E. (2002). Age differences and the identity negative priming effect: An updated meta-analysis. *Psychology and Aging 17*: 525–531.

Gazzaley, A. (2011). Influence of early attentional modulation on working memory. *Neuropsychologia 49*: 1410–1423.

Gazzaley, A. (2012). Top-down modulation deficit in the aging brain: An emerging theory of cognitive aging. In D. T. Stuss and R. T. Knight (eds.), *Principles of Frontal Lobe Function*, 2nd edn. (pp. 593–608). New York: Oxford University Press.

Gazzaley, A., Clapp, W., Kelley, J., McEvoy, K., Knight, R., and D'Esposito, M. (2008). Age-related top-down suppression deficit in the early stages of cortical visual memory processing. *Proceedings of the National Academy of Sciences USA 105*: 13122–13126.

Gazzaley, A., Cooney, J. W., Rissman, J., and D'Esposito, M. (2005). Top-down suppression deficit underlies working memory impairment in normal aging. *Nature Neuroscience 8*: 1298–1300.

Gazzaley, A. and Nobre, A. C. (2012). Top-down modulation: Bridging selective attention and working memory. *Trends in Cognitive Sciences 16*: 129–135.

Gazzaley, A., Rissman, J., Cooney, J., Rutman, A., Seibert, T., Clapp, W., and D'Esposito, M. (2007). Functional interactions between prefrontal and visual association cortex contribute to top-down modulation of visual processing. *Cerebral Cortex 17*: I125–I135.

Giambra, L. M. (1993). Sustained attention in older adults: Performance and processes. In J. Cerella, J. Rybash, W. Hoyer, and M. L. Commons (eds.), *Adult Information Processing: Limits on Loss* (pp. 259–272). San Diego: Academic Press.

Giambra, L. M. (1997). Sustained attention and aging: Overcoming the decrement? *Experimental Aging Research 23*: 145–161.

Glass, J. M., Schumacher, E. H., Lauber, E. J., Zurbriggen, E. L., Gmeindl, L., Kieras, D. E., and Meyer, D. E. (2000). Aging and the psychological refractory period: Task-coordination strategies in young and old adults. *Psychology and Aging 15*: 571–595.

Glisky, E. L. (2007). Changes in cognitive function in human aging. In D. R. Riddle (ed.), *Brain Aging: Models, Methods, and Mechanisms* (pp. 3–20). Boca Raton, Fla.: CRC Press.

Goffaux, P., Phillips, N. A., Sinai, M., and Pushkar, D. (2008). Neurophysiological measures of task-set switching: Effects of working memory and aging. *Journals of Gerontology B: Psychological Sciences and Social Sciences 63*: P57–P66.

Gooch, C. M., Stern, Y., and Rakitin, B. C. (2009). Evidence for age-related changes to temporal attention and memory from the choice time production task. *Neuropsychology, Development, and Cognition B: Aging, Neuropsychology, and Cognition 16*: 285–310.

Gootjes, L., Scheltens, P., Van Strien, J. W., and Bouma, A. (2007). Subcortical white matter pathology as a mediating factor for age-related decreased performance in dichotic listening. *Neuropsychologia 45*: 2322–2332.

Gootjes, L., Van Strien, J. W., and Bouma, A. (2004). Age effects in identifying and localising dichotic stimuli: A corpus callosum deficit? *Journal of Clinical and Experimental Neuropsychology 26*: 826–837.

Gottlob, L. R. and Madden, D. J. (1998). Time course of allocation of visual attention after equating for sensory differences: An age-related perspective. *Psychology and Aging* 13: 138–149.

Grady, C. L., Maisog, J. M., Horwitz, B., Ungerleider, L. G., Mentis, M. J., Salerno, J. A., Pietrini, P., Wagner, E., and Haxby, J. V. (1994). Age-related changes in cortical blood flow activation during visual processing of faces and location. *Journal of Neuroscience* 14: 1450–1462.

Grady, C. L., Protzner, A. B., Kovacevic, N., Strother, S. C., Afshin-Pour, B., Wojtowicz, M., Anderson, J. A. E., Churchill, N., and McIntosh, A. R. (2010). A multivariate analysis of age-related differences in default mode and task-positive networks across multiple cognitive domains. *Cerebral Cortex* 20: 1432–1447.

Guerreiro, M. J. S., Murphy, D. R., and Van Gerven, P. W. M. (2010). The role of sensory modality in age-related distraction: A critical review and a renewed view. *Psychological Bulletin* 136: 975–1022.

Guerreiro, M. J. and Van Gerven, P. W. (2011). Now you see it, now you don't: Evidence for age-dependent and age-independent cross-modal distraction. *Psychology and Aging* 26: 415–426.

Gunstad, J., Cohen, R. A., Paul, R. H., Luyster, F. S., and Gordon, E. (2006). Age effects in time estimation: Relationship to frontal brain morphometry. *Journal of Integrative Neuroscience* 5: 75–87.

Gusnard, D. A., Akbudak, E., Shulman, G. L., and Raichle, M. E. (2001). Medial prefrontal cortex and self-referential mental activity: Relation to a default mode of brain function. *Proceedings of the National Academy of Sciences USA* 98: 4259–4264.

Hahn, M., Falkenstein, M., and Wild-Wall, N. (2010). Age-related performance differences in compensatory tracking under a dual task condition. *Occupational Ergonomics* 9: 75–8686.

Hahn, S. and Kramer, A. F. (1995). Attentional flexibility and aging: You don't need to be 20 years of age to split the beam. *Psychology and Aging* 10: 597–609.

Hallgren, M., Larsby, B., Lyxell, B., and Arlinger, S. (2001). Cognitive effects in dichotic speech testing in elderly persons. *Ear and Hearing* 22: 120–129.

Hampshire, A., Gruszka, A., Fallon, S. J., and Owen, A. M. (2008). Inefficiency in self-organized attentional switching in the normal aging population is associated with decreased activity in the ventrolateral prefrontal cortex. *Journal of Cognitive Neuroscience* 20: 1670–1686.

Handy, T. C., Soltani, M., and Mangun, G. R. (2001). Perceptual load and visuocortical processing: Event-related potentials reveal sensory-level selection. *Psychological Science* 12: 213–218.

Hanslmayr, S., Aslan, A., Staudigl, T., Klimesch, W., Herrmann, C. S., and Bauml, K. H. (2007). Prestimulus oscillations predict between and within subjects. *NeuroImage* 37: 1465–1473.

Hartley, A. A. (1992). Attention. In F. I. Craik and T. A. Salthouse (eds.), *The Handbook of Aging and Cognition* (pp. 3–50). Hillsdale, N.J.: Lawrence Erlbaum Associates.

Hartley, A. A. (1993). Evidence for the selective preservation of spatial selective attention in old-age. *Psychology and Aging* 8: 371–379.

Hartley, A. A., Jonides, J., and Sylvester, C. Y. C. (2011). Dual-task processing in younger and older adults: Similarities and differences revealed by fMRI. *Brain and Cognition* 75: 281–291.

Hartley, A. A., Kieley, J. M., and Slabach, E. H. (1990). Age differences and similarities in the effects of cues and prompts. *Journal of Experimental Psychology: Human Perception and Performance* 16: 523–537.

Hartley, A. A. and Little, D. M. (1999). Age-related differences and similarities in dual-task interference. *Journal of Experimental Psychology: General* 128: 416–449.

Hasbroucq, T. and Guiard, Y. (1992). The effects of intensity and irrelevant location of a tactile stimulation in a choice reaction-time-task. *Neuropsychologia* 30: 91–94.

Hasher, L., Lustig, C., and Zacks, J. M. (2007). Inhibitory mechanisms and the control of attention. In A. Conway, C. Jarrold, M. Kane, A. Miyake, and J. Towse (eds.), *Variation in Working Memory* (pp. 227–249). New York: Oxford University Press.

Hasher, L., Stoltzfus, E. R., Zacks, R. T., and Rypma, B. (1991). Age and inhibition. *Journal of Experimental Psychology: Learning, Memory, and Cognition* 17: 163–169.

Hasher, L. and Zacks, R. T. (1988). Working memory, comprehension and aging: A review and a new view. In G. H. Bower (ed.), *The Psychology of Learning and Motivation* (pp. 193–225). New York: Academic Press.

Hasher, L., Zacks, R. T., and May, C. P. (1999). Inhibitory control, circadian arousal, and age. In D. Gopher and A. Koriat (eds.), *Attention and Performance: Cognitive Regulation of Performance—Interaction of Theory and Application* (vol. 15, pp. 653–675). Cambridge, Mass.: MIT Press.

Hawkins, H. L., Kramer, A. F., and Capaldi, D. (1992). Aging, exercise, and attention. *Psychology and Aging* 7: 643–653.

Helfer, K. S., Chevalier, J., and Freyman, R. L. (2010). Aging, spatial cues, and single- versus dual-task performance in competing speech perception. *Journal of the Acoustical Society of America* 128: 3625–3633.

Helfer, K. S. and Freyman, R. L. (2008). Aging and speech-on-speech masking. *Ear and Hearing* 29: 87–98.

Hillyard, S. A. (1969). Relationships between contingent negative variation (CNV) and reaction time. *Physiology & Behavior* 4: 351.

Hommel, B., Li, K. Z. H., and Li, S. C. (2004). Visual search across the life span. *Developmental Psychology* 40: 545–558.

Hommet, C., Mondon, K., Berrut, G., Gouyer, Y., Isingrini, M., Constans, T., and Belzung, C. (2010). Central auditory processing in aging: The dichotic listening paradigm. *Journal of Nutrition, Health & Aging* 14: 751–756.

Hugenschmidt, C. E., Peiffer, A. M., McCoy, T. P., Hayasaka, S., and Laurienti, P. J. (2009). Preservation of crossmodal selective attention in healthy aging. *Experimental Brain Research* 198: 273–285.

Humes, L. E., Lee, J. H., and Coughlin, M. P. (2006). Auditory measures of selective and divided attention in young and older adults using single-talker competition. *Journal of the Acoustical Society of America* 120: 2926–2937.

Iarocci, G., Enns, J. T., Randolph, B., and Burack, J. A. (2009). The modulation of visual orienting reflexes across the lifespan. *Developmental Science* 12: 715–724.

James, W. (1890). *The Principles of Psychology*. New York: Holt.

Johannsen, P., Jakobsen, J., Bruhn, P., Hansen, S. B., Gee, A., Stodkilde-Jorgensen, H., and Gjedde, A. (1997). Cortical sites of sustained and divided attention in normal elderly humans. *NeuroImage* 6: 145–155.

Johnson, R. C., Cole, R. E., Bowers, J. K., Foiles, S. V., Nikaido, A. M., Patrick, J. W., and Woliver, R. E. (1979). Hemispheric efficiency in middle and later adulthood. *Cortex* 15: 109–119.

Juncos-Rabadán, O., Pereiro, A. X., and Facal, D. (2008). Cognitive interference and aging: Insights from a spatial stimulus-response consistency task. *Acta Psychologica* 127: 237–246.

Juola, J. F., Koshino, H., Warner, C. B., M.Mckell, M., and Peterson, M. (2000). Automatic and voluntary control of attention in young and older adults. *American Journal of Psychology* 113: 159–178.

Kalkstein, J., Checksfield, K., Bollinger, J., and Gazzaley, A. (2011). Diminished top-down control underlies a visual imagery deficit in normal aging. *Journal of Neuroscience* 31: 15768–15774.

Kamijo, K., Hayashi, Y., Sakai, T., Yahiro, T., Tanaka, K., and Nishihira, Y. (2009). Acute effects of aerobic exercise on cognitive function in older adults. *Journals of Gerontology B: Psychological Sciences and Social Sciences* 64: 356–363.

Kawai, N. and Kubo-Kawai, N. (2010). Elimination of the enhanced Simon effect for older adults in a three-choice situation: Ageing and the Simon effect in a go/no-go Simon task. *Quarterly Journal of Experimental Psychology* 63: 452–464.

Kenemans, J. L., Smulders, F. T. Y., and Kok, A. (1995). Selective processing of 2-dimensional visual-stimuli in young and old subjects: Electrophysiological analysis. *Psychophysiology* 32: 108–120.

Kerr, B., Condon, S. M., and McDonald, L. A. (1985). Cognitive spatial processing and the regulation of posture. *Journal of Experimental Psychology: Human Perception and Performance* 11: 617–622.

Keskinen, E., Ota, H., and Katila, A. (1998). Older drivers fail in intersections: Speed discrepancies between older and younger male drivers. *Accident: Analysis and Prevention* 30: 323–330.

Kim, S., Hasher, L., and Zacks, R. T. (2007). Aging and a benefit of distractibility. *Psychonomic Bulletin & Review* 14: 301–305.

Kimberg, D. Y., Aguirre, G. K., and D'Esposito, M. (2000). Modulation task-related neural activity in task-switching: An fMRI study. *Cognitive Brain Research* 10: 189–196.

Klein, M., Ponds, R. W. H. M., Houx, P. J., and Jolles, J. (1997). Effect of test duration on age-related differences in Stroop interference. *Journal of Clinical and Experimental Neuropsychology* 19: 77–82.

Koch, W., Teipel, S., Mueller, S., Buerger, K., Bokde, A. L. W., Hampel, H., Coates, U., Reiser, M., and Meindl, T. (2010). Effects of aging on default mode network activity in resting state fMRI: Does the method of analysis matter? *NeuroImage* 51: 280–287.

Kok, A. (2000). Age-related changes in involuntary and voluntary attention as reflected in components of the event-related potential (ERP). *Biological Psychology* 54: 107–143.

Kosslyn, S. M., Pascual-Leone, A., Felician, O., Camposano, S., Keenan, J. P., Thompson, W. L., Ganis, G., Sukel, K. E., and Alpert, N. M. (1999). The role of area 17 in visual imagery: Convergent evidence from PET and rTMS. *Science* 284: 167–170.

Kosslyn, S. M., Thompson, W. L., and Alpert, N. M. (1997). Neural systems shared by visual imagery and visual perception: A positron emission tomography study. *NeuroImage* 6: 320–334.

Kramer, A. F., Hahn, S., and Gopher, D. (1999a). Task coordination and aging: Explorations of executive control processes in the task switching paradigm. *Acta Psychologica* 101: 339–378.

Kramer, A. F., Hahn, S., Irwin, D. E., and Theeuwes, J. (1999b). Attentional capture and aging: Implications for visual search performance and oculomotor control. *Psychology and Aging* 14: 135–154.

Kramer, A. F., Hahn, S., Irwin, D. E., and Theeuwes, J. (2000). Age differences in the control of looking behavior: Do you know where your eyes have been? *Psychological Science* 11: 210–217.

Kramer, A. F., Humphrey, D. G., Larish, J. F., Logan, G. D., and Strayer, D. L. (1994). Aging and inhibition: Beyond a unitary view of inhibitory processing in attention. *Psychology and Aging* 9: 491–512.

Kramer, A. F. and Larish, J. (1996). Aging and dual-task performance. In W. R. Rogers, A. D. Fisk, and N. Walker (eds.), *Aging and Skilled Performance* (pp. 83–112). Hillsdale, N.J.: Lawrence Erlbaum Associates.

Kramer A. F. and Madden D. J. (2008). Attention. In F. I. Craik and T. A. Salthouse (eds.), *The Handbook of Aging and Cognition*, 3rd edn. (pp. 189–250). New York: Psychology Press.

Kray, J. (2006). Task-set switching under cue-based versus memory-based switching conditions in younger and older adults. *Brain Research 1105*: 83–92.

Kray, J., Li, K. Z. H., and Lindenberger, U. (2002). Age-related changes in task-switching components: The role of task uncertainty. *Brain and Cognition 49*: 363–381.

Kray, J. and Lindenberger, U. (2000). Adult age differences in task switching. *Psychology and Aging 15*: 126–147.

Langley, L. K., Friesen, C. K., Saville, A. L., and Ciernia, A. T. (2011). Timing of reflexive visuospatial orienting in young, young-old, and old-old adults. *Attention, Perception, & Psychophysics 73*: 1546–1561.

Laurienti, P. J., Burdette, J. H., Maldjian, J. A., and Wallace, M. T. (2006). Enhanced multisensory integration in older adults. *Neurobiology of Aging 27*: 1155–1163.

Lavie, N., Hirst, A., de Fockert, J. W., and Viding, E. (2004). Load theory of selective attention and cognitive control. *Journal of Experimental Psychology: General 133*: 339–354.

Lavie, N. and Tsal, Y. (1994). Perceptual load as a major determinant of the locus of selection in visual-attention. *Perception & Psychophysics 56*: 183–197.

Leber, A. B. and Egeth, H. E. (2006). It's under control: Top-down search strategies can override attentional capture. *Psychonomic Bulletin & Review 13*: 132–138.

Leuthold, H. and Schroter, H. (2006). Electrophysiological evidence for response priming and conflict regulation in the auditory Simon task. *Brain Research 1097*: 167–180.

Li, L., Daneman, M., Qi, J. G., and Schneider, B. A. (2004). Does the information content of an irrelevant source differentially affect spoken word recognition in younger and older adults? *Journal of Experimental Psychology: Human Perception and Performance 30*: 1077–1091.

Li, S. C. (2005). Neurocomputational perspectives linking neuromodulation, processing noise, representational distinctiveness, and cognitive aging. In R. Cabeza, L. Nyberg, and D. Park (eds.), *Cognitive Neuroscience of Aging: Linking Cognitive and Cerebral Aging* (pp. 354–379). New York: Oxford University Press.

Li, S. C., Lindenberger, U., and Sikstrom, S. (2001). Aging cognition: From neuromodulation to representation. *Trends in Cognitive Sciences 5*: 479–486.

Lincourt, A. E., Folk, C. L., and Hoyer, W. J. (1997). Effects of aging on voluntary and involuntary shifts of attention. *Aging, Neuropsychology, and Cognition 4*: 290–303.

Lindenberger, U. and Baltes, P. B. (1994). Sensory functioning and intelligence in old age: A strong connection. *Psychology and Aging 9*: 339–355.

Lindenberger, U., Kliegl, R., and Baltes, P. B. (1992). Professional expertise does not eliminate age differences in imagery-based memory performance during adulthood. *Psychology and Aging 7*: 585–593.

Lorenzo-Lopez, L., Amenedo, E., and Cadaveira, F. (2008a). Feature processing during visual search in normal aging: Electrophysiological evidence. *Neurobiology of Aging 29*: 1101–1110.

Lorenzo-Lopez, L., Amenedo, E., Pascual-Marqui, R. D., and Cadaveira, F. (2008b). Neural correlates of age-related visual search decline: A combined ERP and sLORETA study. *NeuroImage 41*: 511–524.

Lorenzo-Lopez, L., Doallo, S., Vizoso, C., Amenedo, E., Holguin, S. R., and Cadaveira, F. (2002). Covert orienting of visuospatial attention in the early stages of aging. *NeuroReport 13*: 1459–1462.

Lustig, C. (2003). Grandfather's clock: Attention and interval timing in older adults. In W. H. Meck (ed.), *Functional and Neural Mechanisms of Interval Timing* (pp. 261–293). Boca Raton, Fla.: CRC Press.

Lustig, C., Snyder, A. Z., Bhakta, M., O'Brien, K. C., McAvoy, M., Raichle, M. E., Morris, J. C., and Buckner, R. L. (2003). Functional deactivations: Change with age and dementia of the Alzheimer type. *Proceedings of the National Academy of Sciences USA 100*: 14504–14509.

McDowd, J.M. and Craik, F. I. (1988). Effects of aging and task difficulty on divided attention performance. *Journal of Experimental Psychology: Human Perception and Performance 14*: 267–280.

McDowd, J. M. and Shaw, R. J. (2000). Attention and aging: A functional perspective. In F. I. Craik and T. A. Salthouse (eds.), *Handbook of Aging and Cognition*, 2nd edn. (pp. 221–292). Hillsdale, N.J.: Lawrence Erlbaum Associates.

McLaughlin, P. M., Szostak, C., Binns, M. A., Craik, F. I. M., Tipper, S. P., and Stuss, D. T. (2010). The effects of age and task demands on visual selective attention. *Canadian Journal of Experimental Psychology/Revue Canadienne de Psychologie Experimentale 64*: 197–207.

Madden, D. J. (2007). Aging and visual attention. *Current Directions in Psychological Science 16*: 70–74.

Madden, D. J., Blumenthal, J. A., Allen, P. A., and Emery, C. F. (1989). Improving aerobic capacity in healthy older adults does not necessarily lead to improved cognitive performance. *Psychology and Aging 4*: 307–320.

Madden, D. J., Costello, M. C., Dennis, N. A., Davis, S. W., Shepler, A. M., Spaniol, J., Bucur, B., and Cabeza, R. (2010). Adult age differences in functional connectivity during executive control. *NeuroImage 52*: 643–657.

Madden, D. J. and Gottlob, L. R. (1997). Adult age differences in strategic and dynamic components of focusing visual attention. *Aging, Neuropsychology, and Cognition 4*: 185–210.

Madden, D. J. and Langley, L. K. (2003). Age-related changes in selective attention and perceptual load during visual search. *Psychology and Aging 18*: 54–67.

Madden, D. J., Spaniol, J., Bucur, B., and Whiting, W. L. (2007a). Age-related increase in top-down activation of visual features. *Quarterly Journal of Experimental Psychology 60*: 644–651.

Madden, D. J., Spaniol, J., Whiting, W. L., Bucur, B., Provenzale, J. M., Cabeza, R., White, L. E., and Huettel, S. A. (2007b). Adult age differences in the functional neuroanatomy of visual attention: A combined fMRI and DTI study. *Neurobiology of Aging 28*: 459–476.

Madden, D. J., Turkington, T. G., Provenzale, J. M., Denny, L. L., Langley, L. K., Hawk, T. C., and Coleman, R. E. (2002). Aging and attentional guidance during visual search: Functional neuroanatomy by positron emission tomography. *Psychology and Aging 17*: 24–43.

Madden, D. J. and Whiting, W. L. (2004). Age-related changes in visual attention. In P. T. Costa and I. C. Siegler (eds.), *Recent Advances in Psychology and Aging* (pp. 41–88). Amsterdam: Elsevier.

Madden, D. J., Whiting, W. L., Cabeza, R., and Huettel, S. A. (2004). Age-related preservation of top-down attentional guidance during visual search. *Psychology and Aging 19*: 304–309.

Madden, D. J., Whiting, W. L., Spaniol, J., and Bucur, B. (2005). Adult age differences in the implicit and explicit components of top-down attentional guidance during visual search. *Psychology and Aging 20*: 317–329.

Malouin, F., Richards, C. L., Jackson, P. L., Dumas, F., and Doyon, J. (2003). Brain activations during motor imagery of locomotor-related tasks: A PET study. *Human Brain Mapping 19*: 47–62.

Mani, T. M., Bedwell, J. S., and Miller, L. S. (2005). Age-related decrements in performance on a brief continuous performance test. *Archives of Clinical Neuropsychology* 20: 575–586.

Mapstone, M., Dickerson, K., and Duffy, C. J. (2008). Distinct mechanisms of impairment in cognitive ageing and Alzheimer's disease. *Brain* 131: 1618–1629.

Martin, J. S. and Jerger, J. F. (2005). Some effects of aging on central auditory processing. *Journal of Rehabilitation Research and Development* 42: 25–44.

Mason, M. F., Norton, M. I., Van Horn, J. D., Wegner, D. M., Grafton, S. T., and Macrae, C. N. (2007). Wandering minds: The default network and stimulus-independent thought. *Science* 315: 393–395.

Mathewson, K. J., Dywan, J., and Segalowitz, S. J. (2005). Brain bases of error-related ERPs as influenced by age and task. *Biological Psychology* 70: 88–104.

Maylor, E. A. and Lavie, N. (1998). The influence of perceptual load on age differences in selective attention. *Psychology and Aging* 13: 563–573.

Mayr, U. and Kliegl, R. (2000). Task-set switching and long-term memory retrieval. *Journal of Experimental Psychology: Learning, Memory, and Cognition* 26: 1124–1140.

Mayr, U. and Liebscher, T. (2001). Is there an age deficit in the selection of mental sets? *European Journal of Cognitive Psychology* 13: 47–69.

Mechelli, A., Price, C. J., Friston, K. J., and Ishai, A. (2004). Where bottom-up meets top-down: Neuronal interactions during perception and imagery. *Cerebral Cortex* 14: 1256–1265.

Meijer, W. A., de Groot, R. H. M., Van Boxtel, M. P. J., Van Gerven, P. W. M., and Jolles, J. (2006). Verbal learning and aging: Combined effects of irrelevant speech, interstimulus interval, and education. *Journals of Gerontology B: Psychological Sciences and Social Sciences* 61: P285–P294.

Miniussi, C., Wilding, E. L., Coull, J. T., and Nobre, A. C. (1999). Orienting attention in time: Modulation of brain potentials. *Brain* 122: 1507–1518.

Mouloua, M. and Parasuraman, R. (1995). Aging and cognitive vigilance: Effects of spatial uncertainty and event rate. *Experimental Aging Research* 21: 17–32.

Munsell, O. S. (1873). *Psychology; or, The Science of Mind*. New York: D. Appleton.

Nagamatsu, L. S., Carolan, P., Liu-Ambrose, T. Y. L., and Handy, T. C. (2011). Age-related changes in the attentional control of visual cortex: A selective problem in the left visual hemifield. *Neuropsychologia* 49: 1670–1678.

Nagamatsu, L. S., Liu-Ambrose, T. Y. L., Carolan, P., and Handy, T. C. (2009). Are impairments in visual-spatial attention a critical factor for increased falls risk in seniors? An event-related potential study. *Neuropsychologia* 47: 2749–2755.

Neider, M. B., Gaspar, J. G., McCarley, J. S., Crowell, J. A., Kaczmarski, H., and Kramer, A. F. (2011). Walking and talking: Dual-task effects on street crossing behavior in older adults. *Psychology and Aging* 26: 260–268.

Nissen, M. J. and Corkin, S. (1985). Effectiveness of attentional cueing in older and younger adults. *Journal of Gerontology* 40: 185–191.

Nobre, A. C., Correa, A., and Coull, J. T. (2007). The hazards of time. *Current Opinion in Neurobiology* 17: 465–470.

Nobre, A. C., Rao, A. L., and Chelazzi, L. (2006). Selective attention to specific features within objects: Behavioral and electrophysiological evidence. *Journal of Cognitive Neuroscience* 18: 539–561.

Northoff, G., Heinzel, A., Greck, M., Bennpohl, F., Dobrowolny, H., and Panksepp, J. (2006). Self-referential processing in our brain: A meta-analysis of imaging studies on the self. *NeuroImage* 31: 440–457.

O'Craven, K. M. and Kanwisher, N. (2000). Mental imagery of faces and places activates corresponding stimulus-specific brain regions. *Journal of Cognitive Neuroscience* 12: 1013–1023.

Olk, B., Cameron, B., and Kingstone, A. (2008). Enhanced orienting effects: Evidence for an interaction principle. *Visual Cognition* 16: 979–1000.

Parasuraman, R. (1998). The attentive brain: Issues and prospects. In R. Parasuraman (ed.), *The Attentive Brain* (pp. 3–15). Cambridge, Mass.: MIT Press.

Parasuraman, R. and Giambra, L. (1991). Skill development in vigilance: Effects of event rate and age. *Psychology and Aging* 6: 155–169.

Parasuraman, R., Nestor, P., and Greenwood, P. (1989). Sustained-attention capacity in young and older adults. *Psychology and Aging* 4: 339–345.

Park, D. C., Polk, T. A., Park, R., Minear, M., Savage, A., and Smith, M. R. (2004). Aging reduces neural specialization in ventral visual cortex. *Proceedings of the National Academy of Sciences USA 101*: 13091–13095.

Park, D. C. and Reuter-Lorenz, P. (2009). The adaptive brain: Aging and neurocognitive scaffolding. *Annual Review of Psychology 60*: 173–196.

Peiffer, A. M., Hugenschmidt, C. E., Maldjian, J. A., Casanova, R., Srikanth, R., Hayasaka, S., Burdette, J. H., Kraft, R. A., and Laurienti, P. J. (2009). Aging and the interaction of sensory cortical function and structure. *Human Brain Mapping 30*: 228–240.

Peiffer, A. M., Mozolic, J. L., Hugenschmidt, C. E., and Laurienti, P. J. (2007). Age-related multisensory enhancement in a simple audiovisual detection task. *NeuroReport 18*: 1077–1081.

Persson, J., Lustig, C., Nelson, J. K., and Reuter-Lorenz, P. A. (2007). Age differences in deactivation: A link to cognitive control? *Journal of Cognitive Neuroscience 19*: 1021–1032.

Pick, D. F. and Proctor, R. W. (1999). Age differences in the effects of irrelevant location information. In M. Scerbo and M. W. Mouloua (eds.), *Automation Technology and Human Performance* (pp. 258–261). Mahwah, N.J.: Lawrence Erlbaum Associates.

Plude, D. J. and Doussard-Roosevelt, J. A. (1989). Aging, selective attention, and feature integration. *Psychology and Aging 4*: 98–105.

Posner, M. I. (1980). Orienting of attention. *Quarterly Journal of Experimental Psychology* 32: 3–25.

Praamstra, P., Kourtis, D., Kwok, H. F., and Oostenveld, R. (2006). Neurophysiology of implicit timing in serial choice reaction-time performance. *Journal of Neuroscience 26*: 5448–5455.

Pratt, J. and Bellomo, C. N. (1999). Attentional capture in younger and older adults. *Aging, Neuropsychology, and Cognition 6*: 19–31.

Proctor, R. W., Pick, D. F., Vu, K. P. L., and Anderson, R. E. (2005). The enhanced Simon effect for older adults is reduced when the irrelevant location information is conveyed by an accessory stimulus. *Acta Psychologica 119*: 21–40.

Quigley, C., Andersen, S. K., Schulze, L., Grunwald, M., and Muller, M. M. (2010). Feature-selective attention: Evidence for a decline in old age. *Neuroscience Letters 474*: 5–8.

Rabbitt, P., Lunn, M., Pendleton, N., Horan, M., Scott, M., Thacker, N., Lowe, C., and Jackson, A. (2007a). White matter lesions account for all age-related declines in speed but not in intelligence. *Neuropsychology 21*: 363–370.

Rabbitt, P., Mogapi, O., Scott, M., Thacker, N., Lowe, C., Horan, M., Pendleton, N., Jackson, A., and Lunn, D. (2007b). Effects of global atrophy, white matter lesions, and cerebral blood flow on age-related changes in speed, memory, intelligence, vocabulary, and frontal function. *Neuropsychology 21*: 684–695.

Raz, N., Briggs, S. D., Marks, W., and Acker J. D. (1999). Age-related deficits in generation and manipulation of mental images. II: The role of dorsolateral prefrontal cortex. *Psychology and Aging* 14: 436–444.

Rees, G., Frith, C. D., and Lavie, N. (1997). Modulating irrelevant motion perception by varying attentional load in an unrelated task. *Science* 278: 1616–1619.

Reuter-Lorenz, P. A. and Cappell, K. A. (2008). Neurocognitive aging and the compensation hypothesis. *Current Directions in Psychological Science* 17: 177–182.

Reuter-Lorenz, P. A., Jonides, J., Smith, E. E., Hartley, A., Miller, A., Marshuetz, C., and Koeppe, R. A. (2000). Age differences in the frontal lateralization of verbal and spatial working memory revealed by PET. *Journal of Cognitive Neuroscience* 12: 174–187.

Reuter-Lorenz, P. A. and Lustig, C. (2005). Brain aging: Reorganizing discoveries about the aging mind. *Current Opinion in Neurobiology* 15: 245–251.

Reuter-Lorenz, P. A. and Mikels, J. A. (2006). The aging mind and brain: Implication of enduring plasticity for behavioral and cultural change. In P. Baltes, P.A. Reuter-Lorenz, and F. Roesler (eds.), *Lifespan Development and the Brain: The Perspective of Biocultural Co-constructivism* (pp. 255–276). Cambridge: Cambridge University Press.

Ristic, J. and Kingstone, A. (2006). Attention to arrows: Pointing to a new direction. *Quarterly Journal of Experimental Psychology* 59: 1921–1930.

Rodriguez, V., Valdes-Sosa, M., and Freiwald, W. (2002). Dividing attention between form and motion during transparent surface perception. *Cognitive Brain Research* 13: 187–193.

Rogers, R. D., Sahakian, B. J., Hodges, J. R., Polkey, C. E., Kennard, C., and Robbins, T. W. (1998). Dissociating executive mechanisms of task control following frontal lobe damage and Parkinson's disease. *Brain* 121: 815–842.

Rogers, W. (2000). Attention and aging. In D. Park and N. Schwarz (eds.), *Cognitive Aging: A Primer* (pp. 57–73). New York: Psychology Press.

Rorden, C., Guerrini, C., Swainson, R., Lazzeri, M., and Baylis, G. C. (2008). Event related potentials reveal that increasing perceptual load leads to increased responses for target stimuli and decreased responses for irrelevant stimuli. *Frontiers in Human Neuroscience* 2: 4. doi: 10.3389/neuro.09.004.2008.

Rosselli, M. and Salvatierra, J. L. (2011). The effect of bilingualism and age on inhibitory control. *International Journal of Bilingualism* 15: 26–37.

Rossi-Katz, J. and Arehart, K. H. (2009). Message and talker identification in older adults: Effects of task, distinctiveness of the talkers' voices, and meaningfulness of the competing message. *Journal of Speech, Language, and Hearing Research* 52: 435–453.

Rouleau, N. and Belleville, S. (1996). Irrelevant speech effect in aging: An assessment of inhibitory processes in working memory. *Journals of Gerontology B: Psychological Sciences and Social Sciences* 51: P356–P363.

Rushworth, M. F. S., Hadland, K. A., Paus, T., and Sipila, P. K. (2002). Role of the human medial frontal cortex in task switching: A combined fMRI and TMS study. *Journal of Neurophysiology* 87: 2577–2592.

Rypma, B. and D'Esposito, M. (2000). Isolating the neural mechanisms of age-related changes in human working memory. *Nature Neuroscience* 3: 509–515.

Salthouse, T. A. (1985). Speed of behavior and its implications for cognition. In J. E. Birren and K. W. Schaie (eds.), *Handbook of the Psychology of Aging* (pp. 400–426). New York: Van Nostrand Reinhold.

Salthouse, T. A. (1996). The processing-speed theory of adult age differences in cognition. *Psychological Review* 103: 403–428.

Salthouse, T. A. (2000). Aging and measures of processing speed. *Biological Psychology* 54: 35–54.

Salthouse, T. A., Fristoe, B. N., and Rhee, S. H. (1996a). How localized are age-related effects on neuropsychological measures? *Neuropsychology* 10: 272–285.

Salthouse, T. A., Hancock, H. E., Meinz, E. J., and Hambrick, D. Z. (1996b). Interrelations of age, visual acuity, and cognitive functioning. *Journals of Gerontology B: Psychological Sciences and Social Sciences* 51: P317–330.

Salthouse, T. A. and Madden, D. J. (2007). Information processing speed and aging. In J. Deluca and J. Kalmar (eds.), *Information Processing Speed in Clinical Populations* (pp. 221–241). New York: Psychology Press.

Salthouse, T. A. and Meinz, E. J. (1995). Aging, inhibition, working-memory, and speed. *Journals of Gerontology B: Psychological Sciences and Social Sciences* 50: P297–P306.

Salthouse, T. A., Rogan, J. D., and Prill, K. A. (1984). Division of attention: Age differences on a visually presented memory task. *Memory & Cognition* 12: 613–620.

Salthouse, T. A., Toth, J., Daniels, K., Parks, C., Pak, R., Wolbrette, M., and Hocking, K. J. (2000). Effects of aging on efficiency of task switching in a variant of the trail making test. *Neuropsychology* 14: 102–111.

Samanez-Larkin, G. R., Robertson, E. R., Mikels, J. A., Carstensen, L. L., and Gotlib, I. H. (2009). Selective attention to emotion in the aging brain. *Psychology and Aging* 24: 519–529.

Sambataro, F., Murty, V. P., Callicott, J. H., Tan, H. Y., Das, S., Weinberger, D. R., and Mattay, V. S. (2010). Age-related alterations in default mode network: Impact on working memory performance. *Neurobiology of Aging* 31: 839–852.

Sarter, M. and Bruno, J. P. (2004). Developmental origins of the age-related decline in cortical cholinergic function and associated cognitive abilities. *Neurobiology of Aging* 25: 1127–1139.

Schmitz, T. W., Cheng, F. H. T., and De Rosa, E. (2010). Failing to ignore: Paradoxical neural effects of perceptual load on early attentional selection in normal aging. *Journal of Neuroscience* 30: 14750–14758.

Schneider, B. A. and Pichora-Fuller, M. K. (2000). Implication of perceptual deterioration for cognitive aging research. In F. I. Craik and T. A. Salthouse (eds.), *The Handbook of Aging and Cognition*, 2nd edn. (pp. 155–219). Mahwah, N.J.: Lawrence Erlbaum Associates.

Schooler, C., Neumann, E., Caplan, L. J., and Roberts, B. R. (1997). Continued inhibitory capacity throughout adulthood: Conceptual negative priming in younger and older adults. *Psychology and Aging* 12: 667–674.

Sekuler, R., McLaughlin, C., and Yotsumoto, Y. (2008). Age-related changes in attentional tracking of multiple moving objects. *Perception* 37: 867–876.

Sheridan, P. L. and Hausdorff, J. M. (2007). The role of higher-level cognitive function in gait: Executive dysfunction contributes to fall risk in Alzheimer's disease. *Dementia and Geriatric Cognitive Disorders* 24: 125–137.

Simon, J. R. (1969). Reactions toward the source of stimulation. *Journal of Experimental Psychology* 81: 174–176.

Simon, J. R., Craft, J. L., and Webster, J. B. (1971). Reaction time to onset and offset of lights and tones: Reactions toward changed element in a 2-element display. *Journal of Experimental Psychology* 89: 197–202.

Simon, J. R. and Pouraghabagher, A. R. (1978). The effect of aging on the status of processing in a choice reaction time task. *Journal of Gerontology* 33: 553–561.

Simone, P. M. and McCormick, E. B. (1999). Effect of a defining feature on negative priming across the life span. *Visual Cognition* 6: 587–606.

Singh, G., Pichora-Fuller, M. K., and Schneider, B. A. (2008). The effect of age on auditory spatial attention in conditions of real and simulated spatial separation. *Journal of the Acoustical Society of America* 124: 1294–1305.

Smith, E. E., Geva, A., Jonides, J., Miller, A., Reuter-Lorenz, P., and Koeppe, R. A. (2001). The neural basis of task-switching in working memory: Effects of performance and aging. *Proceedings of the National Academy of Sciences USA* 98: 2095–2100.

Solbakk, A. K., Alpert, G. F., Furst, A. J., Hale, L. A., Oga, T., Chetty, S., Pickard, N., and Knight, R. T. (2008). Altered prefrontal function with aging: Insights into age-associated performance decline. *Brain Research* 1232: 30–47.

Somberg, B. L. and Salthouse, T. A. (1982). Divided attention abilities in young and old adults. *Journal of Experimental Psychology: Human Perception and Performance* 8: 651–663.

Sommers, M. S. (1996). The structural organization of the mental lexicon and its contribution to age-related declines in spoken-word recognition. *Psychology and Aging* 11: 333–341.

Sommers, M. S. and Danielson, S. M. (1999). Inhibitory processes and spoken word recognition in young and older adults: The interaction of lexical competition and semantic context. *Psychology and Aging* 14: 458–472.

Sommers, M. S. and Huff, L. M. (2003). The effects of age and dementia of the Alzheimer's type on phonological false memories. *Psychology and Aging* 18: 791–806.

Spieler, D. H., Balota, D. A., and Faust, M. E. (1996). Stroop performance in healthy younger and older adults and in individuals with dementia of the Alzheimer's type. *Journal of Experimental Psychology: Human Perception and Performance* 22: 461–479.

Stegemoller, E. L., Simuni, T., and MacKinnon, C. D. (2009). The effects of Parkinson's disease and age on syncopated finger movements. *Brain Research* 1290: 12–20.

Stern, Y. (2002). What is cognitive reserve? Theory and research application of the reserve concept. *Journal of the International Neuropsychological Society* 8: 448–460.

Stern, Y., Habeck, C., Moeller, J., Scarmeas, N., Anderson, K. E., Hilton, H. J., Flynn, J., Sackeim, H., and van Heertum, R. (2005). Brain networks associated with cognitive reserve in healthy young and old adults. *Cerebral Cortex* 15: 394–402.

Stormer, V. S., Li, S. C., Heekeren, H. R., and Lindenberger, U. (2011). Feature-based interference from unattended visual field during attentional tracking in younger and older adults. *Journal of Vision* 11(2): 1.1–12

Strong, R. (1988). Regionally selective manifestations of neostriatal aging. *Annals of the New York Academy of Sciences* 515: 161–177.

Stroop, J. R. (1935). Studies of interference in serial verbal reactions. *Journal of Experimental Psychology* 18: 643–662.

Sullivan, M. P., Faust, M. E., and Balota, D. (1995). Identity negative priming in older adults and individuals with dementia of the Alzheimer-type. *Neuropsychology* 9: 537–555.

Tales, A., Muir, J. L., Bayer, A., and Snowden, R. J. (2002). Spatial shifts in visual attention in normal ageing and dementia of the Alzheimer type. *Neuropsychologia* 40: 2000–2012.

Talsma, D., Kok, A., and Ridderinkhof, K. R. (2006). Selective attention to spatial and non-spatial visual stimuli is affected differentially by age: Effects on event-related brain potentials and performance data. *International Journal of Psychophysiology* 62: 249–261.

Theeuwes, J., Kramer, A. F., Hahn, S., and Irwin, D. E. (1998). Our eyes do not always go where we want them to go: Capture of the eyes by new objects. *Psychological Science* 9: 379–385.

Tipper, S. P. (1991). Less attentional selectivity as a result of declining inhibition in older adults. *Bulletin of the Psychonomic Society* 29: 45–47.

Townsend, J., Adamo, M., and Haist, F. (2006). Changing channels: An fMRI study of aging and cross-modal attention shifts. *NeuroImage* 31: 1682–1692.

Trick, L. M., Perl, T., and Sethi, N. (2005). Age-related differences in multiple-object tracking. *Journals of Gerontology B: Psychological Sciences and Social Sciences 60*: P102–P105.

Tsang, P. S. and Shaner, T. L. (1998). Age, attention, expertise, and time-sharing performance. *Psychology and Aging 13*: 323–347.

Tun, P. A., O'Kane, G., and Wingfield, A. (2002). Distraction by competing speech in young and older adult listeners. *Psychology and Aging 17*: 453–467.

Tun, P. A. and Wingfield, A. (1999). One voice too many: Adult age differences in language processing with different types of distracting sounds. *Journals of Gerontology B: Psychological Sciences and Social Sciences 54*: P317–P327.

Turken, A. U., Whitfield-Gabrieli, S., Bammer, R., Baldo, J. V., Dronkers, N. F., Gabrieli, J. D. E. (2008). Cognitive processing speed and the structure of white matter pathways: Convergent evidence from normal variation and lesion studies. *NeuroImage 42*: 1032–1044.

Ulbrich, P., Churan, J., Fink, M., and Wittmann, M. (2009). Perception of temporal order: The effects of age, sex, and cognitive factors. *Aging, Neuropsychology, and Cognition 16*: 183–202.

Vallesi, A., McIntosh, A. R., and Stuss, D. T. (2009). Temporal preparation in aging: A functional MRI study. *Neuropsychologia 47*: 2876–2881.

Van der Lubbe, R. H. J. and Verleger, R. (2002). Aging and the Simon task. *Psychophysiology 39*: 100–110.

Van Gerven, P. W. M., Meijer, W. A., Vermeeren, A., Vuurman, E. F., and Jolles, J. (2007). The irrelevant speech effect and the level of interference in aging. *Experimental Aging Research 33*: 323–339.

Van Rooij, J. C. G. M. and Plomp, R. (1991). Auditive and cognitive factors in speech-perception by elderly listeners. *Acta Oto-Laryngologica 111*: 177–181.

Vecchi, T. and Cornoldi, C. (1999). Passive storage and active manipulation in visuo-spatial working memory: Further evidence from the study of age differences. *European Journal of Cognitive Psychology 11*: 391–406.

Verhaeghen, P. and Cerella, J. (2002). Aging, executive control, and attention: A review of meta-analyses. *Neuroscience & Biobehavioral Reviews 26*: 849–857.

Verhaeghen, P. and De Meersman, L. (1998). Aging and the negative priming effect: A meta-analysis. *Psychology and Aging 13*: 435–444.

Verhaeghen, P., Steitz, D. W., Sliwinski, M. J., and Cerella, J. (2003). Aging and dual-task performance: A meta-analysis. *Psychology and Aging 18*: 443–460.

Vu, K. P. L. and Proctor, R. W. (2008). Age differences in response selection for pure and mixed stimulus-response mappings and tasks. *Acta Psychologica 129*: 49–60.

Wascher, E., Falkenstein, M., and Wild-Wall, N. (2011). Age related strategic differences in processing irrelevant information. *Neuroscience Letters 487*: 66–69.

Wasylyshyn, C., Verhaeghen, P., and Sliwinski, M. J. (2011). Aging and task switching: A meta-analysis. *Psychology and Aging 26*: 15–20.

Wecker, N. S., Kramer, J. H., Wisniewski, A., Delis, D. C., and Kaplan, E. (2000). Age effects on executive ability. *Neuropsychology 14*: 409–414.

Welford, A. T. (1981). Signal, noise, performance, and age. *Human Factors 23*: 97–109.

Wenk, G. L., Pierce, D. J., Struble, R. G., Price, D. L., and Cork, L. C. (1989). Age-related changes in multiple neurotransmitter systems in the monkey brain. *Neurobiology of Aging 10*: 11–19.

West, R. and Bowry, R. (2005). The aging of cognitive control. In R. W. Engle, G. Sedek, U. von Hecker, and D. N. McIntosh (eds.), *Cognitive Limitations in Aging and Psychopathology* (pp. 97–121). Cambridge: Cambridge University Press.

West, R. and Schwarb, H. (2006). The influence of aging and frontal function on the neural cor-relates of regulative and evaluative aspects of cognitive control. *Neuropsychology 20*: 468–481.

West, R. and Travers, S. (2008). Differential effects of aging on processes underlying task switch-ing. *Brain and Cognition 68*: 67–80.

West, R. L. (1996). An application of prefrontal cortex function theory to cognitive aging. *Psychological Bulletin 120*: 272–292.

Whiting, W. L., Madden, D. J., and Babcock, K. J. (2007). Overriding age differences in atten-tional capture with top-down processing. *Psychology and Aging 22*: 223–232.

Whiting, W. L., Madden, D. J., Pierce, T. W., and Allen, P. A. (2005). Searching from the top down: Ageing and attentional guidance during singleton detection. *Quarterly Journal of Experimental Psychology A: Human Experimental Psychology 58*: 72–97.

Wild-Wall, N. and Falkenstein, M. (2010). Age-dependent impairment of auditory process-ing under spatially focused and divided attention: An electrophysiological study. *Biological Psychology 83*: 27–36.

Wild-Wall, N., Hahn, M., and Falkenstein, M. (2011). Preparatory processes and compensatory effort in older and younger participants in a driving-like dual task. *Human Factors 53*: 91–102.

Wild-Wall, N., Willemssen, R., and Falkenstein, M. (2009). Feedback-related processes during a time-production task in young and older adults. *Clinical Neurophysiology 120*: 407–413.

Wilson, R. H. and Jaffe, M. S. (1996). Interactions of age, ear, and stimulus complexity on dichotic digit recognition. *Journal of the American Academy of Audiology 7*: 358–364.

Woodrow, H. (1914). The measurement of attention. *Psychological Monographs 17*: 1–158.

Woollacott, M. and Shumway-Cook, A. (2002). Attention and the control of posture and gait: A review of an emerging area of research. *Gait & Posture 16*: 1–14.

Wright, L. L. and Elias, J. W. (1979). Age-differences in the effects of perceptual noise. *Journal of Gerontology 34*: 704–708.

Yamaguchi, S., Tsuchiya, H., and Kobayashi, S. (1995). Electrophysiologic correlates of age effects on visuospatial attention shift. *Cognitive Brain Research 3*: 41–49.

Yogev-Seligmann, G., Hausdorff, J. M., and Giladi, N. (2008). The role of executive function and attention in gait. *Movement Disorders 23*: 329–342.

Zanto, T. P., Hennigan, K., Ostberg, M., Clapp, W. C., and Gazzaley, A. (2010a). Predictive knowledge of stimulus relevance does not influence top-down suppression of irrelevant information in older adults. *Cortex 46*: 561–574.

Zanto, T. P., Toy, B., and Gazzaley, A. (2010b). Delays in neural processing during working memory encoding in normal aging. *Neuropsychologia 48*: 13–25.

Zanto, T. P., Pan, P., Liu, H., Bollinger, J., Nobre, A. C., and Gazzaley, A. (2011). Age-related changes in orienting attention in time. *Journal of Neuroscience 31*: 12461–12470.

Zeef, E. J. and Kok, A. (1993). Age-related differences in the timing of stimulus and response processes during visual selective attention: Performance and psychophysiological analyses. *Psychophysiology 30*: 138–151.

Zeef, E. J., Sonke, C. J., Kok, A., Buiten, M. M., and Kenemans, J. L. (1996). Perceptual factors affecting age-related differences in focused attention: Performance and psychophysiological analyses. *Psychophysiology 33*: 555–565.

CHAPTER 33

....

UNILATERAL SPATIAL NEGLECT

....

GIUSEPPE VALLAR AND NADIA BOLOGNINI

INTRODUCTION

....

THE syndrome of unilateral spatial neglect (neglect) and related disorders first appeared in the medical literature in the second half of the nineteenth century (Jackson 1932; Pick 1898). In the first half of the twentieth century in the visual domain a unilateral 'hemi-anopic weakness of attention', particularly under conditions of double simultaneous stimulation of the two sides of the visual field (see Benton 1956, for an historical review; Oppenheim 1885), was described in patients with unilateral lesions (Poppelreuter 1917; Scheller and Seidemann 1931), but no hemispheric asymmetries were noted. An association between right-brain damage and various manifestations of extra-personal and personal neglect was made in the following years (Brain 1941; Paterson and Zangwill 1944). The deficit was classified under the rubric of the agnosias and visuo-constructive disorders: 'syndrome of apractognosia' (Hécaen et al. 1956), 'unilateral spatial agnosia' (Battersby et al. 1956; Hécaen and Albert 1978, for review). The terms 'hemi-inattention' was then introduced, emphasizing the role of defective attentional mechanisms (Friedland and Weinstein 1977). Unilateral 'spatial neglect' is currently the most frequently used term (Critchley 1953; Jeannerod 1987; Lawson 1962).

At the beginning of the twenty-first century, 'neglect' is one of the more extensively investigated conditions in neuropsychology (Marshall and Vallar 2004), and it enlists interest in disciplines unrelated to its original discovery and study, such as philosophy, for issues including consciousness and the self (Churchland 1986; Dennett 1991; Gallagher 2000).

In a nutshell, the basic minimal defining feature of neglect is the patients' inability to report sensory events occurring in one side of space, in most patients contralateral to the side of the cerebral lesion (contralesional), and to perform actions in that portion of space. The interest of neglect for cognitive neuroscience and, more generally, for students of the structure of the mind is at least twofold. First, patients with neglect may show selective impairments. Neglect may concern near extra-personal space or the body (Vallar and Mancini 2010); physical objects or internally generated images (Guariglia et al. 1993; Ortigue et al. 2006); a specific type of stimulus, such as words (Vallar et al. 2010, for review); portions of space along the left–right horizontal, but also the upper–lower altitudinal, dimension (Rapcsak et al. 1988). These dissociations suggest that the internal representation of the space around us (Merleau-Ponty 1945), far from being unitary, as our phenomenal experience may suggest, includes a number of discrete though related components, with partly different neural correlates (Rizzolatti et al. 1997; Vallar 1998). Secondly, the investigation of patients with neglect has shown that a great deal of the processing of events taking place in the space around us occurs in the absence of perceptual awareness (Berti 2002). These unconscious levels, preserved in neglect patients, range from basic processing of elementary stimuli (Mancini et al. 2011; Vallar and Daini 2006) to the computation of extent, as indexed by illusory effects, and lexical and semantic information (Berti 2002; Làdavas et al. 1997a, 1997b; Marshall and Halligan 1988; McGlinchey-Berroth 1997; McGlinchey-Berroth et al. 1993; Vallar et al. 2010, 1996a).

In sum, these observations suggest, on the one hand, a multi-component account of our conscious experience of space and of our body as an object in that space, and, on the other hand, that most of the information processing concerning sensory events does not require spatial awareness.

This chapter reviews the syndrome of neglect in its extra-personal, imaginal, and personal ('personal neglect', 'hemiasomatognosia') aspects. The related deficits of 'anosognosia for hemiplegia', 'hemianopia', and 'hemianesthesia' are reviewed by Prigatano (2010), 'somatoparaphrenia' by Vallar and Ronchi (2009), 'extinction to double simultaneous stimulation' (both in a single modality, and with the stimuli in two different modalities: 'cross-modal extinction') by Brozzoli, Dematté, Pavani et al. (2006), Oliveri and Caltagirone (2006), and Driver and Vuilleumier (2001).

CLINICAL PRESENTATION

Observing neglect

Particularly in the acute phase of a disease such as a stroke, the examiner, most frequently a medical doctor, particularly a neurologist, may readily diagnose the presence of neglect. Observing the patients' behaviour during the routine neurological exam, or spontaneous activities, may reveal the deficit. Since full-fledged neglect is usually the consequence of a lesion located in the right hemisphere, the clinical picture which follows refers to neglect of the left side of space (Bisiach and Vallar 2000; Critchley 1953; Heilman 1979; Mesulam 1985).

Patients with neglect may show a more-or-less complete deviation of the head and eyes towards the right side, ipsilateral to the side of the hemispheric lesion (ipsilesional). Addressed by the examiner from the left (contralesional) side, patients with severe neglect may fail to respond or may look for the speaker in the right side of the room, turning head and eyes more and more to the right. Frequently, these patients do not pick up food from the left half of the plate. Given a crossword puzzle, they may complete only the squares to the right. If walking is not prevented by left hemiparesis, patients with neglect may lose their bearings, since they do not make use of left-sided cues, and turn systematically to the right (see one such case in De Renzi 1977). Neglect may involve internally generated visuospatial representations, such as hallucinations confined to the right side of the room, for instance threatening individuals or spider webs (Mesulam 1981; Perani et al. 1987; Silberpfennig 1941). Patients with neglect may not utilize the contralesional limbs ('motor neglect'; see Laplane and Degos 1983), even though no major motor deficits are present, and may disregard them (hemiasomatognosia, unilateral asomatognosia, or personal neglect; see Bisiach and Vallar 2000; Hécaen and Albert 1978). Neglect for the contralesional side of the body may interfere with a variety of everyday activities, including dressing and shaving.

Neglect and primary sensorimotor deficits

The neurological exam shows that patients with neglect typically fail to respond to visual stimuli presented in the contralesional half-field, and to tactile stimuli delivered to the contralesional limbs. Hemianopia and hemianaesthesia are primarily due, wholly or in part, to the presence of primary sensory disorders, and therefore, in themselves, do not represent unambiguous indicators of neglect. Much less frequently, patients with neglect fail to respond to left-sided auditory stimuli, although they may search for them in the right side of space.

Although frequently associated, primary sensory deficits may occur independent of neglect both in the visual (Cassidy et al. 1999; Daini et al. 2002; Doricchi and Angelelli 1999; Halligan et al. 1990; Vallar and Perani 1986) and in the tactile (Bisiach et al. 1986a; Vallar et al. 1993b) modality. Clinically relevant primary auditory deficits are not usually associated with unilateral hemispheric lesions, due to the bilateral cortical representation of auditory signals (Ropper and Samuels 2009).

Sensory deficits in the left visual half-field (hemianopia) and in the left side of the body (hemianaesthesia), as well as motor deficits of the left limbs (hemiparesis and hemiplegia), caused by right-brain damage, are more frequent than sensorimotor disorders involving the right side of the body or the right visual half-field, caused by left-brain damage (Sterzi et al. 1993). This asymmetry of putatively primary sensorimotor deficits may be due to the additive effect of left neglect (Halligan and Marshall 2002), which is closely associated with a damage to the right hemisphere (Heilman 1995). These manifestations of spatial neglect may even masquerade as primary sensorimotor deficits: 'visual inattention' or 'pseudohemianopia', 'tactile inattention' or 'pseudohemianesthesia'

(Heilman 1995), and 'motor neglect' (Castaigne et al. 1972; Laplane and Degos 1983; Mark et al. 1996).

The differential diagnosis may begin with some clinical observations. The visual behaviour of neglect patients is characterized by defective orientation towards and exploration of the contralesional side of space; these patients are also typically unaware of their neglect (Berti et al. 1996). Conversely, in hemianopia eye, head, and body movements may compensate for the actual loss of the contralesional visual half-field. Drawing from memory is preserved in hemianopia, but may be defective in neglect patients (Kerkhoff and Schindler 1997). Consistent with this behaviour, patients with hemianopia without neglect are usually aware of their visual deficits (Ting et al. 2011). Hemianopic patients may be unaware of the visual disorder, but this anosognosia is frequently associated with neglect, and with lesions typically extending anterior to the occipital cortex, in parietal and frontal regions (Bisiach et al. 1986b; Celesia et al. 1997; Koehler et al. 1986).

At a standard visual field perimetry (i.e. a test consisting in the detection of visual stimuli at various locations in the visual field, while maintaining fixation), a failure to report contralesional stimuli is considered to reflect a field defect. Also, neglect is characterized by the failure to respond to stimuli presented in the contralesional side of space. However, there are differences between the behaviours of neglect and hemianopic patients. The visual field defect is usually characterized by a strict demarcation at the vertical meridian in both eyes in hemianopic, but not in neglect, patients. In visual search tasks, neglect, but not hemianopic, patients show an ipsilesional rightward bias, when the central fixation point disappears. Also, a distractor in the intact hemifield can diminish the report of left-sided stimuli by neglect, but not by hemianopic, patients, with an extinction-like effect (Müller-Oehring et al. 2003).

As shown by saccadic eye movement recording, patients with hemianopia may explore the whole visual display, finding targets in the blind field, although visual scanning may be disorganized, not only in the affected, but, to a minor extent, also in the intact half-field (Machner et al. 2009a, 2009b; Pambakian et al. 2000; Zihl 1995). Conversely, visual search by neglect patients shows a left–right gradient, and may be confined to the ipsilesional right side of space (Behrmann et al. 1997; Husain et al. 2001; Mort and Kennard 2003).

Components related to neglect and primary sensorimotor deficits may be disentangled by showing largely preserved early-evoked potentials in the sensory cortices (Angelelli et al. 1996; Vallar et al. 1991b), with longer latencies (Angelelli et al. 1996) and abnormalities in late potentials in the parietal cortex (Di Russo et al. 2008). A behavioural method to distinguish the two components consists in showing a recovery of hemianopia or hemianaesthesia when the sensory stimulus is presented in the non-neglected side of egocentric space. Manoeuvres such as looking rightwards (Kooistra and Heilman 1989; Nadeau and Heilman 1991), and placing the left hand in the right side of egocentric space (Smania and Aglioti 1995), dissociate sensory (retinotopic and somatotopic) from egocentric reference frames.

The presence of a lesion involving the visual pathways, projecting to the primary striate occipital cortex (Zihl and Kennard 1996), suggests the presence of a primarily sensory visual disorder. Instead, with respect to hemianaesthesia, the differential diagnosis between a sensory and a neglect-related deficit, on the basis of the site of the lesion, is more difficult, since a main correlate of neglect is a posterior parietal cortical damage, close to the anterior parietal somatosensory cortex (Ropper and Samuels 2009).

The role of neglect in the manifestation of sensorimotor deficits is also suggested by the finding that the physiological stimulations (see section 'Modulation of Neglect–Physiological stimulations'), which temporarily improve neglect, also decrease hemianaesthesia (Bottini et al. 1995; Vallar et al. 1996b, 1993b) and hemiplegia (Rode et al. 1998; Vallar et al. 2003, 1997a). These effects of physiological stimulations may presumably operate by reorienting attention towards the neglected side of extra-personal and bodily space, and by restoring a conscious representation of it, through modulations of higher-level neural systems involved in spatial processing, and of sensorimotor regions.

Psychometric Assessment

Neglect is found in over 40% of right-brain-damaged patients and in about 20% of left-brain-damaged patients, although there is a wide variability across studies (about 10–80%), which likely reflects differences in the sensitivity of the tests and batteries used to detect the disorder (Bowen et al. 1999; Buxbaum et al. 2004; Pedersen et al. 1997), as well as in the time of testing with reference to the onset of the cerebrovascular disease. After the acute post-stroke phase, the symptoms of neglect may not be immediately apparent to the examiner, and a psychometric assessment is required for diagnosing its presence and quantifying its severity.

By and large, tests used to assess the presence of neglect require the processing of stimuli presented in the two sides of extra-personal space, within hand reach. They may be broadly subdivided into four main groups, involving: (1) a sequential motor exploration of the spatial working space: cancellation and drawing tasks; (2) perceptual processing, including spatial extent: line bisection, straight ahead, and perceptual judgements; (3) imagery tasks; (4) reading tests. (5) Finally, scales assessing neglect-related deficits in an ecological perspective, and activities of daily living are increasingly used.

When motor responses are required, patients typically use the unaffected ipsilesional arm and hand. While performing these clinical tests, patients are also typically free to move their head and eyes. These features of the diagnostic tasks are aimed at minimizing the confounding effects of primary sensorimotor deficits.

Cancellation tasks

In the most frequently used motor-exploratory tasks, patients are required to cross out target stimuli (Fig. 33.1), such as circles (Vallar and Perani 1986), lines (Albert 1973),

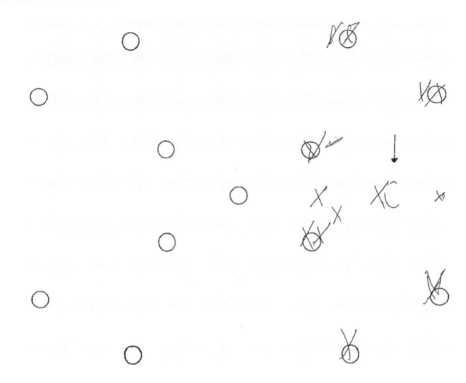

FIGURE 33.1   Left neglect in a cancellation task; perseveration behaviour with repeated crossing and gratuitous drawing of a target subsequently crossed out. Reprinted from *Neuropsychologia*, 40(6), Maria Luisa Rusconi, Angelo Maravita, Gabriella Bottini, and Giuseppe Vallar, Is the intact side really intact? Perseverative responses in patients with unilateral neglect: a productive manifestation, pp. 594–404, figure 4a Copyright (2002), with permission from Elsevier.

letters (Diller and Weinberg 1977), stars (Wilson et al. 1987), bells (Gauthier et al. 1989), or other symbols (Mesulam 1985). Targets may be the only type of stimulus in the display, or distractors may be present, more or less similar to the target. The number of targets appears to be a relevant factor, with more targets bringing about more omission errors by neglect patients (Chatterjee et al. 1992a, 1992b). Cancellation tasks require the programming and executing of a sequence of exploratory movements, and pose demands to spatial working memory, since patients need to keep track of the explored portion of space (i.e. crossed out targets), and to executive resources, since exploratory strategies are to be set up (Husain et al. 2001; Wojciulik et al. 2001). The time-honoured cancellation tasks are frequently used in paper-and-pencil versions, which are very flexible in many clinical settings, such as a stroke unit. At present, a number of computerized versions using touch screen technology have been developed. These computer-based tasks allow recording and computing a variety of performance measures, in addition to the standard number of omitted targets/correct responses; these include total and target-by-target latencies and exploratory pathways (e.g. Rabuffetti et al. 2002). Data from cancellation tasks also enable computing measures (in cm²) of the neglected area (Pia et al. 2013; Ricci et al. 2004), and of the centre of cancellation (namely, the mean horizontal coordinate for the detected items: see Binder et al. 1992; Rorden and Karnath 2010). Patients typically omit targets in the contralesional side of the display; in patients with a severe neglect, the explored area may be limited to the far right-hand side of the working space. Exploratory tasks are typically presented in the visual modality, but tactile versions have also been used (Gentilini et al. 1989; Vallar et al. 1991a).

Drawing tasks

Patients are required to copy meaningless or meaningful drawings, depicting single objects (e.g. a daisy; Rode et al. 2006), or multiple object arrays (a row of objects such as some trees, a house, a fence: see Gainotti et al. 1972 and Fig. 33.2; two daisies: see Marshall and Halligan 1993). Tracing the contours of a figure is an easier task, which may minimize the confounding role of visuospatial and visuo-constructional deficits (Trojano and Conson 2008); patients may show a largely preserved tracing, while exhibiting left neglect in an identification task (Fig. 33.3). In drawing from memory tasks, patients receive verbal instructions to draw objects such as a clock, a daisy, or a butterfly (Bisiach and Vallar 2000; Rode et al. 2006). Patients with neglect typically fail to draw left-sided details of objects. In multiple object displays, patients may either omit left-hand-side objects with reference to the mid-sagittal plane of the body ('egocentric' neglect), or left-hand-side details of each object, with reference to the object's axis: 'object'-based neglect (Walker 1995).

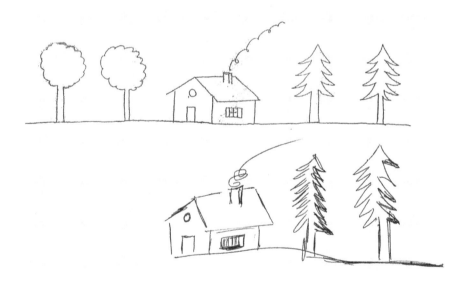

FIGURE 33.2   Left neglect in copying a complex drawing. Reprinted from *Cortex*, 45(3), Roberta Ronchi, Lucio Posteraro, Paola Fortis, Emanuela Bricolo, and Giuseppe Vallar, Perseveration in left spatial neglect: Drawing and cancellation tasks, pp. 300–12, Copyright (2009), with permission from Elsevier.

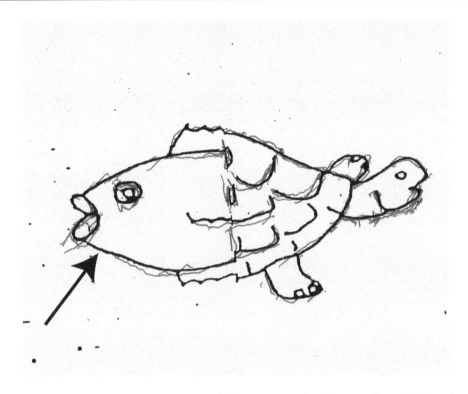

FIGURE 33.3   Largely preserved tracing of the contours of a chimeric figure (fish-turtle; a minor omission in the left lower contour of the fish, indicated by an arrow), identified by the patient as a 'turtle' (the right-hand side of the chimera. Reproduced from Vallar, G., Rusconi, M. L., and Bisiach, E. (1994). Awareness of contralesional information in unilateral neglect: effects of verbal cueing, tracing and vestibular stimulation. In C. Umiltà & M. Moscovitch (Eds.), *Attention and Performance XV. Conscious and Nonconscious Information Processing*, pp. 377–91. ©MIT, published by MIT Press Journals.

Visuomotor cancellation and drawing tasks may reveal perseveration behaviour (see Fig. 33.1), including repeated marks and the gratuitous drawing of objects unrelated to the task's demands. Drawing perseveration, however, is not systematically associated with neglect (Na et al. 1999; Nys et al. 2006; Ronchi et al. 2012, 2009; Rusconi et al. 2002), and is not modulated by factors such as target density, which in turn affects neglect (Pia et al. 2013; Ricci et al. 2004).

Line bisection

In line bisection tasks (Axenfeld 1894; Kerkhoff and Bucher 2008) patients are required to set the perceived mid-point of a horizontal segment (Fig. 33.4). At variance with cancellation and drawing tasks, the motor component is comparatively minor, being confined to pointing to the perceived centre. Furthermore, some versions of the bisection task (Landmark: see Bisiach et al. 1998; Milner et al. 1993) ask patients for a perceptual

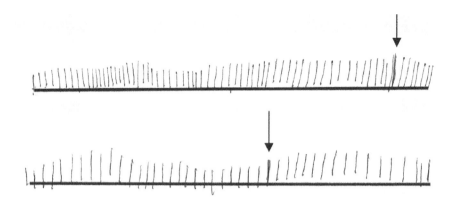

FIGURE 33.4   Left neglect in line bisection (red mark), with a rightward error; preserved left-to-right segmentation of the line. This dissociation between bisection and segmentation may be traced back to impaired 'global' ('bisection') and preserved 'local' ('segmentation') processing in neglect. Reproduced from A. Gallace, E. Imbornone, G. Vallar, *Journal of Neuropsychology*, When the whole is more than the sum of the parts: Evidence from visuospatial neglect, 2(2), pp. 387–413, figure 3 © 2008, The British Psychological Society.

judgement about the two halves of pre-bisected segments (i.e. 'which is longer/shorter?' with no motor component). The Landmark task provides a means of distinguishing 'perceptual/input' vs 'premotor/output' biases: in the former, the judgement is biased by the perceived extent of the segment, with an underestimation of the contralesional side; in the latter an ipsilesional response bias is systematically observed, independent of perceived extent. Line bisection allows the evaluation of the role of a number of variables, including the length of the to-be-bisected lines, their position with respect to the mid-sagittal plane of the body, and the role of cues placed at the ends of the segment (Heilman and Valenstein 1979; Mennemeier et al. 1997; Riddoch and Humphreys 1983; Vallar et al. 2000). Patients with left neglect typically make a rightward error, which increases with line length, and is reduced, though not abolished, when the line is placed on the right-hand side with respect to the mid-sagittal plane of the body. As for exploratory tasks, visual and tactile versions of line bisection have been used (Chokron et al. 2002; Fujii et al. 1991; Hjaltason et al. 1993; Mancini et al. 2011).

In bisection tasks, hemianopic patients bisect the line slightly towards the contralesional side (leftwards in left hemianopia), possibly because they are aware of their visual deficit and attempt to compensate for it (Barton and Black 1998; Kerkhoff and Schenk 2011; see also Machner et al. 2009a, 2009b, for an absence of the contralesional bias in the acute post-stroke phase; Schuett et al. 2011). By contrast, patients with left neglect exhibit an ipsilesional rightward bias (Bisiach et al. 1983, 1976; Daini et al. 2002; Schenkenberg et al. 1980), which may be increased by the co-occurrence of hemianopia (D'Erme et al. 1987; Daini et al. 2002; Doricchi and Angelelli 1999).

Recently, the bisection task has been used to investigate the representation of the extent of body parts such as the left forearm, showing a rightward shift in right-brain-damaged patients with left neglect; the deficit appears independent of the bias concerning extra-personal objects, such as a cylinder (Bolognini et al. 2012; Sposito et al. 2010).

Perceptual judgements

Other perceptual tasks require the identification or same/different judgements about chimeric meaningful stimuli (Vallar et al. 1994b, see Fig. 33.3; Young et al. 1992) and non-symmetrical patterns (Massironi et al. 1988), with patients with neglect making errors involving the left-hand side of them. Patients may be able to trace accurately left-sided details of stimuli they fail to report (Vallar et al. 1994b; Young et al. 1992). Perceptual factors such as the connectedness between the two stimuli modulate the deficit, with a gap improving neglect (Buxbaum and Coslett 1994; Tian et al. 2011). One single case study suggests that the deficit may be domain-specific, involving the left half of faces ('facial neglect'), while sparing objects (Young et al. 1990).

Subjective straight ahead

Patients with left neglect may show a rightward ipsilesional bias, when setting the subjective straight ahead through pointing or adjusting its visual position (Heilman et al. 1983; Karnath 1994). This deviation, however, has not been systematically found in neglect patients, and appears to be unrelated to the main clinical manifestations of the syndrome (Chokron and Bartolomeo 1997; Chokron 2003; Farnè et al. 1998). As in line bisection, patients with hemianopia may show a contralesional deviation of the subjective straight ahead (Kerkhoff 1993; Lewald et al. 2009; but see Saj et al. 2010, for an ipsilesional deviation as in neglect patients, although minor). When the two disorders (neglect and hemianopia) are associated, the evidence is controversial: the two opposite biases may neutralize each other (Ferber and Karnath 1999), or, as found for line bisection, the ipsilesional bias may increase (Saj et al. 2012a, 2010).

Imagery tasks

Patients may be required to recall items in a spatial egocentric frame, such as buildings and other elements in a familiar square from a given imagined vantage point (Bisiach and Luzzatti 1978; Bisiach et al. 1981; Guariglia et al. 1993; see also Meador et al. 1987), or cities in a map (France, see Rode and Perenin 1994). In another task, patients may be asked to compare imagined angles of the hands of clocks' faces (Grossi et al. 1989). Evidence for imaginal neglect is also provided by the rightward error committed by neglect patients in setting the midpoint of a numerical interval, along the left-to-right oriented mental number line (Umiltà et al. 2009; Zorzi et al. 2002), and by left-sided errors in auditory spelling tasks (Barbut and Gazzaniga 1987; Baxter and Warrington 1983).

Reading: 'Neglect dyslexia'

Neglect-related errors may occur when patients read letter strings, sentences, or passages of text. In the case of single letter strings, errors include omissions, substitutions, or, less frequently, additions of letters in the left-hand side of the stimulus. In the case of sentences and text, errors involve the left-hand side of the display, mainly with omissions. Stimuli may be single words, pronounceable meaningless letter strings (non-words), or non-pronounceable letter strings. Accordingly, reading tasks allow investigation of the putative relationships between the language system and spatial cognition. The reading performance of neglect patients is typically affected by lexical factors: a main reported effect is the patients' better performance reading words, compared to non-words (Ellis et al. 1987; Friedmann et al. 2011; Kinsbourne and Warrington 1962; review in Vallar et al. 2010).

Personal neglect

As for personal, corporeal space, the diagnostic tasks typically require exploring the contralesional side of the body, reaching the hand and other body parts (Bisiach et al. 1986a; Cocchini et al. 2001; Fortis et al. 2010, for a modified version of Bisiach et al.'s test; Glocker et al. 2006).

Everyday activities and disability scales

There is increasing consensus that neglect should be evaluated not only by psychometric tests, but also by more ecological scales, which assess the impact of the deficit on everyday activities (Bowen and Lincoln 2007). Some widely used batteries with an ecological component and scales are listed in the following:

1 'The Behavioural Inattention Test' (Wilson et al. 1987) comprises conventional psychometric tests (e.g. cancellation, bisection, drawing) and behavioural (ecological) tasks (e.g. 'menu reading', 'telling and setting the time', 'coin sorting').

2 'The Catherine Bergego Scale' (Azouvi et al. 2003) comprises the observation of the patients' behaviour in standardized daily life tasks, and a parallel self-administered

form, designed as a questionnaire for an auto-evaluation made by the patients themselves. The scale is aimed at comparing activities in the right-hand and the left-hand sides of the patient's body (e.g. 'forgets to shave or groom the left part of his or her face') and of extra-personal space (e.g. 'collides with people or objects on the left side'). The difference between the scores recorded in the parallel versions should provide an index of anosognosia for neglect.

3 A neglect-specific assessment battery based upon standardized 'activities of daily living' (Eschenbeck et al. 2010) is a recent tool, which combines, as the 'Behavioural Inattention Test', conventional tests and daily living activities (e.g. address copying, counting money, clock reading).

In general, activities of daily living are sensitive to detect neglect as conventional psychometric tests. In most patients the 'Behavioural Inattention Test' and the 'Catherine Bergego Scale' have proved to be equally effective in detecting neglect, although dissociations have been found (Luukkainen-Markkula et al. 2011). Importantly, it should be noted that some patients may show no neglect in the activities of daily living tasks, but neglect in psychometric tests, and vice versa (Eschenbeck et al. 2010; Hasegawa et al. 2011). It is therefore appropriate to use both conventional psychometric tests and specifically devised activities of daily-living-based tasks.

The Neglect Syndrome

A multi-component deficit

Most patients with neglect exhibit a full-fledged syndrome, showing a defective performance in all of the tasks mentioned above. However, some patients with neglect show selective patterns of impairment. Neglect for extra-personal space and for the contralesional side of the body (*personal neglect*) may occur independently of each other (Bisiach et al. 1986a; Guariglia and Antonucci 1992).

Extra-personal neglect, in turn, is not a monolithic disorder. A number of dissociated deficits have been reported, including: a defective performance in cancellation but not in line bisection tasks, and vice versa (Binder et al. 1992; Marshall and Halligan 1995); visual and not tactile neglect in exploratory tasks, and vice versa (Cubelli et al. 1991; Vallar et al. 1991a); neglect in copying but not in drawing from memory tasks (Halligan et al. 2003); 'neglect dyslexia' without other manifestations of visual neglect, and vice versa (Vallar et al. 2010); neglect for near but not for far space, and vice versa (Berti and Frassinetti 2000; Berti and Rizzolatti 2002; Halligan and Marshall 1991; Vallar and Maravita 2009).

This list of dissociations, very likely to be incomplete, shows that neglect is not a unitary disorder, including instead a number of discrete deficits. In this respect, neglect is to be conceived as a 'weak' syndrome, whose components frequently co-occur, but may manifest in isolation (Vallar 2000). These findings suggest that the neurofunctional systems in which damage brings about neglect are at least partly dissociable in the brain.

Multisensory aspects of neglect

Notwithstanding the complexity of the neglect syndrome, there has been a wealth of research in the visual domain (Brain 1941; McFie et al. 1950), leading to the use of 'visual' neglect and 'visuospatial' neglect as synonyms for neglect in general (Gainotti 2010 for review). Neglect, however, affects also the auditory and tactile modalities, as well as the chemical senses (Brozzoli et al. 2006; Jacobs et al. 2012; Pavani et al. 2003, 2002). In recent years, the mounting knowledge on multisensory mechanisms for spatial processing in the undamaged human brain (Bolognini and Maravita 2011; Calvert et al. 2004; Spence and Driver 2003) has further propelled research in neglect patients. There is now compelling support to the view that neglect can affect various senses, either separately or concurrently.

Regarding the auditory modality, one can start from a clinical observation: neglect patients often fail to respond when addressed verbally from the left, or more commonly behave as if they heard the voice originating from their right (Bender and Diamond 1965; Denny-Brown et al. 1952): 'alloacusis' (Bender and Diamond 1965) or 'allochiria' (Bisiach and Vallar 2000; Brozzoli et al. 2006). These patients show deficits in the localization of auditory stimuli, particularly, but not only, when sounds originate in the contralesional space (Bisiach et al. 1984; Ruff et al. 1981; Vallar et al. 1995b). Deficits also involve detection and identification, mainly of contralesional sounds (Pavani et al. 2004, 2002, 2001). Right-brain-damaged patients without visual neglect may show a rightward bias in the auditory modality (Vallar et al. 1995b).

In the tactile domain (i.e. in the absence of visual control), neglect is usually less severe than in the visual modality (Gainotti 2010). In haptic line bisection, neglect is absent or very mild (Chokron et al. 2002; Fujii et al. 1991; Hjaltason et al. 1993; Mancini et al. 2011; McIntosh et al. 2002, for haptic neglect in a task requiring setting the centre of a circle). In target cancellation, neglect may be present in the visual, in the tactile modality, or in both (Caneman et al. 1992; Cubelli et al. 1991; Gentilini et al. 1989; Schindler et al. 2006; Vallar et al. 1991a).

Neglect in the 'chemical senses' (i.e. olfaction and taste) has been less investigated (Brozzoli et al. 2006). A few studies suggest the existence of left-sided 'olfactory' neglect and extinction in right-brain-damaged patients. Since the olfactory sensory pathways are uncrossed, the finding of right-brain-damaged patients showing left olfactory neglect and extinction supports a 'spatial', rather than 'sensory', interpretation of neglect (Bellas et al. 1989, 1988a, 1988b; see however Berlucchi et al. 2004, for a critical discussion). There is some evidence for a left hemitongue tactile extinction in right-brain-damaged patients, while the evidence for left 'gustatory' extinction is controversial (Andre et al. 2000, for a clinical study; Berlucchi et al. 2004).

The synthesis of information derived from different sensory channels can markedly enhance the detection and identification of external stimuli (Stein 1998). Neglect patients often exhibit spared mechanisms of multisensory integration, namely, the ability to combine multiple sources of information into a unified percept (Bolognini et al. 2013). In neglect patients, multisensory integration has been explored by examining how the deficit affecting a unimodal sensory system (i.e. visual neglect) can be modulated by the concurrent activation of another modality (e.g. audition). Auditory stimuli can improve perception of visual events in the neglected side of space (Frassinetti et al. 2005; Frassinetti et al. 2002c). In keeping with the functional properties of multisensory neurons described in animal studies (Stein 1998), the amelioration of visual neglect by auditory stimulation follows some spatial and temporal constraints, and it is inversely correlated to the severity of the visual deficit (Frassinetti et al. 2005, 2002c) (Fig. 33.5). In a similar vein, the integration of proprioceptive and visual information may improve visual neglect (Frassinetti et al. 2001), and limb activation studies (Robertson and North 1992) may be seen in this perspective. Similarly, vision of the upper limb and hand may improve somatosensory perception in brain-damaged patients (review in Gallace and Spence 2008; Halligan et al. 1997). Finally, neglect patients are able to integrate visual and haptic information in a unitary percept, as shown by a preserved cross-modal illusion (Mancini et al. 2011).

To summarize, neglect can affect every sensory modality, jointly or separately, with the latter findings suggesting the existence of modality-specific *attentional*

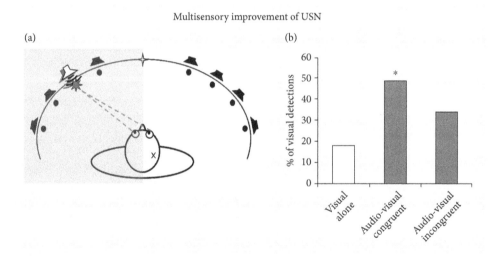

FIGURE 33.5   (a) Bird's-eye schematic view of the experimental set-up used by Frassinetti et al. (2005, 2002b) for the delivery of visual (circles) and auditory (trapezoids) stimuli. All loudspeakers were occluded behind a black panel. (b) Mean percentage of visual detections by neglect patients (without hemianopia) in the 'unimodal' visual and 'bimodal' audio-visual conditions, in which a sound was presented either spatially congruent (i.e. in the same position) or spatially incongruent (i.e. 32° of disparity) with respect to the visual stimulus. The asterisk (*) indicates a significant difference between unimodal and bimodal congruent conditions. Reproduced from Frassinetti, F., Bolognini, N., Bottari, D., Bonora, A., and Làdavas, E. (2005). Audiovisual integration in patients with visual deficit. *Journal of Cognitive Neuroscience*, 17, pp. 1442–52, ©MIT, published by MIT Press Journals.

spatial systems. Nevertheless, some multisensory mechanisms devoted to the integrated coding of spatial information may be preserved, providing potential compensatory mechanisms for the modality-specific neglect symptoms (Bolognini et al. 2013).

MODULATION OF NEGLECT

Physiological stimulations

The first observations that lateralized or directional physiological stimulation may modulate neglect date back to the first half of the twentieth century, with the finding that 'vestibular caloric stimulation' may temporarily improve the deficit (Silberpfennig 1941). These results have been replicated many times (Marshall and Maynard 1983; Rubens 1985), showing effects not only on extra-personal, personal (Cappa et al. 1987), and representational (Rode and Perenin 1994) neglect, but also on related disorders such as anosognosia for hemiplegia (Cappa et al. 1987), somatoparaphrenia (Bisiach et al. 1991; Rode et al. 1992), as well as the neglect-related components of hemiplegia (Rode et al. 1992; Vallar et al. 2003) and somatosensory deficits (Bottini et al. 2005; Vallar et al. 1993b). The effective caloric stimulation is the one which brings about leftward ocular movements (slow phase of nystagmus), according to the type of stimulus (warm, cold water), and the irrigated ear (left, right); conversely, a stimulation causing a rightward slow phase of nystagmus worsens left neglect (Rubens 1985; review in Vallar et al. 1997b). Vestibular galvanic stimulation has overall similar effects (Rorsman et al. 1999; Utz et al. 2011).

Other stimulations may affect neglect in a fashion broadly similar to the caloric vestibular one. Visual 'optokinetic' stimulation with a leftward movement of the luminous dots causes a leftward nystagmus (slow phase): it improves temporarily extra-personal neglect (Pizzamiglio et al. 1990, line bisection) and the neglect-related component of the deficit of limb position sense (Vallar et al. 1995a, 1993a); a stimulation with a rightward movement of the dots worsens these deficits. Slow leftward visual motion and moving background have similar effects on visual neglect, as assessed by line bisection (Choi et al. 2007; Mattingley et al. 1995). Leftward dot motion also improves the representational deficit shown by neglect patients on the mental number line (Salillas et al. 2009).

By and large, similar effects are produced by 'mechanical vibration of the left neck muscles' (Karnath et al. 1993), by 'transcutaneous electrical nerve stimulation' of the left neck and hand (Guariglia et al. 2000, 1998; Vallar et al. 1995c), and by 'limb activation' through active (Gainotti et al. 2002; Robertson and North 1993, 1992) and passive movement of the left upper limb. Transcutaneous electrical nerve stimulation also improves the putatively neglect-related component of left hemianaesthesia (Vallar et al. 1996b).

A related form of modulation of neglect by limb movements ('space remapping training') is based on evidence that tool use can induce a 'virtual' extension of body space, which, in turn, allows a remapping of far space as near space (Maravita and Iriki 2004). This goal can be achieved by using 'virtual' reality methods (Tsirlin et al. 2009). Neglect patients may be trained to reach and grasp a real object in the right side of space with the right hand, while simultaneously observing a 'virtual' hand grasping a 'virtual' object located in the left side of space. The training induces an improvement in grasping accuracy for the left side of space, possibly because the virtual hand is incorporated, through the training procedure, as part of the body, so that the representation of space extends to the virtual space, including the real, neglected side (Ansuini et al. 2006; Castiello et al. 2004).

Finally, the rightward lateral displacement of the visual scene induced by 'optical prisms' brings about, after a period of motor activity such as pointing to visual targets, an improvement of many manifestations of left neglect. The rightward displacement during the pointing activity reduces over the course of the participant's exposure to the prisms ('prism adaptation'). After prism removal, participants make a pointing error in a leftward direction ('after-effects') opposite to the prism-induced rightward displacement (Redding and Wallace 2006; Redding et al. 2005; Rode et al. 2003; Rossetti and Rode 2002). Prism adaptation improves visual (Farnè et al. 2002; Rossetti et al. 1998), haptic (McIntosh et al. 2002), auditory (as indexed by a dichotic listening deficit; see Jacquin-Courtois et al. 2010), and representational neglect (assessed by a number bisection task; see Rossetti et al. 2004). Also the putatively neglect-related component of somatosensory deficits (Maravita et al. 2003), the rightward bias in forearm bisection (Bolognini et al. 2012), and postural imbalance (Tilikete et al. 2001) are improved by prism adaptation.

To summarize, a variety of lateralized and non-symmetrical sensory stimulations may improve (or worsen) many manifestations of neglect. The effects cannot be explained at a lower level of sensorimotor integration, including the restoration of movements (eye, limbs) towards the neglected side or cueing by a peripheral left-sided input. Representational neglect is improved (Geminiani and Bottini 1992; Rode and Perenin 1994; Rossetti et al. 2004), and some effective stimulations are right-sided, such as the irrigation of the right ear with cold water, which brings about leftward eye movements (Rubens 1985). Furthermore, effects on non-visual modalities make unlikely interpretations in terms of an improvement of visual exploration of the neglected left side of space through eye movements (haptic forearm bisection, see Bolognini et al. 2012; personal neglect, see Cappa et al. 1987).

The effects of these stimulations can involve deficits in modalities different from the stimulated sense. Some examples include the effects of caloric vestibular stimulation on left somatosensory deficits (Vallar et al. 1993b), of optokinetic stimulation on proprioceptive deficits (Vallar et al. 1993a), of prism adaptation on left dichotic listening deficits (Jacquin-Courtois et al. 2010), and on the rightward bias in haptic forearm bisection (Bolognini et al. 2012). These observations suggest that the involved mechanisms of 'cross-modal' integration are preserved in neglect patients.

In conclusion, the effective stimulations are likely to exert their effects on higher-level spatial attentional/representational systems, which, in neglect patients, are biased ipsilesionally/corrupted contralesionally, and may be temporarily restored, reducing the contralesional bias. These findings, on the whole, suggest that higher-level spatial systems are open to modulation by sensorimotor loops (Pizzamiglio et al. 1997).

Non-invasive brain stimulation

The chance of modulating visuospatial functions by non-invasive brain stimulation has considerably refined our understanding of the physiopathological mechanisms underlying neglect (Fierro et al. 2006; Hesse et al. 2011). Overall, results from studies using non-invasive brain stimulation are consistent with models of inter-hemispheric relationships where a deficit caused by a unilateral lesion, such as neglect, but also sensorimotor disorders and aphasia, is produced by a twofold mechanism: (1) a direct effect of the unilateral lesion, with damage to brain areas committed to the function of interest; (2) a maladaptive activity of the contralateral undamaged hemisphere, which may inhibit the damaged hemisphere, resulting from a breakdown of the physiological dynamic modulatory (inhibitory) balance between the two hemispheres (Fregni and Pascual-Leone 2007; Kinsbourne 1977, for a seminal model of hemispheric rivalry; Rossi and Rossini 2004). Within this framework, non-invasive brain stimulations have been used to restore the balance of hemispheric activity following stroke. A re-equilibrium of the inter-hemispheric imbalance can be achieved in two main ways: either by up-regulating excitability of the damaged hemisphere or down-regulating it in the intact hemisphere (Miniussi and Vallar 2011). Two techniques of non-invasive brain stimulation are available to this purpose. Transcranial magnetic stimulation (TMS) relies upon the properties of electromagnetic induction: a rapidly changing magnetic field is generated when a high voltage current is passed through a coil. When the coil is held in close proximity to any electrically conducting medium, such as the brain, this time-varying magnetic field induces electrical current that is capable of depolarizing neurons (Wassermann et al. 2008). Transcranial electrical stimulation (tES) delivers weak polarizing currents to the cortex via two electrodes placed on the scalp, which induce sustained changes in the membrane potential of neurons (Nitsche et al. 2008; Paulus 2011). Depending on the stimulation protocol, TMS and tES can have opposite effects on the underlying brain tissue: low-frequency repetitive TMS (<1Hz), continuous Theta Burst TMS, as well as cathodal tES, decrease cortical excitability; high-frequency repetitive (r) TMS (>1Hz), intermittent Theta Burst TMS, and anodal tES primarily enhance excitability. The main differences between tES and TMS include putative mechanisms of action and their spatial and temporal resolution, which is higher for TMS (Nitsche et al. 2008; Wassermann et al. 2008). Despite these differences, both techniques can induce after-effects on cortical excitability, which may translate into behavioural changes (Bolognini and Ro 2010; Vallar and Bolognini 2011).

So far, the most widely used approach has been to inhibit the contralesional hemisphere: low frequency rTMS or cathodal tES delivered to the unaffected left posterior parietal cortex transiently improves contralesional visual neglect (Brighina et al. 2003; Oliveri et al. 2001; Sparing et al. 2009). This evidence supports the view that the dysfunction underlying neglect involves a relative hyperactivity of the unaffected hemisphere, likely due to release from reciprocal inhibition by its twin. A reduction of left neglect in right-brain-damaged patients has also been obtained through the normalization, achieved by 1-Hz rTMS delivered to the left undamaged hemisphere, of a pathologically increased intra-cortical excitability of the posterior parietal-primary motor cortex circuitry in the left hemisphere, as assessed by a double TMS approach (Koch et al. 2008).

Facilitatory protocols, such as anodal tES targeting the posterior parietal cortex of the ipsilesional hemisphere, can also ameliorate neglect (Bestmann et al. 2008; Sparing et al. 2009).

INTERPRETATION

Lower-level interpretations

These interpretations were put forward particularly in the mid-1950s of the twentieth century.

1. 'Defective sensory input from the contralesional side'. This hypothesis posits a 'defective sensory input, primarily visual', though 'superimposed upon a background of altered mental functioning' (Battersby et al. 1956: 92). However, patients may show neglect without visual half-field, somatosensory, or motor deficits. This indicates that a defective sensory input is not a basic pathological mechanism of neglect.

2. 'Defective lower-level sensory integration'. Two main interpretations have been proposed. (i) According to the 'amorphosynthesis' hypothesis (Denny-Brown et al. 1952), neglect, namely the patient's 'failure to attend to the left side of herself or of space, can…be viewed as a disturbance of synthesis of multiple sensory data' (Denny-Brown et al. 1952: 452). This hypothesis has been recently revived, assigning a main role to the temporo-parietal cortex of the right hemisphere (Brandt et al. 2009). (ii) According to the 'extinction' hypothesis, 'When patients with unilateral spatial deficits are required to perform a complex task such as drawing or reading, the multiple sensory input which is of necessity bilateral and simultaneous, interacts between the two sides in which the stimuli on the normal side "extinguish" those arising from the defective side' (Battersby et al. 1956: 91).

    One problem with these interpretations, which posit a deficit at lower levels of sensory integration, is their inability to account for the hemispheric asymmetry of neglect, although one recent such account suggests a main role of the right hemisphere in multisensory integration (Brandt et al. 2009). Furthermore, contrary to the 'amorphosynthesis' hypothesis and to other similar interpretations (Brandt et al. 2009), multisensory integration is largely preserved in neglect patients (Frassinetti et al. 2005, 2002c; Mancini et al. 2011; Van Vleet and Robertson 2006). As for an interpretation of neglect in terms of sensory extinction to double stimulation from the two sides of space (Battersby et al. 1956), there is wide evidence that the two deficits may occur independently of each other (Smania et al. 1998; Vallar et al. 1994a; Vallar and Perani 1986; Vossel et al. 2011).

3. 'Lower-level motor interpretations'. This account of the mechanisms of neglect has been couched primarily in terms of defective ocular movements towards the contralesional, neglected, side of space (De Renzi 1982: 106; Schott et al. 1966). However, while patients with neglect may show such defective ocular movements (Barton et al. 1998; Chedru et al. 1973; Girotti et al. 1983; Ishiai et al. 1989; Karnath and Fetter 1995; Malhotra et al. 2006), saccade deficits after cortical lesions can occur independently of neglect (Pierrot-Deseilligy and Müri 1997). These eye-movement deficits may be interpreted as behavioural motor indexes of the impairment of the higher-level mechanisms (such as attention), which bring about neglect, rather than the primary cause of it (Müri et al. 2009; Pierrot-Deseilligny et al. 2004). In line with these conclusions, impairment of conjugate ocular movements towards the side contralateral to the lesion, with an ipsilesional gaze deviation, is more frequently associated with right-hemisphere, than with left-hemisphere, damage (De Renzi 1982; Marquardsen 1969; Ringman et al. 2005; Tjissen et al. 1991) and has been related to neglect (Becker and Karnath 2010; Fruhmann Berger et al. 2006).

4. 'Defective coordinate frames'. At the upper end of lower-level interpretations, one may posit accounts of neglect in terms of rotation (Karnath 1994; Kerkhoff et al. 2006; Ventre et al. 1984, for the first proposal of this hypothesis) or translation (Saj et al. 2010; Vallar et al. 1995b) of basic coordinate frames, such as the egocentric reference, indexed by an ipsilesional deviation of the subjective straight ahead (Heilman et al. 1983; Karnath 1994). A unilateral cerebral lesion of the parietal lobe or the superior colliculus unbalances a bilateral cortico-subcortical neural system, affecting orienting behaviour and bringing about an ipsilesional bias in neglect patients (Ventre et al. 1984; see also, in the following section, the partly similar, though higher-level, account of Kinsbourne). This ipsilesional bias, shown by patients with parieto-occipital lesions, had been interpreted in terms of defective cortical integration of vestibular inputs (Hécaen et al. 1951; see also Karnath and Dieterich 2006, for a recent account of neglect as a vestibular disorder). However, patients with neglect may show no impairments of the straight ahead (Farnè et al. 1998), making it unlikely that a shift of the egocentric reference frame provides a comprehensive account of the complex phenomenology of the disorder. Finally, the original hypothesis of defective coordinate frames (Ventre et al. 1984) does not readily explain the hemispheric asymmetry of neglect.

Higher-order interpretations of neglect

Attentional interpretations

Higher-order accounts of neglect share the view that defective sensory input from the contralesional side cannot account for the phenomenology of the disorder, in line with the finding that sensorimotor processing, as well as multisensory integration, may be spared in neglect patients, as previously discussed.

The German psychologist and physician Poppelreuter (1917), who examined brain-injured soldiers of the First World War, described a deficit termed 'hemianopic weakness of attention', whereby patients fail to report stimuli presented in the affected hemifield, particularly under conditions of bilateral simultaneous stimulation. Poppelreuter distinguished between 'passive' and 'active' attention: the latter could be preserved, with the patient's performance improving with external cueing. 'Hemianopic weakness of attention' is a significant impairment in everyday life. One patient (HA) 'bumped into people on his right side. Because he omitted to give a military salute when officers approached him on his right side we had to provide him with a written excuse. These cases should be assessed as disabled, therefore, in the same way as are hemianopic cases' (Poppelreuter 1917: 97). In the 1950s, the British neurologist Critchley and co-workers made general suggestions that tactile and visual extinction to double simultaneous stimulation (termed 'inattention' by Critchley) after lesions of either hemisphere, although with a possible greater role of right-brain damage, and left unilateral neglect after right-brain damage could be due to attentional deficits (Critchley 1953; Critchley et al. 1951).

More recent attentional interpretations of neglect include three main hypotheses.

1. 'Deficit of the spatial orienting response'. Patients with neglect may fail to orient towards external contralesional stimuli (Heilman and Watson 1977; Heilman 1979).
2. 'Damage to an attentional vector'. The vector model by Kinsbourne (1993, 1977, 1970) assumes the existence of two antagonistic lateral vectors, which direct attention to the two opposite sides of egocentric space, with the rightward (left-hemisphere-dependent) vector being more focused and prevailing physiologically over the more panoramic leftward (right-hemisphere-dependent) vector in right-handers (see Bisiach and Vallar 2000, for a discussion of this assumption). Damage to one hemisphere impairs the contralaterally oriented vector, therefore releasing the competitor from inhibition. The model also assumes that the selective engagement of either hemisphere in activities of its specific competence energizes the vector pointing towards the opposite side. By postulating a left–right asymmetry of the two attentional vectors, the model explains the asymmetry of neglect resulting from left- and right-hemisphere damage. It also implies that following a unilateral lesion, the attentional imbalance between two separate points on the left–right dimension is preserved whatever the absolute location of these points on that dimension, accounting for the finding that the divide between the neglected and

the preserved side of space is not systematically referred to the mid-sagittal plane of the trunk (see, e.g., Bisiach et al. 1984; Smania et al. 1998). A third prediction of this model is that verbal stimuli, activating the left hemisphere, bring about a more severe left neglect, but the evidence about this effect is controversial (Caplan 1985; Gainotti et al. 2002; Heilman and Watson 1978; Weintraub and Mesulam 1988). One aspect of Kinsbourne's model, namely, the view that the two hemisphere-based vectors are antagonistic, has been strongly supported by transcranial stimulation studies (TMS, tES), showing that not only neglect, but also aphasia and basic neurological deficits, such as unilateral motor disorders, may be improved both by excitatory stimulation of the damaged hemisphere, and by inhibitory stimulation of the unaffected contralateral hemisphere. These effects appear to result from a pathological maladaptive activity in the undamaged hemisphere, due to a disproportionate reduction of a physiological transcallosal modulation by the damaged hemisphere. This basic principle of interhemispheric balance, which applies to both elementary sensorimotor and cognitive functions, has important implications for rehabilitation (Fregni and Pascual-Leone 2007; Miniussi and Vallar 2011; Rossi and Rossini 2004).

3. 'Deficit of attention towards the contralesional side of space' (Heilman et al. 2003, 1993, 1985). This hypothesis accounts for the hemispheric asymmetry of neglect, assuming that the right cerebral hemisphere is able to orient attention not only contralaterally, namely leftwards, but also ipsilaterally (rightwards), with a panoramic distribution across space; the left hemisphere, conversely, possesses the capacity of a contralateral orientation only (Mesulam 2002, 1981). This attentional model, which, unlike Kinsbourne's account, originally implied a sharp dichotomy between the 'neglected' and the 'preserved' space, with reference to the mid-sagittal plane, may be couched in terms of a distribution of spatial attention, with a lateral gradient whereby the contribution of each hemisphere increases from the ipsilateral to the contralateral side (Bisiach and Vallar 2000).

With reference to the specific component of spatial attention damaged in neglect patients, the suggestion has been made that the automatic rather than the voluntary component may be primarily, though not exclusively, defective (Gainotti 2010, 1996; see Poppelreuter 1917 for an early suggestion of this distinction). A role of a deficit of the disengagement of attention from ipsilesional stimuli has also been suggested (Posner et al. 1984, 1982), accounting for the finding that the performance of neglect patients improves on a cancellation task if they are required to erase (rather than mark) targets over the stimulus array, reducing therefore the ipsilesional stimulation (Mark et al. 1988). The rightward bias in line bisection may be reduced in the dark (Gassama et al. 2011; Hjaltason and Tegner 1992; but see Pizzamiglio et al. 1997), in line with the hypothesis of a defective disengagement of spatial attention. Neglect, however, is not completely abolished, and an ipsilesional bias, as indexed by ocular movements, has been found also in the dark, in the absence of visual stimuli (Hornak 1992; Karnath 1997). These findings undermine also the 'extinction' interpretation discussed previously.

Finally, there is some evidence for a disproportionate ipsilesional (rightward in right-brain-damaged patients) attentional bias ('hyperattention'; see De Renzi et al.

1989; Làdavas 1990; Làdavas et al. 1990), rather than a defective leftward orientation, with faster response latencies towards the more peripheral positions in the ipsilesional, spared, side of space (Smania et al. 1998).

Representational interpretations

The view that neglect reflects an impairment of the conscious representation of space was primarily prompted by the observation that the deficit may also involve the contralesional side of internally generated images (conscious internal representations) and not only physical objects (Bisiach and Luzzatti 1978; Bisiach et al. 1981, 1979). Notwithstanding the ambiguities related to the very concept of 'attention' (Anderson 2011), most of the putative differences between 'attentional' and 'representational' interpretations may be overcome (Benke et al. 2004). In an attentional framework, spatial attention supports perceptual awareness and conscious spatial representations. Accordingly, a unilateral deficit of spatial attention (Umiltà 2001) may affect perception of both contralesional external physical objects *and* the contralesional side of each object (i.e. 'extra-personal' neglect). By a similar attentional mechanism, neglect patients may also fail to attend contralesional internally generated images and the contralesional side of each image (i.e. 'representational' neglect).

There is, however, one aspect of the representational view that is not readily accounted for by attentional interpretations (i.e. defective contralesional orientation or ipsilesional bias of spatial attention), namely: some paradoxical manifestations of the neglect syndrome in the contralesional, putatively 'neglected', side of space. These include 'productive' rather than 'defective' (Vallar 1998) behaviours, such as delusional views concerning the contralesional side of the body (somatoparaphrenia; see Vallar and Ronchi 2009) and paradoxical biases towards the neglected side of space (Bisiach et al. 1996, 1994) in tasks such as line extension or, in some patients, drawing (Rode et al. 2008, 2006). The term 'dyschiria', originally proposed by Zingerle (1913) (see Benke et al. 2004, for an abridged translation of this seminal paper), with reference to a disordered representation of one side of the body, was resumed and used by Bisiach and his co-workers (Berti 2004; Bisiach and Berti 1987) to refer to the complex phenomenology of neglect.

The 'dyschiria' interpretation (Bisiach and Vallar 2000) hypothesizes a lesion-induced pathological release of neural subassemblies ('non-veridical', variably unrelated to the content of sensory information), which may bring about the variety of productive manifestations of neglect, ranging from somatoparaphrenia (Vallar and Ronchi 2009) to drawing perseveration (Ronchi et al. 2012, 2009). This account of productive manifestations in terms of the pathological release of the activity of systems otherwise appropriately operating under condition of no brain damage (see Denny-Brown and Chambers 1958, for an early such view) is not a main feature of attentional hypotheses, which focus on lateral biases and defective symptoms.

Multi-component interpretations: Deconstructing neglect

All of the interpretations discussed in the previous sections consider spatial neglect to be a basically unitary deficit (Corbetta and Shulman 2011; see recent accounts of spatial

Table 33.1 Some main dimensions of neglect.

Defective Manifestations

Input Modality

- Visual
- Auditory
- Tactile
- Olfactory

Type of Task

- Motor exploratory: target cancellation
- Computation of lateral extent: line bisection
- Drawing: copy, from memory
- Reading
- ...

Type of Stimulus

- Written material ('neglect dyslexia')
- Faces ('facial neglect')
- ...

Sector of Space

- External (physical objects)
  - Personal, bodily
  - Extrapersonal
    - Near vs far
- Internal (imagined objects)

Reference Frame

- Egocentric
- Allocentric: 'Object-based', 'Object-centred'

Input/Output

- Defective planning/initiation/execution of movements towards the contralesional side: 'premotor neglect'
- Defective awareness of contralesional stimuli: 'perceptual neglect'
- Defective movements by the contralesional limbs: 'motor neglect'

Productive Manifestations
Extrapersonal Space

- Avoidance
- Perseveration and gratuitous productions
- Disproportionate bias towards the ipsilesional 'undamaged' side of space

Personal Space

- Somatoparaphrenia and related disorders

This material has been adapted from Vallar, G. and Mancini, F., Mapping the neglect syndrome onto neurofunctional streams, In N. Gangopadhyay, M. Madary, and F. Spicer (eds), Perception, Action, and Consciousness: Sensorimotor Dynamics and Two Visual Systems, p. 187, table 11.1 (c) 2010, Oxford University Press and has been reproduced by permission of Oxford University Press http://ukcatalogue.oup.com/product/9780199551118.do#.UIKFhFMt2H8. For permission to reuse this material, please visit http://www.oup.co.uk/academic/rights/permissions.

neglect in terms of an egocentric bias in Karnath and Rorden 2012, who also distinguish between the egocentric 'core' and 'satellite' deficits, such as 'allocentric', 'object-based' impairments). There is definite and wide evidence, however, that unilateral spatial neglect and the attentional/representational systems in the brain which support spatial cognition (Vallar and Mancini 2010; Vallar and Maravita 2009) may present with dissociated patterns of impairment (Barbieri and De Renzi 1989; Vallar 1998). These double dissociations (Vallar 2000) have led to a fractionation of neglect, analogously to other neuropsychological syndromes, such as the dyslexias (Coltheart et al. 1980; Patterson et al. 1985). Their main dimensions are shown in Table 33.1.

The observed dissociations differ in important respects. Some of them are mainly empirical, being primarily related to the different clinical tasks used to assess neglect, such as target cancellation vs line bisection (Binder et al. 1992; Halligan and Marshall 1992), and only subsequently interpreted as involving different processes, including sensorimotor exploration and computation of lateral extent. Other dissociations refer to the specificity of neglect, as related to the modality of the sensory input, with the deficit being more frequent and severe in the visual than in the tactile modality (Gainotti 2010), but with a double dissociation between visual and tactile neglect in exploratory tasks (Cubelli et al. 1991; Mancini et al. 2011; Vallar et al. 1991a).

Neglect manifestations may also dissociate with reference to the affected sector of space ('personal vs extrapersonal'; see Bisiach et al. 1986a), and, within extrapersonal space, 'near' vs 'far' (see review in Berti and Rizzolatti 2002), and to the frames of reference (Klatzky 1998; Lacquaniti 1997), in which the sensory event is encoded. Accordingly, the neglected left side of the stimulus may be defined by an 'egocentric reference', including the mid-sagittal plane of the body, or the sagittal planes of other body parts such as the head and the hand (Moscovitch and Behrmann 1994; Bisiach et al. 1985; Vallar et al. 1995a), or the retina (Làdavas 1987). The neglected side may be defined also by an 'allocentric reference', namely: the centre of the object and its axes (Chatterjee 1994; Driver and Halligan 1991; Halligan and Marshall 1993; reviews may be found in Mozer 2002, and Walker 1995). The suggestion has been made that both patterns of impairment may be explained by an 'egocentric' deficit, assuming a continuous, right-to-left gradient of impairment, so that each position, e.g. in a retinal representation, is relatively more neglected than the contiguous right-sided position (Driver and Pouget 2000; Kinsbourne 1993; Pouget and Driver 2000). The independence of the two types of representations is however suggested by instances of double dissociation between 'egocentric' and 'allocentric' neglect (Chatterjee 1994; Kleinman et al. 2007; Marsh and Hillis 2008; Ota et al. 2001).

In the domain of reading, the existence of a canonical orientation of a letter string in the reading system (left-to-right in languages such as English, Italian, French, German) has allowed distinguishing different patterns of 'neglect dyslexia' (and underlying representations): egocentric ('viewer-centred', 'retinocentric') and allocentric, the latter including 'stimulus/object-based' and 'graphemic' or 'word-based'. In a 'word-based' format the two sides of the string are defined with reference to their canonical representation in the reading system, and not to the physical arrangement of the letter string (Hillis and Caramazza 1995; Vallar et al. 2010). The finding that patients may exhibit 'neglect dyslexia' without other manifestations of visuospatial neglect (Vallar et al. 2010 for review) indicates that the deficit may be domain-specific. The report of a patient showing left 'facial neglect' supports this conclusion (Young et al. 1990).

Manifestations of extra-personal neglect, as assessed by target cancellation/detection and line bisection tasks, may be distinguished as primarily caused by 'perceptual' (namely, a deficit of a conscious representation, supported by spatial attention), or by 'premotor' (namely, a deficit of programming and executing movements towards the neglected side of space) impairments. There is evidence for a double dissociation between these two types of neglect, with the perceptual pathological component being the prevailing pattern in right-brain-damaged neglect patients (review in Vallar and Mancini 2010).

While the evidence suggesting that neglect is a multi-component deficit is now conclusive (Barbieri and De Renzi 1989; Vallar 1998), these multiple spatial impairments appear to share the pathological mechanisms discussed in the preceding sections, be they attentional or representational, defective or productive in nature. Also, the building up and updating of these multiple spatial systems is modulated by sensory inputs in a broadly similar fashion. Seen in this perspective, the different putative pathological mechanisms of neglect, suggested by proponents of unitary accounts (Bisiach and Vallar 2000; Bisiach 1993; Heilman et al. 2003; Kinsbourne 1993), may apply to multiple spatial systems (Mesulam 1999).

Finally, within a multi-component account, the manifold manifestations of neglect may be shaped, and, in most instances, made more severe in specific aspects, by associated deficits caused by right-hemispheric damage, which do not constitute its core pathological mechanisms. These include: hypo-arousal (Heilman et al. 1978; Husain and Rorden 2003); deficits of spatial short-term/working memory, with effects on visuospatial search (Husain et al. 2001; Wojciulik et al. 2001); hemianopia, with effects on line bisection (Daini et al. 2002; Doricchi and Angelelli 1999).

NEUROPATHOLOGICAL CORRELATES

The more frequently reported aetiology of neglect is stroke. The deficit recovers spontaneously, though often not completely, and may be found months and years after stroke onset (Appelros et al. 2004; Colombo et al. 1982; Farnè et al. 2004; Hier et al. 1983b; Rengachary et al. 2011; Zarit and Kahn 1974). Neglect has also been reported in patients with brain tumours (Battersby et al. 1956; Shallice et al. 2010; Vallar and Perani 1987), or with neurodegenerative disorders, such as Alzheimer's disease (Ishiai et al. 2000; Venneri et al. 1998), posterior cortical atrophy, cortico-basal degeneration, fronto-temporal dementia (Andrade et al. 2010; Kleiner-Fisman et al. 2003; Silveri et al. 2011), and Huntington's disease (Ho et al. 2003, one patient).

Neglect may be brought about by a variety of lesion sites. Historically, the first suggested neural correlate of neglect was the inferior parietal lobule, at the temporo-parietal junction (Critchley 1953; Hécaen et al. 1956), with neglect being considered a 'parietal syndrome' (Jewesbury 1969). This early localization has been repeatedly confirmed (Heilman and Valenstein 1972a; Mort et al. 2003; Vallar and Perani 1986; Verdon et al. 2010). Neglect may be also caused by damage to the lateral frontal (ventral premotor and dorsolateral prefrontal) cortex (Committeri et al. 2007; Heilman and Valenstein 1972b; Husain and Kennard 1996; Vallar and Perani 1986; Verdon et al. 2010). Lesions of the posterior superior and middle temporal gyri (Karnath et al. 2011, 2001; Saj et al. 2012b), the insular (Berthier et al. 1987; Committeri et al. 2007; Karnath et al. 2004; Manes et al. 1999), and the cingulate (Watson et al. 1973) cortices have been associated with neglect.

The lesion localization in neglect patients discussed above focuses on cortical regions. However, these lesions are typically not confined to the cortical grey matter, involving also subcortical fibre tracts. A number of studies have highlighted the role of damage to the temporo-parietal paraventricular white matter (Samuelsson et al. 1997), the parieto-frontal connections, particularly the superior (Doricchi and Tomaiuolo 2003; Leibovitch et al. 1998; Thiebaut de Schotten et al. 2005), and the inferior (Bird et al. 2006; Leibovitch et al. 1998) longitudinal fasciculi; the role of these fibre tracts, particularly the superior longitudinal fasciculus, is also suggested by a recent meta-analysis (Chechlacz et al. 2012). The superior longitudinal fasciculus is the largest of the fibre bundles that connect the perisylvian frontal, parietal, and temporal cortices (Dejerine 1892); the inferior longitudinal fasciculus connects the parahippocampal gyrus with the posterior part of the inferior parietal lobule (Rushworth et al. 2006). Other relevant fibre tracts, whose damage may be associated with neglect, include the superior (Verdon et al. 2010) and the inferior (Urbanski et al. 2008) fronto-occipital fasciculi, as well as the anterior segment of the arcuate fasciculus (Urbanski et al. 2011), which links the inferior parietal lobule with the ventral premotor cortex. In patients with chronic neglect (Karnath et al. 2011), damage to the uncinate fasciculus, which connects the anterior part of the temporal lobe with the orbital and polar frontal cortices (Catani et al. 2002; Schmahmann et al. 2007), may be relevant.

Neglect may be also caused by damage confined to subcortical grey nuclei (reviews in Cappa and Vallar 1992; Vallar 2008). Lesion sites include the thalamus (Cambier et al. 1980; Vallar and Perani 1986; Watson and Heilman 1979), particularly its posterior (pulvinar, see Karnath et al. 2002) and medial (Watson et al. 1981) nuclei and the basal ganglia (Damasio et al. 1980; Healton et al. 1982; Karnath et al. 2002, the putamen and, to a lesser extent, the caudate nucleus; Vallar and Perani 1986).

Subcortical lesions confined to the white matter are rarely associated with neglect (Cappa and Vallar 1992; Vallar and Perani 1986). There are however a few reports of neglect patients with damage to the posterior limb of the internal capsule (Ferro and

Kertesz 1984; Vallar et al. 1990, patient #2) and to the subcortical white matter (Ciaraffa et al. 2012).

Taken together, these findings indicate that the neural underpinnings of neglect comprise a complex and extensive neural network including cortical regions, subcortical grey nuclei, and white matter fibre tracts. Notably, this network does not include the primary sensory and motor cortices, suggesting, also from a neuro-pathological perspective, that neglect is not caused by primary sensory and motor impairments. Patients with neglect, furthermore, have on average larger lesions than patients without neglect, suggesting that the network discussed above operates to some extent in an integrated fashion, and may compensate for partial damage, so that larger lesions are more likely to bring about neglect (Hier et al. 1983a, 1983b; Leibovitch et al. 1998; Vallar and Perani 1986). Finally, it should be considered that focal lesions may disrupt the operation of regions structurally not damaged, through remote effects, such as hypoperfusion (Hillis et al. 2002, 2000; Perani et al. 1987). Activation studies in which patients with left neglect are engaged in spatial tasks show a reduced activation in a posterior parietal-frontal premotor network and in the lateral occipital cortex (Umarova et al. 2011).

Within the network, there also seems to be some specificity related to the tasks used to assess neglect. Impairments in motor-exploratory tasks have been associated with anterior damage, involving particularly the frontal (premotor and prefrontal) cortex (Binder et al. 1992; Committeri et al. 2007; Verdon et al. 2010). Impairments in more perceptual tasks, such as line bisection and reading, are associated with posterior lesions, involving the inferior parietal lobule and the parieto-occipital regions (Baier et al. 2010; Binder et al. 1992; Daini et al. 2002; Lee et al. 2009; Verdon et al. 2010). However, some investigations are not in line with these conclusions. Neglect, as assessed by visuo-motor exploratory tasks, has been associated with damage to the inferior parietal lobule: the supramarginal gyrus and the temporo-parietal junction (Doricchi and Tomaiuolo 2003; Heilman et al. 1994; Vallar and Perani 1986), the angular gyrus (Molenberghs et al. 2012; Mort et al. 2003), and the superior temporal gyrus (Committeri et al. 2007; Karnath et al. 2001). As for the damage to the temporal lobe, some anatomo-clinical correlation studies report an association between 'allocentric', object-based, neglect and damage to a deep region (Verdon et al. 2010), close to the parahippocampal gyrus, which, in turn, has been reported to be a neuropathological correlate of neglect in general (see also Bird et al. 2006; Mort et al. 2004). Data based on perfusion measures in acute stroke patients, suggest an association between 'egocentric' neglect and posterior inferior parietal lobe dysfunction (angular gyrus), and between 'allocentric' neglect and superior temporal gyrus dysfunction (Hillis et al. 2005). A recent meta-analysis (Chechlacz et al. 2012) shows that the 'egocentric' component of neglect is associated with damage to a perisylvian network (pre- and post-central, supramarginal, and superior temporal gyri), the 'allocentric' component to posterior lesions (angular, middle temporal, and middle occipital gyri).

Finally, infarction in the vascular territory of the posterior cerebral artery (which supplies the occipital and inferomedial temporal regions and thalamic nuclei including the ventral posterolateral), with no frontal structural damage, leads to impairment both in visuomotor exploratory and line bisection tasks (Bird et al. 2006; Chambers et al. 1991; Park et al. 2006; Vallar and Perani 1986).

When more focused tasks, which specifically aim at dissociating the 'perceptual' vs 'premotor' components of neglect, are used, the former mechanisms are associated with posterior damage, the latter with damage involving the frontal regions and the basal ganglia (Bisiach et al. 1990; Sapir et al. 2007, putamen and frontal white matter; Tegnér and Levander 1991; Vallar and Mancini 2010, for review; Vossel et al. 2010a, caudate nucleus).

Brain-damaged patients suffering from successive lesions are rare, but they provide very useful information for the understanding of the neurofunctional organization of spatial attentional systems. One patient showed left neglect in visuomotor exploratory tasks and no sensory extinction after an infarct in the right frontal lobe. After two weeks and a partial recovery from neglect, she suffered a second stroke in the right posterior parietal region, which brought about multimodal extinction and worsening of left neglect (Daffner et al. 1990). These findings are compatible with the view that the anterior regions of the right hemisphere are more involved in the motor-exploratory aspects of spatial cognition (Vallar and Mancini 2010), in the context of a wide right-hemispheric fronto-parietal network.

Another patient (Vuilleumier et al. 1996) showed left neglect after a right-hemisphere lesion in the inferior parietal lobule (angular gyrus). The deficit disappeared after a second left-hemispheric lesion in the frontal lobe (frontal eye fields, BA 8). These findings support the hemispheric rivalry model, where the two hemispheres exert reciprocal inhibitory influences (Kinsbourne 1977; Rossi and Rossini 2004). If one pathological mechanism of neglect is a disproportionate dysfunction of the left hemisphere, released by the right-hemispheric damage, which unbalances spatial systems towards the right side, a subsequent left-hemispheric lesion is expected to restore the balance.

However, bi-parietal lesions cause bilateral deficits, such as spatial disorientation (Kase et al. 1977; Wilson et al. 2005), and the Balint's syndrome (Rizzo and Vecera 2002; Vallar 2007), suggesting that reciprocal inhibition is not the only mechanism that governs the distribution of spatial attention, and the construction of conscious spatial representations.

In sum (Fig. 33.6), the available evidence suggests that damage to different components of an extensive right dorso-lateral frontal (premotor and prefrontal), posterior inferior-parietal, and superior temporal, including the temporo-parietal junction, hemispheric network may bring about the manifold manifestations of the syndrome (Bartolomeo et al. 2012; Corbetta and Shulman 2011; Heilman et al. 2003; Mesulam 2002). However, the association between the various components of neglect, clearly dissociable at the behavioural level, and damage to distinct neural components within the system, is at present much less well understood. This is so, at least in part, because many anatomo-clinical correlation studies use clinical tests as target cancellation (Saj et al. 2012b; Verdon et al. 2010), which do not disentangle the specific (i.e. 'perceptual' vs 'premotor') components involved in the task of interest (Sapir et al. 2007). Damage to the primary sensory and motor cortices does not appear to play a major role, although

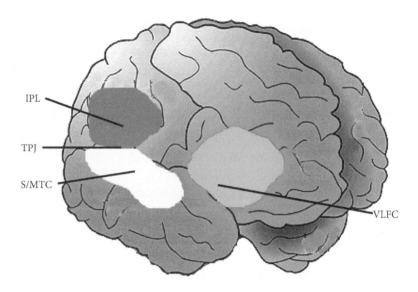

FIGURE 33.6   Main cortical right-hemispheric regions whose damage may cause left neglect: inferior parietal lobule (IPL: angular, BA 39, and supramarginal, BA 40, gyri, blue), temporo-parietal junction (TPJ), superior/middle temporal cortices (S/MTC: yellow), and lateral premotor and prefrontal cortices (VLFC: green).

there are some reports of neglect associated with occipital damage (Bird et al. 2006; Park et al. 2006; Saj et al. 2012b; related evidence in Umarova et al. 2011). Suggestions have been made that additional damage to the splenium of the corpus callosum may be also relevant, preventing access of visual information to the right hemisphere (Park et al. 2006, 2005; Tomaiuolo et al. 2010).

Lesions of the middle and anterior portions (trunk, genu) of the corpus callosum may cause left neglect for the right hand and in verbal tasks (Goldenberg 1986; Kashiwagi et al. 1990). Complex patterns of bias have also been described in line bisection, using manual responses: leftward for the left hand, rightward for the right hand (Goldenberg 1986; Heilman et al. 1984; Kashiwagi et al. 1990; Wolk and Coslett 2004). These findings are compatible with the view that the left hemisphere is primarily, if not exclusively, concerned with the contralateral side of space, and that in the absence of the integration provided by the corpus callosum, such patients may show left neglect when the task of interest is performed by the left hemisphere (right hand, verbal task, see also Kinsbourne 1970). One patient with a right frontal tumour, treated with surgery and radiation, and with no evidence of neglect, underwent a complete section of the corpus callosum ten years later; one year after the section she showed left neglect (Heilman and Adams 2003). Taken together, these findings suggest that the role of the left hemisphere may be compensatory (Heilman and Adams 2003), rather than inhibitory (Rossi and Rossini 2004). In these patients, the role of additional damage to the medial frontal lobe should also be considered (Goldenberg 1986; Heilman et al. 1984; Kashiwagi et al. 1990; Wolk and Coslett 2004).

Damage to the superior parietal lobule is also not a major correlate of neglect (but see the recent direct electrical stimulation study by Vallar et al. 2013), although suggestions have been made that this region may be dysfunctional in neglect patients (Corbetta and Shulman 2011; Szczepanski et al. 2010). Lesions of the superior parietal lobule are, instead, a correlate of a distinct neuropsychological syndrome, 'optic ataxia' (Coulthard et al. 2006; Rossetti et al. 2010), a reaching disorder which is not characterized by the fundamental deficit of neglect, namely a spatially asymmetric processing of sensory events. Finally, lesions involving the middle and inferior temporal regions have not been associated with neglect.

REHABILITATION

Among impairments following stroke, left neglect is recognized as a significant disabling deficit. Indeed, although some spontaneous recovery occurs in the majority of patients in a few months after stroke, left neglect may persist chronically (Colombo et al. 1982; Hier et al. 1983b; Zarit and Kahn 1974). The presence of neglect is associated with poor outcome measures on functional activities following stroke, and it poses considerable obstacles to successful rehabilitation (Di Monaco et al. 2011; Farnè et al. 2004; Katz et al. 1999; Paolucci et al. 2001). The many different available rehabilitation approaches can be broadly divided into two main groups, involving different mechanisms: methods using 'top-down', goal-driven, vs 'bottom-up', stimulus-based, techniques.

Top-down approaches

Top-down approaches were the first developed to rehabilitate neglect (Diller and Weinberg 1977; Lawson 1962). These methods require agency, and taking an active role by the patient in implementing newly learned behaviours and strategies to compensate for the spatial bias, whichever the specific pathological mechanisms involved. According to views interpreting neglect primarily as a disorder of the automatic component of attention (Gainotti 2010, 1996), top-down approaches capitalize on comparatively spared (controlled, voluntary) resources.

The more widely used treatment involves visual scanning training. This method is aimed at eliciting compensatory behaviours in order to bring about a reorientation of visual exploration towards the neglected side of space, by means of training programmes based on explicit instructions (verbal insight-oriented, incidental to eye movements, and motor habit learning) (Pizzamiglio et al. 2006; Weinberg et al. 1979; Young et al. 1983). Treatment programmes are typically progressive, with increasing task difficulty and feedback provided to the patient; tasks used include visual–spatial scanning, reading and copying tasks, figure description (Pizzamiglio et al. 2006). A successful visual scanning training requires many sessions (e.g. 40 for eight weeks) in order to achieve high levels of learning (Pizzamiglio et al. 2006; a negative result in Schröder et al. 2008, with a shorter four-week treatment). Another top-down but less well-investigated approach involves visual and motor imagery, aimed at reducing the left-sided representational impairment (Smania et al. 1997; Welfringer et al. 2011).

A main limitation of top-down approaches is their dependence on the patients' awareness of their deficit. The frequent presence of anosognosia for neglect (Berti et al. 1996) may reduce the utility of these methods for many patients, interfering with the implementation of the newly learned cognitive strategies, also for generalization of the improvement achieved with the training. Notably, indifference and anosognosia for the scanning impairment improves during the training in most patients, who become more conscious of their deficit (Pizzamiglio et al. 2006).

Bottom-up approaches

Bottom-up treatments are, by and large, based on interpretations of neglect as an attentional/representational imbalance, with an ipsilesional bias. This may be reduced by asymmetrical stimulations (see section 'Modulation of Neglect'), which, in turn, may induce an automatic, bottom-up behavioural change or recalibration of the recruited sensorimotor mechanisms that does not depend upon patients adopting new top-down, controlled strategies, in order to look leftwards and to explore the left-hand side of space.

A number of bottom-up treatments have been used in rehabilitation settings.

1. 'Prism adaptation' is so far the most promising and widely investigated bottom-up intervention. In rehabilitation settings, a two-week (20 sessions) treatment improves neglect in right-brain-damaged patients (Fortis et al. 2010, using also an 'ecological' visuomotor adaptation method; Frassinetti et al. 2002a; Serino et al. 2009, 2007, 2006, using a pointing adaptation method; Shiraishi et al. 2008, with effects on postural balance). Negative results, however, have also been noted (Turton et al. 2010), possibly due, at least in part, to differences in the prism adaptation methods used (Fortis et al. 2010).
2. 'Optokinetic stimulation' with a leftward movement of the luminous dots for a three-week period (Schröder et al. 2008; Thimm et al. 2009) improves left neglect (see however Pizzamiglio et al. 2004).
3. 'Eye patching' involves the partial or complete suppression of sensory inputs from the ipsilesional right hemifield, by requiring patients to wear spectacles containing a right monocular patch or right half-field patches (Barrett and Burkholder 2006; Beis et al. 1999; Zeloni et al. 2002, a one-week treatment). By occluding the right eye, or the right hemifields of both eyes, the residual visual input converges, primarily or entirely, on the right superior colliculus, which generates leftward saccades. Accordingly, the orienting of attention and gaze towards the contralesional, neglected, side of space is facilitated. The approach

appears promising, but the available evidence is limited (review in Ogourtsova et al. 2010).

4. 'Limb activation' is aimed at enhancing a poorly attended representation of the body, by requiring patients to execute movements with the contralesional limbs in the left-hand side of the space. This, in turn, may activate the orientation of attention towards (or the internal representation of) close regions of extra-personal space (Frassinetti et al. 2001; Robertson and North 1993). Activation of left limbs in the left side of space in right brain-damaged patients may also take advantage of inter-hemispheric inhibitory processes, since its beneficial effects can be eliminated by the simultaneous movement of the right limbs (Robertson and North 1994). Contralesional limb activation requires relatively preserved motor skills, and the frequent association of neglect with left hemiparesis and sensory loss limits its use.

5. 'Attention training and pharmacological treatments'. Some rehabilitation strategies are aimed at improving non-lateralized alerting deficits that are also present in neglect patients (Coslett et al. 1987; Heilman et al. 1978; Robertson et al. 1997). Sustained attention trainings are based on the functional interaction between arousal/alertness and selective spatial attention. Basically, the stimulation of arousal through external alerting stimuli can enhance the impaired spatial attentional system, improving neglect (Robertson et al. 1995; Sturm et al. 2006; Thimm et al. 2006). The spatial and non-spatial attentional deficits of neglect patients have also been treated through pharmacological interventions, by modulating noradrenergic and cholinergic systems (review in Adair and Barrett 2008; Singh-Curry et al. 2011; Vossel et al. 2010b).

6. 'Non-invasive peripheral nerve and brain stimulation techniques' have been used for the rehabilitation of neglect with positive results (rTMS: see Brighina et al. 2003, review in Fierro et al. 2006; transcutaneous electrical nerve stimulation—TENS: see Schröder et al. 2008), in light of current models of inter-hemispheric relationships and of neuroplasticity after stroke (Fregni and Pascual-Leone 2007; Hesse et al. 2011). A recent randomized double-blind study (Cazzoli et al. 2012) shows that delivering theta-burst TMS for two weeks to the left posterior parietal cortex improves neglect, as assessed by a daily-living disability scale (Catherine Bergego Scale; see Azouvi et al. 2003).

In conclusion, the available evidence suggests that a number of 'top-down' (visual scanning training) and 'bottom-up' (prism adaptation, optokinetic stimulation) methods may improve the neglect syndrome; non-invasive peripheral (transcutaneous electrical nerve stimulation) and central (rTMS, theta-burst TMS) neural stimulations also appear to be effective (Cicerone et al. 2005; Làdavas et al. 2012; Pierce and Buxbaum 2002; Rohling et al. 2009). Critical issues for future research include the search for treatments which affect not only performance on tests assessing neglect, but also disability in daily-life activities (Bowen and Lincoln 2007). There is some recent evidence that a prism adaptation treatment (Fortis et al. 2010; Mizuno et al. 2011; Shiraishi et al. 2010) improves also the patients' disability, assessed by the Catherine Bergego scale (Azouvi et al. 2003) and by the Functional Independence Measure (FIM$_{TM}$; see Tesio et al. 2002), or Activities of Daily Living (Lawton and Brody 1969; Mahoney and Barthel 1965) scales. There is also a growing need to compare the long-term effects and the cost/effort effectiveness of the different treatments.

References

Adair, J. C. and Barrett, A. M. (2008). Spatial neglect: Clinical and neuroscience review: A wealth of information on the poverty of spatial attention. *Annals of the New York Academy of Sciences* 42: 21–43.

Albert, M. L. (1973). A simple test of visual neglect. *Neurology 23*: 658–664.

Anderson, B. (2011). There is no such thing as attention. *Frontiers in Psychology 2*: 246.

Andrade, K., Samri, D., Sarazin, M., de Souza, L. C., Cohen, L., Thiebaut de Schotten, M., Dubois, B., and Bartolomeo, P. (2010). Visual neglect in posterior cortical atrophy. *BMC Neurology 10*: 68.

Andre, J. M., Beis, J. M., Morin, N., and Paysant, J. (2000). Buccal hemineglect. *Archives of Neurology 57*: 1734–1741.

Angelelli, P., De Luca, M., and Spinelli, D. (1996). Early visual processing in neglect patients: A study with steady-state VEPs. *Neuropsychologia 34*: 1151–1157.

Ansuini, C., Pierno, A. C., Lusher, D., and Castiello, U. (2006). Virtual reality applications for the remapping of space in neglect patients. *Restorative Neurology & Neuroscience 24*: 431–441.

Appelros, P., Nydevik, I., Karlsson, G. M., Thorwalls, A., and Seiger, A. (2004). Recovery from unilateral neglect after right-hemisphere stroke. *Disability and Rehabilitation 26*: 471–477.

Axenfeld, D. (1894). Eine einfache Methode Hemianopsie zu constatiren. *Neurologisches Centralblatt 13*: 437–438.

Azouvi, P., Olivier, S., de Montety, G., Samuel, C., Louis-Dreyfus, A., and Tesio, L. (2003). Behavioral assessment of unilateral neglect: Study of the psychometric properties of the Catherine Bergego Scale. *Archives of Physical Medicine and Rehabilitation 84*: 51–57.

Baier, B., Mueller, N., Fechir, M., and Dieterich, M. (2010). Line bisection error and its anatomic correlate. *Stroke 41*: 1561–1563.

Barbieri, C. and De Renzi, E. (1989). Patterns of neglect dissociation. *Behavioural Neurology 2*: 13–24.

Barbut, D. and Gazzaniga, M. S. (1987). Disturbances in conceptual space involving language and speech. *Brain 110*: 1487–1496.

Barrett, A. M. and Burkholder, S. (2006). Monocular patching in subjects with right-hemisphere stroke affects perceptual-attentional bias. *Journal of Rehabilitation Research and Development 43*: 337–346.

Bartolomeo, P., Thiebaut de Schotten, M., and Chica, A. B. (2012). Brain networks of visuospatial attention and their disruption in visual neglect. *Frontiers in Human Neuroscience 6*: 110.

Barton, J. J., Behrmann, M., and Black, S. (1998). Ocular search during line bisection: The effects of hemi-neglect and hemianopia. *Brain 121*: 1117–1131.

Barton, J. J. S. and Black, S. E. (1998). Line bisection in hemianopia. *Journal of Neurology, Neurosurgery & Psychiatry 64*: 660–662.

Battersby, W. S., Bender, M. B., Pollack, M., and Kahn, R. L. (1956). Unilateral 'spatial agnosia' ('inattention') in patients with cerebral lesions. *Brain 79*: 68–93.

Baxter, D. M. and Warrington, E. K. (1983). Neglect dysgraphia. *Journal of Neurology, Neurosurgery & Psychiatry 46*: 1073–1078.

Becker, E. and Karnath, H.-O. (2010). Neuroimaging of eye position reveals spatial neglect. *Brain 133*: 909–914.

Behrmann, M., Watt, S., Black, S. E., and Barton, J. J. (1997). Impaired visual search in patients with unilateral neglect: An oculographic analysis. *Neuropsychologia 35*: 1445–1458.

Beis, J. M., Andre, J. M., Baumgarten, A., and Challier, B. (1999). Eye patching in unilateral spatial neglect: Efficacy of two methods. *Archives of Physical Medicine and Rehabilitation 80*(1): 71–76.

Bellas, D. N., Eskenazi, B., and Wasserstein, J. (1988a). The nature of unilateral neglect in the olfactory sensory system. *Neuropsychologia 26*: 45–52.

Bellas, D. N., Novelly, R. A., Eskenazi, B., and Wasserstein, J. (1988b). Unilateral displacement in the olfactory sense: A manifestation of the unilateral neglect syndrome. *Cortex 24*: 267–275.

Bellas, D. N., Novelly, R. A., and Eskenazi, B. (1989). Olfactory lateralization and identification in right hemisphere lesion and control patients. *Neuropsychologia 27*: 1187–1191.

Bender, M. B. and Diamond, S. P. (1965). An analysis of auditory perceptual defects with observations on the localization of dysfunction. *Brain 88*: 675–686.

Benke, T., Luzzatti, C., and Vallar, G. (2004). Hermann Zingerle's 'Impaired perception of the own body due to organic brain disorders': An introductory comment and an abridged translation. *Cortex 40*: 265–274.

Benton, A. L. (1956). Jacques Loeb and the method of double stimulation. *Journal of the History of Medicine and Allied Sciences 11*: 47–53.

Berlucchi, G., Moro, V., Guerrini, C., and Aglioti, S. M. (2004). Dissociation between taste and tactile extinction on the tongue after right brain damage. *Neuropsychologia 42*: 1007–1016.

Berthier, M., Starkstein, S., and Leiguarda, R. (1987). Behavioral effects of damage to the right insula and surrounding regions. *Cortex 23*: 673–678.

Berti, A., Làdavas, E., and Della Corte, M. (1996). Anosognosia for hemiplegia, neglect dyslexia and drawing neglect: Clinical findings and theoretical considerations. *Journal of the International Neuropsychological Society 2*: 426–440.

Berti, A., and Frassinetti, F. (2000). When far becomes near: Remapping of space by tool use. *Journal of Cognitive Neuroscience 12*: 415–420.

Berti, A. (2002). Unconscious processing in neglect. In H.-O. Karnath, A. D. Milner, and G. Vallar (eds.), *The Cognitive and Neural Bases of Spatial Neglect* (pp. 313–326). Oxford: Oxford University Press.

Berti, A. and Rizzolatti, G. (2002). Coding near and far space. In H. O. Karnath, A. D. Milner, and G. Vallar (eds.), *The Cognitive and Neural Bases of Spatial Neglect* (pp. 119–129). Oxford: Oxford University Press.

Berti, A. (2004). Cognition in dyschiria: Edoardo Bisiach's theory of spatial disorders and consciousness. *Cortex 40*: 275–280.

Bestmann, S., Ruff, C. C., Blankenburg, F., Weiskopf, N., Driver, J., and Rothwell, J. C. (2008). Mapping causal interregional influences with concurrent TMS-fMRI. *Experimental Brain Research 191*(4): 383–402. doi:10.1007/s00221-008-1601-8.

Binder, J., Marshall, R., Lazar, R., Benjamin, J., and Mohr, J. P. (1992). Distinct syndromes of hemineglect. *Archives of Neurology 49*: 1187–1194.

Bird, C. M., Malhotra, P., Parton, A., Coulthard, E., Rushworth, M. F., and Husain, M. (2006). Visual neglect after right posterior cerebral artery infarction. *Journal of Neurology, Neurosurgery & Psychiatry 77*: 1008–1012.

Bisiach, E., Capitani, E., Colombo, A., and Spinnler, H. (1976). Halving a horizontal segment: A study on hemisphere-damaged patients with cerebral focal lesions. *Schweizer Archiv für Neurologie und Psychiatrie 118*: 199–206.

Bisiach, E. and Luzzatti, C. (1978). Unilateral neglect of representational space. *Cortex 14*: 129–133.

Bisiach, E., Luzzatti, C., and Perani, D. (1979). Unilateral neglect, representational schema and consciousness. *Brain 102*: 609–618.

Bisiach, E., Capitani, E., Luzzatti, C., and Perani, D. (1981). Brain and conscious representation of outside reality. *Neuropsychologia 19*: 543–551.

Bisiach, E., Bulgarelli, C., Sterzi, R., and Vallar, G. (1983). Line bisection and cognitive plasticity of unilateral neglect of space. *Brain and Cognition 2*: 32–38.

Bisiach, E., Cornacchia, L., Sterzi, R., and Vallar, G. (1984). Disorders of perceived auditory lateralization after lesions of the right hemisphere. *Brain 107*: 37–52.

Bisiach, E., Capitani, E., and Porta, E. (1985). Two basic properties of space representation in the brain: Evidence from unilateral neglect. *Journal of Neurology, Neurosurgery & Psychiatry 48*: 141–144.

Bisiach, E., Perani, D., Vallar, G., and Berti, A. (1986a). Unilateral neglect: Personal and extrapersonal. *Neuropsychologia 24*: 759–767.

Bisiach, E., Vallar, G., Perani, D., Papagno, C., and Berti, A. (1986b). Unawareness of disease following lesions of the right hemisphere: Anosognosia for hemiplegia and anosognosia for hemianopia. *Neuropsychologia 24*: 471–482.

Bisiach, E. and Berti, A. (1987). Dyschiria: An attempt at its systemic explanation. In M. Jeannerod (ed.), *Neurophysiological and Neuropsychological Aspects of Spatial Neglect* (pp. 183–201). Amsterdam: North Holland.

Bisiach, E., Geminiani, G., Berti, A., and Rusconi, M. L. (1990). Perceptual and premotor factors of unilateral neglect. *Neurology 40*: 1278–1281.

Bisiach, E., Rusconi, M. L., and Vallar, G. (1991). Remission of somatoparaphrenic delusion through vestibular stimulation. *Neuropsychologia 29*: 1029–1031.

Bisiach, E. (1993). Mental representation in unilateral neglect and related disorders: The twentieth Bartlett Memorial Lecture. *Quarterly Journal of Experimental Psychology 46A*: 435–461.

Bisiach, E., Rusconi, M. L., Peretti, V., and Vallar, G. (1994). Challenging current accounts of unilateral neglect. *Neuropsychologia 32*: 1431–1434.

Bisiach, E., Pizzamiglio, L., Nico, D., and Antonucci, G. (1996). Beyond unilateral neglect. *Brain 119*: 851–857.

Bisiach, E., Ricci, R., Lualdi, M., and Colombo, M. R. (1998). Perceptual and response bias in unilateral neglect: Two modified versions of the Milner landmark task. *Brain and Cognition 37*: 369–386.

Bisiach, E. and Vallar, G. (2000). Unilateral neglect in humans. In F. Boller, J. Grafman, and G. Rizzolatti (eds.), *Handbook of Neuropsychology*, 2nd edn. (vol. 1, pp. 459–502). Amsterdam: Elsevier Science, B.V.

Bolognini, N. and Ro, T. (2010). Transcranial magnetic stimulation: Disrupting neural activity to alter and assess brain function. *Journal of Neuroscience 30*: 9647–9650.

Bolognini, N. and Maravita, A. (2011). Uncovering multisensory processing through non-invasive brain stimulation. *Frontiers in Psychology 2*: 46.

Bolognini, N., Casanova, D., Maravita, A., and Vallar, G. (2012). Bisecting real and fake body parts: Effects of prism adaptation after right brain damage. *Frontiers in Human Neuroscience 6*: 154.

Bolognini, N., Convento, S., Rossetti, A., and Merabet, L. B. (2013). Multisensory processing after a brain damage: Clues on post-injury crossmodal plasticity from neuropsychology. *Neuroscience & Biobehavioral Reviews 37*: 269–278.

Bottini, G., Paulesu, E., Sterzi, R., Warburton, E., Wise, R. J. S., Vallar, G., Frackowlak, R. S. J., and Frith, C. D. (1995). Modulation of conscious experience by peripheral sensory stimuli. *Nature 376*(6543): 778–781.

Bottini, G., Paulesu, E., Gandola, M., Loffredo, S., Scarpa, P., Sterzi, R., Santilli, I., Defanti, C. A., Scialfa, G., Fazio, F., and Vallar, G. (2005). Left caloric vestibular stimulation ameliorates right hemianesthesia. *Neurology 65*: 1278–1283.

Bowen, A., McKenna, K., and Tallis, R. C. (1999). Reasons for variability in the reported rate of occurrence of unilateral spatial neglect after stroke. *Stroke 30*: 1196–1202.

Bowen, A. and Lincoln, N. B. (2007). Cognitive rehabilitation for spatial neglect following stroke. *Cochrane Database of Systematic Reviews*: Art. No. CD003586.

Brain, W. R. (1941). Visual disorientation with special reference to lesions of the right cerebral hemisphere. *Brain 64*: 244–272.

Brandt, T., Glasauer, S., Strupp, M., and Dieterich, M. (2009). Spatial neglect: Hypothetical mechanisms of disturbed interhemispheric crosstalk for orientation. *Annals of the New York Academy of Sciences 1164*: 216–221.

Brighina, F., Bisiach, E., Oliveri, M., Piazza, A., La Bua, V., Daniele, O., and Fierro, B. (2003). 1 Hz repetitive transcranial magnetic stimulation of the unaffected hemisphere ameliorates contralesional visuospatial neglect in humans. *Neuroscience Letters 336*: 131–133.

Brozzoli, C., Demattè, M. L., Pavani, F., Frassinetti, F., and Farnè, A. (2006). Neglect and extinction: Within and between sensory modalities. *Restorative Neurology & Neuroscience 24*: 217–232.

Buxbaum, L. J. and Coslett, H. B. (1994). Neglect of chimeric figures: Two halves are better than a whole. *Neuropsychologia 32*: 275–288.

Buxbaum, L. J., Ferraro, M. K., Veramonti, T., Farnè, A., Whyte, J., Làdavas, E., Frassinetti, F., and Coslett, H. B. (2004). Hemispatial neglect: Subtypes, neuroanatomy, and disability. *Neurology 62*: 749–756.

Calvert, G. A., Spence, C., and Stein, B. E. (eds.) (2004). *The Handbook of Multisensory Processes*. Cambridge, Mass.: MIT Press.

Cambier, J., Elghozi, D., and Strube, E. (1980). Lésion du thalamus droit avec syndrome de l'hémisphère mineur: Discussion du concept de négligence thalamique. *Revue Neurologique (Paris) 136*: 105–116.

Caneman, G., Levander, M., and Tegnér, R. (1992). A tactile maze test in unilateral spatial neglect: The influence of vision and recording technique. *Journal of Neurology 239*: 273–276.

Caplan, B. (1985). Stimulus effects in unilateral neglect. *Cortex 21*: 69–80.

Cappa, S. F., Sterzi, R., Vallar, G., and Bisiach, E. (1987). Remission of hemineglect and anosognosia during vestibular stimulation. *Neuropsychologia 25*: 775–782.

Cappa, S. F. and Vallar, G. (1992). Neuropsychological disorders after subcortical lesions: Implications for neural models of language and spatial attention. In G. Vallar, S. F. Cappa, and C. W. Wallesch (eds.), *Neuropsychological Disorders Associated with Subcortical Lesions* (pp. 7–41). Oxford: Oxford University Press.

Cassidy, T. P., Bruce, D. W., Lewis, S., and Gray, C. S. (1999). The association of visual field deficits and visuo-spatial neglect in acute right-hemisphere stroke patients. *Age and Ageing 28*: 257–260.

Castaigne, P., Laplane, D., and Degos, J.-D. (1972). Trois cas de négligence motrice par lésion frontale pré-rolandique. *Revue Neurologique 126*: 5–15.

Castiello, U., Lusher, D., Burton, C., Glover, S., and Disler, P. (2004). Improving left hemispatial neglect using virtual reality. *Neurology 62*: 1958–1962.

Catani, M., Howard, R. J., Pajevic, S., and Jones, D. K. (2002). Virtual in vivo interactive dissection of white matter fasciculi in the human brain. *NeuroImage 17*: 77–94.

Cazzoli, D., Müri, R. M., Schumacher, R., von Arx, S., Chaves, S., Gutbrod, K., Bohlhalter, S., Bauer, D., Vanbellingen, T., Bertschi, M., Kipfer, S., Rosenthal, C. R., Kennard, C., Bassetti, C. L., and Nyffeler, T. (2012). Theta burst stimulation reduces disability during the activities of daily living in spatial neglect. *Brain 135*: 3426–39.

Celesia, G. G., Brigell, M. G., and Vaphiades, M. S. (1997). Hemianopic anosognosia. *Neurology 49*: 88–97.

Chambers, B. R., Brooder, R. J., and Donnan, G. A. (1991). Proximal posterior cerebral artery occlusion simulating middle cerebral artery occlusion. *Neurology 41*: 385–390.

Chatterjee, A., Mennemeier, M., and Heilman, K. M. (1992a). Search patterns and neglect: A case study. *Neuropsychologia 30*: 657–672.

Chatterjee, A., Mennemeier, M., and Heilman, K. M. (1992b). A stimulus-response relationship in unilateral neglect: The power function. *Neuropsychologia 30*: 1101–1108.

Chatterjee, A. (1994). Picturing unilateral spatial neglect: Viewer versus object-centred reference frames. *Journal of Neurology, Neurosurgery & Psychiatry 57*: 1236–1240.

Chechlacz, M., Rotshtein, P., and Humphreys, G. W. (2012). Neuroanatomical dissections of unilateral visual neglect symptoms: ALE meta-analysis of lesion-symptom mapping. *Frontiers in Human Neuroscience 6*: 230.

Chedru, F., Leblanc, M., and Lhermitte, F. (1973). Visual searching in normal and brain-damaged subjects (contribution to the study of unilateral inattention). *Cortex 9*: 94–111.

Choi, K. M., Lee, B. H., Lee, S. C., Ku, B. D., Kim, E. J., Suh, M. K., Jeong, Y., Heilman, K. M., and Na, D. L. (2007). Influence of moving background on line bisection performance in the normal elderly versus patients with hemispatial neglect. *American Journal of Physical Medicine & Rehabilitation 86*: 515–526.

Chokron, S., and Bartolomeo, P. (1997). Patterns of dissociation between left hemineglect and deviation of the egocentric reference. *Neuropsychologia 35*: 1503–1508.

Chokron, S., Colliot, P., Bartolomeo, P., Rhein F., Eusop, E., Vassel, P., and Ohlmann, T. (2002). Visual, proprioceptive and tactile performance in left neglect patients. *Neuropsychologia 40*: 1965–1976.

Chokron, S. (2003). Right parietal lesions, unilateral spatial neglect, and the egocentric frame of reference. *NeuroImage 20*: S75–S81.

Churchland, P. S. (1986). *Neurophilosophy*. Cambridge, Mass.: MIT Press.

Ciaraffa, F., Castelli, G., Parati, E. A., Bartolomeo, P., and Bizzi, A. (2012). Visual neglect as a disconnection syndrome? A confirmatory case report. Neurocase, 2 May. [Epub ahead of print.]

Cicerone, K. D., Dahlberg, C., Malec, J. F., Langenbahn, D. M., Felicetti, T., Kneipp, S., Ellmo, W., Kalmar, K., Giacino, J. T., Harley, J. P., Laatsch, L., Morse, P. A., and Catanese, J. (2005). Evidence-based cognitive rehabilitation: Updated review of the literature from 1998 through 2002. *Archives of Physical Medicine and Rehabilitation 86*: 1681–1692.

Cocchini, G., Beschin, N., and Jehkonen, M. (2001). The Fluff Test: A simple task to assess body representation neglect. *Neuropsychological Rehabilitation 11*: 17–31.

Colombo, A., De Renzi, E., and Gentilini, M. (1982). The time course of visual hemi-inattention. *Archiv für Psychiatrie und Nervenkrankheiten 231*: 539–546.

Coltheart, M., Patterson, K., and Marshall, J. C. (eds.) (1980). *Deep Dyslexia*. London: Routledge & Kegan Paul.

Committeri, G., Pitzalis, S., Galati, G., Patria, F., Pelle, G., Sabatini, U., Castriota-Scanderbeg, A., Piccardi, L., Guariglia, C., and Pizzamiglio, L. (2007). Neural bases of personal and extrapersonal neglect in humans. *Brain 130*: 431–441.

Corbetta, M. and Shulman, G. L. (2011). Spatial neglect and attention networks. *Annual Review of Neuroscience 34*: 569–599.

Coslett, H. B., Bowers, D., and Heilman, K. M. (1987). Reduction in cerebral activation after right hemisphere stroke. *Neurology 37*: 957–962.

Coulthard, E., Parton, A., and Husain, M. (2006). Action control in visual neglect. *Neuropsychologia 44*: 2717–2733.

Critchley, M., Russell, W. R., and Zangwill, O. L. (1951). Discussion on parietal lobe syndromes. *Proceedings of the Royal Society of Medicine 44*: 337–346.

Critchley, M. (1953). *The Parietal Lobes*. New York: Hafner.

Cubelli, R., Nichelli, P., Bonito, V., De Tanti, A., and Inzaghi, M. G. (1991). Different patterns of dissociation in unilateral spatial neglect. *Brain and Cognition 15*: 139–159.

D'Erme, P., De Bonis, C., and Gainotti, G. (1987). Influenza dell'emi-inattenzione e dell'emianopsia sui compiti di bisezione di linee nei pazienti cerebrolesi. *Archivio di Psicologia, Neurologia e Psichiatria 48*: 193–207.

Daffner, K. R., Ahern, G. L., Weintraub, S., and Mesulam, M.-M. (1990). Dissociated neglect behavior following sequential strokes in the right hemisphere. *Annals of Neurology 28*: 97–101.

Daini, R., Angelelli, P., Antonucci, G., Cappa, S. F., and Vallar, G. (2002). Exploring the syndrome of spatial unilateral neglect through an illusion of length. *Experimental Brain Research 144*: 224–237.

Damasio, A. R., Damasio, H., and Chang Chui, H. (1980). Neglect following damage to frontal lobe or basal ganglia. *Neuropsychologia 18*: 123–132.

De Renzi, E. (1977). Le amnesie. In E. Bisiach, F. Denes, E. De Renzi, et al. (eds.), *Neuropsicologia clinica* (pp. 199–246). Milano: Franco Angeli.

De Renzi, E. (1982). *Disorders of Space Exploration and Cognition*. Chichester: John Wiley.

De Renzi, E., Faglioni, P., Gentilini, M., and Barbieri, C. (1989). Attentional shift towards the rightmost stimuli in patients with left visual neglect. *Cortex 25*: 231–237.

Dejerine, J. (1892). Contribution à l'étude anatomo-pathologique et clinique des différentes variétés de cécité verbale. *Mémoires de la Societé Biologique 4*: 61–90.

Dennett, D. C. (1991). *Consciousness Explained*. London: Allen Lane, Penguin Press.

Denny-Brown, D., Meyer, J. S., and Horenstein, S. (1952). The significance of perceptual rivalry resulting from parietal lesion. *Brain 75*: 433–471.

Denny-Brown, D. and Chambers, R. A. (1958). The parietal lobe and behavior. *Association for Research in Nervous and Mental Disease 36*: 35–117.

Di Monaco, M., Schintu, S., Dotta, M., Barba, S., Tappero, R., and Gindri P. (2011). Severity of unilateral spatial neglect is an independent predictor of functional outcome after acute inpatient rehabilitation in individuals with right hemispheric stroke. *Archives of Physical Medicine and Rehabilitation 92*: 1250–1256.

Di Russo, F., Aprile, T., Spitoni, G., and Spinelli, D. (2008). Impaired visual processing of contralesional stimuli in neglect patients: A visual-evoked potential study. *Brain 131*: 842–854.

Diller, L. and Weinberg, J. (1977). Hemi-inattention in rehabilitation: The evolution of a rational remediation program. In E. A. Weinstein, and R. P. Friedland (eds.), *Hemi-inattention and Hemisphere Specialization* (pp. 62–82). New York: Raven Press.

Doricchi, F. and Angelelli, P. (1999). Misrepresentation of horizontal space in left unilateral neglect: Role of hemianopia. *Neurology 52*: 1845–1852.

Doricchi, F. and Tomaiuolo, F. (2003). The anatomy of neglect without hemianopia: A key role for parietal-frontal disconnection? *NeuroReport 14*: 2239–2243.

Driver, J. and Halligan, P. W. (1991). Can visual neglect operate in object-centered co-ordinates? An affirmative single case study. *Cognitive Neuropsychology 8*: 475–496.

Driver, J. and Pouget, A. (2000). Object-centered visual neglect, or relative egocentric neglect? *Journal of Cognitive Neuroscience 12*: 542–545.

Driver, J. and Vuilleumier, P. (2001). Perceptual awareness and its loss in unilateral neglect and extinction. *Consciousness and Cognition 79*: 39–88.

Ellis, A. W., Flude, B. M., and Young, A. W. (1987). 'Neglect dyslexia' and the early visual processing of letters in words and nonwords. *Cognitive Neuropsychology 4*: 439–464.

Eschenbeck, P., Vossel, S., Weiss, P. H., Saliger, J., Karbe, H., and Fink, G. R. (2010). Testing for neglect in right-hemispheric stroke patients using a new assessment battery based upon standardized activities of daily living (ADL). *Neuropsychologia 48*: 3488–3496.

Farnè, A., Buxbaum, L. J., Ferraro, M., Frassinetti, F., Whyte, J., Veramonti, T., Angeli, V., Coslett, H. B., and Làdavas, E. (2004). Patterns of spontaneous recovery of neglect and associated disorders in acute right brain-damaged patients. *Journal of Neurology, Neurosurgery & Psychiatry 75*: 1401–1410.

Farnè, A., Ponti, F., and Ladavas, E. (1998). In search for biased egocentric reference frames in neglect. *Neuropsychologia 36*: 611–623.

Farnè, A., Rossetti, Y., Toniolo, S., and Ladavas, E. (2002). Ameliorating neglect with prism adaptation: Visuo-manual and visuo-verbal measures. *Neuropsychologia 40*: 718–729.

Ferber, S. and Karnath, H. O. (1999). Parietal and occipital lobe contributions to perception of straight-ahead orientation. *Journal of Neurology, Neurosurgery & Psychiatry 67*: 572–578.

Ferro, J. M. and Kertesz, A. (1984). Posterior internal capsule infarction associated with neglect. *Archives of Neurology 41*: 422–424.

Fierro, B., Brighina, F., and Bisiach, E. (2006). Improving neglect by TMS. *Behavioural Neurology 17*: 169–176.

Fortis, P., Maravita, A., Gallucci, M., Ronchi, R., Grassi, E., Senna, I., Olgiati, E., Perucca, L., Banco, E., Posteraro, L., Tesio, L., and Vallar, G. (2010). Rehabilitating patients with left spatial neglect by prism exposure during a visuomotor activity. *Neuropsychology 24*: 681–697.

Frassinetti, F., Rossi, M., and Làdavas, E. (2001). Passive limb movements improve visual neglect. *Neuropsychologia 39*: 725–733.

Frassinetti, F., Angeli, V., Meneghello, F., Avanzi, S., and Làdavas, E. (2002a). Long-lasting amelioration of visuospatial neglect by prism adaptation. *Brain 125*: 608–623.

Frassinetti, F., Bolognini, N., and Làdavas, E. (2002b). Enhancement of visual perception by crossmodal visuo-auditory interaction. *Experimental Brain Research 147*: 332–343.

Frassinetti, F., Pavani, F., and Làdavas, E. (2002c). Acoustical vision of neglected stimuli: Interaction among spatially converging audiovisual inputs in neglect patients. *Journal of Cognitive Neuroscience 14*: 62–69.

Frassinetti, F., Bolognini, N., Bottari, D., Bonora, A., and Làdavas, E. (2005). Audiovisual integration in patients with visual deficit. *Journal of Cognitive Neuroscience 17*: 1442–1452.

Fregni, F. and Pascual-Leone, A. (2007). Technology insight: Noninvasive brain stimulation in neurology: Perspectives on the therapeutic potential of rTMS and tDCS. *Nature Clinical Practice Neurology 3*: 383–393.

Friedland, R. P. and Weinstein, E. A. (1977). Hemi-inattention and hemisphere specialization: Introduction and historical review. In E. A. Weinstein, and R. P. Friedland (eds.),

Advances in Neurology: Hemi-inattention and Hemisphere Specialization (vol. 18, pp. 1–31). New York: Raven Press.

Friedmann, N., Tzailer-Gross, L., and Gvion, A. (2011). The effect of syntax on reading in neglect dyslexia. *Neuropsychologia 49*: 2803–2816.

Fruhmann Berger, M., Pross, R. D., Ilg, U. J., and Karnath, H.-O. (2006). Deviation of eyes and head in acute cerebral stroke. *BMC Neurology 6*: 23.

Fujii, T., Fukatsu, R., Kimura, I., Saso, S., and Kogure, K. (1991). Unilateral spatial neglect in visual and tactile modalities. *Cortex 27*: 339–343.

Gainotti, G., Messerli, P., and Tissot, R. (1972). Qualitative analysis of unilateral spatial neglect in relation to laterality of cerebral lesions. *Journal of Neurology, Neurosurgery & Psychiatry 35*: 545–550.

Gainotti, G. (1996). Lateralization of brain mechanisms underlying automatic and controlled forms of spatial orienting of attention. *Neuroscience & Biobehavioral Reviews 20*: 617–622.

Gainotti, G., Perri, R., and Cappa, A. (2002). Left-hand movements and right hemisphere activation in unilateral spatial neglect: A test of the interhemispheric imbalance hypothesis. *Neuropsychologia 40*: 1350–1355.

Gainotti, G. (2010). The role of automatic orienting of attention towards ipsilesional stimuli in non-visual (tactile and auditory) neglect: A critical review. *Cortex 46*: 150–160.

Gallace, A., Imbornone, E., and Vallar, G. (2008). When the whole is more than the sum of the parts: Evidence from visuospatial neglect. *Jounal of Neuropsychology 2*: 387–413.

Gallace, A. and Spence, C. (2008). The cognitive and neural correlates of 'tactile consciousness': A multisensory perspective. *Consciousness and Cognition 17*: 370–407.

Gallagher, S. (2000). Philosophical conceptions of the self: Implications for cognitive science. *Trends in Cognitive Sciences 4*: 14–21.

Gassama, S., Deplancke, A., Saj, A., Honoré, J., and Rousseaux, M. (2011). Do supine position and deprivation of visual environment influence spatial neglect? *Journal of Neurology 258*: 1288–1294.

Gauthier, L., Dehaut, F., and Joanette, Y. (1989). The Bells Test: A quantitative and qualitative test for visual neglect. *International Journal of Clinical Neuropsychology 11*: 49–54.

Geminiani, G. and Bottini, G. (1992). Mental representation and temporary recovery from unilateral neglect after vestibular stimulation. *Journal of Neurology, Neurosurgery & Psychiatry 55*: 332–333.

Gentilini, M., Barbieri, C., De Renzi, E., and Faglioni, P. (1989). Space exploration with and without the aid of vision in hemisphere-damaged patients. *Cortex 25*: 643–651.

Girotti, F., Casazza, M., Musicco, M., and Avanzini, G. (1983). Oculomotor disorders in cortical lesions in man: The role of unilateral neglect. *Neuropsychologia 21*: 543–553.

Glocker, D., Bittl, P., and Kerkhoff, G. (2006). Construction and psychometric properties of a novel test for body representational neglect (Vest Test). *Restorative Neurology & Neuroscience 24*: 303–317.

Goldenberg, G. (1986). Neglect in a patient with partial callosal disconnection. *Neuropsychologia 24*: 397–403.

Grossi, D., Modaferri, A., Pelosi, L., and Trojano, L. (1989). On the different roles of the cerebral hemispheres in mental imagery: The 'O'Clock Test' in two clinical cases. *Brain and Cognition 10*: 18–27.

Guariglia, C. and Antonucci, G. (1992). Personal and extrapersonal space: A case of neglect dissociation. *Neuropsychologia 30*: 1001–1009.

Guariglia, C., Padovani, A., Pantano, P., and Pizzamiglio, L. (1993). Unilateral neglect restricted to visual imagery. *Nature 364*: 235–237.

Guariglia, C., Lippolis, G., and Pizzamiglio, L. (1998). Somatosensory stimulation improves imagery disorders in neglect. *Cortex 34*: 233–241.

Guariglia, C., Coriale, G., Cosentino, T., and Pizzamiglio, L. (2000). TENS modulates spatial reorientation in neglect patients. *NeuroReport 11*: 1945–1948.

Halligan, P. W., Marshall, J. C., and Wade, D. T. (1990). Do visual field deficits exacerbate visuo-spatial neglect? *Journal of Neurology, Neurosurgery & Psychiatry 53*: 487–491.

Halligan, P. W. and Marshall, J. C. (1991). Left neglect for near but not far space in man. *Nature 350*: 498–500.

Halligan, P. W. and Marshall, J. C. (1992). Left visuo-spatial neglect: A meaningless entity? *Cortex 28*: 525–535.

Halligan, P. W. and Marshall, J. C. (1993). When two is one: A case study of spatial parsing in visual neglect. *Perception 22*: 309–312.

Halligan, P. W., Marshall, J. C., Hunt, M., and Wade, D. T. (1997). Somatosensory assessment: Can seeing produce feeling. *Journal of Neurology 244*: 199–203.

Halligan, P. W. and Marshall, J. C. (2002). Primary sensory deficits after right-brain damage—an attentional disorder by any other name? In H.-O. Karnath, A. D. Milner, and G. Vallar (eds.), *The Cognitive and Neural Bases of Spatial Neglect* (pp. 327–330). Oxford: Oxford University Press.

Halligan, P. W., Fink, G. R., Marshall, J. C., and Vallar, G. (2003). Spatial cognition: Evidence from visual neglect. *Trends in Cognitive Sciences 7*: 125–133.

Hasegawa, C., Hirono, N., and Yamadori, A. (2011). Discrepancy in unilateral spatial neglect between daily living and neuropsychological test situations: A single case study. *Neurocase 17*: 518–526.

Healton, E. B., Navarro, C., Bressman, S., and Brust, J. C. (1982). Subcortical neglect. *Neurology 32*: 776–778.

Hécaen, H., de Ajuriaguerra, J., and Massonnet, J. (1951). Les troubles visuo-constructifs par lesion pariéto-occipitale droite. *Role des perturbations vestibulaires: L'Encéphale 40*: 122–179.

Hécaen, H., Penfield, W., Bertrand, C., and Malmo, R. (1956). The syndrome of apractognosia due to lesions of the minor cerebral hemisphere. *Archives of Neurology and Psychiatry 75*: 400–434.

Hécaen, H. and Albert, M. L. (1978). *Human Neuropsychology*. New York: John Wiley.

Heilman, K. M. and Valenstein, E. (1972a). Auditory neglect in man. *Archives of Neurology 26*: 32–35.

Heilman, K. M. and Valenstein, E. (1972b). Frontal lobe neglect in man. *Neurology 22*: 660–664.

Heilman, K. M. and Watson, R. T. (1977). The neglect syndrome: A unilateral defect of the orienting response. In S. R. Harnad, R. W. Doty, L. Goldstein, J. Jaynes, and G. Krauthamer (eds.), *Lateralization in the Nervous System* (pp. 285–302). New York: Academic Press.

Heilman, K. M., Schwartz, H. D., and Watson, R. T. (1978). Hypoarousal in patients with the neglect syndrome and emotional indifference. *Neurology 28*: 229–232.

Heilman, K. M. and Watson, R. T. (1978). Changes in the symptoms of neglect induced by changing task strategy. *Archives of Neurology 35*: 37–49.

Heilman, K. M. (1979). Neglect and related disorders. In K. M. Heilman, and E. Valenstein (eds.), *Clinical Neuropsychology* (pp. 268–307). New York: Oxford University Press.

Heilman, K. M. and Valenstein, E. (1979). Mechanisms underlying hemispatial neglect. *Annals of Neurology 5*: 166–170.

Heilman, K. M., Bowers, D., and Watson, R. T. (1983). Performance on hemispatial pointing task by patients with neglect syndrome. *Neurology 33*: 661–664.

Heilman, K. M., Bowers, D., and Watson, R. T. (1984). Pseudoneglect in a patient with partial callosal disconnection. *Brain 107*: 519–532.

Heilman, K. M., Watson, R. T., and Valenstein, E. (1985). Neglect and related disorders. In K. M. Heilman, and E. Valenstein (eds.), *Clinical Neuropsychology*, 2nd edn. (pp. 243–293). Oxford: Oxford University Press.

Heilman, K. M., Watson, R. T., and Valenstein, E. (1993). Neglect and related disorders. In K. M. Heilman, and E. Valenstein (eds.), *Clinical Neuropsychology*, 3rd edn. (pp. 279–336). New York: Oxford University Press.

Heilman, K. M., Watson, R. T., and Valenstein, E. (1994). Localization of lesions in neglect and related disorders. In A. Kertesz (ed.), *Localization and Neuroimaging in Neuropsychology* (pp. 495–524). San Diego: Academic Press.

Heilman, K. M. (1995). Attentional asymmetries. In R. J. Davidson and K. Hugdal (eds.), *Brain Asymmetry* (pp. 217–234). Boston: MIT Press.

Heilman, K. M. and Adams, D. J. (2003). Callosal neglect. *Archives of Neurology 60*: 276–279.

Heilman, K. M., Watson, R. T., and Valenstein, E. (2003). Neglect and related disorders. In K. M. Heilman and E. Valenstein (eds.), *Clinical Neuropsychology*, 4th edn. (pp. 296–346). New York: Oxford University Press.

Hesse, M. D., Sparing, R., and Fink, G. R. (2011). Ameliorating spatial neglect with non-invasive brain stimulation: From pathophysiological concepts to novel treatment strategies. *Neuropsychological Rehabilitation 21*: 676–702.

Hier, D. B., Mondlock, J., and Caplan, L. R. (1983a). Behavioral abnormalities after right hemisphere stroke. *Neurology 33*: 337–344.

Hier, D. B., Mondlock, J., and Caplan, L. R. (1983b). Recovery of behavioral abnormalities after right hemisphere stroke. *Neurology 33*: 345–350.

Hillis, A. E. and Caramazza, A. (1995). A framework for interpreting distinct patterns of hemispatial neglect. *Neurocase 1*: 189–207.

Hillis, A. E., Barker, P. B., Beauchamp, N. J., Gordon, B., and Wityk, R. J. (2000). MR perfusion imaging reveals regions of hypoperfusion associated with aphasia and neglect. *Neurology 55*: 782–788.

Hillis, A. E., Wityk, R. J., Barker, P. B., Beauchamp, N. J., Gailloud, P., Murphy, K., Cooper, O., and Metter, E. J. (2002). Subcortical aphasia and neglect in acute stroke: The role of cortical hypoperfusion. *Brain 125*: 1094–1104.

Hillis, A. E., Newhart, M., Heidler, J., Barker, P. B., Herskovits, E. H., and Degaonkar, M. (2005). Anatomy of spatial attention: Insights from perfusion imaging and hemispatial neglect in acute stroke. *Journal of Neuroscience 25*: 3161–3167.

Hjaltason, H. and Tegner, R. (1992). Darkness improves line bisection in unilateral spatial neglect. *Cortex 28*: 353–358.

Hjaltason, H., Caneman, G., and Tegner, R. (1993). Visual and tactile rod bisection in unilateral neglect. *Cortex 29*: 583–588.

Ho, A. K., Manly, T., Nestor, P. J., Sahakian, B. J., Bak, T. H., Robbins, T. W., Rosser, A. E., and Barker, R. A. (2003). A case of unilateral neglect in Huntington's disease. *Neurocase 9*: 261–273.

Hornak, J. (1992). Ocular exploration in the dark by patients with visual neglect. *Neuropsychologia 30*: 547–552.

Hughlings Jackson, J. (1876/1932). Case of large cerebral tumour without optic neuritis and with hemiplegia and imperception. In J. Taylor (ed.), *Selected Writings of John Hughlings Jackson* (pp. 146–152). London: Hodder and Stoughton.

Husain, M. and Kennard, C. (1996). Visual neglect associated with frontal lobe infarction. *Journal of Neurology 243*: 652–657.

Husain, M., Mannan, S., Hodgson, T., Wojciulik, E., Driver, J., and Kennard, C. (2001). Impaired spatial working memory across saccades contributes to abnormal search in parietal neglect. *Brain 124*: 941–952.

Husain, M. and Rorden, C. (2003). Non-spatially lateralized mechanisms in hemispatial neglect. *Nature Reviews Neuroscience 4*: 26–36.

Ishiai, S., Furukawa, T., and Tsukagoshi, H. (1989). Visuospatial processes of line bisection and the mechanisms underlying unilateral spatial neglect. *Brain 112*: 1485–1502.

Ishiai, S., Koyama, Y., Seki, K., Orimo, S., Sodeyama, N., Ozawa, E., Lee, E. Y., Takahashi, M., Watabiki, S., Okiyama, R., Ohtake, T., and Hiroki, M. (2000). Unilateral spatial neglect in AD: Significance of line bisection performance. *Neurology 55*: 364–370.

Jacobs, S., Brozzoli, C., and Farnè, A. (2012). Neglect: A multisensory deficit? *Neuropsychologia 50*: 1029–1044.

Jacquin-Courtois, S., Rode, G., Pavani, F., O'Shea, J., Giard, M. H., Boisson, D., and Rossetti, Y. (2010). Effect of prism adaptation on left dichotic listening deficit in neglect patients: Glasses to hear better? *Brain 133*: 895–908.

Jeannerod, M. (ed.) (1987). *Neurophysiological and Neuropsychological Aspects of Spatial Neglect*. Amsterdam: North Holland.

Jewesbury, E. C. O. (1969). Parietal lobe syndromes. In P. J. Vinken, and G. W. Bruyn (eds.), *Handbook of Clinical Neurology* (vol. 2, pp. 680–699). Amsterdam: North Holland.

Karnath, H.-O., Christ, K., and Hartje, W. (1993). Decrease of contralateral neglect by neck muscle vibration and spatial orientation of trunk midline. *Brain 116*: 383–396.

Karnath, H.-O. (1994). Subjective body orientation in neglect and the interactive contribution of neck muscle proprioception and vestibular stimulation. *Brain 117*: 1001–1012.

Karnath, H.-O., and Fetter, M. (1995). Ocular space exploration in the dark and its relation to subjective and objective body orientation in neglect patients with parietal lesions. *Neuropsychologia 33*: 371–377.

Karnath, H.-O. (1997). Spatial orientation and the representation of space with parietal lobe lesions. *Philosophical Transactions of the Royal Society of London B352*: 1411–1419.

Karnath, H.-O., Ferber, S., and Himmelbach, M. (2001). Spatial awareness is a function of the temporal not the posterior parietal lobe. *Nature 411*: 950–953.

Karnath, H.-O., Himmelbach, M., and Rorden, C. (2002). The subcortical anatomy of human spatial neglect: Putamen, caudate nucleus and pulvinar. *Brain 125*: 350–360.

Karnath, H.-O., Fruhmann Berger, M., Küker, W., and Rorden, C. (2004). The anatomy of spatial neglect based on voxelwise statistical analysis: A study of 140 patients. *Cerebral Cortex 14*: 1164–1172.

Karnath, H.-O., and Dieterich, M. (2006). Spatial neglect—a vestibular disorder? *Brain 129*: 293–305.

Karnath, H.-O., Rennig, S., Johannsen, L., and Rorden, C. (2011). The anatomy underlying acute versus chronic spatial neglect: A longitudinal study. *Brain 134*: 903–912.

Kase, C. S., Troncoso, J. F., Court, J. E., Tapia, J. F., and Mohr, J. P. (1977). Global spatial disorientation: Clinico-pathologic correlations. *Journal of Neurological Sciences 34*: 267–278.

Kashiwagi, A., Kashiwagi, T., Nishikawa, T., Tanabe, H., and Okuda, J. (1990). Hemispatial neglect in a patient with callosal infarction. *Brain 113*: 1005–1023.

Katz, N., Hartman-Maeir, A., Ring, H., and Soroker, N. (1999). Functional disability and rehabilitation outcome in right hemisphere damaged patients with and without unilateral spatial
neglect. *Archives of Physical Medicine and Rehabilitation 80*: 379–384.

Kerkhoff, G. (1993). Displacement of the egocentric visual midline in altitudinal postchiasmatic
scotomata. *Neuropsychologia 31*: 261–265.

Kerkhoff, G. and Schindler, I. (1997). Hemineglekt versus Hemianopsie: Hinweise zur
Differentialdiagnose. *Fortschritte der Neurologie-Psychiatrie 65*: 278–289.

Kerkhoff, G., Schindler, I., Artinger, F., Zoelch, C., Bublak, P., and Finke, K. (2006). Rotation
or translation of auditory space in neglect? A case study of chronic right-sided neglect.
Neuropsychologia 44: 923–933.

Kerkhoff, G. and Bucher, L. (2008). Line bisection as an early method to assess homonymous
hemianopia. *Cortex 44*: 200–205.

Kerkhoff, G. and Schenk, T. (2011). Line bisection in homonymous visual field defects: Recent
findings and future directions. *Cortex 47*: 53–58.

Kinsbourne, M. and Warrington, E. K. (1962). A variety of reading disability associated with
right hemisphere lesions. *Journal of Neurology, Neurosurgery & Psychiatry 25*: 339–344.

Kinsbourne, M. (1970). A model for the mechanism of unilateral neglect of space. *Transactions
of the American Neurological Association 95*: 143–146.

Kinsbourne, M. (1977). Hemi-neglect and hemisphere rivarly. In E. A. Weinstein and R. P.
Friedland (eds.), *Hemi-inattention and Hemispheric Specialization: Advances in Neurology*
(vol. 18, pp. 41–49). New York: Raven Press.

Kinsbourne, M. (1993). Orientational bias model of unilateral neglect: Evidence from attentional gradients within hemispace. In I. H. Robertson and J. C. Marshall (eds.), *Unilateral
Neglect: Clinical and Experimental Studies* (pp. 63–86). Hove: Lawrence Erlbaum Associates.

Klatzky, R. L. (1998). Allocentric and egocentric spatial representations: Definitions, distinctions, and interconnections. In C. Freksa and C. Habel (eds.), *Spatial Cognition. Lecture Notes
in Computer Science* (vol. 1404, pp. 1–17). Berlin: Springer.

Kleiner-Fisman, G., Black, S. E., and Lang, A. E. (2003). Neurodegenerative disease and the
evolution of art: The effects of presumed corticobasal degeneration in a professional artist.
Movement Disorders 18: 294–302.

Kleinman, J. T., Newhart, M., Davis, C., Heidler-Gary, J., Gottesman, R. F., and Hillis, A. E.
(2007). Right hemispatial neglect: Frequency and characterization following acute left hemisphere stroke. *Brain and Cognition 64*: 50–59.

Koch, G., Oliveri, M., Cheeran, B., Ruge, D., Lo Gerfo, E., Salerno, S., Torriero, S., Marconi, B.,
Mori, F., Driver, J., Rothwell, J. C., and Caltagirone, C. (2008). Hyperexcitability of parietal-
motor functional connections in the intact left-hemisphere of patients with neglect. *Brain
131*: 3147–3155.

Koehler, P. J., Endtz, L. J., Velde, J. T., and Hekster, R. E. M. (1986). Aware or non-aware: On the
significance of awareness for localization of the lesion responsible for homonymous hemianopia. *Journal of the Neurological Sciences 75*: 255–262.

Kooistra, C. A. and Heilman, K. M. (1989). Hemispatial visual inattention masquerading as
hemianopia. *Neurology 39*: 1125–1127.

Lacquaniti, F. (1997). Frames of reference in sensorimotor coordination. In F. Boller and J.
Grafman (eds.), *Handbook of Neuropsychology* (vol. 11, pp. 27–64). Amsterdam: Elsevier.

Làdavas, E. (1987). Is the hemispatial deficit produced by right parietal lobe damage associated
with retinal or gravitational coordinates? *Brain 110*: 167–180.

Làdavas, E. (1990). Selective spatial attention in patients with visual extinction. *Brain 113*:
1527–1538.

Làdavas, E., Petronio, A., and Umiltà, C. (1990). The deployment of visual attention in the intact field of hemineglect patients. *Cortex 26*: 307–317.

Làdavas, E., Shallice, T., and Zanella, M. T. (1997a). Preserved semantic access in neglect dyslexia. *Neuropsychologia 35*: 257–270.

Làdavas, E., Umiltà, C., and Mapelli, D. (1997b). Lexical and semantic processing in the absence of word reading: Evidence from neglect dyslexia. *Neuropsychologia 35*: 1075–1085.

Làdavas, E., Serino, A., Bottini, G., Beschin, N., and Magnotti, L. (2012). Riabilitazione dell'eminattenzione spaziale unilaterale o neglect. In G. Vallar, A. Cantagallo, S. F. Cappa, and P. Zoccolotti (eds.), *La riabilitazione neuro psicologica*: Un'analisi basata sul metodo evidence-based medicine (pp. 35–56). Milano: Springer.

Laplane, D. and Degos, J. D. (1983). Motor neglect. *Journal of Neurology, Neurosurgery & Psychiatry 46*: 152–158.

Lawson, I. R. (1962). Visual-spatial neglect in lesions of the right cerebral hemisphere: A study in recovery. *Neurology 12*: 23–33.

Lawton, M. P. and Brody, E. M. (1969). Assessment of older people: Self-maintaining and instrumental activities of daily living. *Gerontologist 9*: 179–186.

Lee, B. H., Suh, M. K., Kim, E. J., Seo, S. W., Choi, K. M., Kim, G. M., Chung, C. S., Heilman, K. M., and Na, D. L. (2009). Neglect dyslexia: Frequency, association with other hemispatial neglects, and lesion localization. *Neuropsychologia 47*: 704–710.

Leibovitch, F. S., Black, S. E., Caldwell, C. B., Ebert, P. L., Ehrlich, L. E., and Szalai, J. P. (1998). Brain-behavior correlations in hemispatial neglect using CT and SPECT: The Sunnybrook Stroke Study. *Neurology 50*: 901–908.

Lewald, J., Peters, S., Tegenthoff, M., and Hausmann, M. (2009). Dissociation of auditory and visual straight ahead in hemianopia. *Brain Research 1287*: 111–117.

Luukkainen-Markkula, R., Tarkka, I. M., Pitkanen, K., Sivenius, J., and Hamalainen, H. (2011). Comparison of the Behavioural Inattention Test and the Catherine Bergego Scale in assessment of hemispatial neglect. *Neuropsychological Rehabilitation 21*: 103–116.

Machner, B., Sprenger, A., Hansen, U., Heide, W., and Helmchen, C. (2009a). Acute hemianopic patients do not show a contralesional deviation in the line bisection task. *Journal of Neurology 256*: 289–290.

Machner, B., Sprenger, A., Sander, T., Heide, W., Kimmig, H., Helmchen, C., and Kömpf, D. (2009b). Visual search disorders in acute and chronic homonymous hemianopia: Lesion effects and adaptive strategies. *Annals of the New York Academy of Sciences 1164*: 419–426.

Mahoney, F. I. and Barthel, D. W. (1965). Functional evaluation: The Barthel Index. *Maryland State Medical Journal 14*: 61–65.

Malhotra, P., Coulthard, E., and Husain, M. (2006). Hemispatial neglect, balance and eye-movement control. *Current Opinion in Neurology 19*: 14–20.

Mancini, F., Bricolo, E., Mattioli, F. C., and Vallar, G. (2011). Visuo-haptic interactions in unilateral spatial neglect: The crossmodal Müller-Lyer illusion. *Frontiers in Perception Science 2*: 341.

Manes, F., Paradiso, S., Springer, J. A., Lamberty, G., and Robinson, R. G. (1999). Neglect after right insular cortex infarction. *Stroke 30*: 946–948.

Maravita, A., McNeil, J., Malhotra, P., Greenwood, R., Husain, M., and Driver, J. (2003). Prism adaptation can improve contralesional tactile perception in neglect. *Neurology 60*: 1829–1831.

Maravita, A. and Iriki, A. (2004). Tools for the body (schema). *Trends in Cognitive Sciences 8*: 79–86.

Mark, V. W., Kooistra, C. A., and Heilman, K. M. (1988). Hemispatial neglect affected by non-neglected stimuli. *Neurology 38*: 1207–1211.

Mark, V. W., Heilman, K. M., and Watson, R. (1996). Motor neglect: What do we mean? *Neurology 46*: 1492–1493.

Marquardsen, J. (1969). The natural history of acute cerebrovascular disease: A retrospective study of 769 patients. *Acta Neurologica Scandinavica 45*: suppl. 38.

Marsh, E. B. and Hillis, A. E. (2008). Dissociation between egocentric and allocentric visuospatial and tactile neglect in acute stroke. *Cortex 44*: 1215–1220.

Marshall, C. R. and Maynard, F. M. (1983). Vestibular stimulation for supranuclear gaze palsy: A case report. *Archives of Physical Medicine and Rehabilitation 64*: 134–136.

Marshall, J. C. and Halligan, P. (1988). Blindsight and insight in visuo-spatial neglect. *Nature 336*: 766–767.

Marshall, J. C. and Halligan, P. W. (1993). Visuo-spatial neglect: A new copying test to assess perceptual parsing. *Journal of Neurology 240*: 37–40.

Marshall, J. C. and Halligan, P. W. (1995). Within- and between-task dissociations in visuo-spatial neglect: A case study. *Cortex 31*: 367–376.

Marshall, J. C. and Vallar, G. (2004). A Festschrift for Edoardo Bisiach (and spatial neglect). *Cortex 40*: 235–236.

Massironi, M., Antonucci, G., Pizzamiglio, L., Vitale, M. V., and Zoccolotti, P. L. (1988). The Wundt-Jastrow illusion in the study of spatial hemi-inattention. *Neuropsychologia 26*: 161–166.

Mattingley, J. B., Bradshaw, J. L., and Bradshaw, J. A. (1995). Horizontal visual motion modulates focal attention in left unilateral spatial neglect. *Journal of Neurology, Neurosurgery & Psychiatry 57*: 1228–1235.

McFie, J., Piercy, M. F., and Zangwill, O. L. (1950). Visual-spatial agnosia associated with lesions of the right cerebral hemisphere. *Brain 73*: 167–190.

McGlinchey-Berroth, R., Milberg, W. P., Verfaellie, M., Alexander, M., and Kilduff, P. (1993). Semantic processing in the neglected visual field: Evidence from a lexical decision task. *Cognitive Neuropsychology 10*: 79–108.

McGlinchey-Berroth, R. (1997). Visual information processing in hemispatial neglect. *Trends in Cognitive Sciences 1*: 91–97.

McIntosh, R. D., Rossetti, Y., and Milner, A. D. (2002). Prism adaptation improves chronic visual and haptic neglect: A single case study. *Cortex 38*: 309–320.

Meador, K. J., Loring, D. W., Bowers, D., and Heilman, K. M. (1987). Remote memory and neglect syndrome. *Neurology 37*: 522–526.

Mennemeier, M., Vezey, E., Chatterjee, A., Rapcsak, S. Z., and Heilman, K. M. (1997). Contributions of the left and right cerebral hemispheres to line bisection. *Neuropsychologia 35*: 703–715.

Merleau-Ponty, M. (1945). *Phénoménologie de la perception*. Paris: Gallimard.

Mesulam, M. M. (1981). A cortical network for directed attention and unilateral neglect. *Annals of Neurology 10*: 309–325.

Mesulam, M. M. (1985). *Principles of Behavioral Neurology*. Philadelphia: F. A. Davis.

Mesulam, M. M. (1999). Spatial attention and neglect: Parietal, frontal and cingulate contributions to the mental representation and attentional targeting of salient extrapersonal events. *Philosophical Transactions of the Royal Society of London B354*: 1325–1346.

Mesulam, M.-M. (2002). Functional anatomy of attention and neglect: From neurons to networks. In H.-O. Karnath, A. D. Milner, and G. Vallar (eds.), *The Cognitive and Neural Bases of Spatial Neglect* (pp. 33–45). Oxford: Oxford University Press.

Milner, A. D., Harvey, M., Roberts, R. C., and Forster, S. V. (1993). Line bisection errors in visual neglect: Misguided action or size distortion? *Neuropsychologia 31*: 39–49.

Miniussi, C. and Vallar, G. (2011). Brain stimulation and behavioural cognitive rehabilitation: A new tool for neurorehabilitation? *Neuropsychological Rehabilitation 21*: 553–559.

Mizuno, K., Tsuji, T., Takebayashi, T., Fujiwara, T., Hase, K., and Liu, M. (2011). Prism adaptation therapy enhances rehabilitation of stroke patients with unilateral spatial neglect: A randomized, controlled trial. *Neurorehabilitation and Neural Repair 25*: 711–720.

Molenberghs, P. and Sale, M. V. (2011). Testing for spatial neglect with line bisection and target cancellation: Are both tasks really unrelated? *PLoS One 6*: e23017.

Molenberghs, P., Sale, M. V., and Mattingley, J. B. (2012). Is there a critical lesion site for unilateral spatial neglect? A meta-analysis using activation likelihood estimation. *Frontiers in Human Neuroscience, 6*.

Mort, D. J. and Kennard, C. (2003). Visual search and its disorders. *Current Opinion in Neurology 16*: 51–57.

Mort, D. J., Malhotra, P., Mannan, S. K., Rorden, C., Pambakian, A., Kennard, C., and Husain, M. (2003). The anatomy of visual neglect. *Brain 126*: 1986–1997.

Mort, D. J., Malhotra, P., Mannan, S. K., Pambakian, A., Kennard, C., and Husain, M. (2004). Using SPM normalization for lesion analysis in spatial neglect. *Brain 127*: E11.

Moscovitch, M. and Behrmann, M. (1994). Coding of spatial information in the somatosensory system: Evidence from patients with neglect following parietal lobe damage. *Journal of Cognitive Neuroscience 6*: 151–155.

Mozer, M. C. (2002). Frames of reference in unilateral neglect and visual perception: A computational perspective. *Psychological Review 109*: 156–185.

Müller-Oehring, E. M., Kasten, E., Poggel, D. A., Schulte, T., Strasburger, H., and Sabel, B. A. (2003). Neglect and hemianopia superimposed. *Journal of Clinical and Experimental Neuropsychology 25*: 1154–1168.

Müri, R. M., Cazzoli, D., Nyffeler, T., and Pflugshaupt, T. (2009). Visual exploration pattern in hemineglect. *Psychological Research 73*: 147–157.

Na, D. L., Adair, J. C., Kang, Y., Chung, C. S., Lee, K. H., and Heilman, K. M. (1999). Motor perseverative behavior on a line cancellation task. *Neurology 52*: 1569–1576.

Nadeau, S. E. and Heilman, K. M. (1991). Gaze-dependent hemianopia without hemispatial neglect. *Neurology 41*: 1244–1250.

Nitsche, M. A., Cohen, L. G., Wassermann, E. M., Priori, A., Lang, N., Antal, A., Paulus, W., Hummel, F., Boggio, P. S., Fregni, F., and Pascual-Leone, A. (2008). Transcranial direct current stimulation: State of the art 2008. *Brain Stimulation 1*: 206–223.

Nys, G. M., van Zandvoort, M. J., van der Worp, H. B., Kappelle, L. J., and de Haan, E. H. F. (2006). Neuropsychological and neuroanatomical correlates of perseverative responses in subacute stroke. *Brain 129*: 2148–2157.

Ogourtsova, T., Korner-Bitensky, N., and Ptito, A. (2010). Contribution of the superior colliculi to post-stroke unilateral spatial neglect and recovery. *Neuropsychologia 48*: 2407–2416.

Oliveri, M., Bisiach, E., Brighina, F., Piazza, A., La Bua, V., Buffa, D., and Fierro, B. (2001). rTMS of the unaffected hemisphere transiently reduces contralesional visuo-spatial hemineglect. *Neurology 57*: 1338–1340.

Oliveri, M., and Caltagirone, C. (2006). Suppression of extinction with TMS in humans: From healthy controls to patients. *Behavioral Neurology 17*: 163–167.

Oppenheim, H. (1885). Über eine durch eine klinisch bisher nicht verwerthete Untersuchungsmethode ermittelte Form der Sensibilitätsstörung bei einseitigen Erkrankungen des Grosshirns. *Neurologische Zentralblatt 4*: 529–533.

Ortigue, S., Mégevand, P., Perren, F., Landis, T., and Blanke, O. (2006). Double dissociation between representational personal and extrapersonal neglect. *Neurology 66*: 1414–1417.

Ota, H., Fujii, T., Suzuki, K., Fukatsu, R., and Yamadori, A. (2001). Dissociation of body-centered and stimulus-centered representations in unilateral neglect. *Neurology 57*: 2064–2069.

Pambakian, A. L., Wooding, D. S., Patel, N., Morland, A. B., Kennard, C., and Mannan, S. K. (2000). Scanning the visual world: A study of patients with homonymous hemianopia. *Journal of Neurology, Neurosurgery & Psychiatry 69*: 751–759.

Paolucci, S., Antonucci, G., Grasso, M. G., and Pizzamiglio, L. (2001). The role of unilateral spatial neglect in rehabilitation of right-brain-damaged ischemic stroke patients: A matched comparison. *Archives of Physical Medicine and Rehabilitation 82*: 743–749.

Park, K. C., Jeong, Y., Lee, B. H., Kim, E. J., Kim, G. M., Heilman, K. M., and Na, D. L. (2005). Left hemispatial visual neglect associated with a combined right occipital and splenial lesion: Another disconnection syndrome. *Neurocase 11*: 310–318.

Park, K. C., Lee, B. H., Kim, E. J., Shin, M. H., Choi, K. M., Yoon, S. S., Kwon, S. U., Chung, C. S., Lee, K. H., Heilman, K. M., and Na, D. L. (2006). Deafferentation-disconnection neglect induced by posterior cerebral artery infarction. *Neurology 66*: 56–61.

Paterson, A. and Zangwill, O. L. (1944). Disorders of visual space perception associated with lesions of the right cerebral hemisphere. *Brain 67*: 331–335.

Patterson, K. E., Marshall, J. C., and Coltheart, M. (eds.) (1985). *Surface Dyslexia:* Neuropsychological and Cognitive Studies of Phonological Reading. London: Lawrence Erlbaum Associates.

Paulus, W. (2011). Transcranial electrical stimulation (tES—tDCS; tRNS, tACS) methods. *Neuropsychological Rehabilitation 21*: 602–617.

Pavani, F., Meneghello, F., and Ladavas, E. (2001). Deficit of auditory space perception in patients with visuospatial neglect. *Neuropsychologia 39*: 1401–1409.

Pavani, F., Ladavas, E., and Driver, J. (2002). Selective deficit of auditory localisation in patients with visuospatial neglect. *Neuropsychologia 40*: 291–301.

Pavani, F., Làdavas, E., and Driver, J. (2003). Auditory and multisensory aspects of visuospatial neglect. *Trends in Cognitive Sciences 9*: 407–414.

Pavani, F., Husain, M., Ladavas, E., and Driver, J. (2004). Auditory deficits in visuospatial neglect patients. *Cortex 40*: 347–365.

Pedersen, P. M., Jørgensen, H. S., Nakayama, H., Raaschou, H. O., and Olsen, T. S. (1997). Hemineglect in acute stroke—incidence and prognostic implications: The Copenhagen stroke study. *American Journal of Physical Medicine & Rehabilitation 76*: 122–127.

Perani, D., Vallar, G., Cappa, S., Messa, C., and Fazio, F. (1987). Aphasia and neglect after subcortical stroke: A clinical/cerebral perfusion correlation study. *Brain 110*: 1211–1229.

Pia, L., Ricci, R., Gindri, P., and Vallar, G. (2013). Drawing perseveration in neglect: Effects of target density. *Journal of Neuropsychology 7*: 45–57.

Pick, A. (1898). Über Allgemeine Dedächtnisschwäche als Unmittelbare Folge Cerebraler Herderkrankung. Belträge zur Pathologie und Pathologische Anatomie des Centralnervensystems mit Bemerkungen zur Normalen Anatomie Desselben. Berlin: Karger.

Pierce, S. R. and Buxbaum, L. J. (2002). Treatments of unilateral neglect: A review. *Archives of Physical Medicine and Rehabilitation 83*: 256–268.

Pierrot-Deseilligy, C. and Müri, R. (1997). Posterior parietal cortex control of saccades in humans. In P. Thier, and H.-O. Karnath (eds.), *Parietal Lobe Contributions to Orientation in 3D Space* (pp. 135–148). Heidelberg: Springer-Verlag.

Pierrot-Deseilligny, C., Milea, D., and Müri, R. M. (2004). Eye movement control by the cerebral cortex. *Current Opinion in Neurobiology 17*: 17–25.

Pizzamiglio, L., Frasca, R., Guariglia, C., Incoccia, C., and Antonucci, G. (1990). Effect of optokinetic stimulation in patients with visual neglect. *Cortex 26*: 535–540.

Pizzamiglio, L., Vallar, G., and Doricchi, F. (1997). Gravitational inputs modulate visuospatial neglect. *Experimental Brain Research 117*: 341–345.

Pizzamiglio, L., Fasotti, L., Jehkonen, M., Antonucci, G., Magnotti, L., Boelen, D., and Asa, S. (2004). The use of optokinetic stimulation in rehabilitation of the hemineglect disorder. *Cortex 40*: 441–450.

Pizzamiglio, L., Guariglia, C., Antonucci, G., and Zoccolotti, P. (2006). Development of a rehabilitative program for unilateral neglect. *Restorative Neurology & Neuroscience 24*: 337–345.

Poppelreuter, W. (1917). *Die psychischen Shädigungen durch Kopfschuß im Kriege 1914/16.* Leipzig: Verlag von Leopold Voss. Trans. J. Zihl and L. Weiskrantz (1990), *Disturbances of Lower and Higher Visual Capacities Caused by Occipital Damage.* Oxford: Clarendon Press.

Posner, M. I., Cohen, Y., and Rafal, R. D. (1982). Neural systems control of spatial orienting. *Philosophical Transactions of the Royal Society of London B298*: 187–198.

Posner, M. I., Walker, J. A., Friedrich, F. J., and Rafal, R. D. (1984). Effects of parietal injury on covert orienting of attention. *Journal of Neuroscience 4*: 1863–1874.

Pouget, A. and Driver, J. (2000). Relating unilateral neglect to the neural coding of space. *Current Opinion in Neurobiology 10*: 242–249.

Prigatano, G. P. (ed.) (2010). *The Study of Anosognosia.* Oxford: Oxford University Press.

Prinz, J. (2000). A neurofunctional theory of visual consciousness. *Consciousness and Cognition 9*: 243–259.

Rabuffetti, M., Ferrarin, M., Spadone, R., Pellegatta, D., Gentileschi, V., Vallar, G., and Pedotti, A. (2002). Touch-screen system for assessing visuo-motor exploratory skills in neuropsychological disorders of spatial cognition. *Medical & Biological Engineering & Computing 40*: 675–686.

Rapcsak, S. Z., Cimino, C. R., and Heilman, K. M. (1988). Altitudinal neglect. *Neurology 38*: 277–281.

Redding, G. M., Rossetti, Y., and Wallace, B. (2005). Applications of prism adaptation: A tutorial in theory and method. *Neuroscience & Biobehavioral Reviews 29*: 431–444.

Redding, G. M. and Wallace, B. (2006). Prism adaptation and unilateral neglect: Review and analysis. *Neuropsychologia 44*: 1–20.

Rengachary, J., He, B. J., Shulman, G. L., and Corbetta, M. (2011). A behavioral analysis of spatial neglect and its recovery after stroke. *Frontiers in Human Neuroscience 5*: 29.

Ricci, R., Pia, L., and Gindri, P. (2004). Effects of illusory spatial anisometry in unilateral neglect. *Experimental Brain Research 154*: 226–237.

Riddoch, M. J. and Humphreys, G. W. (1983). The effect of cueing on unilateral neglect. *Neuropsychologia 21*: 589–599.

Ringman, J. M., Saver, J. L., Woolson, R. F., and Adams, H. P. (2005). Hemispheric asymmetry of gaze deviation and relationship to neglect in acute stroke. *Neurology 65*: 1661–1662.

Rizzo, M. and Vecera, S. P. (2002). Psychoanatomical substrates of Balint's syndrome. *Journal of Neurology, Neurosurgery & Psychiatry 72*: 162–178.

Rizzolatti, G., Fadiga, L., Fogassi, L., and Gallese, V. (1997). The space around us. *Science 277*: 190–191.

Robertson, I. H. and North, N. (1992). Spatio-motor cueing in unilateral left neglect: The role of hemispace, hand and motor activation. *Neuropsychologia 30*: 553–563.

Robertson, I. H. and North, N. (1993). Active and passive activation of left limbs: Influence on visual and sensory neglect. *Neuropsychologia 31*: 293–300.

Robertson, I. H. and North, N. (1994). One hand is better than two: Motor extinction of left-hand advantage in unilateral neglect. *Neuropsychologia 32*: 1–11.

Robertson, I. H., Tegnér, R., Tham, K., Lo, A., and Nimmo-Smith, I. (1995). Sustained attention training for unilateral neglect: Theoretical and rehabilitation inplications. *Journal of Clinical and Experimental Neuropsychology 17*: 416–430.

Robertson, I. H., Manly, T., Beschin, N., Daini, R., Haeske-Dewick, H., Hömberg, V., Jehkonen, M., Pizzamiglio, L., Shiel, A., and Weber, E. (1997). Auditory sustained attention is a marker of unilateral spatial neglect. *Neuropsychologia 35*: 1527–1532.

Rode, G., Charles, N., Perenin, M. T., Vighetto, A., Trillet, M., and Aimard, G. (1992). Partial remission of hemiplegia and somatoparaphrenia through vestibular stimulation in a case of unilateral neglect. *Cortex 28*: 203–208.

Rode, G. and Perenin, M. T. (1994). Temporary remission of representational hemineglect through vestibular stimulation. *NeuroReport 5*: 869–872.

Rode, G., Perenin, M. T., Honoré, J., and Boisson, D. (1998). Improvement of the motor deficit of neglect patients through vestibular stimulation: Evidence for a motor neglect component. *Cortex 34*: 253–261.

Rode, G., Pisella, L., Rossetti, Y., Farnè, A., and Boisson, D. (2003). Bottom-up transfer of sensory-motor plasticity to recovery of spatial cognition: Visuomotor adaptation and spatial neglect. *Progress in Brain Research 142*: 273–287.

Rode, G., Michel, C., Rossetti, Y., Boisson, D., and Vallar, G. (2006). Left size distortion (hyperschematia) after right brain damage. *Neurology 67*: 1801–1808.

Rode, G., Revol, P., Rossetti, Y., and Vallar, G. (2008). 3D left hyperschematia after right brain damage. *Neurocase 14*: 369–377.

Rohling, M. L., Faust, M. E., Beverly, B., and Demakis, G. (2009). Effectiveness of cognitive rehabilitation following acquired brain injury: A meta-analytic re-examination of Cicerone et al.'s (2000, 2005) systematic reviews. *Neuropsychology 23*: 20–39.

Ronchi, R., Posteraro, L., Fortis, P., Bricolo, E., and Vallar, G. (2009). Perseveration in left spatial neglect; Drawing and cancellation tasks. *Cortex 45*: 300–312.

Ronchi, R., Algeri, L., Chiapella, L., Spada, M. S., and Vallar, G. (2012). Spatial neglect and perseveration in visuo-motor exploration. *Neuropsychology 26*: 588–603.

Ropper, A. H. and Samuels, M. A. (eds.) (2009). *Adams & Victor's Principles of Neurology.*. New York: McGraw-Hill Companies, Inc.

Rorden, C. and Karnath, H.-O. (2010). A simple measure of neglect severity. *Neuropsychologia 48*: 2758–2763.

Rorsman, I., Magnusson, M., and Johansson, B. B. (1999). Reduction of visuo-spatial neglect with vestibular galvanic stimulation. *Scandinavian Journal of Rehabilitation Medicine 31*: 117–124.

Rossetti, Y., Rode, G., Pisella, L., Farnè, A., Li, L., Boisson, D., and Perenin, M. T. (1998). Prism adaptation to a rightward optical deviation rehabilitates left hemispatial neglect. *Nature 395*: 166–169.

Rossetti, Y. and Rode, G. (2002). Reducing spatial neglect by visual and other sensory manipulations: Non-cognitive (physiological) routes to the rehabilitation of a cognitive disorder. In H.-O. Karnath, A. D. Milner, and G. Vallar (eds.), *The Cognitive and Neural Bases of Spatial Neglect* (pp. 375–396). Oxford: Oxford University Press.

Rossetti, Y., Jacquin-Courtois, S., Rode, G., Ota, H., Michel, C., and Boisson, D. (2004). Does action make the link between number and space representation? Visuo-manual adaptation improves number bisection in unilateral neglect. *Psychological Science 15*: 426–430.

Rossetti, Y., Ota, H., Blangero, A., Vighetto, A., and Pisella, L. (2010). Why does the perception-action functional dichotomy not match the ventral-dorsal stream's anatomical segregation: Optic ataxia and the function of the dorsal stream. In N. Gangopadhyay,

M. Madary, and F. Spicer (eds.), *Perception, Action, and Consciousness: Sensorimotor Dynamics and Two Visual Systems* (pp. 163–181). Oxford: Oxford University Press.

Rossi, S. and Rossini, P. M. (2004). TMS in cognitive plasticity and the potential for rehabilitation. *Trends in Cognitive Sciences 8*: 273–279.

Rubens, A. B. (1985). Caloric stimulation and unilateral visual neglect. *Neurology 35*: 1019–1024.

Ruff, R. M., Hersh, N. A., and Pribram, K. H. (1981). Auditory spatial deficits in the personal and extrapersonal frames of reference due to cortical lesions. *Neuropsychologia 19*: 435–443.

Rusconi, M. L., Maravita, A., Bottini, G., and Vallar, G. (2002). Is the intact side really intact? Perseverative responses in patients with unilateral neglect: A productive manifestation. *Neuropsychologia 40*: 594–604.

Rushworth, M. F., Behrens, T. E., and Johansen-Berg, H. (2006). Connection patterns distinguish 3 regions of human parietal cortex. *Cerebral Cortex 16*: 1418–1430.

Saj, A., Honoré, J., Richard, C., Bernati, T., and Rousseaux, M. (2010). Hemianopia and neglect influence on straight-ahead perception. *European Neurology 64*: 297–303.

Saj, A., Honoré, J., Braem, B., Bernati, T., and Rousseaux, M. (2012a). Time since stroke influences the impact of hemianopia and spatial neglect on visual-spatial tasks. *Neuropsychology 26*: 37–44.

Saj, A., Verdon, V., Vocat, R., and Vuilleumier, P. (2012b). The anatomy underlying acute versus chronic spatial neglect also depends on clinical tests. *Brain 135*: e207.

Salillas, E., Granà, A., Juncadella, M., Rico, I., and Semenza, C. (2009). Leftward motion restores number space in neglect. *Cortex 45*: 730–737.

Samuelsson, H., Jensen, C., Ekholm, S., Naver, H., and Blomstrand, C. (1997). Anatomical and neurological correlates of acute and chronic visuospatial neglect following right hemisphere stroke. *Cortex 33*: 271–285.

Sapir, A., Kaplan, J. B., He, B. J., and Corbetta, M. (2007). Anatomical correlates of directional hypokinesia in patients with hemispatial neglect. *Journal of Neuroscience 27*: 4045–4051.

Scheller, H. and Seidemann, H. (1931). Zur Frage der optisch-räumlichen Agnosie (Zugleich ein Beitrag zur Dyslexie). *Monatsschrift für Psychiatrie und Neurologie 81*: 97–188.

Schenkenberg, T., Bradford, D. C., and Ajax, E. T. (1980). Line bisection and unilateral visual neglect in patients with neurologic impairment. *Neurology 30*: 509–517.

Schindler, I., Clavagnier, S., Karnath, H.-O., Derex, L., and Perenin, M. T. (2006). A common basis for visual and tactile exploration deficits in spatial neglect? *Neuropsychologia 44*: 1444–1451.

Schmahmann, J. D., Pandya, D. N., Wang, R., Dai, G., D'Arceuil, H. E., Crespigny, A. J. de, and Wedeen, V. J. (2007). Association fibre pathways of the brain: Parallel observations from diffusion spectrum imaging and autoradiography. *Brain 130*: 630–653.

Schott, B., Jeannerod, M., and Zahin, M. Z. (1966). L'agnosie spatiale unilatérale: Perturbation en secteur des mécanismes d'exploration et de fixation du regard. *Le journal de médicine de Lyon 47*: 169–195.

Schröder, A., Wist, E. R., and Hömberg, V. (2008). TENS and optokinetic stimulation in neglect therapy after cerebrovascular accident: A randomized controlled study. *European Journal of Neurology 15*: 922–927.

Schuett, S., Dauner, R., and Zihl, J. (2011). Line bisection in unilateral homonymous visual field defects. *Cortex 47*: 47–52.

Serino, A., Angeli, V., Frassinetti, F., and Làdavas, E. (2006). Mechanisms underlying neglect recovery after prism adaptation. *Neuropsychologia 44*: 1068–1078.

Serino, A., Bonifazi, S., Pierfederici, L., and Làdavas, E. (2007). Neglect treatment by prism adaptation: What recovers and for how long. *Neuropsychological Rehabilitation 17*: 657–687.

Serino, A., Barbiani, M., Rinaldesi, M. L., and Làdavas, E. (2009). Effectiveness of prism adaptation in neglect rehabilitation: A controlled trial study. *Stroke 40*: 1392–1398.

Shallice, T., Mussoni, A., D'Agostino, S., and Skrap, M. (2010). Right posterior cortical functions in a tumour patient series. *Cortex 46*: 1178–1188.

Shiraishi, H., Yamakawa, Y., Itou, A., Muraki, T., and Asada, T. (2008). Long-term effects of prism adaptation on chronic neglect after stroke. *NeuroRehabilitation 23*: 137–151.

Shiraishi, H., Muraki, T., Ayaka Itou, Y. S., and Hirayama, K. (2010). Prism intervention helped sustainability of effects and ADL performances in chronic hemispatial neglect: A follow-up study. *Neurorehabilitation and Neural Repair 27*: 165–172.

Silberpfennig, J. (1941). Contributions to the problem of eye movements, III: Disturbances of ocular movements with pseudohemianopsia in frontal lobe tumors. *Confinia Neurologica 4*: 1–13.

Silveri, M. C., Ciccarelli, N., and Cappa, A. (2011). Unilateral spatial neglect in degenerative brain pathology. *Neuropsychology 25*: 554–566.

Singh-Curry, V., Malhotra, P., Farmer, S. F., and Husain, M. (2011). Attention deficits following ADEM ameliorated by guanfacine. *Journal of Neurology, Neurosurgery & Psychiatry 82*: 688–690.

Smania, N. and Aglioti, S. (1995). Sensory and spatial components of somaesthetic deficits following right brain damage. *Neurology 45*: 1725–1730.

Smania, N., Bazoli, F., Piva, D., and Guidetti, G. (1997). Visuomotor imagery and rehabilitation of neglect. *Archives of Physical Medicine and Rehabilitation 78*: 430–436.

Smania, N., Martini, M. C., Gambina, G., Tomelleri, G., Palamara, A., Natale, E., and Marzi, C. A. (1998). The spatial distribution of visual attention in hemineglect and extinction patients. *Brain 121*: 1759–1770.

Sparing, R., Thimm, M., Hesse, M. D., Küst, J., Karbe, H., and Fink, G. R. (2009). Bidirectional alterations of interhemispheric parietal balance by non-invasive cortical stimulation. *Brain 132*: 3011–3020.

Spence, C. and Driver, J. (eds.) (2003). *Crossmodal Space and Crossmodal Attention.* Oxford: Oxford University Press.

Sposito, A. V., Bolognini, N., Vallar, G., Posteraro, L., and Maravita, A. (2010). The spatial encoding of body parts in patients with neglect and neurologically unimpaired participants. *Neuropsychologia 48*: 334–340.

Stein, B. E. (1998). Neural mechanisms for synthesizing sensory information and producing adaptive behaviors. *Experimental Brain Research 123*: 124–135.

Sterzi, R., Bottini, G., Celani, M. G., Righetti, E., Lamassa, M., Ricci, S., and Vallar, G. (1993). Hemianopia, hemianaesthesia, and hemiplegia after left and right hemisphere damage: A hemispheric difference. *Journal of Neurology, Neurosurgery & Psychiatry 56*: 308–310.

Sturm, W., Thimm, M., Küst, J., Karbe, H., and Fink, G. R. (2006). Alertness-training in neglect: Behavioral and imaging results. *Restorative Neurology & Neuroscience 24*: 371–384.

Szczepanski, S. M., Konen, C. S., and Kastner, S. (2010). Mechanisms of spatial attention control in frontal and parietal cortex. *Journal of Neuroscience 30*: 148–160.

Tegnér, R. and Levander, M. (1991). Through a looking glass: A new technique to demonstrate directional hypokinesia in unilateral neglect. *Brain 114*: 1943–1951.

Tesio, L., Granger, C. V., Perucca, L., Franchignoni, F. P., Battaglia, M. A., and Russell, C. F. (2002). The FIM instrument in the United States and Italy: A comparative study. *American Journal of Physical Medicine & Rehabilitation 81*: 168–176.

Thiebaut de Schotten, M., Urbanski, M., Duffau, H., Volle, E., Levy, R., Dubois, B., and Bartolomeo, P. (2005). Direct evidence for a parietal-frontal pathway subserving spatial awareness in humans. *Science* 309: 2226–2228.

Thimm, M., Fink, G. R., Küst, J., Karbe, H., and Sturm, W. (2006). Impact of alertness training on spatial neglect: A behavioural and fMRI study. *Neuropsychologia* 44: 1230–1246.

Thimm, M., Fink, G. R., Küst, J., Karbe, H., Willmes, K., and Sturm, W. (2009). Recovery from hemineglect: Differential neurobiological effects of optokinetic stimulation and alertness training. *Cortex* 45: 850–862.

Tian, Y., Huang, Y., Zhou, K., Humphreys, G. W., Riddoch, M. J., and Wang, K. (2011). When connectedness increases hemispatial neglect. *PLoS One* 6: e24760.

Tilikete, C., Rode, G., Rossetti, Y., Pichon, J., Li, L., and Boisson, D. (2001). Prism adaptation to rightward optical deviation improves postural imbalance in left-hemiparetic patients. *Current Biology* 11: 524–528.

Ting, D. S. J., Pollock, A., Dutton, G. N., Doubal, F. N., Thompson, M., and Dhillon, B. (2011). Visual neglect following stroke: Current concepts and future focus. *Survey of Ophthalmology* 56: 114–134.

Tjissen, C. C., van Gisbergen, J. A. and Schulte, B. P. (1991). Conjugate eye deviation: Site, side and size of the hemispheric lesion. *Neurology* 41: 846–850.

Tomaiuolo, F., Voci, L., Bresci, M., Cozza, S., Posteraro, F., Oliva, M., and Doricchi, F. (2010). Selective visual neglect in right brain damaged patients with splenial interhemispheric disconnection. *Experimental Brain Research* 206: 209–217.

Trojano, L. and Conson, M. (2008). Visuospatial and visuoconstructive deficits. In G. Goldenberg and B. Miller (eds.), *Handbook of Clinical Neurology* (vol. 88, 373–391): *Neuropsychology and Behavioral Neurology*. Amsterdam: Elsevier.

Tsirlin, I., Dupierrix, E., Chokron, S., Coquillart, S., and Ohlmann, T. (2009). Uses of virtual reality for diagnosis, rehabilitation and study of unilateral spatial neglect: Review and analysis. *CyberPsychology & Behavior* 12: 175–181.

Turton, A. J., O'Leary, K., Gabb, J., Woodward, R., and Gilchrist, I. D. (2010). A single blinded randomised controlled pilot trial of prism adaptation for improving self-care in stroke patients with neglect. *Neuropsychological Rehabilitation* 20: 180–196.

Umarova, R. M., Saur, D., Kaller, C. P., Vry, M. S., Glauche, V., Mader, I., Hennig, J., and Weiller, C. (2011). Acute visual neglect and extinction: Distinct functional state of the visuospatial attention system. *Brain* 134: 3310–3325.

Umiltà, C. (2001). Mechanisms of attention. In B. Rapp (ed.), *The Handbook of Cognitive Neuropsychology* (pp. 135–158). Philadelphia: Psychology Press.

Umiltà, C., Priftis, K., and Zorzi, M. (2009). The spatial representation of numbers: Evidence from neglect and pseudoneglect. *Experimental Brain Research* 192: 561–569.

Urbanski, M., Thiebaut de Schotten, M., Rodrigo, S., Catani, M., Oppenheim, C., Touzé, E., Chokron, S., Méder, J. F., Lévy, R., Dubois, B., and Bartolomeo, P. (2008). Brain networks of spatial awareness: Evidence from diffusion tensor imaging tractography. *Journal of Neurology, Neurosurgery & Psychiatry* 79: 598–601.

Urbanski, M., Thiebaut de Schotten, M., Rodrigo, S., Oppenheim, C., Touzé, E., Méder, J. F., Moreau, K., Loeper-Jeny, C., Dubois, B., and Bartolomeo, P. (2011). DTI-MR tractography of white matter damage in stroke patients with neglect. *Experimental Brain Research* 208: 491–505.

Utz, K. S., Keller, I., Kardinal, M., and Kerkhoff, G. (2011). Galvanic vestibular stimulation reduces the pathological rightward line bisection error in neglect: A sham stimulation-controlled study. *Neuropsychologia* 49: 1219–1225.

Vallar, G. and Perani, D. (1986). The anatomy of unilateral neglect after right hemisphere stroke lesions: A clinical/CT scan correlation study in man. *Neuropsychologia* 24: 609–622.

Vallar, G. and Perani, D. (1987). The anatomy of spatial neglect in humans. In M. Jeannerod (ed.), *Neurophysiological and Neuropsychological Aspects of Spatial Neglect* (pp. 235–258). Amsterdam: Elsevier Science Publishers B. V., North Holland.

Vallar, G., Sterzi, R., Bottini, G., Cappa, S., and Rusconi, M. L. (1990). Temporary remission of left hemianaesthesia after vestibular stimulation. *Cortex* 26: 123–131.

Vallar, G., Bottini, G., Sterzi, R., Passerini, D., and Rusconi, M. L. (1991a). Hemianesthesia, sensory neglect and defective access to conscious experience. *Neurology* 41: 650–652.

Vallar, G., Rusconi, M. L., Geminiani, G., Berti, A., and Cappa, S. F. (1991b). Visual and nonvisual neglect after unilateral brain lesions: Modulation by visual input. *International Journal of Neuroscience* 61: 229–239.

Vallar, G., Antonucci, G., Guariglia, C., and Pizzamiglio, L. (1993a). Deficits of position sense, unilateral neglect, and optokinetic stimulation. *Neuropsychologia* 31: 1191–1200.

Vallar, G., Bottini, G., Rusconi, M. L., and Sterzi, R. (1993b). Exploring somatosensory hemineglect by vestibular stimulation. *Brain* 116: 71–86.

Vallar, G., Rusconi, M. L., Bignamini, L., Geminiani, G., and Perani, D. (1994a). Anatomical correlates of visual and tactile extinction in humans: A clinical CT scan study. *Journal of Neurology, Neurosurgery & Psychiatry* 57: 464–470.

Vallar, G., Rusconi, M. L., and Bisiach, E. (1994b). Awareness of contralesional information in unilateral neglect: Effects of verbal cueing, tracing and vestibular stimulation. In C. Umiltà and M. Moscovitch (eds.), *Attention and Performance XV: Conscious and Nonconscious Information Processing* (pp. 377–391). Cambridge, Mass.: MIT Press.

Vallar, G., Guariglia, C., Magnotti, L., and Pizzamiglio, L. (1995a). Optokinetic stimulation affects both vertical and horizontal deficits of position sense in unilateral neglect. *Cortex* 31: 669–683.

Vallar, G., Guariglia, C., Nico, D., and Bisiach, E. (1995b). Spatial hemineglect in back space. *Brain* 118: 467–472.

Vallar, G., Rusconi, M. L., Barozzi, S., Bernardini, B., Ovadia, D., Papagno, C., and Cesarani, A. (1995c). Improvement of left visuo-spatial hemineglect by left-sided transcutaneous electrical stimulation. *Neuropsychologia* 33: 73–82.

Vallar, G., Guariglia, C., Nico, D., and Tabossi, P. (1996a). Left neglect dyslexia and the processing of neglected information. *Journal of Clinical and Experimental Neuropsychology* 18: 733–746.

Vallar, G., Rusconi, M. L., and Bernardini, B. (1996b). Modulation of neglect hemianesthesia by transcutaneous electrical stimulation. *Journal of the International Neuropsychological Society* 2: 452–459.

Vallar, G., Guariglia, C., Nico, D., and Pizzamiglio, L. (1997a). Motor deficits and optokinetic stimulation in patients with left hemineglect. *Neurology* 49: 1364–1370.

Vallar, G., Guariglia, C., and Rusconi, M. L. (1997b). Modulation of the neglect syndrome by sensory stimulation. In P. Thier and H.-O. Karnath (eds.), *Parietal Lobe Contributions to Orientation in 3D Space* (pp. 555–578). Heidelberg: Springer-Verlag.

Vallar, G. (1998). Spatial hemineglect in humans. *Trends in Cognitive Sciences* 2: 87–97.

Vallar, G. (2000). The methodological foundations of human neuropsychology: Studies in brain-damaged patients. In F. Boller, J. Grafman, and G. Rizzolatti (eds.), *Handbook of Neuropsychology*, 2nd edn. (vol. 1, pp. 305–344). Amsterdam: Elsevier.

Vallar, G., Daini, R., and Antonucci, G. (2000). Processing of illusion of length in spatial hemineglect: A study of line bisection. *Neuropsychologia* 38: 1087–1097.

Vallar, G., Bottini, G., and Sterzi, R. (2003). Anosognosia for left-sided motor and sensory deficits, motor neglect, and sensory hemiinattention: Is there a relationship? *Progress in Brain Research* 142: 289–301.

Vallar, G. and Daini, R. (2006). Visual perceptual processing in unilateral spatial neglect: The case of visual illusions. In T. Vecchi and G. Bottini (eds.), *Imagery and Spatial Cognition: Methods, Models and Cognitive Assessment* (pp. 337–362). Amsterdam and Philadelphia: John Benjamins.

Vallar, G. (2007). Spatial neglect, Balint-Homes' and Gerstmann's syndrome, and other spatial disorders. *CNS Spectrum* 12: 527–536.

Vallar, G. (2008). Subcortical neglect. In P. Märien and J. Abutalebi (eds.), *Neuropsychological Research: A Review* (pp. 307–330). Hove: Psychology Press.

Vallar, G. and Maravita, A. (2009). Personal and extra-personal spatial perception. In G. G. Berntson and J. T. Cacioppo (eds.), *Handbook of Neuroscience for the Behavioral Sciences* (vol. 1, pp. 322–336). New York: John Wiley & Sons.

Vallar, G. and Ronchi, R. (2009). Somatoparaphrenia—a body delusion: A review of the neuropsychological literature. *Experimental Brain Research* 192: 533–551.

Vallar, G., Burani, C., and Arduino, L. S. (2010). Neglect dyslexia: A review of the neuropsychological literature. *Experimental Brain Research* 206: 219–235.

Vallar, G. and Mancini, F. (2010). Mapping the neglect syndrome onto neurofunctional streams. In N. Gangopadhyay, M. Madary, and F. Spicer (eds.), *Perception, Action, and Consciousness: Sensorimotor Dynamics and Two Visual Systems* (pp. 183–215). Oxford: Oxford University Press.

Vallar, G. and Bolognini, N. (2011). Behavioural facilitation following brain stimulation: Implications for neurorehabilitation. *Neuropsychological Rehabilitation* 21: 618–649.

Vallar, G., Bello, L., Bricolo, E., Castellano, A., Casarotti, A., Falini, A., Riva, M., Fava E., and Papagno, C. (2013). Cerebral correlates of visuospatial neglect: A direct cerebral stimulation study. *Human Brain Mapping*.

Van Vleet, T. M. and Robertson, L. C. (2006). Cross-modal interactions in time and space: Auditory influence on visual attention in hemispatial neglect. *Journal of Cognitive Neuroscience* 18: 1368–1379.

Venneri, A., Pentore, R., Cotticelli, B., and Della Sala, S. (1998). Unilateral spatial neglect in the late stage of Alzheimer's disease. *Cortex* 34: 743–752.

Ventre, J., Flandrin, J. M., and Jeannerod, M. (1984). In search for the egocentric reference: A neurophysiological hypothesis. *Neuropsychologia* 22: 797–806.

Verdon, V., Schwartz, S., Lovblad, K. O., Hauert, C. A., and Vuilleumier, P. (2010). Neuroanatomy of hemispatial neglect and its functional components: A study using voxel-based lesion-symptom mapping. *Brain* 133: 880–894.

Vossel, S., Eschenbeck, P., Weiss, P. H., and Fink, G. R. (2010a). The neural basis of perceptual bias and response bias in the Landmark task. *Neuropsychologia* 48: 3949–3954.

Vossel, S., Kukolja, J., Thimm, M., Thiel, C. M., and Fink, G. R. (2010b). The effect of nicotine on visuospatial attention in chronic spatial neglect depends upon lesion location. *Journal of Psychopharmacology* 24: 1357–1365.

Vossel, S., Eschenbeck, P., Weiss, P. H., Weidner, R., Saliger, J., Karbe, H., and Fink, G. R. (2011). Visual extinction in relation to visuospatial neglect after right-hemispheric stroke: Quantitative assessment and statistical lesion-symptom mapping. *Journal of Neurology, Neurosurgery & Psychiatry* 82: 862–868.

Vuilleumier, P., Hester, D., Assal, G., and Regli, F. (1996). Unilateral spatial neglect recovery after sequential strokes. *Neurology* 46: 184–189.

Walker, R. (1995). Spatial and object-based neglect. *Neurocase* 1: 371–383.

Wassermann, E. M., Epstein, C. M., Ziemann, U., Walsh, V., Paus, T., and Lisanby, S. H. (eds.) (2008). *The Oxford Handbook of Transcranial Stimulation.* New York: Oxford University Press.

Watson, R. T., Valenstein, E., and Heilman, K. M. (1981). Thalamic neglect: Possible role of the medial thalamus and nucleus reticularis in behavior. *Archives of Neurology 38*: 501–506.

Watson, R. T., Heilman, K. M., Cauthen, J. C., and King, F. A. (1973). Neglect after cingulectomy. *Neurology 23*: 1003–1007.

Watson, R. T. and Heilman, K. M. (1979). Thalamic neglect. *Neurology 29*: 690–694.

Weinberg, J., Diller, L., Gordon, W. A., Gerstman, L. J., Lieberman, A., Lakin, P., Hodges, G., and Ezrachi, O. (1979). Training sensory awareness and spatial organization in people with right brain damage. *Archives of Physical Medicine and Rehabilitation 60*: 491–496.

Weintraub, S. and Mesulam, M. M. (1988). Visual hemispatial inattention: Stimulus parameters and exploratory strategies. *Journal of Neurology, Neurosurgery & Psychiatry 51*: 1481–1488.

Welfringer, A., Leifert-Fiebach, G., Babinsky, R., and Brandt, T. (2011). Visuomotor imagery as a new tool in the rehabilitation of neglect: A randomised controlled study of feasibility and efficacy. *Disability and Rehabilitation 33*: 2033–2043.

Wilson, B., Cockburn, J., and Halligan, P. W. (1987). *Behavioural Inattention Test.* Titchfield, Hants: Thames Valley Test Company.

Wilson, B. A., Berry, E., Gracey, F., Harrison, C., Stow, I., Macniven, J., Weatherley, J., and Young, A. W. (2005). Egocentric disorientation following bilateral parietal lobe damage. *Cortex 41*: 547–554.

Wojciulik, E., Husain, M., Clarke, K., and Driver, J. (2001). Spatial working memory deficit in unilateral neglect. *Neuropsychologia 39*: 390–396.

Wolk, D. A. and Coslett, H. B. (2004). Hemispheric mediation of spatial attention: Pseudoneglect after callosal stroke. *Annals of Neurology 56*: 434–436.

Young, G. C., Collins, D., and Hren, M. (1983). Effect of pairing scanning training with block design training in the remediation of perceptual problems in left hemiplegics. *Journal of Clinical Neuropsychology 5*: 201–212.

Young, A. W., Haan, E. H. F. de, Newcombe, F., and Day, D. C. (1990). Facial neglect. *Neuropsychologia 28*: 391–415.

Young, A. W., Hellawell, D. J., and Welch, J. (1992). Neglect and visual recognition. *Brain 115*: 51–71.

Zarit, S. H. and Kahn, R. L. (1974). Impairment and adaptation in chronic disabilities: Spatial inattention. *Journal of Nervous and Mental Disease 159*: 63–72.

Zeloni, G., Farne, A., and Baccini, M. (2002). Viewing less to see better. *Journal of Neurology, Neurosurgery & Psychiatry 73*: 195–198.

Zihl, J. (1995). Visual scanning behavior in patients with homonymous hemianopia. *Neuropsychologia 33*: 287–303.

Zihl, J. and Kennard, C. (1996). Disorders of higher visual function. In T. Brandt, L. R. Caplan, J. Dichgans, H. C. Diener, and C. Kennard (eds.), *Neurological Disorders: Course and Treatment* (pp. 201–212). San Diego, Calif.: Academic Press.

Zingerle, H. (1913). Über Störungen der Wahrnehmung des eigenen Körpers bei organischen Gehirnerkrankungen. *Monatsschrift für Psychiatrie und Neurologie 34*: 13–36.

Zorzi, M., Priftis, K., and Umiltà, C. (2002). Brain damage: Neglect disrupts the mental number line. *Nature 417*: 138–139.

CHAPTER 34

NEUROLOGICAL DISORDERS OF ATTENTION

SANJAY MANOHAR, VALERIE BONNELLE, AND MASUD HUSAIN

INTRODUCTION

It is now relatively well accepted that attention is not a unitary process but rather can be fractionated into subcomponents such as selective, sustained, divided, and executive attention (Leclercq and Zimmermann 2002; Petersen and Posner 2012). The identification of specific disruptions in these different subcomponents is necessary to indicate appropriate treatment for neurological conditions with attentional deficits. Many models have been proposed to describe these attentional components and their underlying neural structure. These were largely driven by lesion studies and, later, by functional imaging (Desimone and Duncan 1995; Corbetta and Shulman 2002; Husain and Rorden 2003; Posner 2003). Although they have played an important role in the evolution of modern clinical neuroscience, a potential limitation of these previous 'localizationist' approaches is that they often consider the function of one particular brain region in isolation from the rest of the brain. However, the emergence of new theories of the brain as being organized into large-scale networks proposes that the transfer of information between distinct regions also plays a critical role in efficient attentional processing (Mesulam 1981, 1990; Corbetta and Shulman 2002; Posner and Rothbart 2007).

Consequently, in principle, there are three main mechanisms by which a neurological disorder can affect the function of these networks: either via direct damage to network 'nodes' (e.g. focal lesions or neurodegenerative conditions), damage to the network connections (e.g. axonal injury in traumatic head injury, multiple sclerosis, and neurodegenerative conditions), and/or dysfunction of neurotransmitter systems supporting the function of these networks. This chapter aims to provide an overview of how such mechanisms might be disrupted in neurological conditions and the impact they can have in patients. We focus on three key disorders which serve as important models for understanding attention deficits across a range of conditions: focal brain lesions (other than those causing neglect or extinction which are reviewed by Vallar and Bolognini (chapter 33, this volume), traumatic brain injury, and Parkinson's disease. First, we briefly introduce four attentional processes around which this chapter is structured, and consider some of the brain regions and neural networks that have been proposed to underpin them. Characterization of such structure–function correlations is in its infancy and by no means established. Here, we present the reader with emerging views regarding the functions of attention networks and their disruption in brain disorders, but would urge caution since these concepts are likely to evolve considerably over the next few years.

Selective attention

Selective or focused attention refers to the ability to attend selectively to information that is relevant to a task while ignoring irrelevant and distracting information. Selective attention deficits might be evident when a response produced by automatic processing interferes with a response produced by controlled processing. For example, Posner's covert orienting of attention task (Posner 1980) has been used extensively to investigate discrete attentional deficits in a number of neurological disorders. In this paradigm, healthy subjects typically show a benefit in reaction time (RT) to targets appearing at a validly cued location, and an RT cost when targets appear at an unexpected location. This suggests that attention can be captured by a cue so that visual processing is selectively oriented towards it, thereby improving performance if a target subsequently appears at that location. Other important probes of selective attention include measures of visual search (Mack and Eckstein 2011; Davis and Palmer 2004) and attentional dwell time (Dux and Marois 2009).

Previous neuroimaging and lesion studies consistently identified a bilateral network of fronto-parietal regions as supporting this type of selective attention (Gitelman et al. 1999; Nobre et al. 1997; Nobre 2001; Yantis and Serences 2003; Hopfinger et al. 2001; Kastner and Ungerleider 2000). Core regions of this so-called 'orienting' or 'dorsal attention' network (DAN) include parts of the dorsal frontal cortex, along the precentral sulcus, close or at the frontal eye field (FEF), and regions of the dorsal parietal cortex, particularly the intraparietal sulcus (IPS) and superior parietal lobule (Fig. 34.1). It has been proposed that a primary function of this network is to generate and maintain endogenous ('top-down') signals based on current goals and pre-existing information about likely future events. The selection of information that guides attention may also occur in a 'bottom-up' fashion, that is, driven by competition between sensory inputs. Corbetta and Shulman (2002) proposed that such stimulus-driven attention is supported by a right lateralized, ventral attentional network (VAN) comprising regions of the right inferior frontal cortex and the temporo-parietal junction (Fig. 34.1).

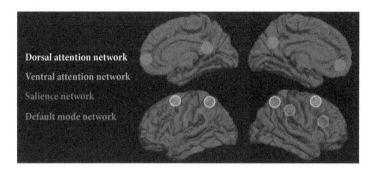

FIGURE 34.1 Four brain networks involved in different aspect of attentions. Core regions of the dorsal attention network include regions of the dorsal frontal cortex, along the precentral sulcus, close or at the frontal eye field, and regions of the dorsal parietal cortex, particularly the intraparietal sulcus and superior parietal lobule. Core regions of the ventral attention network include the right inferior frontal gyrus and the right temporoparietal junction. The Salience network comprises a set of paralimbic structures, most prominently the anterior cingulate cortex, the pre-supplementary motor area and bilateral orbitofrontal insula. The two major nodes of the default mode network (DMN) are the precuneus/posterior cingulate cortex and the ventro-medial prefrontal cortex. The DMN comprises other regions not represented on this figure such as the inferior parietal lobes and the parahippocampal gyri.

According to their proposal, this network would serve as an alerting system that acts as a circuit breaker of ongoing cognitive activity when salient, unexpected, or low frequency stimuli are detected.

Sustained attention

Sustained attention refers to the ability to maintain attention on task requirements. Some authors have distinguished this function from 'phasic alertness': processes underlying the ability to improve performance following a warning signal, for example an auditory tone or visual cue (Posner 2008). Deficits in sustained attention can be considered to comprise two distinct components: vigilance level and vigilance decrement over time (Sarter, Givens, and Bruno 2001). A decrease in vigilance level leads to lapses in attention, often associated with momentary fluctuations in RT or response errors (Robertson et al. 1997) which can be indexed by intra-individual variability (IIV). Vigilance tasks typically require the participant to monitor a series of stimuli in order to detect infrequent targets. A vigilance decrement corresponds to the inability to maintain attention over a prolonged period of time, and is characterized by increased RT and/or error rate with time on task (Mackworth 1948). In general, such decrements in performance have been more frequently observed under conditions of high cognitive load or attentional demand, such as when stimuli are presented at a high event rate (for a review, see Sarter et al. 2001).

Previous lesions and neuroimaging studies have consistently documented a critical role for a right hemispheric ventral fronto-parietal system in sustaining attention (Wilkins, Shallice, and McCarthy 1987; Pardo, Fox, and Raichle 1991; Coull, Frackowiak, and Frith 1998; Posner and Rothbart 2007; Robertson 2001; Husain and Rorden 2003; Singh-Curry and Husain 2009). Thus the VAN appears to be involved in both stimulus-driven attention and sustained attention, potentially allowing functional interaction between stimulus-driven attention and internally maintained sustained attention (Coull 1998). Consistent with this proposal, deactivation observed in the VAN as vigilance decreases over time is opposed by the demand to respond to intermittent target objects (Coull et al. 1998). Furthermore, exogenous stimuli have been found to activate and improve vigilant attention (Manly et al. 2002; O'Connor et al. 2004), demonstrating that stimulus-driven attention can modulate cortical systems supporting sustained attention.

Recent neuroimaging and electrophysiological studies suggest that the right VAN might not be the only system involved in sustained attention. Indeed, it has recently become apparent that brain activity within the default mode network (DMN) also tracks fluctuations in attention (Weissman et al. 2006; Sonuga-Barke and Castellanos 2007; Hayden, Smith, and Platt 2009) (Fig. 34.1). In contrast to the right lateralized fronto-parietal VAN system, the DMN shows a *reduction* in activation during externally oriented attentionally demanding tasks (Raichle et al. 2001). This anticorrelation has been proposed to reflect the dichotomy between tasks requiring internally oriented versus externally oriented attentional modes (Fransson 2005). As the attention demands of a cognitive task increase, this dichotomy becomes more pronounced, and the strength of the anticorrelation has been found to be associated with increased vigilance level (Kelly et al. 2008). It has been proposed that increasing attention may be accomplished either by predominantly boosting fronto-parietal network activity (i.e. regions of the DAN and VAN), deactivating the DMN, or a combination of the two (Lawrence et al. 2003).

Executive control of attention

Current views of 'executive control' generally refer to cognitive processes that allow the production of adaptive and flexible behaviour, such as monitoring for situations where automatic actions need to be suppressed or changed, inhibiting or changing those actions, monitoring performance outcome and adjusting behaviour when needed. They stem from concepts that have emerged from Norman and Shallice's model of a 'supervisory attention system' (Norman and Shallice 1986). Executive control of attention has often been studied using paradigms that involve conflict, such as the Stroop task in which conflict or interference occurs when the colour word name differs from the colour of the ink. In the modern literature, executive control is also sometimes referred to as 'cognitive control'.

Inhibitory control, defined as the ability to suppress inappropriate or no longer required responses, is another important aspect of executive attention that is frequently impaired in many neurological disorders. It has been extensively studied both in healthy volunteers and clinical populations using the stop-signal task (Logan, Cowan, and Davis 1984). This task is based on a simple choice reaction-time task, but at irregular intervals and unpredictably for the participants, the Go stimulus is followed by a stop signal (e.g. flashing visual shape), which instructs subjects to withhold their response. The time it takes for a subject to inhibit a response can be estimated by the stop-signal reaction time (SSRT).

While it is clear that regions of the frontal lobes are strongly involved in executive control of attention, the way dorsal and ventral frontal areas interact with each other, as well as with more posterior regions, remains less well understood. There is a long history of lesion and imaging research that has implicated dorsolateral prefrontal cortex (DLPFC) in executive control, such as maintaining task sets and switching flexibly to new task sets when required (Shallice 1988; Fuster 1997). More recently, medial frontal regions such as the anterior cingulate cortex (ACC) and the pre-supplementary motor area (pre-SMA) have been implicated in conflict detection, error monitoring, and inhibition or change of motor plans (Botvinick et al. 2001; Garavan et al. 2003; Nachev et al. 2007; Sharp et al. 2010; Rushworth 2008; Rushworth et al. 2007). The ACC often co-activates with insular cortex across a variety of tasks (Dosenbach et al. 2006). These regions are both functionally and structurally connected (Seeley et al. 2007; van den Heuvel et al. 2009) and have been referred to as the 'Core' or 'Salience' network (Fig. 34.1) which is anatomically distinct from the VAN or DAN. It has been proposed that activity within this network is not task-specific but rather *salience-driven*, regardless of whether such salience is cognitive, emotional, or homeostatic (Seeley et al. 2007), providing stable 'set-maintenance' over entire task periods (Dosenbach et al. 2006, 2008).

Divided attention

Divided attention refers to the ability to process simultaneously more than one source of information at a time. This aspect of attention is directly linked to the concept of attentional resource, which assumes that attention processing capacity is limited (Kahneman 1973). As a consequence, allocating additional resources to one task can improve performance on that task, but it depletes attentional resources available for other concurrent tasks (Luck et al. 1996). Divided attention deficits have often been studied using dual-task paradigms, under conditions of high cognitive load. The observation that simultaneously performing two well learnt, relatively automatic tasks (with minimal demand on executive attention) does not generally lead to performance impairment suggests that impairments in divided attention might reflect a limitation of executive attention resources. Few studies have attempted to map divided attention onto a specific brain system. In general, fMRI studies have shown that divided attention is associated with increased recruitment of brain networks supporting selective and executive attention (Hahn et al. 2008; Loose et al. 2003; Vohn et al. 2007), potentially reflecting demand on these systems to selectively process information from two different tasks, implement rules and select appropriate responses.

ATTENTION DEFICITS AFTER FOCAL
BRAIN LESIONS

Introduction

Focal lesions that cause deficits of attention provide an important opportunity to study the role of brain regions in directing attention. Although some of the most striking effects are observed in the syndromes of unilateral neglect or extinction (reviewed in Vallar and Bolognini (chapter 33), this volume), many other deficits in several different aspects of attention occur following focal brain injury. Below we review some key findings, excluding investigations of patients who suffer from neglect or extinction. Many of these studies focus on parietal and frontal regions which are part of the DAN, VAN, or Salience network that have been implicated in imaging studies of attention in healthy individuals (Corbetta and Shulman 2002; Singh-Curry and Husain 2009).

Selective attention

Mild lateralized effects in selective attention, worse to the contralesional side, are common following unilateral brain lesions. In fact, in the classical study of Posner and his colleagues, often cited as demonstrating in parietal neglect patients a deficit in disengaging and shifting attention contralesionally, five of the thirteen cases had no demonstrable signs of visual extinction or neglect (Posner et al. 1984). The key finding in that study was that parietal lesions can lead to a directional deficit in deploying attention from an invalidly cued location on the Posner exogenous orienting task. By contrast, thalamic lesions lead to difficulty in engaging attention to the contralesional side, resulting in slow RTs for targets on the side contralateral to the lesion, regardless of whether attention is pre-cued to that location (Rafal and Posner 1987).

The precise location within parietal cortex where damage leads to selective attention deficits has been the subject of some debate (reviewed in Vandenberghe, Molenberghs, and Gillebert 2012). Recent studies of patients with extremely focal lesions involving the IPS and superior parietal lobe (SPL) suggest these regions play a critical role, consistent with functional imaging results from healthy individuals. Gillebert et al. (2011) found that their patient with damage to the left posterior IPS showed a deficit only for invalidly (centrally) cued contralesional targets, an effect that was amplified when an irrelevant, ipsilesional distractor was presented in competition with a valid contralesional target. By contrast, a patient with a very small lesion of the right middle IPS, extending into the SPL, demonstrated a bilateral impairment on invalidly cued trials. These effects have been interpreted in terms of possible different roles of posterior and middle IPS in compiling a 'priority map' of items in visual space (Vandenberghe et al. 2012; see also Bisley and Goldberg 2010).

Patients with prefrontal lesions also show selective attention deficits, missing more items and showing increased RTs to detected targets presented contralesionally (Barceló, Suwazono, and Knight 2000). Using a whole-report paradigm and analysis based on Bundesen's Theory of Visual Attention (in chapter 37, this volume), Habekost and Bundesen (2003) have reported slowing of attention for left-sided stimuli (as measured by a lower capacity of entry into working memory) following right frontal damage. Further studies, conducted on a group of patients with focal lesions using this methodology, revealed that parietal damage, particularly involving the temporal-parietal junction (TPJ), reduced processing speed and visual short-term memory capacity (Peers et al. 2005). By contrast, measures of attention weighting (directional bias and 'top-down' filtering ability) were best predicted by total volume of lesion—not simply frontal involvement. These results correspond well to the findings using the Posner task, demonstrating that directional biases in deploying attention are not confined to patients with clinical neglect or extinction (Posner et al. 1984).

In addition to directional biases in attention, prefrontal lesions can also produce *bilateral* deficits as demonstrated with endogenous cueing. Vecera and Rizzo (2004) used a central cueing task to show that a frontal lesion impaired voluntary attention shifts, but with preserved exogenous orienting. Similarly, frontal lobe resection impaired the ability to utilize informative spatial pre-cues, presented in the form of arrows pointing to the most likely location of an upcoming target (Koski, Paus, and Petrides 1998). These findings are supported by the results of electrophysiological studies that show frontal lesions attenuate neural correlates of attention in both auditory and visual domains. For example, Woods and Knight (1986) reported that patients with left prefrontal lesions lack ERP evidence of attentional selection in dichotic listening, while Barceló et al. (2000) reported that even early visual processing in extrastriate regions (<125 ms) is reduced by prefrontal damage.

Some authors have also investigated the effects of focal lesions on global vs. local attention, or the ability to shift attention from a wide to a tight attention focus. These studies have often used Navon figures: large, 'global' letters made up of small, 'local' letters (Navon 1977). In normal healthy people, RTs are generally faster in the globally directed condition than the local one (Navon 1977). In addition, RTs to the local level are longer—demonstrating interference—when the letters at the two levels are different (e.g. local 'S's forming a global 'H') compared to when they were the same (e.g. local 'S's forming a global 'S'). In contrast, patients with posterior lesions centred on the posterior superior temporal gyrus and adjacent caudal inferior parietal lobe showed no interference (Lamb, Robertson, and Knight 1989), suggesting these regions normally play a role in integration of and/or attention to local- and global-level information. Left and right hemisphere lesions appeared to affect attention deployment differentially, with a local advantage following right TPJ lesions and a global advantage following left superior temporal gyrus lesions (Robertson, Lamb, and Knight 1988). Other investigators have observed that patients with ventral lesions to extrastriate cortex have a global bias for Navon figures, whereas dorsal lesions lead to a local bias (Riddoch et al. 2008).

Müller-Plath and colleagues (2010) have developed an attractive method to study neuropsychological effects of attention. Their search task varies set-size and target-distractor similarity independently, and using a model of serial vs. parallel visual search, they decomposed performance into three components: size of attention focus, dwell time, and movement time. In patients with unilateral focal lesions, these authors reported that damage to the DLPFC reduced the focus of attention while temporal lesions enlarged it, consistent with studies using Navon figures. Lesions involving the FEF, SPL, and parieto-occipital cortex significantly increased attention movement time, consistent with views of the SPL being involved in shifting attention (see Vandenberghe et al. 2012). Attention dwell time was significantly reduced in patients with damage to the anterior insula as well as the SPL.

Sustained attention

Several studies have implicated right inferior frontal regions—typically involving frontal regions of the VAN—in playing a key role in sustaining attention over time. Wilkins et al. (1987) first noted that right frontal patients were impaired at counting stimuli—auditory or tactile—when presented slowly (1 item/second) but not quickly (7/second). Clearly, such a deficit might be interpreted in many ways, including distractibility, memory interference, alertness, motivation, or fatigue. Subsequent studies have tried to narrow the interpretation. Godefroy et al. (1994) demonstrated that neither fatigability, nor practice or motivation was specifically worse in frontal patients.

The Sustained Attention to Response Task (SART) is similar to the simple reaction-time studies mentioned above, but also requires selectivity: responding to pre-specified target items and withholding responses to other, distracting items. Frontal patients demonstrate increased commission errors on the SART (Robertson et al. 1997). A voxelwise lesion analysis of 41 patients on SART demonstrated that commission errors correlate strongly with right inferior frontal gyrus (RIFG) damage (Molenberghs et al. 2009). Reduced post-error slowing correlated with right inferior frontal sulcus damage, comparable with findings in the go/no-go task (see below). Right prefrontal patients also show deficits on versions of the continuous performance task (CPT) with worsening effects as target complexity increased (Glosser and Goodglass 1990; Rueckert and Grafman 1996; Wilkins et al. 1987; Woods and Knight 1986), as well as demonstrating a vigilance decrement, performing slower with time on task (Rueckert and Grafman 1996; Wilkins et al. 1987).

Frontal patients also demonstrate slowing (Howes and Boller 1975; Rueckert and Grafman 1996) and increased variability (Picton et al. 2006) of simple RTs. With respect to alerting, Alivisatos and Milner used a warning-signal task to show that right and left frontal patients are unable to utilize a 'get-ready' signal to speed subsequent responses (Alivisatos and Milner 1989). In fact, frontal patients may show a reversed foreperiod effect, slowing down with longer delay periods (Stuss et al. 2005).

Although most studies have implicated right inferior frontal regions, there is also some evidence for a role of right dorsomedial regions (also part of the Salience network), with some investigators arguing for a role of these areas in *energizing* attention for responses (Alexander et al. 2005). Lesions here lead to progressive slowing of response times. Regardless of the interpretation, lesion data confirm the key role played by the right inferior and dorsomedial frontal cortices in sustaining attention over time.

Divided and executive attention

Divided attention has perhaps been probed most simply by comparing RTs in a task with only one stimulus modality versus two possible modalities (Godefroy and Rousseaux 1996). Patients with lesions involving the left prefrontal cortex and head of the caudate were unduly slow on the dual-modality task. Further evidence pointing to a deficit in dividing attention in prefrontal patients comes also from bedside tasks such as the trail-making test. In Part B of this test, participants have to search in alternating fashion for letters and numbers, joining them up as they find them. Thus this test also potentially assesses the ability to switch tasks and might not be simply a measure of divided attention. Patients with dorsolateral prefrontal lesions of either hemisphere and paramedian thalamic damage are most likely to be impaired, while those with inferomedial thalamic damage seem not to be (Stuss et al. 1988, 2001). Similarly, on multi-target visual search tasks, patients with frontal damage are specifically slowed when trying to find more than one type of target among distractors compared to searching for a single target (Richer et al. 1993).

In clinical studies, the Wisconsin Card-Sorting Test (WCST) is one of the most common tests used for executive attention in patients, but clearly there might be several reasons why patients might fail on this task, including keeping in mind task rules and previous outcomes. Damage to many areas impairs performance, including basal ganglia (Eslinger and Grattan 1993), DLPFC (Demakis 2003), thalamus, and even cerebellum, according to some authors (Mukhopadhyay et al. 2008). Patients with frontal lesions have deficits on the related stimulus-classification task from the CANTAB battery, specifically when switching to a previously irrelevant dimension (Owen et al. 1991). However, a review of 25 lesion studies concluded that although the WCST is a sensitive test of frontal lobe damage, it is by no means specific (Alvarez and Emory 2006). A recent lesion analysis found only a very mild effect of lesion location on task performance, with moderate localization to left prefrontal areas (Jodzio and Biechowska 2010). Other studies comparing subregions of the right frontal lobe have found no evidence of specificity of localization within the frontal lobe (Alvarez and Emory 2006; Davidson et al. 2007).

Problems in inhibition are characteristic of frontal lesions, including bedside tests of delayed alternation and interference (Roca et al. 2010). Right IFG lesions have been particularly implicated, with increased commission errors on the stop-signal task (Aron et al. 2003) and go/no-go task (Picton et al. 2007). In addition, some authors have presented evidence for a role of right dorsomedial areas in response inhibition (Floden and Stuss 2006; Picton et al. 2007), consistent with the view that the pre-SMA and right IFG form critical nodes of a stopping network (Aron et al. 2007).

Frontal lesions also lead to deficits on tasks that produce stimulus or response conflict such as the Stroop or Eriksen flanker (Swick and Turken 2002; Ullsperger and von Cramon 2006; Coulthard, Nachev, and Husain 2008). Some authors who have reviewed the lesion evidence for localization of Stroop deficits conclude that lateral and dorsomedial prefrontal, but not orbitofrontal damage, is associated with performance impairments (Alvarez and Emory 2006). However, the results are inconsistent and, while some studies find no differences between lesion locations, others have reported quite specific differences between lesions to different frontal areas. For example, damage to the left ventrolateral region produced an increased number of incorrect responses to distractors, while right dorsomedial lesions (including ACC, SMA, and pre-SMA) and dorsolateral prefrontal areas, were associated with a slow RT and a decreased number of correct responses to targets on the Stroop (Alexander et al. 2007). Impaired Stroop performance has also been associated with thalamic lesions (Annoni et al. 2003; Ghika-Schmid and Bogousslavsky 2000).

This brief review of the effects of focal brain lesions on attention functions demonstrates how diverse findings might be organized in terms of a framework of selective, sustained, divided, and executive attention. Next, we consider an important example of brain damage that often has its greatest impact on the connections between brain regions that serve key roles in directing attention.

ATTENTIONAL DEFICITS AFTER TRAUMATIC BRAIN INJURY (TBI)

Introduction

TBI produces a complex combination of focal lesions and traumatic axonal injury (Gentry, Godersky, and Thompson 1988) both of which can have an important impact on attention (for reviews on attention deficits after TBI, see Niemann, Ruff, and Kramer 1996; Cossa and Fabiani 1999; Chan 2001; Mathias and Wheaton 2007). While the way focal lesions affect these processes via, for example, direct damage to the frontal lobes, has been extensively described (for a review see Stuss and Knight 2002; Stuss 2011), the impact of traumatic axonal injury remains less clear. One key reason for focusing on TBI in this review is that this condition can provide important information on attention deficits due to disruption of white matter pathways in brains that usually had no pre-existing neuropathology.

Traumatic axonal injury is the most common pathological feature of TBI, found in almost three quarters of patients with moderate to severe injury (Smith, Meaney, and Shull 2003; Skandsen et al. 2010). However, it is likely to have been underestimated until recently, due to the lack of imaging techniques sensitive to identify axonal injury (for a review on techniques to characterize axonal injury see Sharp and Ham 2011). Diffusion tensor imaging (DTI) is a relatively recent MRI modality that provides a particularly useful way to help understand TBI white matter pathology (Niogi and Mukherjee 2010; Zappalà, Thiebaut de Schotten, and Eslinger 2012). Frontal and temporal white matter structures (e.g. anterior corona radiata, uncinate fasciculus, superior longitudinal fasciculus, and fronto-occipital fasciculus), midline structures such as the corpus callosum and cingulum bundles, as well as cortical–subcortical connections, are the most frequently damaged (Rutgers et al. 2008; Niogi and Mukherjee 2010). White matter damage predicts functional outcome better than the presence, location, or volume of focal lesions (Benson et al. 2007; Sidaros et al. 2008; Kinnunen et al. 2011). It is observable even in patients with no visible focal lesions or microbleeds, and correlates with TBI severity (Nakayama et al. 2006; Kinnunen et al. 2011) and cognitive impairment following TBI (Salmond et al. 2006; Kraus et al. 2007; Niogi et al. 2008b; Little et al. 2010; Kinnunen et al. 2011).

Selective attention

On Posner's covert orienting of attention task, a normal cost but reduced or absent benefit in RT to targets at expected locations has been observed both in acute and chronic moderate to severe TBI patients, suggesting an impairment in the ability to pre-engage attention to a cued location (Cremona-Meteyard et al. 1992; Cremona-Meteyard and Geffen 1994). However, this result was not replicated in a later study investigating a larger cohort of patients with severe TBI (Bate, Mathias, and Crawford 2001). More recently, Halterman et al. (2006) have reported findings using the Attentional Network Test, which attempts to separate three components of attention described by Posner, namely alerting, orienting, and executive control in the face of conflict (Fan et al. 2002). The results demonstrated that orienting and executive attention were impaired two days post-TBI, but only deficits in executive attention remained after a month (Halterman et al. 2006). In general, there does not seem to be strong evidence for persistent selective attention deficits after TBI. Rather, Stuss et al. (1989) suggested that TBI patients may have a relatively intact ability to focus attention, but that this might be achieved at a cost and could not be maintained by all patients, possibly as a result of limited available attention resources.

The frontal and parietal areas implicated in selective and sustained attention are richly interconnected via fibre tracts passing through the superior longitudinal fasciculus (SLF) (Schmahmann and Pandya 2006). Structural integrity of the SLF has been related to attention performance, both in healthy people (Bennett et al. 2012), and stroke patients with neglect (He et al. 2007; Doricchi et al. 2008; Bartolomeo, Thiebaut de Schotten, and Doricchi 2007). Although some studies have reported damage within the SLF after TBI (Messe et al. 2011; Kraus et al. 2007; Bendlin et al. 2008), this is not a consistent finding (Bonnelle et al. 2012) (Fig. 34.2: panels a and b (4) and (5)).

Other white matter tracts are also likely to be important for selective attention, but have not been extensively investigated in TBI. For example, a recent study in normal subjects using the Attentional Network Task (ANT) related orienting of attention performance to structural integrity of the splenium of the corpus callosum (Niogi et al.

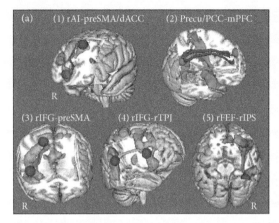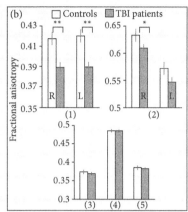

FIGURE 34.2 Comparison of white matter structure between TBI patients (N=57) and controls (N=25) in key white matter tracts. (a) White matter tracts between local maxima of brain activation (red spheres) or deactivation (blue spheres) during response inhibition represented in 3D on the MNI-152 T1 1mm brain 3D template. Tracts are shown for the connections between (1) the right anterior insula (rAI) and the anterior cingulate cortex (ACC) (**Salience network**), (2) the precuneus (Precu) and medial prefrontal cortex (mPFC) bilaterally (**Default mode network**), (3) the right pre-supplementary motor area (pre-SMA) and right inferior frontal gyrus (IFG), (4) the right IFG and the right temporo-parietal junction (TPJ) (**VAN**) and (5) the right frontal eye field (FEF) and inferior parietal sulcus (IPS) (**DAN**). White matter tracts were generated using probabilistic tractography in a group of ten young healthy volunteers. (b) The bar charts show fractional anisotropy (FA) ± SEM within each tract compared between patients (grey) and age-matched controls (white). $*p<0.05$, $**p<0.005$ statistical significance. R: Right, L: Left. Lower FA reflects lower structural integrity. Reproduced from Bonnelle, V, Ham, TE, Leech, R, Kinnunen, KM, Mehta, MA, Greenwood, RJ and Sharp, DJ Salience network integrity predicts default mode network function after traumatic brain injury, *Proceedings of the National Academy of Sciences of the United States of America*, 109(12), pp. 4690–4695. Copyright © 2012, The National Academy of Sciences, USA.

2010), a region which is frequently damaged after TBI (Kraus et al. 2007; Rutgers et al. 2008; Sharp et al. 2011).

Sustained attention

TBI patients often suffer from sustained attention deficits, which manifest themselves as increased distractibility, poor concentration and a decreased ability to maintain attention focused over a long period of time, suggesting both a decrease in vigilance level and a vigilance decrement over time (Stuss et al. 1989; Whyte et al. 1995; Dockree et al. 2004). These impairments have been found to be closely related to other executive function deficits in these patients, such as performance monitoring (McAvinue et al. 2005; O'Keeffe et al. 2007) and inhibitory control (Robertson et al. 1997).

A number of studies have used measures of vigilance level such as variability in RTs (Stuss et al. 1994; Whyte et al. 1995) or increased error rates (Robertson et al. 1997) to investigate sustained attention deficits after TBI. However, a possible limitation of these measures is that RT inconsistencies or errors could also reflect difficulties due to the specific cognitive demands of the task and are not necessarily due to sustained attention deficits (Malhotra, Coulthard, and Husain 2009). Impairment of sustained attention might thus be best demonstrated through decline in performance (RT and/or accuracy) over the duration of a task that patients are initially able to perform well. In keeping with that, many studies investigating groups of moderate to severe TBI have observed that patients often perform tasks well initially, but fail to maintain their attention focused toward the end, leading to impaired performance over time (Loken et al. 1995; Whyte et al. 1995; Bonnelle et al. 2011) (Fig. 34.3a). However, this vigilance decrement is not a consistent finding (Parasuraman, Mutter, and Molloy 1991). This might be due to differences in paradigms used; studies using tasks where the response can become automated over time might fail to observe a performance decrement.

Previous neuroimaging and lesion studies proposed that a predominantly right-lateralized fronto-parietal system supports sustained attention (Wilkins et al. 1987; Pardo et al. 1991; Rueckert and Grafman 1996; Coull et al. 1998). Nonetheless, no studies to date have described a relationship between sustained attention deficits and white matter integrity in the right SLF after TBI. However, increased activation within

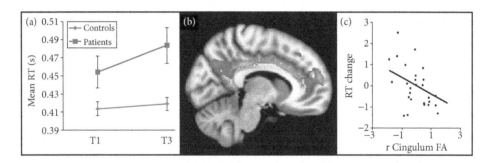

FIGURE 34.3 Vigilance decrement deficits after TBI are associated with changes in DMN function and structure. (a) Mean reaction time (RT) during the first (T1) and the last third (T3) of a simple choice reaction time task, plotted for TBI patients in orange and age matched controls in blue. (b) Sagittal view of the brain regions showing increase activation over time in patients with high change in RT compared to patients in low change in RT (red-yellow). The right cingulum bundle connecting the posterior and anterior parts of the DMN is shown in green (from the JHU White Matter Tractography Atlas). (c) Fractional anisotropy (FA) of the cingulum bundle in patients is plotted against the change in RT between the first and the last part of the task (N=28). Measures are age-normalized, i.e. age was regressed out from the measures using a linear regression, where residuals were saved as standardized values. Adapted from Bonnelle, V., Leech, R., Kinnunen, K. M., Ham, T. E., Beckmann, C. F., De Boissezon, X., Greenwood, R. J., and Sharp, D. J., Default mode network connectivity predicts sustained attention deficits after traumatic brain injury, *Journal of Neuroscience*, 31(38), pp. 13442–13451 © 2011, The Society for Neuroscience.

the DMN has been associated with vigilance decrement in TBI patients (Bonnelle et al. 2011) (Fig. 34.3b). The cingulum bundles, which are the major tracts connecting the anterior and posterior parts of the DMN (Greicius et al. 2009) (Fig. 34.3b), have consistently been found to be damaged after TBI (Kraus et al. 2007; Niogi et al. 2008b; Bonnelle et al. 2011, 2012). Decreased structural integrity of the right cingulum bundle has been associated with greater vigilance decrement in TBI patients (Bonnelle et al. 2011) (Fig. 34.3c), and has also been implicated in individual differences in sustained attention in the normal brain (Takahashi et al. 2010).

Divided and executive attention

Most evidence for impaired divided attention in TBI patients comes from studies investigating dual-task performance. In general, patients' deficits in divided attention tend to manifest under conditions of high cognitive load rather than when tasks are relatively simple and automatic (Park, Moscovitch, and Robertson 1999; Leclercq et al. 2000; Brouwer et al. 2001; Azouvi et al. 2004). These deficits do not appear to be due to impairments of strategic allocation of attention, switching between tasks or working memory. Indeed, a dual-task performance decrement, with preserved ability to allocate attention resources preferentially to one task or the other according to instructions, has been described after TBI (Azouvi et al. 2004). The difficulty in dealing with two tasks at a time might result from limited attention resources, consistent with the high frequency of fatigue complaints after TBI, perhaps resulting from additional mental effort required by patients to manage a complex task and compensate for lower attention resources (Belmont et al. 2006; Belmont, Agar, and Azouvi 2009; Ashman et al. 2008).

Divided attention does not appear to be associated with one specific brain system. The increased attention resource recruitment characteristic of divided attention has often been associated with increased recruitment of contralateral brain regions. For instance, when gradually increasing difficulty level on a visual attention task, easier conditions typically begin with mainly right-sided activity, but as conditions become more difficult, left-lateralized homologue areas activate (Nebel et al. 2005). One prediction would therefore be that the structural integrity of the corpus callosum, consistently found to be damaged after TBI (Kraus et al. 2007; Kumar et al. 2009; Niogi et al. 2008b), might play an important role in supporting the need for an increase in attention resource. However, most TBI studies have failed to relate white matter integrity within the corpus callosum to specific attention measures (Mathias et al. 2004; Little et al. 2010). Furthermore, although divided attention deficits after TBI have been extensively investigated behaviourally, no study to our knowledge has specifically investigated the relationship between divided attention and white matter damage in TBI patients.

Deficits in many aspects of executive functions, such as conflict and error monitoring or inhibitory control, have been reported in TBI (Hart et al. 1998; O'Keeffe, Dockree, and Robertson 2004; Larson et al. 2007; Dimoska-Di Marco et al. 2011). However, it is not always clear whether executive functions are directly impaired, or whether these deficits are the consequence of other attention impairments. Consider the case of inhibitory control, which has been extensively studied in healthy volunteers using the stop-signal task (Logan et al. 1984). Several studies found evidence for inhibitory impairment in TBI patients, as reflected by longer stop-signal reaction-time measures (for a review, see Dimoska-Di Marco et al. 2011). However, this behavioural measure has been found to be influenced by other factors including focused and sustained attention, or motivation (Boehler et al. 2010; Leotti and Wager 2010).

Interestingly, comparison of the pattern of brain activation during the stop-signal task in TBI and control subjects revealed no difference in frontal regions considered to be involved in inhibitory control or attention capture, but major differences were observed in the DMN (Bonnelle et al. 2012). This was the result of patients showing less DMN deactivation on stop trials (Fig. 34.4b). This decrease in DMN deactivation was associated with poorer inhibitory performance, suggesting that, similarly to what has been observed in ADHD (Liddle et al. 2011), a deficit in attention regulation, or more generally a failure of task engagement, rather than a deficit in motor response inhibition, underlies inhibitory control deficit in TBI patients.

It has recently been proposed that the Salience network, and more particularly the right anterior insula, might play an important role in rapidly and dynamically 'switching' between other large-scale networks (including the DMN) to facilitate rapid access to attention resources when a salient stimulus is detected (Sridharan, Levitin, and Menon 2008; Menon and Uddin 2010). In keeping with this proposal, white matter connections between regions of this network have been found to be particularly damaged after TBI (Fig. 34.2, panels a and b (1), rAI-dACC/preSMA connection), and importantly this has been associated with changes in DMN function as well as impaired inhibitory performance (Bonnelle et al. 2012) (Fig. 34.4b and c).

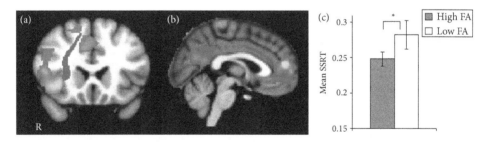

FIGURE 34.4 White matter damage between the right anterior insula and the ACC/pre-SMA relates to DMN deactivation and inhibitory performance during the stop-signal task. (a) Coronal view of the white matter connection between rAI and (blue) overlaid on the activation map for the contrast comparing successful inhibition to go trials in patients (orange), superimposed on the MNI 152 T1 1mm brain template. (b) Sagittal view of the brain regions showing negatively correlated activation with FA measures within the rAI-pre-SMA/dACC tract for StC relative to Go trials, superimposed on the MNI 152 T1 2mm brain template. Cluster corrected Z=2.3, p <0.05. (c) Comparison of stop signal reaction times (SSRT) between TBI patients with low (white) and high (grey) fractional anisotropy (FA) within the raI- pre-SMA/dACC tract.

Executive dysfunctions after TBI are also likely to be the result of structural discon-nections between ACC and other frontal and parietal brain regions. For example, the corona radiata, which connects ACC to DLPFC, is one of the most frequently damaged white matter tracts after TBI (Niogi and Mukherjee 2010). The structural integrity of this tract has often been related to executive functions, especially conflict monitoring, both in healthy individuals (Niogi et al. 2010) and in TBI patients (Kraus et al. 2007; Niogi et al. 2008a). The cingulum bundle constitutes another important pathway via which the ACC connects with posterior regions of the brain. Damage within the cingulum bun-dles has been associated with lower cognitive performance on the Eriksen flanker task, measuring interference and conflict processing (Wilde et al. 2010). Performance on the Stroop test has also been used as a measure of executive attention in TBI, but results have not always been consistent (Ponsford and Kinsella 1992; Chan 2002). A potential limi-tation, just as for other measures, is that performance might reflect deficits in speed of information processing as well as several executive functions (Spikman, van Zomeren, and Deelman 1996; Rios, Perianez, and Munoz-Cespedes 2004; Ben-David, Nguyen, and van Lieshout 2011).

To conclude, it is difficult to generalize on the impact of TBI on attention at the group level because of the heterogeneity of this clinical population (each patient presents with a unique combination of focal and diffuse injury). Recent studies suggest that the dis-ruption of specific white matter tracts might explain the occurrence of specific types of attentional deficits. However, further research is required to clarify the impact of axonal injury on the different aspects of attention.

ATTENTION DEFICITS IN PARKINSON'S DISEASE

The previous sections have dealt with the effects of focal lesions on the cortical nodes of attention networks and the effects of TBI, focusing largely on its effects on white matter connections of attention networks. By the very nature of the underlying pathologies, most of those studies have investigated patients with abrupt, acquired brain damage. Parkinson's disease (PD), by contrast, is a slowly progressive neurodegenerative dis-order, traditionally characterized by difficulty in initiating movements, motor slow-ing, stiffness, and sometimes tremor. It is associated with destruction of dopaminergic neurons in the substantia nigra pars compacta with a pathological signature of accu-mulation of cytoplasmic protein aggregates known as Lewy bodies. In addition, there is substantial cholinergic denervation which is evident even in early PD (Bohnen and Albin 2011).

Over the last three decades, it has become clear that PD is not just a motor disor-der. Many patients develop cognitive deficits, including deficits of attention. Indeed, recent imaging studies have revealed that cortical hypometabolism in PD patients with cognitive impairment involves regions within medial and lateral parietal and frontal cortex (Huang et al. 2007) that have been identified as critical nodes in attention networks (cf. Fig. 34.5a and Fig. 34.1). Furthermore, cognitive impairment is associated with white matter changes as indexed by diffusion tensor imaging in a large series of patients (Hattori et al. 2012) (Fig. 34.5b, c, and d). Thus PD is associated with slow degeneration of both attentional networks' nodes and white matter connections, and thus serves as an important model of neurodegeneration affecting these networks to compromise function. In addition, neurochemical alterations in the degenerating PD brain, particularly dopaminergic and cholinergic depletion, provide important insights into neuromodulation of attention in normal brains.

In PD with established motor symptoms and signs, cognitive impairments may eventually lead to dementia or Parkinson's disease with dementia (PDD). Alternatively, dementia may be evident before or occur simultaneously with motor deficits, leading to a diagnosis of dementia with Lewy bodies (DLB). PDD and DLB are probably different manifestations of the same underlying pathological process (McKeith and Mosimann 2004). Both cortical and white matter changes increase in PDD patients compared to those with PD without dementia (e.g. see Fig. 34.5c). For example, among other tracts, the superior longitudinal fasciculus has been found to be disrupted in PDD patients, correlating with patients' cognitive performance (Hattori et al. 2012) (Fig. 34.5d).

Selective attention

Although there have been several studies of selective attention in PD, the findings have been variable. On the one hand, deficits in covert exogenous orienting of attention have been reported in some patients (see Nys, Santens, and Vingerhoets 2010). However, several studies have demonstrated *excessive* exogenous orienting compared to healthy controls. For example, Briand et al. (2001) showed that exogenous non-predictive cues in a Posner task give a bigger initial facilitation in PD. Similarly, Wright et al. (1990) reported that although Parkinson's patients are slower overall, they incur smaller costs for invalid pre-cues (at 1100 ms). The interpretation of these investigators was that PD patients disengage from attended locations more readily. Using the Attentional Network Task protocol, Zhou et al. (2012) also documented that patients have stronger exogenous orienting than controls, but no difference in flanker conflict or alerting.

On visual search, Troscianko and Calvert (1993) first demonstrated impairments in pop-out search but no impairment on serial or conjunction search in PD (but see Berry et al. 1999). Similarly, Filoteo et al. (1997) showed deficits on a simple visual search task, but *less* slowing than controls on the conjunction task. The conclusion from a series of visual search tasks that altered attention demands was that PD patients were most impaired on so-called 'preattentive tasks', requiring significantly greater orientation differences between target and distractors or longer stimulus durations to find stimuli (Lieb et al. 1999), perhaps reflecting impaired low-level saliency processing (Mannan et al. 2008). DLB patients, who by definition have more advanced cognitive impairment, have been

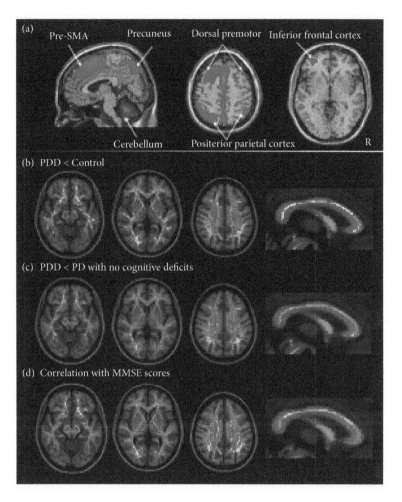

FIGURE 34.5   Changes in brain metabolism and white matter structure in Parkinson's disease. (a) Parkinson's disease-related cognitive pattern identified by spatial covariance analysis of FDG PET scans is characterized by co-varying bilateral metabolic reductions in the rostral supplementary motor area (pre-SMA) and precuneus, the dorsal premotor cortex, and the inferior parietal lobule, as well as in the left prefrontal region (blue) and metabolic increases in the cerebellar vermis and dentate nuclei. Adapted from Huang et al. 2007. Comparison of white matter structure between PD patients with dementia (PDD) and controls (b), and PDD patients and PD patients with no evidence of cognitive deficits (c). White matter tracts highlighted in yellow have significantly reduced fractional anisotropy in PDD. (d) Fractional anisotropy within the white matter sections highlighted in yellow are significantly correlated with Mini-Mental State Examination (MMSE) scores. Adapted from Takaaki Hattori, Satoshi Orimo, Shigeki Aoki, Kenji Ito, Osamu Abe, Atsushi Amano, Ryo Sato, Kasumi Sakai, and Hidehiro Mizusawa, Cognitive status correlates with white matter alteration in Parkinson's disease, *Human Brain Mapping*, 33(3), pp. 727–39 © 2011, Wiley Periodicals, Inc., with permission from John Wiley & Sons.

reported to be bad at both pop-out and serial search, compared to PD patients without dementia and individuals with Alzheimer's disease (Cormack et al. 2004). Thus deficits in more demanding conjunction search are evident with greater cognitive deficits in PD.

Indeed, Horowitz et al. (2006) found deficits in both parallel and conjunction search in PD patients without dementia when the search target was unknown, as well as when stimulus-driven information decreased in salience. They interpreted this as evidence for deficits at a higher level than salience processing. Evidence that attention deficits in PD may also occur at later stages comes from findings that patients fail to learn from contextual cues in visual search (van Asselen et al. 2009).

There has also been much controversy about inhibition of previously selected attended locations in PD (Kingstone et al. 2002; Yamaguchi and Kobayashi 1998). One group has claimed that although the benefit of exogenous, non-predictive cues is negatively correlated with disease severity, inhibition of return is positively correlated (Briand et al. 2001). Poliakoff et al. (2003) have reviewed the data on inhibition of return in PD, considering reasons for the contradictory results. They concluded that tactile inhibition of return is reduced in PD patients, and suggest that this might be due to general impairments of inhibitory control, rather than specific attention processes.

Sustained attention

An important clinical feature that has long been recognized in DLB and PDD is fluctuations of attention over even short periods of time. When tested using experimental batteries that include simple or choice reaction time and digit vigilance (rapid serial visual presentation), patients with PDD/DLB have large fluctuations in choice RT and poor vigilance (Ballard et al. 2002). Slow responses in a vigilance task have been correlated with bilateral prefrontal atrophy (Brück et al. 2004). More recently, it has been reported that vigilance is impaired especially in those PD patients who suffer visual hallucinations (Koerts et al. 2010). Although Zhou et al. (2012) found no effect of warning signals on the ANT protocol, other investigators have reported that warning signals have a more transient (though equally strong) alerting effect than in controls on a simple reaction time task (Bloxham, Dick, and Moore 1987). Gait problems and falling in PD are strongly correlated with attention, as measured by sustained reaction speed and RT variability (Allcock et al. 2009). In one study, measures of sustained attention accounted for 10% of the variance in gait speed in PD patients (Lord et al. 2010).

Divided and executive attention

Several studies have reported deficits of divided attention or on dual tasks in PD. For example, PD patients are impaired compared to healthy controls on detection of targets if two auditory streams have to be attended simultaneously (Sharpe 1996). Moreover, using the dual task methodology employed by Baddeley and his colleagues to investigate the 'central executive', some authors have demonstrated that PD patients have a significant decline in performance on a visuomotor tracking task while recalling digit span forward sequences, whereas controls showed no such change (Dalrymple-Alford et al. 1994). Such dual-task deficits can have significant effects on function in everyday life for PD patients, with concurrent tasks significantly slowing gait speed and reducing mean step length (Rochester et al. 2004; Lord et al. 2010; but see Smulders et al. 2012).

Although early studies were inconclusive (Weingartner et al. 1984; Taylor, Saint-Cyr, and Lang 1987), more recent research has revealed that some the greatest impairments of PD patients on a cognitive battery include performance on the trail-making test, consistent with a problem in dividing and/or switching attention (Elgh et al. 2009). The same study also demonstrated that another key performance indicator is the Wisconsin Card-Sorting Test. It has long been known that PD patients are impaired on this task (Bowen et al. 1975; Lees and Smith 1983) with particular difficulty in switching their sorting strategy (Cools et al. 1984). Specifically, extradimensional shifts, i.e. switching classification to be a previously irrelevant stimulus dimension, appear to be particularly difficult (Downes et al. 1989).

Price and colleagues (2009) have recently extensively reviewed studies of categorization tasks such as the Wisconsin Card-Sorting Test, and by fractionating the task components, concluded that under-medicated patients have difficulty in rule shifting (particularly to a previously irrelevant dimension) but are less distractible when required to continue the current rule. In their view, when over-medicated, patients are improved at set shifting, but have difficulty generating rules and cannot effectively use negative feedback to select new rules. Interestingly, deep brain stimulation (DBS) to the subthalamic nucleus (STN)—a treatment option for some patients with PD—also improves performance on the Wisconsin Card-Sorting Test (Jahanshahi et al. 2000).

Some attention deficits in PD may be explainable as a failure of 'braking' or inhibition. PD increases errors on go/no-go tasks in a complexity-dependent manner (Cooper et al. 1994). A recent study has revealed that early PD patients who perform within normal limits on a go/no-go task nevertheless have increased prefrontal and basal ganglia activation compared to healthy people, suggesting greater involvement of these structures is necessary to exert similar levels of control (Baglio et al. 2011). On the stop-signal task, PD patients have increased stop-signal reaction times, independent of their 'go' reaction times (Gauggel, Rieger, and Feghoff 2004; Obeso et al. 2011). Deep brain stimulation to the subthalamic nucleus (STN) can also increase stop-signal reaction times on the stop-signal task (Ray et al. 2009), although the opposite effect has also been observed (Mirabella et al. 2012). Deep brain stimulation may give varying effects on inhibition depending on the exact site being stimulated, with ventral but not dorsal STN stimulation leading to worse inhibitory control (Hershey et al. 2010). This intervention has also been shown to increase the speed of responses on a go/no-go task, while increasing commission errors (Ballanger et al. 2009).

On the Stroop test, PD patients are worse when task type (ink-naming vs. word-reading) has to be remembered through a block, but not when it changes from trial to trial (Brown and Marsden 1988). Thus, one potential cause for impaired performance on the Stroop might be a deficit in maintaining task set, particularly when no exogenous cues are available. However, Obeso et al. (2011) interpret such deficits in the context of other tests of inhibitory control, including prolonged SSRT and go/no-go task impairments, pointing to a general disorder of inhibition underlying several aspects of executive attention impairment in PD.

CONCLUSION

Deficits in directing attention are a major cause of everyday problems and functional impairment across many brain disorders. Here we have focused on patients with focal brain lesions, traumatic brain injury, and Parkinson's disease to bring out common themes and principles that cut across different underlying pathological processes. We have tried to frame the findings in terms of deficits in selective, sustained, divided, and executive attention. In many ways, of course, this may be an artifice, but such a conceptual framework nevertheless provides a useful means to organize the extensive empirical data that have now emerged from studies of neurological patients. The challenge will be to use this information to develop effective treatments, an area of research that is currently in its infancy.

REFERENCES

Alexander, M. P., Stuss, D. T., Picton, T. W., Shallice, T., and Gillingham, S. (2007). Regional frontal injuries cause distinct impairments in cognitive control. *Neurology* 68(18): 1515–1523.

Alexander, M. P., Stuss, D. T., Shallice, T., Picton, T. W., and Gillingham, S. (2005). Impaired concentration due to frontal lobe damage from two distinct lesion sites. *Neurology* 65(4): 572–579.

Alivisatos, B. and Milner, B. (1989). Effects of frontal or temporal lobectomy on the use of advance information in a choice reaction time task. *Neuropsychologia* 27(4): 495–503.

Allcock, L. M., Rowan, E. N., Steen, I. N., Wesnes, K., Kenny, R. A., and Burn, D. J. (2009). Impaired attention predicts falling in Parkinson's disease. *Parkinsonism & Related Disorders* 15(2): 110–115.

Alvarez, J. A. and Emory, E. (2006). Executive function and the frontal lobes: A meta-analytic review. *Neuropsychology Review* 16(1): 17–42.

Annoni, J.-M., Khateb, A., Gramigna, S., Staub, F., Carota, A., Maeder, P., and Bogousslavsky, J. (2003). Chronic cognitive impairment following laterothalamic infarcts: A study of 9 cases. *Archives of Neurology* 60(10): 1439–1443.

Aron, A. R., Durston, S., Eagle, D. M., Logan, G. D., Stinear, C. M., and Stuphorn, V. (2007). Converging evidence for a fronto-basal-ganglia network for inhibitory control of action and cognition. *Journal of Neuroscience* 27(44): 11860–11864.

Aron, A. R., Fletcher, P. C., Bullmore, E. T., Sahakian, B. J., and Robbins, T. W. (2003). Stop-signal inhibition disrupted by damage to right inferior frontal gyrus in humans. *Nature Neuroscience* 6(2): 115–116.

Ashman, T. A., Cantor, J. B., Gordon, W. A., Spielman, L., Egan, M., Ginsberg, A., Engmann, C., Dijkers, M., and Flanagan, S. (2008). Objective measurement of fatigue following traumatic brain injury. *Journal of Head Trauma Rehabilitation* 23(1): 33–40.

Azouvi, P., Couillet, J., Leclercq, M., Martin, Y., Asloun, S., and Rousseaux, M. (2004). Divided attention and mental effort after severe traumatic brain injury. *Neuropsychologia* 42(9): 1260–1268.

Baglio, F., Blasi, V., Falini, A., Farina, E., Mantovani, F., Olivotto, F., Scotti, G., Nemni, R., and Bozzali, M. (2011). Functional brain changes in early Parkinson's disease during motor response and motor inhibition. *Neurobiology of Aging* 32(1): 115–124.

Ballanger, B., van Eimeren, T., Moro, E., Lozano, A. M., Hamani, C., Boulinguez, P., Pellecchia, G., Houle, S., Poon, Y. Y., Lang, A. E., and Strafella, A. P. (2009). Stimulation of the subthalamic nucleus and impulsivity: Release your horses. *Annals of Neurology* 66(6): 817–824.

Ballard, C. G., Aarsland, D., McKeith, I., O'Brien, J., Gray, A., Cormack, F., Burn, D., Cassidy, T., Starfeldt, R., Larsen, J.-P., Brown, R., and Tovee, M. (2002). Fluctuations in attention PD dementia vs DLB with Parkinsonism. *Neurology* 59(11): 1714–1720.

Barceló, F., Suwazono, S., and Knight, R. T. (2000). Prefrontal modulation of visual processing in humans. *Nature Neuroscience* 3(4): 399–403.

Bartolomeo, P., Thiebaut de Schotten, M., and Doricchi, F. (2007). Left unilateral neglect as a disconnection syndrome. *Cerebral Cortex* 17(11): 2479–2490.

Bate, A. J., Mathias, J. L., and Crawford, J. R. (2001). The covert orienting of visual attention following severe traumatic brain injury. *Journal of Clinical and Experimental Neuropsychology* 23(3): 386–398.

Belmont, A., Agar, N., and Azouvi, P. (2009). Subjective fatigue, mental effort, and attention deficits after severe traumatic brain injury. *Neurorehabilitation and Neural Repair* 23(9): 939–944.

Belmont, A., Agar, N., Hugeron, C., Gallais, B., and Azouvi, P. (2006). Fatigue and traumatic brain injury. *Annales de Réadaptation et de Médecine Physique* 49(6): 283–288, 370–374.

Ben-David, B. M., Nguyen, L. L., and van Lieshout, P. H. (2011). Stroop effects in persons with traumatic brain injury: Selective attention, speed of processing, or color-naming? A meta-analysis. *Journal of the International Neuropsychological Society* 17(2): 354–363.

Bendlin, B. B., Ries, M. L., Lazar, M., Alexander, A. L., Dempsey, R. J., Rowley, H. A., Sherman, J. E., and Johnson, S. C. (2008). Longitudinal changes in patients with traumatic brain injury assessed with diffusion-tensor and volumetric imaging. *NeuroImage* 42(2): 503–514.

Bennett, I. J., Motes, M. A., Rao, N. K., and Rypma, B. (2012). White matter tract integrity predicts visual search performance in young and older adults. *Neurobiology of Aging* 33(2): 433. e21–31.

Benson, R. R., Meda, S. A., Vasudevan, S., Kou, Z., Govindarajan, K. A., Hanks, R. A., Millis, S. R., Makki, M., Latif, Z., Coplin, W., Meythaler, J., and Haacke, E. M. (2007). Global white matter analysis of diffusion tensor images is predictive of injury severity in traumatic brain injury. *Journal of Neurotrauma* 24(3): 446–459.

Berry, E. L., Nicolson, R. I., Foster, J. K., Behrmann, M., and Sagar, H. J. (1999). Slowing of reaction time in Parkinson's disease: The involvement of the frontal lobes. *Neuropsychologia* 37(7): 787–795.

Bisley, J. W. and Goldberg, M. E. (2010). Attention, intention, and priority in the parietal lobe. *Annual Review of Neuroscience* 33(1): 1–21.

Bloxham, C. A., Dick, D. J., and Moore, M. (1987). Reaction times and attention in Parkinson's disease. *Journal of Neurology, Neurosurgery & Psychiatry* 50(9): 1178–1183.

Boehler, C. N., Appelbaum, L. G., Krebs, R. M., Hopf, J. M., and Woldorff, M. G. (2010). Pinning down response inhibition in the brain: Conjunction analyses of the stop-signal task. *NeuroImage* 52(4): 1621–1632.

Bohnen, N. I. and Albin, R. L. (2011). The cholinergic system and Parkinson disease. *Behavioural Brain Research* 221(2): 564–573.

Bonnelle, V., Ham, T. E., Leech, R., Kinnunen, K. M., Mehta, M. A., Greenwood, R. J., and Sharp, D. J. (2012). Salience network integrity predicts default mode network function after traumatic brain injury. *Proceedings of the National Academy of Sciences USA* 109(12): 4690–4695.

Bonnelle, V., Leech, R., Kinnunen, K. M., Ham, T. E., Beckmann, C. F., De Boissezon, X., Greenwood, R. J., and Sharp, D. J. (2011). Default mode network connectivity predicts sustained attention deficits after traumatic brain injury. *Journal of Neuroscience: The Official Journal of the Society for Neuroscience* 31(38): 13442–13451.

Botvinick, M. M., Braver, T. S., Barch, D. M., Carter, C. S., and Cohen, J. D. (2001). Conflict monitoring and cognitive control. *Psychological Review* 108(3): 624–652.

Bowen, F. P., Kamienny, R. S., Burns, M. M., and Yahr, M. (1975). Parkinsonism: Effects of levodopa treatment on concept formation. *Neurology* 25(8): 701–704.

Briand, K. A., Hening, W., Poizner, H., and Sereno, A. B. (2001). Automatic orienting of visuospatial attention in Parkinson's disease. *Neuropsychologia* 39(11): 1240–1249.

Brouwer, W., Verzendaal, M., van der Naalt, J., Smit, J., and van Zomeren, E. (2001). Divided attention years after severe closed head injury: The effect of dependencies between the subtasks. *Brain and Cognition* 46(1–2): 54–56.

Brown, R. G. and Marsden, C. D. (1988). Internal versus external cues and the control of attention in Parkinson's disease. *Brain* 111(2): 323–345.

Brück, A., Kurki, T., Kaasinen, V., Vahlberg, T., and Rinne, J. O. (2004). Hippocampal and prefrontal atrophy in patients with early non-demented Parkinson's disease is related to cognitive impairment. *Journal of Neurology, Neurosurgery & Psychiatry* 75(10): 1467–1469.

Chan, R. C. (2001). Attentional deficits in patients with post-concussion symptoms: A componential perspective. *Brain Injury* 15(1): 71–94.

Chan, R. C. (2002). Attentional deficits in patients with persisting postconcussive complaints: A general deficit or specific component deficit? *Journal of Clinical and Experimental Neuropsychology* 24(8): 1081–1093.

Cools, A. R., van den Bercken, J. H., Horstink, M. W., van Spaendonck, K. P., and Berger, H. J. (1984). Cognitive and motor shifting aptitude disorder in Parkinson's disease. *Journal of Neurology, Neurosurgery & Psychiatry* 47(5): 443–453.

Cooper, J. A., Sagar, H. J., Tidswell, P., and Jordan, N. (1994). Slowed central processing in simple and go/no-go reaction time tasks in Parkinson's disease. *Brain: A Journal of Neurology* 117(3): 517–529.

Corbetta, M. and Shulman, G. L. (2002). Control of goal-directed and stimulus-driven attention in the brain. *Nature Reviews Neuroscience* 3(3): 201–215.

Cormack, F., Gray, A., Ballard, C., and Tovée, M. J. (2004). A failure of 'pop-out' in visual search tasks in dementia with Lewy Bodies as compared to Alzheimer's and Parkinson's disease. *International Journal of Geriatric Psychiatry* 19(8): 763–772.

Cossa, F. M. and Fabiani, M. (1999). Attention in closed head injury: A critical review. *Italian Journal of Neurological Sciences* 20(3): 145–153.

Coull, J. T. (1998). Neural correlates of attention and arousal: Insights from electrophysiology, functional neuroimaging and psychopharmacology. *Progress in Neurobiology* 55(4): 343–361.

Coull, J. T., Frackowiak, R. S., and Frith, C. D. (1998). Monitoring for target objects: Activation of right frontal and parietal cortices with increasing time on task. *Neuropsychologia* 36(12): 1325–1334.

Coulthard, E. J., Nachev, P., and Husain, M. (2008). Control over conflict during movement preparation: Role of posterior parietal cortex. *Neuron* 58(1): 144–157.

Cremona-Meteyard, S. L., Clark, C. R., Wright, M. J., and Geffen, G. M. (1992). Covert orientation of visual attention after closed head injury. *Neuropsychologia* 30(2): 123–132.

Cremona-Meteyard, S. L. and Geffen, G. M. (1994). Persistent visuospatial attention deficits following mild head injury in Australian rules football players. *Neuropsychologia* 32(6): 649–662.

Dalrymple-Alford, J. C., Kalders, A. S., Jones, R. D., and Watson, R. W. (1994). A central executive deficit in patients with Parkinson's disease.. *Journal of Neurology, Neurosurgery & Psychiatry* 57(3): 360–367.

Davidson, P. S. R., Gao, F. Q., Mason, W. P., Winocur, G., and Anderson, N. D. (2007). Verbal fluency, trail making, and Wisconsin Card Sorting Test performance following right frontal lobe tumor resection. *Journal of Clinical and Experimental Neuropsychology* 30(1): 18–32.

Davis, E. T. and Palmer, J. (2004). Visual search and attention: An overview. *Spatial Vision* 17(4–5): 249–255.

Demakis, G. J. (2003). A meta-analytic review of the sensitivity of the Wisconsin Card Sorting Test to frontal and lateralized frontal brain damage. *Neuropsychology* 17(2): 255–264.

Desimone, R. and Duncan, J. (1995). Neural mechanisms of selective visual attention. *Annual Review of Neuroscience* 18: 193–222.

Dimoska-DiMarco, A., McDonald, S., Kelly, M., Tate, R., and Johnstone, S. (2011). A meta-analysis of response inhibition and Stroop interference control deficits in adults with traumatic brain injury (TBI). *Journal of Clinical and Experimental Neuropsychology* 33(4): 471–485.

Dockree, P. M., Kelly, S. P., Roche, R. A., Hogan, M. J., Reilly, R. B., and Robertson, I. H. (2004). Behavioural and physiological impairments of sustained attention after traumatic brain injury. *Brain Research* 20(3): 403–414.

Doricchi, F., Thiebaut de Schotten, M., Tomaiuolo, F., and Bartolomeo, P. (2008). White matter (dis)connections and grey matter (dys)functions in visual neglect: Gaining insights into the brain networks of spatial awareness. *Cortex* 44(8): 983–995.

Dosenbach, N. U., Fair, D. A., Cohen, A. L., Schlaggar, B. L., and Petersen, S. E. (2008). A dual-networks architecture of top-down control. *Trends in Cognitive Sciences* 12(3): 99–105.

Dosenbach, N. U., Visscher, K. M., Palmer, E. D., Miezin, F. M., Wenger, K. K., Kang, H. C., Burgund, E. D., Grimes, A. L., Schlaggar, B. L., and Petersen, S. E. (2006). A core system for the implementation of task sets. *Neuron* 50(5): 799–812.

Downes, J. J., Roberts, A. C., Sahakian, B. J., Evenden, J. L., Morris, R. G., and Robbins, T. W. (1989). Impaired extra-dimensional shift performance in medicated and unmedicated Parkinson's disease: Evidence for a specific attentional dysfunction. *Neuropsychologia* 27(11–12): 1329–1343.

Dux, P. E. and Marois, R. (2009). The attentional blink: A review of data and theory. *Attention, Perception, & Psychophysics* 71(8): 1683–1700.

Elgh, E., Domellöf, M., Linder, J., Edström, M., Stenlund, H., and Forsgren, L. (2009). Cognitive function in early Parkinson's disease: A population-based study. *European Journal of Neurology* 16(12): 1278–1284.

Eslinger, P. J. and Grattan, L. M. (1993). Frontal lobe and frontal-striatal substrates for different forms of human cognitive flexibility. *Neuropsychologia* 31(1): 17–28.

Fan, J., McCandliss, B. D., Sommer, T., Raz, A., and Posner, M. I. (2002). Testing the efficiency and independence of attentional networks. *Journal of Cognitive Neuroscience* 14(3): 340–347.

Filoteo, J. V., Williams, B. J., Rilling, L. M., and Roberts, J. W. (1997). Performance of Parkinson's disease patients on the visual search and attention test: Impairment in single-feature but not dual-feature visual search. *Archives of Clinical Neuropsychology* 12(7): 621–634.

Floden, D. and Stuss, D. T. (2006). Inhibitory control is slowed in patients with right superior medial frontal damage. *Journal of Cognitive Neuroscience* 18(11): 1843–1849.

Fransson, P. (2005). Spontaneous low-frequency BOLD signal fluctuations: An fMRI investigation of the resting-state default mode of brain function hypothesis. *Human Brain Mapping* 26(1): 15–29.

Fuster, J. M. (1997). *The Prefrontal Cortex: Anatomy, Physiology and Neuropsychology of the Frontal Lobe*, 3rd revised edn. Philadelphia: Lippincott Williams and Wilkins.

Garavan, H., Ross, T. J., Kaufman, J., and Stein, E. A. (2003). A midline dissociation between error-processing and response-conflict monitoring. *NeuroImage* 20(2): 1132–1139.

Gauggel, S., Rieger, M., and Feghoff, T. (2004). Inhibition of ongoing responses in patients with Parkinson's disease. *Journal of Neurology, Neurosurgery & Psychiatry* 75(4): 539–544.

Gentry, L. R., Godersky, J. C., and Thompson, B. (1988). MR imaging of head trauma: Review of the distribution and radiopathologic features of traumatic lesions. *American Journal of Roentgenology* 150(3): 663–672.

Ghika-Schmid, F. and Bogousslavsky, J. (2000). The acute behavioral syndrome of anterior thalamic infarction: A prospective study of 12 cases. *Annals of Neurology* 48(2): 220–227.

Gillebert, C. R., Mantini, D., Thijs, V., Sunaert, S., Dupont, P., and Vandenberghe, R. (2011). Lesion evidence for the critical role of the intraparietal sulcus in spatial attention. *Brain: A Journal of Neurology* 134(6): 1694–1709.

Gitelman, D. R., Nobre, A. C., Parrish, T. B., LaBar, K. S., Kim, Y. H., Meyer, J. R., and Mesulam, M. (1999). A large-scale distributed network for covert spatial attention: Further anatomical delineation based on stringent behavioural and cognitive controls. *Brain: A Journal of Neurology* 122(6): 1093–1106.

Glosser, G. and Goodglass, H. (1990). Disorders in executive control functions among aphasic and other brain-damaged patients. *Journal of Clinical and Experimental Neuropsychology* 12(4): 485–501.

Godefroy, O., Cabaret, M., and Rousseaux, M. (1994). Vigilance and effects of fatigability, practice and motivation on simple reaction time tests in patients with lesion of the frontal lobe. *Neuropsychologia* 32(8): 983–990.

Godefroy, O. and Rousseaux, M. (1996). Divided and focused attention in patients with lesion of the prefrontal cortex. *Brain and Cognition* 30(2): 155–174.

Greicius, M. D., Supekar, K., Menon, V., and Dougherty, R. F. (2009). Resting-state functional connectivity reflects structural connectivity in the default mode network. *Cerebral Cortex* 19(1): 72–78.

Habekost, T. and Bundesen, C. (2003). Patient assessment based on a theory of visual attention (TVA): Subtle deficits after a right frontal-subcortical lesion. *Neuropsychologia* 41(9): 1171–1188.

Hahn, B., Wolkenberg, F. A., Ross, T. J., Myers, C. S., Heishman, S. J., Stein, D. J., Kurup, P. K., and Stein, E. A. (2008). Divided versus selective attention: Evidence for common processing mechanisms. *Brain Research* 1215: 137–146.

Halterman, C. I., Langan, J., Drew, A., Rodriguez, E., Osternig, L. R., Chou, L. S., and van Donkelaar, P. (2006). Tracking the recovery of visuospatial attention deficits in mild traumatic brain injury. *Brain* 129(3): 747–753.

Hart, T., Giovannetti, T., Montgomery, M. W., and Schwartz, M. F. (1998). Awareness of errors in naturalistic action after traumatic brain injury. *Journal of Head Trauma Rehabilitation* 13(5): 16–28.

Hattori, T., Orimo, S., Aoki, S., Ito, K., Abe, O., Amano, A., Sato, R., Sakai, K., and Mizusawa, H. (2012). Cognitive status correlates with white matter alteration in Parkinson's disease. *Human Brain Mapping* 33(3): 727–739.

Hayden, B. Y., Smith, D. V., and Platt, M. L. (2009). Electrophysiological correlates of default-mode processing in macaque posterior cingulate cortex. *Proceedings of the National Academy of Sciences USA* 106(14): 5948–5953.

He, B. J., Shulman, G. L., Snyder, A. Z., and Corbetta, M. (2007). The role of impaired neuronal communication in neurological disorders. *Current Opinion in Neurology* 20(6): 655–660.

Hershey, T., Campbell, M. C., Videen, T. O., Lugar, H. M., Weaver, P. M., Hartlein, J., Karimi, M., Tabbal, S. D., and Perlmutter, J. S. (2010). Mapping go-no-go performance within the subthalamic nucleus region. *Brain: A Journal of Neurology* 133(12): 3625–3634.

Hopfinger, J. B., Woldorff, M. G., Fletcher, E. M., and Mangun, G. R. (2001). Dissociating top-down attentional control from selective perception and action. *Neuropsychologia* 39(12): 1277–1291.

Horowitz, T. S., Choi, W. Y., Horvitz, J. C., Côté, L. J., and Mangels, J. A. (2006). Visual search deficits in Parkinson's disease are attenuated by bottom-up target salience and top-down information. *Neuropsychologia* 44(10): 1962–1977.

Howes, D. and Boller, F. (1975). Simple reaction time: Evidence for focal impairment from lesions of the right hemisphere. *Brain: A Journal of Neurology* 98(2): 317–332.

Huang, C., Mattis, P., Tang, C., Perrine, K., Carbon, M., and Eidelberg, D. (2007). Metabolic brain networks associated with cognitive function in Parkinson's disease. *NeuroImage* 34(2): 714–723.

Husain, M. and Rorden, C. (2003). Non-spatially lateralized mechanisms in hemispatial neglect. *Nature Reviews Neuroscience* 4(1): 26–36.

Jahanshahi, M., Ardouin, C. M., Brown, R. G., Rothwell, J. C., Obeso, J., Albanese, A., Rodriguez-Oroz, M. C., Moro, E., Benabid, A. L., Pollak, P., and Limousin-Dowsey, P. (2000). The impact of deep brain stimulation on executive function in Parkinson's disease. *Brain: A Journal of Neurology* 123(6): 1142–1154.

Jodzio, K. and Biechowska, D. (2010). Wisconsin Card Sorting Test as a measure of executive function impairments in stroke patients. *Applied Neuropsychology* 17(4): 267–277.

Kahneman, D. (1973). *Attention and Effort*. Englewood Cliffs, N.J.: Prentice Hall.

Kastner, S. and Ungerleider, L. G. (2000). Mechanisms of visual attention in the human cortex. *Annual Review of Neuroscience* 23: 315–341.

Kelly, A. M., Uddin, L. Q., Biswal, B. B., Castellanos, F. X., and Milham, M. P. (2008). Competition between functional brain networks mediates behavioral variability. *NeuroImage* 39(1): 527–537.

Kingstone, A., Klein, R., Morein-Zamir, S., Hunt, A., Fisk, J., and Maxner, C. (2002). Orienting attention in aging and Parkinson's disease: Distinguishing modes of control. *Journal of Clinical and Experimental Neuropsychology* 24(7): 951–967.

Kinnunen, K. M., Greenwood, R., Powell, J. H., Leech, R., Hawkins, P. C., Bonnelle, V., Patel, M. C., Counsell, S. J., and Sharp, D. J. (2011). White matter damage and cognitive impairment after traumatic brain injury. *Brain* 134(2): 449–463.

Koerts, J., Borg, M. A. J. P., Meppelink, A. M., Leenders, K. L., van Beilen, M., and van Laar, T. (2010). Attentional and perceptual impairments in Parkinson's disease with visual hallucinations. *Parkinsonism & Related Disorders* 16(4): 270–274.

Koski, L. M., Paus, T., and Petrides, M. (1998). Directed attention after unilateral frontal excisions in humans. *Neuropsychologia* 36(12): 1363–1371.

Kraus, M. F., Susmaras, T., Caughlin, B. P., Walker, C. J., Sweeney, J. A., and Little, D. M. (2007). White matter integrity and cognition in chronic traumatic brain injury: A diffusion tensor imaging study. *Brain* 130(10): 2508–2519.

Kumar, R., Gupta, R. K., Husain, M., Chaudhry, C., Srivastava, A., Saksena, S., and Rathore, R. K. (2009). Comparative evaluation of corpus callosum DTI metrics in acute mild and moderate traumatic brain injury: Its correlation with neuropsychometric tests. *Brain Injury* 23(7): 675–685.

Lamb, M. R., Robertson, L. C., and Knight, R. T. (1989). Attention and interference in the processing of global and local information: Effects of unilateral temporal-parietal junction lesions. *Neuropsychologia* 27(4): 471–483.

Larson, M. J., Kaufman, D. A., Schmalfuss, I. M., and Perlstein, W. M. (2007). Performance monitoring, error processing, and evaluative control following severe TBI. *Journal of the International Neuropsychological Society* 13(6): 961–971.

Lawrence, N. S., Ross, T. J., Hoffmann, R., Garavan, H., and Stein, E. A. (2003). Multiple neuronal networks mediate sustained attention. *Journal of Cognitive Neuroscience* 15(7): 1028–1038.

Leclercq, M., Couillet, J., Azouvi, P., Marlier, N., Martin, Y., Strypstein, E., and Rousseaux, M. (2000). Dual task performance after severe diffuse traumatic brain injury or vascular prefrontal damage. *Journal of Clinical and Experimental Neuropsychology* 22(3): 339–350.

Leclercq, M. and Zimmermann, P. (eds.) (2002). *Applied Neuropsychology of Attention: Theory, Diagnosis and Rehabilitation.* London: Psychology Press.

Lees, A. J. and Smith, E. (1983). Cognitive deficits in the early stages of Parkinson's disease. *Brain: A Journal of Neurology* 106 (2): 257–270.

Leotti, L. A. and Wager, T. D. (2010). Motivational influences on response inhibition measures. *Journal of Experimental Psychology* 36(2): 430–447.

Liddle, E. B., Hollis, C., Batty, M. J., Groom, M. J., Totman, J. J., Liotti, M., Scerif, G., and Liddle, P. F. (2011). Task-related default mode network modulation and inhibitory control in ADHD: Effects of motivation and methylphenidate. *Journal of Child Psychology and Psychiatry and Allied Disciplines* 52(7): 761–771.

Lieb, K., Brucker, S., Bach, M., Lücking, C., and Greenlee, M. (1999). Impairment in preattentive visual processing in patients with Parkinson's disease. *Brain* 122(2): 303–313.

Little, D. M., Kraus, M. F., Joseph, J., Geary, E. K., Susmaras, T., Zhou, X. J., Pliskin, N., and Gorelick, P. B. (2010). Thalamic integrity underlies executive dysfunction in traumatic brain injury. *Neurology* 74(7): 558–564.

Logan, G. D., Cowan, W. B., and Davis, K. A. (1984). On the ability to inhibit simple and choice reaction time responses: A model and a method. *Journal of Experimental Psychology: Human Perception and Performance* 10(2): 276–291.

Loken, W. J., Thornton, A. E., Otto, R. L., and Long, C. J. (1995). Sustained attention after severe closed head injury. *Neuropsychology* 9(4): 592–598.

Loose, R., Kaufmann, C., Auer, D. P., and Lange, K. W. (2003). Human prefrontal and sensory cortical activity during divided attention tasks. *Human Brain Mapping* 18(4): 249–259.

Lord, S., Rochester, L., Hetherington, V., Allcock, L. M., and Burn, D. (2010). Executive dysfunction and attention contribute to gait interference in 'off' state Parkinson's disease. *Gait & Posture* 31(2): 169–174.

Luck, S. J., Hillyard, S. A., Mouloua, M., and Hawkins, H. L. (1996). Mechanisms of visual-spatial attention: Resource allocation or uncertainty reduction? *Journal of Experimental Psychology: Human Perception and Performance* 22(3): 725–737.

McAvinue, L., O'Keeffe, F. M., McMackin, D., and Robertson, I. H. (2005). Impaired sustained attention and error awareness in traumatic brain injury: Implications for insight. *Neuropsychological Rehabilitation* 15(5): 569–587.

Mack, S. C. and Eckstein, M. P. (2011). Object co-occurrence serves as a contextual cue to guide and facilitate visual search in a natural viewing environment. *Journal of Vision* 11(9): 1–16.

McKeith, I. G. and Mosimann, U. P. (2004). Dementia with Lewy Bodies and Parkinson's disease. *Parkinsonism & Related Disorders* 10(Suppl. 1): S15–S18.

Mackworth, N. H. (1948). The breakdown of vigilance during prolonged visual search. *Quarterly Journal of Experimental Psychology* 1(1): 6–21.

Malhotra, P., Coulthard, E. J., and Husain, M. (2009). Role of right posterior parietal cortex in maintaining attention to spatial locations over time. *Brain* 132(3): 645–660.

Manly, T., Hawkins, K., Evans, J., Woldt, K., and Robertson, I. H. (2002). Rehabilitation of executive function: Facilitation of effective goal management on complex tasks using periodic auditory alerts. *Neuropsychologia* 40(3): 271–281.

Mannan, S. K., Hodgson, T. L., Husain, M., and Kennard, C. (2008). Eye movements in visual search indicate impaired saliency processing in Parkinson's disease. *Progress in Brain Research* 171: 559–562.

Mathias, J. L., Bigler, E. D., Jones, N. R., Bowden, S. C., Barrett-Woodbridge, M., Brown, G. C., and Taylor, D. J. (2004). Neuropsychological and information processing performance and its relationship to white matter changes following moderate and severe traumatic brain injury: A preliminary study. *Applied Neuropsychology* 11(3): 134–152.

Mathias, J. L. and Wheaton, P. (2007). Changes in attention and information-processing speed following severe traumatic brain injury: A meta-analytic review. *Neuropsychology* 21(2): 212–223.

Menon, V. and Uddin, L. Q. (2010). Saliency, switching, attention and control: A network model of insula function. *Brain Structure & Function* 214(5–6): 655–667.

Messe, A., Caplain, S., Paradot, G., Garrigue, D., Mineo, J. F., Soto Ares, G., Ducreux, D., Vignaud, F., Rozec, G., Desal, H., Pelegrini-Issac, M., Montreuil, M., Benali, H., and Lehericy, S. (2011). Diffusion tensor imaging and white matter lesions at the subacute stage in mild traumatic brain injury with persistent neurobehavioral impairment. *Human Brain Mapping* 32(6): 999–1011.

Mesulam, M. M. (1981). A cortical network for directed attention and unilateral neglect. *Annals of Neurology* 10(4): 309–325.

Mesulam, M. M. (1990). Large-scale neurocognitive networks and distributed processing for attention, language, and memory. *Annals of Neurology* 28(5): 597–613.

Mirabella, G., Iaconelli, S., Romanelli, P., Modugno, N., Lena, F., Manfredi, M., and Cantore, G. (2012). Deep brain stimulation of subthalamic nuclei affects arm response inhibition in Parkinson's patients. *Cerebral Cortex* 22(5): 1124–1132.

Molenberghs, P., Gillebert, C. R., Schoofs, H., Dupont, P., Peeters, R., and Vandenberghe, R. (2009). Lesion neuroanatomy of the sustained attention to response task. *Neuropsychologia* 47(13): 2866–2875.

Mukhopadhyay, P., Dutt, A., Kumar Das, S., Basu, A., Hazra, A., Dhibar, T., and Roy, T. (2008). Identification of neuroanatomical substrates of set-shifting ability: Evidence from patients with focal brain lesions. *Progress in Brain Research* 168: 95–104.

Müller-Plath, G., Ott, D. V. M., and Pollmann, S. (2010). Deficits in subprocesses of visual feature search after frontal, parietal, and temporal brain lesions: A modeling approach. *Journal of Cognitive Neuroscience* 22(7): 1399–1424.

Nachev, P., Wydell, H., O'Neill, K., Husain, M., and Kennard, C. (2007). The role of the pre-supplementary motor area in the control of action. *NeuroImage* 36(Suppl. 2): T155–T163.

Nakayama, N., Okumura, A., Shinoda, J., Yasokawa, Y.-T., Miwa, K., Yoshimura, S.-I., and Iwama, T. (2006). Evidence for white matter disruption in traumatic brain injury without macroscopic lesions. *Journal of Neurology, Neurosurgery & Psychiatry* 77(7): 850–855.

Navon, D. (1977). Forest before trees: The precedence of global features in visual perception. *Cognitive Psychology* 9: 353–383.

Nebel, K., Wiese, H., Stude, P., de Greiff, A., Diener, H.-C., and Keidel, M. (2005). On the neural basis of focused and divided attention. *Brain Research: Cognitive Brain Research* 25(3): 760–776.

Niemann, H., Ruff, R. M., and Kramer, J. H. (1996). An attempt towards differentiating attentional deficits in traumatic brain injury. *Neuropsychology Review* 6(1): 11–46.

Niogi, S. N. and Mukherjee, P. (2010). Diffusion tensor imaging of mild traumatic brain injury. *Journal of Head Trauma Rehabilitation* 25(4): 241–255.

Niogi, S. N., Mukherjee, P., Ghajar, J., Johnson, C. E., Kolster, R. A., Lee, H., Suh, M., Zimmerman, R. D., Manley, G. T., and McCandliss, B. D. (2008a). Structural dissociation of attentional control and memory in adults with and without mild traumatic brain injury. *Brain* 131(12): 3209–3221.

Niogi, S. N., Mukherjee, P., Ghajar, J., Johnson, C. E., Kolster, R. A., Sarkar, R., Lee, H., Meeker, M., Zimmerman, R. D., Manley, G. T., and McCandliss, B. D. (2008b). Extent of microstructural white matter injury in postconcussive syndrome correlates with impaired cognitive reaction time: A 3T diffusion tensor imaging study of mild traumatic brain injury. *American Journal of Neuroradiology* 29(5): 967–973.

Niogi, S. N., Mukherjee, P., Ghajar, J., and McCandliss, B. D. (2010). Individual differences in distinct components of attention are linked to anatomical variations in distinct white matter tracts. *Frontiers in Neuroanatomy* 4(2). doi: 10.3389/neuro.05.002.2010.

Nobre, A. C. (2001). The attentive homunculus: Now you see it, now you don't. *Neuroscience & Biobehavioral Reviews* 25(6): 477–496.

Nobre, A. C., Sebestyen, G. N., Gitelman, D. R., Mesulam, M. M., Frackowiak, R. S., and Frith, C. D. (1997). Functional localization of the system for visuospatial attention using positron emission tomography. *Brain: A Journal of Neurology* 120(3): 515–533.

Norman, D. A. and Shallice, T. (1986). Attention to action: Willed and automatic control of behavior. In R. J. Davidson, G. E. Schwartz, and D. Shapiro (eds.), *Consciousness and Self-Regulation* (pp. 376–390). New York: Plenum Press.

Nys, G. M. S., Santens, P., and Vingerhoets, G. (2010). Horizontal and vertical attentional orienting in Parkinson's disease. *Brain and Cognition* 74(3): 179–185.

O'Connor, C., Manly, T., Robertson, I. H., Hevenor, S. J., and Levine, B. (2004). An fMRI of sustained attention with endogenous and exogenous engagement. *Brain and Cognition* 54(2): 133–135.

O'Keeffe, F. M., Dockree, P. M., Moloney, P., Carton, S., and Robertson, I. H. (2007). Characterising error-awareness of attentional lapses and inhibitory control failures in patients with traumatic brain injury. *Experimental Brain Research/Experimentelle Hirnforschung/Expérimentation Cérébrale* 180(1): 59–67.

O'Keeffe, F. M., Dockree, P. M., and Robertson, I. H. (2004). Poor insight in traumatic brain injury mediated by impaired error processing? Evidence from electrodermal activity. *Brain Research* 22(1): 101–112.

Obeso, I., Wilkinson, L., Casabona, E., Bringas, M. L., Álvarez, M., Álvarez, L., Pavón, N., Rodríguez-Oroz, M.-C., Macías, R., Obeso, J. A., and Jahanshahi, M. (2011). Deficits in inhibitory control and conflict resolution on cognitive and motor tasks in Parkinson's disease. *Experimental Brain Research/Experimentelle Hirnforschung/Expérimentation Cérébrale* 212(3): 371–384.

Owen, A. M., Roberts, A. C., Polkey, C. E., Sahakian, B. J., and Robbins, T. W. (1991). Extra-dimensional versus intra-dimensional set shifting performance following frontal lobe excisions, temporal lobe excisions or amygdalo-hippocampectomy in man. *Neuropsychologia* 29(10): 993–1006.

Parasuraman, R., Mutter, S. A., and Molloy, R. (1991). Sustained attention following mild closed-head injury. *Journal of Clinical and Experimental Neuropsychology* 13(5): 789–811.

Pardo, J. V., Fox, P. T., and Raichle, M. E. (1991). Localization of a human system for sustained attention by positron emission tomography. *Nature* 349(6304): 61–64.

Park, N. W., Moscovitch, M., and Robertson, I. H. (1999). Divided attention impairments after traumatic brain injury. *Neuropsychologia* 37(10): 1119–1133.

Peers, P. V., Ludwig, C. J. H., Rorden, C., Cusack, R., Bonfiglioli, C., Bundesen, C., Driver, J., Antoun, N., and Duncan, J. (2005). Attentional functions of parietal and frontal cortex. *Cerebral Cortex* 15(10): 1469–1484.

Petersen, S. E. and Posner, M. I. (2012). The attention system of the human brain: 20 years after. *Annual Review of Neuroscience* 35: 73–89.

Picton, T. W., Stuss, D. T., Alexander, M. P., Shallice, T., Binns, M. A., and Gillingham, S, (2007). Effects of focal frontal lesions on response inhibition. *Cerebral Cortex* 17(4): 826–838.

Picton, T. W., Stuss, D. T., Shallice, T., Alexander, M. P., and Gillingham, S. (2006). Keeping time: Effects of focal frontal lesions. *Neuropsychologia* 44(7): 1195–1209.

Poliakoff, E., O'Boyle, D. J., Moore, A. P., McGlone, F. P., Cody, F. W. J., and Spence, C. (2003). Orienting of attention and Parkinson's disease: Tactile inhibition of return and response inhibition. *Brain* 126(9): 2081–2092.

Ponsford, J. and Kinsella, G. (1992). Attentional deficits following closed-head injury. *Journal of Clinical and Experimental Neuropsychology* 14(5): 822–838.

Posner, M. I. (1980). Orienting of attention. *Quarterly Journal of Experimental Psychology* 32(1): 3–25.

Posner, M. I. (2003). Imaging a science of mind. *Trends in Cognitive Sciences* 7(10): 450–453.

Posner, M. I. (2008). Measuring alertness. *Annals of the New York Academy of Sciences* 1129: 193–199.

Posner, M. I. and Rothbart, M. K. (2007). Research on attention networks as a model for the integration of psychological science. *Annual Review of Psychology* 58: 1–23.

Posner, M. I., Walker, J. A., Friedrich, F. J., and Rafal, R. D. (1984). Effects of parietal injury on covert orienting of attention. *The Journal of Neuroscience: The Official Journal of the Society for Neuroscience* 4(7): 1863–1874.

Price, A., Filoteo, J. V., and Maddox, W. T. (2009). Rule-based category learning in patients with Parkinson's disease. *Neuropsychologia* 47(5): 1213–1226.

Rafal, R. D. and Posner, M. I. (1987). Deficits in human visual spatial attention following thalamic lesions. *Proceedings of the National Academy of Sciences USA* 84(20): 7349–7353.

Raichle, M. E., MacLeod, A. M., Snyder, A. Z., Powers, W. J., Gusnard, D. A., and Shulman, G. L. (2001). A default mode of brain function. *Proceedings of the National Academy of Sciences USA* 98(2): 676–682.

Ray, N. J., Jenkinson, N., Brittain, J., Holland, P., Joint, C., Nandi, D., Bain, P. G., Yousif, N., Green, A., Stein, J. S., and Aziz, T. Z. (2009). The role of the subthalamic nucleus in response inhibition: Evidence from deep brain stimulation for Parkinson's disease. *Neuropsychologia* 47(13): 2828–2834.

Richer, F., Décary, A., Lapierre, M. F., Rouleau, I., Bouvier, G., and Saint-Hilaire, J. M. (1993). Target detection deficits in frontal lobectomy. *Brain and Cognition* 21(2): 203–211.

Riddoch, M. J., Humphreys, G. W., Akhtar, N., Allen, H., Bracewell, R. M., and Schofield, A. J. (2008). A tale of two agnosias: Distinctions between form and integrative agnosia. *Cognitive Neuropsychology* 25(1): 56–92.

Rios, M., Perianez, J. A., and Munoz-Cespedes, J. M. (2004). Attentional control and slowness of information processing after severe traumatic brain injury. *Brain Injury* 18(3): 257–272.

Robertson, I. H. (2001). Do we need the 'lateral' in unilateral neglect? Spatially nonselective attention deficits in unilateral neglect and their implications for rehabilitation. *NeuroImage* 14(1 Pt. 2): S85–S90.

Robertson, I. H., Manly, T., Andrade, J., Baddeley, B. T., and Yiend, J. (1997). 'Oops!': Performance correlates of everyday attentional failures in traumatic brain injured and normal subjects. *Neuropsychologia* 35(6): 747–758.

Robertson, L. C., Lamb, M. R., and Knight, R. T. (1988). Effects of lesions of temporal-parietal junction on perceptual and attentional processing in humans. *The Journal of Neuroscience: The Official Journal of the Society for Neuroscience* 8(10): 3757–3769.

Roca, M., Parr, A., Thompson, R., Woolgar, A., Torralva, T., Antoun, N., Manes, F., and Duncan, J. (2010). Executive function and fluid intelligence after frontal lobe lesions. *Brain* 133(1): 234–247.

Rochester, L., Hetherington, V., Jones, D., Nieuwboer, A., Willems, A.-M., Kwakkel, G., and Van Wegen, E. (2004). Attending to the task: Interference effects of functional tasks on walking in Parkinson's disease and the roles of cognition, depression, fatigue, and balance. *Archives of Physical Medicine and Rehabilitation* 85(10): 1578–1585.

Rueckert, L. and Grafman, J. (1996). Sustained attention deficits in patients with right frontal lesions. *Neuropsychologia* 34(10): 953–963.

Rushworth, M. F. S. (2008). Intention, choice, and the medial frontal cortex. *Annals of the New York Academy of Sciences* 1124: 181–207.

Rushworth, M. F. S., Buckley, M. J., Behrens, T. E. J., Walton, M. E., and Bannerman, D. M. (2007). Functional organization of the medial frontal cortex. *Current Opinion in Neurobiology* 17(2): 220–227.

Rutgers, D. R., Toulgoat, F., Cazejust, J., Fillard, P., Lasjaunias, P., and Ducreux, D. (2008). White matter abnormalities in mild traumatic brain injury: A diffusion tensor imaging study. *American Journal of Neuroradiology* 29(3): 514–519.

Salmond, C. H., Menon, D. K., Chatfield, D. A., Williams, G. B., Pena, A., Sahakian, B. J., and Pickard, J. D. (2006). Diffusion tensor imaging in chronic head injury survivors: Correlations with learning and memory indices. *NeuroImage* 29(1): 117–124.

Sarter, M., Givens, B., and Bruno, J. P. (2001). The cognitive neuroscience of sustained attention: Where top-down meets bottom-up. *Brain Research: Brain Research Reviews* 35(2): 146–160.

Schmahmann, J. D. and Pandya, D. N. (2006). *Fiber Pathways of the Brain*. New York: Oxford University Press.

Seeley, W. W., Menon, V., Schatzberg, A. F., Keller, J., Glover, G. H., Kenna, H., Reiss, A. L., and Greicius, M. D. (2007). Dissociable intrinsic connectivity networks for salience processing and executive control. *Journal of Neuroscience* 27(9): 2349–2356.

Shallice, T. (1988). *From Neuropsychology to Mental Structure.* Cambridge: Cambridge University Press.

Sharp, D. J., Beckmann, C. F., Greenwood, R., Kinnunen, K. M., Bonnelle, V., De Boissezon, X., Powell, J. H., Counsell, S. J., Patel, M. C., and Leech, R. (2011). Default mode network functional and structural connectivity after traumatic brain injury. *Brain* 134(8): 2233–2247.

Sharp, D. J., Bonnelle, V., De Boissezon, X., Beckmann, C. F., James, S. G., Patel, M. C., and Mehta, M. A. (2010). Distinct frontal systems for response inhibition, attentional capture, and error processing. *Proceedings of the National Academy of Sciences USA* 107(13): 6106–6111.

Sharp, D. J. and Ham, T. E. (2011). Investigating white matter injury after mild traumatic brain injury. *Current Opinion in Neurology* 24(6): 558–563.

Sharpe, M. H. (1996). Is there a divided attention deficit in patients with early Parkinson's disease? *Cortex* 32(4): 747–753.

Sidaros, A., Engberg, A. W., Sidaros, K., Liptrot, M. G., Herning, M., Petersen, P., Paulson, O. B., Jernigan, T. L., and Rostrup, E. (2008). Diffusion tensor imaging during recovery from severe traumatic brain injury and relation to clinical outcome: A longitudinal study. *Brain* 131(2): 559–572.

Singh-Curry, V. and Husain, M. (2009). The functional role of the inferior parietal lobe in the dorsal and ventral stream dichotomy. *Neuropsychologia* 47(6): 1434–1448.

Skandsen, T., Kvistad, K. A., Solheim, O., Strand, I. H., Folvik, M. and Vik, A. (2010). Prevalence and impact of diffuse axonal injury in patients with moderate and severe head injury: A cohort study of early magnetic resonance imaging findings and 1-year outcome. *Journal of Neurosurgery* 113(3): 556–563.

Smith, D. H., Meaney, D.,F., and Shull, W. H. (2003). Diffuse axonal injury in head trauma. *Journal of Head Trauma Rehabilitation* 18(4): 307–316.

Smulders, K., Esselink, R. A. J., Weiss, A., Kessels, R. P. C., Geurts, A. C. H., and Bloem, B. R. (2012). Assessment of dual tasking has no clinical value for fall prediction in Parkinson's disease. *Journal of Neurology* 259(9): 1840–1847.

Sonuga-Barke, E. J. and Castellanos, F. X. (2007). Spontaneous attentional fluctuations in impaired states and pathological conditions: A neurobiological hypothesis. *Neuroscience & Biobehavioral Reviews* 31(7): 977–986.

Spikman, J. M., van Zomeren, A. H., and Deelman, B. G. (1996). Deficits of attention after closed-head injury: Slowness only? *Journal of Clinical and Experimental Neuropsychology* 18(5): 755–767.

Sridharan, D., Levitin, D. J., and Menon, V. (2008). A critical role for the right fronto-insular cortex in switching between central-executive and default-mode networks. *Proceedings of the National Academy of Sciences USA* 105(34): 12569–12574.

Stuss, D. T. (2011). Traumatic brain injury: Relation to executive dysfunction and the frontal lobes. *Current Opinion in Neurology* 24(6): 584–589.

Stuss, D. T., Alexander, M. P., Shallice, T., Picton, T. W., Binns, M. A., Macdonald, R., Borowiec, A., and Katz, D. I. (2005). Multiple frontal systems controlling response speed. *Neuropsychologia* 43(3): 396–417.

Stuss, D. T., Bisschop, S. M., Alexander, M. P., Levine, B., Katz, D., and Izukawa, D. (2001). The trail making test: A study in focal lesion patients. *Psychological Assessment* 13(2): 230–239.

Stuss, D. T., Guberman, A., Nelson, R., and Larochelle, S. (1988). The neuropsychology of para-median thalamic infarction. *Brain and Cognition* 8(3): 348–378.

Stuss, D. T. and Knight, R. T. (eds.) (2002). *Principles of Frontal Lobe Function*. New York: Oxford University Press.

Stuss, D. T., Pogue, J., Buckle, L., and Bondar, J. (1994). Characterization of stability of performance in patients with traumatic brain injury: Variability and consistency on reaction time tests. *Neuropsychology* 8(3): 316–324.

Stuss, D. T., Stethem, L. L., Hugenholtz, H., Picton, T. W., Pivik, J., and Richard, M. T. (1989). Reaction time after head injury: Fatigue, divided and focused attention, and consistency of performance. *Journal of Neurology, Neurosurgery & Psychiatry* 52(6): 742–748.

Swick, D. and Turken, U. (2002). Dissociation between conflict detection and error monitoring in the human anterior cingulate cortex. *Proceedings of the National Academy of Sciences USA* 99(25): 16354–16359.

Takahashi, M., Iwamoto, K., Fukatsu, H., Naganawa, S., Iidaka, T., and Ozaki, N. (2010). White matter microstructure of the cingulum and cerebellar peduncle is related to sustained attention and working memory: A diffusion tensor imaging study. *Neuroscience Letters* 477(2): 72–76.

Taylor, A. E., Saint-Cyr, J. A., and Lang, A. E (1987). Parkinson's disease: Cognitive changes in relation to treatment response. *Brain: A Journal of Neurology* 110(1): 35–51.

Troscianko, T. and Calvert, J. (1993). Impaired parallel visual search mechanisms in Parkinson's disease: Implications for the role of dopamine in visual attention. *Clinical Vision Sciences* 8(3): 281–287.

Ullsperger, M. and von Cramon, D. Y. (2006). The role of intact frontostriatal circuits in error processing. *Journal of Cognitive Neuroscience* 18(4): 651–664.

van Asselen, M., Almeida, I., Andre, R., Januário, C., Gonçalves, A. F., and Castelo-Branco, M. (2009). The role of the basal ganglia in implicit contextual learning: A study of Parkinson's disease. *Neuropsychologia* 47(5): 1269–1273.

Vandenberghe, R., Molenberghs, P. and Gillebert, C. R. (2012). Spatial attention deficits in humans: The critical role of superior compared to inferior parietal lesions. *Neuropsychologia* 50(6): 1092–1103.

van den Heuvel, M. P., Mandl, R. C., Kahn, R. S., and Hulshoff Pol, H. E. (2009). Functionally linked resting-state networks reflect the underlying structural connectivity architecture of the human brain. *Human Brain Mapping* 30(10): 3127–3141.

Vecera, S. P. and Rizzo, M. (2004). What are you looking at? Impaired 'social attention' following frontal-lobe damage. *Neuropsychologia* 42(12): 1657–1665.

Vohn, R., Fimm, B., Weber, J., Schnitker, R., Thron, A., Spijkers, W., Willmes, K., and Sturm, W. (2007). Management of attentional resources in within-modal and cross-modal divided attention tasks: An fMRI study. *Human Brain Mapping* 28(12): 1267–1275.

Weingartner, H., Burns, S., Diebel, R., and LeWitt, P. A. (1984). Cognitive impairments in Parkinson's disease: Distinguishing between effort-demanding and automatic cognitive processes. *Psychiatry Research* 11(3): 223–235.

Weissman, D. H., Roberts, K. C., Visscher, K. M., and Woldorff, M. G. (2006). The neural bases of momentary lapses in attention. *Nature Neuroscience* 9(7): 971–978.

Whyte, J., Polansky, M., Fleming, M., Coslett, H. B., and Cavallucci, C. (1995). Sustained arousal and attention after traumatic brain injury. *Neuropsychologia* 33(7): 797–813.

Wilde, E. A., Ramos, M. A., Yallampalli, R., Bigler, E. D., McCauley, S. R., Chu, Z., Wu, T. C., Hanten, G., Scheibel, R. S., Li, X., Vasquez, A. C., Hunter, J. V., and Levin, H. S. (2010).

Diffusion tensor imaging of the cingulum bundle in children after traumatic brain injury. *Developmental Neuropsychology* 35(3): 333–351.

Wilkins, A. J., Shallice, T., and McCarthy, R. (1987). Frontal lesions and sustained attention. *Neuropsychologia* 25(2): 359–365.

Woods, D. L. and Knight, R. T. (1986). Electrophysiologic evidence of increased distractibility after dorsolateral prefrontal lesions. *Neurology* 36(2): 212–216.

Wright, M. J., Burns, R. J., Geffen, G. M., and Geffen, L. B. (1990). Covert orientation of visual attention in Parkinson's disease: An impairment in the maintenance of attention. *Neuropsychologia* 28(2): 151–159.

Yamaguchi, S. and Kobayashi, S. (1998). Contributions of the dopaminergic system to voluntary and automatic orienting of visuospatial attention. *The Journal of Neuroscience: The Official Journal of the Society for Neuroscience* 18(5): 1869–1878.

Yantis, S. and Serences, J. T. (2003). Cortical mechanisms of space-based and object-based attentional control. *Current Opinion in Neurobiology* 13(2): 187–193.

Zappalà, G., Thiebaut de Schotten, M., and Eslinger, P. J. (2012). Traumatic brain injury and the frontal lobes: What can we gain with diffusion tensor imaging? *Cortex* 48(2): 156–165.

Zhou, S., Chen, X., Wang, C., Yin, C., Hu, P., and Wang, K. (2012). Selective attention deficits in early and moderate stage Parkinson's disease. *Neuroscience Letters* 509(1): 50–55.

CHAPTER 35

··

BALINT'S SYNDROME AND THE STUDY OF ATTENTION

··

LYNN C. ROBERTSON

BALINT's syndrome is a clinical neuropsychology classification describing a number of classic symptoms that occur together: simultanagnosia, optic apraxia, and optic ataxia. Simultanagnosia in Balint's syndrome is a problem in seeing more than one object at any given time. The object (or sometimes part of an object) that is perceived may be large or small, simple or complex, but the patient's attention seems to be captured by that object, sometimes even for several minutes. Optic ataxia refers to inaccurate and basically random performance in reaching for or pointing to the location of the perceived object. Optic apraxia is a problem in controlling eye movements (but with no evidence of oculomotor paralysis) which often leads to a fixation of gaze (Rafal 2001) or to random eye movements over the visual field (Luria et al. 1963).

The three symptoms together were first described by a Hungarian neurologist named Rezso Balint in 1909 (see Hussain and Stein 1988) in a patient under his care.[1] He attributed the cluster of symptoms to a restricted 'psychic field of view' that reduced the patient's attention to only one (or at most two) objects at any given time and suggested that this was due to a disconnection between visual and motor systems. He also concluded that association areas of the cortex, particularly the occipital-parietal lobes, were the underlying locus of the problems. However, it was not until Holmes and Horrax (1919) provided several additional cases that the symptoms as a cluster of deficits produced through bilateral occipito-parietal involvement solidified. These authors also suggested that spatial disorientation was the source of all three symptoms, although each symptom has been reported independently of the others since that time (Kinsbourne and Warrington 1962, 1963; Perenin and Vighetto 1988; Rizzo and Robin 1990; Stark et al. 1996). As with Balint's original patient, their patients did not know where the object they perceived was located in the world, which could also explain inaccuracies in moving their eyes or hands to its correct location. If a person does not know where to move his or her eyes, the best option may be not to move them at all. Again, as with Balint's original case, their patients could not navigate from one place to another without help, could not read or write normally, and could not find needed objects set in front of them (e.g. a fork for eating). For every practical purpose, they were functionally blind.[2]

Fortunately, Balint's syndrome is relatively rare, as it leaves a patient's perceptual world in chaos with objects appearing and disappearing without warning, and features moving in and out of awareness. Its rarity, however, has made it more difficult to study the mechanisms that cause it. Despite the small numbers, its relevance for issues in the study of perception, attention, and consciousness in general has grown. The present chapter provides an overview of this relevance and describes some of the evidence that has emerged that affects the study of attention but, as importantly, has also helped in understanding the perceptual world that the patients themselves experience.

BALINT'S SIMULTANAGNOSIA

Balint's simultanagnosia is a particular type of simultanagnosia that is associated with bilateral brain damage in the dorsal cortical stream of processing (Farah 1990). Other variants of simultanagnosia have been observed in many patients who do not have bilateral lesions or occipito-parietal lobe involvement. In fact, the term was introduced by Wolpert in 1924 to refer to problems in integrating multiple objects in a visual scene to form a coherent, meaningful whole. His patient could see multiple objects and was able to point to each of them, but was not able to relate them to each other in a larger semantic framework. For instance, if shown the drawing in Fig. 35.1 and asked to describe what the picture conveys, a patient might name different objects in the scene (little boy, mother, cookie jar) but not see them as telling the story of a boy stealing cookies while his mother is distracted. Although Balint's patients will fail in the same way, it might be for a different reason; specifically, they can get stuck on one object in the scene and see no others.

Another form of simultanagnosia is associated with left occipital-temporal lesions and may be due to an overall slowing of visual processing. For instance, Kinsbourne and Warrington (1962) used the term to describe a deficit in the ability to recognize single objects presented in rapid sequential order; which may not occur in Balint's patients (see Costlett and Saffron 1991). These different uses of the term have caused some confusion in the literature, but for our purposes, the form of simultanagnosia that is observed in Balint's syndrome presents more as a hyperattention to an object without the voluntary control to switch attention away from it.

OBJECT-BASED ATTENTION

The very existence of Balint's simultanagnosia is consistent with behavioural and neuro-biological evidence for a distinction between object-based and space-based attention (see

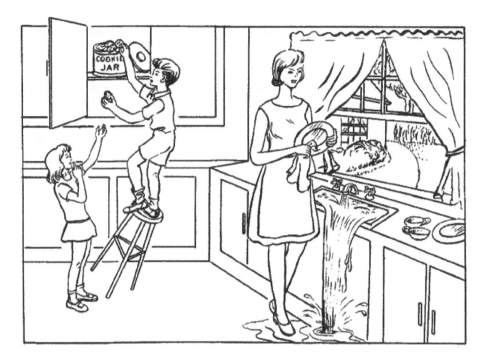

FIGURE 35.1 The Cookie Theft Picture from Boston Diagnostic Aphasia Examination—Third Edition (BDAE-3), by H. Goodglass in collaboration with E. Kaplan and B. Barresi, 2001, Austin, TX: PRO-ED. Copyright 2001 by PRO-ED, Inc. Reprinted with permission.

Serences and Kastner (chapter 4), this volume; Treue (chapter 21), this volume). Theories of object-based attention originally argued that attentional selection was for objects with space-based effects mainly involved in object individuation. They assumed that stimuli were automatically parsed into 'objects' through bottom-up mechanisms that were then candidates for selection. Yet, this begs the question of how stimulus information gets parsed into object candidates to begin with (i.e. what is an object?). This is especially problematic when, in most natural settings, objects are embedded in other objects (e.g. leaves on a tree). With spatial abilities all but absent in Balint's syndrome and attention stuck on one object at a time, it seems that evidence from patients with Balint's syndrome could help address the question of what an object might be. However, on the surface, this seems entirely circular. That is, since Balint's patients see only one object, an object is whatever a Balint's patient sees. Nevertheless, by manipulating the stimulus and/or task, studies have shown that the object a Balint patient perceives follows principles of perceptual organization that govern what normal perceivers will report as an object. For instance, a line that connects one item in a visual display to another may influence what the patient will perceive. Shown two circles separated on a page, the patient may only report that there is one, yet when the circles are connected by a single line, the same patient may then see two circles that are parts of a single object, for example seeing 'spectacles' (Luria et al. 1958).

Closure is another especially strong cue for perceptual organization. For instance, in Fig. 35.2, the two rectangular shapes on the left are closed figures because the contour that

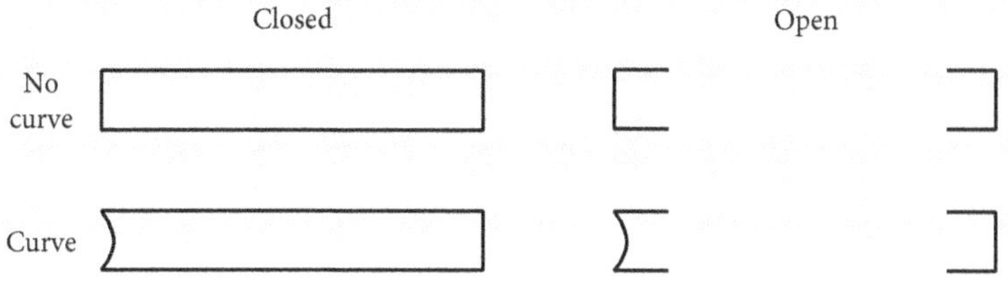

FIGURE 35.2 The figures on the left are 'closed' and form a single object, while those on the right are open and do not. A patient with Balint's simultanagnosia will detect the curve more accurately when there is closure than when there is not. Adapted from Attending to space within and between objects: Implications from a patient with Balint's syndrome, Lynn C. Robertson and Anne Treisman, *Cognitive Neuropsychology*, 23 (3) © 2006, Taylor & Francis, reprinted by permission of the publisher (Taylor & Francis Ltd, http://www.tandf.co.uk/journals).

defines them is continuous and isolates a space that then belongs to the object, separate from its background. The contours of the figures on the right are broken by a large gap that interrupts closure. The result is that the patterns on the right are not seen as a single object separated from a background, but are more likely to be perceived as two separate sketched lines (i.e. two objects) in normal perception. Robertson and Treisman (2006) presented stimuli like these in the middle of a computer screen to a patient with Balint's simultanagnosia, and had him report whether a particular feature (curved line) was present or not in each display and if the feature was reported as present, where the feature was located. They found that integrating the two sides of the object through closure improved feature detection but did not improve the perception of where the feature was located.

More specifically, on each trial one of the four patterns shown in Fig. 35.2 would appear centred on a computer screen, and the patient was asked to report whether or not there was a curve in the stimulus (bottom patterns), and if he reported that there was, to say where it was located (the response was to say whether the feature was on the left, right, top, or bottom of the screen). If closure made the rectangle more likely to be perceived as a single object, then curve detection should be better in the closed than the open case, and indeed it was substantially better (90% compared to 75% for the closed and open case, respectively). However, closure had no effect on knowing where the curve was located (64% in each case). The space within the object did not stabilize in perception to any greater extent than space as a whole.

Other studies have shown that both top-down and bottom-up information can affect perceptual organization in Balint's syndrome. For instance, Shaliv and Humphreys (2002) presented an oval with two rectangular shapes in what would be in the eye position if the stimulus were represented as a face (Fig. 3a). When the patient was told that the rectangles represented eyes compared to when he was not given this prior information, he reported a face when the rectangles were properly positioned in the oval but not when they were not. In other words, when he was primed with information that there could be eyes, his visual system responded to the stimulus as a whole. Adding line place holders in the nose and mouth positions (Fig. 3b) increased his accuracy to almost perfect. Thus, both top-down and bottom-up information that taps into the spatial

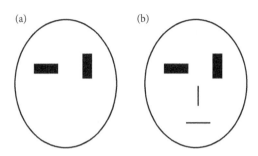

FIGURE 35.3 The rectangles are in the eyes position of a face (a) but a patient with Balint's simultanagnosia will not see them as such unless told that there might be faces in a stimulus display. Their representation as eyes is more salient when supported by other features in the correct position (b) and patients automatically see it as a face. Adapted from Implicit Location Encoding Via Stored Representations Of Familiar Objects: Neuropsychological Evidence, Lilach Shalev and Glyn W. Humphreys, *Cognitive Neuropsychology*, 19 (8) © 2002, Taylor & Francis, reprinted by permission of the publisher (Taylor & Francis Ltd, http://www.tandf.co.uk/journals).

description of a familiar object such as a face will increase coherence and draw attention to that object in perception.

These and other studies of perceptual organization in Balint's simultanagnosia (Boutsen and Humphreys 1999; Cooper and Humphreys 2000; Humphreys 1998) are consistent with the literature on normal visual perception and show that a spatial description of familiar object structure remains relatively intact. These studies have shown that grouping, familiarity, similarity, connectedness, etc., that contribute to normal integration of a set of parts into a perceptual whole can be achieved, while spatially individuating one object from another in perception can be all but destroyed.

The spatial problems observed in Balint's simultanagnosia occur when objects are located on a single surface but also when they are located in the same retinal coordinates but appear in normal perception on different planes in depth. This was first reported by Holmes (1918) in patients who, as he also showed, had normal stereoscopic fusion. In fact, depth location problems can be easily observed in clinical evaluation. Such patients cannot report how far away an object that they see may be from their own body or whether it is moved towards or away from them by the examiner. They also do not show a normal reflexive blink response when an object looms towards them, consistent with the view that the object's location in depth is not detected (Rafal 2001). Somewhat paradoxically, their visual system does respond to depth cues implicitly in other situations. For instance, in a study reported by Humphreys (1998) occlusion was introduced and a patient with Balint's simultanagnosia was asked to report how many black squares were in the stimulus (see Fig. 4). When a single oval was placed such that it appeared as an occluder, connecting the two squares behind it in depth (Fig. 4a), both squares were reported 80% of the time (well above chance). However, when the oval was offset and no longer suggested that the two squares were connected in the background plane (Fig. 4b), the patient reported that there was only one square most of the time (36% correct). This accuracy rate was about the same as when the two black squares were presented alone

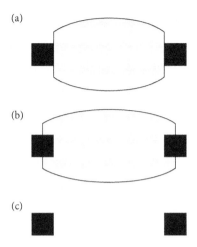

FIGURE 35.4 For normal perceivers the two black squares can be seen as a long rectangle connected behind the curved oblong (a). In (b) they appear as two squares in front of the oblong or as simply two squares when no oblong is present (c). Patients with Balint's simultanagnosia are also influenced by the relationship between the oblong and the square.

(Fig. 4c—30% correct). Thus, cues that would change normal perception of objects in depth also affected Balint's simultanagnosia. The visual system implicitly organized these depth cues.

In Balint's simultanagnosia attention becomes attracted to objects, and it is clear that rather high-level object representations are involved, but why does attention become stuck on a single object? Humphreys (1998) argued that although multiple object representations may occur, each representation must be serially selected for grasping and manipulation. One of the prerequisites for voluntarily grasping an object would be to select it first. He argued that when selective attention is used for this purpose, one object will be selected among all the others. But when moving attention from a selected object is no longer possible and location information is absent, then there is only one place for attention to go, and that is to an object. The argument is that the object that 'wins' the competition for attention is the only one that rises to perceptual awareness in classic Balint's syndrome.

Evidence from cognitive neuroscience is consistent with this idea and has shown that voluntarily shifting attention between objects that are thought to be represented by different ventral cortical systems (e.g. houses and faces) produces transient activity in the same area of the parietal cortex as shifting attention between spatial locations (Serences et al. 2004). Although there is ample evidence that object representations and spatial representations can be dissociated, the voluntary shift of attention from one object to another or one location to another appears to require a signal that is generated by more dorsal systems. Object representation itself is argued to emerge from the connectivity between neurons in distributed visual areas that are related in time to form a 'coherence field' (Rensink 2000; Serences and Yantis 2006). In other words, synchronous oscillations between distributed neurons form a temporal–spatial pattern that is differ-ent for each object. In order to switch from one coherence field to another, a switch in attention is necessary, and this switch transiently activates a dorsal network thought to be necessary for voluntarily switching attention. It follows that lesions in parietal areas would disrupt this network and impair switching, leaving the system in a state similar to that described in Balint's simultanagnosia where moving attention is not under vol-untary control. There would obviously be noise in the system that could perturb one coherence field in favour of another, which could result in objects abruptly appearing and disappearing from view.

It should be emphasized that Balint's simultanagnosia demonstrates that not all top-down signals need be attentional in nature. Being told that two rectangles in a stim-ulus display represent eyes (top-down knowledge) improves detecting the figure as a face-like whole (bottom-up), and it is the whole that attracts attention under these cir-cumstances. Without that knowledge, the rectangular parts are the objects that attract attention. If coherence fields are the neural representation of objects that compete for attention, then the field that 'wins' may be a local object (a rectangle) or a more global object (a face) which may be different under different conditions. The source of this contextual type of top-down influence is not clear, but it is a reminder that 'top-down' and 'attention' are not necessarily synonymous. Familiar structural descriptions of objects such as faces that are presumably stored in long-term memory can also have an influence.

FEATURES AND BINDING

The previous section described evidence showing that integration of visual features such as lines and angles of a single object are relatively intact in patients with Balint's syndrome, while binding the objects to spatial locations is absent or severely impaired. However, there are other integration problems in these patients that do affect how objects are perceived. For instance, the colour or motion from one object that has been missed entirely can be mis-combined in perception with the object that attracts atten-tion (Bernstein and Robertson 1998; Friedman-Hill et al. 1995; Humphreys et al. 2000). The colour and shape form an 'illusory conjunction' (Treisman and Schmidt 1982). A patient with severe Balint's symptoms who is shown a stimulus with just two objects, say a red square and a blue circle, might see only the square (due to Balint's simultana-gnosia), but is nearly as likely to report its colour as blue or red. These reports are made with high confidence by the patients, and they occur whether the stimulus is on the screen for a short period of time (less than a second) or up to 10 seconds.

Colour/shape binding errors can also be observed in normal perception (Treisman and Schmidt 1982) when the stimuli are presented very briefly and spa-tial attention is diverted. For instance, if a display similar to that shown in Fig. 35.5 is presented for a brief period of time and participants are instructed that their

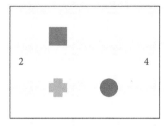

FIGURE 35.5 An example of the type of display that might be used in an experiment to test for illusory conjunctions in normal perceiving participants. The primary task would be to report the numbers at the right and left of the coloured display and then report the shape and colour at a cued location.

primary task is to report the two numbers that are present on the right and left sides of the display, spatial attention will be distributed across the display in order to report the numbers. After the numbers are reported correctly, participants are asked to report a shape at a cued location and its colour. Under such conditions, they may report the triangle as green or the plus as red, inaccurately binding the colour to the shape. Models applied to data derived from such studies using stringent guessing assumptions have supported the reality of illusory conjunctions in normal perception (Ashby et al. 1996). Such models have been applied to the data from Balint's patients as well, and again support illusory conjunctions as a real perceptual problem (Robertson et al. 1997).

These findings are consistent with an influential theory of attention proposed by Treisman and Gelade in 1980 known as Feature Integration Theory (see Wolfe, chapter 2, this volume). In fact, the theory motivated the prediction that such binding errors would be observed under free viewing conditions when spatial attention was severely impaired. Feature Integration Theory (FIT) proposed that basic features such as colour, orientation, size, etc. were encoded in separate 'feature maps', and that spatial attention was necessary to accurately bind the features together. It was originally based on the finding that individual features would 'pop out' of a multi-item display independent of the number of distractors in the display, while detecting an item with the correct combination of features (e.g. colour and shape) depended on the number of distractors. Search was slower when there were more distractors than when there were fewer, and search rates increased linearly with the number of items in the display. Treisman and Gelade proposed that conjunction detection required an attentional search through the display. The theory predicted that illusory conjunctions should arise when attention was stressed, and this prediction was confirmed in patients with Balint's syndrome.

Note that from the beginning FIT was more than a theory of attention. It was a theory of how attention interacts with basic features coded in parallel, and at least partially separately, in the visual system. It also predicted that if a person could not move attention from one place to another, illusory conjunctions would happen and that conjunction search (but not feature search) would be nearly impossible. Taking away space in normal perceiving individuals is of course a monumental challenge, if not impossible, but this is exactly what nature does in the case of Balint's syndrome. Thus, FIT predicted that illusory conjunctions would occur under free viewing conditions, and they do. Consistently, visual search is also affected in the ways predicted by the theory. Conjunction search is extremely poor, even in displays of three, four, or five items (see Fig. 6a) but feature search is very good, even in displays of 40 items (see Fig. 6b). Although features are encoded more slowly, the search rates can be unaffected by the number of distractors (at least for colour), while search for a conjunction is highly impaired even for small set sizes. Perhaps equally important, when features pop out of a feature search display, and thus grab attention of a person with Balint's simultanagnosia, the feature's location is unknown (Robertson et al. 1997). They are not bound to their locations in perception.

One early explanation for illusory conjunctions in Balint's syndrome was that simultanagnosia extends to features. That is, if there is a red square and blue circle in a display, attention may be limited to one shape and one colour at any given time and the only binding possible is between these two values. There are some reasons to question this explanation, with perhaps the most convincing being that most patients can report many colours in a display even when they only report one shape. To test this experimentally, Marcia Grabowecky (unpublished data) showed displays similar to those in Fig. 35.7 to a patient with Balint's simultanagnosia who had a high rate of illusory conjunctions. The displays were composed of nine circles and seven of them were always

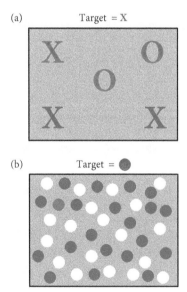

FIGURE 35.6 The top figure (a) represents a conjunction search display with a set size of 5, while the bottom figure (b) represents a feature search display with a set size of 40. Patients with Balint's simultanagnosia detect the target easily in 6b but not 6a.

green. The other two circles could both be red or both blue, or one could be red and the other blue as in Fig. 35.7a. When asked to report whether there was one or two odd colours, the patient performed very well and when asked to report all the colours present he said red, blue, and green for Fig. 35.7a and red and green for Fig. 35.7b. However, he could not say whether there was more green than red and could not report the number of circles, typically saying he saw only one with the different colours appearing simultaneously on it.

Although seeing different colours on the same shape seems impossible, there are people with certain forms of colour-grapheme synaesthesia whose brains are structurally intact who experience this type of perception all the time. The letter S may always appear as red, but it also appears in its print colour as well (see Robertson and Sagiv 2005). For instance, if it is presented in, say. blue ink, a synaesthete might report seeing the S as both red and blue at the same time and in the same place. More interesting for the present purposes is that synaesthetes show increased parietal and temporal (V4) activity in imaging studies when shown shapes that induce synaesthesia compared to those that do not (see Alvarez and Robertson, 2013, for a review). Furthermore, their synaesthetic colour can be disrupted briefly by a TMS pulse to inferior parietal lobe (Esterman et al. 2006). A model proposed by Robertson (2003) explained both the reduced colour/shape binding in Balint's syndrome and the increased colour/shape binding in synaesthesia by suggesting that the parietal lobes are directly involved in synchronizing neural activity between ventral areas of the visual cortex that register different features such as colour and shape. If synchrony is not established between these areas because of parietal damage, features will continue to signal their presence and are more likely to result in illusory conjunctions, as observed in Balint's patients. Conversely when parietal signals are overactive as in colour-grapheme synaesthesia, synchrony can be established between two colour codes (one from wavelength and one synaesthetic) within the same feature domain. In this way, more dorsal activity is necessary to form the correct binding between two colours and one shape, resulting in the conscious perception of the shape as two colours simultaneously.

It is clear from the above discussion that different theoretical approaches have been proposed to account for why bilateral parietal-occipital damage produces binding problems across feature domains. Although resolution of this question is not yet at hand, the evidence discussed in this section demonstrates that binding problems are real when

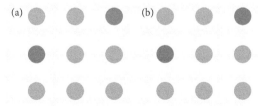

FIGURE 35.7 Representation of displays presented to the patient. One task was to report whether the two unique circles were both the same colour (b) or two different colours (a).

such damage is present and there are candidate cognitive and neurobiological mechanisms that may make their occurrence in perception less mysterious.

Implicit (Pre-attentive) Spatial Coding

It has long been thought that spatial information in Balint's syndrome was absent. However, other studies of this syndrome suggest that the bottleneck that allows conscious access to space is rather late in visual processing. This claim receives support from findings showing that the locations of objects are implicitly coded even when explicit location information is absent. The first evidence for at least a rough implicit spatial map came from a study in which a Balint's patient was asked to read a single word that appeared on a computer screen (Robertson et al. 1997). The word was either 'up' or 'down' and it appeared either towards the top or bottom of a large vertical rectangle centred on the screen (Fig. 8). When asked to report the location of the word in the rectangle, the patient was resistant to respond, saying things like 'you know I don't know where it is', and his performance was at chance when requested to guess. However, when asked simply to voice the word that appeared on the screen on each trial, the task was easy. (Single words attract attention in Balint's simultanagnosia just as single objects do; see Baylis et al. 1994.) Voice response time was recorded and it was reliably faster when the word's meaning and its location were congruent ('up' at the top, 'down' at the bottom as in Fig. 8a) than when they were incongruent ('down' at the top, 'up' at the bottom as in Fig. 8b). These effects were later replicated and extended in other Balint's patients (see Cinel and Humphreys 2006).

Another study demonstrated that although the location of features in a feature search display (e.g. Fig. 6b) is not explicitly known to such patients, their location is coded implicitly. Kim and Robertson (2001) presented displays such as that shown in Fig. 35.9 in which four elements (one in each quadrant) were presented with one being a different colour than the other three, thus a feature display. Consistent with previous findings, the distinct colour popped out of the display, but its location could not be reported above chance levels. However, in another block of trials the same stimuli were presented and the colours were irrelevant. The task was now to respond as rapidly as possible whether a shape that appeared at central fixation was an arrow or not. The results showed that response time to detect an arrow at fixation was dependent on the location of the irrelevant features. When the arrow pointed to the unique colour as in Fig. 35.9, response time to detect the arrow was faster than when it pointed to any of the other colours, and in fact, it was slowest when it pointed to the item opposite to the unique feature. These results demonstrated that the location of all the items in the irrelevant display were implicitly encoded, not just the location of the unique feature itself, as there was

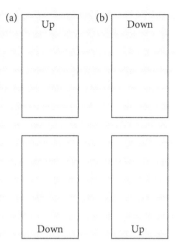

FIGURE 35.8 Example of words that are congruent with their location (a) or incongruent with their location (b).

a difference in response time between non-unique features (green items in Fig. 9) depending on where they were located in the display.

Other more complex spatial organizations continue to be processed as well in patients with Balint's simultanagnosia. For instance, in a display like that shown in Fig. 35.10, where the repetition and spatial arrangement of one shape (local) produces another shape (global), Balint's simultanagnosia results in the local shape almost always being reported, while the global shape is almost always missed (Jackson et al. 2004; Karnath et al. 2000; Huberle and Karnath 2006).

Despite problems in perceiving the global shapes explicitly in Balint's simultanagnosia, they are implicitly represented. Even when such patients are at chance levels in detecting the global shape, reaction times to name the local shape (the shape they do perceive) are faster when the global shape is consistent with the local compared to when it is inconsistent (Egly et al. 1995; Karnath et al. 2000). Electrophysiological measures have also shown that the ERP response is influenced by the consistency between

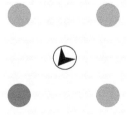

FIGURE 35.9 Representation of the stimuli. The red and green items were irrelevant, and the task was to respond as quickly as possible whether the pattern in the middle was an arrow or not. In this case it is an arrow and the arrow is pointing to the unique feature.

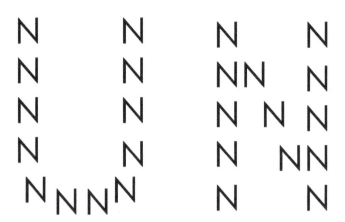

FIGURE 35.10 An example of hierarchically structured stimuli with a global U created from local Ns on the left (incongruent) and a global N created from local Ns on the right (congruent). The task for the patient was to report the local letter as rapidly as possible.

the local and global shapes, again, even under conditions when the patient could only report the identity of the local shape (Jackson et al. 2004). Specifically, when the global shape was different (e.g. a global U made from local Ns) ERP amplitude was greater over occipital-temporal scalp sites than when it was the same (e.g. a global N made from local Ns). This difference was evident as early as 160 milliseconds after stimulus onset. Note that global shapes in these types of displays are defined by the spatial position of the local elements, thus the spatial representation must be precise enough for a global shape representation to emerge.

In sum, there is good evidence for implicit spatial representation across various stimulus displays and tasks. There is also evidence that the features that inhabit that space are coded implicitly as well. If features and shapes in different locations are implicitly coded, it follows that co-location of shape and feature may be implicitly coded as well. That is, there could be implicit binding, and the next section makes the case that there is.

FEATURE BINDING AND ATTENTION

It is clear from evidence discussed in the section on features and binding that binding errors are common in classic Balint's syndrome. However, as with space itself, there is now good evidence that features are bound implicitly with each other, even in patients with Balint's syndrome, meaning that binding of distributed features such as colour and shape occurs without conscious spatial attention.

The first evidence that binding in Balint's syndrome was possible was reported by Wojciulik and Kanwisher in 1998 and later replicated by Cinel and Humphreys (2006) using a standard Stroop colour naming task, but with two words and two colours rather than the standard one colour/word on each trial (Table 35.1). In the normal Stroop task

Table 35.1 Dual word task.

Both Congruent (a)	Distractor Incongruent (b)	Distractor Congruent (c)	Both Incongruent (d)
PURPLE	PURPLE	YELLOW	YELLOW
PURPLE	YELLOW	PURPLE	YELLOW

a single colour word is printed either in a colour congruent with the word (the word PURPLE in purple ink) or incongruent with the word (the word PURPLE in yellow ink), and the participant is asked to name the ink colour as rapidly as possible. Hundreds of studies have shown that response time is consistently faster when the print and word colour are congruent than when they are incongruent. As would be expected, this is also the case in Balint's syndrome when the normal Stroop task is administered (there is one word and one colour in each stimulus). But the question addressed by the dual word stimuli as shown in Table 35.1 is whether the colours are correctly bound to the correct word.

To address this question in Balint's syndrome two colour words (with one word coloured and the other not) were paired in four different conditions. In one condition the two words were both congruent (e.g. PURPLE with one word printed in purple ink and the other achromatic, Table 35.1a). In another, both words were incongruent with the colour (YELLOW with one word printed in purple ink and the other achromatic, Table 35.1d). The task was to name the ink colour as rapidly as possible, which is an easy task for a patient with Balint's syndrome. These two conditions are similar to the standard one-word, one-colour Stroop task, and response time should be longer in the condition in which both words are incongruent than when both are congruent, and this was indeed the case.

The critical comparison was between conditions in which the target (the coloured word) and distractor (the achromatic word) were combined differently with the distractor being incongruent with the ink colour in one case and congruent with it in another (Table 35.1b and c, respectively). Note that the features in these displays are the same (there are the words PURPLE and YELLOW and there is the colour purple), but they are bound in the stimulus in different ways. Since the task was to name the ink colour, there should be Stroop interference in both conditions (compared to when both words were congruent, Table 35.1a), and indeed there was. But if the ink colour is not bound to the appropriate word in perception, then Stroop interference should be the same in these two conditions. This was not the case. Instead responses were slower when the distractor was congruent than when it was incongruent with the ink, meaning the visual system knew which was which even if the patient did not. It is important to note that this was found under conditions when explicit report of which word was coloured was at chance performance. Only one of the two words in the display was reported, and it was as likely to be the coloured as the achromatic word. Nevertheless, implicit measures, as in the Stroop test, demonstrate that both words were encoded, but more importantly for the question of implicit binding, the evidence showed that the colour was assigned to the correct word at an implicit level.

If colour and shape are already bound during initial visual processing, why do patients with Balint's syndrome experience illusory conjunctions? In fact, why do normal perceivers experience illusory conjunctions under impoverished stimulus conditions or when attention is diverted? Do features become unbound during visual processing but somehow leave a residual of their earlier bound selves? This is a possibility, but it is also possible that multiple bindings occur between features, and the role of attention is to select the right combination. In fact, Treisman (2006) incorporated the evidence for implicit binding in Balint's patients and revised feature integration theory in just this way. The original premise that features are encoded in different feature maps remained (and continues to be supported by more recent studies, e.g. see Bodelon, Fallah, and Reynolds 2007; Vul and Rich 2010), but the relationship between attention and binding errors changed, while focused attention at a given location was the means for binding features together in the original version. The revised theory claims that binding between features such as colour and shape produces multiple bound representations during pre-attentive processing, and attention selects from among this set.

In this version, a plausible neurobiological account is also described. Early vision feeds different features forward through the ventral visual stream that are reiteratively tuned by feedback from higher areas within that stream. Consistently, electrophysiological recordings from monkey have shown numerous times that neurons that prefer one colour over another (as in area V4) have receptive fields that cover large areas of the visual field, and receptive field size gets larger as information is transmitted forward. Thus, during feedforward processing of visual information (through ventral, temporal areas) one would expect large spatial overlap between different features such as colour values and shapes, but of course this is not what we perceive. At this stage a stimulus that was a red square and blue circle would produce four possible combinations; red square, blue square, red circle, and blue circle according to the revised version of FIT. However, in normal perception colour is confined within the boundaries of a shape. One way this is hypothesized to happen is via feedback from higher visual areas that tune the receptive fields in earlier visual areas through re-entry signals (e.g. Ahissar and Hochstein 2004). As the earlier areas receive more and more of these feedback signals the system is thought to settle into an oscillitatory network that connects different neurons with the same firing patterns. If visual processing is halted or disrupted in some way before the system settles into this pattern (e.g. masked exposure, brain injury) then attention may not be focused sufficiently and select an incorrectly bound shape from the multiple representations that are produced during the feedforward response. The role of attention in the newer version of FIT is not directly involved in binding per se, but rather in selection of the most likely bound representation for perceptual awareness. In this more recent version, illusory conjunctions in Balint's simultanagnosia would occur due to an error in selecting the properly bound representation from a set of possible bindings.

Attention in normal perception selects the correct representation when time is sufficient and spatial location is unambiguous.

An alternative theory to that put forward in revised FIT was offered by Humphreys
and Riddoch (2012). In both versions, perception needs time to correctly bind features for perceptual awareness, but Humphreys and Riddoch's conclusions differ in
terms of the stages that are involved. Rather than having multiple parallel bindings,
in their view bindings are unstable during initial visual coding which limits or slows
access to a final representation stored in short-term visual memory. In their account,
they rely on neurobiological evidence that shows that the parietal cortex feeds back
to primary visual cortex (V1) and suggest that this feedback is then involved in consolidation of visual information through the ventral system into a stored memory
representation. They argue that without parietal feedback into primary visual centres
consolidation of information across different feature domains (e.g. colour and shape)
is less likely to occur, and the proper features are incorrectly bound even at long display presentation times.

Another, related argument is that dorsal attentional functions contribute to ventral
stream processing more directly, both during feedforward and feedback within that
stream. In this view, parietal signals stabilize oscillatory patterns between distributed
feature maps in ventral cortex directly with a limited number of features being passed
from earlier to later visual areas. Although electrophysiological evidence in animals
suggests that features are fed forward in a 'winner-take-all' fashion (see review by Fries
2009), there would likely be noise in the system, such that some features are passed
forward while others are not. Within a framework such as this, attentional functions
of the dorsal stream would be involved in limiting what features are fed forward and
also in the selection of the resulting combinations during and after coherence between
areas became stable (Robertson 2012). If posterior occipital-parietal input is not available (as in Balint's syndrome) all features would continue to be processed through the
ventral stream without modulation and result in an explosion of feature combinations.
As voluntary attention from one combination to another may be nearly impossible in
Balint's syndrome, involuntary attention would be attracted to different combinations at
different times without cognitive control. The perceptual chaos that would result could
account for many of the perceived outcomes in Balint's syndrome (most specifically illusory conjunctions).

Summary

In conclusion, the study of Balint's syndrome has been greatly influenced by attentional theories that were derived from cognitive psychology, and in turn has contributed to revisions in attentional theories as the field advanced. This is especially evident
in accounts of how attention interacts with different features to produce a reasonably

accurate representation of the visual world. It is still an open question as to why certain features require dorsal stream input to be bound correctly in perceptual awareness (e.g. colour, motion, shape) while others do not (e.g. T junctions, common onset, closure). But, it is clear from studies of neuropsychological patients with Balint's syndrome that this is the case. The findings, in turn, have contributed substantially to our understanding of how perception and attention may interact and their relationship to underlying neurobiological functions.

NOTES

1. The cluster of symptoms was first referred to as Balint's syndrome by Hecaen and Ajuriaguerra (1954).
2. One of the most complete early descriptions of the cluster of symptoms was provided by Holmes and Horrax (1919) in a series of individual cases.

REFERENCES

Ahissar, M. and Hochstein, S. (2004). The reverse hierarchy theory of visual perceptual learning. *Trends in Cognitive Sciences 8*: 457–464.

Alvarez, B. and Robertson, L. C. (2013). Synesthesia and binding. In S. Jools and E. Hubbard (eds.), *The Oxford Handbook of Synesthesia*. New York: Oxford University Press.

Ashby, F. G., Prinzmetal, W., Ivry, R., and Maddox, T. (1996). A formal theory of feature binding in object perception. *Psychological Review 103*: 165–192.

Balint, R. (1909). Seelenlahmung des 'Schauens', optische Ataxie, raumliche Storung der Aufmerksamkeit. *Monatshrift für Psychiatrie und Neurologie 25*: 5–81 (translated in *Cognitive Neuropsychology 12* (1995): 265–281).

Baylis, G. C., Driver, J., Baylis, L. L., and Rafal, R. D. (1994). Perception of letters and words in Balint's syndrome: Evidence for the unity of words. *Neuropsychologia 32*: 1273–1286.

Bernstein, L. J. and Robertson, L. C. (1998). Independence between illusory conjunctions of color and motion with shape following bilateral parietal lesions. *Psychological Science 9*: 167–175.

Bodelòn, C., Fallah, M., and Reynolds, J. H. (2007) Temporal resolution for the perception of features and conjunctions. *Journal of Neuroscience, 27*: 725–730.

Boutsen, L. and Humphreys, G. W. (1999). Axis-alignment affects perceptual grouping: Evidence from simultaneous agnosia. *Cognitive Neuropsychology 16*: 655–672.

Cinel, C. and Humphreys, G. W. (2006). On the relationship between implicit and explicit binding: Evidence from Balint's syndrome. *Cognitive, Affective, & Behavioral Neuroscience 6*: 127–140.

Cooper, C. G. and Humphreys, G. W. (2000). Coding space within but not between objects: Evidence from Balint's syndrome. *Neuropsychologia 38*: 723–733.

Costlett, H. B. and Saffran, E. (1991). Simultaneous agnosia: To see but not two see. *Brain 113*: 1523–1545.

Egly, R., Robertson, L. C., Rafal, R., and Grabowecky, M. (November, 1995). Implicit processing of unreportable objects in Balint's syndrome. Paper presented at the 36th Annual Meeting of the Psychonomic Society, Los Angeles.

Esterman, M., Verstynen, T., Ivry, R. B., and Robertson, L. C. (2006). Coming unbound: Disrupting automatic integration of synesthetic color and graphemes by TMS of the parietal lobe. *Journal of Cognitive Neuroscience 18*: 1–7.

Farah, M. J. (1990). *Visual Agnosia: Disorders of Object Recognition and What They Tell Us about Normal Vision*. Cambridge, Mass.: MIT Press.

Flevaris, A. V., Bentin, S., and Robertson, L. C. (2010). Local or global? Attentional selection of spatial frequencies binds shapes to hierarchical levels. *Psychological Science 21*: 424–431.

Friedman-Hill, S., Robertson, L. C., and Treisman, A. (1995). Parietal contributions to visual feature binding: Evidence from a patient with bilateral lesions. *Science 269*: 853–855.

Fries, P. (2009). Neuronal gamma-band synchronization as a fundamental process in cortical computation. *Annual Review of Neuroscience 32*: 209–224.

Hecaen, H. and Ajuriaguerra, J. (1954). Balint syndrome (psychic paralysis of visual fixation) and its minor forms. *Brain 77*: 373–400.

Holmes, G. (1918). Disturbances of visual orientation. *British Journal of Ophthalmology 2*: 449–468.

Holmes, G. and Horrax, G. (1919). Disturbances of spatial orientation and visual attention without loss of stereoscopic vision. *Archives of Neurology and Psychiatry 1*: 385–407.

Huberle, E. and Karnath, H.-O. (2006). Global shape recognition is modulated by the spatial distance of local elements: Evidence from simultanagnosia. *Neuropsychologia 44*: 905–911.

Humphreys, G. W. (1998). Neural representation of objects in space: A dual coding account. *Philosophical Transactions of the Royal Society B: Biological Sciences 353*: 1341–1351.

Humphreys, G. W., Cincel, C., Wolfe, J., Olson, A., and Klempers, N. (2000). Fractionating the binding process: Neuropsychological evidence distinguishing binding of form from binding of surface features. *Vision Research 40*: 1569–1596.

Humphreys, G. W. and Riddoch, J. M. (2012). There's binding and there's binding, or is there just binding? Neuropsychological insights from Balint's syndrome. In J. Wolfe and L. C. Robertson (eds.), *From Perception to Consciousness: Searching With Anne Treisman* (pp. 324–327). New York: Oxford University Press.

Husain, M. and Stein, J. (1988). Rezso Balint and his most celebrated case. *Archives of Neurology 45*: 89–93.

Jackson, G. M., Swainson, R., Mort, D., Husain, M., and Jackson, S. R. (2004). Implicit processing of global information in Balint's syndrome. *Cortex 40*: 179–180.

Karnath, H.-O., Ferber, S., Rorden, C., and Driver, J. (2000). The fate of global information in dorsal simultanagnosia. *Neurocase 6*: 295–306.

Kim, M. S. and Robertson, L. C. (2001). Implicit representations of visual space after bilateral parietal damage. *Journal of Cognitive Neuroscience 13*: 1080–1087.

Kinsbourne, M. and Warrington, E. K. (1962). A disorder of simultaneous form perception. *Brain 85*: 461–486.

Kinsbourne, M. and Warrington, E. K. (1963). The localizing significance of limited simultaneous visual form perception. *Brain 86*: 697–702.

Luria, A. R. (1958). Disorders of 'simultaneous perception' in a case of bilateral occipito-parietal brain injury. *Brain 83*: 437–449.

Luria, A. R., Pravdina-Vinarskaya, E. N., and Yarbus, A. L. (1963). Disorders of ocular movement in a case of simultaneous agnosia. *Brain 86*: 219–228.

Perenin, M.-T. and Vighetto, A. (1988). Optic ataxia: A specific disruption in the visuomotor mechanisms. I: Different aspects of the deficit in reaching for objects. *Brain 111*: 643–674.

Phan, M. L., Schendel, K. L., Recanzone, G. H., and Robertson, L. C. (2000). Auditory and visual spatial localization deficits following bilateral parietal lobe lesions in a patient with Balint's syndrome. *Journal of Cognitive Neuroscience* 12: 583–600.

Rafal, R. (2001). Balint's syndrome. In M. Behrmann (ed.), *Disorders of Visual Behavior* (pp. 121–142). Amsterdam: Elsevier Science.

Rensink, R. A. (2000). Seeing, sensing and scrutinizing. *Vision Research* 40: 1469–1487.

Rizzo, M. and Robin, D. A. (1990). Simultaneous agnosia: A deficit of sustained attention yields insights on visual information processing. *Neurology* 40: 447–455.

Rizzo, M. and Vecera, S. P. (2002). Psychoanatomical substrates of Balint's syndrome. *Journal of Neurology, Neurosurgery & Psychiatry* 72: 162–178.

Robertson, L. C. (2003). Binding, spatial attention and perceptual awareness. *Nature Reviews Neuroscience* 4: 93–102.

Robertson, L. C. (2004). *Space, Objects, Minds and Brains*. Hove: Psychology Press.

Robertson, L. C. (2012). Spatial deficits and feature integration theory. In J. Wolfe and L. C. Robertson (eds.), *From Perception to Consciousness: Searching with Anne Treisman* (pp. 318–323). New York: Oxford University Press.

Roberson, L. C. and Sagiv, N. (eds.) (2005). *Synesthesia: Perspectives from Cognitive Neuroscience*. New York: Oxford University Press.

Robertson, L. C. and Treisman, A. (2006). Attending to space within and between objects: Implications from a patient with Balint's syndrome. *Cognitive Neuropsychology* 23: 448–462.

Robertson, L. C., Treisman, A., Friedman-Hill, S., and Grabowecky, M. (1997). The interaction of spatial and object pathways: Evidence from Balint's syndrome. *Journal of Cognitive Neuroscience* 9: 295–317.

Serences, J. T., Schwarzback, J., Courtney, S. M., Golay, X., and Yantis, S. (2004). Control of object-based attention in human cortex. *Cerebral Cortex* 14: 1346–1357.

Serences, J. T. and Yantis, S. (2006). Selective visual attention and perceptual coherence. *Trends in Cognitive Sciences* 10: 38–45.

Shalev, L. and Humphreys, G. W. (2002). Implicit location encoding via stored representations of familiar objects: Neuropsychological evidence. *Cognitive Neuropsychology* 19: 721–744.

Stark, M., Coslett, H. B., and Saffran, E. (1996). Impairment of an egocentric map of locations: Implications for perception and action. *Cognitive Neuropsychology* 13: 481–523.

Treisman, A. M. and Gelade, G. (1980). A feature-integration theory of attention. *Cognitive Psychology* 12: 97–136.

Treisman, A. M. and Schmidt, H. (1982). Illusory conjunctions in perception of objects. *Cognitive Psychology* 14: 107–141.

Vul, E. and Rich, A. N. (2010). Independent sampling of features enables conscious perception of objects. *Psychological Science* 21: 1168–1175.

Wojciulik, E. and Kanwisher, N. (1998). Implicit but not explicit feature binding in a Balint's patient. *Visual Cognition* 5: 157–181.

CHAPTER 36

....

REHABILITATION OF ATTENTION FUNCTIONS

....

IAN H. ROBERTSON AND REDMOND G. O'CONNELL

INTRODUCTION
....

ATTENTION is what allows one stream of information from the internal or external environment to be selected over others and therefore pervades almost any thought or action we take in our daily lives. It is little wonder then that deficient attention, a common feature of many disorders of the brain (see Manohar, Bonnelle and Hunter (chapter 34), this volume; Vallar and Bolognini (chapter 33), this volume), can produce such profound functional impairments. With the benefit of accumulated knowledge from cognitive science, neuropsychology, and neuroimaging, it is now abundantly clear that attention is not a simple unitary process. In addition to being able to *select stimuli* for preferential processing according to some attribute (selective attention), we must also be able to sustain that selectivity, particularly in conditions of monotony or repetition (sustained attention), and further, we must have the capacity to change the selection from one feature or stream to another (attention switching) (Posner and Petersen 1990; Robertson et al. 1996). Our ever-increasing understanding of how attention is instantiated in the brain is directly fuelling the development of new treatment strategies that can target specific attention subsystems (Posner and Petersen 1990). The field of cognitive rehabilitation has received a boost in recent years with a number of computer-based training studies reporting promising results. For the most part these studies have addressed deficits in working memory (Jaeggi et al. 2008; Klingberg 2010). In the present chapter we look at the current state of play in the effort to treat deficits in attention. In so doing we adopt the three-component framework of Posner and Rothbart by reviewing studies that have specifically targeted selective attention, sustained attention, and attentional control or switching.

There is rather strong evidence for the effectiveness of rehabilitation of classically 'executive' functions such as initiation, planning, and problem solving (Von Cramon et al. 1991; Levine et al. 2000, 2007, 2011; Fish et al. 2007; Basak et al. 2008; Chen et al. 2011). However, these are not reviewed here as these cognitive abilities do not fall under the scope of 'attentional functions' as we define them in this chapter. Finally, this chapter does not cover deficits of spatial attention such as unilateral neglect and their rehabilitation (see Vallar and Bolognini (chapter 33), this volume).

REHABILITATION OF ATTENTIONAL SELECTIVITY

Some of the strongest evidence for the considerable plasticity of the selective attention system comes from an unusual source: action video game players. In one of the first studies in this area, Green and Bavelier (2003) showed that habitual players had significantly enhanced visual selective attention abilities on untrained tasks, which had never been practised. Furthermore, individuals who did not regularly play video games also showed strong improvements in attentional selectivity when they were given extended practice, confirming that the game playing has a causal role in enhancing attentional selectivity (Green and Bavelier 2003). Importantly, the benefits of video game playing have also been shown to transfer to complex real-world tasks such as piloting procedures (Gopher et al. 1994).

Specifically, video game practice has been shown to affect fundamental mechanisms of visual attention including inhibition of return (Castel et al. 2005), and the resolution of spatial-attentional (Green and Bavelier 2007) and backward masking effects (Li et al. 2010). A recent electrophysiological study that compared frequent video game players with controls recorded steady-state visual evoked potentials (SSVEPs) while participants monitored for targets in a multi-stimulus display consisting of rapid sequences of alphanumeric stimuli presented at rates of 8.6/12 Hz in the left/right peripheral visual fields, with a central square at fixation flashing at 5.5 Hz and a letter sequence flashing at 15 Hz at an upper central location. Cued to attend to one of the peripheral or central stimulus sequences, video game players detected targets with greater speed and accuracy than non-players. These benefits seemed to be achieved in two ways: (a) an increased suppression of SSVEP amplitudes to unattended peripheral sequences in the context of equivalent SSVEPs to attended-to streams in the two groups; (b) greater P3 amplitudes by the video game group to targets in the alphanumeric streams. The authors suggest that the behavioural improvements in attentional selectivity that many studies have now demonstrated are attributable in part to better inhibition of irrelevant information and also more effective perceptual decision-making processes. Comparable ERP effects on inhibition of irrelevant stimuli and enhanced processing of targets following attention training in healthy participants were obtained by Melara and colleagues (Melara et al. 2002). A likely reason that action video games are so effective is that they are specifically designed to be entertaining and immersive, while their fast pace, increasing difficulty, and unpredictability place substantial demands on attentional control. Many games also include the element of adaptive training, with difficulty altering in line with performance, a crucial element of the success of other types of cognitive training including working memory training (Klingberg 2010).

There have been fewer studies of selective attention training with individuals suffering from brain lesions or disease, but those studies which have been carried out have been broadly consistent with studies of healthy participants using commercial video games. Sturm and his colleagues in Aachen, Germany (Sturm et al. 1997), developed computerized training programmes which targeted either alertness/sustained attention or selective/divided attention, using a progressive shaping procedure where tasks became more challenging as performance improved (adaptive training). Patients with vascular lesions and associated attentional impairments showed training-specific (14 one-hour sessions) improvements on untrained tasks, with the selective/divided attention training programmes improving only on selective attention measures and not on the sustained attention/vigilance measures, and vice versa. Similarly specific improvement in test-measured attention performance has been found in patients with multiple sclerosis (Plohmann et al. 1998) trained for 12 hours on computerized attention training programmes aimed at different attentional functions, with selectivity showing improvements following selective attention training. Age-related selective attention deficits have also been successfully improved using progressive training in maintaining attention to stimuli in the face of auditory or visual distractors (Mozolic et al. 2011).

A more general computerized attention training which addressed a range of different attention functions but which included a selectivity component also yielded specific improvements in attention in a group of 29 traumatic brain injured patients (Niemann et al. 1990) and other studies have shown similarly promising results with this patient group (e.g. Ruff et al. 1994). General attentional training programmes have also shown promising effects following stroke (Barker-Collo et al. 2009). A systematic review of the literature by the Cochrane group, however, concluded that while there was evidence of the effectiveness of attentional training, there was insufficient evidence of generalizability to real-life function (Lincoln et al. 2008).

Training on tasks that are more ecologically valid may be one way of achieving greater transfer to real-life function. For example, an early single case study with a patient suffering from severe distractibility following a traumatic brain injury showed significant increases in the amount of text he could read by practising at home reading against distracting verbal auditory stimuli—this behavioural goal was important for this person's college studies (Wilson and Robertson 1992). We recently completed a study with traumatic brain injured patients with self-reported difficulties in attending against background noise and conversations could be trained to improve their selective attention to, and consequent memory for, spoken material, by applying a behavioural shaping method similar to that devised by Wilson and Robertson (1992) (Dundon et al. in preparation). Patients listened to spoken text in one ear, against initially low volume competing text in the other. Gradually the volume of the competing text was increased. After training, patients showed better memory for the target text. Furthermore, patients with the greatest amount of pre-training self-reported distractibility and associated stress showed the greatest improvements in memory post-training. The trained group also showed evidence of generalized attentional selectivity improvements on an untrained oddball auditory attention task: the trained group showed a specific increase in the amplitude of the ERP P3b response to targets, without any change in the ERP P3a response (see Fig. 36.1).

In summary, there is clear evidence that training in selective attention can improve attentional selectivity in both healthy and brain-impaired individuals, though the evidence for the generalization of these effects to real-life function is still lacking, in the main. The mechanisms by which selective attention training operates are not clear, except that both inhibitory and selective processes appear to be upregulated, down to quite low levels of perceptual processing (e.g. inhibition of return and backward masking). A key ingredient of the training methods that have proved successful is the use of *adaptive training*, namely increasing the difficulty level of the selective attention challenge in line with progression in performance, a method which has also been used successfully with working memory training (see Klingberg 2010).

With respect to the second set of attentional functions (sustained attention and attention switching), however, the range of approaches has been more varied, and hence the theoretical basis for them requires some elaboration.

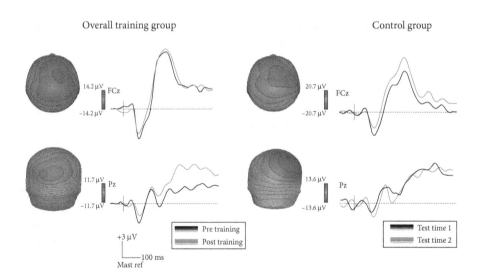

FIGURE 36.1 ERPs derived from a 3-stimulus oddball task. The overall training group demonstrated no training related change in the P3a component but a post-training increase in the P3b component. By contrast, the control group (receiving no intervening training between test and retest) did not show reliable change in either the P3b or P3a components.

REHABILITATION OF SUSTAINED ATTENTION/ALERTNESS

Human beings find it surprisingly difficult to deploy the top-down aspects enhancing selectivity to unchanging, or unchallenging repetitive stimuli and responses for extended periods of time. This already fragile ability to sustain goal-directed attention is very sensitive to disorders and damage to the brain, and can be a major source of impairment in everyday life in conditions such as traumatic brain injury (Robertson et al. 1997a), attention-deficit hyperactivity disorder (ADHD) (Bellgrove et al. 2005a, 2005b), and tauopathy-related neurodegeneration (O'Keeffe et al. 2007). It is also interesting to note that the ability to sustain attention is an important factor in determining recovery of motor and other functions following stroke (Ben-Yishay et al. 1968; Blanc-Garin 1994). Motor recovery following right hemisphere stroke over a two-year period was significantly predicted by measures of sustained attention taken two months after right hemisphere stroke (Robertson et al. 1997b). This is perhaps not surprising in light of the fact that learning any skill typically requires many hundreds, even thousands, of trials, which is particularly true for the re-learning underpinning recovery following brain damage. As mentioned above, attention is the capacity to allocate processing resources selectively to particular stimuli or classes of stimuli, and as Blake et al. (Blake et al. 2006) showed, this is a critical element in experience-dependent plasticity. If plastic reorganization requires attention to mediate the effects of rehabilitative experience, then the capacity to deploy attention over relatively long periods to relatively unchanging and monotonous stimuli is likely to be a strong predictor of successful recovery. This sustained component of attention has tended to be neglected in the literature but recent research is pointing to new avenues towards its enhancement.

Imaging studies have indicated that this type of attention is controlled by a right lateralized cortical network, including the anterior cingulate gyrus, the right dorsolateral prefrontal cortex, and the inferior parietal lobule, which regulates activity within subcortical arousal structures (Robertson and Garavan 2004). Posner and Petersen (Posner and Petersen 1990) identified the midbrain locus coeruleus (LC) as the critical arousal hub supporting the alert state by increasing perceptual signal-to-noise ratios via the neurotransmitter noradrenaline. The influence of the locus coeruleus system in humans was demonstrated by Smith and Nutt (Smith and Nutt 1996), who reported that suppressing the release of noradrenaline through clonidine administration resulted in the sorts of attentional lapses that are characteristic of diminished vigilant attention. Pharmacological studies have found similarly close links between noradrenergic function and vigilant attention (Coull 1995). More recently, our group has demonstrated a specific linkage in humans between noradrenaline activity and performance on a vigilant attention task in healthy adults who differ in a genotype that codes for an enzyme (dopamine ß-hydroxylase) controlling the availability of noradrenaline in the brain.

Individuals whose genotype was associated with relatively low noradrenergic avail-ability showed significantly increased errors of commission (Greene et al. 2009) and we showed similar results in children diagnosed with ADHD (Bellgrove et al. 2006).

Anyone who has worked in a rehabilitation hospital will be familiar with the differ-ence between the responses of many individuals—those who have suffered a stroke for instance—first thing in the morning, versus in the early afternoon. Even in those of us who have not suffered an adverse neurological event but who have had to catch an early morning flight or two, it is not uncommon to find that our arousal levels can be so low at certain times of the day that cognitive function becomes severely compromised. Yerkes and Dodson famously studied the effects of different degrees of arousal (by varying the degree of shock) on the ability of mice to learn discriminations between the luminance of two compartments (Yerkes and Dodson 1908). They found that where lightness levels were easily discriminated, the mice performed better at high levels of arousal, whereas difficult light discriminations were best learned at low levels of arousal. On the basis of these experiments, they formulated the Yerkes–Dodson law. This law proposed that any task will have an optimal level of arousal below and beyond which performance will decline; they hypothesized this optimal level is lower in challenging tasks than in routine tasks. Similarly, Broadbent (Broadbent 1971) showed that while stress can improve performance on routine, non-demanding tasks, the same levels of stress can impair performance on more complex and demanding tasks. In a comprehensive review of catecholamine modulation of prefrontal cognitive function, Arnsten highlighted that many studies show a Yerkes–Dodson type inverted-U relationship between levels of noradrenaline release on the one hand, and behavioural performance on the other (Arnsten 1998). These studies, suggesting an interaction between arousal levels, opti-mal performance, and degree of challenge in a task, mesh well with the notion of exog-enous modulation of arousal as previously discussed. They also suggest, however, that the relationship between the system for sustaining attention and that of arousal may not be a simple one of mutual facilitation, and a number of other more recent studies sup-port such a view. Nevertheless, the above research tells us that without adequate levels of arousal, attention will not function well.

As mentioned above, vigilant attention can be impaired through administration of drugs—for instance clonidine—that inhibit noradrenaline release and reduce arousal, as described above in the study by Smith and Nutt (Smith and Nutt 1996). What they also showed, however, was that the deleterious effects of clonidine were much attenu-ated when the participants were exposed to loud white noise while performing the task. This suggests that external stimuli can induce 'bottom-up' or exogenous modulation of the cortical systems for vigilant attention. Coull and her colleagues confirmed that this is indeed the case (Coull 1995), showing that clonidine-induced noradrenergic suppres-sion impaired vigilant attention performance much more when the task was familiar than when it was unfamiliar—and thus more arousing.

Sustained attention is a fundamental cognitive function that underpins many other more complex functions. While Smith and Nutt showed that externally arousing white noise could mitigate the effects of an arousal-depleting drug, we for instance showed some time ago that left spatial neglect in patients with large right hemisphere strokes could be briefly alleviated—and on average, abolished for a very brief period—by being exposed to a moderately loud and somewhat unexpected tone (Robertson et al. 1998). The intervention derived from Michael Posner's observation of a close linkage between the right fronto-parietal 'alertness' attentional system on the one hand, and a spatial selective attention 'orientation' system on the other: he predicted that the former could modulate the latter (Posner 1993). George et al. (George et al. 2008) demonstrated that externally imposed time pressure could have a similar effect, based on the observation that perceived time pressure is associated with moderate increases in arousal (Slobounov et al. 2000). George et al. asked patients with left spatial neglect to find and cross out visual targets scattered over a sheet of paper. As predicted by the Yerkes–Dodson effect, when the patients thought they were acting under time pressure they missed significantly *fewer* targets than under open-ended testing conditions.

Based on these observations of the interplay between attention and arousal we showed that patients suffering left spatial neglect could learn to 'self-alert' and hence improve both left neglect and their sustained attention (Robertson et al. 1995).Their arousal was first increased by a loud noise—a hand clap—and their attention drawn to their temporarily more alert state. Using a graded self-instructional strategy, patients learned to replace the external stimulus with a simple, internally generated 'self-alert' instruction—a word or phrase which to them signified alertness, and which they applied periodically—and eventually spontaneously—to voluntarily increase arousal. Significant improvements were observed in eight patients, using a carefully controlled multiple-baseline by subject design. Patients were not simply externally alerted, but they were also given a metacognitive strategy with which the temporary arousal could be linked, and hence re-evoked periodically to produce enduring, rather than temporary effects. We further developed these methods with patients suffering from impaired executive function.

Shallice and Burgess (Shallice and Burgess 1991) developed the 6-Element test, where participants were asked to attempt six simple tasks. They were told that they would not have time to complete all of the items in every test. To meet the main requirement (i.e. to do something from all six), participants had to switch spontaneously between the tasks during the 15 minutes available to them. Despite being tested on their comprehension of the rules before and after the test, and their above average IQ scores, the patients with frontal lesions showed a strong tendency to get caught up in one or other of the tasks to the detriment of the overall goal. This may be in part because the ability to maintain the salience of an overarching goal is heavily dependent on sustained attention. Manly and colleagues (Manly et al. 2002) tested whether patients with traumatic brain injury who showed executive problems could improve through a simple manipulation which had elements of the arousal-inducing methods just described. The task was a variant of the 6-Element test, the Hotel Test, in which participants were asked to sample a series of simple tasks involved in running a hotel, such as sorting conference labels into alphabetical order and looking up telephone numbers. As with the 6-Element test, they were told that they could not complete even one of the tasks during the 15 minutes. In the standard condition, the patients were significantly worse than IQ-matched controls—they missed on average one whole task, and deviated significantly from the optimal time allocation on all the others. However, in a condition in which they were asked to 'think about what they were doing' in response to each of six tones presented at random intervals, their performance improved significantly relative to that of the healthy controls.

Jessica Fish et al. (Fish et al. 2007) extended this approach to realizing goals (making phone calls at certain times) that needed to be executed by patients during normal daily life over a period of two weeks. In training, a particular cue phrase ('STOP': Stop Think Organize Plan) was associated with reviewing one's intentions. Over the study phase, 'STOP' text (SMS) messages were sent to the patient participants' mobile phones on half of the days selected at random. The messages were sent at random times during the working day but, crucially, not within half an hour of the time a call was due. Despite this, success in the telephone task was substantially greater on days with cues than days without. Even given the delay between a cue and the execution of the intention, this periodic interruption/review facilitated performance. Further work is required looking at the persistence and generality of this effect. A merit of the approach, however, lies in its potential flexibility. It does not require intentions to be pre-specified. The aim is to assist patients to manage actively their *own* goals, however recently these were formed.

Our research group has also applied very similar principles to treating the deficits in sustained attention that are characteristic of ADHD (O'Connell et al. 2008). Again, participants learned to produce self-generated increases in alertness first in response to a periodic auditory cue and later in response to an internally generated cue. In order to strengthen the training effect participants were provided with visual feedback conveying the magnitude of each self-alert event via online changes in electrodermal activity (EDA), an index of autonomic arousal. In the first trial of this brief training protocol, neurologically healthy participants who implemented this strategy showed increased arousal levels (as indexed by EDA) during the performance of an untrained sustained attention task and made significantly fewer errors. In the second trial, we found the same pattern of improvement in a group of adults diagnosed with ADHD.

The sustained attention/alertness function has also been tackled using the relatively non-strategic adaptive training methods which have been used with some success in selective attention and working memory training. These have also had significant, sustained-attention-specific effects using computerized adaptive training methods (Longoni et al. 1999; Sturm et al. 1997, 2004), confirmed by a Cochrane Review (Lincoln et al. 2008) which highlighted the effectiveness of such training for sustained attention/alertness, albeit without evidence of generalization to real-life function.

In summary, as with selective attention, there is evidence for promising effects of training aimed at the sustained attention/alertness system.

TRAINING OF ATTENTIONAL SWITCHING/CONTROL

Training of this third set of attentional processes has been less commonly carried out and so the evidence of its effectiveness is very limited. Art Kramer and his colleagues in Michigan have been the main researchers in this area, focusing on elderly cognition, producing promising results albeit without evidence of generalization to everyday function (Kramer et al. 1995). They observed that elderly people had particular difficulties in performing two tasks concurrently, particularly when the two tasks require similar motor responses. But Kramer and his colleagues found that both older and younger adults can learn to perform such tasks more accurately, and that these improvements are associated with cortical reorganization measured by fMRI (Erickson et al. 2007a, 2007b). The results of a number of studies suggested that both older and younger adults showed substantial gains in performance after training, and that the improvement generalized to new task combinations involving new stimuli. The authors conclude that such attentional control skills can be improved in older people and thus that cognitive plasticity in attentional control is possible.

CONCLUSION

The attentional systems of the brain appear to have a significant capacity for plastic reorganization, though the real-life benefits of attentional training remain to be demonstrated. The effectiveness of such training may in future be enhanced by combining training with non-invasive brain stimulation and/or pharmacological methods. The results of attentional training are sufficiently promising to justify a large programme of research into the clinical viability and applicability of these methods, and we hope that such a programme, currently in its very early stages, will accelerate.

REFERENCES

Arnsten, A. F. T. (1998). Catecholamine modulation of prefrontal cortical cognitive function. *Trends in Cognitive Sciences* 2(11): 436–447.

Barker-Collo, S. L., Feigin, V. L., Lawes, C. M. M., Parag, V., Senior, H., and Rodgers, A. (2009). Reducing attention deficits after stroke using attention process training. *Stroke* 40(10): 3293–3298.

Basak, C., Boot, W. R., Voss, M. W., and Kramer, A. F. (2008). Can training in a real-time strategy video game attenuate cognitive decline in older adults? *Psychology and Aging* 23(4): 765–777.

Bellgrove, M. A., Gill, M., Hawi, Z., Kirley, A., and Robertson, I. H. (2005a). Dissecting the attention deficit hyperactivity disorder (ADHD) phenotype: Sustained attention, response variability and spatial attentional asymmetries in relation to dopamine transporter (DAT1) genotype. *Neuropsychologia* 43(13): 1847–1857.

Bellgrove, M. A., Domschke, K., Hawi, Z., Kirley, A., Mullins, C., Robertson, I. H., and Gill, M., (2005b). The methionine allele of the COMT polymorphism impairs prefrontal cognition in children and adolescents with ADHD. *Experimental Brain Research* 163(3): 352–360.

Bellgrove, M. A., Hawi, Z., Gill, M., and Robertson, I. H. (2006). The cognitive genetics of attention deficit hyperactivity disorder (ADHD): Sustained attention as a candidate phenotype. *Cortex* 42(6): 838–845.

Ben-Yishay, Y., Diller, L., Gerstman, L., and Haas, A. (1968). The relationship between impersistence, intellectual function and outcome of rehabilitation in patients with left hemiplegia. *Neurology* 18(9): 852–861.

Blake, D. T., Heiser, M. A., Caywood, M., and Merzenich, M. M. (2006). Experience-dependent adult cortical plasticity requires cognitive association between sensation and reward. *Neuron* 52(2): 371–381.

Blanc-Garin, J. (1994). Patterns of recovery from hemiplegia following stroke. *Neuropsychological Rehabilitation* 4(4): 359–385.

Broadbent, D. E. (1971). *Decision and Stress.* London: Academic Press.

Castel, A. D., Pratt, J., and Drummond, E. (2005). The effects of action video game experience on the time course of inhibition of return and the efficiency of visual search. *Acta Psychologica (Amsterdam)* 119(2): 217–230. Epub 2005 Mar 23.

Chen, A. J. W., Novakovic-Agopian, T., Nycum, T. J., Song, S., Turner, G. R., Hills, N. K., Rome, S., Abrams, G. M., and D-Esposito, M. (2011). Training of goal-directed attention regulation enhances control over neural processing for individuals with brain injury. *Brain* 134(5): 1541–1554.

Coull, J. (1995). Monoaminergic modulation of human attentional and executive function. Unpublished Ph.D., Cambridge University.

Dundon, N., Korpelainen, S. P., Robertson, I. H., Lalor, E. C., Clarke, S., Buckley, V., et al. (in preparation). Training attentional filtering in patients with traumatic brain injury.

Erickson, K. I., Colcombe, S. J., Wadhwa, R., Bherer, L., Peterson, M. S., Scalf, P. E., Kim, J. S., Alvarado, M., and Kramer, A. F. (2007a). Training-induced functional activation changes in dual-task processing: An fMRI study. *Cerebral Cortex* 17(1): 192–204.

Erickson, K. I., Colcombe, S. J., Wadhwa, R., Bherer, L., Peterson, M. S., Scalf, P. E., Kim, J. S., Alvarado, M., and Kramer, A. F. (2007b). Training-induced plasticity in older adults: Effects of training on hemispheric asymmetry. *Neurobiology of Aging* 28(2): 272–283.

Fish, J., Evans, J. J., Nimmo, M., Martin, E., Kersel, D., Bateman, A., Wilson, B. A., and Manly, T. (2007). Rehabilitation of executive dysfunction following brain injury: 'Content-free' cueing improves everyday prospective memory performance. *Neuropsychologia* 45(6): 1318–1330.

George, M. S., Mercer, J. S., Walker, R., and Manly, T. (2008). A demonstration of endogenous modulation of unilateral spatial neglect: The impact of apparent time-pressure on spatial bias. *Journal of the International Neuropsychological Society* 14(1): 33–41.

Gopher, D., Weil, M., and Bareket, T. (1994). Transfer of skill from a computer game trainer to flight. *Human Factors* 36: 387–405.

Green, C. S. and Bavelier, D. (2003). Action video game modifies visual selective attention. *Nature* 423(6939): 534–537.

Green C. S. and Bavelier D. (2007). Action-video-game experience alters the spatial resolution of vision. *Psychological Science* 18(1): 88–94. PMID: 17362383 [PubMed - indexed for MEDLINE] Free PMC Article.

Greene, C., Bellgrove, M. A., Gill, M., and Robertson, I. H. (2009). Noradrenergic genotype predicts lapses in sustained attention. *Neuropsychologia* 47(2): 591–594.

Jaeggi, S. M., Buschkuehl, M., Jonides, J., and Perrig, W. J. (2008). Improving fluid intelligence with training on working memory. *Proceedings of the National Academy of Sciences USA* 105(19): 6829–6833.

Klingberg, T. (2010). Training and plasticity of working memory. *Trends in Cognitive Sciences* 14(7): 317–324.

Kramer, A. F., Larish, J. F., and Strayer, D. L. (1995). Training for attentional control in dual task settings: A comparison of young and old adults. *Journal of Experimental Psychology: Applied* 1(1): 50–76.

Levine, B., Robertson, I., Clare, L., Carter, G., Hong, J., Wilson, B. A., Duncan, J., and Stuss, D. T. (2000). Rehabilitation of executive functioning: An experimental-clinical validation of goal management training. *Journal of the International Neuropsychological Society* 6(3): 299–312.

Levine, B., Schweizer, T. A., O'Connor, C., Turner, G., Gillingham, S., Stuss, D. T., Manly, T., and Robertson, I. H. (2011). Rehabilitation of executive functioning in patients with frontal lobe brain damage with goal management training. *Frontiers in Human Neuroscience* 5: 1–9.

Levine, B., Stuss, D. T., Winocur, G., Binns, M., Fahy, L., Mandic, M., Bridges, K., and Robertson, I. H. (2007). Cognitive rehabilitation in the elderly: Effects on strategic behaviour in relation to goal management. *Journal of the International Neuropsychological Society* 13(1): 143–152.

Li, R., Polat, U., Scalzo, F., and Bavelier, D. (2010). Reducing backward masking through action game training. *Journal of Vision* 10(14): article 33.

Lincoln, N., Majid, M., and Weyman, N. (2008). Cognitive rehabilitation for attention deficits following stroke. In C. S. Group (ed.), *Cochrane Database of Systematic Reviews* (pp. 1–11). New York: John Wiley.

Longoni, F., Weis, S., Specht, K., Holtel, C., Herzog, H., Achten, B., et al. (1999). Functional reorganisation after training of alertness. Paper presented at the 17th European Workshop on Cognitive Neuropsychology, Bressanone, Italy, January.

Manly, T., Hawkins, K., Evans, J., Woldt, K., and Robertson, I. H. (2002). Rehabilitation of executive function: Facilitation of effective goal management on complex tasks using periodic auditory alerts. *Neuropsychologia* 40(3): 271–281.

Melara, R. D., Rao, A., and Tong, Y. (2002). The duality of selection: Excitatory and inhibitory processes in auditory selective attention. *Journal of Experimental Psychology: Human Perception and Performance* 28(2): 279–306.

Mozolic, J. L., Long, A. B., Morgan, A. R., Rawley-Payne, M., and Laurienti, P. J. (2011). A cognitive training intervention improves modality-specific attention in a randomized controlled trial of healthy older adults. *Neurobiology of Aging* 32(4): 655–668.

Niemann, H., Ruff, R. M., and Baser, C. A. (1990). Computer-assisted attention retraining in head-injured individuals: A controlled efficacy study of an outpatient program. *Journal of Consulting and Clinical Psychology* 58(6): 811–817.

O'Connell, R. G., Bellgrove, M. A., Dockree, P. M., Lau, A., Fitzgerald, M., and Robertson, I. H. (2008). Self-alert training: Volitional modulation of autonomic arousal improves sustained attention. *Neuropsychologia* 46(5): 1379–1390.

O'Keeffe, F. M., Murray, B., Coen, R. F., Dockree, P. M., Bellgrove, M. A., Garavan, H., Lynch, T., and Robertson, I. H. (2007). Loss of insight in frontotemporal dementia, corticobasal degeneration and progressive supranuclear palsy. *Brain* 130(3): 753–764.

Plohmann, A. M., Kappos, L., Ammann, W., Thordai, A., Wittwer, A., Huber, S., Bellaiche, Y., and Lechner-Scott, J. (1998). Computer assisted retraining of attentional impairments in patients with multiple sclerosis. *Journal of Neurology, Neurosurgery & Psychiatry* 64(4): 455–462.

Posner, M. I. (1993). Interaction of arousal and selection in the posterior attention network. In A. Baddeley and L. Weiskrantz (eds.), *Attention: Selection, Awareness and Control* (pp. 390–405). Oxford: Clarendon Press.

Posner, M. I. and Petersen, S. E. (1990). The attention system of the human brain. *Annual Review of Neuroscience* 13: 25–42.

Posner, M. I. and Rothbart, M. K. (1998). Attention, self-regulation and consciousness. *Philosophical Transactions of the Royal Society B: Biological Sciences* 353(1377): 1915–1927. Review.

Robertson, I. H. and Garavan, H. (2004). Vigilant attention. In M. S. Gazzaniga (ed.), *The Cognitive Neurosciences*, 3rd edn. (pp. 563–578). Cambridge, Mich.: MIT Press.

Robertson, I. H., Manly, T., Andrade, J., Baddeley, B. T., and Yiend, J. (1997a). Oops!: Performance correlates of everyday attentional failures in traumatic brain injured and normal subjects: The Sustained Attention to Response Task (SART). *Neuropsychologia* 35(6): 747–758.

Robertson, I. H., Mattingley, J. B., Rorden, C., and Driver, J. (1998). Phasic alerting of neglect patients overcomes their spatial deficit in visual awareness. *Nature* 395(10): 169–172.

Robertson, I. H., Ridgeway, V., Greenfield, E., and Parr, A. (1997b). Motor recovery after stroke depends on intact sustained attention: A two-year follow-up study. *Neuropsychology* 11(2): 290–295.

Robertson, I. H., Tegner, R., Tham, K., Lo, A., and Nimmo-Smith, I. (1995). Sustained attention training for unilateral neglect: Theoretical and rehabilitation implications. *Journal of Clinical and Experimental Neuropsychology* 17(3): 416–430.

Robertson, I. H., Ward, T., Ridgeway, V., and Nimmo-Smith, I. (1996). The structure of normal human attention: The Test of Everyday Attention. *Journal of the International Neuropsychological Society* 2(6): 525–534.

Ruff, R., Mahaffey, R., Engel, J., Farrow, C., Cox, D., and Karzmark, P. (1994). Efficacy study of Thinkable in the attention and memory retraining of traumatically head-injured patients. *Brain Injury* 8(1): 3–14.

Shallice, T. and Burgess, P. (1991). Deficit in strategy application following frontal lobe damage in man. *Brain* 114(2): 727–741.

Slobounov, S. M., Fukada, K., Simon, R., Rearick, M., and Ray, W. (2000). Neurophysiological and behavioural indices of time pressure effects on visuomotor task performance. *Cognitive Brain Research* 9(3): 287–298.

Smith, A. and Nutt, D. (1996). Noradrenaline and attention lapses. *Nature* 380(6572): 291.

Sturm, W., Longoni, F., Weis, S., Specht, K., Herzog, H., Vohn, R., Thimm, M., and Willmes, K. (2004). Functional reorganisation in patients with right hemisphere stroke after training of alertness: A longitudinal PET and fMRI study in eight cases. *Neuropsychologia* 42(4): 434–450.

Sturm, W., Willmes, K., Orgass, B., and Hartje, W. (1997). Do specific attention deficits need specific training? *Neuropsychological Rehabilitation* 7(2): 81–176.

Von Cramon, D. Y., Cramon, G. M.-von, and Mai, N. (1991). Problem solving deficits in brain injured patients: A therapeutic approach. *Neuropsychological Rehabilitation* 1(1): 45–64.

Wilson, C. and Robertson, I. H. (1992). A home-based intervention for attentional slips during reading following head injury: A single case study. *Neuropsychological Rehabilitation* 2(3): 193–205.

Yerkes, R. M. and Dodson, J. D. (1908). The relation of strength of stimulus to rapidity of habit-formation. *Journal of Comparative and Neurological Psychology* 18(5): 459–482.

PART G

COMPUTATIONAL MODELS

···

CHAPTER 37

THEORY OF VISUAL ATTENTION (TVA)

···

CLAUS BUNDESEN AND THOMAS HABEKOST

THIS chapter is a review of the theory of visual attention (TVA). The first version of TVA (Bundesen 1990) was a formal computational theory that accounted for attentional effects in mind and behaviour reported in the psychological literature. TVA seems to have been the first theory of attention based on the principle that Desimone and Duncan (1995) in a later, highly influential article called 'biased competition'. Thus, in TVA, all possible visual categorizations ascribing features to objects *compete* (race) to become encoded into visual short-term memory before it is filled up. Each possible categorization is supported by the sensory evidence that the categorization is true. However, the competition is *biased* by attentional weights and perceptual biases, so that certain objects and categorizations have higher probabilities of being consciously perceived. The way sensory evidence and attentional biases interact is specified in two equations: the rate and weight equations of TVA. Thus, TVA represents a mathematical formalization of the biased competition principle.

Bundesen (1990) showed how TVA can account for many psychological findings (reaction times and error rates) in the field of visual attention. Duncan et al. (1999) showed how TVA provides a method to quantify individual variation in attentional abilities, which has been used to study many normal and clinical populations. More recently TVA was extended by Bundesen et al. (2005) and Bundesen and Habekost (2008) into a neural theory of visual attention (NTVA). By use of essentially the same equations as the original TVA model, NTVA accounts for many effects of attention observed in firing rates of single cells in the visual system of primates.

In this chapter we first describe TVA as a formal theory of visual attention and summarize applications of TVA to performance in normal human subjects. We then present the neural interpretation of TVA, NTVA, and review some examples of how NTVA accounts for findings from single-cell studies in primates. Finally, we review how TVA has been applied to study attentional functions in neuropsychological, pharmacological, and genetic research.

A Formal Theory of Visual Attention (TVA)

Basic assumptions

In attention research there is a long-standing debate on whether selection takes place before or after perceptual recognition (early vs. late selection; see, e.g., Bundesen and Habekost 2008). TVA takes a different view and assumes that the two processes occur simultaneously. According to TVA, both recognition and selection of objects in the visual field consist in making *visual categorizations*. A visual categorization has the form 'object x has feature i' or, equivalently, 'object x belongs to category i'. The categorization is *made* (or, equivalently, *selected*) when the categorization is encoded into visual short-term memory (VSTM). When the categorization is made, object x is said both to be selected and to be recognized as a member of category i. This way selection and recognition are viewed as two aspects of the same process.

When a visual categorization of an object completes processing, the categorization enters VSTM if memory space for the categorization is available in this system. Usually the capacity of VSTM is assumed to be limited to K different objects, where K is about 4 (cf. Luck and Vogel 1997). K varies from individual to individual and is one of the main parameters of TVA. Clearing VSTM starts a race among objects in the visual field to become encoded into VSTM. An object is encoded in VSTM if, and only if, some categorization of the object is encoded in VSTM. Each object x may be represented in the encoding race by all possible categorizations of the object.

Rate equation

By the rate equation of TVA, the rate, $v(x, i)$, at which a particular visual categorization, 'x belongs to i', is encoded into VSTM is given by a product of three terms:

$$v(x,i) = \eta(x,i)\beta_i \frac{w_x}{\displaystyle\sum_{z \in S} w_z} \qquad (1)$$

The first term, $\eta(x, i)$, is the strength of the sensory evidence that x belongs to category i. The second term, β_i, is a perceptual decision bias associated with category i ($0 \le \beta_i \le 1$). The third term is the relative attentional weight of object x—that is, the weight of object x, w_x, divided by the sum of weights across all objects in the visual field, S.

The total visual processing speed, C, is defined as the sum of all v values across all perceptual categorizations of all elements in the visual field:

$$C = \Sigma_{x \in S}\, v(x) = \Sigma_{x \in S} \Sigma_{i \in R}\, v(x, i) \qquad (2)$$

Weight equation

The attentional weights in the rate equation of TVA are derived from *pertinence* values. Every visual category j is supposed to have a pertinence, π_j, which is a non-negative real number. The pertinence of category j is a measure of the momentary importance of attending to objects that belong to category j. The attentional weight of an object x in the visual field is given by the weight equation of TVA,

$$w_x = \Sigma_{j \in R}\, \eta(x, j)\, \pi_j, \tag{3}$$

where R is the set of all visual categories, $\eta(x, j)$ is the strength of the sensory evidence that object x belongs to category j, and π_j is the pertinence of category j. By Equation 3, the attentional weight of an object is a weighted sum of pertinence values. The pertinence of a given category enters the sum with a weight equal to the strength of the sensory evidence that the object belongs to the category.

In some situations (e.g. visual search tasks) the visual stimuli fall into two categories: targets (i.e. elements to be reported or otherwise responded to) and distractors (elements to be ignored), such that every target has approximately the same attentional weight as any other target, and every distractor has approximately the same attentional weight as any other distractor. In such cases, the efficiency of top-down selection can be defined as the ratio, α, between the attentional weights of a distractor and a target:

$$\alpha = w_{\text{distractor}}/w_{\text{target}} \tag{4}$$

Mechanisms of selection

Taken together, the rate and weight equations of TVA describe two mechanisms of selection: a mechanism for selection of objects (filtering) and a mechanism for selection of categories (pigeonholing). The *filtering* mechanism is represented by pertinence values and attentional weights. If selection of objects with feature j is desired, the pertinence of feature j should be high. The weight equation implies that when feature j has a high pertinence, objects possessing feature j get high attentional weights. Accordingly, by the rate equation, processing of objects with feature j is fast, so objects with this feature are likely to win the processing race and be encoded into VSTM.

The *pigeonholing* mechanism is represented by perceptual decision bias parameters. Pertinence values determine which objects are selected (*filtering*), but perceptual biases determine how the objects are categorized (*pigeonholing*). If particular types of categorizations must be reported or otherwise responded to, the bias values of the corresponding categories should be high so that the desired types of categorizations are likely to be made (cf. Equation 1).

When the selection system is coupled to a sensory system that supplies appropriate η values, and when pertinence and bias parameters have been set, both filtering and pigeonholing are accomplished by an encoding race between visual categorizations whose rate parameters are determined through the simple algebraic operations of the rate and weight equations. Thus the theory yields a truly computational account of selective attention in vision.

Applications to basic studies of human performance

TVA has been applied to findings from a broad range of paradigms concerned with single-stimulus identification and selection from multielement displays in normal subjects. In addition, the scope of the theory has been extended to other cognitive domains such as memory and executive control.

Single-stimulus identification

For single-stimulus identification, TVA provides a mathematical derivation of the classical biased-choice model of Luce (1963) (see Bundesen 1990, 1993). The biased-choice model has been successful in explaining many experimental findings on effects of visual discriminability and bias (see, e.g. Townsend and Ashby 1982; Townsend and Landon 1982).

TVA also provides predictions of the time taken to recognize a singly-presented simple stimulus. The v value in Equation 1 is a hazard rate. Specifically, at any time t, the instantaneous value of $v(x, i)$ is the conditional probability density that the categorization that object x belongs to category i is encoded into VSTM at time t, given that the categorization has not been encoded before time t, and given that storage space for the categorization is available in VSTM. This assumption implies that, if $v(x, i) = 0$ until time t_0, and $v(x, i)$ is kept constant for times $t > t_0$, the probability $p(t)$ of making the categorization 'x belongs to i' at or before time t is given by

$$p(t) = 1 - \exp[-v(x, i)(t - t_0)] \tag{5}$$

When guessing and perceptual confusions among stimuli (i.e. incorrect perceptual categorizations) can be neglected, $p(t)$ equals the probability of recognizing x as a member of i from a postmasked presentation with an exposure duration of t, given that t_0 equals the longest ineffective exposure duration.

Equation 5 has yielded close and useful fits to empirical data, including data from patient studies based on TVA (see Habekost and Starrfelt 2009, for a review). The equation presupposes that perceptual confusions among stimuli can be neglected, but Kyllingsbæk et al. (2012) recently showed how the time course of visual recognition of mutually confusable stimuli can be analysed by use of TVA (also see Logan 1996). Kyllingsbæk et al. proposed and tested a Poisson counter model of visual recognition of briefly presented, mutually confusable single stimuli in pure accuracy tasks. The model implies that during stimulus analysis, tentative categorizations that stimulus x belongs to category i are made at a constant Poisson rate, $v(x, i)$. The analysis is continued until the stimulus disappears, and the overt response is based on the categorization made the greatest number of times. The model provided a close fit to individual data on identification of digits and an apparently perfect fit to data on identification of Landolt rings.

Temporal attention in single-stimulus identification

Vangkilde et al. (2013) extended TVA to temporal attention (also see Matthias et al. 2009, 2010). In a dynamic world, temporal expectations guide our attention in time (see, e.g., Nobre 2001, 2010). Beneficial effects of valid temporal expectations on motoric responses have been demonstrated repeatedly over the last century (Woodrow 1914; for reviews see Los 2010; Niemi and Näätänen 1981). Vangkilde et al. explored effects of temporal expectation on *visual* processing speed in a cued single-stimulus recognition paradigm with briefly presented, postmasked stimuli. Different hazard rate functions for the cue-stimulus foreperiod were used to manipulate temporal expectations. For example, in one experiment, the length of the foreperiod from the cue to the stimulus was distributed exponentially. For each block of trials, the participants knew which of two exponential distributions with different hazard rates the foreperiods would be drawn from. The hazard rate could be either high (1.33 s^{-1}) or low (0.22 s^{-1}) corresponding to mean foreperiods of 750 ms and 4 500 ms, respectively. In either condition, the probability $p(t)$ of correct report as a function of the stimulus duration (t) was well described by Equation 5, t_0 being the threshold of conscious perception (the longest ineffective exposure duration), and $v(x, i)$ being the speed of encoding into VSTM at times $t > t_0$. As manipulated by the hazard rate, temporal expectation had no effect on the threshold of conscious perception but strong effect on the speed of subsequent encoding into VSTM. Averaged across participants, the speed of encoding was lowered by 30% in the low hazard rate condition. This effect was found even though no general decrease in processing speed with time-on-task occurred. Thus, the effect was independent of the actual duration of the foreperiod on a given trial, but depended entirely on expectation. Vangkilde et al. explained the effect in terms of TVA by assuming that temporal expectations affect perception by changing perceptual biases (values of β parameters). Specifically, a strong expectation that a stimulus letter will appear at the next moment should yield an increase in the β values of letter types, which should speed the recognition of the stimulus letter if it appears when it is highly expected.

Selection from multielement displays

For selection from multielement displays, TVA provides a mathematical derivation of the fixed-capacity independent race model (FIRM) of Shibuya and Bundesen (1988). FIRM describes the processing of a stimulus display as a two-stage process. At the first stage of processing, an attentional weight is computed for each element in the display. The attentional weight is a measure of the strength of the sensory evidence that the element is a target. At the second stage of processing, the race between the elements takes place. The total processing capacity at this stage of the system is assumed to be a constant, C elements per second, which is a basic parameter of FIRM. The processing capacity is distributed across the elements in proportion to their weights. Thus, every element in the display is allocated a certain fraction of the total processing capacity; the fraction equals the attentional weight of the element divided by the sum of the attentional weights across all of the elements in the display.

The amount of processing capacity that is allocated to an element determines how fast the element can be encoded into VSTM. Specifically, the time taken to encode an element is assumed to be exponentially distributed with a rate parameter equal to the amount of processing capacity that is allocated to the element. Encoding times for different elements are stochastically independent, and the elements actually selected are those elements whose encoding processes complete before the stimulus presentation terminates and before VSTM has been filled up.

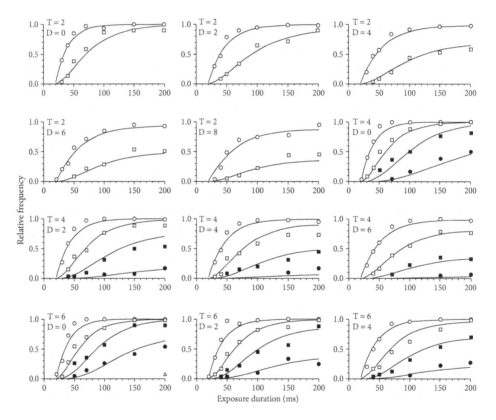

FIGURE 37.1 Relative frequency of scores of *j* or more (correctly reported targets) as a function of exposure duration with *j*, number of targets *T*, and number of distractors *D* as parameters in partial report experiment of Shibuya and Bundesen (1988). Data are shown for Subject MP. Parameter *j* varies within panels; *j* is 1 (open circles), 2 (open squares), 3 (solid squares), 4 (solid circles), or 5 (triangle). *T* and *D* vary among panels. Smooth curves represent a theoretical fit to the data by the FIRM model. For clarity, observed frequencies less than .02 were omitted from the figure. Adapted from H. Shibuya and C. Bundesen, Visual Selection From Multielement Displays: Measuring and Modeling Effects of Exposure Duration, *Journal of Experimental Psychology: Human Perception and Performance*, 14, p. 595. Copyright 1988 the American Psychological Association.

FIRM predicts effects of variations in the exposure duration of the stimuli. Shibuya and Bundesen (1988) tested such predictions in a comprehensive study of partial report of digits from mixtures of letters and digits. Exposure durations ranged from 10 ms up to 200 ms, and each display was terminated by a pattern mask. Fig. 37.1 shows the probability distribution of the number of correctly reported targets as a function of the exposure duration, the number of targets (T), and the number of distractors (D) in the display for one representative subject. Each panel shows the results for a particular combination of T and D. The top curve in the panel shows the probability of reporting at least 1 element correct as a function of exposure duration, the second curve from the top shows the probability of reporting at least 2 elements correct, etc. The fit shown by the smooth curves was obtained with VSTM capacity K at a value of 3.7 elements, total processing capacity C at 49 elements per second, parameter α (the weight ratio of a distractor to a target) at 0.40, and longest ineffective exposure duration t_0 at 19 ms. As can be seen, the fit was strikingly close.

Other well-established results closely fitted by TVA include effects of object integrality (Duncan 1984) and findings of stochastic independence (Bundesen et al. 2003; Kyllingsbæk and Bundesen 2007) in processing of multiple features, effects of the spatial position of targets in studies of divided attention (e.g. Sperling 1967; Posner et al. 1978), effects of selection criterion and effects of the number of distractors in studies of focused attention (e.g. Bundesen and Pedersen 1983; Estes and Taylor 1964; Treisman and Gelade 1980; Treisman and Gormican 1988), and effects of consistent practice in search (Schneider and Fisk 1982; also see Kyllingsbæk et al. 2001).

Relation to other cognitive domains

Logan (1996) proposed a combination of TVA with the contour detector (CODE) theory of perceptual grouping by proximity (van Oeffelen and Vos 1982, 1983): the CODE theory of visual attention (CTVA). CTVA explains a wide range of spatial effects in visual attention (see Logan 1996; Logan and Bundesen 1996; see Bundesen 1998, for a formalization of CVTA). Logan and Gordon (2001) extended CTVA into a theory of executive control in dual-task situations. The theory, ECTVA, accounts for crosstalk, set-switching cost, and concurrence costs. ECTVA assumes that executive processes control subordinate processes by manipulating their parameters. TVA is used as the theory of subordinate processes, and a task set is defined as a set of TVA parameters that is sufficient to configure TVA to perform a task. Set switching is viewed as a change in one or more of these parameters, and the time taken to change a task set is assumed to depend on the number of parameters to be changed. Logan (2002) proposed a wide-ranging instance theory of attention and memory (ITAM) combining ECTVA with the exemplar-based random walk model of categorization proposed by Nosofsky and Palmeri (1997). The exemplar-based random walk model is itself a combination of Nosofsky's (1986) generalized context model of categorization and Logan's (1988) instance theory of automaticity. By integrating theories of attention, categorization, and memory, the development of ITAM seems to be a major step toward a unified account of visual cognition.

A NEURAL INTERPRETATION OF TVA (NTVA)

Two selection mechanisms at the single-cell level

The NTVA model by Bundesen et al. (2005) provides a neural interpretation of the two central equations of TVA, the rate and weight equations. Together, these equations describe two mechanisms of attentional selection: one for selection of objects and one for selection of features. NTVA describes how the mechanisms work at the single-cell level: filtering changes the number of cortical neurons in which an object is represented, and pigeonholing changes the rate of firing in cortical neurons coding for particular features (see Fig. 37. 2). Specifically, the total neural activation representing a visual categorization of the form 'object x has feature i' is directly proportional to (a) the number of neurons representing the categorization, which is controlled by filtering, and (b) the level of activation of the individual neurons representing the categorization, which is controlled by pigeonholing.

Filtering makes the number of cells in which an object is represented increase with the behavioural importance of the object. Thus, in NTVA visual processing is assumed to occur in parallel and with differential allocation of resources so that important objects are represented in many cells. More specifically, the probability that a cortical neuron represents a particular object in its classical receptive field equals the attentional weight of the object divided by the sum of the attentional weights across all objects in the neuron's receptive field.

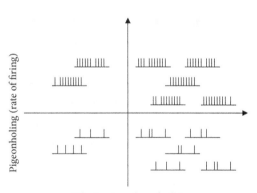

Filtering (number of cells)

FIGURE 37.2 Attentional selection in NTVA: Combined effects of filtering (selection of objects) and pigeonholing (selection of features) on the set of cortical spike trains representing a particular visual categorization of the form 'object x has feature i'. The 4 conditions (quadrants) correspond to the factorial combinations of 2 levels of filtering (weak vs. strong support to object x) by 2 levels of pigeonholing (weak vs. strong support to feature i). Filtering changes the number of cortical neurons in which an object is represented. Pigeonholing changes the rate of firing of cortical neurons coding for a particular feature. From C. Bundesen, T. Habekost, and S. Kyllingsbæk, A Neural Theory of Visual Attention: Bridging Cognition and Neurophysiology, *Psychological Review*, 112, p. 292, Copyright 2005, the American Psychological Association.

The *weight equation* of TVA describes the computation of attentional weights. Logically the weights must be computed before processing resources (cells) can be distributed in accordance with the weights. Therefore, in NTVA, a normal perceptual cycle consists of two waves: a wave of unselective processing, in which attentional weights are computed, and a wave of selective processing, in which processing resources have been allocated in accordance with the weights. During the first wave, cortical processing resources are distributed at random (unselectively) across the visual field. At the end of the first wave, an attentional weight has been computed for each object in the visual field and the weight has been stored in a priority map. The weights are used for reallocation of attention (visual processing capacity) by *dynamic remapping* of receptive fields of cortical neurons. The remapping of receptive fields makes the number of neurons allocated to an object increase with the attentional weight of the object. Thus, during the second wave, cortical processing is selective in the sense that the amount of processing resources allocated to an object (the number of neurons that represent the properties of the object) varies with the attentional weight of the object. Because more processing resources are devoted to behaviourally important objects than to less important ones, the important objects are processed faster, and are therefore more likely to become encoded into visual short-term memory (VSTM). The VSTM system is conceived as a feedback mechanism that sustains activity in the neurons that have won the attentional competition, making the information represented by these neurons available for other cognitive processes.

NTVA assumes that a typical neuron in the visual system is specialized to represent a single feature. The feature for which the neuron is specialized can be a more or less simple 'physical feature' or it can be a 'microfeature' in a distributed representation (Hinton et al. 1986). NTVA further assumes that a visual neuron responds to the properties of only one object at any given time. In the first wave of processing the object is selected at random among the ones in the neuron's classical receptive field. In the second wave of processing, the probability that the neuron represents a particular object equals the attentional weight of the object divided by the sum of the attentional weights across all objects in the receptive field.

NTVA defines the *activation* of a neuron by the appearance of an object in its receptive field as the increase in firing rate above a baseline rate representing the undriven activity of the neuron. If the baseline rate is zero, the activation is just the firing rate. Regardless of how neurons are distributed among objects (i.e. independently of filtering), the activation in neurons representing particular features (say, the activation in the set of neurons representing feature i) can be scaled up or down. This scaling of firing rates corresponds to varying β_i in TVA (i.e. the pigeonholing mechanism). In this neural interpretation, the rate equation of TVA:

$$v(x,i) = \eta(x,i)\beta_i \frac{w_x}{\sum_{z \in S} w_z}$$

describes the combined effects of filtering and pigeonholing on the total activation of the population of neurons that represents the categorization 'object x has feature i'. The

v value on the left-hand side of the rate equation is the total activation of the neurons that represent this particular categorization at the level of processing in the brain where objects compete for entrance into VSTM. At this level in the visual system, the classical receptive fields of neurons are assumed to be so large that each one covers the entire visual field. On the right-hand side of the equation, both the bias for categorizing objects as having feature i, β_i, and the relative attentional weight of object x:

$$\frac{w_x}{\displaystyle\sum_{z \in S} w_z}$$

range between 0 and 1. This implies that the strength of the sensory evidence that x is an i, $\eta(x, i)$, equals the highest possible value of $v(x, i)$. Thus, $\eta(x, i)$ equals the total activation of the set of all neurons coding feature i when all of these cells represent object x (say, when x is the only object in the visual field) and when the featural bias in favour of i is maximal (i.e., $\beta_i = 1$). When the proportion of feature-i coding neurons representing object x:

$$\frac{w_x}{\displaystyle\sum_{z \in S} w_z}$$

is less than 1, then the total activation representing the categorization 'object x has feature i' is scaled down by multiplication with this factor on the right-hand side of the equation. The total activation representing the categorization also depends on the level of activation of the individual neurons representing the categorization. The bias parameter β_i is a scale factor that multiplies activations of all feature-i coding neurons, so the total activation representing the categorization 'object x has feature i' is also directly proportional to β_i.

This way, in the neural interpretation of TVA's rate equation, the total activation representing the categorization 'object x has feature i' is directly proportional to (a) the number of neurons representing the categorization, and (b) the level of activation of the individual neurons representing the categorization. The number of neurons is controlled by the relative attentional weight of x (filtering) and the activation of the individual neurons is controlled by β_i (pigeonholing).

Related models

The core of TVA is the rate equation, which summarizes the way the strength $\eta(x, i)$ of the sensory evidence supporting the categorization 'object x has feature i' interacts with two types of biases: the perceptual bias associated with feature i, β_i, and the relative attentional weight of object x:

$$\frac{w_x}{\displaystyle\sum_{z \in S} w_z}$$

in determining the total competitive strength $v(x, i)$ of the given categorization. As suggested in the introduction, the rate equation makes TVA a theory of *biased competition* in the general sense of Desimone and Duncan (1995). However, TVA is special in assuming two different types of biases (one associated with features and one with objects) and also in being formalized.

TVA is not only a theory of biased competition, but also a *feature similarity gain model* in the sense of Treue and Martinez-Trujillo (1999). A gain model of attention is a model in which attention works by multiplicative scaling of neuronal responses by a certain gain factor (see McAdams and Maunsell 1999). Treue and Martinez-Trujillo proposed the *feature similarity gain principle*, that the gain factor of a neuron increases with increasing similarity between the sensory selectivity (the stimulus preferences) of the neuron and the currently attended features. Thus, assuming that a neuron encodes those features it prefers, attention to feature i should increase the responses of neurons encoding feature i or features similar to feature i. In terms of TVA, the gain factor in question is the multiplicative perceptual bias β_i, which is applied to neurons that are specialized for signalling feature i.

Finally TVA is closely related to the *normalization models* of Lee and Maunsell (2009) and Reynolds and Heeger (2009). For example, in the model of Reynolds and Heeger, neuronal responses are normalized by being divided by a measure of 'the sum total stimulus drive across a population of neurons' (Reynolds and Heeger 2009: 170). The effect of the normalization is akin to the effect of using relative (i.e. normalized) instead of absolute attentional weights in the rate equation of TVA.

The VSTM system

A main purpose of the VSTM system is to keep visual information available for other cognitive processes—further perceptual analysis, thinking, or permanent storage—after the immediate sensory stimulation has disappeared. In modelling visual short-term memory, NTVA follows a general idea dating back to Hebb (1949). Hebb suggested that short-term memory works by sustaining the activity of neurons representing the selected information in a positive feedback loop. This way information is kept active in a reverberating circuit that outlasts the original sensory stimulation. Hebb's notion of short-term memory has now gained wide acceptance in cognitive neuroscience. The feedback mechanism is often assumed to depend on interactions between prefrontal and posterior cortical areas (Fuster 1997; Goldman-Rakic 1995) but thalamo-cortical loops are also a main candidate (cf. Fig. 37.3).

In NTVA the short-term memory mechanism depends on a topographically organized map of the objects in the visual field. The map does not in itself represent the features of the selected objects, but rather functions as a pointer to their locations. The neurons representing objects at the pointed-to locations are kept active beyond the immediate sensory stimulation by reciprocal connections to the corresponding parts of the VSTM map. Thus, NTVA assumes that visual short-term memory is constituted by a feedback interaction between sensory neurons and the VSTM map of locations, making it possible for visual representations to outlast the original sensory stimulation.

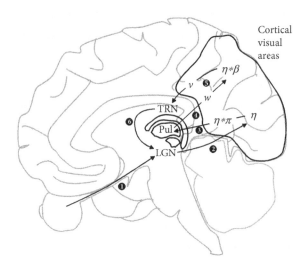

FIGURE 37.3 Possible distribution of visual processing across the human brain. Visual information from the eye enters the lateral geniculate nucleus (LGN) of the thalamus (1) and is transmitted to striate and extrastriate cortical areas where η values (strengths of evidence that objects at particular scales and positions have particular features) are computed (2). The η values are multiplied by π (pertinence) values, and the products are transmitted from the cortex to a saliency map in the pulvinar (Pul) nucleus of the thalamus, where the products are summed up as attentional weights of the stimulus objects (3). After the first (unselective) wave of processing, cortical processing capacity is redistributed by means of attentional weight signals (w) from the pulvinar to the cortex, so that during the second (selective) wave of processing, objects with high attentional weights are processed by many neurons (4). The resulting η values are multiplied by β (bias) values, and the products are transmitted from the cortex to a multiscale VSTM map of locations, which is tentatively localized in the thalamic reticular nucleus (TRN) (5). When the VSTM map is initialized, objects in the visual field effectively start a race to become encoded into VSTM. In this race, each object is represented by all possible categorizations of the object, and each possible categorization participates with an activation (v value) proportional to the corresponding η value multiplied by the corresponding β value. For the winners of the race, the TRN gates activation representing a categorization back to some of those cells in LGN whose activation supported the categorization (6). Thus activity in neurons representing winners of the race is sustained by positive feedback. From C. Bundesen, T. Habekost, and S. Kyllingsbæk, A Neural Theory of Visual Attention: Bridging Cognition and Neurophysiology, *Psychological Review*, 112, p. 295, Copyright 2005, the American Psychological Association.

The process of encoding information into VSTM starts each time the map of locations is initialized (i.e. cleared of previous activity). This is assumed to happen immediately after attentional weights have been computed for a new sensory impression, when the visual system is optimally tuned to select the most relevant information. Following TVA's race model framework, the selection process is assumed to function in a winner-take-all manner in which the first activated object representations in the

VSTM map block later ones from entering. The winner-take-all property can occur in a network where all nodes excite themselves (when externally triggered) while inhibiting the other nodes (Grossberg 1976, 1980). Thus, once a node has been triggered by external stimulation, its activity will tend to sustain itself while inhibiting the other nodes to the point where they can no longer be activated by external signals. In the VSTM map of locations the inhibitory connections are configured such that when fewer than K objects are active, an external signal can still overcome the inhibition from the objects that are already encoded. However, when K units are active, external stimulation representing a new object (an object at a new location or a different scale) can no longer activate a new object node ('K-winners-take-all network'). This mechanism provides a simple explanation of the limited storage capacity of VSTM, where only K objects can be active at the same time. Note that the network is limited in terms of the number of objects in the VSTM map, but not necessarily in the number of features related to each of the selected objects. Once an object has established itself in VSTM, many different categorizations can be attached to it.

It is not currently clear which type of neural signal is needed to capture a slot in the VSTM map. The simplest possibility is the very first spike from one of the many visual neurons that project to the map. If neural activity is viewed as inherently noisy, this may seem like a highly unreliable mechanism. However, there is evidence to suggest that single spikes can in fact have profound effects on the cognitive processes of the whole organism (Parker and Newsome 1998). Alternatively a stronger signal from multiple neurons may be needed, perhaps a volley of at least n synchronized spikes, n being a number substantially greater than one. However the effective signal is defined, NTVA assumes that the VSTM system is configured so that the first such impulse to the VSTM map activates the winner-take-all network. Assuming that signals for different categorizations as well as repeated signals for a given categorization occur independently of each other, this is mathematically equivalent to an exponential race model. That is, NTVA implies that selection is determined by a parallel processing race among categorizations, a race in which processing times for individual categorizations are mutually independent, exponentially distributed random variables. Such a model is completely in line with the original TVA model.

Functional anatomy

NTVA is a general neurocomputational model that does not depend critically on a particular anatomical localization of the proposed computations. However, we have suggested some plausible ways in which visual processing may be distributed across the human brain. One possibility is the so-called *thalamic version* of NTVA, which is illustrated in Fig. 37.3. For further discussions of the functional anatomy of the processes described in TVA, see below, as well as Bundesen et al. (2005) and Habekost and Starrfelt (2009).

Applications to single-cell studies

NTVA can provide quantitative explanations of a wide range of attentional effects observed in single-cell studies: effects on the rate of firing with multiple stimuli in the receptive field of a cell, effects on the rate of firing with a single stimulus in the receptive field, effects on baseline firing, and effects on neural synchronization (see Bundesen et al. 2005; Bundesen and Habekost 2008). Central examples of simple, qualitative applications to classical studies are presented below, separately for the filtering and pigeonholing mechanisms.

Neural filtering

NTVA's notion of attentional filtering by dynamic remapping of receptive fields was originally inspired by a study of Moran and Desimone (1985). Moran and Desimone presented macaque monkeys with stimuli at two locations in the visual field. The monkeys were trained to attend only to stimuli presented at one of the locations and ignore any stimuli shown at the other location. The monkeys performed a match-to-sample task, in which they were to encode a sample stimulus shown at the attended location, retain it in memory for a brief delay period, and then compare it to a test stimulus shown at the same location. During the presentation of both the sample and test displays, Moran and Desimone recorded the responses of single neurons to the stimuli in cortical areas V1, V4, and IT. Their main result was that, when the target and distractor stimuli were both present within the receptive field of the recorded cell in visual areas V4 or IT, the cell's rate of firing depended on the properties of the target object, but not the distractor. For example, they recorded the responses of individual cells to a pair of stimuli consisting of (a) a stimulus that produced a high rate of firing when the stimulus was presented alone (an effective sensory stimulus) and (b) a stimulus that had little or no effect on the rate of firing when presented alone (an ineffective sensory stimulus). On trials in which the effective stimulus was the target and the ineffective stimulus was the distractor, the cell showed a high rate of firing. However, on trials in which the ineffective stimulus was the target and the effective stimulus was the distractor, the cell's firing rate was low. Moran and Desimone remarked that the typical cell responded 'as if the receptive field had contracted around the attended stimulus'.

Notably, the effect only occurred when both the target and the distractor were located within the recorded neuron's receptive field. In cortical area IT the receptive fields were very large, covering at least the central 12 degrees of both the contralateral and ipsilateral visual field; for neurons in this area, the distractors were always located inside the receptive field. In contrast, in area V1 only one stimulus could be fitted into each neuron's receptive field. In this case, no significant effects of attention were found. Also in area V4, no effect of attention was found when only a single stimulus was placed in the receptive field. These negative findings fit well with the predictions of NTVA: If a neuron's receptive field contains only one stimulus, the neuron should always represent the properties of this object, regardless of whether it is a target or a distractor. Overall, the results of Moran and Desimone clearly support NTVA's notion of filtering, and in fact suggested the interpretation in the first place.

Reynolds et al. (1999) corroborated and extended the findings of Moran and Desimone (1985). Recording from neurons in cortical areas V2 and V4, they found that the mean firing rate of a cell to a pair of stimuli in its receptive field approximated a weighted average of the firing rates of the cell to each of the stimuli in the pair when they were presented alone. When the monkey's attention was directed to one of the stimuli in the pair, this increased the weight on the target stimulus so that the mean response of the neuron was driven (up or down) toward the response elicited when the target stimulus was presented alone. The results fit in with the dual conjectures that (a) at any time, a cell was driven by only one of the stimuli in its receptive field, and (b) the probability that the cell was driven by a given stimulus equalled the attentional weight of the stimulus divided by the sum of the attentional weights of all stimuli in the receptive field of the cell. This is exactly what is predicted by NTVA.

Neural pigeonholing

Whereas NTVA's filtering mechanism affects the number of neurons in which an object x is represented, the *pigeonholing* mechanism affects the strength of the response in each of those neurons that are allocated to the object. The activation in a neuron representing the categorization that object x has feature i is assumed to be proportional to the perceptual bias, β_i, which is applied to neurons that are specialized for signalling feature i. Recordings from single cells in the visual system of monkeys have provided evidence of such a mechanism: a *feature-based* mechanism of attention that selects groups of neurons with similar stimulus preferences for a multiplicative enhancement in response strength.

Treue and Martinez-Trujillo (1999; also see Martinez-Trujillo and Treue 2004) recorded from cortical area MT, which contains cells that are selective to the direction of motion. In the basic task, Treue and Martinez-Trujillo presented monkeys with two coherently moving random dot patterns, one placed inside the receptive field of the neuron being recorded and the other one in the opposite visual hemifield (see Fig. 37.4). At the start of each trial, the monkey was shown a cue at one of the two locations. Following this, the two random dot patterns appeared and the monkey was required to detect small changes in the speed or direction of movement of the pattern at the cued location. These motion changes occurred after a random delay ranging between a few hundred milliseconds and several seconds.

In one of their experiments, Treue and Martinez-Trujillo demonstrated an effect of pigeonholing with respect to a given direction of movement ('feature-based attention'). This was probably the first clear demonstration of pigeonholing in the single-cell literature. In this experiment, the recorded neuron's receptive field was stimulated by a pattern moving in the direction preferred by this particular neuron. Outside the receptive field a pattern was presented that moved either in the same direction or in the opposite (non-preferred) direction. The crucial finding was that when the monkey

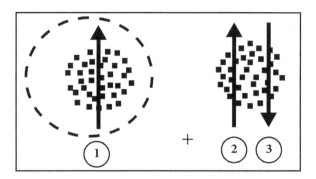

FIGURE 37.4 Stimuli used by Treue and Martinez-Trujillo (1999). The random dot pattern inside the receptive field (dashed circle) always moved in the cell's preferred direction (upward pointing arrow, (1)); the stimulus outside moved in either the same (2) or the opposite direction (3). Reprinted by permission from Macmillan Publishers Ltd: *Nature*, 399 (6736), Feature-based attention influences motion processing gain in macaque visual cortex, Stefan Treue and Julio C. Martinez Trujillo, copyright 1999, Nature Publishing Group.

attended to the pattern outside the receptive field, the response of the recorded neuron varied with the direction of movement being attended: The firing rate went up when the attended pattern (outside the receptive field of the recorded neuron) moved in the preferred direction of the recorded neuron. Conversely, the firing rate went down when the attended pattern moved in the direction opposite to the preferred direction of the recorded neuron. Since the spatial location of the attended pattern was exactly the same in the two conditions, a non-spatial, feature-based mechanism of attention seemed to be at work: pigeonholing.

The result can be explained in the following way by NTVA. When the monkey attended to movement in a particular direction, the β value for movement in that direction was high while the β value for movement in the opposite direction was low. As the monkey was monitoring the pattern for hundreds to thousands of milliseconds, there should be plenty of time to adjust the β values in accordance with the display. Consider the situation in which the preferred movement of the recorded neuron was upwards but the monkey attended to movement in the opposite direction (downwards), trying to detect a small change in the movement of the pattern to be attended. Perceptual bias should generally reflect expectations, and since the monkey had learned that only small changes in the direction of movement of the target would occur (and the target pattern was moving downwards) $\beta_{upwards}$ should be low. Because the activation of the recorded cell should be proportional to $\beta_{upwards}$, the recorded activation should also be low. By contrast, when the monkey attended to movement in the preferred direction of the recorded cell, β values should be high for upwards and nearby directions. In this case, $\beta_{upwards}$ being high, the activation of the recorded neuron also should be high.

TVA-based Assessment

TVA is a general theory of the mechanisms involved in visual attention, but the model can also be used to quantify individual differences in attention abilities. According to TVA, the efficiency of a person's visual attention system can be characterized by the values of a few basic parameters: the speed of visual processing, C, the storage capacity of the VSTM system, K, and the efficiency of top-down selectivity, α. As detailed below, these parameters can be measured by a combination of two simple experimental tasks, whole and partial report. These tasks also allow for estimation of the individual's perception threshold, t_0, which can be defined as the longest visual exposure duration at which processing is still ineffective. By comparing attentional weights in different parts of the visual field it is also possible to test if there is a tendency to encode objects from particular parts of the display (the w_{index} parameter). Following the pioneering study by Duncan et al. (1999), many research groups have taken up TVA-based assessment for studying attention deficits in various neurological and psychiatric conditions. Recently the scope of the research has been widened to include genetic and pharmacologically based studies of healthy participants, including children. This section gives an overview of the rapidly developing field of TVA-based assessment.

The test method

Whole and partial report

TVA can be used to analyse data from many experimental paradigms, but the most direct way to estimate the basic parameters of the model is to combine *whole report* and *partial report* tasks. The fundamental method was established by Duncan et al. (1999), and the experimental design and data analysis have later been refined. The details of the report tasks vary from study to study, but share the same basic design: an array of simple visual objects (from one to six) is displayed on a computer screen; see Fig. 37.5 for an example. The stimuli of choice are typically letters, but digits and faces have also been used (e.g. Peers et al. 2005; Starrfelt et al. 2009). The presentation of the items is shorter than the reaction time for eye movements (i.e. at most 200 ms) and the display is followed by either a set of pattern masks or a blank screen. In case of a blank screen, an afterimage of the display persists for some time in the visual system (the 'iconic memory' phenomenon, see Sperling 1960), which effectively prolongs the exposure duration. In whole report only target items are presented and the task is to verbally report the identity of as many items as possible without guessing. In partial report the display is a mixture of targets and distractors (e.g. red and blue letters) and the task is to report the identity of only the target items (e.g. the red letters).

For the best measurement of the TVA parameters the exposure duration must be systematically varied to cover the full range from the individual's perception threshold to

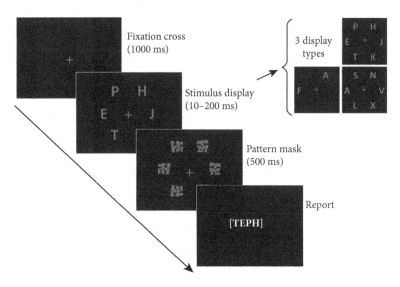

FIGURE 37.5 A typical example of whole and partial report tasks used for TVA-based assessment (the CombiTVA paradigm used by Vangkilde et al. 2011). The outline of a single trial is shown, as well as three types of stimulus displays: 6-target whole report (red letters), 2-target whole report (red letters), and 2-target + 4-distractor partial report (red and blue letters).

near-ceiling performance. Also, to obtain reliable estimates of the TVA parameters each display condition must be repeated many times. The number of repetitions per condition depends on the purpose of the assessment (e.g. clinical or research) but is typically between 25 and 100; however, as few as 10 repetitions per condition may produce reasonably valid data (see Finke et al. 2005, for a discussion).

Parameter estimation

The performance in whole report (the mean number of items correctly reported) increases as a function of the exposure duration in a characteristic way (see Fig. 37.6). When the exposure duration is shorter than the tested person's perception threshold, t_0, the score is zero. After the threshold has been passed, the score rises abruptly. The slope of the curve at the point where the exposure duration equals t_0 corresponds to the individual's visual processing speed, C. Over the course of a few hundred milliseconds the mean score gradually levels off to approach an asymptotic value representing the maximum storage capacity of visual short-term memory, K. If distractor elements are added to the display (i.e. partial report) the parameter α can be measured by comparing the accuracy reduction in this condition to trials without distractor elements. The spatial bias, w_{index}, can be quantified by comparing attentional weights for objects in different parts of the visual field.

Whole and partial report experiments typically include a large set of observations (e.g. 432 trials) for each participant. Given a psychometric model (such as TVA) of the probability distributions underlying these test data, the unknown parameters of the

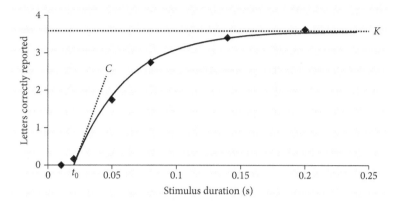

FIGURE 37.6 Typical performance in a whole report experiment. Dots represent observed mean scores and the curve shows the maximum likelihood fit to these observations based on the TVA equations. Estimates of visual short-term memory capacity, K, and visual threshold, t_0, are marked out. The slope of the curve at $t = t_0$ represents the visual processing speed, C.

distributions (e.g. the individual's K and C values) can be inferred. The standard mathematical procedure for this estimation is the maximum likelihood method. Basically this is a computational algorithm that searches the parameter space for the set of values that maximizes the probability of obtaining the actual set of observations (Kyllingsbæk 2006). Dyrholm et al. (2011) have recently developed a very effective fitting algorithm for this procedure. Compared to previous methods for TVA analysis, Dyrholm et al.'s fitting procedure includes two new assumptions that provide additional robustness for the parameter analysis: (a) the visual threshold t_0 is not necessarily fixed across the experiment, but may vary from trial to trial (following a Gaussian distribution), and (b) the capacity of visual short-term memory K, which was previously assumed to vary between just two neighbouring integers from trial to trial, is now derived from a broader distribution of values. Based on a large data set from hundreds of normal participants, Dyrholm et al. demonstrated how these new assumptions lead to very precise and reliable model fits of whole and partial report data.

Test qualities

A main quality of the TVA-based test method is its *specificity*. Main parameters like t_0, C, and K reflect specific features of the observed data (in simple cases, t_0 is a specific zero-intercept, C a specific slope, and K a specific asymptote), and the feature reflected by a particular parameter is relatively easy to distinguish from the features reflected by other main parameters. Also, TVA-based assessment is currently the only way of estimating K without presupposing that C is so high that at a given exposure duration, VSTM is filled up with items. Further, unlike reaction time based tests of attention, TVA-based measurement is not significantly influenced by motor factors: Report is unspeeded and accuracy is the only important performance variable. This makes the measurements quite specific to processes in the visual system. Another important quality of TVA-based assessment is *sensitivity*. By using near-threshold stimulation, the report tasks are so demanding that subtle impairments of visual function that are not evident on standard clinical tests have repeatedly been demonstrated in brain damaged participants (Habekost and Bundesen 2003; Habekost and Rostrup 2006; Habekost and Starrfelt 2006). A third test quality is *reliability*: TVA-based parameter estimates generally have low measurement error (as measured, e.g., by bootstrap statistics, see Habekost and Bundesen 2003). For example, in a typical whole report experiment with 25 repetitions per condition, the standard measurement error related to the C and K estimates were only about 10% and 3%, respectively (Habekost and Rostrup 2006). Finally, TVA-based assessment has high *validity* by being grounded in a theoretical framework that accounts for large parts of the psychological and neurophysiological literature on visual attention. This ensures that the measured parameters relate directly to general theoretical constructs rather than to particular aspects of the (whole/partial report) test situation.

Clinical neuropsychology

A main application of TVA-based assessment is to study the clinical effects, that is, patterns of attention deficits, after different types of brain damage. So far, three main types of neurological disorders have been investigated: (a) neglect and related disorders after stroke (Duncan et al. 1999, 2003; Habekost and Rostrup 2006, 2007; Peers et al. 2005), (b) neurodegenerative diseases (Bublak et al. 2006, 2011; Finke et al. 2006, 2007; Redel et al. 2012; Sorg et al., 2012), and (c) reading disturbances following stroke in the posterior left hemisphere (Habekost and Starrfelt 2006; Starrfelt et al. 2009, 2010). A general feature of these studies is the strong specificity provided by TVA-based assessment, which allows for separate measurement of different aspects of visual attention. As a result, many interesting mixtures of preserved and impaired attentional functions have been found in diverse patient groups. For example, the pioneering study by Duncan et al. (1999) showed that patients with neglect after stroke in the right hemisphere had bilateral reductions in visual processing capacity, but preserved selectivity in both visual fields (besides the expected attentional bias towards stimuli in the right hemifield). Bublak et al. (2006) showed a similar deficit pattern in two neurological syndromes that are normally regarded as very different from neglect, Huntington's and Alzheimer's disease. In both groups of patients there was a strong leftward bias of spatial attention in addition to the (expected) general reduction in visual processing speed. The analytical specificity of TVA has also been useful for studies of reading disturbances after brain damage. For example, competing theories hold that patients with pure alexia either have difficulties with simultaneous perception of letters (corresponding to the K parameter) or visual form recognition of single letters (corresponding to the C parameter). Starrfelt et al. (2009), however, found that patients with pure alexia are impaired in terms of both of these visual capacity parameters, and that the deficits generalize to a different stimulus category than letters, namely digits.

The lesion anatomy of the TVA parameters

A number of studies have compared the effects of lesions in different parts of the brain to map the anatomy of specific TVA parameters. Lesions in a broad range of brain areas have been investigated, including the thalamus, extrastriate cortex, parietal cortex, frontal cortex, and the basal ganglia. The two main parameters of visual capacity, C and K, seem to depend on a large network of brain areas, where a lesion in each part can lead to impairments. The network includes the extrastriate cortex (Starrfelt et al. 2009, 2010), the parietal cortex (Duncan et al. 1999; Peers et al. 2005), and the frontal cortex/basal ganglia (Habekost and Rostrup 2006; Finke et al. 2006). The anatomical networks for C and K seem to be largely overlapping, which explains why brain damage seldom leads to selective impairment in only one of these capacity parameters.

The efficiency of top-down selection, α, also may not be strictly localized, but depend on a number of different brain areas. Peers et al. (2005) found that the volume of damaged tissue, not the exact location of the lesion, correlated significantly with poor α values in patients who had focal lesions in the parietal or frontal cortex. This finding is in line with the influential theoretical notion that attentional control depends on multiple brain areas organized in large fronto-parietal networks (e.g. Hopfinger et al., 2000). Other studies have targeted specific components of these fronto-parietal networks. In a study using transcranial magnetic stimulation (TMS) of healthy participants Hung et al. (2005) found that stimulation of the right posterior parietal cortex diminished visual selectivity (as measured by the α parameter) in the left hemifield, but increased it in the right hemifield. No effect on α was found by stimulating the homologous area in the left hemisphere. Hung et al. (2011) recently followed up on this study and reported that TMS of the right, but not the left, frontal eye fields significantly impaired visual selectivity in both hemifields. Both TMS studies indicate that fronto-parietal structures in the right hemisphere have a special importance for the α parameter, at least when selection is based on colour.

Another issue concerns the spatial distribution of attentional weights, measured by the w_{index} parameter. Peers et al. (2005) found that large lesions to one hemisphere typically led to lower attentional weights for stimuli in the contralesional visual field, relatively independently of lesion location. Habekost and Rostrup (2006) also found that large lesions of the right hemisphere were generally related to low weighting of the left hemifield. However, Habekost and Rostrup found an important exception to this 'mass effect' of unilateral brain damage, namely asymmetric attentional weights after focal damage in the right thalamus. Interestingly, this performance pattern was only found if the lesion included the pulvinar. The result corresponds well with the anatomical model of NTVA suggested in Fig. 37.3, where attentional weights are computed in the pulvinar nucleus: damage to one side of this brain area should specifically reduce attentional weights for the opposite visual hemifield.

New research directions

In the first decade after the original study by Duncan et al. (1999), TVA-based assessment was almost exclusively used for studies of adults with brain damage. However, the research focus is widening. For example, studies of children with congenital brain damage (Caspersen and Habekost 2013), dyslexia (Dubois et al. 2010; Stenneken et al. 2011), and ADHD (McAvinue et al. 2012) are beginning to appear (for a study on adults with ADHD, see Finke et al. 2011). Testing children poses special challenges, but the general method has worked well with children as young as 9 years old, and work is in progress to adapt the experimental design to even younger children. Another main development is that TVA-based assessment is now being used for cognitive pharmacology, that is, to study how neurochemical substances impair or improve attentional function in healthy participants. Drugs so far investigated include modafinil and methylphenidate (Finke et al. 2010) as well as nicotine (Vangkilde et al. 2011); all three substances were found to influence specific TVA parameters. The pharmacological research approach potentially links well with genetic studies, and TVA-based assessment is currently being used in two large-scale investigations of behavioural genetics (the Betula study in Sweden and the NCNG study in Norway). Other researchers have used TVA-based assessment to study how attentional function can be improved by cognitive means, for example using meditation (Jensen et al. 2012) and self-alerting techniques (McAvinue et al. 2012). All in all, TVA-based investigations have been taken up in many novel research contexts in the last few years, and the list is still growing.[1]

CONCLUDING REMARKS

In this chapter we have presented TVA as a formal theory of visual attention with applications to human perception and performance. We have also presented the neural interpretation of TVA, NTVA, and provided examples of how NTVA accounts for findings from single-cell studies in primates. Finally, we have reviewed how TVA has been applied to study attentional functions in neuropsychological, pharmacological, and genetic research. The prospects seem highly encouraging.

ACKNOWLEDGEMENTS

This work was supported by a grant from the University of Copenhagen Programme of Excellence to Claus Bundesen. We thank Signe Vangkilde for producing Figs. 37.5 and 37.6.

NOTE

1. Despite their varied interests all of the involved researchers use the same basic methods, and an international network (ITVA) has been established to coordinate the research activities.

REFERENCES

Bublak, P., Redel, P., and Finke, K. (2006). Spatial and non-spatial attention deficits in neuro-degenerative diseases: Assessment based on Bundesen's theory of visual attention (TVA). *Restorative Neurology & Neuroscience 24*: 287–301.

Bublak, P., Redel, P., Sorg, C., Kurz, A., Förstl, H., Müller, H. J., Schneider, W. X., and Finke, K. (2011). Staged decline of visual processing capacity in mild cognitive impairment and Alzheimer's disease. *Neurobiology of Aging 32*: 1219–1230.

Bundesen, C. (1990). A theory of visual attention. *Psychological Review 97*: 523–547.

Bundesen, C. (1993). The relationship between independent race models and Luce's choice axiom. *Journal of Mathematical Psychology 37*: 446–471.

Bundesen, C. (1998). A computational theory of visual attention. *Philosophical Transactions of the Royal Society B: Biological Sciences 353*: 1271–1281.

Bundesen, C. and Habekost, T. (2008). *Principles of Visual Attention: Linking Mind and Brain*. Oxford: Oxford University Press.

Bundesen, C., Habekost, T., and Kyllingsbæk, S. (2005). A neural theory of visual attention: Bridging cognition and neurophysiology. *Psychological Review 112*: 291–328.

Bundesen, C., Kyllingsbæk, S., and Larsen, A. (2003). Independent encoding of colors and shapes from two stimuli. *Psychonomic Bulletin & Review 10*: 474–479.

Bundesen, C. and Pedersen, L. F. (1983). Color segregation and visual search. *Perception & Psychophysics 33*: 487–493.

Caspersen, I. C. and Habekost, T. (2013). Selective and sustained attention in children with spina bifida myelomeningocele. *Child Neuropsychology 19*: 55–57.

Desimone, R. and Duncan, J. (1995). Neural mechanisms of selective visual attention. *Annual Review of Neuroscience 18*: 193–222.

Dubois, M., Kyllingsbæk, S., Prado, C., Musca, S. C., Peiffer, E., Lassus-Sangosse, D., and Valdois, S. (2010). Fractionating the multi-character processing deficit in developmental dyslexia: Evidence from two case studies. *Cortex 46*: 717–738.

Duncan, J. (1984). Selective attention and the organization of visual information. *Journal of Experimental Psychology: General 113*: 501–517.

Duncan, J., Bundesen, C., Olson, A., Humphreys, G., Chavda, S., and Shibuya, H. (1999). Systematic analysis of deficits in visual attention. *Journal of Experimental Psychology: General 128*: 450–478.

Duncan, J., Bundesen, C., Olson, A., Humphreys, G., Ward, R., Kyllingsbæk, S., van Raamsdonk, M., Rorden, C., and Chavda, S. (2003). Dorsal and ventral simultanagnosia. *Cognitive Neuropsychology 20*: 675–701.

Dyrholm, M., Kyllingsbæk, S., Espeseth, T., and Bundesen, C. (2011). Generalizing parametric models by introducing trial-by-trial parameter variability: The case of TVA. *Journal of Mathematical Psychology 55*: 416–429.

Estes, W. K. and Taylor, H. A. (1964). A detection method and probabilistic models for assessing information processing from brief visual displays. *Proceedings of the National Academy of Sciences USA 52*: 446–454.

Finke, K., Bublak, P., Dose, M., Müller, H. J., and Schneider, W. X. (2006). Parameter-based assessment of spatial and non-spatial attentional deficits in Huntington's disease. *Brain 129*: 1137–1151.

Finke, K., Bublak, P., Krummenacher, J., Kyllingsbæk, S., Müller, H. J., and Schneider, W. X. (2005). Usability of a theory of visual attention (TVA) for parameter-based measurement of attention I: Evidence from normal subjects. *Journal of the International Neuropsychological Society 11*: 832–842.

Finke, K., Dodds, C. M., Bublak, P., Regenthal, R., Baumann, F., Manly, T., and Müller, U. (2010). Effects of modafinil and methylphenidate on visual attention capacity: A TVA-based study. *Psychopharmacology 210*: 317–329.

Finke, K., Schneider, W. X., Redel, P., Dose, M., Kerkhoff, G., Müller, H. J., et al. (2007). The capacity of attention and simultaneous perception of objects: A group study of Huntington's disease patients. *Neuropsychologia 45*: 3272–3284.

Finke, K., Schwarzkopf, W., Müller, U., Frodl, T., Müller, H. J., Schneider, W. X., Engel, R. R., Riedel, M., Möller, H.-J., and Hennig-Fast, K. (2011). Disentangling the adult attention-deficit hyperactivity disorder endophenotype: Parametric measurement of attention. *Journal of Abnormal Psychology 120*: 890–901.

Fuster, J. M. (1997). *The Prefrontal Cortex: Anatomy, Physiology, and Neuropsychology of the Frontal Lobe*. New York and Philadelphia: Lippincott-Raven.

Goldman-Rakic, P. S. (1995). Cellular basis of working memory. *Neuron 14*: 477–485.

Grossberg, S. (1976). Adaptive pattern classification and universal recoding: I. Parallel development and coding of neural feature detectors. *Biological Cybernetics 23*: 121–134.

Grossberg, S. (1980). How does a brain build a cognitive code? *Psychological Review 87*: 1–51.

Habekost, T. and Bundesen, C. (2003). Patient assessment based on a theory of visual attention (TVA): Subtle deficits after a right frontal-subcortical lesion. *Neuropsychologia 41*: 1171–1188.

Habekost, T. and Rostrup, E. (2006). Persisting asymmetries of vision after right side lesions. *Neuropsychologia 44*: 876–895.

Habekost, T. and Rostrup, E. (2007). Visual attention capacity after right hemisphere lesions. *Neuropsychologia 45*: 1474–1488.

Habekost, T. and Starrfelt, R. (2006). Alexia and quadrant-amblyopia: Reading disability after a minor visual field deficit. *Neuropsychologia 44*: 2465–2476.

Habekost, T. and Starrfelt, R. (2009). Visual attention capacity: A review of TVA-based patient studies. *Scandinavian Journal of Psychology 50*: 23–32.

Hebb, D. O. (1949). *Organization of Behavior*. New York: Wiley.

Hinton, G. E., McClelland, J. L., and Rumelhart, D. E. (1986). Distributed representations. In D. E. Rumelhart and J. L. McClelland (eds.), *Parallel Distributed Processing* (vol. 1, pp. 77–109). Cambridge, Mass.: MIT Press.

Hopfinger, J. B., Buonocore, M. H., and Mangun, G. R. (2000). The neural mechanisms of top-down attentional control. *Nature Neuroscience 3*: 284–291.

Hung, J., Driver, J., and Walsh, V. (2005). Visual selection and posterior parietal cortex: Effects of repetitive transcranial magnetic stimulation on partial report analyzed by Bundesen's theory of visual attention. *Journal of Neuroscience 25*: 9602–9612.

Hung, J., Driver, J., and Walsh, V. (2011). Visual selection and the human frontal eye fields: Effects of frontal transcranial magnetic stimulation on partial report analyzed by Bundesen's theory of visual attention. *Journal of Neuroscience 31*: 15904–15913.

Jensen, C. G., Vangkilde, S., Frøkjær, V., and Hasselbalch, S. G. (2012). Mindfulness training affects attention—or is it attentional effort? *Journal of Experimental Psychology: General* *141*: 106–123.

Kyllingsbæk, S. (2006). Modeling visual attention. *Behavior Research Methods 38*: 123–133.

Kyllingsbæk, S. and Bundesen, C. (2007). Parallel processing in a multi-feature whole-report paradigm. *Journal of Experimental Psychology: Human Perception and Performance 33*: 64–82.

Kyllingsbæk, S., Markussen, B., and Bundesen, C. (2012). Testing a Poisson counter model for visual identification of briefly presented, mutually confusable single stimuli in pure accuracy tasks. *Journal of Experimental Psychology: Human Perception and Performance 38*: 628–642.

Kyllingsbæk, S., Schneider, W. X., and Bundesen, C. (2001). Automatic attraction of attention to former targets in visual displays of letters. *Perception & Psychophysics 63*: 85–98.

Lee, J. and Maunsell, J. H. R. (2009). A normalization model of attentional modulation of single unit responses. *PLoS One 4*(2): e4651.

Logan, G. D. (1988). Toward an instance theory of automatization. *Psychological Review* *95*: 492–527.

Logan, G. D. (1996). The CODE theory of visual attention: An integration of space-based and object-based attention. *Psychological Review 103*: 603–649.

Logan, G. D. (2002). An instance theory of attention and memory. *Psychological Review* *109*: 376–400.

Logan, G. D. and Bundesen, C. (1996). Spatial effects in the partial report paradigm: A challenge for theories of visual spatial attention. In D. L. Medin (ed.), *The Psychology of Learning and Motivation* (vol. *35*, pp. 243–282). San Diego, Calif.: Academic Press.

Logan, G. D. and Gordon, R. D. (2001). Executive control of visual attention in dual-task situations. *Psychological Review 108*: 393–434.

Los, S. A. (2010). Foreperiod and sequential effects: theory and data. In A. C. Nobre and J. T. Coull (eds.), *Attention and Time* (pp. 289–302). Oxford: Oxford University Press.

Luce, R. D. (1963). Detection and recognition. In R. D. Luce, R. R. Bush, and E. Galanter (eds.), *Handbook of Mathematical Psychology* (vol. 1, pp. 103–189). New York: Wiley.

Luck, S. J. and Vogel, E. K. (1997). The capacity of visual working memory for features and conjunctions. *Nature 390*: 279–281.

McAdams, C. J. and Maunsell, J. H. R. (1999). Effects of attention on orientation-tuning functions of single neurons in macaque cortical area V4. *Journal of Neuroscience 19*: 431–441.

McAvinue, L. P., Vangkilde, S., Johnson, K. A., Habekost, T., Kyllingsbæk, S., Bundesen, C., and Robertson, I. H. (2012). A componential analysis of visual attention in children with ADHD. *Journal of Attention Disorders,* Nov 27 [Epub ahead of print].

McAvinue, L. P., Vangkilde, S., Johnson, K. A., Habekost, T., Kyllingsbæk, S., Robertson, I. H., and Bundesen, C. (2012). The relationship between sustained attention, attentional selectivity, and capacity. *Journal of Cognitive Psychology 24*: 313–328.

Martinez-Trujillo, J. C. and Treue, S. (2004). Feature-based attention increases the selectivity of population responses in primate visual cortex. *Current Biology 14*: 744–751.

Matthias, E., Bublak, P., Costa, A., Müller, H. J., Schneider W. X., and Finke, K. (2009). Attentional and sensory effects of lowered levels of intrinsic alertness. *Neuropsychologia 47*: 3255–3264.

Matthias, E., Bublak, P., Müller, H. J., Schneider, W. X., Krummenacher, J., and Finke, K. (2010). The influence of alertness on spatial and nonspatial components of visual attention. *Journal of Experimental Psychology: Human Perception and Performance 36*: 38–56.

Moran, J. and Desimone, R. (1985). Selective attention gates visual processing in the extrastriate cortex. *Science 229*: 782–784.

Niemi, P. and Näätänen, R. (1981). Foreperiod and simple reaction time. *Psychological Bulletin* 89: 133–162.

Nobre, A. C. (2001). Orienting attention to instants in time. *Neuropsychologia 39*: 1317–1328.

Nobre, A. C. (2010). How can temporal expectations bias perception and action? In A. C. Nobre and J. T. Coull (eds.), *Attention and Time* (pp. 371–392). Oxford: Oxford University Press.

Nosofsky, R. M. (1986). Attention, similarity, and the identification–categorization relationship. *Journal of Experimental Psychology: General 115*: 39–57.

Nosofsky, R. M. and Palmeri, T. J. (1997). An exemplar-based random walk model of speeded classification. *Psychological Review 104*: 266–300.

Parker, A. J. and Newsome, W. T. (1998). Sense and the single neuron: Probing the physiology of perception. *Annual Review of Neuroscience 21*: 227–277.

Peers, P. V., Ludwig, C. J., Rorden, C., Cusack, R., Bonfiglioli, C., Bundesen, C., et al. (2005). Attentional functions of parietal and frontal cortex. *Cerebral Cortex 15*: 1469–1484.

Posner, M. I., Nissen, M. J., and Ogden, W. C. (1978). Attended and unattended processing modes: the role of set for spatial location. In H. L. Pick and I. J. Saltzman (eds.), *Modes of Perceiving and Processing Information* (pp. 137–157). Hillsdale, N.J.: Lawrence Erlbaum Associates.

Redel, P., Bublak, P., Sorg, C., Kurz, A., Förstl, H., Müller, H. J., Schneider, W. X., Perneczky, R., and Finke, K. (2012). Deficits of spatial and task-related attentional selection in mild cognitive impairment and Alzheimer's disease. *Neurobiology of Aging 33*: e27–e42.

Reynolds, J. H., Chelazzi, L., and Desimone, R. (1999). Competitive mechanisms subserve attention in macaque areas V2 and V4. *Journal of Neuroscience 19*: 1736–1753.

Reynolds, J. H. and Heeger, D. J. (2009). The normalization model of attention. *Neuron* 61: 168–185.

Schneider, W. and Fisk, A. D. (1982). Degree of consistent training: Improvements in search performance and automatic process development. *Perception & Psychophysics 31*: 160–168.

Shibuya, H. and Bundesen, C. (1988). Visual selection from multielement displays: Measuring and modeling effects of exposure duration. *Journal of Experimental Psychology: Human Perception and Performance 14*: 591–600.

Sorg, C., Myers, N., Redel, P., Bublak, P., Riedl, V., Manoliu, A., Perneczky, R., Grimmer, T., Kurz, A., Förstl, H., Drzezga, A., Müller, H. J., Wohlschläger, A.M., and Finke, K. (2012). Asymmetric loss of parietal activity causes spatial bias in prodromal and mild Alzheimer's disease. *Biological Psychiatry 71*: 798–804.

Sperling, G. (1960). The information available in brief visual presentations. *Psychological Monographs 74* (11, Whole No. 498).

Sperling, G. (1967). Successive approximations to a model for short-term memory. *Acta Psychologica 27*: 285–292.

Starrfelt, R., Habekost, T., and Gerlach, C. (2010). Visual processing in pure alexia: A case study. *Cortex 46*: 242–255.

Starrfelt, R., Habekost, T., and Leff, A. P. (2009). Too little, too late: Reduced visual span and speed characterize pure alexia. *Cerebral Cortex 19*: 2880–2890.

Stenneken, P., Egetemeir, J., Schulte-Körne, G., Müller, H. J., Schneider, W. X., and Finke K. (2011). Slow perceptual processing at the core of developmental dyslexia: A parameter-based assessment of visual attention. *Neuropsychologia 49*: 3454–3465.

Townsend, J. T. and Ashby, F. G. (1982). Experimental test of contemporary mathematical models of visual letter recognition. *Journal of Experimental Psychology: Human Perception and Performance 8*: 834–864.

Townsend, J. T. and Landon, D. E. (1982). An experimental and theoretical investigation of the constant-ratio rule and other models of visual letter confusion. *Journal of Mathematical Psychology* 25: 119–162.

Treisman, A. M. and Gelade, G. (1980). A feature-integration theory of attention. *Cognitive Psychology* 12: 97–136.

Treisman, A. M. and Gormican, S. (1988). Feature analysis in early vision: Evidence from search asymmetries. *Psychological Review* 95: 15–48.

Treue, S. and Martinez-Trujillo, J. C. M. (1999). Feature-based attention influences motion processing gain in macaque visual cortex. *Nature* 399: 575–579.

van Oeffelen, M. P. and Vos, P. G. (1982). Configurational effects on the enumeration of dots: Counting by groups. *Memory & Cognition* 10: 396–404.

van Oeffelen, M. P. and Vos, P. G. (1983). An algorithm for pattern description on the level of relative proximity. *Pattern Recognition* 16: 341–348.

Vangkilde, S., Coull, J. T., and Bundesen, C. (2012). Great expectations: Temporal expectation modulates perceptual processing speed. *Journal of Experimental Psychology: Human Perception and Performance* 38: 1183–1191.

Vangkilde, S., Coull, J. T., and Bundesen, C. (2013). Great expectations: Temporal expectation modulates perceptual processing speed. *Journal of Experimental Psychology: Human Perception and Performance*. doi: 10.1037/a0026343.

Woodrow, H. (1914). The measurement of attention. *Psychological Monographs* 17(5, Whole No. 76): 1–158.

CHAPTER 38

COMPUTATIONAL MODELS: BOTTOM-UP AND TOP-DOWN ASPECTS

LAURENT ITTI AND ALI BORJI

PRELIMINARIES AND DEFINITIONS

COMPUTATIONAL models of visual attention have become popular over the past decade, we believe primarily for two reasons: First, models make testable predictions that can be explored by experimentalists as well as theoreticians; second, models have practical and technological applications of interest to the applied science and engineering communities. In this chapter, we take a critical look at recent attention modelling efforts. We focus on *computational models of attention* as defined by Tsotsos and Rothenstein (2011): Models which can process any visual stimulus (typically, an image or video clip), which can possibly also be given some task definition, and which make predictions that can be compared to human or animal behavioural or physiological responses elicited by the same stimulus and task. Thus, we here place less emphasis on abstract models, phenomenological models, purely data-driven fitting or extrapolation models, or models specifically designed for a single task or for a restricted class of stimuli. For theoretical models, we refer the reader to a number of previous reviews that address attention theories and models more generally (Itti and Koch 2001a; Paletta et al. 2005; Frintrop et al. 2010; Rothenstein and Tsotsos 2008; Gottlieb and Balan 2010; Toet 2011; Borji and Itti 2012b).

To frame our narrative, we embrace a number of notions that have been popularized in the field, even though many of them are known to only represent coarse approximations to biophysical or psychological phenomena. These include the *attention spotlight* metaphor (Crick 1984), the role of focal attention in binding features into coherent representations (Treisman and Gelade 1980), and the notions of an *attention bottleneck*, a *nexus*, and an *attention hand* as embodiments of the attentional selection process (Rensink 2000; Navalpakkam and Itti 2005). Further, we cast the problem of modelling attention computationally as comprising at least three facets: *guidance* (that is, which computations are involved in deciding where or what to attend to next?), *selection* (how is attended information segregated out of other incoming sensory information?), and *enhancement* (how is the information selected by attention processed differently than non-selected information?). While different theories and models have addressed all three aspects, most computational models as defined above have focused on the initial and primordial problem of guidance. Thus guidance is our primary focus, and we refer the reader to previous reviews on selection and enhancement (Allport et al.1993; Desimone and Duncan 1995; Reynolds and Desimone 1999; Driver and Frith 2000; Robertson 2003; Carrasco 2011). Note that guidance of attention is often thought of as involving *pre-attentive* computations to attract the focus of attention to the next most behaviourally relevant location (hence, attention guidance models might—strictly speaking—be considered pre-attention rather than attention models).

We explore models for exogenous (or bottom-up, stimulus-driven) attention guidance as well as for endogenous (or top-down, context-driven, or goal-driven) attention guidance. Bottom-up models process sensory information primarily in a feed-forward manner, typically applying successive transformations to visual features received over the entire visual field, so as to highlight those locations which contain the most interesting, important, conspicuous, or so-called *salient* information (Koch and Ullman 1985; Itti and Koch 2001a). Many, but not all, of these bottom-up models embrace the concept of a topographic saliency map, which is a spatial map where the map value at every location directly represents visual salience, abstracted from the details of why a location is salient or not (Koch and Ullman 1985). Under the saliency map hypothesis, the task of a computational model is then to transform an image into its spatially corresponding saliency map, possibly also taking into account temporal relations between successive video frames of a movie (Itti et al. 1998). Many models thus attempt to provide an operational definition of salience in terms of some image transform or some importance operator that can be applied to an image and that directly returns salience at every location, as we further examine below.

By far, the bottom-up, stimulus-driven models of attention have been more developed, probably because they are task-free, and thus often require no learning, training, or tuning to open-ended task or contextual information. This makes the definition of a purely bottom-up importance operator tractable. Another attractive aspect of bottom-up models—and especially saliency map models—is that, once implemented, they can easily be applied to any image and yield some output that can be tested against human or animal experimental data. Thus far, the most widely used test to validate predictions of attention models has been direct comparison between model output and eye movements recorded from humans or animals watching the same stimuli as given to the models (see, for example, among many others, Parkhurst et al. 2002; Itti 2006; Le Meur et al. 2006). Recently, several standard benchmark image and video datasets with corresponding eye movement recordings from pools of observers have been adopted, which greatly facilitates quantitative comparisons of computational models (Carmi and Itti 2006; Judd et al.

2009; Toet 2011; Li et al. 2011; Borji et al. 2012b). It is important to note, however, that several alternative measures have been employed as well (e.g. mouse clicks, search efficiency, reaction time, optimal information gain, scanpath similarity; see Eckstein et al. 2009; Borji and Itti 2012b). One caveat of metrics that compare model predictions to eye movements is that the distinction between covert and overt attention is seldom explicitly addressed by computational models: models usually produce as their final result a saliency map without further concern for how such map may give rise to an eye movement scanpath (Noton and Stark 1971) (but see Itti et al.2003; Ma and Deng 2009; Sun et al. 2012; and active vision/robotics systems like Orabona et al. 2005; Frintrop 2006; Belardinelli et al. 2006; Ajallooeian et al. 2009). Similarly, biases in datasets, models, and/or behaviour may affect the comparison results (Tatler and Vincent 2009; Tseng et al. 2009; Bonev et al.2012). While these are important for specialist audiences, here we should just remember that quantitative model evaluation metrics based on eye movements exist and are quite well established, although they remain approximate and should be used with caution (Tatler et al. 2005). Beyond metric issues, one last important consideration to ensure a valid direct comparison between model and eye movements is that conditions should be exactly matched between the model run and the experimental participants, which has not always been the case in previous work, as we discuss below.

While new bottom-up attention models are constantly proposed which rely on novel ways of analysing images to determine the most interesting or salient locations (we list over 50 of them below), several research efforts have also started to address the more complex problem of building top-down models that are tractable and can be implemented computationally. In the early days, top-down models have been mostly descriptive as they operated at the level of conceptual entities (e.g. collections of objects present in a scene, to be evaluated in terms of a mental model of which objects might be more important to a particular task of interest (Ballard et al. 1995)), and hence have lacked generalized computational implementations (because, for example, algorithms that can robustly recognize objects in scenes were not available). As some of these hurdles have been alleviated by the advent of powerful new theories and algorithms for object recognition, scene classification, decision-making under uncertainty, machine learning, and formal description languages that can capture task descriptions and background knowledge, exciting new models are beginning to emerge which significantly surpass purely bottom-up approaches in their ability to predict attention behaviour in complex situations. Implementing complete, autonomous computational models of top-down attention is particularly important to our theoretical understanding of task and context effects on attention, as these implementations remind us that some assumptions often made to develop abstract models may not give rise to tractable computational models (e.g. it is easy to note how humans are able to directly fixate a jar of jam when it is the next object required to make a sandwich (Land and Hayhoe 2001)—but how did they know that a jar is present and where it is located, if not through some previous bottom-up analysis of the visual environment?). As we further discuss in this chapter, these new computational models also often blur the somewhat artificial dichotomy between bottom-up and top-down processing, since the so-called top-down models do rely to a large extent on a bottom-up flow of incoming information that is merged with goals and task demands to give rise to the decision of where to attend next.

To frame the concepts exposed so far into a broader picture, we refer to Fig. 38.1 as a possible anchor to help organize our thoughts and discussions of how different elements of a visual scene understanding system may work together in the primate brain. In practice, few system-level efforts have included all components mentioned in Fig. 38.1, and most of our discussion will focus on computational models that implement parts of such a system.

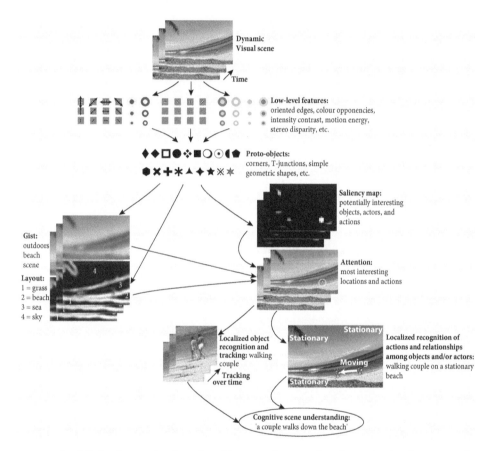

FIGURE 38.1 Minimal attention-based architecture for complex dynamic visual scene understanding. This diagram augments the triadic architecture of Rensink (2000), which identified three key components of visual processing: volatile (instantaneous) and parallel pre-attentive processing over the entire visual field, from the lowest-level features up to slightly more complex proto-object representations (top), identification of the setting (scene gist and layout; left), and attentional vision including detailed and more persistent object recognition within the spatially circumscribed focus of attention (right). Here we have extended Rensink's architecture to include a saliency map to guide attention bottom-up towards salient image locations, and action recognition in dynamic scenes. Reprinted from *Vision Research*, 45(2), Vidhya Navalpakkam and Laurent Itti, Modeling the influence of task on attention, pp. 205-31, Fig. 1, Copyright (2005), with permission from Elsevier.

In what follows, we first examine in more details the key concepts of early bottom-up attention models, and then provide an overview and comparison of many subsequent models that have provided new exciting insights into defining and computing bottom-up salience and attention. We then turn to top-down models, first motivating them from experimental evidence, and then examining in turn top-down models that modulate feature gains, that derive spatial priors from the gist of the visual scene, and that implement more complex information foraging and decision-making schemes. Finally, we discuss lessons learned from these models, including on the nature and interaction between bottom-up and top-down processes, and promising directions towards the creation of even more powerful combined bottom-up and top-down models.

EARLY BOTTOM-UP ATTENTION CONCEPTS AND MODELS

Early attention models have been primarily influenced by the Feature Integration Theory (Treisman and Gelade 1980), according to which incoming visual information is first analysed by early visual neurons which are sensitive to elementary visual features of the stimulus (e.g. colours, orientations, etc.). This analysis, operated in parallel over the entire visual field and at multiple spatial and temporal scales, gives rise to a number of cortical feature maps, where each map represents the amount of a given visual feature at any location in the visual field. Attention is then the process by which a region in space is selected and features within that region are reassembled or bound back together to yield more complex object representations (Fig. 38.2a). Koch and Ullman (1985) extended the theory by advancing the concept of a single topographic and scalar saliency map, receiving inputs from the feature maps, as a computationally efficient representation upon which to operate the selection of where to attend next: A simple maximum-detector or *winner-take-all* neural network (Arbib and Didday 1971) was proposed which would simply pick the next most salient location as the next attended one, while an active *inhibition-of-return* (Posner 1980) mechanism would later inhibit that location and thereby allow attention to shift as the winner-take-all network would pick the next most salient location (Fig. 38.2b). From these ideas, a number of fully computational models started to be developed (e.g. Fig. 38.2c, d).

At the core of these early models is the notion of visual salience, a signal that is computed in a stimulus-driven manner and which indicates that some location is significantly different from its surroundings and is worthy of attention. Early models computed visual salience from bottom-up features in several feature maps, including luminance contrast, red–green and blue–yellow colour opponency, and oriented edges (Itti et al. 1998). While visual salience is sometimes carelessly described as a physical property of a visual stimulus, it is important to remember that salience is the consequence of an

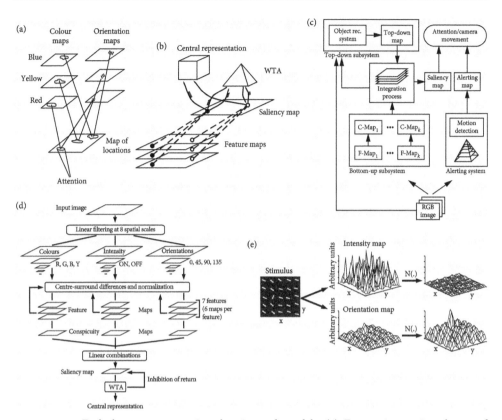

FIGURE 38.2 Early bottom-up attention theories and models. (a) Feature integration theory of Treisman and Gelade (1980) posits several feature maps, and a focus of attention that scans a map of locations and collects and binds features at the currently attended location. Adapted from Treisman, A., and Souther, J., Search asymmetry: A diagnostic for preattentive processing of seperable features, *Journal of Experimental Psychology*: General, 114(3), pp. 285-310, Copyright 1985, the American Psychological Association. (b) Koch and Ullman (1985) introduced the concept of a saliency map receiving bottom-up inputs from all feature maps, where a winner-take-all (WTA) network selects the most salient location for further processing. Reproduced from *Human Neurobiology* 4(4), Joch, C. and Ullman, S., Shifts in selective visual attention: towards the underlying neural circuitry, pp. 219-27, copyright 1985, *Journal of Human Neurobiology*. (c) Milanese et al. (1994) provided one of the earliest computational models. They included many elements of the Koch and Ullman framework, and added new components, such as an alerting subsystem (motion-based saliency map) and a top-down subsystem (which could modulate the saliency map based on memories of previously recognized objects). © 1998 IEEE. Reprinted, with permission, from Proceedings of IEEE Conference on Computer Vision and Pattern Recognition, Milanese, R., Wechsler, H., Gill, S., Bost, J.M., & Pun, T., Integration of bottom-up and top-down cues for visual attention using non-linear relaxation, pp. 781–785. (d) Itti et al. (1998) proposed a complete computational implementation of a purely bottom-up and task-independent model based on Koch and Ullman's theory, including multiscale feature maps, saliency map, winner-take-all, and inhibition of return. © 1998 IEEE. Reprinted, with permission, from IEEE *Transactions on Pattern Analysis and Machine Intelligence*, 20(11) Itti, L.; Koch, C. and Niebur, E., A model of saliency-based visual attention for rapid scene analysis. (e) One of the key elements of Itti et al.'s model is to clearly define an attention interest operator, here denoted N(.), whereby the weight

interaction of a stimulus with other stimuli, as well as with a visual system (biological or artificial). For example, a colour-blind person will have a dramatically different experience of visual salience than a person with normal colour vision, even when both look at exactly the same colourful physical scene. Nevertheless, because visual salience is believed to primarily arise from fairly low-level and stereotypical computations in the early stages of visual processing, the factors contributing to salience are generally quite comparable from one observer to the next, leading to similar experiences across a range of observers and of viewing conditions.

The essence of salience lies in enhancing the neural and perceptual representation of locations whose local visual statistics significantly differ from the broad surrounding image statistics, in some behaviourally relevant manner. This basic principle is intuitively motivated as follows. Imagine a simple search array as depicted in Fig. 38.2e, where one bar pops-out because of its unique orientation. Now imagine examining a feature map which is tuned to stimulus intensity (luminance) contrast: because there are many white bars on a black background, early visual neurons sensitive to local intensity contrast will respond vigorously to each of the bars (distractors and target alike, since all have identical intensity). Based on the pattern of activity in this map, in which essentially every bar elicits a strong peak of activity, one would be hard pressed to pick one location as being clearly more interesting and worthy of attention than any of the others. Intuitively, hence, one might want to apply some normalization operator N(.) which would give a very low overall weight to this map's contribution to the final saliency map. The situation is quite different when examining a feature map where neurons are tuned to local vertical edges. In this map, one location (where the single roughly vertical bar is) would strongly excite the neural feature detectors, while all other locations would elicit much weaker responses. Hence, one location clearly stands out and hence becomes an obvious target for attention. It would be desirable in this situation that the normalization operator N(.) give a high weight to this map's contribution to the final saliency map (Itti et al. 1998; Itti and Koch 2000, 2001a).

Early bottom-up attention models have created substantial interest and excitement in the community, especially as they were shown to be applicable to an unconstrained variety of stimuli, as opposed to more traditional computer vision approaches at the time, which often had been designed to solve a specific task in a specific environment (e.g. detect human faces in photographs taken from a standing human viewpoint (Viola

---

by which each feature map contributes to the final saliency map depends on how busy the feature map is. This embodies the idea that feature maps where one location significantly stands out from all others (as is the case in the orientation map shown) should strongly contribute to salience because they clearly vote for a particular location in space as the next focus of attention. In contrast, feature maps where many locations elicit comparable responses (e.g. intensity map shown) should not strongly contribute because they provide no clear indication of which location should be looked at next. © 1998 IEEE. Reprinted, with permission, from *IEEE Transactions on Pattern Analysis and Machine Intelligence*, 20(11) Itti, L.; Koch, C. and Niebur, E., A model of saliency-based visual attention for rapid scene analysis.

and Jones 2001)). Indeed, no parameter tuning nor any prior knowledge related to the contents of the images or video clips to be processed was necessary for any of many early results, as the exact same model processed psychophysical stimuli, filmed outdoors scenes, Hollywood movie footage, video games, and robotic imagery. This gave rise to model prediction results that included, for example, the reproduction by Itti et al.'s model of human behaviour in visual search tasks (e.g. pop-out versus conjunctive search (Itti and Koch 2000)); demonstration of strong robustness to image noise (Itti et al. 1998); automatic detection of traffic signs and other salient objects in natural environments filmed by a consumer-grade colour video camera (Itti and Koch 2001b); the detection of pedestrians in natural scenes (Miau et al. 2001); and of military vehicles in overhead imagery (Itti et al. 2001); and—most importantly—the widely demonstrated ability of the model to predict where humans look when freely viewing images or videos that range from search arrays to fractals to satellite images to everyday indoors and outdoors scenes (Parkhurst et al. 2002; Peters et al. 2005).

FLOURISHING OF BOTTOM-UP MODELS

Following initial success, many research groups started exploring the notions of bottom-up attention and visual salience, which has given rise to many new computational models. We summarize 53 bottom-up models along 13 different factors in Fig. 38.3. A thorough examination of all models is certainly not feasible in this limited space. Instead, we highlight below the main trends in seven categories that span from strong inspiration from biological vision to more abstract mathematical definitions and implementations of the concept of saliency. Models can coarsely be categorized as follows (but also see Tsotsos and Rothenstein 2011) for another possible taxonomy). Please note that some models fall under more than one category.

Cognitive models. Research into saliency modelling escalated after Itti et al.'s (1998) implementation of Koch and Ullman's (1985) computational architecture based on the Feature Integration Theory (Treisman and Gelade 1980). In cognitive models, which were the first ones to approach the problem of algorithmically computing saliency in arbitrary digital images, an input image is decomposed into a set of feature maps across spatial scales which are then linearly or non-linearly normalized and combined to form a master saliency map. An important element of this theory is the idea of centre-surround which defines saliency as distinctiveness of an image region in relation to its immediate surroundings. Almost all saliency models are directly or indirectly inspired by cognitive concepts of visual attention (e.g. Le Meur et al. 2006; Marat et al. 2009).

Information-theoretic models. Stepping back from biological implementation machinery, models in this category are based on the premise that localized saliency computations serve to maximize information sampled from one's environment. These models assign higher saliency values to scene regions with rare features. Information of visual feature F is $I(F) = -\log p(F)$ which is inversely proportional to the likelihood

	No	Model	Year	f1	f2	f3	f4	f5	f6	f7	f8	f9	f10	f11	f12	f13
Bottom-up visual saliency models for fixation prediction or salient region detection	1	Itti et al.	1998	+	-		-	+	-	-	+	f	+	CIO	C	-	-
	2	Privitera & Stark	2000	+	-		-	+	-	-	+	f	+	-	O	-	Stark and Choi
	3	Salah et al.	2002	+	+		-	+	-	-	+	-	+	O	G	DR	Digit & Face
	4	Itti et al.	2003	+	-	+	+	+	+	+	f	+	CIOFM	C	-	-
	5	Torralba	2003	+	+		-	+	-	-	+	s	-	CI	B	DR	Torralba et al.
	6	Sun & Fisher	2003	+	-		-	+	-	-	+	-	-	CIO	G	-	-
	7	Gao & Vasconcelos	2004	+	+		-	+	-	-	+	s	-	DCT	D	DR	Brodatz, Caltech
	8	Ouerhani et al.	2004	+	-		-	+	-	-	+	f	+	CIO+Corner	C	CC	Ouerhani
	9	Boccignone & Ferraro	2004	+	-		-	+	-	-	+	f	-	Optical Flow	B	-	BEHAVE
	10	Frintrop	2005	+	+	+	+	+	+	+	f/s	+/-	CIOM	C	-	-
	11	Itti & Baldi	2005	+	-	+	+	+	+	-	f	+	CIOFM	B	KL, AUC	ORIG-MTV
	12	Ma et al.	2005	+	-	+	-	-	-	+	f	+	M*	O	-	-
	13	Bruce & Tsotsos	2006	+	-		-	-	+	+	f	+	DOG, ICA	I	KL, ROC	Bruce and Tsotsos
	14	Navalpakkam & Itti	2006	+	+		-	+	-	+	+	s	+	CIO	C	-	-
	15	Zhai & Shah	2006	+	-	+	+	+	-	-	+	f	+	SIFT	O	-	-
	16	Harel et al.	2006	+	-		-	+	-	-	+	f	+	IO	G	AUC	Bruce and Tsotsos
	17	Le Meur et al.	2006	+	-		-	+	-	-	+	f	+	LM*	C	CC, KL	Le Meur et al.
	18	Walther & Koch	2006	+	-		-	+	-	+	+	f	+/-	CIO	C	-	-
	19	Peters & Itti	2007	+	+	+	+	+	-	-	i	+	CIOFM	P	KL, NSS	Peters and Itti
	20	Liu et al.	2007	+	-		-	+	-	-	+	f	-	Liu*	G	F-measure	Regional
	21	Shic & Scassellati	2007	+	-	+	+	+	-	+	f	+	CIOM	C	ROC	Shic and Scassellati
	22	Hou & Zhang	2007	+	-		-	+	-	+	+	f	+	FFT, DCT	S	NSS	DB of Hou and Zhang, 2007
	23	Cerf et al.	2007	+	+		-	+	-	+	+	f/s	+	CIO :)	C	AUC	Cerf et al.
	24	Le Meur et al.	2007	+	-	+	+	+	-	-	+	f	+	LM*	C	CC, KL	Le Meur et al.
	25	Mancas	2007	+	-	+	+	+	+	-	+	f	+	CI	I	CC	Le Meur et al.
	26	Guo et al.	2008	+	-		-	+	-	-	+	f	+	CIO	D	CC	Self data
	27	Zhang et al.	2008	+	-		-	+	-	+	+	f	+	DOG, ICA	B	KL, AUC	Bruce and Tsotsos
	28	Hou & Zhang	2008	+	-	+	+	+	-	+	f	+	ICA	I	AUC, KL	Bruce and Tsotsos, ORIG
	29	Pang et al.	2008	+	+		-	+	+	-	+	f	+	CIOM	G	NSS	ORIG, Self data
	30	Kootstra et al.	2008	+	-		-	+	-	-	+	f	+	Symmetry	C	CC	Kootstra et al.
	31	Ban et al.	2008	+	-	+	+	+	-	+	f	+	CIO+SYM	I	-	-
	32	Rajashekar et al.	2008	+	-		-	+	-	-	+	f	+	R*	S	CC	Rajashekar et al.
	33	Aziz and Mertsching	2008	+	-		-	+	-	+	+	f	+	CO, size, sym	I	-	-
	34	Kienzle et al.	2009	+	-		-	+	-	-	+	f	+	I	P	K*	Kienzle et al.
	35	Marat et al.	2009	+	-	+	-	+	-	+	f	+	SM*	C	NSS	Marat et al.
	36	Judd et al.	2009	+	-		-	+	-	-	+	f	+	J*	P	AUC	Judd et al.
	37	Seo & Milanfar	2009	+	-	+	+	+	+	+	f	+	LSK	I	AUC, KL	Bruce and Tsotsos, ORIG
	38	Rosin	2009	+	-		-	+	-	-	+	f	+	C+ Edge	O	PR, F-measure	DB of Liu et al, 2007
	39	Yin Li et al.	2009	-	+	+	+	+	+	+	s	+	RGB	S	DR	DB of Hou and Zhang, 2007
	40	Bian & Zhang	2009	+	-	+	+	-	+	+	f	+	FFT	S	AUC	Bruce and Tsotsos
	41	Diaz et al.	2009	+	-		-	+	-	-	+	f	+	CIO	O	AUC	Bruce and Tsotsos
	42	Zhang et al.	2009	+	-	+	-	+	-	+	f	+	DOG, ICA	B	KL, AUC	Bruce and Tsotsos
	43	Achanta et al.	2009	+	-		-	+	-	-	+	f	+	DOG	S	PR	DB of Liu et al, 2007
	44	Gao et al.	2009	+	-	+	+	+	-	+	f	+	CIO	D	AUC	Bruce and Tsotsos
	45	Chikkerur et al.	2010	+	+		-	+	-	+	+	f/s	+/-	CIO	B	AUC	Bruce and Tsotsos, Chikkerur
	46	Mahadaven & Vasconcelos	2010	+	-	+	-	+	-	+	f	+	I	D	DR, AUC	SVCL background data
	47	Avraham & Lindenbaum	2010	+	+		-	+	-	+	+	f/s	+/-	CIO	G	DR, CC	UWGT, Ouerhani et al.
	48	Jia Li et al.	2010	-	+	+	+	+	-	+	f	+	CIO	B	AUC	RSD, MTV, ORIG, Peters and Itti
	49	Guo et al.	2010	+	-	+	+	+	+	+	f/s	+/-	FFT	S	DR	Self data
	50	Borji et al.	2010	+	-		-	+	-	+	+	s	+/-	CIO	O	DR	-
	51	Goeferman et al.	2010	+	-		-	+	-	-	+	-	+	C :)	O	AUC	DB of Hou and Zhang, 2007
	52	Murray et al.	2011	+	-		-	+	-	-	+	f	+	CIO	C	AUC, KL	Bruce and Tsotsos, Judd et al.
	53	Wang et al.	2011	+	-		-	+	-	-	+	f	+	ICA	I	AUC	Self data
Top-down (general models)	54	McCallum	1995	-	+		-	+	-	+	-	i	+	-	R	-	Self data
	55	Rao et al.	1995	-	+		-	+	-	-	+	s	+	CIO	O	-	Self data
	56	Ramstrom & Christiansen	2002	-	+		-	+	-	-	+	-	+	CI	O	-	-
	57	Sprague & Ballard	2003	-	+	+	-	+	+	+	i	-	S*	R	-	-
	58	Renninger et al.	2004	-	+		-	+	-	+	-	s	-	Edgelet	I	DR	Self data
	59	Navalpakkam & Itti	2005	-	+		-	+	-	+	+	-	+	CIO	C	-	-
	60	Paletta et al.	2005	-	+		-	+	-	-	+	-	-	SIFT	R	DR	COIL-20, TSG-20
	61	Jodogne & Piater	2007	-	+		-	+	-	-	+	i	-	SIFT	R	-	-
	62	Butko & Movellan	2009	-	+	+	+	+	+	+	s	-	-	R	-	-
	63	Verma & McOwan	2009	+	-		-	+	-	+	-	s	-	CIO	O	-	-
	64	Borji et al.	2010	-	+		-	+	-	-	+	i	-	CIO	R	-	self data
	65	Borji et al.	2012	-	+		-	+	+	-	+	i	-	CIO	B	AUC, NSS	self data

FIGURE 38.3 Survey of bottom-up and top-down computational models, classified according to 13 factors. Factors in order are: Bottom-up (f_1), Top-down (f_2), Spatial (-)/Spatiotemporal (+) (f_3), Static (f_4), Dynamic (f_5), Synthetic (f_6) and Natural (f_7) stimuli, Task-type (f_8), Space-based(+)/Object-based(-) (f_9), Features (f_{10}), Model type (f_{11}), Measures (f_{12}), and Used dataset (f_{13}). In Task type (f_8) column: free-viewing (f); target search (s); interactive (i). In Features (f_{10}) column: CIO: colour, intensity, and orientation saliency; CIOFM: CIO plus flicker and motion saliency; M* = motion saliency, static saliency, camera motion, object (face) and aural saliency (Speech-music); LM* = contrast sensitivity, perceptual decomposition, visual masking and centre–surround interactions; Liu* = centre–surround histogram, multi-scale contrast and colour spatial-distribution; R* = luminance, contrast, luminance-bandpass, contrast-bandpass; SM* = orientation and motion; J* = CIO, horizontal line, face, people detector, gist, etc.; S* = colour matching, depth and lines; :) = face. In Model type (f_{11}) column, R means that a model is based RL. In Measures (f_{12}) column: K* = used

of observing F (i.e. $p(F)$). By fitting a distribution $P(F)$ to features (e.g. using Gaussian Mixture Model or Kernels), rare features can be immediately found by computing $P(F)^{-1}$ in an image. While in theory using any feature space is feasible, usually these models (inspired by efficient coding representations in visual cortex) utilize a sparse set of basis functions (using independent component analysis (ICA) filters) learned from a repository of natural scenes. Some basic approaches in this domain are AIM (Bruce and Tsotsos 2005), Rarity (Mancas 2007), LG (Local + Global image patch rarity) (Borji and Itti 2012a), and incremental coding length models (Hou and Zhang 2008).

Graphical models. Graphical models are generalized Bayesian models which have been employed for modelling complex attention mechanisms over space and time. Torralba (2003) proposed a Bayesian approach for modelling contextual effects on visual search which was later adopted in the SUN model (Zhang et al. 2008) for fixation prediction in free viewing. Itti and Baldi (Itti and Baldi 2005) defined surprising stimuli as those which significantly change beliefs of an observer. Harel et al. (2007) propagated similarity of features in a fully connected graph to build a saliency map. Avraham and Lindenbaum (2010), Li and Fei-Fei (2010), and Rezazadegan Tavakoli et al. (2011) have also exploited Bayesian concepts for saliency modelling.

Decision-theoretic models. This interpretation states that attention is driven optimally with respect to the end task. Gao and Vasconcelos (2004) argued that for recognition, salient features are those that best distinguish a class of objects of interest from all other classes. Given some set of features $X = \{X_1, \cdots, X_d\}$, at locations l, where each location is assigned a class label Y with $Y_l = 0$ corresponding to background and $Y_l = 1$ indicates objects of interest, saliency is then a measure of mutual information (usually Kullback-Leibler divergence (KL)), computed as $I(X, Y) = \sum_{i=1}^{d} (X_i, Y)$. Besides having good accuracy in predicting eye fixations, these models have been very successful in computer vision applications (e.g. anomaly detection and object tracking).

Spectral-analysis models. Instead of processing an image in the spatial domain, these models derive saliency in the frequency domain. This way, there is no need for image processing operations such as centre-surround or segmentation. Hou and Zhang (2007) derive saliency for an image with amplitude $A(f)$ and phase $P(f)$ as follows: The log spectrum $L(f)$ is computed from the down-sampled image. From $L(f)$, the spectral residual $R(f)$ is obtained by multiplying $L(f)$ with $h_n(f)$ which is an $n \times n$ local average filter and subtracting the result from itself. Saliency map is then the inverse Fourier transform of the exponential of amplitude plus phase (i.e. $S(x) = F^{-1}[\exp(R(f) + P(f))]$). The saliency of each point is squared to indicate the estimation error and is then smoothed with

---

Wilcoxon–Mann–Whitney test (the probability that a random chosen target patch receives higher saliency than a randomly chosen negative one); DR means that models have used a measure of detection/classification rate to determine how successful a model was. PR stands for Precision-Recall. In dataset (f_{13}) column: Self data means that authors gathered their own data. For detailed definition of these factors please refer to Borji and Itti (2012b).

a Gaussian filter for better visual effect. Bian and Zhang (2009) and Guo and Zhang (2010) proposed spatio-temporal models in the spectral domain.

Pattern classification models. Models in this category use machine learning techniques to learn 'stimuli-saliency' mappings from image features to eye fixations. They estimate saliency s; $p(s|f)$ where f is a feature vector which could be the contrast of a location and its surrounding neighbourhood. Kienzle et al. (2007), Peters and Itti (2007), and Judd et al. (2009) used image patches, scene gist, and a vector of several features at each pixel, respectively, and used classical support vector machine (SVM) and regression classifiers for learning saliency. In an extension of Judd's model, Borji (2012) showed that using a richer set of features, including bottom-up saliency maps of other models and within-object regions (e.g. eye within faces) along with a boosting classifier, leads to higher fixation predicting accuracy. Rezazadegan Tavakoli et al. (2011) used sparse sampling and kernel density estimation to estimate the above probability in a Bayesian framework. Note that some of these models may not be purely bottom-up since they use features that guide top-down attention, for example faces or text (Cerf et al. 2008; Judd et al. 2009).

Other models. Some other models exist that do not easily fit into our categorization. For example, Seo and Milanfar (2009) proposed self-resemblance of local image structure for saliency detection. The idea of decorrelation of neural response was used for a normalization scheme in the Adaptive Whitening Saliency (AWS) model (Garcia-Diaz et al. 2009). Kootstra et al. (2008) developed symmetry operators for measuring saliency and Goferman et al. (2010) proposed a context-aware saliency detection model with successful applications in re-targeting and summarization.

An important trend to consider is that over the past years starting from Liu et al. (2007), models have begun to diverge into two different classes: models of *fixation prediction* and models of *salient region detection*. While the goal of the former models is to predict locations that grab attention, the latter models attempt to segment the most salient object or region in a scene. A saliency operator is usually used to estimate the extent of the object that is predicted to be the most likely first attended object. Evaluation is often done by measuring precision-recall of saliency maps of a model against ground-truth data (explicit saliency judgements of subjects by annotating salient objects or clicking on locations). Some models in two categories have compared themselves against each other, without being aware of the distinction.

Fig. 38.3 shows a list of models and their properties according to thirteen qualitative criteria derived from behavioural and computational studies. The majority (53 out of 65) of covered attention models consists of bottom-up models, indicating that at least from a computational perspective it is easier to formulate attention guidance mechanisms based on low-level image features. This is reinforced by the existence of several established benchmark datasets and standard evaluation scores for bottom-up models. The situation is the opposite for top-down attention modelling although we have recently initiated an effort to share data and code (Borji et al. 2012a, 2012c).

A brief comparison of saliency maps of 26 models on a few test images (Fig. 38.4) shows large differences in appearance of the maps generated by different models. Some models generate very sparse maps while others are smoother. This makes fair model comparison a challenge since some scores may be influenced by smoothness of a map

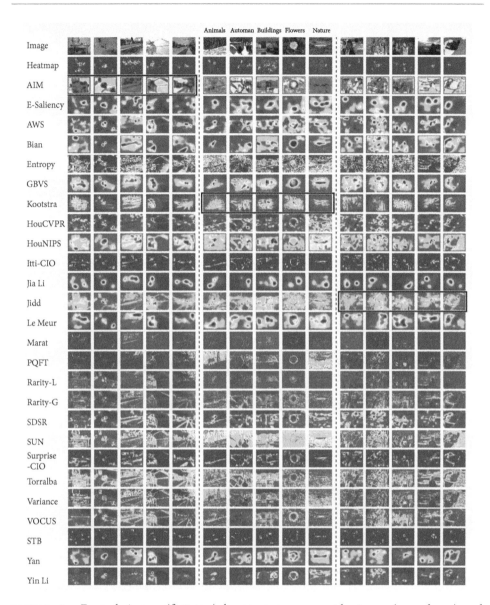

Animals Automan Buildings Flowers Nature

Image
Heatmap
AIM
E-Saliency
AWS
Bian
Entropy
GBVS
Kootstra
HouCVPR
HouNIPS
Itti-CIO
Jia Li
Jidd
Le Meur
Marat
PQFT
Rarity-L
Rarity-G
SDSR
SUN
Surprise-CIO
Torralba
Variance
VOCUS
STB
Yan
Yin Li

FIGURE 38.4 Example images (first row), human eye movement heatmaps (second row), and saliency maps from 26 computational models. The three vertical dashed lines separate the three datasets used (Bruce and Tsotsos 2005; and Judd et al. 2009). Black rectangles indicate the model originally associated with a given image dataset. See Borji et al. (2012b) for additional details.

(Tatler et al. 2005). Recently, Borji et al. (2012b) performed a detailed investigation of models to quantify their correlations with human attentional behaviour. This study suggests that so far the so-called 'shuffled AUC (Area Under the ROC Curve)' score (Zhang et al. 2008) is the most robust (this score uses distributions of human fixations on other stimuli than the one being scored to establish a baseline, which attenuates the effects of certain biases in eye movements datasets, the strongest being a bias towards looking

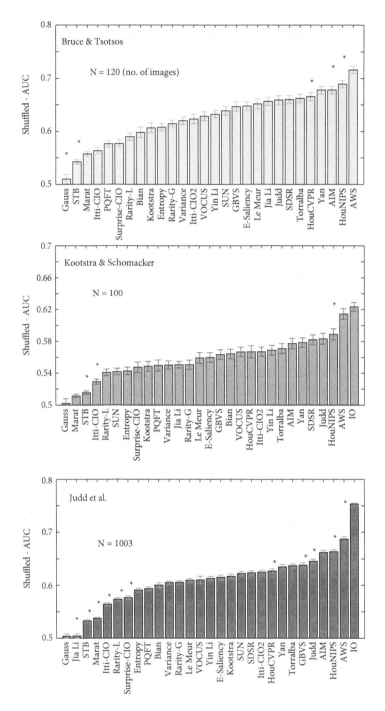

FIGURE 38.5 Ranking visual saliency models over three image datasets. Left column: Bruce and Tsotsos (2005), Middle column: Kootstra et al. (2008), and Right column: Judd et al. (2009) using shuffled AUC score. Stars indicate statistical significance using t-test (95%, $p \leq 0.05$) between consecutive models. Error bars indicate standard error of the mean (SEM): $\frac{\sigma}{\sqrt{N}}$, where

preferentially near the centre of any image). Results are shown in Fig. 38.5. This model evaluation shows a gap between current models and human performance. This gap is smaller for some datasets, but overall exists. Discovering and adding more top-down features to models will hopefully boost their performance. The analysis also shows that some models are very effective (e.g. HouNIPS, Bian, HouCVPR, Torralba, and Itti-CIO2 in Fig. 38.5) and also very fast, providing a trade-off between accuracy and speed necessary for many applications.

Despite past progress in bottom-up saliency modelling and fixation prediction while freely viewing natural scenes, several open questions remain that should be answered in the future. The most confusing one is that of 'centre bias', whereby humans often appear to preferentially look near an image's centre. It is believed to be largely caused by stimulus bias (e.g. photographer bias, whereby photographers tend to frame interesting objects near the image centre). Collecting fixation datasets with no or less centre bias, and studying its role on model evaluation needs to be addressed with natural scenes (see, for example, Parkhurst et al. 2002 and Peters et al. 2005 for unbiased artificial datasets of fractal images). As opposed to saliency modelling on static scenes, the domain of spatio-temporal attention remains less explored (see Dorr et al. 2010 and Wang et al. 2012 for examples). Emphasis should be on finding cognitive factors (e.g. actor, non-actor) rather than simple bottom-up features (e.g. motion, flicker, or focus of expansion), and some of the top-down models discussed below have started to explore how more semantic scene analysis can influence attention. Another aspect is the study of attention on affective and emotional stimuli. Although a database of fixations on emotional images has been gathered by Ramanathan et al. (2010), it is still not clear whether current models can be extended to explain such fixations.

Top-Down Guidance of Attention by Task Demands

Research towards understanding the mechanisms of top-down attention has given rise to two broad classes of models: models which operate on semantic content, and models

---

σ is the standard deviation and N is the number of images. The Judd model uses centre feature, gist and horizon line, and object detectors for cars, faces, and human body. Itti-CIO2 is the approach proposed by Itti et al. (1998) that uses a normalization scheme known as Maxnorm: For each feature map, find the global max M and find the average m of all other local maxima. Then just weight the map by $(M - m)^2$. In the Itti-CIO method (Itti and Koch 2000), normalization is: Convolve each map by a Difference of Gaussian (DoG) filter, cut off negative values, and iterate this process for a few times. As results show the Maxnorm normalization scheme performs better. In the literature, the majority of models have been compared against the Itti-CIO model. See Borji et al. (2012b) for additional details on these results.

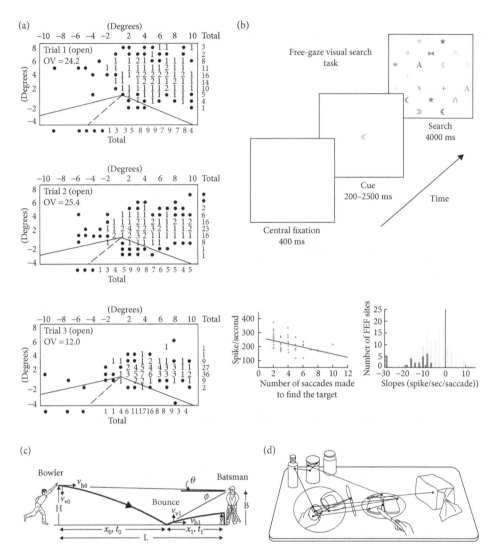

FIGURE 38.6 Experimental motivation to explore spatial biases, feature biases, and more complex semantic top-down models. (a) Percentage of fixations onto different road locations while human drivers drove at 50 miles/hour on an open road three times (once each panel; dots indicate non-zero percentages smaller than 1). We can see that over the three repetitions (top to bottom panels), eye fixations started clustering more tightly around the left side of the horizon line. This motivates top-down models to learn over time how a task may induce some spatial biases in the deployment of attention. Reproduced from Ronald R. Mourant and Thomas H. Rockwell, *Human Factors* 12(1), Mapping Eye-Movement Patterns to the Visual Scene in Driving: An Exploratory Study, pp. 81–7, copyright© 1970 by Sage Publications. Reprinted by Permission of SAGE Publications. (b) Neural recordings in the frontal eye fields (FEF) as monkeys searched from a cued target among various distractors reveal that the number of saccades the animal made to find the target is negatively correlated with neural firing at the target location around (±50ms) the onset of the first saccade (scatter plot shows examples, one dot per trial, from one recording site, and the negatively sloped

which operate on raw pixels and images. Models in the first category are not fully computational in the sense used in the present chapter, in that they require that an external expert (typically, one or more humans) first pre-processes raw experimental recordings, often to create semantic annotations (e.g. translate from recorded video frames and gaze positions into sequences that describe which objects were being looked at). For example, in a block copying task (Ballard et al. 1995), the observers' algorithm for completing the task was revealed by their pattern of eye movements: first select a target block in the model by fixating it, then find a matching block in the resource pool, then revisit the model to verify the block's position, then fixate the workspace to place the new block in the corresponding position. Other studies have used naturalistic interactive or immersive environments to give high-level accounts of gaze behaviour in terms of objects, agents, 'gist' of the scene, and short-term memory (Yarbus 1967; Henderson and Hollingworth 1999; Rensink 2000; Land and Hayhoe 2001; Sodhi et al.2002; Hayhoe et al. 2003) to describe, for example, how task-relevant information guides eye movements while subjects make a sandwich (Land and Hayhoe 2001; Hayhoe et al. 2003) or how distractions such as setting the radio or answering a phone affect eye movements while driving (Sodhi et al. 2002).

While such perceptual studies have provided important constraints regarding goal-oriented high-level vision, additional work is needed to translate these descriptive results into fully automated computational models that can be used in the application domains mentioned above. That is, although the block copying task reveals observers' algorithm for completing the task, it does so only in the high-level language of 'workspace' and 'blocks' and 'matching'. In order for a machine vision system to

---

linear regression; histogram shows distributions of slopes over all recording sites, with the significant ones in black and all others in grey). This suggests that top-down models can also exploit biasing for specific features of a search target to attempt to guide attention faster towards the target. Reprinted from *Neuron* 70, (6), Huihui Zhou and Robert Desimone, Feature-Based Attention in the Frontal Eye Field and Area V4 during Visual Search, pp. 1205–17, Copyright (2011), with permission from Elsevier. (c) Eye movement recordings of cricket batsmen revealed that their 'eye movements monitor the moment when the ball is released, make a predictive saccade to the place where they expect it to hit the ground, wait for it to bounce, and follow its trajectory for 100–200 ms after the bounce'. Reproduced from Nature Neuroscience, 3(12), Michael F. Land & Peter McLeod, From eye movements to actions: how batsmen hit the ball, pp. 1340–1345, © 2000, Nature Publishing Group. This suggests that some knowledge of physics, gravity, bouncing, etc. may be necessary to fully understand human gaze behaviour in this more complex scenario. (d) Eye movement recordings while making a sandwich are clearly aimed towards the next required item during the unfolding of the successive steps required by the task, with very little searching or exploration. Reprinted from Vision Research, 41 (25–26), Michael F. Land and Mary Hayhoe, In what ways do eye movements contribute to everyday activities?, pp. 3559–3565, Fig. 38.1b, Copyright (2001), with permission from Elsevier. Thus, recognition and memorization of objects in the scene are also likely to be required of top-down models to tackle such more complex scenarios.

replicate human observers' ability to understand, locate, and exploit such visual concepts, we need a 'compiler' to translate such high-level language into the assembly language of vision—that is, low-level computations on a time-varying array of raw pixels. Unfortunately, a general computational solution to this task is tantamount to solving computer vision.

From behavioural and in particular eye-tracking experiments during execution of real-world tasks, several key computational factors can be identified which can be implemented in computational models (Fig. 6):

- *Spatial biases*, whereby a given high-level task or top-down set may make some region of space more likely to contain relevant information. For example, when the task is to drive, it is important to keep our eyes on the road (Fig. 38.6a). We describe below how bottom-up attention models can be enhanced by considering such task-driven spatial constraints, for example to suppress salient stimuli that lie outside the task-relevant region of visual space. These models are motivated by both psychophysical and physiological evidence of spatial biasing of attention based on both short-term and long-term top-down cues (Chun and Jiang 1998; Summerfield et al. 2011), resulting in enhancement of attended visual regions and suppression of the unattended ones (Brefczynski and DeYoe 1999; Kastner et al. 1999).
- *Feature biases*, whereby the task may dictate that some visual features (e.g. some colours) are more likely associated with items of interest than other features (Fig. 38.6b). Bottom-up models can also be enhanced to account for feature biases, for example by modulating according to top-down goals the relative weights by which different feature maps contribute to a saliency map (e.g. when searching for a blue item, increase the gain of blue-selective feature maps). These models also are motivated by experimental studies of so-called feature-based attention (Treue and Martinez Trujillo 1999; Saenz et al. 2002; Zhou and Desimone 2011; Martinez-Trujillo 2011) and, in particular, recent theories and experiments investigating the role of the pulvinar nucleus in carrying out such biases (Baluch and Itti 2011; Saalmann et al. 2012).
- *Object-based and cognitive biases*, whereby knowing about objects, about how they may interact with each other, and about how they obey the laws of physics such as gravity and friction, may help humans make more efficient decisions of where to attend next to achieve a certain top-down goal (e.g. playing cricket, Fig. 6c, or making a sandwich, Fig. 6d). Models can be taught how to recognize objects and possibly other aspects of the world, to enable semantic reasoning that may give rise to these more complex top-down attention behaviours. These models are also motivated by recent experimental findings (Võ and Henderson 2009; Schmidt and Zelinsky 2009; Hwang et al. 2011).

We review top-down models that have implemented these strategies below. Although spatial biases have historically been studied first, we start with feature biasing models as those are conceptually simpler extensions to the bottom-up models described in the previous sections.

Top-down biasing of bottom-up feature gains

A simple strategy to include top-down influences in a computational attention model is to modulate the low levels of visual processing of the model according to the top-down task demands. This embodies the concept of *feature-based attention*, whereby increased neural response can be detected in monkeys and humans to visual locations which contain features that match a feature of current behavioural interest (e.g. locations that contain upward moving dots when the animal's task is to monitor upward motion; Treue and Martinez Trujillo 1999; Saenz et al. 2002; Zhou and Desimone 2011).

While the idea of top-down feature biases was already present in early conceptual models like the *Guided Search* theory (Wolfe 1994) and *FeatureGate* (Cave 1999), the question for computational modellers has been how exactly the feature gains should be adjusted to yield optimal expected enhancement of a desired target among unwanted distractors (Fig. 38.7). Earlier models have used supervised learning techniques to compute feature gains from example images where targets of interest had been manually indicated (Itti and Koch 2001b; Frintrop et al. 2005; Borji et al. 2011). A more recent approach uses eye movement recordings to determine these weights (Zhao and Koch 2011). Interestingly, it has recently been proposed that an optimal set of weight can be computed in closed form given distributions of expected features for both targets of interest to the task and irrelevant clutter or distractors. In this approach, each feature map is characterized by a target-to-distractor response ratio (or signal-to-noise ratio, SNR), and feature maps are simply assigned a weight that is inversely proportional to their SNR (Navalpakkam and Itti 2006; Navalpakkam and Itti 2007). In addition to giving rise to a fully computational model, this theory has also been found to explain many aspects of human guided search behaviour (Navalpakkam and Itti 2007; Serences and Saproo 2010).

Note how the models of Fig. 38.7 start introducing a blur between the notions of bottom-up and top-down processing. In these models, indeed, the effect of top-down knowledge is to modulate the way in which bottom-up computations are carried out. This opens the question of whether a pure bottom-up state may ever exist, and what the corresponding gain values may be (e.g. unity as has been assumed in many models?). These questions are also being raised by a number of recent experiments (Theeuwes 2010; Awh et al. 2012), and are further discussed below.

Spatial priors and scene context

In a recent model, Ehinger et al. (2009) investigated whether a model that, in addition to a bottom-up saliency map, learns spatial priors about where people may

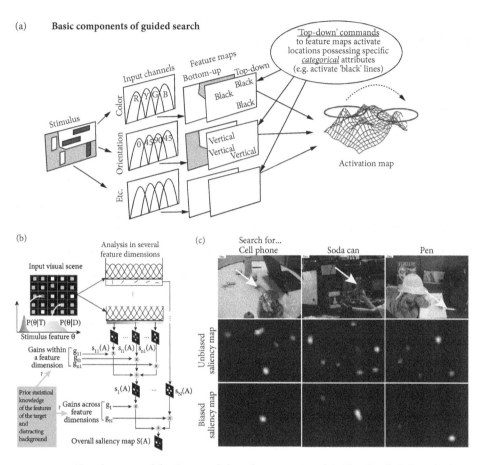

FIGURE 38.7 Top-down models that modulate feature gains. (a) The Guided Search theory of Wolfe (1994) predicted that bottom-up feature maps can be weighted and modulated by top-down commands. Reproduced from Psychonomic Bulletin & Review, 1(2), pp. 202–238, Guided Search 2.0 A revised model of visual search, Jeremy M. Wolfe, Fig. 38.2, ©1994, Springer Science and Business Media. With kind permission from Springer Science and Business Media. (b) Computational framework to optimally compute the weight of each feature map, given top-down knowledge of the expected distribution of feature values θ for both target objects ($P(\theta|T)$) and distractors ($P(\theta|D)$). The gain of each feature is set inversely proportionally to the expected target-to-distractor signal-to-noise ratio given these distributions. ©2006, IEEE. Reprinted, with permission, from Navalpakkam, V. and Itti, L., An Integrated Model of Top-Down and Bottom-Up Attention for Optimizing Detection Speed, IEEE Proceedings, 2, pp. 2049–2056. (c) Examples of images (top row), naive unweighted saliency maps (middle row), and optimally biased saliency maps based on feature distributions gathered from sample training images (bottom row). Although the object of interest was not the most salient according to a purely bottom-up model in these examples, it becomes the most salient once the model is biased using top-down gains computed from the target and distractor feature distributions. © 2006, IEEE. Reprinted, with permission, from Navalpakkam, V. and Itti, L., An Integrated Model of Top-Down and Bottom-Up Attention for Optimizing Detection Speed, IEEE Proceedings, 2, pp. 2049–2056.

appear and a feature prior about what people may look like would better predict gaze patterns of humans searching for people. Indeed, several earlier studies had suggested that bottom-up models, while widely demonstrated to correlate with human fixations during free viewing, may not well predict fixations of participants once they are given a top-down task, for example a search task (Zelinsky et al. 2006; Foulsham and Underwood 2007; Henderson et al. 2007; Einhäuser et al. 2008). One may argue, however, especially in the light of our above discussion of whether pure bottom-up salience is a valid concept, that in these experiments the models were at an unfair disadvantage: Human participants had been provided with some information which had not been communicated to models (e.g. search for a specific target, shown for 1 second before the search (Zelinsky et al. 2006); search of objects in a category or for a specific object (Foulsham and Underwood 2007); search for a small bulls-eye pattern or for a local higher-contrast region (Einhäuser et al. 2008); or count people (Henderson et al. 2007)). Ehinger et al. addressed this by proposing a model that combines three sources of information (Fig. 38.8a): First, a 'scene context' map was derived from learning the associations between holistic or global scene features (coarsely capturing the gist of the scene (Torralba, 2003)) and the locations where humans appeared in scenes with given holistic features (trained over 1,880 example images). This map, which is of central interest to this section of our chapter, thus learned the typical locations where humans were expected to appear in different views of street scenes. This learning step produces a prior on locations that can be used to filter out salient responses in locations that are highly unlikely to contain the target (e.g. in the sky, assuming that no human was seen flying in the training dataset). Second, a person detector was run in a sliding window manner over the entire image, creating a 'target features' map that highlighted locations that closely look like humans. This provides an alternative to learning feature gains as discussed above; instead, an object detector algorithm is trained for the desired type of target. While possibly more efficient than gain modulation, this approach suffers from lower biological plausibility (see Rao et al. 2002 and Orabona et al. 2005 for related models). Third and finally, a standard bottom-up 'saliency map' provided additional candidate locations (also see Oliva et al. 2003 for earlier related work, integrating only saliency and scene context). Ehinger et al. found that the model which combined all three maps outperformed any of the three component models taken alone (Fig. 8b).

In a related model, Peters and Itti (2007) also used a combination of bottom-up saliency maps and top-down spatial maps derived from the holistic gist of the scene, but their top-down maps were directly learned from eye movements of human observers, playing the same 3D video games as would be used for testing (games included driving, exploration, flight combat, etc.; note that since players control the game's virtual camera viewpoint, each run of such games gives rise to a unique set of viewpoints and of generated scenes). The bottom-up component of this model is based on the Itti–Koch saliency model (Itti et al. 1998), which predicts interesting locations based on low-level visual features such as luminance contrast, colour contrast, orientation, and motion. The top-down component is based on the idea of 'gist', which in psychophysical terms is the ability of people to roughly describe the type and overall layout of an image after only a very brief presentation

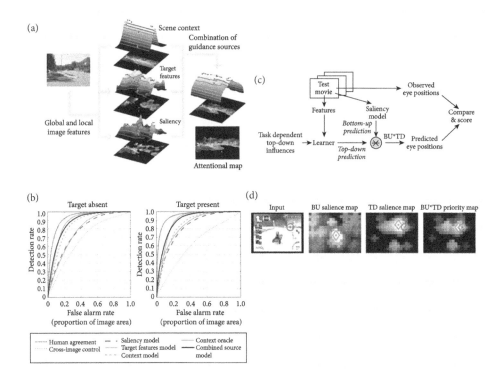

FIGURE 38.8 Top-down models that involve spatial modulation. (a) Model of Ehinger at al. (2009) where an attention map is informed by three guidance sources, given the task of finding people: (1) a spatial map that, based on the coarse scene structure, provides a spatial prior on where humans might appear in the given scene (e.g. they might appear on pavements); (2) a map that indicates where visual features in the image that resemble the features of the desired targets are observed; (3) a bottom-up saliency map. Reproduced from Krista A. Ehinger, Barbara Hidalgo-Sotelo, Antonio Torralba et al., Modelling search for people in 900 scenes: A combined source model of eye guidance, Visual Cognition, 17 (6–7), pp. 945–78 © 2009, Taylor & Francis with permission. http://www.informaworld.com. (b) The combined-source model performs best and significantly better than any of the three component models taken alone and also performs better than an empirical context oracle (where a set of humans manually indicated where humans might appear in the given scenes). (c) A model that learns top-down priors from human gaze behaviour while engaged in complex naturalistic tasks, such as driving. A task-dependent learner component builds, during a training phase, associations between distinct coarse types of scenes and observed eye movements (e.g. drivers tend to look to the left when the road turns left). During testing, exposure to similar scenes gives rise to a top-down salience map, which is combined with a standard bottom-up salience map to give rise to the final (BU*TD) priority map that guides attention. (d) Example results from the model of (c) applied to a driving video game. Blue diamonds represent the peak location in each map and orange circles represent the current eye position of the human driver. Here the bottom-up (BU) salience map considers that the main character is the most interesting scene element, but, as more correctly predicted by the top-down (TD) map, the driver is looking into the road's turn and on the horizon line. © 2007 IEEE. Reprinted, with permission, Peters, R. J. and Itti, L., Beyond bottom-up: Incorporating task-dependent influences into a computational model of spatial attention, IEEE Conference on Computer Vision and Pattern Recognition, pp. 1–8.

(Li et al. 2002), and to use this information to guide subsequent target searches (Torralba 2003). This model (Fig. 38.8c) decomposes each video frame into a low-level image signature intended to capture some of the properties of 'gist' (Siagian and Itti 2007), and learns to pair the low-level signatures from a series of video clips with the corresponding eye positions; once trained, it generates predicted gaze density maps from the gist signatures of previously unseen video frames. To test these bottom-up and top-down components, we compared their predicted gaze density maps with the actual eye positions recorded while people interactively played video games (Fig. 8d).

More complex top-down models

Many top-down models have been proposed which include higher degrees of cognitive scene understanding. Already in the late 1990s several models included a top-down component that decided where to look next based on what had been observed so far (e.g. Rybak et al. 1998; Schill et al. 2001; also see Itti and Koch 2001a for review). In robotics, the notion of combining or alternating between different behaviours (such as exploration versus search, or bottom-up versus top-down) has also led to several successful models (Sprague and Ballard 2003; Forssén et al. 2008; Burattini et al. 2010; Xu et al. 2010). More recently, and our focus here, probabilistic inference and reasoning techniques, very popular in computer vision, have started to be used in attention models.

In many recent models, the saliency map of bottom-up models is conserved as a data-driven source of information for an overarching top-down system (more complicated than the feature or spatial biasing described above). For example, Boccignone and Ferraro (2004) developed an overt attention system where the top-down component is a random walker that follows an information foraging strategy over a bottom-up saliency map. They demonstrate simulated gaze patterns that better match human distributions (Tatler et al. 2011). Interesting related models have been proposed where bottom-up and top-down attention interact through object recognition (Ban et al. 2010; Lee et al. 2011), or by formulating a task as a classification problem with missing features, with top-down attention then providing a choice process over the missing features (Hansen et al. 2011).

Of growing recent interest is the use of probabilistic reasoning and graphical models to explore how several sources of bottom-up and top-down information may combine in a Bayesian-optimal manner. For example, the model of Akamine et al. (2012) (also see Kimura et al. 2008) employs probabilistic graphical modelling techniques and considers the following factors, interacting in a dynamic Bayesian network (Fig. 38.9a): On the one hand, input video frames give rise to deterministic saliency maps. These are converted into stochastic saliency maps via a random process that affects the shape of salient blobs over time (e.g. dynamic Markov random field (Kimura et al. 2008)). An eye focusing map is then created which highlights maxima in the stochastic saliency map, additionally integrating top-down influences from an eye movement pattern (a stochastic selection between passive and active state with a learned transition probability

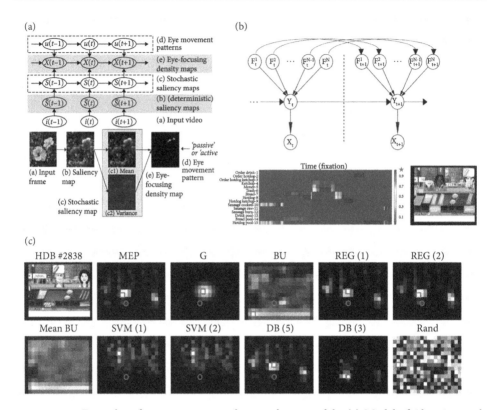

FIGURE 38.9 Examples of recent more complex top-down models. (a) Model of Akamine et al. (2012) which combines bottom-up saliency influences and top-down active/passive state influences over space and time using a dynamic Bayesian network. Although the top-down state is quite simple in this model (active vs. passive), the proposed mathematical framework could easily extend to more complex top-down influences. This material was originally published in The Computer Journal, 55(1), Fully Automatic Extraction of Salient Objects from Videos in Near Real Time, Kazuma Akamine, Ken Fukuchi, Akisato Kimura, and Shigeru Takagi, pp. 3–14, Fig. 38.4 © 2012, Oxford University Press and has been reproduced by permission of Oxford University Press http://comjnl.oxfordjournals.org/content/55/1/3.full.pdf+html. For permission to reuse this material, please visit http://www.oup.co.uk/academic/rights/permissions. (b) Graphical representation of the DBNs approach of Borji et al. (2012a) unrolled over two time-slices. X_t is the current saccade position, Y_t is the currently attended object, and F_t^i is the function that describes object i at the current scene. All variables are discrete. It also shows a time series plot of probability of objects being attended and a sample frame with tagged objects and eye fixation overlaid. (c) Sample predicted saccade maps of the DBN model (shown in b). Each red circle indicates the observer's eye position superimposed with each map's peak location (blue squares). Smaller distance indicates better prediction. Images from top-left to bottom-right are: a sample frame from the hot-dog bush game where the player has to serve customers food and drink; MEP stands for the mean eye position over all frames during the game play; G is just a trivial Gaussian map at the image centre; BU is the bottom-up saliency map of the Itti model; REG(1) is a regression model which maps the previous attended object to the current attended object and fixation location; REG(2) is similar to REG(1) but the input vector consists of the available objects at the scene augmented with the previously attended object; SVM(1) and SVM(2)

matrix). The authors use a particle filter with Markov chain Monte Carlo (MCMC) sampling to estimate the parameters; this technique, often used in machine learning, allows for fast and efficient estimation of unknown probability density functions. Although the top-down component is quite simple in this version of the model, it is easy to see how more sophisticated top-down and contextual influences could be integrated into the dynamic Bayesian network framework of Kimura et al. Several additional recent related models using graphical models have been proposed (e.g. Chikkerur et al. 2010).

Although few have been implemented as fully computational models, several efforts have started to develop models that perform reasoning over objects or other scene elements to make a cognitive decision of where to look next (Navalpakkam and Itti 2005; Yu et al. 2008; Beuter et al. 2009; Yu et al. 2012).

As a recent example, using probabilistic reasoning and inference tools, Borji et al. (2012a) introduced a framework to model top-down overt visual attention based on reasoning, in a task-dependent manner, about objects present in the scene and about previous eye movements. They designed a Dynamic Bayesian Network (DBN) that infers probability distributions over attended objects and spatial locations directly from observed data. Two basic concepts in this model are: (1) taking advantage of the sequence structure of tasks, which allows prediction of the future fixations from past fixations and knowledge about objects present in the scene. Graphical models have indeed been very successful in the past to model sequences with applications in different domains, including biology, time series modelling, and video processing, and (2) computing attention at the object level. Since objects are essential building blocks in scenes, it is reasonable to assume that humans have instantaneous access to task-driven object-level variables (as opposed to only gist-like, scene-global, representations). Briefly, the model works by defining a Bayesian network over object variables that matter for the task. For example, in a video game where one runs a hot-dog stand and has to serve multiple hungry customers while managing the grill, those include raw sausages, cooked sausages, buns, ketchup, etc. (Fig. 9b). Then, existing objects in the scene, as well as the previous attended object, provide evidence towards the next attended object (Fig. 38.9b). The model also allows one to read out which spatial location will be attended, thus allowing one to verify its accuracy against the next actual fixation of the human player. The parameters of the network are learned directly from training data in the same form as the test data (human players playing the game). This object-based model was significantly more predictive of eye fixations compared to simpler classifier-based models, also developed by the same authors, that map a signature of a scene to eye positions, several state-of-the-art bottom-up saliency

---

correspond to REG(1) and REG(2) but using an SVM classifier, Mean BU is the average BU map showing which regions are salient throughout the game course. Similarly, DBN(1) and DBN(2) correspond to REG(1) and REG(2) meaning that in DBN(1) each network slice consists of just one node for previously attended object while in DBN(2) each network slice consists of the previously attended object as well as information of the previous objects in the scene and finally, Rand is a white noise random map.

models, as well as brute-force algorithms such as mean eye position (Fig. 9c). This points towards the efficacy of this class of models for modelling spatio-temporal visual data in presence of a task and hence a promising direction for the future. Probabilistic inference in this model is performed over object-related functions which are fed from manual annotations of objects in video scenes or by state-of-the-art object detection models. (Also see Sun and Fisher 2003 and Sun et al. 2008 for models that consider objects, although they do not reason about object identities and task-dependent roles.)

Finally, several computational models have started to explore making predictions that go beyond simply the next attended location. For example, Peters and Itti (2008) developed a model that monitors in an online manner video frames and eye gaze of humans engaged in 3D video games, computing instantaneous measures of how well correlated the eye is with saliency predictions and with gist-based top-down predictions. They then learn to detect specific patterns in these instantaneous measures, which allows them to predict—up to several seconds in advance—when players are about to fire a missile in a flight combat game, or to shift gears in a driving game. This model hence in essence estimates the intentions and predicts the future actions of the player. A related recent model was proposed by Doshi and Trivedi (2010) for active vehicle safety and driver monitoring. The system both computes bottom-up and top-down saliency maps from a video feed of the driver's view, and monitors the eye movements of the driver to better predict driver attention and gaze by estimating online the cognitive state and level of distraction of the driver. Using similar principles and adding pattern classification techniques, Tseng et al. (2009) have recently introduced a model that uses machine learning to classify, from features collected at the point of gaze over a few minutes of television viewing, control subjects from patients with disorders that affect the attention and oculomotor systems. The model has been successfully applied to elderly subjects (classifying patients with Parkinson's disease vs. controls) as well as children (classifying children with Attention Deficit Hyperactivity Disorder vs. Foetal Alcohol Spectrum Disorder vs. controls well above chance). These recent efforts suggest that eye movement patterns in complex scenes do contain—like a drop of saliva—latent individual biomarkers, which the latest attention modelling and pattern classification techniques are now beginning to reliably decode.

DISCUSSION AND OUTLOOK

Our review shows that tremendous progress has been made in modelling both bottom-up and top-down aspects of attention computationally. Tens of new models have been developed, each bringing new insight into the question of what makes some stimuli more important to visual observers than other stimuli.

Our quantitative comparison of many existing computational models on three standard datasets (Fig. 5) prompts at least two reactions: First, it is encouraging to see that several models perform significantly better than trivial models (e.g. a central Gaussian blob) or than older models (e.g. Itti-CIO2 model in Fig. 38.5). Second, however, it is surprising that the ranking of model scores is quite substantially different from the chronological order in which models were published. Indeed, one would typically expect that for a new model to be recognized, it should demonstrate superior performance compared to the state of the art, and actually often this is the case—just using possibly different datasets, scoring metrics, etc. Thus one important conclusion of our study is that carrying out standardized evaluations is important to ensure that the field keeps moving forward (see Borji 2010 for a web-based effort in this direction).

Another important aspect of model evaluation is that currently almost all model comparisons and scoring are based on average performance over a dataset of images or video clips, where often the dataset has been hand-picked and may contain significant biases (Torralba and Efros 2011). It may be more fruitful in the future to focus scoring on the most dramatic mistakes a model might make, or the worst-case disagreement between model and human observers. Indeed, average measures can easily be dominated by trivial cases if those happen often (e.g. we discussed earlier the notion of centre bias and how a majority of saccades which humans make are aimed towards the centres of images), and models may be developed which perform well in these cases but miss conceptually important understanding of how attention may operate in the minority of non-trivial cases. In addition, departure from average performance measures may provide richer information about which aspects of attention are better captured by a given model (e.g. some models may perform better on some sub-categories or even instances of images than others).

As we described more models, and in particular started moving from bottom-up models to those which include top-down biases, the question arose of whether purely bottom-up models are indeed relevant to real life. In other words, is there such a state of human cognition where a default or unbiased form of salience may be computed and may guide gaze. Many experiments have assumed that free viewing, just telling observers to 'watch and enjoy' stimuli presented to them, might be an acceptable approximation to this canonical unbiased state. However, it is trivially clear from introspection that cognition is not turned off during free viewing, and that what we look at in one instant triggers a range of memories, emotions, desires, cognitive inferences, etc. which all will ultimately influence where we look next. In this regard, it has been recently suggested that maybe only the initial volley of activity through visual cortex following stimulus onset may represent such canonical bottom-up saliency representation (Theeuwes 2010). If such is the case, then maybe comparing model predictions to sometimes rather long sequences of eye movements may be not be the best measure of how well a model captures this initial purely bottom-up attention.

Models where top-down influences serve to bias the bottom-up processing stages have also blurred the line between bottom-up and top-down. In fact, this is an important reminder that bottom-up and top-down influences are not mutually exclusive and do not sum to give rise to attention control (Awh et al. 2012). Instead, bottom-up and top-down often agree: The actor cognitively identified as the protagonist in a video clip may also move in such ways that he is the most salient. In fact, today's bottom-up may be nothing more than our former generations' top-down. Indeed, some bottom-up models have successfully integrated high-level features such as human face detectors into their palette of feature maps (Judd et al. 2009), which blurs again the line between bottom-up and top-down (these features are computed in a bottom-up manner from the image, but their very presence in a model is based on top-down knowledge that humans do strongly tend to look at faces in images (Cerf et al. 2009)).

When there is a task, top-down influences on attention are often believed to dominate, though this remains controversial and depends both on the task and on the quantification method used (Zelinsky et al. 2006; Foulsham and Underwood 2007; Henderson et al. 2007; Einhäuser et al. 2008; Greene et al. 2012). In human vision, we should not forget the following: Purely top-down attention (i.e. making a purely volitional eye movement unrelated to any visual stimulus) is not a generally viable model, except perhaps in blind persons. Others may make pure top-down eye movements from time to time, but certainly not always—that is, no matter how strongly one believes that top-down influences dominate, in the end controlling visual attention is a visually guided behaviour, and, as such, it is dependent on visual stimuli. This is important for future modelling efforts, as they attempt to tackle more complex tasks and situations, such as making a sandwich (Fig. 38.6d): A person may indeed look at the jar of jam because it is the next required object for the task (top-down guidance towards the jam). However, how did that person know where the jam is? In most cases, some bottom-up analysis (maybe in the past) must have provided that information (except perhaps if the person was told where the jam is). Thus, modelling human behaviour in complex tasks will likely require very careful control over the experimental setup, so that human participants are not given more information or additional priors that are not communicated to models (e.g. let a person look around before the task begins; see Foulsham 2012 for recent relevant data). This consideration echoes our earlier remark about making fair comparisons: If a model is not given the same information as a human participant (e.g. the model is not biased towards a search target or is not allowed to explore a scene before the task begins), likely the model will not perform as well, but we will also learn very little from such an experiment.

Another important challenge for models briefly mentioned above is dealing with sequence in eye movement data (i.e. scanpath) and with how to capture temporality in saccades. When comparing models, a model might be favoured not only if it can predict exact saccade locations, but also their ordering and their individual times of occurrence. In free viewing, in spite of past efforts (Privitera and Stark 2000), it is still not clear whether such sequential information is a strong factor of attention control and to what extent it depends on the subject or the asked question (Yarbus 1967). Despite this, recently some researchers (e.g. Wang et al. 2011) have tried to develop models and scores to explain sequences of saccades. As opposed to free viewing, it seems that there is much more temporal information in saccades in the presence of a task. For instance, assume an observer is viewing videos of two different tasks such as sandwich making or driving. It probably should not be very difficult to decode the task just from the sequential pattern of eye movements. This means that the task governs sequence of saccades when there is a task. In free viewing, however, when subjects are asked to watch a static scene freely there might not be a unique instruction making them saccade sequentially to certain places. Even if subjects are asked to watch the scene under different questions, the chances are that sequence may not help to decode the task (Greene et al. 2012).

Our survey shows that the remaining gap between man and machine seems to a large extent to be in 3D+time scene understanding, which includes reconstruction of the 3D geometry of the scene, understanding temporal sequences of events, simulation and extrapolation of physics over time in that 3D environment (e.g. to extrapolate the trajectory of a ball as in Fig. 38.6c), and so on. This requires some degree of machine vision and scene understanding which is not yet solved in the general case. This means that future computational models of attention will need to bring to bear sophisticated machine vision algorithms for scene understanding to provide the necessary parsing of visual inputs into tokens that can be reasoned upon and prioritized by attention.

Acknowledgements

Supported by the National Science Foundation (grant numbers BCS-0827764 and CMMI-1235539), the Army Research Office (W911NF-11-1-0046 and 62221-NS), the U.S. Army (W81XWH-10-2-0076), and Google. The authors affirm that the views expressed herein are solely their own, and do not represent the views of the United States government or any agency thereof.

References

Ajallooeian, M., Borji, A., Araabi, B. N., Ahmadabadi, M. N., and Moradi, H. (2009). Fast hand gesture recognition based on saliency maps: An application to interactive robotic marionette playing. In *18th IEEE International Symposium on Robot and Human Interactive Communication, 2009* (pp. 841–847). New York: IEEE.

Akamine, K., Fukuchi, K., Kimura, A., and Takagi, S. (2012). Fully automatic extraction of salient objects from videos in near real time. *The Computer Journal* 55(1): 3–14.

Allport, A., Meyer, D. E., and Kornblum, S. (1993). Attention and control: Have we been asking the wrong questions? A critical review of twenty-five years. In D. E. Meyer and S. Kornblum (eds.), *Attention and Performance XIV: Synergies in Experimental Psychology, Artificial Intelligence, and Cognitive Neuroscience* (pp. 183–218). Cambridge: Mass.: MIT Press.

Arbib, M. A. and Didday, R. L. (1971). The organization of action-oriented memory for a perceiving system. Part I: The basic model. *Journal of Cybernetics* 1(1): 3–18.

Avraham, T. and Lindenbaum, M. (2010). Esaliency (extended saliency): Meaningful attention using stochastic image modeling. *IEEE Transactions on Pattern Analysis and Machine Intelligence* 32(4): 693–708.

Awh, E., Belopolsky, A. V., and Theeuwes, J. (2012). Top-down versus bottom-up attentional control: A failed theoretical dichotomy. *Trends in Cognitive Sciences* 16(8): 437–443.

Ballard, D. H., Hayhoe, M. M., and Pelz, J. B. (1995). Memory representations in natural tasks. *Journal of Cognitive Neuroscience* 7(1): 66–80.

Baluch, F. and Itti, L. (2011). Mechanisms of top-down attention. *Trends in Neurosciences* 34(4): 210–224.

Ban, S. W., Kim, B., and Lee, M. (2010). Top-down visual selective attention model combined with bottom-up saliency map for incremental object perception. In *2010 International Joint Conference on Neural Networks* (pp. 1–8). New York: IEEE.

Belardinelli, A., Pirri, F., and Carbone, A. (2006). Robot task-driven attention. In *Proceedings of the 2006 International Symposium on Practical Cognitive Agents and Robots* (pp. 117–128). New York: Association for Computing Machinery.

Beuter, N., Lohmann, O., Schmidt, J., and Kummert, F. (2009). Directed attention: A cognitive vision system for a mobile robot. In *18th IEEE International Symposium on Robot and Human Interactive Communication, 2009* (pp. 854–860). New York: IEEE.

Bian, P. and Zhang, L. (2009). Biological plausibility of spectral domain approach for spatiotemporal visual saliency. *Advances in Neuro-Information Processing* 5506: 251–258.

Boccignone, G. and Ferraro, M. (2004). Modelling gaze shift as a constrained random walk. *Physica A: Statistical Mechanics and its Applications* 331(1): 207–218.

Bonev, B., Chuang, L. L., and Escolano, F. (2012). How do image complexity, task demands and looking biases influence human gaze behavior? *Pattern Recognition Letters* 34(7): 723–730.

Borji, A. (2010). Saliency evaluation project <https://sites.google.com/site/saliencyevaluation/>.

Borji, A. (2012). Boosting bottom-up and top-down visual features for saliency estimation. In *IEEE Conference on Computer Vision and Pattern Recognition, 2012. CVPR 2012* (pp. 438–445). New York: IEEE.

Borji, A., Ahmadabadi, M. N., and Araabi, B. N. (2011). Cost-sensitive learning of top-down modulation for attentional control. *Machine Vision and Applications* 22(1): 61–76.

Borji, A., Ahmadabadi, M. N., Araabi, B. N., and Hamidi, M. (2010). Online learning of task-driven object-based visual attention control. *Image and Vision Computing* 28(7): 1130–1145.

Borji, A. and Itti, L. (2012a). Exploiting local and global patch rarities for saliency detection. In *IEEE Conference on Computer Vision and Pattern Recognition, 2012. CVPR 2012* (pp. 478–485). New York: IEEE.

Borji, A. and Itti, L. (2012b). State-of-the-art in visual attention modeling. *IEEE Transactions on Pattern Analysis and Machine Intelligence* 35(1): 185–207.

Borji, A., Sihite, D. N., and Itti, L. (2012a). An object-based Bayesian framework for top-down visual attention. In *26th AAAI Conference on Artificial Intelligence, 2012* (pp. 1529–1535). Palo Alto, Calif.: Association for the Advancement of Artificial Intelligence.

Borji, A., Sihite, D. N., and Itti, L. (2012b). Quantitative analysis of human-model agreement in visual saliency modeling: A comparative study. *IEEE Transactions on Image Processing* 22(1): 55–69.

Borji, A., Sihite, D. N., and Itti, L. (2012c). What/where to look next? Modeling top-down visual attention in complex interactive environments. *IEEE Transactions on Systems, Man, and Cybernetics, Part A: Systems and Humans.* Available at: <http://ilab.usc.edu/publications/doc/Borji_etal12smc.pdf>.

Brefczynski, J. A. and DeYoe, E. A. (1999). A physiological correlate of the 'spotlight' of visual attention. *Nature Neuroscience* 2(4): 370–374.

Bruce, N. D. B. and Tsotsos, J. K. (2005). Saliency based on information maximization. *Advances in Neural Information Processing Systems* 18: 155–62.

Burattini, E., Rossi, S., Finzi, A., and Staffa, M. (2010). Attentional modulation of mutually dependent behaviors. In *From Animals to Animats 11: Proceedings of the 11th International Conference on Simulation of Adaptive Behavior* (pp. 283–292). New York: Springer.

Carmi, R. and Itti, L. (2006). The role of memory in guiding attention during natural vision. *Journal of Vision* 6(9): 898–914.

Carrasco, M. (2011). Visual attention: The past 25 years. *Vision Research* 51: 1484–1525.

Cave, K. R. (1999). The FeatureGate model of visual selection. *Psychological Research* 62(2–3): 182–194.

Cerf, M., Frady, E. P., and Koch, C. (2009). Faces and text attract gaze independent of the task: Experimental data and computer model. *Journal of Vision* 9(12): 1–15.

Cerf, M., Harel, J., Einhauser, W., and Koch, C. (2008). Predicting human gaze using low-level saliency combined with face detection. *Advances in Neural Information Processing Systems* 20: 241–248.

Chikkerur, S., Serre, T., Tan, C., and Poggio, T. (2010). What and where: A Bayesian inference theory of attention. *Vision Research* 50(22): 2233–2247.

Chun, M. M. and Jiang, Y. (1998). Contextual cueing: Implicit learning and memory of visual context guides spatial attention. *Cognitive Psychology* 36(1): 28–71.

Crick, F. (1984). Function of the thalamic reticular complex: The searchlight hypothesis. *Proceedings of the National Academy of Sciences USA* 81(14): 4586–4590.

Desimone, R. and Duncan, J. (1995). Neural mechanisms of selective visual attention. *Annual Review of Neuroscience* 18(1): 193–222.

Dorr, M., Martinetz, T., Gegenfurtner, K. R., and Barth, E. (2010). Variability of eye movements when viewing dynamic natural scenes. *Journal of Vision* 10(10): Article 28.

Doshi, A. and Trivedi, M. M. (2010). Attention estimation by simultaneous observation of viewer and view. In *2010 IEEE Computer Society Conference on Computer Vision and Pattern Recognition Workshops (CVPRW)* (pp. 21–27). New York: IEEE.

Driver, J. and Frith, C. (2000). Shifting baselines in attention research. *Nature Reviews Neuroscience* 1(2): 147–148.

Eckstein, M. P., Peterson, M. F., Pham, B. T., and Droll, J. A. (2009). Statistical decision theory to relate neurons to behavior in the study of covert visual attention. *Vision Research* 49(10): 1097–1128.

Ehinger, K. A., Hidalgo-Sotelo, B., Torralba, A., and Oliva, A. (2009). Modelling search for people in 900 scenes: A combined source model of eye guidance. *Visual Cognition* 17(6–7): 945–978.

Einhäuser, W., Rutishauser, U., and Koch, C. (2008). Task-demands can immediately reverse the effects of sensory-driven saliency in complex visual stimuli. *Journal of Vision* 8(2): Article 2.

Forssén, P. E., Meger, D., Lai, K., Helmer, S., Little, J. J., and Lowe, D. G. (2008). Informed visual search: Combining attention and object recognition. In *IEEE International Conference on Robotics and Automation. ICRA 2008* (pp. 935–942). New York: IEEE.

Foulsham, T. (2012). 'Eyes closed' and 'eyes open' expectations guide fixations in real-world search. In *Proceedings of the Cognitive Science Society* (CogSci), 34th Annual Meeting, Saporo, Japan (pp. 1–6). Austin, Tex.: Cognitive Science Society.

Foulsham, T. and Underwood, G. (2007). How does the purpose of inspection influence the potency of visual salience in scene perception? *Perception* 36(8): 1123–1138.

Frintrop, S. (2006). *VOCUS: A Visual Attention System for Object Detection and Goal-Directed Search*. Lecture Notes in Computer Science (vol. 3899). New York and Berlin: Springer-Verlag.

Frintrop, S., Backer, G., and Rome, E. (2005). Goal-directed search with a top-down modulated computational attention system. In W. Kropatsch, R. Sablatnig, and A. Hanbury (eds.), *Pattern Recognition*. Lecture Notes in Computer Science (vol. 3663, pp. 117–124). New York and Berlin: Springer-Verlag.

Frintrop, S., Rome, E., and Christensen, H. I. (2010). Computational visual attention systems and their cognitive foundations: A survey. *ACM Transactions on Applied Perception* 7(1): Article 6.

Gao, D., Han, S., and Vasconcelos, N. (2009). Discriminant saliency, the detection of suspicious coincidences, and applications to visual recognition. *IEEE Transactions on Pattern Analysis and Machine Intelligence* 31(6): 989–1005.

Gao, D. and Vasconcelos, N. (2004). Discriminant saliency for visual recognition from cluttered scenes. *Advances in Neural Information Processing Systems* 17(1): 481–488.

Garcia-Diaz, A., Fdez-Vidal, X., Pardo, X., and Dosil, R. (2009). Decorrelation and distinctiveness provide with human-like saliency. In J. Blanc-Talon, W. Philips, D. Popescu, and P. Scheunders (eds.), *Advanced Concepts for Intelligent Vision Systems* (pp. 343–354). Heidelberg: Springer-Verlag.

Goferman, S., Zelnik-Manor, L., and Tal, A. (2010). Context-aware saliency detection. In *IEEE Conference on Computer Vision and Pattern Recognition. CVPR 2010* (pp. 2376–2383). New York: IEEE.

Gottlieb, J. and Balan, P. (2010). Attention as a decision in information space. *Trends in Cognitive Sciences* 14(6): 240–248.

Greene, M. R., Liu, T., and Wolfe, J. M. (2012). Reconsidering Yarbus: A failure to predict observers task from eye movement patterns. *Vision Research* 62: 1–8.

Guo, C., Ma, Q., and Zhang, L. (2008). Spatio-temporal saliency detection using phase spectrum of quaternion fourier transform. In *IEEE Conference on Computer Vision and Pattern Recognition, 2008. CVPR 2008* (pp. 1–8). New York: IEEE.

Guo, C. and Zhang, L. (2010). A novel multiresolution spatiotemporal saliency detection model and its applications in image and video compression. *IEEE Transactions on Image Processing* 19(1): 185–198.

Hansen, L. K., Karadogan, S., and Marchegiani, L. (2011). What to measure next to improve decision making? On top-down task driven feature saliency. In *IEEE Symposium on Computational Intelligence, Cognitive Algorithms, Mind, and Brain. CCMB 2011* (pp. 1–7). New York: IEEE.

Harel, J., Koch, C., and Perona, P. (2007). Graph-based visual saliency. *Advances in Neural Information Processing Systems* 19: 545–552.

Hayhoe, M. M., Shrivastava, A., Mruczek, R., and Pelz, J. B. (2003). Visual memory and motor planning in a natural task. *Journal of Vision* 3(1): 49–63.

Henderson, J. M., Brockmole, J. R., Castelhano, M. S., and Mack, M. (2007). Visual saliency does not account for eye movements during visual search in real-world scenes. In R. P. G. Van Gompel, M. H. Fischer, W. S. Murray, and R. L. Hill (eds.), *Eye Movements: A Window on Mind and Brain* (pp. 537–562). Oxford: Elsevier.

Henderson, J. M. and Hollingworth, A. (1999). High-level scene perception. *Annual Review of Psychology* 50(1): 243–271.

Hou, X. and Zhang, L. (2007). Saliency detection: A spectral residual approach. In *IEEE Conference on Computer Vision and Pattern Recognition. CVPR 2007* (pp. 1–8). New York: IEEE.

Hou, X. and Zhang, L. (2008). Dynamic visual attention: Searching for coding length increments. *Advances in Neural Information Processing Systems* 21: 681–688.

Hwang, A. D., Wang, H. C., and Pomplun, M. (2011). Semantic guidance of eye movements in real-world scenes. *Vision Research* 51(10): 1192–1205.

Itti, L. (2006). Quantitative modeling of perceptual salience at human eye position. *Visual Cognition* 14(4–8): 959–984.

Itti, L. and Baldi, P. F. (2005). A principled approach to detecting surprising events in video. In *IEEE Conference on Computer Vision and Pattern Recognition. CVPR 2005* (pp. 631–637). New York: IEEE.

Itti, L., Dhavale, N., and Pighin, F. (2003). Realistic avatar eye and head animation using a neurobiological model of visual attention. In B. Bosacchi, D. Fogel, and J. C. Bezdek (eds.), *Proceedings of the SPIE 48th Annual International Symposium on Optical Science and Technology* (vol. 5200, pp. 64–78). Bellingham, Wash.: SPIE Press.

Itti, L., Gold, C., and Koch, C. (2001). Visual attention and target detection in cluttered natural scenes. *Optical Engineering* 40(9): 1784–1793.

Itti, L. and Koch, C. (2000). A saliency-based search mechanism for overt and covert shifts of visual attention. *Vision Research* 40(10–12): 1489–1506.

Itti, L. and Koch, C. (2001a). Computational modelling of visual attention. *Nature Reviews Neuroscience* 2(3): 194–203.

Itti, L. and Koch, C. (2001b). Feature combination strategies for saliency-based visual attention systems. *Journal of Electronic Imaging* 10(1): 161–169.

Itti, L., Koch, C., and Niebur, E. (1998). A model of saliency-based visual attention for rapid scene analysis. *IEEE Transactions on Pattern Analysis and Machine Intelligence* 20(11): 1254–1259.

Judd, T., Ehinger, K., Durand, F., and Torralba, A. (2009). Learning to predict where humans look. In *IEEE 12th International Conference on Computer Vision, 2009* (pp. 2106–2113). New York: IEEE.

Kastner, S., Pinsk, M. A., De Weerd, P., Desimone, R., and Ungerleider, L. G. (1999). Increased activity in human visual cortex during directed attention in the absence of visual stimulation. *Neuron* 22(4): 751–761.

Kienzle, W., Wichmann, F., Schölkopf, B., and Franz, M. (2007). A nonparametric approach to bottom-up visual saliency. *Advances in Neural Information Processing Systems* 19: 1–8.

Kimura, A., Pang, D., Takeuchi, T., Yamato, J., and Kashino, K. (2008). Dynamic Markov random fields for stochastic modeling of visual attention. In *IEEE 19th International Conference on Pattern Recognition. ICPR 2008* (pp. 1–5). New York: IEEE.

Koch, C. and Ullman, S. (1985). Shifts in selective visual attention: Towards the underlying neural circuitry. *Human Neurobiology* 4(4): 219–27.

Kootstra, G., Nederveen, A., and De Boer, B. (2008). Paying attention to symmetry. In M. Everingham, C. J. Needham, and R. Fraile (eds.), *Proceedings of the British Machine Vision Conference (BMVC 2008)* (pp. 1115–1125). Manchester: British Machine Vision Association.

Land, M. F. and Hayhoe, M. (2001). In what ways do eye movements contribute to everyday activities? *Vision Research* 41(25–26): 3559–3565.

Land, M. F. and McLeod, P. (2000). From eye movements to actions: How batsmen hit the ball. *Nature Neuroscience* 3(12): 1340–1345.

Le Meur, O., Le Callet, P., Barba, D., and Thoreau, D. (2006). A coherent computational approach to model bottom-up visual attention. *IEEE Transactions on Pattern Analysis and Machine Intelligence* 28(5): 802–817.

Lee, S., Oh, J., Park, J., Kwon, J., Kim, M., and Yoo, H. J. (2011). A 345 mW heterogeneous many-core processor with an intelligent inference engine for robust object recognition. *IEEE Journal of Solid-State Circuits* 46(1): 42–51.

Li, F. F., VanRullen, R., Koch, C., and Perona, P. (2002). Rapid natural scene categorization in the near absence of attention. *Proceedings of the National Academy of Sciences USA* 99(14): 9596.

Li, J., Tian, Y., Huang, T., and Gao, W. (2011). Multi-task rank learning for visual saliency estimation. *IEEE Transactions on Circuits and Systems for Video Technology* 21(5): 623–636.

Li, L. J. and Fei-Fei, L. (2010). Optimol: Automatic online picture collection via incremental model learning. *International Journal of Computer Vision 88*(2): 147–168.

Li, Y., Zhou, Y., Yan, J., Niu, Z., and Yang, J. (2010). Visual saliency based on conditional entropy. In *Computer Vision–ACCV 2009*. Lecture Notes in Computer Science (vol. 5994, pp. 246–257). New York and Berlin: Springer-Verlag.

Liu, T., Sun, J., Zheng, N., Tang, X., and Shum, H. (2007). Learning to detect a salient object. In *IEEE Conference on Computer Vision and Pattern Recognition. CVPR 2007*. New York: IEEE.

Ma, X. and Deng, Z. (2009). Natural eye motion synthesis by modeling gaze-head coupling. In *IEEE Conference on Virtual Reality, 2009. VR 2009* (pp. 143–150). New York: IEEE.

Mancas, M. (2007). *Computational Attention Towards Attentive Computers*. Louvain-la-Neuve: Presses Universitaires de Louvain.

Marat, S., Ho Phuoc, T., Granjon, L., Guyader, N., Pellerin, D., and Guérin-Dugué, A. (2009). Modelling spatio-temporal saliency to predict gaze direction for short videos. *International Journal of Computer Vision 82*(3): 231–243.

Martinez-Trujillo, J. (2011). Searching for the neural mechanisms of feature-based attention in the primate brain. *Neuron 70*(6): 1025–1028.

Miau, F., Papageorgiou, C., and Itti, L. (2001). Neuromorphic algorithms for computer vision and attention. In B. Bosacchi, D. B. Fogel, and J. C. Bezdek (eds.), *Proceedings of the SPIE 46th Annual International Symposium on Optical Science and Technology* (vol. 4479, pp. 12–23). Bellingham, Wash.: SPIE Press.

Milanese, R., Wechsler, H., Gill, S., Bost, J. M., and Pun, T. (1994). Integration of bottom-up and top-down cues for visual attention using non-linear relaxation. In *IEEE Computer Society Conference on Computer Vision and Pattern Recognition. CVPR 1994* (pp. 781–785). New York: IEEE.

Mourant, R. R. and Rockwell, T. H. (1970). Mapping eye-movement patterns to the visual scene in driving: An exploratory study. *Human Factors: The Journal of the Human Factors and Ergonomics Society 12*(1): 81–87.

Murray, N., Vanrell, M., Otazu, X., and Parraga, C. A. (2011). Saliency estimation using a non-parametric low-level vision model. In *IEEE Conference on Computer Vision and Pattern Recognition. CVPR 2011* (pp. 433–440). New York: IEEE.

Navalpakkam, V., Arbib, M. A., and Itti, L. (2005). Attention and scene understanding. In L. Itti, G. Rees, and J. K. Tsotsos (eds.), *Neurobiology of Attention* (pp. 197–203). San Diego, Calif.: Elsevier.

Navalpakkam, V. and Itti, L. (2005). Modeling the influence of task on attention. *Vision Research 45*(2): 205–231.

Navalpakkam, V. and Itti, L. (2006). An integrated model of top-down and bottom-up attention for optimal object detection. In *IEEE Conference on Computer Vision and Pattern Recognition. CVPR 2006* (pp. 2049–2056). New York: IEEE.

Navalpakkam, V. and Itti, L. (2007). Search goal tunes visual features optimally. *Neuron 53*(4): 605–617. Commentary/preview: Paying attention to neurons with discriminating taste (A. Pouget and D. Bavelier). *Neuron 53*(4): 473–475.

Noton, D. and Stark, L. (1971). Scanpaths in eye movements during pattern perception. *Science 171*(968): 308–11.

Oliva, A., Torralba, A., Castelhano, M. S., and Henderson, J. M. (2003). Top-down control of visual attention in object detection. In *IEE International Conference on Image Processing. ICIP 2003.* (vol. 1, pp. 253–256). New York: IEEE.

Orabona, F., Metta, G., and Sandini, G. (2005). Object-based visual attention: A model for a behaving robot. In *IEEE Computer Society Conference on Computer Vision and Pattern Recognition Workshops* (pp. 1–89). New York: IEEE.

Ouerhani, N. and Hügli, H. (2003). Real-time visual attention on a massively parallel SIMD architecture. *Real-Time Imaging* 9(3): 189–196.

Paletta, L., Rome, E., and Buxton, H. (2005). Attention architectures for machine vision and mobile robots. In L. Itti, G. Rees, and J. K. Tsotsos (eds.), *Neurobiology of Attention* (pp. 642–648). San Diego, Calif.: Elsevier.

Pang, D., Kimura, A., Takeuchi, T., Yamato, J., and Kashino, K. (2008). A stochastic model of selective visual attention with a dynamic Bayesian network. In *IEEE International Conference on Multimedia and Expo. ICME 2008* (pp. 1073–1076). New York: IEEE.

Parkhurst, D., Law, K., and Niebur, E. (2002). Modeling the role of salience in the allocation of overt visual attention. *Vision Research* 42(1): 107–123.

Peters, R. J. and Itti, L. (2007). Beyond bottom-up: Incorporating task-dependent influences into a computational model of spatial attention. In *IEEE Conference on Computer Vision and Pattern Recognition. CVPR 2007* (pp. 1–8). New York: IEEE.

Peters, R. J. and Itti, L. (2008). Congruence between model and human attention reveals unique signatures of critical visual events. *Advances in Neural Information Processing Systems* 20: 1145–1152.

Peters, R. J., Iyer, A., Itti, L., and Koch, C. (2005). Components of bottom-up gaze allocation in natural images. *Vision Research* 45(8): 2397–2416.

Posner, M. I. (1980). Orienting of attention. *Quarterly Journal of Experimental Psychology* 32(1): 3–25.

Privitera, C. M. and Stark, L.W. (2000). Algorithms for defining visual regions-of-interest: Comparison with eye fixations. *IEEE Transactions on Pattern Analysis and Machine Intelligence* 22(9): 970–982.

Rajashekar, U., van der Linde, I., Bovik, A. C., and Cormack, L. K. (2008). GAFFE: A gaze-attentive fixation finding engine. *IEEE Transactions on Image Processing* 17(4): 564–573.

Ramanathan, S., Katti, H., Sebe, N., Kankanhalli, M., and Chua, T. S. (2010). An eye fixation database for saliency detection in images. In K. Danilidis, P. Maragos, and N. Paragios (eds.), *Computer Vision–ECCV 2010*. Lecture Notes in Computer Science (vol. 6312, pp. 30–43). New York and Berlin: Springer-Verlag.

Ramström, O. and Christensen, H. (2002). Visual attention using game theory. In H. H. Bülthoff, C. Wallraven, S.-W. Lee, and T. A. Poggio (eds.), *Biologically Motivated Computer Vision*. Lecture Notes in Computer Science (vol. 2525, pp. 462–471). New York and Berlin: Springer-Verlag.

Rao, R. P. N., Hayhoe, M. M., Zelinsky, G. J., and Ballard, D. H. (1996). Modeling saccadic targeting in visual search. *Advances in Neural Information Processing Systems* 8: 830–836.

Rao, R. P. N., Zelinsky, G. J., Hayhoe, M. M., and Ballard, D. H. (2002). Eye movements in iconic visual search. *Vision Research* 42(11): 1447–1463.

Renninger, L. W., Coughlan, J., Verghese, P., and Malik, J. (2005). An information maximization model of eye movements. *Advances in Neural Information Processing Systems* 17: 1121–1128.

Rensink, R. A. (2000). The dynamic representation of scenes. *Visual Cognition* 7(1–3): 17–42.

Reynolds, J. H. and Desimone, R. (1999). The role of neural mechanisms of attention in solving the binding problem. *Neuron* 24(1): 19–29, 111–25.

Rezazadegan Tavakoli, H., Rahtu, E., and Heikkilä, J. (2011). Fast and efficient saliency detection using sparse sampling and kernel density estimation. In A. Heyden and F. Kahl (eds.),

Image Analysis. Lecture Notes in Computer Science (vol. 6688, pp. 666–675). New York and Berlin: Springer-Verlag.

Robertson, L. C. (2003). Binding, spatial attention and perceptual awareness. *Nature Reviews Neuroscience* 4(2): 93–102.

Rosin, P. L. (2009). A simple method for detecting salient regions. *Pattern Recognition* 42(11): 2363–2371.

Rothenstein, A. L. and Tsotsos, J. K. (2008). Attention links sensing to recognition. *Image and Vision Computing* 26(1): 114–126.

Rybak, I. A., Gusakova, V. I., Golovan, A. V., Podladchikova, L. N., and Shevtsova, N. A. (1998). A model of attention-guided visual perception and recognition. *Vision Research* 38(15–16): 2387–2400.

Saalmann, Y. B., Pinsk, M. A., Wang, L., Li, X., and Kastner, S. (2012). The pulvinar regulates information transmission between cortical areas based on attention demands. *Science* 337(6095): 753–756.

Saenz, M., Buracas, G. T., and Boynton, G. M. (2002). Global effects of feature-based attention in human visual cortex. *Nature Neuroscience* 5(7): 631–632.

Salah, A. A., Alpaydin, E., and Akarun, L. (2002). A selective attention-based method for visual pattern recognition with application to handwritten digit recognition and face recognition. *IEEE Transactions on Pattern Analysis and Machine Intelligence* 24(3): 420–425.

Schill, K., Umkehrer, E., Beinlich, S., Krieger, G., and Zetzsche, C. (2001). Scene analysis with saccadic eye movements: Top-down and bottom-up modeling. *Journal of Electronic Imaging* 10(1): 152–160.

Schmidt, J. and Zelinsky, G. J. (2009). Search guidance is proportional to the categorical specificity of a target cue. *Quarterly Journal of Experimental Psychology* 62(10): 1904–1914.

Seo, H. and Milanfar, P. (2009). Static and space-time visual saliency detection by self-resemblance. *Journal of Vision* 9(12): 1–27.

Serences, J. T. and Saproo, S. (2010). Population response profiles in early visual cortex are biased in favor of more valuable stimuli. *Journal of Neurophysiology* 104(1): 76–87.

Shic, F. and Scassellati, B. (2007). A behavioral analysis of computational models of visual attention. *International Journal of Computer Vision* 73(2): 159–177.

Siagian, C. and Itti, L. (2007). Rapid biologically-inspired scene classification using features shared with visual attention. *IEEE Transactions on Pattern Analysis and Machine Intelligence* 29(2): 300–312.

Sodhi, M., Reimer, B., Cohen, J. L., Vastenburg, E., Kaars, R., and Kirschenbaum, S. (2002). On-road driver eye movement tracking using head-mounted devices. In *Proceedings of the 2002 Symposium on Eye Tracking Research and Applications* (pp. 61–68). New York: Association for Computing Machinery.

Sprague, N. and Ballard, D. (2003). Eye movements for reward maximization. *Advances in Neural Information Processing Systems* 16: 1467–1474.

Summerfield, J. J., Rao, A., Garside, N., and Nobre, A. C. (2011). Biasing perception by spatial long-term memory. *Journal of Neuroscience* 31(42): 14952–14960.

Sun, X., Yao, H., and Ji, R. (2012). What are we looking for? Towards statistical modeling of saccadic eye movements and visual saliency. In *IEEE Conference on Computer Vision and Pattern Recognition. CVPR 2012* (pp. 1552–1559). New York: IEEE.

Sun, Y. and Fisher, R. (2003). Object-based visual attention for computer vision. *Artificial Intelligence* 146(1): 77–123.

Sun, Y., Fisher, R., Wang, F., and Gomes, H. M. (2008). A computer vision model for visual-object-based attention and eye movements. *Computer Vision and Image Understanding* 112(2): 126–142.

Tatler, B. W., Baddeley, R. J., and Gilchrist, I. D. (2005). Visual correlates of fixation selection: effects of scale and time. *Vision Research* 45(5): 643–659.

Tatler, B. W., Hayhoe, M. M., Land, M. F., and Ballard, D. H. (2011). Eye guidance in natural vision: Reinterpreting salience. *Journal of Vision* 11(5): 1–23.

Tatler, B. W. and Vincent, B. T. (2009). The prominence of behavioural biases in eye guidance. *Visual Cognition* 17(6–7): 1029–1054.

Theeuwes, J. (2010). Top-down and bottom-up control of visual selection. *Acta Psychologica* 135(2): 77–99.

Toet, A. (2011). Computational versus psychophysical bottom-up image saliency: A comparative evaluation study. *IEEE Transactions on Pattern Analysis and Machine Intelligence* 33(11): 2131–2146.

Torralba, A. (2003). Modeling global scene factors in attention. *Journal of the Optical Society of America A* 20(7): 1407–1418.

Torralba, A. and Efros, A.A. (2011). Unbiased look at dataset bias. In *IEEE Conference on Computer Vision and Pattern Recognition. CVPR 2011* (pp. 1521–1528). New York: IEEE.

Treisman, A. M. and Gelade, G. (1980). A feature-integration theory of attention. *Cognitive Psychology* 12(1): 97–136.

Treisman, A. and Souther, J. (1985). Search asymmetry: A diagnostic for preattentive processing of separable features. *Journal of Experimental Psychology: General* 114(3): 285–310.

Treue, S. and Martinez Trujillo, J. C. (1999). Feature-based attention influences motion processing gain in macaque visual cortex. *Nature* 399(6736): 575–579.

Tseng, P. H., Carmi, R., Cameron, I. G. M., Munoz, D. P., and Itti, L. (2009). Quantifying center bias of observers in free viewing of dynamic natural scenes. *Journal of Vision* 9(7).

Tsotsos, J. K. and Rothenstein, A. (2011). Computational models of visual attention. *Scholarpedia* 6(1): 6201.

Verma, M. and McOwan, P. W. (2009). Generating customised experimental stimuli for visual search using genetic algorithms shows evidence for a continuum of search efficiency. *Vision Research* 49(3): 374–382.

Viola, P. and Jones, M. (2001). Rapid object detection using a boosted cascade of simple features. In *IEEE Computer Society Conference on Computer Vision and Pattern Recognition. CVPR 2001* (vol. 1, pp. 511–518). New York: IEEE.

Võ, M. L. H. and Henderson, J. M. (2009). Does gravity matter? Effects of semantic and syntactic inconsistencies on the allocation of attention during scene perception. *Journal of Vision* 9(3).

Walther, D. and Koch, C. (2006). Modeling attention to salient proto-objects. *Neural Networks* 19(9): 1395–1407.

Wang, H. X., Freeman, J., Merriam, E. P., Hasson, U., and Heeger, D. J. (2012). Temporal eye movement strategies during naturalistic viewing. *Journal of Vision* 12(1).

Wang, W., Chen, C., Wang, Y., Jiang, T., Fang, F., and Yao, Y. (2011). Simulating human saccadic scanpaths on natural images. In *IEEE Conference on Computer Vision and Pattern Recognition. CVPR 2011* (pp. 441–448). New York: IEEE.

Wolfe, J. M. (1994). Guided search 2.0. A revised model of visual search. *Psychonomic Bulletin & Review* 1(2): 202–238.

Xu, T., Kuhnlenz, K., and Buss, M. (2010). Autonomous behavior-based switched top-down and bottom-up visual attention for mobile robots. *IEEE Transactions on Robotics* 26(5): 947–954.

Yarbus, A. (1967). *Eye Movements and Vision*. New York: Plenum Press.

Yu, Y., Mann, G. K. I., and Gosine, R. G. (2008). An object-based visual attention model for robots. In *IEEE International Conference on Robotics and Automation, 2008. ICRA 2008* (pp. 943–948). New York: IEEE.

Yu, Y., Mann, G. K. I., and Gosine, R. G. (2012). A goal-directed visual perception system using object-based top-down attention. *IEEE Transactions on Autonomous Mental Development* 4(1): 87–103.

Zelinsky, G., Zhang, W., Yu, B., Chen, X., and Samaras, D. (2006). The role of top-down and bottom-up processes in guiding eye movements during visual search. *Advances in Neural Information Processing Systems* 18: 1569–1576.

Zhai, Y. and Shah, M. (2006). Visual attention detection in video sequences using spatiotemporal cues. In *Proceedings of the 14th Annual ACM International Conference on Multimedia* (pp. 815–824). New York: Association for Computing Machinery.

Zhang, L., Tong, M. H., and Cottrell, G. W. (2009). SUNDAy: Saliency using natural statistics for dynamic analysis of scenes. In *Proceedings of the Cognitive Science Society* (CogSci), 34th Annual Meeting, Amsterdam (pp. 2944–2949). Austin, Tex.: Cognitive Science Society.

Zhang, L., Tong, M. H., Marks, T. K., Shan, H., and Cottrell, G. W. (2008). SUN: A Bayesian framework for saliency using natural statistics. *Journal of Vision* 8(7).

Zhao, Q. and Koch, C. (2011). Learning a saliency map using fixated locations in natural scenes. *Journal of Vision* 11(3).

Zhou, H. and Desimone, R. (2011). Feature-based attention in the frontal eye field and area V4 during visual search. *Neuron* 70(6): 1205–1217.

....

CHAPTER 39

BAYESIAN MODELS
OF ATTENTION

....

ANGELA J. YU

INTRODUCTION

....

OUR senses are constantly bombarded by a rich stream of complex and noisy inputs. Selectively filtering these sensory inputs and maintaining useful interpretations for them are important computational tasks faced by the brain. Traditionally, the process of attentional selection has commonly been associated with the metaphor of a 'bottle-neck': limited processing resources giving rise to the exclusion or attenuation of certain aspects or components of sensory inputs (Broadbent 1958; Deutsch and Deutsch 1963; Treisman 1969; Norman 1968). This ongoing debate has focused on whether the 'unat-tended' stimuli are totally ignored (Broadbent 1958) or merely attenuated (Treisman 1969); whether the selection process happens early on, such that semantic processing is only applied to the attended stimuli (Broadbent 1958), or much later on, after seman-tic analysis has been applied and before reaching consciousness (Deutsch and Deutsch 1963); whether the filter operates only on physical features of the stimuli (Broadbent 1958), or depends on top-down contextual influences (Deutsch and Deutsch 1963); and whether a discrete bottleneck, through which only one item is selected, or a spatially embedded 'spotlight' (LaBerge 1983; Eriksen and St James 1986), privileging all stimuli within a spatial region, is the more apt analogy.

Instead of trying to characterize the exact capacity and limitation of attentional selection, a number of recent modelling papers have focused on the *computational goals* of selective processing, i.e. a normative framework for 'why' attentional selec-tion behaves the way it does in different context, instead of a descriptive picture of 'how' it operates. For example, selective filtering may arise because certain aspects or components of the sensory landscape are more *relevant* for the observer's current behavioural goals, and the remaining components, if included for processing, may be confusing or even detrimental to the task at hand. Thus, selective processing could be useful for *computational optimality*, beyond any resource limitation considerations. To motivate the selection-for-computation perspective on attentional selection, it is instructive to recall an early insight articulated by Hermann von Helmholtz. He was among the first to recognize that sensory processing involves an active *inductive process* of 'unconscious inference', which combines remembered ideas arising from past sensory experiences with fresh sense impressions, in order to arrive at 'conclusions' about the sensory world (Helmholtz 1878). From this perspective, the concept of selection-for-computation arises quite naturally: different pieces of information, whether from immediate sensory inputs or past knowledge, must be combined according to their respective relevance and informativeness, as part of the inductive process. In other words, selection-for-computation concretely implies selection for optimizing the inductive process. Notably, it has long been known that human sensory processing manifests many types of inductive biases. Indeed, many of the Gestalt laws of psychophysics formulated in the early twentieth century can also be interpreted this way (Elder and Goldberg 2002).

A number of recent theoretical models, based on Bayesian probability theory, have formalized the need of attentional selection to be shaped by computational desiderata (Dayan and Zemel 1999; Dayan and Yu 2002; Yu and Dayan 2005a, 2005b; Yu et al. 2009). Bayesian probability theory is a powerful and increasingly prevalent ideal observer (Green and Swets 1966) framework for understanding selective processing, as it provides a set of statistically optimal tools for the quantification and integration of imperfect information sources. It has been successfully applied to explain human and animal behaviour in a number of cognitive tasks, including perceptual inference (Grenander 1976–81; Bolle and Cooper 1984; Geman and Geman 1984; Marroquin et al. 1987; Szeliski 1989; Clark and Yuille 1990; Knill and Richards 1996), multi-modal sensory integration (Jacobs 1999; Ernst and Banks 2002; Battaglia et al. 2003; Dayan et al. 2000; Körding and Wolpert 2004; Shams et al. 2005; Körding et al. 2007a), reward learning (Behrens et al. 2007), and motor adaptation (Körding et al. 2007b).

In the following, we will review recently proposed Bayesian models of attention for learning, covert spatial attention, and overt spatial attention.

ATTENTION FOR LEARNING

In the Bayesian framework, the two main computational tasks under conditions of uncertainty are inductive *inference* and *learning*. Inference refers to the computation of an 'interpretation' or 'representation' for sensory inputs based on an internal model of how events and properties of our external environment 'generate' these observations, while learning deals with a longer timescale process through which sensory experiences get incorporated into the internal representations of how entities in the environment interact and generate sensory observations. In the context of attentional selection, inference and learning both assign weight to a piece of information according to its associated uncertainty, but they require precisely the *opposite* pattern of prioritization as a function of uncertainty. For *inference*, sensory inputs associated with greater uncertainty are accorded relatively less weight so that more informative inputs are selectively processed; for *learning*, cues associated with greater uncertainty are accorded greater weights, so that learning focuses on less well-known aspects of the environment.

As an illustrative example of attention for learning, we first consider a simple classical conditioning learning scenario that we previously modelled as a Kalman filter (Dayan and Yu 2003). This example demonstrates that when multiple sources of noisy information are available, an ideal observer should 'attend' more to the more reliable sources of information. Moreover, such uncertainty, if reducible through experience, should encourage the observer to 'attend' to the most uncertain aspects of the environment in order to reduce uncertainty.

The field of classical conditioning probes the way that animals learn and utilize predictive relationships in the world, between initially neutral stimuli such as lights and tones, and reinforcers such as food, water, or small electric shocks (Dickinson 1980; Mackintosh 1983). In these experiments, the animals are thought to be 'reverse-engineering' the arbitrary predictive relationships set by the experimenter (Sutton 1992). Figure 39.1 graphically illustrates these ideas.

One statistical formulation of the 'true' underlying stimulus–reinforcer relationship, constituting the *generative model*, is to assume that the stimuli x_t (e.g. light, tone) on trial t stochastically determine the reward (or punishment) r_t, through a linear relationship:

$$r_t = x_t \cdot w + \eta_t \tag{1}$$

Here, each x_t^i in $x_t = \{x_t^i, ..., x_t^n\}$ is a binary variable representing whether stimulus i is present or not on trial t, $\cdot$ denotes the dot product, $w = \{w_1, ..., w_n\}$ are the weights that specify how each stimulus x_i contributes to the reward outcome, and $\eta_t \sim N(0, \tau^2)$ is a noise term following a Gaussian (normal) distribution with zero mean and variance τ^2. The task for the animal on each trial is to predict the amount of reinforcer given the stimuli, based on the learned relationship between stimuli and reinforcer, and to update those relationships according to the observation of a new pair of x_t, r_t on each trial.

Let us consider the simple case of there being two stimuli, $i = 1, 2$, and that it is known that only the first stimulus is present on trial 1, $x_1 = (1, 0)$, and both are present on trial 2, $x_2 = (1, 1)$.

Before any observations, we assume that the prior distributions of w_1 and w_2 are independent and Gaussian: $w_i \sim \mathcal{N}(w_0, \sigma_0^2)$, for $i = 1, 2$. After observing the first set of (x_1, r_1), the distribution over w_2 is still just the prior distribution $\mathcal{N}(w_0, \sigma_0^2)$, since stimulus 2 was not present. The distribution over w_1 takes the following form:

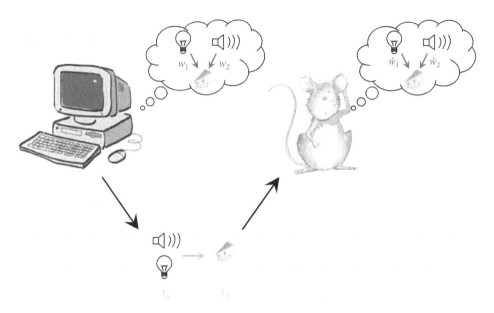

FIGURE 39.1 Inference and learning in classical conditioning. The experimenter, typically using a computer, would set the weights $\{w_i\}$ that specify how stimuli combine to predict the reinforcement outcome (see Eq. 1). Based on these relationships, the subject is shown one or more stimuli (e.g. light or tone), followed by the appropriate reward, and then the presentation is repeated, with either the same set of stimuli, or a different set. Based on these stimulus–reward pairings, the subject learns the weights that parameterize the stimulus–reward relationships, and uses them to make predictions about future rewards based on stimulus presentations.

$$p\left(w_{1}\,|\,\mathbf{x}_{1},r_{1}\right)=\frac{p\left(r_{1},\mathbf{x}_{1}\,|\,\mathbf{w}\right)p\left(\mathbf{w}\right)}{p\left(\mathbf{x}_{1},r_{1}\right)}$$

$$\propto \mathcal{N}\!\left(\frac{1/\tau^{2}}{1/\tau^{2}+1/\sigma_{0}^{2}}\,r_{1}+\frac{1/\sigma_{0}^{2}}{1/\tau^{2}+1/\sigma_{0}^{2}}\,w_{0},\frac{1}{1/\tau^{2}+1/\sigma_{0}^{2}}\right) \qquad (2)$$

The first part of the equation is just an instantiation of Bayes' Rule (Bayes 1763), which states that the *posterior* distribution of a variable (w_1) after observations $(x_1,$ $r_1)$ is proportional to the *likelihood* of the data $(p(r_1, x_1|w))$ times the *prior* $(p(w))$. The distribution is normalized by the constant $p(x_1, r_1)$. The second part, where $\propto$ denotes 'proportional to', shows that the posterior distribution is also Gaussian. It has a mean estimate that is a linear combination of the observed reinforcer for cue 1 and the prior mean w_0, where the weight assigned to each is determined by the relative *precision* (1/variance) of each—thus, the information source that is less noisy/uncertain is given proportionally greater weight. The precision of the posterior distribution is the sum of the individual precisions of the prior and likelihood distributions, reflecting the fact that combining multiple sources of information ultimately results in greater precision (less uncertainty) than having only one of them.

On the second trial, when both stimuli are presented, we can again apply Bayes' Rule to obtain a new posterior distribution in the weights, $p(w_1, w_2 | x_1, r_1, x_2, r_2)$, where now the prior distribution is the posterior from the previous trial. If we make the simplifying assumption that the correlation between w_1 and w_2 is 0, then it can be shown using a set of iterative Bayesian computations, known as the Kalman filter (Anderson and Moore 1979), that the posterior distribution is Gaussian with mean $\hat{\mathbf{w}}_t = \left\{ \hat{w}_t^1, \hat{w}_t^2 \right\}$ and diagonal variance $\left\{ \left(\sigma_t^1\right)^2, \left(\sigma_t^2\right)^2 \right\}$, where for $i = 1, 2$,

$$\hat{w}_t^i = \hat{w}_{t-1}^i + \frac{\left(\sigma_{t-1}^i\right)^2}{\sum_j \left(\sigma_{t-1}^j\right)^2 + \tau^2} \left(r_t - \mathbf{x}_t \cdot \hat{\mathbf{w}}_t\right) \tag{3}$$

$$\left(\sigma_t^i\right)^2 = \left(\sigma_{t-1}^i\right)^2 \left(\frac{\tau^2}{\left(\sigma_{t-1}^i\right)^2 + \tau^2} \right) \tag{4}$$

Eq. 3 says that the new estimate w_t^i is just the old one plus the prediction error $r_t - \mathbf{x}_t \cdot \hat{\mathbf{w}}_t$ times a coefficient, called the *Kalman gain*, which depends on the uncertainty associated with each weight estimate relative to the observation noise. The Kalman gain indicates a *competitive* allocation between the stimuli, so that the stimulus associated with the larger uncertainty σ_i gets the bigger share. On trial 2, because $\left(\sigma_2^2\right)^2 = \sigma_0^2$ and $\left(\sigma_1^1\right)^2 < \sigma_0^2$, $\hat{w}^2$ would be accorded relatively faster learning. In addition, large observation noise τ^2 would result in slower learning for all weights, as the inputs are known to be unreliable indicators of the underlying weights, and small τ^2 leads to faster learning. Eq. 4 indicates that the uncertainty associated with each stimulus is also reduced faster when the observation noise τ^2 is relatively small.

In the computation of the new weight estimate, larger prior uncertainty $\left(\sigma_t^i\right)^2$ (relative to observation noise) leads to greater weight placed on the observation, and lower prior uncertainty limits the impact of the observation. This again demonstrates the principle that in probabilistic inference, more uncertain information sources have *less* influence in the information integration process. Notice that the uncertainty $\left(\sigma_t^i\right)^2$ in Eq. 4 gradually reduces as a function of the number of times that the stimulus x^i has been observed, but not on the actual observations. This is a quirk of the simple linear-Gaussian generative (Kalman filter) model that we consider here. Critically, learning rate is parcelled out among cues differentially in this normative framework, such that the cue whose predictive consequences are least well known is accorded the greatest 'attention' during the learning process.

While this simple conditioning example demonstrates that uncertainty plays important roles in various aspects of selective attention in learning, it is overly simplistic in several respects. Firstly, it conflates the inference and learning problems by having a single kind of hidden variable, w. Under more realistic circumstances, there would be noise associated with any sensory inputs (both stimuli and reward), whether at the receptor level, generated in the cortex, or due to true stochasticity within the external

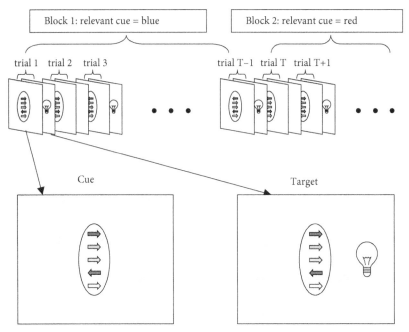

FIGURE 39.2 Example of an extended Posner task involving differently colour cue stimuli: (1) red, (2) green, (3) blue, (4) purple, (5) yellow. This is just for illustrative purposes—
experimental concerns have been omitted for clarity. Each trial consists of a cue frame
followed by a target frame after a variable delay. The subject must report the target onset as
quickly as possible. The first block has $T-1$ trials, during which the blue arrow predicts the
target location with a constant cue validity ($\gamma_1 = \ldots = \gamma_{T-1}$), and the arrows of all other colours are irrelevant (each on average points toward the target on half of the trials by chance).
In the second block, starting on trial T, the red arrow becomes the predictive cue, but with
a different cue validity $\gamma_T = \gamma_{T+1} = \ldots$

environment itself. If x_t and r_t were not observed directly but induce noisy sensory
inputs, then computing a distribution over potential values of x_t and r_t would be part of
the inference problem, whereas the computation about the weights can be considered a
learning problem. Secondly, the 'hidden' relationships in the world (parameterized by
w) are assumed to be constant over time. What if these predictive relationships can actually fundamentally change at times, as for instance through the common experimental
manipulations of reversal or extinction? Clearly, the simple linear-Gaussian model that
we have proposed would be inadequate, since it cannot capture such discrete, abrupt
changes. One consequence of dramatic changes in the parameters of an environmen-
tally specified generative model is the need for a measure of *unexpected uncertainty*,
which monitors gross discrepancy between predictions made by the internal model and
actual observations. This unexpected uncertainty measures the amount of 'surprise' in
addition to any expected stochasticity within the (learned) behavioural environment.
We call this latter form of well-known stochasticity *expected uncertainty*, which should
be encoded in the internal model for the current environment. Jumps in unexpected

uncertainty would signal that there may have been dramatic changes in the statistical contingencies governing the behavioural environment, and should alert the system to a possible need to overhaul the internal model.

What should we expect of the neural realization of expected and unexpected uncertainty signals? First, both should have the effect of suppressing internal, expectation-driven information relative to external, sensory-induced signals, as well as promoting learning about lesser-known aspects of the environment. Second, they should be differentially involved in tasks engaging just one or the other form of uncertainty. A wide variety of experimental evidence suggests that the cholinergic (ACh) and noradrenergic (NE) neuromodulatory systems satisfy these conditions (Robbins and Everitt 1995; Posner and Petersen 1990; Sarter and Bruno 1997; Baxter and Chiba 1999; Gu 2002). We reviewed much of the supporting experimental evidence in Yu and Dayan (2002) and Yu and Dayan (2005b), and proposed a Bayesian model of expected and unexpected uncertainty, respectively signalled by ACh and NE (Yu and Dayan 2005b).

To understand the concrete roles of expected uncertainty and unexpected uncertainty in inference and learning, we examined their computational roles in a novel, hypothesized experimental task (Fig. 39.2) (Yu and Dayan 2005b) that generalizes a discrimination variant of the original Posner spatial cueing task (Posner 1980), and an attention-shifting task (Devauges and Sara 1990). In this generalized task, subjects observe a sequence of trials, each containing a set of cue stimuli (the coloured arrows, pointing left or right), preceding a target stimulus (the light bulb) after a variable delay, and must respond as soon as they detect the target. The directions of the coloured arrows are randomized independently of each other on every trial, but one of them, the

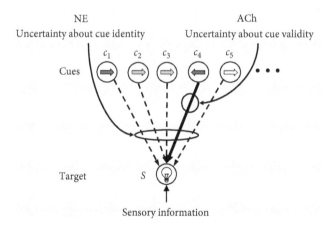

FIGURE 39.3 Schematic of the inference method. ACh and NE report expected and unexpected uncertainty, and jointly control the balance between top-down and bottom-up information processing in cortical inference and learning. The statistical contingencies in the combined attention task are captured in a common framework. On trial t, one single cue colour (among the many) is actually predictive of target location. ACh reports the estimated invalidity of the presumed cue; NE reports on the uncertainty associated with the identity (i.e. colour) of the informative cue.

cue, specified by its colour, predicts the location of the subsequent target with a significant probability (*cue validity* $\gamma > 0.5$); the rest of the arrows are irrelevant distractors. On each trial, the cue is correct (*valid*) with probability γ, and incorrect (*invalid*) with probability $1 - \gamma$ (cue *invalidity*). The colour of the cue arrow (the 'relevant' colour) and the cue validity persist over many trials, defining a relatively stable *context*. However, the experimenter can suddenly change the behavioural context by changing the relevant cue colour and cue validity, without informing the subject. The subject's implicit probabilistic task on each trial is to predict the likelihood of the target appearing on the left versus on the right given the set of cue stimuli on that trial. Doing this correctly requires the subject to infer the identity (colour) of the currently relevant arrow and estimate its validity. In turn, the subject must accurately detect the infrequent and unsignalled switches in the cue identity (and the context).

This novel task generalizes probabilistic cueing tasks, which typically have a predictive cue with fixed *identity*, but whose *validity* is explicitly manipulated. The task also generalizes attention-shifting tasks, for which the *identity* of the relevant cue stimulus is experimentally manipulated, but whose *validity* is fixed at being perfectly correct. In this generalized task, unsignalled changes in the cue identity result in observations about the cue and target that are atypical for the learned behavioural context. They give rise to unexpected uncertainty, and should therefore engage NE. Within each context, the cue has a fixed invalidity, which would give rise to expected uncertainty, and should therefore engage ACh.

Despite the apparent simplicity of the cue–target contingency in this novel task, achieving these computational goals is difficult due to the noise and non-stationarity underlying the cue–target relationship. The mathematically optimal *ideal learner* algorithm imposes rather high computational and representational costs, so that biological implementation of its exact form is unlikely. Nevertheless, the brain seems quite capable of solving similar, and much more difficult, problems. Therefore, we propose that the brain may be implementing an alternative algorithm (sketched in Fig. 39.3) that *approximates* the ideal one (Yu and Dayan 2005b). More detailed discussion of the model can be found in Yu and Dayan (2005b), along with a discussion of the circumstances under which the performance of the approximate algorithm closely tracks that of the ideal learner.

Specifically, the approximation we propose bases all estimates on just a single assumed relevant cue colour, rather than maintaining the full probability distribution over all potential cue colours. NE reports the estimated *lack of confidence* as to the particular colour that is currently believed to be relevant. This signal is driven by any unexpected cue–target observations on recent trials, and is the signal implicated in controlling learning following cue shift in the maze navigation task (Devauges and Sara 1990). ACh reports the estimated *invalidity* of the colour that is assumed to be relevant, and is the signal implicated in controlling the performance impact of cueing in the spatial cueing task, measured in validity effect, or the difference between reaction time or accuracy between validly and invalidly cued trials (Phillips et al. 2000). These two sources of uncertainty cooperate to determine how the subjects perform the trial-by-trial prediction task of estimating the likelihood that the target will appear on the left versus the right. Either form of uncertainty reduces the attention paid to the target location predicted by the assumed cue, since it reduces the degree to which that cue can be trusted. Validity effect in our model is therefore assumed to be proportional to $(1-ACh)(1-NE)$, though other formulations inversely related to each type of the uncertainties signalled by ACh and NE would produce qualitatively similar results. This is consistent with the observed ability of both ACh and NE to suppress top-down, intracortical information (associated with the cue), relative to bottom-up, input-driven sensory processing (associated with the target) (Gil et al. 1997; Hasselmo et al. 1996; Hsieh et al. 2000; Kimura et al. 1999; Kobayashi 2000).

In addition to the uncertainties signalled by ACh and NE, two other pieces of information are necessary for the appropriate updating of the internal model after each cue–target observation. One is the identity of the cue that is currently perceived to be relevant, which is critical for predicting target locations. The other is the estimate of the number of trials in the current context (since this colour first became relevant), which controls how much the estimated cue validity is influenced by the outcome of a single trial (analogous to the simple Kalman filter model discussed above). More details about these quantities, and their roles in the approximate algorithm, can be found in Yu and Dayan (2005b). We suggested that these two quantities are represented and updated in the prefrontal working memory (Miller and Cohen 2001). The prefrontal cortex has dense reciprocal connections with both the cholinergic (Sarter and Bruno 1997; Zaborszky et al. 1997; Hasselmo and Schnell 1994) and noradrenergic (Sara and Hervé-Minvielle 1995; Jodo et al. 1998) nuclei, in addition to the sensory processing areas, making it well suited to the integration and updating of the various quantities.

Figures 39.4 and 39.5 show comparisons between experimental and simulated data for the specific renditions of Posner's task (Phillips et al. 2000) and the maze navigation task (Devauges and Sara 1990), which we discussed above. We model the Posner task (Phillips et al. 2000) as a restricted version of the general task, for which the identity of the relevant colour does not change and the cue validity is fixed. An iterative algorithm computes expected and unexpected uncertainties and thereby predicts the size of validity effect (Yu and Dayan 2005b). Since there is no unexpected uncertainty, NE is not explicitly involved, and so noradrenergic manipulation is incapable of interfering with performance in this task. This is consistent with experimental data (Witte and Marrocco 1997). However, ACh captures the invalidity of the cue, and so, as in the experimental data (Fig. 39.4a, b), the validity effect depends inversely on boosting (Fig. 39.4c) or suppressing (Fig. 39.4d) ACh.

In contrast to the Posner task, which involves no unexpected uncertainty, the attention-shifting task involves unexpected, but not expected, uncertainty. Within our theoretical framework, such a task explicitly manipulates the identity of the relevant cue, while the cue validity is kept constant (with high validity). Experimentally enhancing NE level (Devauges and Sara 1990) would result in greater unexpected uncertainty and therefore a greater readiness to abandon the current hypothesis and adopt a new model for environmental contingencies. As expected, simulations of our model showed

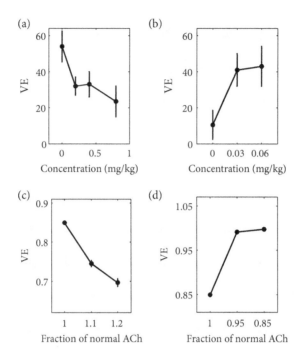

FIGURE 39.4 The Posner task and cholinergic modulation. The validity effect is taken to be the difference in reaction time between invalidly and validly cued trials. (a) Systemic administration of nicotine decreases validity effect in a dose-dependent manner. Adapted from Phillips et al. 2000. (b) Systemic administration of scopolamine increases validity effect in a dose-dependent manner. Adapted from *Psychopharmacology*, 150(1), 2000, pp. 112–6, Cholinergic neurotransmission influences covert orientation of visuospatial attention in the rat, Janice M. Phillips. With kind permission from Springer Science and Business Media. Even though the baselines for the two control groups (with drug concentration equal to 0) in (a) and (b) are not well-matched, the opposite and dose-dependent effects of the bi-directional manipulations are clear. (c, d) Simulation results replicate these trends qualitatively. Error bars: standard errors of the mean over 1000 trials.

an advantage for NE elevation to 10% above normal (Fig. 39.5b), similar to experimental data (Fig. 39.5a) (Devauges and Sara 1990). Our model also predicts a lack of ACh involvement, since the perfect reliability of the cues obviates a role for expected uncertainty, consistent with experimental data (McGaughy et al. 2008).

These results do not imply that increasing NE would create individuals that are generally 'smarter'. In the model, control animals are relatively slow in switching to a new visual strategy because their performance embodies an assumption (which is normally correct) that task contingencies do not easily change. Pharmacologically increasing NE counteracts the conservative character of this internal model, allowing idazoxan animals to learn faster than the control animals under these particular circumstances. The extra propensity of the NE group to consider that the task has changed based on relatively little evidence can also impair their performance in other circumstances, for instance when the underlying statistical contingencies are highly stable.

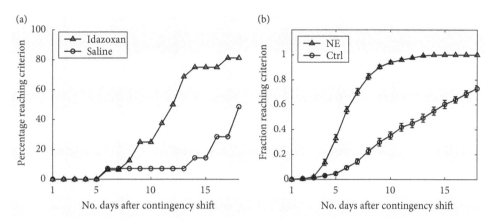

FIGURE 39.5 A maze-navigation task and the effects of NE. (a) The cumulative percentage of idazoxan rats reaching criterion (making no more than one error on two consecutive days) considerably outpaced that of the saline-control group. Adapted from *Behavioural Brain Research*, 39(1), Valerie Devauges and Susan J. Sara, Activation of the noradrenergic system facilitates an attentional shift in the rat, pp. 19–28, Copyright (1990), with permission from Elsevier. (b) In the model, simulated subjects with elevated NE levels (10% greater than normal) also learned the strategy shift considerably faster than controls. Data averaged over 20 simulated experiments of 30 models rats each: 15 NE-enhanced, 15 controls. Error bars: standard errors of the mean.

In the generalized task of Fig. 39.2, both cue identity and validity are explicitly manipulated, and therefore we expect both ACh and NE to play significant roles. The key to solving the full task is the timely and accurate detection of context changes in the face of invalidity. A trial perceived to be valid always increases confidence in the current context, as well as estimated cue validity. But when a trial is apparently invalid, subjects have to decide between maintaining the current context with an increased invalidity, or abandoning it altogether. This decision requires comparing the relative probability of having observed a chance invalid trial given the estimated cue validity, and the probability of the predictive cue identity having changed altogether. As ACh reports the first probability, and NE the second, we can expect there to be a rich interaction between these neuromodulators. In Yu and Dayan (2005b), we showed that near-optimal learning can be approximated by assuming the context to have changed whenever

$$NE > \frac{ACh}{0.5 + ACh}. \tag{5}$$

This inequality points to an *antagonistic* relationship between ACh and NE: the threshold for NE which determines whether or not the context should be assumed to have changed is set monotonically by the level of ACh. Intuitively, when the estimated cue invalidity is low, a single observation of a mismatch between cue and target could signal a context switch. But when the estimated cue invalidity is high, indicating low correlation between cue and target, then a single mismatch would be more likely to be treated as an invalid trial rather than a context switch. This antagonistic relationship

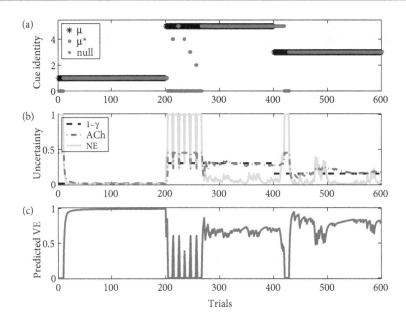

FIGURE 39.6 Typical run of approximate inference on the generalized attention task. (a) Tracking of cue identity. The true underlying context variable μ (in black stars), indicates which one of the $h = 5$ coloured cue stimuli is actually predictive of the target location: $\mu = 1$ for first 200 trials, $\mu = 5$ for the next 200, and $\mu = 3$ for the final 200. The true μ is closely tracked by the estimated μ^* (in magenta circles, mostly overlapping the black stars). The blue dots indicate 'null' trials on which the algorithm has detected a context change but has yet to come up with a new hypothesis for the predictive cue among the h possible cue stimuli. (b) Tracking of cue validity. The black dashed line is $1 - \gamma$, indicating the true cue invalidity: $1 - \gamma$ is 0.01 for the first 200 trials, $1 - \gamma = 0.3$ for the next 200, and $1 - \gamma = 0.15$ for the final 200. Higher values of $1 - \gamma$ result in noisier observations. The red trace indicates the level of ACh, reporting $1 - \gamma^*$, or the estimated probability of invalid cueing in the model. It closely tracks the true value of $1 - \gamma$. The green trace indicates the level of NE, reporting on the approximate algorithm's model uncertainty $1 - \lambda^*$. (c) Predicted validity effect, corresponding to either the difference in accuracy or reaction time between valid and invalid trials. Modelled as proportional to the total confidence in the predictive power of the cue, which depends on both types of uncertainty, validity effect varies inversely with both ACh and NE levels: validity effect = $(1 - \text{ACh})(1 - \text{NE})$.

between ACh and NE in the *learning* of the cue–target relationship over trials contrasts with their chiefly *synergistic* relationship in the *prediction* of the target location on each trial.

Figure 39.6a shows a typical run in the full task that uses differently coloured cue stimuli. The predictive cue stimulus is $\mu = 1$ for the first 200 trials, $\mu = 5$ for the next 200, and $\mu = 3$ for the final 200. The approximate algorithm does a good job of tracking the underlying contextual sequence from the noisy observations. The black dashed line (labelled $1 - \gamma$) in Fig. 39.6b shows the cue invalidities of 1%, 30%, and 15% for the three contexts.

Simulated ACh levels (dashed red trace in Fig. 39.6b) approach these values in each context. The corresponding simulated NE levels (solid green trace in Fig. 39.6b) show that NE generally correctly reports a contextual change when one occurs, though occasionally a false alarm can be triggered by a chance accumulation of unexpected observations, which takes place most frequently when the true cue validity is low. These traces directly give rise to physiological predictions regarding ACh and NE activations, which could be experimentally verified. Psychophysical predictions can also be derived from the model. The validity effect is predicted to exhibit the characteristic pattern shown in Fig. 39.6c, where large transients are mostly dependent on NE activities, while tonic values are more determined by ACh levels. During the task, there is a strong dip in the validity effect just after each contextual change, arising from a drop in model confidence. The asymptotic validity effect within a context, on the other hand, converges to a level that is proportional to the expected probability of valid cues.

It follows from Eq. 5 and the related discussion above, that ACh and NE interact critically to help construct appropriate cortical representations and make correct inferences. Thus, simulated experimental interference with one or both neuromodulatory systems should result in an intricate pattern of impairments. Using simulations, we showed that NE depletion results in the model having excessive confidence in the current cue–target relationship, leading to perseverative behaviour and an impairment in the ability to adapt to environmental changes (Yu and Dayan 2005b), which are also observed in animals with experimentally reduced NE levels (Sara 1998). In addition, the model makes the prediction that this reluctance to adapt to new environments would make the ACh level, which reports expected uncertainty, gradually rise to take into account all the accumulating evidence of deviation from the current model. Conversely, suppressing ACh leads the model to underestimate the amount of variation in a given context (Yu and Dayan 2005b). Consequently, the significance of deviations from the primary location is exaggerated, causing the NE system to overreact and lead to frequent and unnecessary alerts of context switches. Overall, the system exhibits symptoms of 'hyper-distractibility', reminiscent of empirical observations that anti-cholinergic drugs enhance distractibility (Jones and Higgins 1995) while agonists suppress it (Prendergast et al. 1998; Terry et al. 2002; O'Neill et al. 2003).

We also simulated combined ACh and NE depletion (Yu and Dayan, 2005b): it is predicted to lead to inaccurate cholinergic tracking of cue invalidity and a significant increase in false alarms about contextual changes, though it also results in *less severe* impairments than either single depletion: intermediate values of NE depletion, combined with ACh depletion, induce impairments that are significantly less severe than either single manipulation (Yu and Dayan 2005b). Intuitively, since ACh sets the threshold for NE-dependent contextual change (Eq. 5), abnormal suppression of either system can be partially alleviated by directly inhibiting the other. Due to this antagonism, depleting the ACh level in the model has somewhat similar effects to enhancing NE; and depleting NE is similar to enhancing ACh. Intriguingly, Sara and colleagues have found similarly antagonistic interactions between ACh and NE in a series of learning and memory studies (Sara 1989; Ammassari-Teule et al. 1991; Sara et al. 1992;

Dyon-Laurent et al. 1993, 1994). They demonstrated that learning and memory deficits caused by cholinergic lesions can be alleviated by the administration of clonidine (Sara 1989; Ammassari-Teule et al. 1991; Sara et al. 1992; Dyon-Laurent et al. 1993, 1994), a noradrenergic α-2 agonist that decreases the level of NE (Coull et al. 1997).

While we have illustrated our model using a hypothetical task that is a combination of a spatial cueing task and a maze learning task, the key concepts could be equivalently realized by modifying a number of other familiar attention tasks, such as allowing the cue validity to vary in an attention-shifting task. There is also a rich background of experimental data consistent with our uncertainty theory of ACh and NE, which lie outside traditional attentional tasks. For instance, the enhanced learning animals accord to stimuli with uncertain predictive consequences (Bucci et al. 1998), and decreased learning they accord to stimuli with well-known consequences (Baxter et al. 1997), in conditioning tasks (Pearce and Hall, 1980) is critically dependent on the ACh system. Also, recordings of neurons in the locus coeruleus, the source of cortical NE, indicate strong neural response to unexpected external changes such as novelty, the introduction of reinforcement pairing, and the extinction or reversal of these contingencies (Sara and Segal 1991; Vankov et al. 1995; Sara et al. 1994; Aston-Jones et al. 1997). NE has also been observed to modulate the P300 component of ERP (Pineda et al. 1997; Missonnier et al. 1999; Turetsky and Fein 2002), which has been associated with various types of violation of expectations: 'surprise' (Verleger et al. 1994), 'novelty' (Donchin et al. 1978), and 'oddball' (Pineda et al. 1997). These data provide additional evidence that NE reports unexpected global changes in the external environment, and thus serving as an alarm system for contextual switches. In addition, the well-documented ability of ACh and NE to control experience-dependent plasticity in the cortex (Gu 2002) is consistent with their proposed ability to alter sensory processing after the detection of a global contextual change in a fundamental manner.

COVERT ATTENTION IN PERCEPTUAL DECISION-MAKING

In the previous section, we focused on the role of neuromodulatory systems in the representation of uncertainty in inference and learning tasks. In addition to this more macroscopic form of uncertainty, there is a separate body of work on the encoding of *microscopic* form of uncertainty by cortical neuronal populations. This spans a broad spectrum, from distributional codes that can encode mean and variance (Zemel et al. 1998), to more exotic codes that can represent complex distributions (Sahani and Dayan 2003; Barber et al. 2003; Rao 2004; Weiss and Fleet 2002). How microscopic and macroscopic neural representations of uncertainty work together is an important and relatively unexplored area. Another under-explored area of attention is the decision component. For simple binary perceptual decision, an elegant theoretical framework has emerged: lateral intraparietal sulcus (LIP) neurons have been suggested to accumulate sensory information about relevant stimulus properties, such as motion direction in the case of a moving stimulus, until a fixed decision threshold is reached (Gold and Shadlen 2002; Ratcliff 2001; Smith and Ratcliff 2004), in a process computationally reminiscent of the Bayes-optimal statistical decision procedure, the sequential probability ratio test (Wald 1947; Wald and Wolfowitz 1948). However, how sensory information translates into decision in more complex scenarios, such as when there are multiple (greater than two) perceptual outcomes, or when there is a computational need to attend more to some aspect of the sensory environment over the other, is less understood in terms of both the computational and neural principles underlying brain processing. Recently (Yu and Dayan 2005a), we tackled these challenges in the context of a spatial (covert) attention cueing task that we introduced earlier. We used a temporally more detailed model to examine the way neuronal populations interact to filter and accumulate noisy information over time, the influence of attention and neuromodulation on the dynamics of cortical processing, and the process through which perceptual decisions are made (Yu and Dayan 2005a).

One empirically observed consequence of spatial attention is a *multiplicative* increase in the activities of visual cortical neurons (McAdams and Maunsell 1999, 2000). If cortical neuronal populations are coding for uncertainty in the underlying variable, it is of obvious importance to understand how attentional effects on neural response, such as multiplicative modulation, change the implied uncertainty, and what statistical characteristics of attention license this change. One early Bayesian model of spatial attention gave an abstract computational account of this effect (Dayan and Zemel 1999). It was argued that performing an orientation discrimination task on a spatially localized stimulus is equivalent to marginalizing out the spatial uncertainty in the joint posterior over orientation φ and spatial location y given inputs I:

$$p(\phi|I) = \int_y p(\phi, y|I).$$

(6)

If that spatial integration is restricted to a smaller region that contains the visual stimulus, then less irrelevant input (i.e. noise) is integrated into the computation. This in turn leads to more accurate and less uncertain posterior estimates of $\hat{\phi}$. It was proposed that under encoding schemes such as the standard Poisson model, such decrease in posterior uncertainty is equivalent to a *multiplicative* modulation of the orientation tuning curve (Dayan and Zemel 1999), which may be implemented by, for example, a contrast gain mechanism (see also chapter by Maunsell).

Following up on that work, we proposed a more detailed model of neural coding to demonstrate how neuromodulator-mediated spatial attention interacts with cortical probabilistic information to influence the dynamics and semantics of perceptual inference and decision-making (Yu and Dayan 2005a). In this scheme, spatial attention also effects a multiplicative scaling of the orientation tuning function. Compared to the standard Poisson model (Dayan and Abbott 2001), however, this encoding scheme is able to represent a more diverse range of probabilistic distributions over stimulus values. We also examined how information is accumulated over time in such a network, and enables the timely and accurate execution of perceptual decisions (Yu and Dayan 2005a). We review the model and its main implications here.

For concreteness, we again focus on a discrimination variant of the Posner task (Posner 1980), in which a cue predicts the location (left or right, y) of a subsequent target, on which the subject must perform a discrimination task (e.g. orientation, φ). The cue induces a prior distribution over the target location y. However, 'robustness' would require that a sensory stimulus, however improbable under the current top-down model, should get processed to some extent. We therefore model the prior distribution to be a mixture between a peaked cue-induced component and a 'flat' generic component, $p_c(y;c) = \gamma \mathcal{N}(\tilde{y}, v^2) + (1-\gamma)c$. γ parameterizes the relative probability of the cue-induced component being correct, and incorporates factors such as the validity of the cue. Consistent with our theory of neuromodulation outlined in the previous section, we suggest that $1 - \gamma$ should be signalled by ACh. The Gaussian component of the prior comes from a top-down source, perhaps a higher cortical area such as the parietal cortex, and its mean and width, possibly of high spatial precision, should be represented by a cortical population itself.

The neural computations under consideration here involve some intermediate level of processing in the visual pathway, which receives top-down attentional inputs embodied by the prior $p(y; c)$ and noisy sensory inputs $D_t = \{x_1, \ldots, x_t\}$ that are sampled independently and identically (iid) from a stimulus with true location and orientation y^* and φ^*. We model the pattern of activations $x_t = \{x_{ij}(t)\}$ to the stimulus as independent and Gaussian, $x_{ij}(t) \sim N(f_{ij}(y^*, \varphi^*), \sigma_n)$, with variance σ_n^2 around a mean tuning function that is bell-shaped and separable in space and orientation:

$$f_{ij}\left(y^*, \phi^*\right) = z_y \exp\left(-\frac{\left(y_i - y^*\right)^2}{2\sigma_y^2}\right) z_\phi \exp\left(k \cos\left(\phi_j - \phi^*\right)\right). \tag{7}$$

The task involves making explicit inferences about φ and implicit ones about y. The computational steps involved in the inference can be decomposed into the following:

$$p(x_t | y, \varphi) = \Pi_{ij}\, p(x_{ij}(t) | y, \varphi)\, \text{Likelihood}$$

$$p(\varphi | x_t) = \int_{y \in Y} p(y, \varphi)p(x_t | y, \varphi)dy\, \text{Prior-weighted marginalization}$$

$$p(\varphi | D_t) \propto p(\varphi | D_{t-1})p(y, \varphi | x_t)\, \text{Temporal accumulation}$$

Because the marginalization step is weighted by the priors, even though the task is ultimately about the orientation variable φ, the shape of the prior $p(y)$ on the spatial variable can have dramatic effects on the marginalization and the subsequent computations. In particular, if the prior $p(y)$ assigns high probability to the true y^*, then the more 'signal' and less 'noise' would be integrated into the posterior, whereas just the opposite happens if $p(y)$ assigns low probability to the true y^*. This is the computational cost between valid and invalid cueing, a point we will return to later.

To implement the necessary probabilistic computations, we consider a hierarchical neural architecture in which top-down attentional priors are integrated with sequentially sampled sensory input in a sound Bayesian manner, using a direct log probability encoding (Weiss and Fleet 2002; Rao 2004). Fig. 39.7 shows the semantics and architecture of this hierarchical neural network, along with example activities of each layer at one moment in time. The first layer reports likelihood information and represents the activities of early stages in sensory processing (e.g. the retina in the visual system). The second layer represents the next stage of processing that incorporates top-down influence and bottom-up inputs (for instance, visual areas from LGN to MT/MST have all been shown to be significantly modulated by spatial attention (O'Connor et al. 2002); also see chapter by Beck and Kastner). Layer III represents neuronal populations that specialize in a particular aspect of featural processing, as it is well documented that higher visual cortical areas become increasingly specialized. Layer IV represents

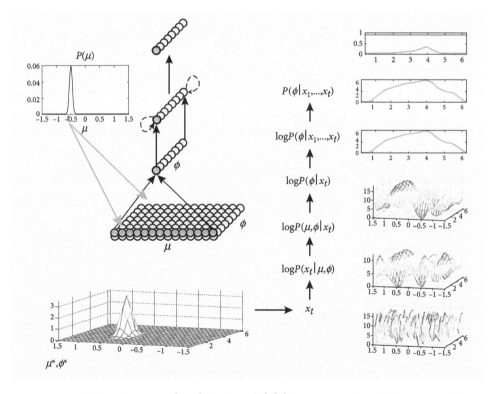

FIGURE 39.7 A Bayesian neural architecture. Solid lines represent excitatory connections, dashed lines represent inhibitory connections. Blue circles illustrate how the activities of one row of inputs in Layer I travel through the hierarchy to affect the final decision layer. Brown circles illustrate how one unit in the spatial prior layer comes into the integration process.

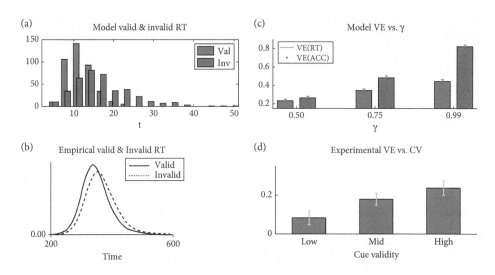

FIGURE 39.8 Validity effect and dependence on γ. (a) The distribution of reaction times for the invalid condition has a greater mean and longer tail than the valid condition in model simulation results. $\gamma = 0.5$. (b) Similar trend in a spatial cueing task in rats. CV $= 0.5$. © 1993, The American Physiological Society (APS). *Journal of Neurophysiology*, 70(1), E. M. Bowman, V. J. Brown, C. Kertzman, U. Schwarz, and D. L. Robinson, Covert orienting of attention in macaques. I. Effects of behavioral context, pp. 431–443. (c) Stimulated validity effect, whether in terms of reaction time (validity effect$_{rt}$ = $(RT_{inv} - RT_{val})/RT_{inv}$) or in error rate (validity effect$_{er}$ = $(ER_{inv} - ER_{val})/ER_{inv}$), increases with increasing cue validity, γ. Error rate is defined as the angular distance between $\hat{\phi}$ and φ^*. Error-bars are standard errors of the mean. Simulation parameters: $\{y_i\} = \{-1.5, -1.4,\ldots,$ 1.4, 1.5\}, $\{\varphi_j\} = \{\pi/8, 2\pi/8,\ldots, 16\pi/8\}$, $\sigma_y = 0.1$, $\sigma_\varphi = \pi/16$, $q = 0.90$, $y^* = 0.5$, $\gamma \in \{0.5, 0.75, 0.99\}$, $v = 0.05$, 300 trials each of valid and invalid trials. 100 trials of each γ value. (d) Validity effect, defined in terms of RT, also increases with cue validity in a human Posner task. Data from Yu, A. J., Bentley, P., Seymour, B., Driver, J., Dolan, R., and Dayan, P.,   Expected and unexpected uncertainties control allocation of attention in a novel attentional learning task, Society for Neuroscience Abstract, pp. 176.17 © 2004, Society for Neuroscience.

neuronal populations that integrate information over time, as for instance seen in the monkey LIP (Gold and Shadlen 2002). And finally, layer V neurons represent those involved in the actual decision-making, presumably in the frontal cortical areas (though some have argued that higher visual cortical areas such as LIP may be responsible for this stage as well (Gold and Shadlen 2002)). At any given time t, a decision is made based on the maximum of the posterior: if it is greater than a decision threshold q, then the observation process is terminated, and the most probable orientation is reported as the estimated $\hat{\phi}$ for the current trial; otherwise, the observation process continues for at least one more time step. This is an n-hypothesis generalization of the sequential probability ratio test for binary decisions (Wald and Wolfowitz 1948), which has also been proposed to explain apparent evidence integration computations in the lateral intraparietal sulcus (Gold and Shadlen 2002).

Figure 39.8 demonstrates that the model indeed exhibits the cue-induced validity effect. That is, mean reaction time and error rates for invalid cue trials are greater than those for valid cue trials. The model 'reaction time' (RT) is the average number of iid samples (presumed to be generated with independent and identical noise conditioned on the stimulus state) necessary to reach the decision threshold q, and 'error rate' is the average angular distance between estimated $\hat{\phi}$ and the true ϕ^*.

Fig. 39.8 shows simulation results for 300 trials each of valid and invalid cue trials, for different values of γ which reflect the model's belief of cue validity. The RT distribution for invalid-cue trials is broader and right-shifted compared to valid-cue trials, consistent with experimental data (Posner 1980; Bowman et al. 1993) (Fig. 39.8b). Fig. 39.8a shows a similar pattern in the distribution of RT obtained in the case of $\gamma = 0.5$. Fig. 39.8c shows that the validity effect increases with increasing perceived cue validity, as parameterized by γ, in both reaction times and error rates. The robust validity effect in both measures excludes the possibility of a simple speed–accuracy trade-off, instead reflecting a real cost of invalid cueing that depends on assumed cue validity.

Since we have an explicit model of not only the 'behavioural responses' on each trial, but the intermediate levels of neural machinery underlying the computations, we can look more closely at the activity patterns in the various neuronal layers and relate them to physiological phenomena. Electrophysiological and functional imaging studies have shown that spatial cueing to one side of the visual field increases stimulus-induced activities in the corresponding part of the visual cortex (Reynolds and Chelazzi 2004; Kastner and Ungerleider 2000). Fig. 39.9a shows that our model can qualitatively reproduce this effect: the cued side is more active than the uncued side. Moreover, the difference

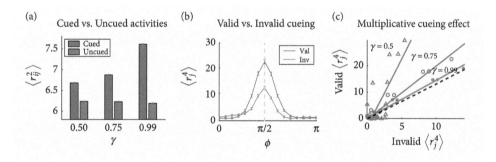

FIGURE 39.9 Multiplicative gain modulation by spatial attention. (a) r_{ij}^2 activities, averaged over the half of layer II where the prior peaks, are greater for valid (blue) than invalid (red) conditions. (b) Effect of spatial cueing on layer IV activities is multiplicative, similar to multiplicative modulation of V4 orientation tuning curves observed experimentally. Data from McAdams, C. J. and Maunsell, J. H. R. (1999). Effects of attention on orientation-tuning functions of single neurons in macaque cortical area V4, Journal of Neuroscience, 19, pp. 431–41 © 1999, Society for Neuroscience. (c) Linear fits to scatter-plot of layer IV activities for valid cue condition vs. invalid cue condition show that the slope is greatest for large γ and smallest for small γ. Magenta: $\gamma = 0.99$, blue: $\gamma = 0.75$, red: $\gamma = 0.5$, dashed black: empirical linear fit in V4 neurons. Data from McAdams, C. J. and Maunsell, J. H. R. (1999). Effects of attention on orientation-tuning functions of single neurons in macaque cortical area V4, Journal of Neuroscience, 19, pp. 431–41 © 1999, Society for Neuroscience. Simulation parameters are same as in Fig. 39.8. Error bars are standard errors of the mean.

increases for increasing γ, the perceived cue validity. Electrophysiological experiments have also shown that spatial attention has an approximately multiplicative effect on orientation tuning responses in visual cortical neurons (McAdams and Maunsell 1999). We see a similar phenomenon in the layer III and IV neurons. Fig. 39.9b shows the layer IV responses averaged over 300 trials of each of the valid and invalid conditions; layer III effects are similar and not shown here. The shape of the average tuning curves and the effect of attentional modulation are qualitatively similar to those observed in spatial attention experiments (McAdams and Maunsell 1999) (also see Maunsell chapter). Fig. 39.9c is a scatter-plot of $\langle r_j^4 \rangle_t$ for the valid condition versus the invalid condition, for various values of γ. The quality of the linear least square error fits is fairly good, and the slope increases with increasing confidence in the cued location (e.g. larger γ). For comparison, the slope fit to the experimental data (McAdams and Maunsell 1999) is shown in black dashed line. In the model, the slope not only depends on γ but also the noise model, the discretization, and so on, so the comparison of Fig. 39.9c should be interpreted loosely.

In valid cases, the effect of attention is to increase the certainty (narrow the width) of the marginal posterior over φ, since the correct prior allows the relative suppression of noisy input from the irrelevant part of space. If the marginal posterior were Gaussian, the increased certainty would translate into a decreased variance. For Gaussian probability distributions, logarithmic coding amounts to something close to a quadratic (adjusted for the circularity of orientation), with the curvature determined by the variance. Decreasing the variance increases the curvature, and therefore has a multiplicative effect on the activities (as in Fig. 39.9). While it is difficult to show the multiplicative modulation rigorously, we proved it for the case where the spatial prior is very sharply peaked at its Gaussian mean $\tilde{y}$ (Yu and Dayan 2005a). The approximate Gaussianity of the marginal posterior comes from the accumulation of many independent samples over time and space, and is related to the central limit theorem. Readers are referred to a standard statistics probability textbook for further reading on this point.

Another interesting aspect of the intermediate representation is the way attention modifies the evidence accumulation process over time. Fig. 39.10 shows the effect of cueing on the activities of neuron $r_{j^*}^5(t)$, or $P(\varphi^*|D_t)$, for all trials with correct responses: i.e. where neuron j^* representing the true underlying orientation φ^* reached decision threshold before all other neurons in layer V. The mean activity trajectory is higher for the valid cue case than the invalid one: in this case, spatial attention mainly acts through increasing the rate of evidence accumulation after stimulus onset (steeper rise). This attentional effect is more pronounced when the system has more confidence about its prior information (A. $\gamma = 0.5$, B. $\gamma = 0.75$, C. $\gamma = 0.99$). It is interesting that changing the perceived validity of the cue affects the validity effect mainly by changing the cost of invalid cues, and not the benefit of the valid cue. This has also been experimentally observed in rat versions of the Posner task (Witte and Marrocco 1997). Crudely, as γ approaches 1, the evidence accumulation rate in valid-cue case saturates due to input noise. But for the invalid-cue case, the near-complete withdrawal of weight on the 'true' signal coming from the uncued location leads to catastrophic consequences. The general effect of increasing γ is similar to increasing input *noise* in invalid trials.

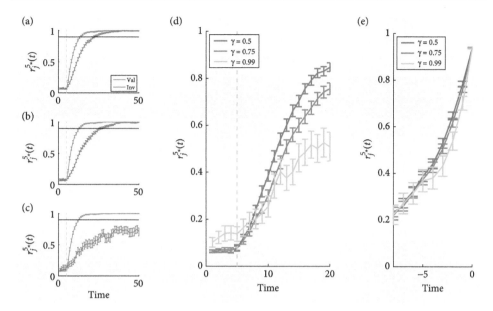

FIGURE 39.10 Accumulation of iid samples in orientation discrimination, and dependence on prior belief about stimulus location. (a–c) Average activity of neuron, r_{j*}^5, which represents $P(\varphi^*|D_t)$, saturates to 100% certainty much faster for valid cue trials (blue) than invalid cue trials (red). The difference is more drastic when γ is larger, or when there is more prior confidence in the cued target location. (a) $\gamma = 0.5$, (b) $\gamma = 0.75$, (c) $\gamma = 0.99$. Cyan dashed line indicates stimulus onset. (d) First 15 time steps (from stimulus onset) of the invalid cue traces from (a–c) are aligned to stimulus onset; cyan line denotes stimulus onset. The differential rates of rise are apparent. (e) Last 8 time steps of the invalid traces from (a–c) are aligned to decision threshold-crossing; there is no clear separation as a function γ. Simulation parameters are same as in Fig. 39.8.

Fig. 39.10d shows the average traces for invalid-cueing trials aligned to the stimulus onset, and Fig. 39.10e to the decision threshold crossing. These results bear remarkable similarities to the LIP neuronal activities recorded during monkey perceptual decision-making (Roitman and Shadlen 2002; Gold and Shadlen 2002). In the stimulus-aligned case, the traces rise linearly at first and then tail off somewhat, and the rate of rise increases for lower (effective) noise. In the decision-aligned case, the traces rise steeply and in sync. Roughly speaking, greater input noise leads to smaller *average* increase of r_j^5 at each time step, but greater *variance*. Because the threshold-crossing event is strongly determined by both the mean and the variance of the random walk, the two effects tend to counteract each other, resulting in similarly steep rise prior to threshold-crossing independent of the underlying noise process. All these characteristics can also be seen in the LIP neural response (Roitman and Shadlen 2002; Gold and Shadlen 2002), where the input noise level was explicitly varied.

This work has various theoretical and experimental implications. The model presents one possible reconciliation of cortical and neuromodulatory representations of uncertainty. The sensory-driven activities (layer I in this model) themselves encode bottom-up uncertainty, including sensory receptor noise and any processing noise that have occurred up until then. The top-down information, which specifies the Gaussian component of the spatial prior $p(y)$, involves two kinds of uncertainty. One determines the locus and spatial extent of visual attention, the other specifies the relative importance of this top-down bias compared to the bottom-up stimulus-driven input. The first is highly specific in modality and featural dimension, presumably originating from higher visual cortical areas (e.g. parietal cortex for spatial attention, inferotemporal cortex for complex featural attention). The second is more generic and may affect different featural dimensions and maybe even different modalities simultaneously, and is thus more appropriately signalled by a diffusely projecting neuromodulator such as ACh. This characterization is also in keeping with our previous models of ACh (Yu and Dayan 2002, 2003) and experimental data showing that ACh selectively suppresses cortico-cortical transmission relative to bottom-up processing in primary sensory cortices (Kimura et al. 1999), as well as pharmacological studies showing an inverse relationship between the cue validity effect and the level of ACh (Phillips et al. 2000).

The results illustrate the important concept that prior belief about one dimension of a stimulus can significantly alter the inferential performance in an independent stimulus dimension (orientation). Increasing y leads to an increased mismatch between the assumed prior distribution (sharply peaked at cued location) and the true generative distribution over space (bimodally–modally peaked at the two locations $\pm y'$). Because the spatial prior affects the marginal posterior over φ by altering the relative importance of joint posterior terms in the marginalization process, overly large y results in undue prominence of the noise samples in the cued location and negligence of samples in the uncued sample. Thus, while a fixed posterior threshold would normally lead to a fixed accuracy level under the correct prior distribution, in this case larger y induces larger mismatch and therefore poor discrimination performance.

In addition to its theoretical implications, this work has interesting bearings on the experimental debate over the target of top-down attention. Earlier studies suggested that spatial attention acts mainly at higher visual areas, that attentional modulation of striate cortical activities is minimal, if at all significant (Moran and Desimone 1985). However, a recent study using more sensitive techniques (O'Connor et al. 2002) has demonstrated that spatial attention alters visual processing not only in primary visual cortex, but also in the lateral geniculate nucleus in the thalamus (see also Beck and Kastner, chapter 9, this volume, Saalmann and Kastner, chapter 14, this volume). In our neural architecture, even though attentional effects are prominent at higher processing layers (III–V), the prior actually comes into the integration process at a lower layer (II). This raises the intriguing possibility that attention directly acts on the lowest level that receives top-down input and is capable of representing the prior information. The attentional modulation observed in higher visual areas may be a consequence of differential bottom-up input rather than direct attentional modulation.

An important question that remains is how the *quality* of the input signal can be detected and encoded. If the stimulus onset time is not precisely known, then naive integration of bottom-up inputs is no longer optimal, because the effective signal/noise ratio of the input changes when the stimulus is turned on (or off). More generally, the signal strength (possibly 0) could be any one of several possibilities, as in the random-dot coherent motion task, in which subjects have to identify the primary direction of motion of a field of moving dots, only a fraction of which are moving coherently in the same direction, the rest flickering randomly (Gold and Shadlen 2002). Optimal discrimination under such conditions requires the inference of both the stimulus strength and its property (e.g. orientation or motion direction). There is some suggestive evidence that the neuromodulator norepinephrine may be involved in such computations. In a version of the Posner task in which cues are presented on both sides (so-called double cueing), and so provide only information about stimulus onset, there is experimental evidence that norepinephrine is involved in optimizing sensory processing (Witte and Marrocco 1997). Based on a slightly different task involving sustained attention or vigilance (Rajkowski et al. 1994), Brown et al. (2004) have recently made the interesting suggestion that one role for noradrenergic neuromodulation is to implement a change in the integration strategy when the stimulus is detected. We have also tackled this issue by ascribing to phasic norepinephrine a related but distinct role in signalling unexpected state uncertainty (Dayan and Yu 2006; Shenoy and Yu 2012).

OVERT SPATIAL ATTENTION

In experimental settings, spatial attention tends to be studied purely in the overt setting, with subjects instructed to resist eye movements. This is in part to allow stability to be established in visual cortical receptive field responses, and in part to simplify the visual processing itself. However, in naturalistic settings, covert and overt attention interact intimately to aid sensory processing (Yantis and Jonides 1984; Rizzolatti et al. 1987; Hoffman and Subramaniam 1995; Moore and Fallah 2001; Stigchel and Theeuwes 2007). Humans and other animals continuously use strategic self-motion to improve sensory information collection, in a manner sensitive to prior knowledge and task goals. Recently, we used a novel visual search task, combined with Bayesian ideal-observer modelling, to examine whether and how the brain internalizes spatial regularities in target location and uses such information to optimize saccadic search strategy for a noisy target (Huang and Yu 2010).

While it has long been known that eye movement patterns are strongly influenced by cognitive factors (Yarbus 1967), such as prior knowledge about target location (He and Kowler 1989), temporal onset (Oswal et al. 2007), and reward probability (Roesch and Olson 2003), it is poorly understood how such contextual knowledge is acquired and how it precisely modulates saccadic choices and perceptual decisions. We recently used a novel visual search task, in which the target stimulus appeared in different locations with different probabilities, to investigate how humans learn and use knowledge about the spatial distribution of targets to control eye movements (Huang and Yu 2010). We formulated several Bayesian ideal observer models (Huang and Yu 2010), based on different hypotheses about statistical learning and decision-making, and compared them to experimental data—in order to identify the learning procedure used by subjects to acquire spatial prior information, and the decision process that they employ to choose sequential fixation locations.

There has been a long history of debate over whether humans and animals *match* (Herrnstein 1961, 1970; Davison and McCarthy 1987) or *maximize* (Hall-Johnson and Poling 1984; Blakely et al. 1988; Poling et al. 2011) in their choice behaviour, where there are multiple options that yield different magnitude or probability or reward. While the maximizing strategy would seem more optimal (greater expected reward), there is an intriguing body of studies suggesting that humans and animals often adopt a matching-like choice policy instead (Herrnstein 1961, 1970; Sugrue et al. 2004) or the related sampling policy (Vul et al. 2009). This debate is relevant for saccadic strategy—in understanding whether subjects first search the most probable location (maximizing), or allocate search fixation proportional to the underlying probability of different locations containing the target (matching). We also explored a third alternative, an algorithmically simple but computationally suboptimal heuristic policy, in which subjects always start searching from the target location of the previous trial, which we call 'follow-last-target' policy. This is related to the classic win-stay-lose-shift policy, first proposed in game theory for games like Prisoner's Dilemma (Rapoport and Chammah 1965; Nowak and Sigmund 1993) and later used to characterize pigeon (Randall and Zentall 1997), monkey (Warren 1966), and human (Frank et al. 2008; Steyvers et al. 2009; Lee et al. 2011; Otto et al. 2011; Scheibehenne et al. 2011; Worthy and Maddox 2012) learning and choice behaviour.

From a different angle, we were also interested in characterizing the dynamic learning procedure humans adopt to learn about spatial regularities in the environment. Specifically, we investigated whether human subjects' learning policy accumulates spatial statistics stably over a long timescale (across a block), or takes into account only the recent trial history. This was motivated by our previous work showing that in serial 2-alternative reaction time tasks, subjects' tendency to exhibit a sequential effect (sensitivity to local runs of repetitions and alternations) (Laming 1968; Soetens et al. 1985; Cho et al. 2002) may arise from Bayesian stimulus expectancy computation based on statistical regularities in recent trial history (Yu and Cohen 2009). Ultimately, subjects' behavioural choices reflect a combination of their internal knowledge about the world (reflecting the learning process) and their saccadic choice based on that knowledge (reflecting the decision policy). We adopted a Bayesian inference and decision modelling framework that allows us to consider different combinations of learning and decision strategies, and differentiate their relevance based on subjects' behaviour (Huang and Yu 2010).

In our visual search task (Huang and Yu 2010), subjects must find a target motion stimulus in one of three possible locations, with the other two locations containing distractor motion stimuli (Fig. 39.11a). In the spatially 'biased condition' (1:3:9 condition), the target location is biased among the three options with 1:3:9 odds. In the 'uniform condition' (1:1:1 condition), the target is distributed uniformly across the three locations. The order of the eight blocks (six biased blocks and two uniform ones, 90 trials per block) are randomized for each subject. To eliminate the complications associated with

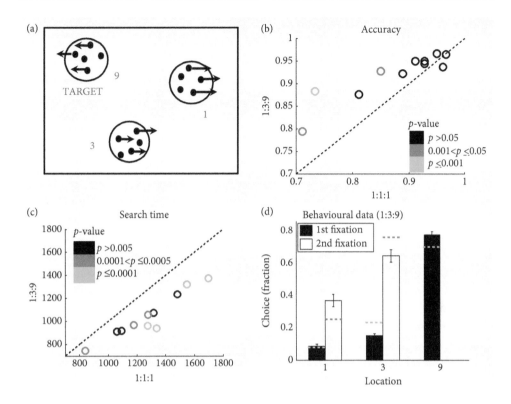

FIGURE 39.11 A motion stimulus search task and behavioural data. (a) Subjects must find the target stimulus (left-moving 12% random-dot motion stimulus for half of the subjects, right-moving for the other half), with the distractor stimulus in the other two possible locations (right-moving for half of the subjects, left-moving for the other half, respectively). The target appears in the three different locations with relative ratio of 1:3:9 in six blocks (random permutation of the six possible configurations), and with equal probability in two other blocks (1:1:1 condition). Stimulus display is gaze-contingent, so that only the fixated location displays the moving stimulus, while the other two are replaced by two small dots at the centre of the circles to indicate saccadic target location. (b) As a group, subjects are more accurate in identifying the target in the 1:3:9 condition than the 1:1:1 condition ($p = 0.0094$), and all but one subject is individually significant. (c) As a group, subjects are faster in responding in the 1:3:9 condition than the 1:1:1 condition ($p = 0.0000016$), and all but four subjects are individually significant. (d) In the 1:3:9 condition, for the first fixation (black), subjects preferentially fixate the most likely location (9) over the second most likely location (3), which in turn was favoured over the least likely location (1); for the second fixation (white), on trials in which subjects fixated the 9 location first and that was *not* the target, subjects then allocated their fixation in favour of the more likely location (3) over the less likely one (1). Green dashed lines indicate the matching probabilities on the first fixation, (1/13, 3/13, 9/13); blue dashed lines indicate matching probabilities on the second fixation, (1/4, 3/4). $n = 11$.

the spatial dynamics of covert attention, the display is gaze-contingent: only the fixated stimulus is visible at any given time, the other two replaced by two small dots indicating available fixation alternatives. Subjects receive feedback about true target location on each trial after making their choice. Other than experiencing training blocks with similar statistics before the main experiments, subjects do not receive any explicit instructions on the spatial distribution of target location. They are only told to find the target quickly and accurately, as they receive performance-contingent pay at the end of the experiment, proportional to points they earn: +50 points for each correct trial, −50 points for each error trial, −12.5 points for each second spent searching, and −25 points for each switch of search location.

We found that human subjects indeed notice and take advantage of the spatial statistics to locate the target stimulus more accurately (Fig. 39.11b) and rapidly (Fig. 39.11c). Underlying this performance improvement is a prioritized search strategy that favours the '9' location over the '3' location, in turn over the '1' location, as the first search location (Fig. 39.11d, black bars). If they first fixated 9 and did not find the target, they favoured the 3 location over the 1 location as the second search location (Fig. 39.11d, white bars). Moreover, average distribution of subjects' first fixation distribution appeared close to a 'matching' strategy (Fig. 39.11d, dashed lines), by allocating choices similar in proportion to the actual underlying statistical frequencies.

The observed 'matching' search strategy suggests that humans can internalize and utilize a *graded* probabilistic representation of potential target location. The most salient interpretation is that subjects stochastically select on each trial the first fixation duration in proportion to that block's target probabilities in the different locations. However, another possibility is that subjects base their beliefs about the configuration of target probabilities *not* on the entire history of experienced trials (we call this the Fixed Belief Model, or FBM), but instead giving more weight to the more recent trials (we call this the Dynamic Belief Model, or DBM). This is motivated by our previous work (Yu and Cohen 2009) showing that subjects often (implicitly) assume that the world is potentially changeable, and therefore the most recent observations ought to be given greater emphasis than more distant ones in predicting future outcomes. Under such a non-stationarity assumption, an accumulation of unexpected outcomes (e.g. target appearing in unexpected locations) suggests a potential shift in underlying environmental statistics, and a rational observer should be willing to update his/her internal world model and recalibrate his/her interactions with the environment, e.g. by favouring a recently frequented target location, instead of choosing purely according to long-term averages. Thus, matching-like search behaviour may arise not from a stochastic choice policy, but rather a limited-memory belief update process, in combination with a *maximizing* choice policy.

A third possibility for matching-like search pattern is that subjects may adopt a follow-last-target heuristic strategy, related to the previously proposed win-stay-lose-shift strategy for binary choices (Rapoport and Chammah 1965; Nowak and Sigmund 1993; Randall and Zentall 1997; Warren 1966; Steyvers et al. 2009; Lee et al. 2011; Otto et al. 2011; Scheibehenne et al. 2011; Worthy and Maddox 2012). That

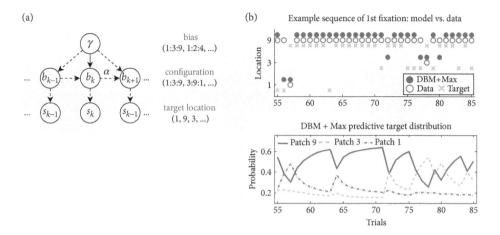

FIGURE 39.12 Dynamic Belief Model (DBM), a Bayesian hidden Markov model for trial-by-trial learning and prediction. (a) DBM generative model: $\gamma = (\gamma_h, \gamma_m)$ specifies the probability of high-probability and medium-probability locations containing the target; it is (9/13, 3/13) by experimental design, but we assume that subjects perform Bayesian inference to learn γ based on experienced trial outcomes. b_k denotes the configuration of location probabilities on trial k—besides the six biased configurations (L:M:H, L:H:M, M:L:H, M:H:L, H:L:M, H:M:L), b_k can also take on a seventh 'uniform' state (1:1:1). α denotes the probability of the configuration *not* changing from trial to trial, and thus $1 - \alpha$ is the probability of it changing, in which case it adopts one of the six biased configurations each with 1/8 probability, and the 1:1:1 configuration with 2/8 probability. By experimental design, the true $\alpha = 1$, as the configuration stayed the same throughout a block; $\alpha = 1$ is a special case of the DBM, which we call the Fixed Belief Model (FBM), in which the ideal observer still has to learn about the underlying bias γ and configuration b, but b does not change over time. s_k denotes the actual target location, which is sampled independently on trial k from the categorical distribution specified by b_k. (b) An example trial sequence (subject 2, block 4, trials 55–85, fitted $\alpha = 0.92$). Given the actual experienced sequence of target location (green crosses in top panel) before trial k, DBM computes the *predictive* probability on trial k of each location containing the target (bottom panel). The model employs a maximizing decision policy in choosing first fixation location (filled blue circle, top panel), which is in good accordance with the subject's actual first fixation location (open blue circle, top panel).

is, subjects could simply be searching first in last trial's target location, in which case the 1:3:9 empirical statistics would naturally result in matching-like behaviour with one-trial lag. This heuristic strategy would not require any explicit or implicit knowledge about spatial distribution of target locations. However, as shown in Fig. 39.14a, while subjects are swayed by last trial target location, their first fixation choice also reflects long-term statistics—thus favouring 9 over 1 and 3.

Figure 39.12a shows the generative model for the DBM; the FBM is just a special case of the dynamic model with $\alpha = 1$. Fig. 39.12b shows a sample run of the DBM, in which the target (green x) mostly appears in location 9, but sometimes in location 3, and occasionally in location 1. The marginalized predictive belief DBM assigns to each of the potential target locations on each trial fluctuates with the prior history of experienced trials. The marginalized predictive belief that the target will appear in location 9 (blue) is highest most of the sequence, but a few trials of location 1 leads to relatively high predictive probability assigned to location 1 (red) early on in the sequence, and several trials of location 3 in the latter half of the sequence sways the DBM to assign higher predictive probability to location 3 (green). Note that the DBM plus a maximizing strategy

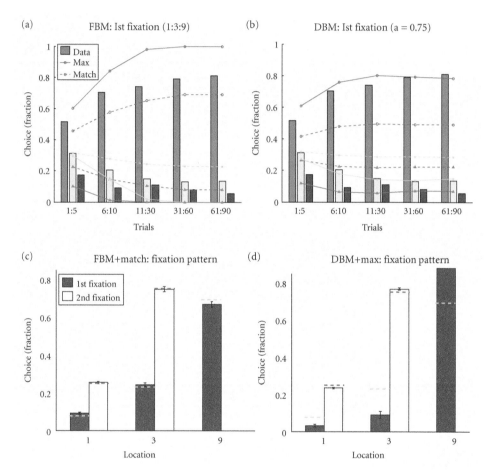

FIGURE 39.13 Model comparison of fixation distributions. (a) Averaged over all six blocks and over all subjects ($n = 11$), first fixation location (coloured bars: blue = 9, green = 3, red = 1) increasingly favour the 9 location over 3, and in turn over 1, for different segments of the 90-trial blocks. FBM+max (solid line) predicts faster learning/over-matching compared to subjects; FBM+match produces predictions more similar to subjects' data. (b) Human data (coloured bars) same as in (a). DBM+max produces predictions similar to subjects' data; DBM+match produces slower learn/under-matching compared to subjects. FBM+match (c) and DBM+max (d) both produce average first (black) and second (white) fixation patterns similar to subjects in Figure 1d, and similar to matching (dashed lines). Error bars = SEM.

produces first fixation predictions that closely correspond to this subject's actual choices (top panel). The rare discrepancies occur when there are unexpected observations and the underlying probabilities are close in magnitude: for example, trials 56, 72, 77, and 80. Other times, the model and the subject concur on switching (57, 78) or staying (64, 76).

To investigate more closely whether subjects employ something akin to the FBM or DBM in learning spatial statistics, and whether they match or maximize in their fixation policy, we examined how subjects' fixation choices evolve over the course of 1:3:9 blocks, and compared their behaviour to four different models: FBM+match (FBM for learning spatial statistics and a matching policy for generating first fixation location based on current beliefs), DBM+match (DBM for learning and a matching fixation policy), FBM+max (FBM for learning and a maximization policy for generating first fixation location based on current beliefs), and DBM+max (DBM for learning and

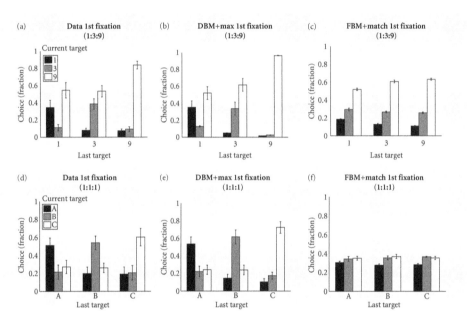

FIGURE 39.14 Data vs. model prediction of first fixation distribution conditioned on last target location. (a) In the 1:3:9 condition, human subjects generally prefer 9 (white) over 1 (black) and 3 (grey) regardless of last trial target location, but location 1 is particularly favoured if the last target location was also 1 (left group), location 2 is particularly favoured if the last target location was also 3 (middle group), and location 9 is particularly favoured if the last target was also 9 (right group). (b) DBM+max produces a conditional distribution very similar to the behavioural data in (a). (c) DBM+match produces a conditional distribution dissimilar to the behavioural data in (a), in particular it is insensitive to last trial target location. (d) In the 1:1:1 condition, human subjects favour last trial target location in the first fixation of the current trial. (b) DBM+max produces a conditional distribution very similar to the behavioural data in (a). (c) DBM+match produces a conditional distribution dissimilar to the behavioural data in (a), in particular it is insensitive to last trial target location. Error bars = SEM.

Table 39.1 Accuracy of different models in predicting subjects' trial–by–trial choice of first fixation. Average predictive accuracy computed for each 1:3:9 or 1:1:1 block, then averaged across all blocks of each condition and all subjects. DBM+max outperforms all other algorithms in both conditions significantly (*, $p < 0.05$) or very significantly (**, $p < 0.001$).

1:3:9 Condition		
Model	Predictive Accuracy	SEM
Follow-last-target	0.7172**	0.0018
FBM+match	0.5770**	0.0250
FBM+max	0.7776*	0.0214
DBM+match	0.5435**	0.0200
DBM+max	0.8086	0.0187
1:1:1 Condition		
Model	Predictive Accuracy	SEM
Follow-last-target	0.5700**	0.0078
FBM+match	0.3508**	0.0129
FBM+max	0.4864**	0.0229
DBM+match	0.3586**	0.0140
DBM+max	0.6495	0.0211

a maximization fixation policy). As we expected, both FBM+match and DBM+max produce learning curves quite similar to the behavioural data (Fig. 39.13a, b), as well as in terms of overall fixation distributions (Fig. 39.13c, d). In contrast, FBM+max over-match (Fig. 39.13a, solid) and DBM+match (Fig. 39.13b, dashed) under-match subjects' behavioural distribution.

While the average statistics cannot distinguish FBM+match or DBM+max in their fit to human behaviour, the conditional distribution of fixation choices as a function of last trial target location reveals some dramatic differences. For both 1:3:9 (Fig. 39.14a) and 1:1:1 (Fig. 39.14d) conditions, DBM+max produced conditional distributions statistically indistinguishable from subjects' first fixation distributions ($p = 0.076$, one-sided t-test of average Kullback–Leibler divergence between subjects' conditional distributions and that of DBM+max), whereas FBM+match produced conditional distributions that are very significantly different from subjects' distributions ($p = 0.00075$). Human subjects and DBM+max both adopt a first fixation policy that combines both long-term (1:3:9) and short-term (last trial) influences, where FBM+match makes fixation choices with little regard to the most recent trial target location.

We then examined how well the various model predict subjects' first fixation choices on a trial-to-trial basis. We found that DBM+max significantly outperformed all four of the other models (DBM+match, FBM+max, FBM+match, Follow-last-target) in both 1:3:9 and 1:1:1 conditions (Table 39.1, $p < 0.05$ for all one-sided paired t-test of

DBM+match versus all the other models). Note that we fit a value for α for each subject that maximized the DBM predictive accuracy of first fixation choice; we fit α separately for 1:3:9 and 1:1:1, and for DBM+match and DBM+max.

To summarize, we showed in this work that humans readily internalize spatial statistics after just a handful of exemplars, and use that information to improve accuracy and efficiency in target search by biasing both saccadic planning and perceptual processing towards the more probable target locations. We found that a combination of optimal fixation decision policy (maximizing accuracy) and suboptimal learning procedure (overestimating the volatility of statistical regularities) gives rise to 'matching' choice behaviour on a longer timescale, a strategy known to be suboptimal but nevertheless often observed in experiments. While the non-stationarity assumption and matching-like behaviour seem suboptimal in our experimental context, it would be a valuable asset in natural environments where statistical regularities do change over time, such as financial and economic markets, seasonal weather patterns, rise and fall in predator and prey populations, and so on. Indeed, few things are entirely constant in life besides gravity—even here, astronauts have shown a large degree of adaptability in outer space. We hypothesize that the apparently irrational matching behaviour is an adaptive response to the inherent non-stationarity in natural environments, and that the variability in how close subjects act like a 'matcher' versus a 'maximizer' may arise from implicit assumptions about the stability of environmental statistics in a particular behavioural context.

The results demonstrate that overt attention, mediated by purposeful eye movements, complements covert attention to play a critical role in the brain's selection and filtering process. While traditionally attentional selection was thought of as arising from limited neuronal resources at perceptual, decisional, and motor levels (Eriksen and Eriksen 1974), more recently formal Bayesian statistical models have suggested covert attentional selection to be computationally desirable beyond any resource limitation considerations (Dayan and Yu 2002; Dayan and Zemel 1999; Yu and Dayan 2005a; Yu and Cohen 2009). This work adds to this 'selection-for-computation' principle of attentional selection by demonstrating that overt attention also contributes to sensory processing efficiency by precisely favouring sensing locations in a manner that is sensitive to environmental statistics and task objectives. Future work is needed to clarify the precise manner in which covert and overt attention interact to mediate efficient sensory processing.

CONCLUSIONS AND DISCUSSION

In this chapter, we reviewed a number of Bayesian models that envision selective attention as selection-for-computation. From this normative viewpoint, we saw that attention for *learning* requires a greater amount of learning be accorded to aspects of the environment that are less well known (Dayan and Yu 2003), but attention for *prediction* and *inference* requires greater emphasis on the most precise sources of information in the environment (Yu and Dayan 2005b). We saw how both expected and unexpected uncertainties play a crucial role in these computations, and discussed their putative neural realization by the cholinergic and noradrenergic neuromodulatory systems (Yu and Dayan 2005b). We saw how cortical representations of uncertainty interact with neuromodulatory uncertainty to modulate visual cortical processing of sequentially processed sensory information (Yu and Dayan 2005a). And finally, we saw how overt attention (Huang and Yu 2010) can be understood within a similar Bayesian normative rubric as covert attention.

A great deal of work still remains in understanding attentional selection in a common theoretical framework. Clearly, more needs to be understood about how the different forms of attention discussed here interact with each other. Our understanding of the underlying neural mechanisms is still in its infancy. So far, there is a rather large disconnect between theoretical models of attentional mechanisms and neurophysiological data. Some of the neural hypotheses proposed here, such as those related to ACh, NE, and cortical neural populations, still need to be experimentally explored and verified. Finally, there are many other aspects of attention that have not yet received a Bayesian treatment, such as the large body of experimental results related to feature integration (Treisman and Gelade 1980) and the binding problem (Zeki 1978; Maunsell and Newsome 1987; Wade and Bruce 2001).

REFERENCES

Ammassari-Teule, M., Maho, C., and Sara, S. J. (1991). Clonidine reverses spatial learning deficits and reinstates θ frequencies in rats with partial fornix section. *Behavioural Brain Research 45*: 1–8.

Anderson, B. D. and Moore, J. B. (1979). *Optimal Filtering*. Eaglewood Cliffs, N.J.: Prentice-Hall.

Aston-Jones, G., Rajkowski, J., and Kubiak, P. (1997). Conditioned responses of monkey locus coeruleus neurons anticipate acquisition of discriminative behavior in a vigilance task. *Neuroscience 80*(3): 697–715.

Barber, M. J., Clark, J. W., and Anderson, C. H. (2003). Neural representation of probabilistic information. *Neural Computation 15*(8): 1843–1864.

Battaglia, P. W., Jacobs, R. A., and Aslin, R. N. (2003). Bayesian integration of visual and auditory signals for spatial localization. *Journal of the Optical Society of America A: Optics, Image Science, and Vision 20*(7): 1391–1397.

Baxter, M. G. and Chiba, A. A. (1999). Cognitive functions of the basal forebrain. *Current Opinion in Neurobiology 9*: 178–183.

Baxter, M. G., Holland, P. C., and Gallagher, M. (1997). Disruption of decrements in conditioned stimulus processing by selective removal of hippocampal cholinergic input. *Journal of Neuroscience 17*(13): 5230–5236.

Bayes, T. (1763). An essay toward solving a problem in the doctrine of chances. *Philosophical Transactions of the Royal Society 53*: 370–418.

Behrens, T. E. J., Woolrich, M. W., Walton, M. E., and Rushworth, M. F. S. (2007). Learning the value of information in an uncertain world. *Nature Neuroscience 10*(9): 1214–1221.

Blakely, E., Starin, S., and Poling, A. (1988). Human performance under sequences of fixed-ratio schedules: Effects of ratio size and magnitude of reinforcement. *Psychological Record* 38: 111–120.

Bolle, R. M. and Cooper, D. B. (1984). Bayesian recognition of local 3-D shape by approximating image intensity functions with quadric polynomials. *IEEE Transactions on Pattern Analysis and Machine Intelligence* 6(4): 418–429.

Bowman, E. M., Brown, V., Kertzman, C., Schwarz, U., and Robinson, D. L. (1993). Covert orienting of attention in Macaques. I: Effects of behavioral context. *Journal of Neurophysiology* 70(1), 431–443.

Broadbent, D. (1958). *Perception and Communication*. Elmsford, N.Y.: Pergamon.

Brown, E., Gilzenrat, M., and Cohen, J. D. (2004). *The Locus Coeruleus, Adaptive Gain, and the Optimization of Simple Decision Tasks* (Technical Report No. 04-01). Princeton, N.J.: Center for the Study of Mind, Brain, and Behavior, Princeton University.

Bucci, D. J., Holland, P. C., and Gallagher, M. (1998). Removal of cholinergic input to rat posterior parietal cortex disrupts incremental processing of conditioned stimuli. *Journal of Neuroscience* 18(19): 8038–8046.

Cho, R. Y., Nystrom, L. E., Brown, E. T., Jones, A. D., Braver, T. S., Holmes, P. J., and Cohen, J. D. (2002). Mechanisms underlying dependencies of performance on stimulus history in a two-alternative forced-choice task. *Cognitive, Affective, & Behavioral Neuroscience* 2(4): 283–299.

Clark, J. J. and Yuille, A. L. (1990). *Data Fusion for Sensory Information Processing Systems*. Boston, Dordrecht, and London: Kluwer Academic Press.

Coull, J. T., Frith, C. D., Dolan, R. J., Frackowiak, R. S., and Grasby, P. M. (1997). The neural correlates of the noradrenergic modulation of human attention, arousal and learning. *European Journal of Neuroscience* 9(3): 589–598.

Davison, M. and McCarthy, D. (1987). *The Matching Law: A Research Review*. Hillsdale, N.J.: Lawrence Erlbaum Associates.

Dayan, P. and Abbott, L. F. (2001). *Theoretical Neuroscience: Computational and Mathematical Modeling of Neural Systems*. Cambridge, Mass.: MIT Press.

Dayan, P., Kakade, S., and Montague, P. R. (2000). Learning and selective attention. *Nature Neuroscience* 3: 1218–1223.

Dayan, P. and Yu, A. J. (2002). ACh, uncertainty, and cortical inference. In T. G. Dietterich, S. Becker, and Z. Ghahramani (eds.), *Advances in Neural Information Processing Systems 14* (pp. 189–196). Cambridge, Mass.: MIT Press.

Dayan, P. and Yu, A. J. (2003). Uncertainty and learning. *IETE Journal of Research* 49: 171–181.

Dayan, P. and Yu, A. J. (2006). Norepinephrine and neural interrupts. In Y. Weiss, B. Schölkopf, and J. Platt (eds.), *Advances in Neural Information Processing Systems 18* (pp. 243–250). Cambridge, Mass.: MIT Press.

Dayan, P. and Zemel, R. S. (1999). Statistical models and sensory attention. In *Proceedings of the 9th International Conference on Artificial Neural Networks* (ICANN) (pp. 1017–1022). Edinburgh, UK.

Deutsch, J. A. and Deutsch, D. (1963). Attention: Some theoretical considerations. *Psychological Review* 87: 272–300.

Devauges, V. and Sara, S. J. (1990). Activation of the noradrenergic system facilitates an attentional shift in the rat. *Behavioural Brain Research* 39(1): 19–28.

Dickinson, A. (1980). *Contemporary Animal Learning Theory*. Cambridge: Cambridge University Press.

Donchin, E., Ritter, W., and McCallum, W. C. (1978). Cognitive psychophysiology: The endogenous components of the ERP. In E. Callaway, P. Tueting, and S. Koslow (eds.), *Event-Related Brain Potentials In Man* (pp. 1–79). New York: Academic Press.

Dyon-Laurent, C., Hervé, A., and Sara, S. J. (1994). Noradrenergic hyperactivity in hippocampus after partial denervation: Pharmacological, behavioral, and electrophysiological studies. *Experimental Brain Research* 99: 259–266.

Dyon-Laurent, C., Romand, S., Biegon, A., and Sara, S. J. (1993). Functional reorganization of the noradrenergic system after partial fornix section: A behavioral and autoradiographic study. *Experimental Brain Research* 96: 203–211.

Elder, J. H. and Goldberg, R. M. (2002). Ecological statistics of gestalt laws for the perceptual organization of contours. *Journal of Vision* 2(4): 324–353.

Eriksen, B. A. and Eriksen, C. W. (1974). Effects of noise letters upon the identification of a target letter in a nonsearch task. *Perception & Psychophysics* 16: 143–149.

Eriksen, C. and St James, J. (1986). Visual attention within and around the field of focal attention: A zoom lens model. *Perception & Psychophysics* 40(4): 225–240.

Ernst, M. O. and Banks, M. S. (2002). Humans integrate visual and haptic information in a statistically optimal fashion. *Nature* 415(6870): 429–433.

Frank, M. J., O'Reilly, R. C., and Curran, T. (2008). When memory fails, intuition reigns: Midazolam enhances implicit inference in humans. *Psychological Science* 17: 700–707.

Geman, S. and Geman, D. (1984). Stochastic relaxation, Gibbs distributions, and the Bayesian restoration of images. *IEEE Transactions on Pattern Analysis and Machine Intelligence* 6: 721–741.

Gil, Z., Conners, B. W., and Amitai, Y. (1997). Differential regulation of neocortical synapses by neuromodulators and activity. *Neuron* 19: 679–686.

Gold, J. I. and Shadlen, M. N. (2002). Banburismus and the brain: Decoding the relationship between sensory stimuli, decisions, and reward. *Neuron* 36: 299–308.

Green, D. M. and Swets, J. A. (1966). *Signal Detection Theory and Psychophysics*. Los Altos, Calif.: Peninsula Publishing.

Grenander, U. (1976–1981). *Lectures in Pattern Theory*. 3 vols.: *Pattern Analysis, Pattern Synthesis, and Regular Structures*. New York: Springer-Verlag.

Gu, Q. (2002). Neuromodulatory transmitter systems in the cortex and their role in cortical plasticity. *Neuroscience* 111: 815–835.

Hall-Johnson, E. and Poling, A. (1984). Preference in pigeons given a choice between sequences of fixed-ratio schedules: Effects of ratio values and duration of food delivery. *Journal of the Experimental Analysis of Behavior* 42: 127–135.

Hasselmo, M. E. and Schnell, E. (1994). Laminar selectivity of the cholinergic suppression of synaptic transmission in rat hippocampal region CA1: Computational modeling and brain slice physiology. *Journal of Neuroscience* 14(6): 3898–3914.

Hasselmo, M. E., Wyble, B. P., and Wallenstein, G. V. (1996). Encoding and retrieval of episodic memories: Role of cholinergic and GABAergic modulation in the hippocampus. *Hippocampus* 6: 693–708.

He, P. Y. and Kowler, E. (1989). The role of location probability in the programming of saccades: Implications for 'center-of-gravity' tendencies. *Vision Research* 29(9): 1165–1181.

Helmholtz, H. L. F. von (1878). The facts of perception. In R. Kahl (ed.), *Selected Writings of Hermann von Helmholtz*. Middletown, Conn.: Wesleyan University Press, 1971 (translated from German original *Die Tatsachen in der Wahrnehmung*).

Herrnstein, R. J. (1961). Relative and absolute strength of responses as a function of frequency of reinforcement. *Journal of the Experimental Analysis of Behaviour* 4: 267–272.

Herrnstein, R. J. (1970). On the law of effect. *Journal of the Experimental Analysis of Behaviour* 13: 243–266.

Hoffman, J. E. and Subramaniam, B. (1995). The role of visual attention in saccadic eye movements. *Perception & Psychophysics* 57(6): 787–795.

Hsieh, C. Y., Cruikshank, S. J., and Metherate, R. (2000). Differential modulation of auditory thalamocortical and intracortical synaptic transmission by cholinergic agonist. *Brain Research* 800(1–2): 51–64.

Huang, H. and Yu, A. J. (2010). Statistical learning across trials and reward-driven decision-making within trials in an active visual search task: Comparison of human behavioral data to Bayes-optimal sensory processing and saccade planning. Paper presented at the Society for Neural Science Annual Meeting, 15 November.

Jacobs, R. A. (1999). Optimal integration of texture and motion cues in depth. *Vision Research* 39: 3621–3629.

Jodo, E., Chiang, C., and Aston-Jones, G. (1998). Potent excitatory influence of prefrontal cortex activity on noradrenergic locus coeruleus neurons. *Neuroscience* 83(1): 63–79.

Jones, D. N. and Higgins, G. A. (1995). Effect of scopolamine on visual attention in rats. *Psychopharmacology* 120(2): 142–149.

Kastner, S. and Ungerleider, L. G. (2000). Mechanisms of visual attention in the human cortex. *Annual Review of Neuroscience* 23: 315–341.

Kimura, F., Fukuada, M., and Tusomoto, T. (1999). Acetylcholine suppresses the spread of excitation in the visual cortex revealed by optical recording: Possible differential effect depending on the source of input. *European Journal of Neuroscience* 11: 3597–3609.

Knill, D. C. and Richards, W. (eds.) (1996). *Perception as Bayesian Inference*. Cambridge: Cambridge University Press.

Kobayashi, M. (2000). Selective suppression of horizontal propagation in rat visual cortex by norepinephrine. *European Journal of Neuroscience* 12(1): 264–272.

Körding, K. P., Beierholm, U., Ma, W., Quartz, S., Tenenbaum, J., and Shams, L. (2007a). Causal inference in cue combination. *PLoS One* 2(9): e943.

Körding, K. P., Tenenbaum, J. B., and Shadmehr, R. (2007b). The dynamics of memory as a consequence of optimal adaptation to a changing body. *Nature Neuroscience* 10(6): 779–786.

Körding, K. P. and Wolpert, D. M. (2004). Bayesian integration in sensorimotor learning. *Nature* 427: 244–247.

LaBerge, D. (1983). Spatial extent of attention to letters and words. *Journal of Experimental Psychology: Human Perception and Performance* 9(3): 371–379.

Laming, D. R. J. (1968). *Information Theory of Choice-Reaction Times*. London: Academic Press.

Lee, M. D., Zhang, S., Munro, M., and Steyvers, M. (2011). Psychological models of human and optimal performance in bandit problems. *Cognitive Systems Research* 12: 164–174.

McAdams, C. J. and Maunsell, J. H. (2000). Attention to both space and feature modulates neuronal responses in macaque area V4. *Journal of Neurophysiology* 83(3): 1751–1755.

McAdams, C. J. and Maunsell, J. H. R. (1999). Effects of attention on orientation-tuning functions of single neurons in macaque cortical area V4. *Journal of Neuroscience* 19: 431–441.

McGaughy, J., Ross, R. S., and Eichenbaum, H. (2008). Noradrenergic, but not cholinergic, deafferentation of prefrontal cortex impairs attentional set-shifting. *Neuroscience* 153: 63–71.

Mackintosh, N. J. (1983). *Conditioning and Associative Learning*. Oxford: Oxford University Press.

Marroquin, J. L., Mitter, S., and Poggio, T. (1987). Probabilistic solution of ill-posed problems in computational vision. *Journal of the American Statistical Association* 82(397): 76–89.

Maunsell, J. H. and Newsome, W. T. (1987). Visual processing in monkey extrastriate cortex. *Annual Review of Neuroscience 10*: 363–401.

Miller, E. K. and Cohen, J. D. (2001). An integrative theory of prefrontal cortex function. *Annual Review of Neuroscience 24*: 167–202.

Missonnier, P., Ragot, R., Derouesné, C., Guez, D., and Renault, B. (1999). Automatic attentional shifts induced by a noradrenergic drug in Alzheimer's disease: Evidence from evoked potentials. *International Journal of Psychophysiology 33*: 243–251.

Moore, T. and Fallah, M. (2001). Control of eye movements and spatial attention. *Proceedings of the National Academy of Sciences USA 98*(3): 1273–1276.

Moran, J. and Desimone, R. (1985). Selective attention gates visual processing in the extrastriate cortex. *Science 229*: 782–784.

Norman, D. A. (1968). Toward a theory of memory and attention. *Psychological Review 75*(6): 522–536.

Nowak, M. and Sigmund, K. (1993). A strategy of win-stay, lose-shift that outperforms tit-for-tat in the prisoner's dilemma game. *Nature 364*: 56–58.

O'Connor, D. H., Fukui, M. M., Pinsk, M. A., and Kastner, S. (2002). Attention modulates responses in the human lateral geniculate nucleus. *Nature Neuroscience 15*(1): 31–45.

O'Neill, J., Siembieda, D. W., Crawford, K. C., Halgren, E., Fisher, A., and Fitten, L. J. (2003). Reduction in distractibility with AF102B and THA in the macaque. *Pharmacology, Biochemistry, and Behavior 76*(2): 306–301.

Oswal, A., Ogden, M., and Carpenter, R. H. S. (2007). The time course of stimulus expectation in a saccadic decision task. *Journal of Neurophysiology 97*: 2722–2730.

Otto, A. R., Taylor, E. G., and Markman, A. B. (2011). There are at least two kinds of probability matching: Evidence from a secondary task. *Cognition 118*: 274–279.

Pearce, J. M. and Hall, G. (1980). A model for Pavlovian learning: Variation in the effectiveness of conditioned but not unconditioned stimuli. *Psychological Review 87*: 532–552.

Phillips, J. M., McAlonan, K., Robb, W. G. K., and Brown, V. (2000). Cholinergic neurotransmission influences covert orientation of visuospatial attention in the rat. *Psychopharmacology 150*: 112–116.

Pineda, J. A., Westerfield, M., Kronenberg, B. M., and Kubrin, J. (1997). Human and monkey P3-like responses in a mixed modality paradigm: Effects of context and context-dependent noradrenergic influences. *International Journal of Psychophysiology 27*: 223–240.

Poling, A., Edwards, T., Weeden, M., and Foster, T. M. (2011). The matching law. *Psychological Record 61*(2): 313–322.

Posner, M. I. (1980). Orienting of attention. *Quarterly Journal of Experimental Psychology 32*: 3–25.

Posner, M. I. and Petersen, S. E. (1990). The attention system of the human brain. *Annual Review of Neuroscience 13*: 25–42.

Prendergast, M. A., Jackson, W. J., Terry, A. V. J., Decker, M. W., Arneric, S. P., and Buccafusco, J. J. (1998). Central nicotinic receptor agonists ABT-418, ABT-089, and (–)-nicotine reduce distractibility in adult monkeys. *Psychopharmacology 136*(1): 50–58.

Rajkowski, J., Kubiak, P., and Aston-Jones, P. (1994). Locus coeruleus activity in monkey: Phasic and tonic changes are associated with altered vigilance. *Synapse 4*: 162–164.

Randall, C. K. and Zentall, T. R. (1997). Win-stay/lose-shift and win-shift/lose-stay learning by pigeons in the absence of overt response mediation. *Behavioural Processes 41*(3): 227–236.

Rao, R. P. (2004). Bayesian computation in recurrent neural circuits. *Neural Computation 16*: 1–38.

Rapoport, A. and Chammah, A. M. (1965). *Prisoner's Dilemma*. Ann Arbor, Mich.: University of Michigan Press.

Ratcliff, R. (2001). Putting noise into neurophysiological models of simple decision making. *Nature Neuroscience* 4: 336–337.

Reynolds, J. H. and Chelazzi, L. (2004). Attentional modulation of visual processing. *Annual Review of Neuroscience* 27: 611–647.

Rizzolatti, G., Riggio, L., Dascola, I., and Umiltá, C. (1987). Reorienting attention across the horizontal and vertical meridians: evidence in favor of a premotor theory of attention. *Neuropsychologia* 25: 31–40.

Robbins, T. W. and Everitt, B. J. (1995). Arousal systems and attention. In M. S. Gazzaniga (ed.), *The Cognitive Neurosciences* (pp. 703–720). Cambridge, Mass.: MIT Press.

Roesch, M. R. and Olson, C. R. (2003). Impact of expected reward on neuronal activity in prefrontal cortex, frontal and supplementary eye fields and premotor cortex. *Journal of Neurophysiology* 90(3): 1766–1789.

Roitman, J. D. and Shadlen, M. N. (2002). Response of neurons in the lateral intraparietal area during a combined visual discrimination reaction time task. *Journal of Neuroscience* 22(21): 9475–9489.

Sahani, M. and Dayan, P. (2003). Doubly distributional population codes: simultaneous representation of uncertainty and multiplicity. *Neural Computation* 15: 2255–2279.

Sara, S. J. (1989). Noradrenergic-cholinergic interaction: Its possible role in memory dysfunction associated with senile dementia. *Archives of Gerontology and Geriatrics, Supplement* 1: 99–108.

Sara, S. J. (1998). Learning by neurons: Role of attention, reinforcement and behavior. *Comptes Rendus de l'Academie des Sciences Série III: Sciences de la Vie/Life Sciences* 321: 193–198.

Sara, S. J., Dyon-Laurent, C., Guibert, B., and Leviel, V. (1992). Noradrenergic hyperactivity after fornix section: Role in cholinergic dependent memory performance. *Experimental Brain Research* 89: 125–132.

Sara, S. J. and Hervé-Minvielle, A. (1995). Inhibitory influence of frontal cortex on locus coeruleus neurons. *Proceedings of the National Academy of Sciences USA* 92: 6032–6036.

Sara, S. J. and Segal, M. (1991). Plasticity of sensory responses of LC neurons in the behaving rat: Implications for cognition. *Progress in Brain Research* 88: 571–585.

Sara, S. J., Vankov, A., and Hervé, A. (1994). Locus coeruleus-evoked responses in behaving rats: A clue to the role of noradrenaline in memory. *Brain Research Bulletin* 35: 457–465.

Sarter, M. and Bruno, J. P. (1997). Cognitive functions of cortical acetylcholine: Toward a unifying hypothesis. *Brain Research Reviews* 23: 28–46.

Scheibehenne, B., Wilke, A., and Todd, P. M. (2011). Expectations of clumpy resources influence predictions of sequential events. *Evolution and Human Behavior* 32(5): 326–333.

Shams, L., Ma, W. J., and Beierholm, U. (2005). Sound-induced flash illusion as an optimal percept. *NeuroReport* 16(17): 1923–1927.

Shenoy, P. and Yu, A. J. (2012). Stimulus expectancy, norepinephrine, and inhibitory control (Under review).

Smith, P. L. and Ratcliff, R. (2004). Psychology and neurobiology of simple decisions. *Trends in Neurosciences* 27(3): 161–168.

Soetens, E., Boer, L. C., and Hueting, J. E. (1985). Expectancy or automatic facilitation? Separating sequential effects in two-choice reaction time. *Journal of Experimental Psychology: Human Perception and Performance* 11: 598–616.

Steyvers, M., Lee, M. D., and Wagenmakers, E. J. (2009). A Bayesian analysis of human decision-making on bandit problems. *Journal of Mathematical Psychology* 53: 168–179.

Stigchel, S. Van der and Theeuwes, J. (2007). The relationship between covert and overt attention in endogenous cuing. *Perception & Psychophysics* 69(5): 719–731.

Sugrue, L. P., Corrado, G. S., and Newsome, W. T. (2004). Matching behavior and the representation of value in the parietal cortex. *Science* 304(5678): 1782–1787.

Sutton, R. S. (1992). Gain adaptation beats least squares? In *Proceedings of the 7th Yale Workshop on Adaptive and Learning Systems* (pp. 161–166).

Szeliski, R. M. (1989). *Bayesian Modeling of Uncertainty in Low-Level Vision*. Norwell, Mass.: Kluwer Academic Press.

Terry, A. V. J., Risbrough, V. B., Buccafusco, J. J., and Menzaghi, F. (2002). Effects of (+/−)-4-[[2-(1-methyl-2-pyrrolidinyl)ethyl]thio]phenol hydrochloride (SIB-1553A), a selective ligand for nicotinic acetylcholine receptors, in tests of visual attention and distractibility in rats and monkeys. *Journal of Pharmacology and Experimental Therapeutics* 301(1): 384–392.

Treisman, A. (1969). Strategies and models of selective attention. *Psychological Review* 76: 282–299.

Treisman, A. G. and Gelade, G. (1980). A feature-integration theory of attention. *Cognitive Psychology* 12(1): 97–136.

Turetsky, B. I. and Fein, G. (2002). α2-noradrenergic effects on ERP and behavioral indices of auditory information processing. *Psychophysiology* 39: 147–157.

Vankov, A., Hervé-Minvielle, A., and Sara, S. J. (1995). Response to novelty and its rapid habituation in locus coeruleus neurons of freely exploring rat. *European Journal of Neuroscience* 109: 903–911.

Verleger, R., Jaskowski, P., and Wauschkuhn, B. (1994). Suspense and surprise: On the relationship between expectancies and P3. *Psychophysiology* 31(4): 359–369.

Vul, E., Goodman, N. D., Griffiths, T. L., and Tenenbaum, J. B. (2009). One and done? Optimal decisions from very few samples. In *Proceedings of the 31st Annual Conference of the Cognitive Science Society*. Amsterdam, Netherlands.

Wade, N. J. and Bruce, V. (2001). Surveying the seen: 100 years of British vision. *British Journal of Psychology* 92: 79–112.

Wald, A. (1947). *Sequential Analysis*. New York: John Wiley and Sons.

Wald, A. and Wolfowitz, J. (1948). Optimal character of the sequential probability ratio test. *Annals of Mathematical Statistics* 19: 326–339.

Warren, J. M. (1966). Reversal learning and the formation of learning sets by cats and rhesus monkeys. *Journal of Comparative and Physiological Psychology* 61(3): 421–428.

Weiss, Y. and Fleet, D. J. (2002). Velocity likelihoods in biological and machine vision. In R. P. N. Rao, B. A. Olshausen, and M. S. Lewicki (eds.), *Probabilistic Models of the Brain: Perception and Neural Function* (pp. 77–96). Cambridge, Mass.: MIT Press.

Witte, E. A. and Marrocco, R. T. (1997). Alteration of brain noradrenergic activity in rhesus monkeys affects the alerting component of covert orienting. *Psychopharmacology* 132: 315–323.

Worthy, D. A. and Maddox, W. T. (2012). Age-based differences in strategy use in choice tasks. *Frontiers in Neuroscience*: doi: 10.3389/fnins.2011.00145.

Yantis, S. and Jonides, J. (1984). Abrupt visual onsets and selective attention: Evidence from visual search. *Journal of Experimental Psychology: Human Perception and Performance* 10(5): 601–621.

Yarbus, A. L. (1967). *Eye Movements and Vision* (B. Haigh, Trans.). New York: Plenum Press.

Yu, A. J., Bentley, P., Seymour, B., Driver, J., Dolan, R., and Dayan, P. (2004). Expected and unexpected uncertainties control allocation of attention in a novel attentional learning task. *Society for Neuroscience Abstracts* 30: 176.17.

Yu, A. J. and Cohen, J. D. (2009). Sequential effects: Superstition or rational behavior? *Advances in Neural Information Processing Systems* 21: 1873–1880.

Yu, A. J. and Dayan, P. (2002). Acetylcholine in cortical inference. *Neural Networks* 15(4/5/6): 719–730.

Yu, A. J. and Dayan, P. (2003). Expected and unexpected uncertainty: ACh and NE in the neocortex. In S. T. S. Becker and K. Obermayer (eds.), *Advances in Neural Information Processing Systems 15* (pp. 157–164). Cambridge, Mass.: MIT Press.

Yu, A. J. and Dayan, P. (2005a). Inference, attention, and decision in a Bayesian neural architecture. In L. K. Saul, Y. Weiss, and L. Bottou (eds.), *Advances in Neural Information Processing Systems 17* (pp. 1577–1584). Cambridge, Mass.: MIT Press.

Yu, A. J. and Dayan, P. (2005b). Uncertainty, neuromodulation, and attention. *Neuron* 46: 681–692.

Yu, A. J., Dayan, P., and Cohen, J. D. (2009). Dynamics of attentional selection under conflict: Toward a rational Bayesian account. *Journal of Experimental Psychology: Human Perception and Performance 35*: 700–717.

Zaborszky, L., Gaykema, R. P., Swanson, D. J., and Cullinan, W. E. (1997). Cortical input to the basal forebrain. *Neuroscience 79*(4): 1051–1078.

Zeki, S. M. (1978). Functional specialization in the visual cortex of the rhesus monkey. *Nature 274*: 423–428.

Zemel, R. S., Dayan, P., and Pouget, A. (1998). Probabilistic interpretation of population codes. *Neural Computation 10*: 403–430.

PART H

EPILOGUE

ATTENTION: TIME CAPSULE 2013

ANNA C. NOBRE AND SABINE KASTNER

In this Handbook, we have pooled together some of the active researchers investigating different aspects of the field to provide a broad coverage and overview of contemporary attention research. Their combination forms a kind of scientific 'time capsule' for attention research today. The various researchers bring along their own assumptions, theories, experimental questions, tasks, methods, and models. Looking at all these elements together, it may be possible to gain clearer and deeper insights into the general principles of attention, as well as an intuition of the trajectory of attention research. In this epilogue, we provide a sketch of the patterns we glimpse in the time capsule.

You may be reading this epilogue because you read some of the chapters in the Handbook already. Or, who knows, like us, you may have read it cover to cover? Or perhaps you are still wondering whether to delve in? We hope you enjoy(ed) your reading. We have both greatly enjoyed working on this laborious project, and we have learned a lot along the way. Of course, we don't agree with everything in the Handbook, nor do we expect you will. But we bring the offerings to the fore to encourage and facilitate the continued active and lively discussion of ideas, issues, and data that is essential for the health of any scientific discipline.

BOTTLENECKS IN PERCEPTION AND COGNITION

Our mental interface with external reality is likely to remain perennially wondrous and puzzling. Over the centuries, we have come to accept that our grasp of our physical surroundings is neither immediate nor complete. Instead, our perception and cognition are highly selective and oriented towards the stimuli and events that are relevant to our current goals. Traditionally, it has been recognized that there are 'limits' to how much of the transduced external energy we can process to guide our conscious awareness, actions, and memories. Bottlenecks along the information-processing stream have been proposed. Their exact nature and location have been the subject of enduring speculation and theorizing.

What exactly is limited? In the 1950s and 1960s, scholars talked of limitations in 'capacity' or 'resources' along a given critical stage of information processing. What was meant by capacity or resources was not always clear, but the terms imply some generic fuel or currency for information processes. Contemporary expressions of this view can still be found. For example, Carrasco (in chapter 7) suggests 'limits are likely imposed by the fixed amount of overall energy available to the brain and by the high-energy cost of the neuronal activity involved in cortical computation'. Furthermore, in the early conceptualizations, single bottlenecks were envisaged. Different theories emphasized limitations in early stages of perceptual analysis (e.g. Broadbent 1958) versus late, post-perceptual stages (e.g. Deutsch and Deutsch 1963). The question regarding the locus of resource limitations framed much of the early empirical work in the field of attention; its seminal role is attested by the many summaries and discussions of this debate in numerous chapters of this handbook (see Lavie and Dalton (in chapter 3); Serences and Kastner (in chapter 4); Nobre and Mesulam (in chapter 5); Theeuwes (in chapter 8); Yu (in chapter 39)).

Over time, we have come to realize that there is much more flexibility in the process of prioritizing relevant information to guide cognition and action. Kahneman and Treisman (1984) took the first important step in pointing out that empirical evidence for early versus late selection coincided with the use of experimental tasks in which there was strong competition among perceptual streams of information (e.g. dichotic listening; Cherry 1953) versus response tendencies (e.g. Stroop task; Stroop 1935). They suggested that bottlenecks might reflect points of competition and thus move in its location depending on task demands. Following on this influential work, Lavie (1995) developed the perceptual load theory, positing a central role for resource limitations at perceptual stages in determining whether early modulation of information processing takes place (see Lavie and Dalton (in chapter 3), this volume).

The consensus in contemporary research is that prioritization of information processing occurs at multiple stages. Many statements to this regard appear throughout the Handbook (see Box 40.1). In addition to revealing where the critical, process-limiting steps are located, current scholars are interested in characterizing the nature of process limitations at the various stages. A full picture is yet to form, but several candidate mechanisms are under investigation. Most researchers recognize that one major type of bottleneck is the competition among multiple stimuli occurring within the receptive fields of individual neurons (Desimone and Duncan 1995; see Serences and Kastner (in chapter 4); Stokes and Duncan (in chapter 6); Beck and Kastner (in chapter 9); Eimer (in chapter 10); Gottlieb (in chapter 12); Saalmann and Kastner (in chapter 14); Pessoa (in chapter 25); Soto and Humphreys (in chapter 26); Miller and Bushman (in chapter 27); Deubel (in chapter 30); Bundesen and Habekost (in chapter 37); Itti and Borji (in chapter 38)). Competitive interactions among stimuli occur throughout the visual system, especially in areas with large receptive fields (Reynolds et al. 1999; see chapters by Cohen and Maunsell (in chapter 11); Treue (in chapter 21)). Though less well studied,

Box 40.1 Quotes from contributors to this volume expressing the view that modulatory mechanisms of attention operate at multiple levels of processing

'As with nearly all dichotomies in psychology, the emerging consensus is that neither extreme is correct. Instead, depending on task demands, the mechanisms of selective attention can flexibly operate on the quality of low-level sensory representations as well as on later stages of semantic analysis and decision making' (Serences and Kastner (in chapter 4)).

'The classical questions about the locus of capacity limitations quickly became obsolete, replaced by the clear realization that modulatory mechanisms operate at multiple levels of analysis in a distributed fashion in the brain...' (Nobre and Mesulam (in chapter 5))

'Neural competition is likely to take many forms throughout the central nervous system...' (Stokes and Duncan (in chapter 6))

'Evidence from functional brain imaging reveals that attention operates at various processing levels within the human visual system and beyond.' (Beck and Kastner (in chapter 9))

'Shifts in spatial attention have been associated with changes in the responses of individual neurons in every visual cortical area that has been examined, including primary visual cortex...' (Cohen and Maunsell (in chapter 11))

'The new consensus is that the locus of attentional selectivity can be shifted flexibly and rapidly between stages and subsystems, in accordance with a variety of factors that include stimulus parameters, current task demands, and top-down selection intentions.' (Eimer (in chapter 10))

'One area of growing research interest relates to the question of how attention spreads across the various modality-specific features of an object...or event as a function of the semantic relationship...between the component parts...' (Spence (in chapter 16))

'the emerging consensus is that feature-based and object-based attentional mechanisms...operate along a continuum and the extent to which selection is based on a specific feature or an object depends on both the complexity of the stimulus array and on the specific behavioral goals of the observer'. (Scolari, Ester and Serences (in chapter 20))

'feature-based and object-based attention are selective modulation processes that, just like spatial attention, affect the responses of sensory neurons throughout the visual cortex of primates'. (Treue (in chapter 21))

'there may be multiple sources of temporal expectation, which can bias multiple stages of stimulus analysis depending on the stages of information-processing that are critical for task performance'. (Nobre and Rohenkohl (in chapter 24))

'Rather, at every stage of memory, processing constraints are present and selection is required...we argue that the ways in which we form, retrieve, and work with our memories largely represent *acts of attention*...' (Kuhl and Chun (in chapter 28))

'attention influences perception, as well as learning and memory'. (Scerif and Wu (in chapter 31))

'In attention research there is a long-standing debate on whether selection takes place before or after perceptual recognition...TVA takes a different view and assumes that the two processes occur simultaneously.' (Bundesen and Habekost (in chapter 37)) stimulus competition within receptive fields is also likely to limit processing in other perceptual systems and at later, post-perceptual stages of analysis (e.g. see Deubel (in chapter 30)). Many other types of process-limiting steps exist beyond receptive-field competition, which could act as targets for modulation. Contributors to the Handbook highlight a few, such as: overcoming the intrinsic noise of sensory neurons (see Serences and Kastner (in chapter 4); Cohen and Maunsell (in chapter 11)), integrating both simple and complex high-level features into coherent object representations (see Wolfe (in chapter 2); Nobre and Mesulam (in chapter 5)), indexing and keeping track of targets (see Cavanagh, Battelli, and Holcombe (in chapter 23)), selecting and executing an appropriate response among competing response tendencies (see Serences and Kastner (in chapter 4)), and encoding information into short-term memory (see Shapiro and Hanslmayr (in chapter 22)).

Defining Attention

The limitations in our perception and cognition, however we come to characterize them, are what bring us to notions of (selective) attention. But getting from notions to crisp definitions has been problematic. The field starts well, with a clear definition by William James that everyone knows (Box 40.2). Perhaps surprisingly, this well-loved definition does not make too many appearances in the Handbook (but see Zanto and Gazzaley (in chapter 32) for its insinuation). This definition emphasizes *functions* of prioritization among various simultaneously competing objects or trains of thought, including both selecting and inhibiting. Many contemporary definitions echo or try to refine this original proposal (see Box 40.2). Indeed, if one were to distil a core definition of attention out of the contemporary literature, it would be something like: the prioritization of processing information that is relevant to current task goals. Some researchers incorporate specific proposed mechanisms of prioritization functions into their conceptualizations. For example, the biased competition framework proposes the raison d'être of attention is to help resolve competitive interactions in perception (Desimone and Duncan 1995), Yu (in chapter 39) proposes a Bayesian computational framework for optimizing learning or prediction and inference, Bundesen and Habekost (in chapter 37) emphasize perceptual categorizations and competition for limited short-term memory capacity. Other researchers argue for consideration of a broader scope of prioritization functions. For example, Nobre and Mesulam (in chapter 5) propose that there may be multiple sources of top-down modulatory signals related not only to task goals, but also to expectations, motivations, and memory (see also Pessoa (in chapter 25); Kuhl and Chun (in chapter 28); Summerfield and Egner (in chapter 29)). Furthermore, a number of researchers also consider other, closely related functions that are not strictly involved with prioritization of information processing to represent other 'kinds' of attention—such as sustained attention and executive control (see Posner, Rothbart, and Rueda (in chapter 19); Robbins (in chapter 18); Zanto and

Box 40.2 Definitions of attention by William James and by contributors to this volume

'Every one knows what attention is. It is the taking possession by the mind, in clear and vivid form, of one out of what seem several simultaneously possible objects or trains of thought. Focalization, concentration, of consciousness are of its essence. It implies withdrawal from some things in order to deal effectively with others...' (William James 1890: 404)

'ability to prioritize relevant over irrelevant information'. (Serences and Kastner (in chapter 4))

'Attention refers to the set of mechanisms that tune psychological and neural processing in order to identify and select the relevant events against all the competing distractions.' (Nobre and Mesulam (in chapter 5))

'Attention allows us to selectively process the vast amount of information with which we are confronted, prioritizing some aspects of information while ignoring others by focusing on a certain location or aspect of the visual scene...' (Carrasco (in chapter 7))

'Visual attention allows people to select information that is relevant for their ongoing behaviour, and ignore information that is irrelevant.' (Theeuwes (in chapter 8))

'Attention is associated with improved performance on perceptual tasks and also with changes in the way that individual neurons in the visual system respond to sensory stimuli.' (Cohen and Maunsell (in chapter 11))

'Covert spatial attention prioritizes the processing of stimuli at a given peripheral location, away from the direction of gaze, and selectively enhances visual discrimination, speed of processing, contrast sensitivity, and spatial resolution at the attended location.' (Clark, Noudoost, Schafer, and Moore (in chapter 13))

'Selective attention attacks this problem, by modulating sensory-evoked neuronal responses so as to enhance the processing of task-relevant stimuli while suppressing that of irrelevant stimuli... This "active control" processing is essential to normal perception and cognition because it enables information processing to adapt to the immediate goals of the observer.' (Schroeder, Herrero, and Haegens (in chapter 17))

'Broadly speaking, the term "selective attention" refers to a collection of mechanisms that insulate patterns of neural activity evoked by relevant stimuli from the deleterious effects of stochastic synaptic transmission and interference generated by other, irrelevant stimuli...' (Scolari, Ester, and Serences (in chapter 20))

'Visual attention... allows us to select a small subset of the information picked up by our eyes and enhance its processing, thus concentrating scant resources onto those aspects of the incoming deluge of sensory data that we momentarily deem most relevant.' (Treue (in chapter 21))

'In order to process the events around us we must select and keep track of the objects of current interest, ignoring others around them. This indexing or individuation of targets is a central function of attention...' (Cavanagh, Battelli, and Holcombe (in chapter 23))

'Selective attention, understood as the processes that focus neural processing in service of current goals and requirements, is inherently and necessarily dynamic.' (Nobre and Rohenkohl (in chapter 24))

'The central challenge of executive control, then, is how finite cognitive resources are brought to bear on the information (sensory inputs, stored memories, action plans, and strategies, etc.) that is currently important for the goal at hand and how potential distractions are excluded. When this is applied to the external world, we call it attention.' (Miller and Buschman (in chapter 27))

'Attention has been defined in a variety of overlapping ways typically in terms of a mechanism that preferentially allocates processing resources to percepts, memories, or tasks on the basis of a current goal... A related definition of attention... is that it constitutes a mechanism by which sensory information is weighted according to its motivational relevance.' (Summerfield and Egner (in chapter 29))

'attention enables us to select relevant objects and locations over less important ones'. (Deubel (in chapter 30))

'attention operates as a set of biases on information processing...' (Scerif and Wu (in chapter 31))

'Selective attention refers to goal-directed focus on task-relevant information while ignoring other irrelevant information.' (Zanto and Gazzaley (in chapter 32))

'Attention is what allows one stream of information from the internal or external environment to be selected over others and therefore pervades almost any thought or action we take in our daily lives.' (Robertson and O'Connell (in chapter 36))

'Selectively filtering these sensory inputs and maintaining useful interpretations for them are important computational tasks faced by the brain.' (Yu (in chapter 39))

Gazzaley (in chapter 32); Manohar, Bonnelle, and Husain (in chapter 34); Robertson and O'Connell (in chapter 36)). Finally, many simply leave the term undefined, relying on a you-know-what-I-mean approach.

Overall, it must be admitted that the field of attention could do better in terms of providing explicit and consistent definitions of its topic. The term 'attention' is often used in a vague manner, or multiple technical meanings can be juggled inconsistently or used incorrectly. Notions from folk psychology also creep in. Across the literature, 'attention' can indicate prioritization, target selection, mental effort, a mental state, the availability of resources, executive control functions, awareness, or simply 'thinking'. In addition to the core concept at stake, many other important concepts remain poorly defined or misused. We have already mentioned 'capacity' and 'resources'. Examples of other terms or concepts that prove challenging are: 'automatic', 'salience', 'relevance', 'top-down', and 'bottom-up'. In some cases, the premature coining of functional or mechanistic labels for phenomena, brain areas, or circuits can also cause confusion, and derail research and theorizing.

Several authors in the Handbook lament the state of our current nomenclature and urge for more care. Developing precise terminology and working towards an accepted taxonomy are important aims for the field at this stage. Clearly stated definitions and concepts would help kick-start the essential iterative process between theory and experimentation—guiding future experimentation and discussion, which in turn leads to refinement of definitions and concepts, which in turn guide experimentation and discussion... Having said this, it is also remarkable how much progress the field has achieved with its flexible and somewhat erratic terminology.

CLASSICAL AND CONTEMPORARY
EXPERIMENTAL QUESTIONS

The questions that have framed and guided 'attention' research have evolved over the years. In addition to questions regarding the locus at which attention operated to overcome capacity limitations, another important question regarded the 'units' of attentional selection. Rival proposals held that attention operated on spatial locations (Posner 1978; Treisman and Gelade 1980) versus on representations of objects (Duncan 1984; Kahneman and Treisman 1984). Subsequent experimentation considered whether modulation could also occur at the level of feature values or dimensions, independently of objects and spatial location (see Scolari, Ester, and Serences (in chapter 20); Treue (in chapter 21)). The close intrinsic relationship between space, objects, and their constituent features naturally gives mileage to such controversies.

Nowadays, we accept a multiplicity of modulatory mechanisms, which can operate upon different types of representations in a non-mutually exclusive manner (see Wolfe (in chapter 2); Nobre and Mesulam (in chapter 5); Scolari, Ester, and Serences (in chapter 20); Treue (in chapter 21); Shapiro and Hanslmayr (in chapter 22); Zanto and Gazzaley (in chapter 32); Bundesen and Habekost (in chapter 37); Itti and Borji (in chapter 38)). It is clearly established that modulatory mechanisms can influence processing according to the various types of properties coded in neuronal receptive fields. Thus, spatial, object-based, and feature-based attention can all occur. Much current research is devoted to understanding the mechanisms of attentional modulation at the cellular level (see Cohen and Maunsell (in chapter 11); Gottlieb (in chapter 12); Clark, Noudoost, Schafer, and Moore (in chapter 13); Saalman and Kastner (in chapter 14); Krauzlis (in chapter 15); Treue (in chapter 21); Miller and Bushman (in chapter 27)). In addition, it is important to recognize that attention can also operate on attributes that may not be directly related to neuronal receptive field properties, such as on the timing of events (see Nobre and Rohenkohl (in chapter 24); Zanto and Gazzaley (in chapter 32); Bundesen and Habekost (in chapter 37)) and meaning representations (Neely 1977; see Nobre and Mesulam (in chapter 5)). Contemporary research is also beginning to investigate the types of modulatory mechanisms that may be involved in these cases (see Schroeder, Herrero, and Haegens (in chapter 17)). There is also increasing interest in linking neuronal mechanisms with specific consequences for behavioural performance on a trial-by-trial basis (see Cohen and Maunsell (in chapter 11); Bundesen and Habekost (in chapter 37)). Typically, the mechanisms related to different types of attention have been studied in isolation. This has proven a pragmatic first step, yielding many relevant and tractable discoveries. However, in the real world, multiple types of attentional bias co-occur (see Itti and Borji (in chapter 38)). Depending on the particular stimulus parameters and task demands, a given type of attention may dominate, or multiple mechanisms may contribute in complementary ways. Moving forward, it will be increasingly important to compare and contrast the mechanisms involved in the different types of attention, and to investigate their interactions (see Cohen and Maunsell (in chapter 11); Scolari, Ester and Serences (in chapter 20); Treue (in chapter 21); Nobre and Rohenkohl (in chapter 24)).

One useful distinction that has emerged is that between mechanisms involved in controlling the shifts of attention (between locations, objects, features, or other attributes) versus those involved in modulating ongoing processing along the information-processing stream (Corbetta 1998). As with all such categorizations, in the limit the boundary between these two aspects can become fuzzy. Nevertheless, separating the 'source' of attention signals from the 'site' where they act has been of great heuristic value for organizing research in the field. In investigating the source of attention control, the focus has moved from individual brain areas to large-scale networks (Mesulam 1981, 1990; see Nobre and Mesulam (in chapter 5); Beck and Kastner (in chapter 9); Vallar and Bolognini (in chapter 33); Manohar, Bonnelle, and Husain (in chapter 34)). Accordingly, studies of the contributions of individual brain areas (see Gottlieb (in chapter 12); Clark, Noudoost, Schafer, and Moore (in chapter 13); Krauzlis (in chapter 15)) are increasingly supplemented by investigations of how information across different network regions is coordinated and integrated (see Saalmann and Kastner (in chapter 14); Spence (in chapter 16); Schroeder, Herrero, and Haegens (in chapter 17); Miller and Buschman (in chapter 27)). Similarly, researchers characterizing mechanisms of modulation at the sites of attention increasingly consider the dynamics of modulation and information flow in neuronal assemblies, between sensory areas, and between sensory and control areas (see Cohen and Maunsell (in chapter 11); Clark, Noudoost, Schafer, and Moore (in chapter 13); Miller and Buschman (in chapter 27)).

Since their earliest descriptions (James 1890), shifts of attention are known to have different possible origins: endogenous/controlled/voluntary/active or exogenous/automatic/reflexive/passive. These shifts are often characterized as involving modulatory signals moving in a *top-down* versus *bottom-up* direction through the processing hierarchy. Understanding the relative contributions of these types of shifts to behavioural performance and charting the overlap, differences, and interactions in their mechanisms, continue to be of great interest (see Wolfe (in chapter 2); Nobre and Mesulam (in chapter 5); Carrasco (in chapter 7); Theeuwes (in chapter 8); Eimer (in chapter 10); Gottlieb (in chapter 12); Clark, Noudoost, Schafer, and Moore (in chapter 13); Miller and Buschman (in chapter 27); Kuhl and Chun (in chapter 28); Zanto and Gazzaley (in chapter 32); Vallar and Bolognini (in chapter 33); Manohar, Bonnelle, and Husain (in chapter 34)).

For researchers of spatial attention, one enduring issue has been the relationship between the mechanisms involved in the control and eye movements and of covert shifts of attention (see Theeuwes (in chapter 8); Gottlieb (in chapter 12); Clark, Noudoost, Schafer, and Moore (in chapter 13); Krauzlis (in chapter 15); Deubel (in chapter 30)). The close relationship in the computational demands and functional dynamics of eye movements and spatial attention has been long noted (Rizzolatti, Riggio, Dascola, and Umiltà 1987). Research has also revealed striking similarities in the brain areas and neuronal mechanisms involved in both cases. Indeed, within network models of attention control, it becomes very difficult to separate signals related to action intention, which can readily enhance perceptual codes of the target items, from signals related to perceptual prioritization, which can readily activate associated action codes (see Nobre and Mesulam (in chapter 5)). Current research employs increasingly shrewd experimental designs and sophisticated methodology to measure and model behavioural performance and brain activity to understand the nature of the relationship between eye movements and spatial attention and the dynamics of their mutual influence (see Theeuwes (in chapter 8); Gottlieb (in chapter 12); Clark, Noudoost, Schafer, and Moore (in chapter 13); Krauzlis (in chapter 15); Deubel (in chapter 30)).

EXPERIMENTAL PARADIGMS AND METHODS

Over the years, the dominant experimental paradigm for attention investigations has moved from dichotic listening (Cherry 1953) to visual spatial orienting (Posner 1978) and visual search (Treisman and Gelade 1980). In orienting tasks, the experimental subject uses predictive or instructive cues to focus on a region of space to identify or discriminate relevant, target stimuli. Variations of this task can be used to investigate the orienting of attention to objects, features, actions, temporal instants, semantic categories, and more. In visual search tasks, participants are required to identify a pre-specified target, or a stimulus with certain pre-specified attributes, among a set of other, distracting stimuli. These tasks can also be modified to investigate attention in other modalities or across multiple sensory modalities. The prevalence of visual studies in attention naturally follows the same prevalence in research concerned with basic perceptual mechanisms. The same bias is reflected in this Handbook. Over the years, it will be imperative to increase efforts in understanding mechanisms of attention and perception in other modalities, as well as their integration across sensory modalities (see Eimer (in chapter 10); Spence (in chapter 16); Zanto and Gazzaley (in chapter 32)).

Methodological tools for investigating cognitive and brain functions have changed radically, probably in unimaginable ways, since the early empirical studies of attention. We have mostly left behind methods of introspection, which admittedly provided an incredibly fertile foundation (James 1890). In developing experimental tasks, scientists built ingenious mechanical devices to control stimulation and measure responses with increasing flexibility and chronometric control. We can now routinely rely on digital control of stimulus presentation and data collection devices—so that the main limit of the quality of the tasks we use and the behavioural data we collect is our own imagination. The most significant advances have been made in our ability to measure brain activity with increasing precision as participants perform attention tasks. In humans, structural imaging methods, such as computerized tomography and magnetic-resonance imaging (MRI), greatly facilitated linking attention-related deficits to sites of neurological lesions in patients. Hemodynamic imaging methods, positron-emission tomography, and then functional MRI (fMRI) revealed networks of brain areas correlated with attention control and modulation in the healthy brain. Event-related potentials provided rich dependent variables enabling the investigation of attention-related modulation at different stages of information processing independently of responses. Time-frequency analysis of the electrocencephalogram is beginning to reveal the role of oscillatory brain activity in coordinating and integrating activity within and between brain areas during attention-related functions. With its increased spatial resolution and sensitivity, magnetoencephalogram is taking these electrophysiological studies to new levels. Non-invasive brain-stimulation methods, such as transcranial magnetic stimulation, provide the means to test the causal involvement and timing of brain areas within attention-related functions. By combining stimulation and correlational imaging studies, researchers can also start to investigate the causal interactions among brain areas and the dynamics of attentional control and modulation. Developments in analysis methods have kept pace with those in data acquisition methods, so that it is routinely possible to investigate fluctuations or influences in brain activity at the single-trial level.

In animal-model studies, the move from anaesthetized preparations that laid the foundations for neurophysiological systems explorations in the 1950s–1970s to awake behaving preparations has paved the way towards developing detailed physiological models for cognitive functions such as attention. Initially, studies focused on recording spiking activity in single neurons from a variety of brain areas. These revealed attentional modulation throughout many cortical and subcortical areas, such as the superior colliculus (Goldberg and Wurtz 1972), frontal eye fields (Bruce and Goldberg 1985), lateral intraparietal area (Robinson et al. 1978), and visual extrastriate cortex (Moran and Desimone 1985). More recently, methodological upgrades enable recordings from neuronal ensembles and from multiple interconnected sites simultaneously (see Saalmann and Kastner (in chapter 14); Schroeder, Herrero, and Haegens (in chapter 17); Miller and Buschman (in chapter 27)). Field-potentials, reflecting the neural activity of local populations, are now routinely recorded. Data analysis has advanced beyond quantifying spike counts and histograms, to consider the timing and variability in spiking, the degree of local and inter-areal synchronization, and statistical measures of causal influences between areas. Microstimulation of individual neurons is also coupled to recordings of neurons with congruent receptive fields in order to investigate causal neural dynamics of attention at the cellular level (see Clark, Noudoost, Schafer, and Moore (in chapter 13)). Increasingly, these properties and effects are considered for different neuronal subtypes, sorted according to their spiking characteristics. The methodological innovations keep coming. We stand at the dawn of optogenetic methods (Deisseroth 2010) being adapted for stimulating individual neurons within local microcircuits in behaving non-human primates in attention tasks (Gerits and Vanduffel 2013). Together, these methods will lead to a thorough understanding of the neural circuitry that subserves attentional selection. Great challenges will remain in relating the different neuronal effects to behavioural performance and in understanding the way information is coded and communicated across cognitive networks. Methods for modelling behavioural and brain activity at the various levels of analysis in humans and in animal models (see Bundesen and Habekost (in chapter 37); Itti and Borji (in chapter 38); Yu (in chapter 39)) will continue to be essential for putting the various findings together, guiding the interpretation of experiments, generating new hypotheses, and building computational theories of attention.

Neural Systems and Mechanisms

Increasingly sophisticated behavioural experimentation has revealed many consequences of focused attention (see Carrasco (in chapter 7); Theeuwes (in chapter 8); Beck and Kastner (in chapter 9)); for example: reduction of spatial or stimulus uncertainty (Eckstein et al. 2002; Palmer 1994), enhancement of signal strength, increased discrimination sensitivity (Lu and Dosher 1998), improved acuity (Carrasco and Yeshurun 1998), increased contrast senstivity (Cameron et al. 2002), increased speed and efficiency of processing (Posner et al. 1980), increased temporal integration (Yeshurun and Marom 2008), suppressed masking of attended stimuli (Enns and Di Lollo 1997), inhibition of distracting information (Shiu and Pashler 1995; Theeuwes 1991), reduction of external noise (Lu et al. 2002), reduction of internal noise (Wyart et al. 2012), reweighting of information used for decision-making (Kinchla et al. 1995), improved encoding into short-term memory (Gazzaley 2011), and effective maintenance in short-term memory (Cowan 1995; Awh and Jonides 2001). Many of these effects are mutually compatible, and may occur simultaneously. Which effects take place may depend on a variety of factors involving stimulus parameters, task demands, and intentions (see Eimer (in chapter 10); Scolari, Ester, and Serences (in chapter 20)). As experimentation continues, it is hoped that these effects become better catalogued and the factors contributing to their occurrence become better understood.

The relentless methodological advances have enabled the field to make enormous progress in characterizing the neural systems and mechanisms involved in attention control and modulation. Converging lines of evidence from the various methods have substantiated network models for the control of attention (Mesulam 1981, 1990). Particularly implicated and heavily investigated are cortical and subcortical areas that are also involved in oculomotor control—posterior parietal area LIP (see Gottlieb (in chapter 12)), frontal eye fields (see Clark, Noudoost, Schafer, and Moore (in chapter 13)), and superior colliculus (see Krauzlis (in chapter 15)). Other frontal and parietal regions may also contribute, and their contributions continue to be parcellated (see Beck and Kastner (in chapter 9)). Subcortical areas in the thalamus and basal ganglia related to the coordination and integration of activity across large-scale neural circuits also play an important role (see Nobre and Mesulam (in chapter 5)). New insights into their role are coming from renewed research efforts fuelled by the interest in network dynamics and the availability of methods with which to investigate them (see Saalmann and Kastner (in chapter 14)). Network investigations are also increasingly considering the contribution of pharmacological agents (see Robbins (in chapter 18); Miller and Buschman (in chapter 27); Scerif and Wu (in chapter 31); Manohar, Bonnelle, and Husain (in chapter 34); Robertson and O'Connell (in chapter 36); Yu (in chapter 39)).

As researchers investigate the physiological properties of neurons and neuronal assemblies in perceptual and attention-control areas, they also reveal an increasing number of modulatory effects that contribute to the prioritization of information processing. In perceptual areas, one of the first attention-related effects described was that competition among stimuli within receptive fields of neurons in extrastriate cortices (areas IT, V4, and V2) became resolved in favour of the task-relevant stimulus (Moran and Desimone 1985). Also reported were increases in firing rates of neurons coding relevant object-related features (Chelazzi et al. 1993) and spatial locations (Luck et al. 1997) in anticipation of their preferred targets and during sustained attention (Motter 1993). These effects suggested that one of the main mechanisms of selective attention was the biasing of competitive perceptual interactions towards relevant stimuli by filtering out the influence of irrelevant, unattended stimuli (biased competition model; Desimone and Duncan 1995). Though biasing competition is undoubtedly an important effect of attention, it is not the only one. Selective attention has been shown to enhance signals related to isolated stimuli, in the absence of competition (see Cohen and Maunsell (in chapter 11); Treue (in chapter 21)). Various types of gain control in firing rates have been reported in different visual areas as well as in the same area across experiments, including changes in response gain, contrast gain, and additive gains. Computational theories, considering the basic perceptual mechanisms of neuronal sization, have been proposed to reconcile the various findings (Boynton 2009; Lee and Maunsell 2009; Reynolds and Heeger 2009; see Cohen and Maunsell (in chapter 11); Treue (in chapter 21)). In addition to changes related to firing rates, recent studies have discovered attention-related changes in the levels of intrinsic and correlated noise of neurons (Cohen and Maunsell 2009; Mitchell et al. 2009; see Cohen and Maunsell (in chapter 11); Serences and Kastner (in chapter 4)).

In control areas, firing is enhanced when stimuli gain behavioural relevance or indicate the focus of attention for responding to subsequent targets (see Colby and Goldberg 1999; Schall 2004; see Gottlieb (in chapter 12); Clark, Noudoost, Schafer, and Moore (in chapter 13); Miller and Buschman (in chapter 27)). Changes in baseline firing rates have also been reported (e.g. Chafee and Goldman-Rakic 1998). The degree of overlap between the cellular mechanisms involved in attention and oculomotor functions continues to be investigated in these regions (see Gottlieb (in chapter 12); Krauzlis (in chapter 15); Clark, Noudoost, Schafer, and Moore (in chapter 13)). Furthermore, neurons in lateral prefrontal cortex flexibly adapt to code task-relevant stimulus attributes to guide top-down biasing signals (Duncan 2001; see Stokes and Duncan (in chapter 6); Miller and Buschman (in chapter 27)).

More recent studies of changes in baseline rates have suggested that these can be extremely dynamic, following spatiotemporally specific patterns of activation (e.g. Crowe et al. 2010; see Stokes and Duncan (in chapter 6)). Current research has also been trying to tease apart whether changes in baseline firing that have commonly been observed in working-memory tasks reflect the maintenance of memoranda, the anticipation of upcoming targets, or the transition between these two states (Lepsien and Nobre 2007; LaRocque et al. 2013; see Soto and Humphreys (in chapter 26); Kuhl and Chun (in chapter 28)). Furthermore, in addition to sustained or dynamic changes in firing rates, short-term synaptic plasticity has also been proposed to play a role in maintaining the content of past experience and rules to guide goal-directed processing (Stokes et al. 2013; see Stokes and Duncan (in chapter 6); Miller and Buschman (in chapter 27)).

Perhaps the most salient new line of investigation in deciphering the mechanisms of attention is aimed at revealing the role of neural oscillations (see Saalman and Kastner (in chapter 14); Schroeder, Herrero, and Haegens (in chapter 17); Shapiro and Hanslmayr (in chapter 22); Rohenkohl and Nobre (in chapter 24); Miller and Buschman (in chapter 27)). There is great interest in forming a cohesive picture of how oscillations contribute to the neural organization of cognitive functions in general, and of selective attention in particular. Though still not fully proven or accepted (e.g. Shadlen and Movshon 1999), many present-day researchers believe that oscillations may provide conduits for the regulation of neural excitability in functional cell assemblies within or between brain areas (see Buzsaki 2009). In a ground-breaking study, Fries and colleagues (2001) showed that spatial attention greatly increased synchronization of neuronal activity in the gamma band. Computational and theoretical models suggest that increased gamma-band synchronization can greatly potentiate the throughput of the signals from the neuronal populations onto their efferent structures (Fries 2009). Many researchers are currently busy trying to extract the general principles through which oscillations aid prioritization and integration of information processing. In attention, a central question is the contribution of different frequency bands to top-down versus bottom-up signals (Buschman and Miller 2009; Bosman et al. 2012; Lee et al. 2013). Of increasing interest is whether and how oscillations may regulate neural excitability according to temporal expectations generated by the temporal regularities or associations of ongoing stimuli (see Schroeder, Herrero, and Haegens (in chapter 17); Nobre and Rohenkohl (in chapter 24)).

As this brief sampling shows, the field has revealed a dizzying collection of attention effects at the behavioural, network, and cellular level. More effects are certain to be reported. As Serences and Kastner (in chapter 4) observe: the 'major challenge for future investigators is to meld the multiple mechanisms that support selective attention into a unified framework'.

ATTENTION AND OTHER COGNITIVE DOMAINS

Attention is not an isolated cognitive domain. Indeed, if we accept the narrow, consensus definition of attention—the prioritization of processing information relevant to current task goals—one can immediately intuit how these functions interface with perception, action control and decision-making, motivation and emotions, memories at different time scales, and awareness. Various chapters in the Handbook consider these relationships. Working across the categorical boundaries in cognitive psychology and neuroscience is fundamental for cross-fertilization of methodological advances and insights, and for reaching a cohesive and well-integrated understanding of the general principles of cognition.

The close relationship between spatial attention and action (and especially oculo-motor) control has already been mentioned (see Theeuwes (in chapter 8); Gottlieb (in chapter 12); Clark, Noudoost, Schafer, and Moore (in chapter 13); Krauzlis (in chapter 15); Deubel (in chapter 30)). The field of action control is being advanced significantly by current efforts to investigate the mechanisms of choice and decision-making. Many of the factors being considered in decision-making research overlap or relate closely to those in attention research, such as notions about prediction, expectation, value, and informativeness of stimuli (see Gottlieb (in chapter 12); Scolari, Ester, and Serences (in chapter 20); Summerfield and Egner (in chapter 29); Yu (in chapter 39)). It will be essential to enhance the dialogue between these fields of research to avoid reinventing or undermining wheels. As Gottlieb (in chapter 12) notes, one 'key question for future [attention] work therefore is to integrate this work with a reinforcement learning frame-work...' It will also be important for researchers coming from the decision-making field to take into account the rich stock of modulatory mechanisms unveiled by attention research in order to broaden and enrich predictive-coding models.

Like attention, motivation and emotion modulate information processing (see Pessoa (in chapter 25); Scerif and Wu (in chapter 31)). Whereas the field of attention tends to home in on the influences on perception, the field of motivation has often considered effects on decision-making and responses, and the field of emotion has emphasized the effects on memory. But these preferences are somewhat arbitrary. Attention, motiva-tion, and emotions probably all influence perception, decision-making, responses, and memories (see Nobre and Mesulam (in chapter 5); Pessoa (in chapter 25)). This realiza-tion prompts reflection into what characterizes the differences among these different types of modulatory mechanisms, the extent to which they are common, or the degree to which they interact with one another to influence ongoing perception and cognition.

Memory is another long acknowledged source of influence on our present perception and cognition. From the time of Helmholtz, memories have been considered funda-mental in shaping and guiding the construction of sensible percepts (Helmholtz 1867). With some notable exceptions, attention research has not traditionally considered the prioritization of information processing by long-term memories, but this is chang-ing (see Nobre and Mesulam (in chapter 5); Kuhl and Chun (in chapter 28); Scerif and Wu (in chapter 31)). Current research is investigating the networks and mechanisms by which memories modulate perception, and looking at the relationship of the net-works and mechanisms associated with attention. Ultimately, memories are also formed about attended events, those that were prioritized for being relevant of interesting at their time. Therefore, there is a continuous, bidirectional interplay between long-term memory and attention (e.g. see Fuster 2009).

Attention also has an intimate relationship with memories on a much shorter time-scale, held in the 'rearward portion of the present space of time' (James 1890: 647).

Many theoretical accounts consider the contents of short-term memory, or working memory—maintained and manipulated to guide future action—to be the vital source of top-down modulatory signals in attention (Desimone and Duncan 1995; see Nobre and Mesulam (in chapter 5); Soto and Humphreys (in chapter 26); Kuhl and Chun (in chapter 28); Zanto and Gazzaley (in chapter 32); Bundesen and Habekost (in chapter 37)).[1] Again, the relationship is not unidirectional, but multifaceted. Attention, in turn, gates what comes to be encoded into short-term memory, helps maintain information in short-term memory, and dynamically modulates the information being maintained (see Kuhl and Chun (in chapter 28); Gazzaley and Nobre 2012). As with long-term memory, a virtuous cycle forms between short-term memory and perception with attention-related modulatory mechanisms facilitating prioritization and selection of relevant information at multiple stages along both directions of influence.

Missing from the Handbook is a chapter on the relationship between attention and conscious awareness. This was not deliberate, but the inevitable misfortune of being let down by a contributor. Attention and awareness are undeniably entwined, but research increasingly suggests that they are not synonymous or always coexistent. Some researchers propose that attention is a prerequisite for conscious awareness, and that the contents of awareness are mainly determined by top-down biasing of competing object representations by frontoparietal networks involved in attention (e.g. Rees 2007; Rees and Frith 2007). But others emphasize functional dissociations between attention and awareness (e.g. Koch and Tsuchiya 2007; Wyart and Tallon-Baudry 2008; Kentridge 2011). For example, Kentridge and colleagues have shown that it is possible to enhance detection and discrimination of unconscious stimuli by attention, such as in the case of blindsight (Kentridge et al. 1999, 2004). Continuing to make progress charting the relationship between these two fundamental but slippery domains will rely on having much clearer and accepted definitions as well as criteria for their measurement.

APPLICATIONS OF ATTENTION RESEARCH

The widespread effects of attention on our cognition are probably evident by now. Prioritization and selection of information influence what we perceive, hold in mind, decide, do, and remember. Arguably, no other cognitive domain has as much reach in terms of applicability to real-world situations. Attention is fundamental to how we navigate through the world, how we learn, how we cope with the multiple demands and distractions as we perform our jobs, and how we focus on the things we enjoy in our moments of leisure. As technology continues to proliferate the amount of stimulation and data that surround us, our attentional mechanisms become more and more essential for coping at every step of life.

Given the pervasive influence of attention in our dealings with the environment, it is vital for the experimental field to step up its engagement with applied fields in education, industry, information and communication technologies, sports, and health. The academic field of attention has amassed tremendous know-how of direct and important practical implications for these diverse sectors of our society. The field also stands to benefit from these various disciplines. They can tell us about particular challenges in improving or maintaining efficient performance under specific contexts. In some cases, the dialogue is beginning. For example, current research is testing the contribution of attention functions to the ability of children to maintain information in mind and to follow instructions in the classroom (see Gathercole and Alloway 2006; see Posner, Rothbart, and Rueda (in chapter 19); Scerif and Wu (in chapter 31)). But there is much further to go in terms of applying attention research to education as well as to other fields. Quick brainstorming should easily bring many areas for potential contributions, for example: design of web and other interfaces, effective advertisement, airport screening, diagnosis in medical images, sensory recognition in robots, cinema and television production, software and game design....

An important first step is for academic researchers to start investigating the dynamics of attention and selection under naturalistic conditions. What happens in the brain when we cross the street and look for cars? Do the mechanisms established using our simplified experimental paradigms apply to complex and ever-changing contexts of natural scenes? Are there important shortcomings in our understanding that we need to address? Recent behavioural and imaging studies have begun to increase ecological validity of experimental paradigms (e.g. Summerfield et al. 2006; Peelen and Kastner 2011) and to tackle questions of attention in real-life contexts (e.g. Ho, Reed, and Spence 2007; Drew, Evans, Võ, Jacobson, and Wolfe 2013; Evans, Birdwell, and Wolfe 2013). To complement studies embracing the complex and dynamic nature of real-life contexts, it will also be important to consider individual differences. Variations in genetics, environmental experience, and their interaction play important roles in how attention functions develop and operate across the lifespan (see Posner, Rothbart, and Rueda (in chapter 19); Scerif and Wu (in chapter 31)).

DEFICITS IN ATTENTION

The importance of attention functions to cognitive health is obvious. Unilateral spatial neglect is the neurological condition that has been most closely associated with deficits in attention. As with our conception of attention functions in the healthy brain, neglect has come to be understood as a syndrome of multiple symptoms related to spatial and non-spatial deficits in different modalities and levels of processing, underpinned by damage to nodes or connections of a large-scale network of brain areas (see Vallar and Bolognini (in chapter 33); Manohar, Bonnelle, and Husain (in chapter 34); Robertson and O'Connell (in chapter 36)). Symptoms in Balint's syndrome are also related to deficits in allocating attention across visual objects (simulanagnosia) and in spatially orienting and organizing eye movements (oculomotor apraxia) and manual responses (optic ataxia) (see Hécaen and De Ajuriaguerra 1954; Robertson (in chapter 35)).

Contemporary work in neurology, psychiatry, and clinical psychology is greatly broadening our understanding of how deficits in attention contribute to cognitive health. In neurological cases, attention deficits do not only result after damage to brain areas caused by stroke, but they can also contribute to behavioural deficits after traumatic brain injury and in neurodegenerative conditions such as Parkinson's and Alzheimer's diseases (see Manohar, Bonnelle, and Husain (in chapter 34)). A number of psychiatric and psychological conditions are also currently believed to include attention-related factors. For example, individuals with anxiety or mood disorders display distorted patterns of attention (see Bar-Haim et al. 2007; MacLeod et al. 2002; Pessoa (in chapter 25)). Accordingly cognitive and behavioural interventions are being developed to redress attentional biases (see Bar-Haim 2010; Browning et al. 2010). The reasons why prioritization and selection of information can become pathological and dysfunctional in certain individuals are many, including genetic predispositions as well as environmental factors. Revealing the interplay of factors in determining individual differences in susceptibility to psychiatric and psychological conditions should prove a fruitful area for research.

Attention can also fail in the healthy brain. We all experience momentary lapses. An important new line of investigation suggests that deficits in attention become more frequent as we age (see Zanto and Gazzaley (in chapter 32))—as implied by the term 'senior moment'. Given the important role that attention plays in supporting cognition, deficits in attention may result in or greatly exacerbate deficits in other psychological functions, such as memory and decision-making. Deficits in attention are also implicated in compromising other psychological functions on the other side of the age spectrum, during early development (see Scerif and Wu (in chapter 31)). These observations suggest that interventions that are effective at enhancing attention-related functions may hold great promise in boosting healthy cognitive development in the early years and in waylaying cognitive decline during ageing (e.g. Anguera et al. 2013; Bavelier et al. 2011; see Zanto and Gazzaley (in chapter 32); Robertson and O'Connell (in chapter 36)). The race is on to devise viable and effective interventions that have reproducible and generalizable benefits.

CONCLUSIONS

As we pack up the attention time capsule and muse over its contents, we cannot help but be impressed by the industry of the field. It is true that some key elements are still missing. The field is still a bit disorganized on the nomenclature and taxonomy front. That makes it difficult to put all the findings and insights in their proper place. But the advances in revealing the mechanisms of attention at the behavioural, systems, and cellular levels remain remarkable nevertheless. Multiple effects have been documented that contribute to the prioritization, selection, and integration of information across all stages of the information-processing stream. Findings have come from convergent methodologies used across species and levels of analysis. The various aspects of the field move ahead in a harmonious fashion. In this sense, 'attention' may be considered a role model within the fields investigating cognitive function.

But, of course, this is still the beginning. One major challenge ahead is weaving together the various findings into a cohesive and comprehensive framework. Although incomplete, our current understanding is ripe for incorporating principles of attention into the investigation of other cognitive domains. The other major challenge is reaching out to real-world applications. The role of attention in maintaining a healthy and balanced cognitive life is beginning to be recognized, and there will be important activity in understanding how best to translate our empirical work to the benefit of individuals. Attention research is poised to contribute to enhancing human experience through open dialogue and collaborative efforts with various other sectors of society.

Beyond this snapshot are so many possibilities... But for now it is a good start.

NOTE

1. Most of these accounts consider the 'content' representations related to the target goal to be doing most of the work during top-down guidance. However, one may also expand this notion by recognizing that representations about the current context, task set, rules, intentions, expectations, etc. are also maintained in short-term memory. These are also likely to exert influence.

REFERENCES

Anguera. J. A., Boccanfuso, J., Rintoul, J. L., Al-Hashimi, O., Faraji, F., Janowich, J., Kong, E., Larraburo, Y., Rolle, C., Johnston, E., and Gazzaley, A. (2013). Video game training enhances cognitive control in older adults. *Nature 501*: 97–101.

Awh, E. and Jonides, J. (2001). Overlapping mechanisms of attention and spatial working memory. *Trends in Cognitive Sciences 5*(3): 119–126.

Bar-Haim, Y. (2010). Research review: Attention bias modification (ABM)—a novel treatment for anxiety disorders. *Journal of Child Psychology and Psychiatry 51*(8): 859–870.

Bar-Haim, Y., Lamy, D., Pergamin, L., Bakermans-Kranenburg, M. J., and van IJzendoorn, M. H. (2007). Threat-related attentional bias in anxious and nonanxious individuals: A meta-analytic study. *Psychological Bulletin 133*(1): 1–24.

Bavelier, D., Green, C. S., Han, D. H., Renshaw, P. F., Merzenich, M. M., and Gentile, D. A. (2011). Brains on video games. *Nature Reviews Neuroscience 12*(12): 763–768.

Bosman, C. A., Schoffelen, J. M., Brunet, N., Oostenveld, R., Bastos, A. M., Womelsdorf, T., Rubehn, B., Stieglitz, T., De Weerd, P., and Fries, P. (2012). Attentional stimulus selection through selective synchronization between monkey visual areas. *Neuron 75*(5): 875–888.

Boynton, G. M. (2009). A framework for describing the effects of attention on visual responses. *Vision Research 49*(10): 1129–1143.

Broadbent, D. E. (1958) *Perception and Communication*. London: Pergamon Press.

Browning, M., Holmes, E. A., and Harmer, C. J. (2010). The modification of attentional bias to emotional information: A review of the techniques, mechanisms, and relevance to emotional disorders. *Cognitive, Affective, & Behavioral Neuroscience 10*(1): 8–20.

Bruce, C. J. and Goldberg, M. E. (1985). Primate frontal eye fields. I: Single neurons discharging before saccades. *Journal of Neurophysiology* 53(3): 603–635.

Buschman, T. J. and Miller, E. K. (2009). Serial, covert shifts of attention during visual search are reflected by the frontal eye fields and correlated with population oscillations. *Neuron* 63(3): 386–396.

Buzsaki, G. (2009). *Rhythms of the Brain*. Oxford: Oxford University Press.

Cameron, E. L., Tai, J. C., and Carrasco, M. (2002). Covert attention affects the psychometric function of contrast sensitivity. *Vision Research* 42(8): 949–967.

Chafee, M. V. and Goldman-Rakic, P. S. (1998). Matching patterns of activity in primate prefrontal area 8a and parietal area 7ip neurons during a spatial working memory task. *Journal of Neurophysiology* 79(6): 2919–2940.

Chelazzi, L., Miller, E. K., Duncan, J., and Desimone, R. (1993). A neural basis for visual search in inferior temporal cortex. *Nature* 363: 345–347.

Cherry, E. C. (1953). Some experiments on the recognition of speech, with one and with two ears. *Journal of the Acoustical Society of America* 25: 975–979.

Cohen, M. R. and Maunsell, J. H. (2009). Attention improves performance primarily by reducing interneuronal correlations. *Nature Neuroscience* 12(12): 1594–1600.

Colby, C. L. and Goldberg, M. E. (1999). Space and attention in parietal cortex. *Annual Review of Neuroscience* 22(1): 319–349.

Corbetta, M. (1998). Frontoparietal cortical networks for directing attention and the eye to visual locations: Identical, independent, or overlapping neural systems? *Proceedings of the National Academy of Sciences USA* 95(3): 831–838.

Cowan, N. (1995). *Attention and Memory*. Oxford: Oxford University Press.

Crowe, D. A., Averbeck, B. B., and Chafee, M. V. (2010). Rapid sequences of population activity patterns dynamically encode task-critical spatial information in parietal cortex. *Journal of Neuroscience* 30(35): 11640–11653.

Deisseroth, K. (2010). Optogenetics. *Nature Methods* 8(1): 26–29.

Desimone, R. and Duncan, J. (1995). Neural mechanisms of selective visual attention. *Annual Review of Neuroscience* 18(1): 193–222.

Deutsch, J. A. and Deutsch, D. (1963). Attention: Some theoretical considerations. *Psychological Review* 70(1): 80–90.

Drew, T., Evans, K., Võ, M. L. H., Jacobson, F. L., and Wolfe, J. M. (2013). Informatics in radiology: What can you see in a single glance and how might this guide visual search in medical images? *Radiographics* 33(1): 263–274.

Duncan, J. (1984). Selective attention and the organization of visual information. *Journal of Experimental Psychology: General* 113(4): 501–517.

Duncan, J. (2001). An adaptive coding model of neural function in prefrontal cortex. *Nature Reviews Neuroscience* 2(11): 820–829.

Eckstein, M. P., Shimozaki, S. S., and Abbey, C. K. (2002). The footprints of visual attention in the Posner cueing paradigm revealed by classification images. *Journal of Vision* 2(1): 25–45.

Enns, J. T. and Di Lollo, V. (1997). Object substitution: A new form of masking in unattended visual locations. *Psychological Science* 8(2): 135–139.

Evans, K. K., Birdwell, R. L., and Wolfe, J. M. (2013). If you don't find it often, you often don't find it: Why some cancers are missed in breast cancer screening. *PloS One* 8(5): e64366.

Fries, P. (2009). Neuronal gamma-band synchronization as a fundamental process in cortical computation. *Annual Review of Neuroscience* 32: 209–224.

Fries, P., Reynolds, J. H., Rorie, A. E., and Desimone, R. (2001). Modulation of oscillatory neuronal synchronization by selective visual attention. *Science* 291(5508): 1560–1563.

Fuster, J. M. (2009). Cortex and memory: Emergence of a new paradigm. *Journal of Cognitive Neuroscience* 21(11): 2047–2072.

Gathercole, S. E. and Alloway, T. P. (2006). Working memory in the classroom. *Sciences* 4: 417–423.

Gazzaley, A. (2011). Influence of early attentional modulation on working memory. *Neuropsychologia* 49(6): 1410–1424.

Gazzaley, A. and Nobre, A. C. (2012). Top-down modulation: Bridging selective attention and working memory. *Trends in Cognitive Sciences* 16(2): 129–135.

Gerits, A. and Vanduffel, W. (2013). Optogenetics in primates: A shining future? *Trends in Genetics* 29(7): 403–411.

Goldberg, M. E. and Wurtz, R. H. (1972). Activity of superior colliculus in behaving monkey. II: Effect of attention on neuronal responses. *Journal of Neurophysiology* 35(4): 560–574.

Hécaen, H. and De Ajuriaguerra, J. (1954). Balint's syndrome (psychic paralysis of visual fixation) and its minor forms. *Brain* 77(3): 373–400.

Helmholtz, H. von (1867). *Handbuch der physiologischen Optik*. Leipzig: L. Voss.

Ho, C., Reed, N., and Spence, C. (2007). Multisensory in-car warning signals for collision avoidance. *Human Factors: The Journal of the Human Factors and Ergonomics Society* 49(6): 1107–1114.

James, W. (1890). *The Principles of Psychology*. New York: Holt.

Kahneman, D. and Treisman, A. (1984). Changing views of attention and automaticity. In R. Parasuraman and D. R. Davies (eds.), *Varieties of Attention* (pp. 29–61). New York: Academic Press.

Kentridge, R. W. (2011). Attention without awareness: A brief review. In C. Mole, D. Smithies, and W. Wu (eds.), *Attention: Philosophical and Psychological Essays* (pp. 228–245). Oxford: Oxford University Press.

Kentridge, R. W., Heywood, C. A., and Weiskrantz, L. (1999). Attention without awareness in blindsight. *Proceedings of the Royal Society of London B: Biological Sciences* 266(1430): 1805–1811.

Kentridge, R. W., Heywood, C. A., and Weiskrantz, L. (2004). Spatial attention speeds discrimination without awareness in blindsight. *Neuropsychologia* 42(6): 831–835.

Kinchla, R. A., Chen, Z., and Evert, D. (1995). Precue effects in visual search: Data or resource limited? *Perception & Psychophysics* 57(4): 441–450.

Koch, C. and Tsuchiya, N. (2007). Attention and consciousness: Two distinct brain processes. *Trends in Cognitive Sciences* 11(1): 16–22.

LaRocque, J. J., Lewis-Peacock, J. A., Drysdale, A. T., Oberauer, K., and Postle, B. R. (2013). Decoding attended information in short-term memory: An EEG study. *Journal of Cognitive Neuroscience* 25(1): 127–142.

Lavie, N. (1995). Perceptual load as a necessary condition for selective attention. *Journal of Experimental Psychology: Human Perception and Performance* 21(3): 451–468.

Lee, J. and Maunsell, J. H. (2009). A normalization model of attentional modulation of single unit responses. *PLoS One* 4(2): e4651.

Lee, J. H., Whittington, M. A., and Kopell, N. J. (2013). Top-down beta rhythms support selective attention via interlaminar interaction: A model. *PLoS Computational Biology* 9(8): e1003164.

Lu, Z.-L., and Dosher, B. A. (1998). External noise distinguishes attention mechanisms. *Vision Research* 38(9): 1183–1198.

Lu Z.-L., Lesmes L. A., and Dosher B. A. (2002). Spatial attention excludes external noise at the target location. *Journal of Vision* 2(4): 312–323.

Luck, S. J., Chelazzi, L., Hillyard, S. A., and Desimone, R. (1997). Neural mechanisms of spatial selective attention in areas V1, V2, and V4 of macaque visual cortex. *Journal of Neurophysiology* 77(1): 24–42.

MacLeod, C., Rutherford, E., Campbell, L., Ebsworthy, G., and Holker, L. (2002). Selective attention and emotional vulnerability: Assessing the causal basis of their association through the experimental manipulation of attentional bias. *Journal of Abnormal Psychology* 111(1): 107–123.

Mesulam, M. (1981). A cortical network for directed attention and unilateral neglect. *Annals of Neurology* 10(4): 309–325.

Mesulam, M. (1990). Large-scale neurocognitive networks and distributed processing for attention, language, and memory. *Annals of Neurology* 28(5): 597–613.

Mitchell, J. F., Sundberg, K. A., and Reynolds, J. H. (2009). Spatial attention decorrelates intrinsic activity fluctuations in macaque area V4. *Neuron* 63(6): 879–888.

Moran, J. and Desimone, R. (1985). Selective attention gates visual processing in the extrastriate cortex. *Science* 229(4715): 782–784.

Motter, B. C. (1993). Focal attention produces spatially selective processing in visual cortical areas V1, V2, and V4 in the presence of competing stimuli. *Journal of Neurophysiology* 70(3): 909–919.

Neely, J. H. (1977). Semantic priming and retrieval from lexical memory: Roles of inhibitionless spreading activation and limited-capacity attention. *Journal of Experimental Psychology: General* 106(3): 226–254.

Palmer, J. (1994). Set-size effects in visual search: The effect of attention is independent of the stimulus for simple tasks. *Vision Research* 34(13): 1703–1721.

Peelen, M. V. and Kastner, S. (2011). A neural basis for real-world visual search in human occipitotemporal cortex. *Proceedings of the National Academy of Sciences USA* 108(29): 12125–12130.

Posner, M. I. (1978). *Chronometric Explorations of Mind*. Mahwah, N.J.: Lawrence Erlbaum.

Posner, M. I., Snyder, C. R., and Davidson, B. J. (1980). Attention and the detection of signals. *Journal of Experimental Psychology: General* 109(2): 160–174.

Rees, G. (2007). Neural correlates of the contents of visual awareness in humans. *Philosophical Transactions of the Royal Society B: Biological Sciences* 362(1481): 877–886.

Rees, G. and Frith, C. (2007). Methodologies for identifying the neural correlates of consciousness. In M. Velmans and S. Schneider (eds.), *The Blackwell Companion to Consciousness* (pp. 551–566). Oxford: Blackwell.

Reynolds, J. H., Chelazzi, L., and Desimone, R. (1999). Competitive mechanisms subserve attention in macaque areas V2 and V4. *Journal of Neuroscience* 19(5): 1736–1753.

Reynolds, J. H. and Heeger, D. J. (2009). The normalization model of attention. *Neuron* 61(2): 168–185.

Rizzolatti, G., Riggio, L., Dascola, I., and Umiltá, C. (1987). Reorienting attention across the horizontal and vertical meridians: Evidence in favor of a premotor theory of attention. *Neuropsychologia* 25(1): 31–40.

Robinson, D. L., Goldberg, M. E., and Stanton, G. B. (1978). Parietal association cortex in the primate: Sensory mechanisms and behavioral modulations. *Journal of Neurophysiology* 41(4): 910–932.

Schall, J. D. (2004). On the role of frontal eye field in guiding attention and saccades. *Vision Research* 44(12): 1453–1467.

Shadlen, M. N. and Movshon, J. A. (1999). Synchrony unbound: A critical evaluation of the temporal binding hypothesis. *Neuron* 24(1): 67–77.

Shiu, L. P. and Pashler, H. (1995). Spatial attention and vernier acuity. *Vision Research* 35(3): 337–343.

Stokes, M. G., Kusunoki, M., Sigala, N., Nili, H., Gaffan, D., and Duncan, J. (2013). Dynamic coding for cognitive control in prefrontal cortex. *Neuron* 78: 364–375.

Stroop, J. R. (1935). Studies of interference in serial verbal reactions. *Journal of Experimental Psychology* 18(6): 643–662.

Summerfield, J. J., Lepsien, J., Gitelman, D. R., Mesulam, M., and Nobre, A. C. (2006). Orienting attention based on long-term memory experience. *Neuron* 49(6): 905–916.

Theeuwes, J. (1991). Exogenous and endogenous control of attention: The effect of visual onsets and offsets. *Perception & Psychophysics* 49(1): 83–90.

Treisman, A. M. and Gelade, G. (1980). A feature-integration theory of attention. *Cognitive Psychology* 12(1): 97–136.

Wyart, V. and Tallon-Baudry, C. (2008). Neural dissociation between visual awareness and spatial attention. *Journal of Neuroscience* 28(10): 2667–2679.

Wyart, V., Nobre, A. C., and Summerfield, C. (2012). Dissociable prior influences of signal probability and relevance on visual contrast sensitivity. *Proceedings of the National Academy of Sciences USA*, 109(9): 3593–3598.

Yeshurun, Y. and Carrasco, M. (1999). Spatial attention improves performance in spatial resolution tasks. *Vision Research* 39(2): 293–306.

Yeshurun, Y. and Marom, G. (2008). Transient spatial attention and the perceived duration of brief visual events. *Visual Cognition* 16(6): 826–848.

INDEX

attention for action 366
attention for learning 366, 1160–72
attention from memory 824–6
Attention Network Test (ANT) 546, 551, 554,
    1038, 1044
attention to memory model 821
attributes 21, 23–7
auditory cortex
    cueing 696–7
    temporal expectations 691
autism spectrum disorder 67
awareness 765–6, 1215

Balint's syndrome 1062–78
    feature binding 1068–72, 1074–7
    first description 1062
    illusory conjunctions 1068, 1070–1, 1076
    implicit spatial coding 1072–4
    object-based attention 1063–8
    simultanagnosia 1062, 1063
basal ganglia 545, 789, 791–5
baseline shift 85, 86, 153, 155, 156, 158, 163,
    173, 261, 264–6, 1212–13
Bayesian models 1131, 1143, 1159–90
    attention for learning 1160–72
    decision-making 854, 1172–81
    overt spatial attention 1181–9
    perceptual load 60–1
Behavioural Inattention Test 982
benzodiazepines 531
beta oscillations
    attentional blink 642
    LGN 405
    relationship with other oscillations 643
    temporal expectations 685
    thalamic reticular nucleus 413–14, 415
biased-choice model 1098
biased competition model 88, 108, 110, 155,
    183–4, 253–4, 255, 290, 355, 358,
    511–12, 608–9, 782, 828, 867, 1095,
    1105, 1212
biases 108–9
    computational models 1138
    slates for 129, 131–3
    sources of 123–7
    top-down/bottom-up 109, 110
    types of 128–9

binding
    Balint's syndrome 1068–72, 1074–7
    crowding 16
    divided attention 810
    illusory conjunctions 15–16
    necessity of 16–18
    property binding 15
    pulvinar 407
    range binding 15
    re-entry 23
    types of 14–15
BOLD, see functional magnetic resonance
    imaging
bootstrapping 795–6
bottleneck 23, 107, 626, 627, 778–80, 1201–4
bottom-up control
    attentional capture 309–13, 782
    biases 109, 110
    computational models 1123, 1126–35
    LIP 358–69, 782–3
    memory encoding 813–14
    neural competition 261–4
    visual search 34, 309–13
brain networks
    alerting 542–3
    development 551–5
    executive attention 544–6, 1032
    genes and experience 555–61
    orienting 543–4
    see also network model
brain oscillations, see neural oscillations
brightness perception 208
bromocriptine 528

caloric stimulation 986
cancellation tasks 976–8
Catherine Bergego Scale 982–3
central performance drop 214
centre bias 1135
change blindness 390–2, 439
children
    attention and learning 910–11
    brain development 546–7
    crossmodal attention 462
    perceptual capacity 67
    theory of visual attention-based
        assessment 1116

cholinergic system, *see* acetylcholine
cingulate cortex 114; *see also* anterior
    cingulate cortex; posterior cingulate
    cortex
cingulate gyrus 110
cingulum bundle 1043
classical conditioning
    1161–3
clonidine 521–2, 1085, 1086
closure 18, 1064–5
CODE theory of visual attention (CTVA) 1101
cognitive ageing 948–53
cognitive biases 1138
cognitive capacity 778–82
cognitive enhancement 530
cognitive models 1129
cognitive reserve 951–2
Colavita effect 459–60
compensation-related utilization of neural
    circuits hypothesis (CRUNCH) 950–1
competition
    crossmodal attention 459–60
    emotion–attention interaction 742, 745
    memory encoding 811–15
    memory retrieval 815–24
    neural 152–3, 258–64
computerized attention training 1083, 1088
COMT 526, 557, 559
conditioned taste aversion 789
conditioning 367–9, 386, 388–90, 1161–3
conflict processing 734–8
conjunction search 14, 19–21, 32
connectivity models 276
conscious awareness 765–6, 1215
context
    context model of ageing 949–50
    scene context 1141
contextual cueing 123–5, 824, 826
contingent capture 242–3, 247–8
contingent negative variation 552, 702, 935
continuous flash suppression 64
continuous performance tasks 551–2, 1035
contrast gain 257, 847, 849
contrast response function 848–9
contrast sensitivity 190–208
    endogenous attention 198–201, 208
    exogenous attention 194–7, 205–8

perceived contrast 205–8
second-order 196–7
corona radiata 1043
corpus callosum 1000
cortical cell classes 339
cortical magnification factor 209, 210
covert attention 184–90, 351, 375
    behavioural studies 188–90
    contrast sensitivity 190–208
    frontal eye fields 376
    mechanisms 187–8
    spatial resolution 208–19
    superior colliculus 436–40
crossmodal attention 446–63
    attending to a sensory modality 447–9
    attentional blink 458
    cue salience 462
    development 462
    endogenous 296–8, 452–6
    ERPs 296–303
    exogenous 298, 449–52
    facilitation versus competition 459–60
    neural substrates 462
    postural changes 456
    temporal orienting 456, 458
    unity assumption 461
crowding 16
CRUNCH model 950–1

d′ 189, 193, 480, 840, 842
decision-making 837–58
    Bayesian models 854, 1172–81
    decision policy 838
    decision threshold bound 838
    decision variable 838
    drift-diffusion model 845
    economic 838
    evidence 838
    expectation 850–1, 854–7
    feature-based attention 581–2
    ideal observer models 842–4
    normative models 838–9
    perceptual 837
    predictive perception 849–51
    principles 838
    serial sampling models 845–6
    signal detection theory 840–2